# 2006

## Leonard L. Lance, RPh, BSPharm
*Senior Editor*
Pharmacist
Lexi-Comp, Inc.
Hudson, Ohio

## Charles F. Lacy, PharmD, FCSHP
*Editor*
Vice President, Information Technologies
Director, Drug Information Services
Professor, Pharmacy Practice
University of Southern Novada
Las Vegas, Nevada

## Morton P. Goldman, PharmD, BCPS, FCCP
*Associate Editor*
Assistant Director, Pharmacotherapy Services
Department of Pharmacy
Cleveland Clinic Foundation
Cleveland, Ohio

## Lora L. Armstrong, PharmD, BCPS
*Associate Editor*
Vice President, Clinical Affairs
Pharmacy & Therapeutics Formulary Process
Clinical Program Oversight
CaremarkRx
Northbrook, Illinois

# NOTICE

This handbook is intended to serve the user as a handy quick reference and not as a complete drug information resource. It does not include information on every therapeutic agent available. The publication covers 1591 commonly used drugs and is specifically designed to present certain important aspects of drug data in a more concise format than is generally found in medical literature or product material supplied by manufacturers.

Although great care was taken to ensure the accuracy of the handbook's content when it went to press, the editors, contributors, and publisher cannot be responsible for the continued accuracy of the supplied information due to ongoing research and new developments in the field. Further, the *Quick Look Drug Book* is not offered as a guide to dosing. The reader, herewith, is advised that information shown under the heading **Usual Dosage** is provided only as an indication of the amount of the drug typically given or taken during therapy. Actual dosing amount for any specific drug should be based on an in-depth evaluation of the individual patient's therapy requirement and strong consideration given to such issues as contraindications, warnings, precautions, adverse reactions, along with the interaction of other drugs. The manufacturers' most current product information or other standard recognized references should always be consulted for such detailed information prior to drug use.

The editors and contributors have written this book in their private capacities. No official support or endorsement by any federal agency or pharmaceutical company is intended or inferred.

This manual was produced using the FormuLex™ Program —
a complete publishing service of Lexi-Comp Inc.

**LEXI-COMP**

1100 Terex Road
Hudson, Ohio 44236
(330) 650-6506

# QUICK LOOK DRUG BOOK

## 2006

### Leonard L. Lance, RPh, BSPharm
*Senior Editor*
Pharmacist
Lexi-Comp, Inc.
Hudson, Ohio

### Charles F. Lacy, PharmD, FCSHP
*Editor*
Vice President, Information Technologies
Director, Drug Information Services
Professor, Pharmacy Practice
University of Southern Nevada
Las Vegas, Nevada

### Morton P. Goldman, PharmD, BCPS, FCCP
*Associate Editor*
Assistant Director, Pharmacotherapy Services
Department of Pharmacy
Cleveland Clinic Foundation
Cleveland, Ohio

### Lora L. Armstrong, PharmD, BCPS
*Associate Editor*
Vice President, Clinical Affairs
Pharmacy & Therapeutics Formulary Process
Clinical Program Oversight
CaremarkRx
Northbrook, Illinois

LIPPINCOTT WILLIAMS & WILKINS

Philadelphia • Baltimore • New York • London
Buenos Aires • Hong Kong • Sydney • Tokyo

# QUICK LOOK
# DRUG BOOK

# TABLE OF CONTENTS

# ABOUT THE AUTHORS

## Leonard L. Lance, RPh, BSPharm

Leonard L. (Bud) Lance has been directly involved in the pharmaceutical industry since receiving his bachelor's degree in pharmacy from Ohio Northern University in 1970. Upon graduation from ONU, Mr Lance spent four years as a navy pharmacist in various military assignments and was instrumental in the development and operation of the first whole hospital I.V. admixture program in a military (Portsmouth Naval Hospital) facility.

After completing his military service, he entered the retail pharmacy field and has managed both an independent and a home I.V. franchise pharmacy operation. Since the late 1970s, Mr Lance has focused much of his interest on using computers to improve pharmacy service. The independent pharmacy he worked for was one of the first retail pharmacies in the State of Ohio to computerize (1977).

His love for computers and pharmacy led him to Lexi-Comp, Inc. in 1988. He developed Lexi-Comp's first drug database in 1989 and was involved in the editing and publishing of Lexi-Comp's first *Drug Information Handbook* in 1990.

As a result of his strong publishing interest, he presently serves in the capacity of pharmacy editor and technical advisor as well as pharmacy (information) database coordinator for Lexi-Comp. Along with the *Quick Look Drug Book*, he provides technical support to Lexi-Comp's *Drug Information Handbook for the Allied Health Professional* and Lexi-Comp's reference publications. Mr Lance also assists approximately 200 major hospitals in producing their own formulary (pharmacy) publications through Lexi-Comp's custom publishing service.

Mr Lance is a member and past president (1984) of the Summit Pharmaceutical Association (SPA). He is also a member of the Ohio Pharmacists Association (OPA), the American Pharmaceutical Association (APhA), and the American Society of Health-System Pharmacists (ASHP).

## Charles F. Lacy, PharmD, FCSHP

Dr Lacy is the Vice President for Information Technologies and Professor of Pharmacy Practice at the University of Southern Nevada. In his capacity at the university, Dr Lacy oversees the directors of the Library and Learning Resources Center, the Computer Information Systems, and the Drug Information Center. This college-based service provides drug use policy services in addition to traditional drug information resources to the college's affiliated institutions. Prior to his promotion, Dr Lacy was the Facilitative Officer for Clinical Programs where he managed the clinical curriculum, clinical faculty activities, student experiential programs, pharmacy residency programs, and the college's continuing education programs. Currently, Dr Lacy is also Director of International Programs for the university, which includes the College of Pharmacy, the College of Business Administration, the College of Nursing, and the Physician Assistant Masters Program.

Prior to co-founding the Nevada College of Pharmacy, Dr Lacy was the Clinical Coordinator for the Department of Pharmacy at Cedars-Sinai Medical Center. With over 19 years of clinical experience at one of the nation's largest teaching hospitals, he developed a reputation as an acknowledged expert in drug information and critical care drug therapy.

Dr Lacy received his doctorate from the University of Southern California School of Pharmacy. Presently, Dr Lacy holds teaching affiliations with the Nevada College of Pharmacy, the University of Southern California School of Pharmacy, the University of the Pacific School of Pharmacy, Western University of Health Sciences School of Pharmacy, and the University of Alberta at Edmonton, School of Pharmacy and Health Sciences.

Dr Lacy is an active member of numerous professional associations including the American Society of Health-System Pharmacists (ASHP), the American College of Clinical Pharmacy (ACCP), the American Society of Consultant Pharmacists (ASCP), the American Association of Colleges of Pharmacy (AACP), American Pharmacists Association (APhA), the Nevada Pharmacy Alliance (NPA), and the California Society of Hospital Pharmacists (CSHP), through which he has chaired many committees and subcommittees.

## Morton P. Goldman, PharmD, BCPS, FCCP

Dr Goldman received his bachelor's degree in pharmacy from the University of Pittsburgh, College of Pharmacy and his Doctor of Pharmacy degree from the University of Cincinnati, Division of Graduate Studies and Research. He completed his concurrent 2-year hospital pharmacy residency at the VA Medical Center in Cincinnati. Dr Goldman is presently the Assistant Director of Pharmacotherapy Services for the Department of Pharmacy at the Cleveland Clinic Foundation (CCF) after having spent over 4 years at CCF as an Infectious Disease pharmacist and 4 years as Clinical Manager. He holds faculty appointments from The University of Toledo, College of Pharmacy and Case Western Reserve University, College of Medicine and is the Pharmacology Curriculum Coordinator for the new Cleveland Clinic Lerner College of Medicine. Dr Goldman is a Board-Certified Pharmacotherapy Specialist (BCPS) with added qualifications in infectious diseases.

In his capacity as Assistant Director of Pharmacotherapy Services at CCF, Dr Goldman remains actively involved in patient care and clinical research with the Department of Infectious Disease, as well as the continuing education of the medical and pharmacy staff. He is an editor of CCF's *Guidelines for Antibiotic Use* and participates in their annual Antimicrobial Review retreat. He is a member of the Pharmacy and Therapeutics Committee and many of its subcommittees. Dr Goldman has authored numerous journal articles and lectures locally and nationally on infectious diseases topics and current drug therapies. He is currently a reviewer for the *Annals of Pharmacotherapy* and the *Journal of the American Medical Association*, an editorial board member of the *Journal of Infectious Disease Pharmacotherapy*, and coauthor of the *Infectious Diseases Handbook*, the *Drug Information Handbook*, and the *Drug Information Handbook for the Allied Health Professional* produced by Lexi-Comp, Inc. He also provides technical support to Lexi-Comp's Clinical Reference Library™ publications.

Dr Goldman is an active member of the Ohio College of Clinical Pharmacy, the Society of Infectious Disease Pharmacists, the American College of Clinical Pharmacy (and is a Fellow of the College), and the American Society of Health-Systems Pharmacists.

## Lora L. Armstrong, PharmD, BCPS

Dr Armstrong received her bachelor's degree in pharmacy from Ferris State University and her Doctor of Pharmacy degree from Midwestern University. Dr Armstrong is a Board-Certified Pharmacotherapy Specialist (BCPS).

In her current position, Dr Armstrong serves as the Director of the Pharmacy & Therapeutics Committee process at Caremark, Inc, Prescription Services Division. Caremark is a prescription benefit management company (PBM). Dr Armstrong is responsible for coordination of the Caremark National Pharmacy & Therapeutics Committee, the Caremark Pharmacy & Therapeutics Subcommittee, and Clinical Program Oversight. Dr Armstrong is also responsible for monitoring the pharmaceutical product pipeline, monitoring drug surveillance, and communicating Pharmacy & Therapeutics Committee Formulary information to Caremark's internal and external customers.

Prior to joining Caremark, Inc, Dr Armstrong served as the Director of Drug Information Services at the University of Chicago Hospitals. She obtained 17 years of experience in a variety of clinical settings including critical care, hematology, oncology, infectious diseases, and clinical pharmacokinetics. Dr Armstrong played an active role in the education and training of medical, pharmacy, and nursing staff. She coordinated the Drug Information Center, the medical center's Adverse Drug Reaction Monitoring Program, and the continuing Education Program for pharmacists. She also maintained the hospital's strict formulary program and was the editor of the University of Chicago Hospitals' *Formulary of Accepted Drugs* and the drug information center's monthly newsletter *Topics in Drug Therapy.*

Dr Armstrong is an active member of the Academy of Managed Care Pharmacy (AMCP), the American Society of Health-Systems Pharmacists (ASHP), the American Pharmaceutical Association (APhA), the American College of Clinical Pharmacy (ACCP), and the Pharmacy & Therapeutics Society (P & T Society). Dr Armstrong wrote the chapter entitled "Drugs and Hormones Used in Endocrinology" in the 4th edition of the textbook *Endocrinology.* She is an Adjunct Clinical Instructor of Pharmacy Practice at Midwestern University. Dr Armstrong currently serves on the Drug Information Advisory Board for pharmacist.com and on the American Pharmaceutical Association Scientific Review Panel for Evaluations of Drug Interactions (EDI).

# EDITORIAL ADVISORY PANEL

# PREFACE

Working with clinical pharmacists, hospital pharmacy and therapeutics committees, and hospital drug information centers, the editors of this handbook have directly assisted in the development and production of hospital-specific formulary documentation for several hundred major medical institutions in the United States and Canada. The resultant documentation provides pertinent detail concerning use of medications within the hospital and other clinical settings. The most current information on medications has been extracted, reviewed, coalesced, and cross-referenced by the editors to create this *Quick Look Drug Book*.

Thus, this handbook gives the user quick access to data on 1591 medications with cross-referencing to 5318 U.S. and Canadian brand or trade names. Selection of the included medications was based on the analysis of those medications offered in a wide range of hospital formularies. The concise standardized format for data used in this handbook was developed to ensure a consistent presentation of information for all medications.

All generic drug names and synonyms appear in lower case, whereas brand or trade names appear in upper/lower case with the proper trademark information. These three items appear as individual entries in the alphabetical listing of drugs and, thus, there is no requirement for an alphabetical index of drugs.

Mailing and WEB site addresses for Pharmaceutical Manufacturers' and Drug Distributors are provided in the appendix section of this book.

The Indication/Therapeutic Category Index is an expedient mechanism for locating the medication of choice along with its classification. This index will help the user, with knowledge of the disease state, to identify medications which are most commonly used in treatment. All disease states are cross-referenced to a varying number of medications with the most frequently used medication(s) noted.

— L.L. Lance

# ACKNOWLEDGMENTS

The *Quick Look Drug Book* exists in its present form as the result of the concerted efforts of the following individuals: Robert D. Kerscher, publisher and president of Lexi-Comp, Inc; Mark Bonfiglio, PharmD, director of pharmacotherapy resources; Stacy S. Robinson, editorial manager; Barbara F. Kerscher, production manager; Cynthia Forney, drug identification database manager; Daniel L. Krinsky, director, pharmacotherapy sales and marketing; Ginger S. Stein, project manager; Alexandra Hart, composition specialist; and David C. Marcus, director of information systems.

Special acknowledgment goes to all Lexi-Comp staff for their contributions to this handbook.

# USE OF THE HANDBOOK

The *Quick Look Drug Book* is organized into a drug information section, an appendix, and an indication/therapeutic category index.

The drug information section of the handbook, wherein all drugs are listed alphabetically, details information pertinent to each drug. Extensive cross-referencing is provided by brand name and synonyms.

Drug information is presented in a consistent format and for quick reference will provide the following:

| | |
|---|---|
| Generic Name | U.S. Adopted Name (USAN) or International Nonproprietary Name (INN) |
| | If a drug product is only available in Canada, a *(Canada only)* will be attached to that product and will appear with every occurrence of that drug throughout the book |
| Pronunciation Guide | Subjective aid for pronouncing drug names |
| Sound-Alike/Look-Alike Issues | Lists drugs with similar sounding names or names that look alike |
| Synonyms | Official names and some slang |
| Tall-Man | "Tall-Man" lettering revisions recommended by the FDA |
| U.S./Canadian Brand Names | Common trade names used in the United States and Canada |
| Therapeutic Category | Lexi-Comp's own system of logical medication classification |
| Controlled Substance | Drug Enforcement Agency (DEA) classification for federally scheduled controlled substances |
| Use | Information pertaining to appropriate use of the drug |
| Usual Dosage | The amount of the drug to be typically given or taken during therapy |
| Dosage Forms | Information with regard to form, strength and availability of the drug |

## Appendix

The appendix offers a compilation of tables, guidelines, and conversion information that can often be helpful when considering patient care.

## Indication/Therapeutic Category Index

This index provides a listing of accepted drugs for various disease states thus focusing attention on selection of medications most frequently prescribed in relation to a clinical diagnosis. Diseases may have other nonofficial drugs for their treatment and this indication/therapeutic category index should not be used by itself to determine the appropriateness of a particular therapy. The listed indications may encompass varying degrees of severity and, since certain medications may not be appropriate for a given degree of severity, it should not be assumed that the agents listed for specific indications are interchangeable. Also included as a valuable reference is each medication's therapeutic category.

# TALL-MAN LETTERS

Confusion between similar drug names is an important cause of medication errors. For years, The Institute for Safe Medication Practices (ISMP), has urged generic manufacturers use a combination of large and small letters as well as bolding (ie, chlorpro**MAZINE** and chlorpro**PAMIDE**) to help distinguish drugs with look-alike names, especially when they share similar strengths. Recently the FDA's Division of Generic Drugs began to issue recommendation letters to manufacturers suggesting this novel way to label their products to help reduce this drug name confusion. Although this project has had marginal success, the method has successfully eliminated problems with products such as diphenhydr**AMINE** and dimenhy**DRINATE**. Hospitals should also follow suit by making similar changes in their own labels, preprinted order forms, computer screens and printouts, and drug storage location labels.

In order for all involved to become more familiar with the FDA's recent suggestion, in this edition of the *Quick Look Drug Book* the "Tall-Man" lettering revisions will be listed in a field called **Tall-Man**.

The following is a list of product names and recommended FDA revisions.

| Drug Product | Recommended Revision |
|---|---|
| acetazolamide | aceta**ZOLAMIDE** |
| acetohexamide | aceto**HEXAMIDE** |
| bupropion | bu**PROP**ion |
| buspirone | bus**PIR**one |
| chlorpromazine | chlorpro**MAZINE** |
| chlorpropamide | chlorpro**PAMIDE** |
| clomiphene | clomi**PHENE** |
| clomipramine | clomi**PRAMINE** |
| cycloserine | cyclo**SERINE** |
| cyclosporine | cyclo**SPORINE** |
| daunorubicin | **DAUNO**rubicin |
| dimenhydrinate | dimenhy**DRINATE** |
| diphenhydramine | diphenhydr**AMINE** |
| dobutamine | **DOBUT**amine |
| dopamine | **DOP**amine |
| doxorubicin | **DOXO**rubicin |
| glipizide | glipi**ZIDE** |
| glyburide | gly**BURIDE** |
| hydralazine | hydr**ALAZINE** |
| hydroxyzine | hydr**OXY**zine |
| medroxyprogesterone | medroxy**PROGESTER**one |
| methylprednisolone | methyl**PREDNIS**olone |
| methyltestosterone | methyl**TESTOSTER**one |
| nicardipine | ni**CAR**dipine |
| nifedipine | **NIFE**dipine |
| prednisolone | predniso**LONE** |
| prednisone | predni**SONE** |

| | |
|---|---|
| sulfadiazine | sulfa**DIAZINE** |
| sulfisoxazole | sulfi**SOXAZOLE** |
| tolazamide | **TOLAZ**amide |
| tolbutamide | **TOLBUT**amide |
| vinblastine | vin**BLAS**tine |
| vincristine | vin**CRIS**tine |

Institute for Safe Medication Practices. "New Tall-Man Lettering Will Reduce Mix-Ups Due to Generic Drug Name Confusion," *ISMP Medication Safety Alert*, September 19, 2001. Available at: http://www.ismp.org.

Institute for Safe Medication Practices. "Prescription Mapping, Can Improve Efficiency While Minimizing Errors With Look-Alike Products," *ISMP Medication Safety Alert*, October 6, 1999. Available at: http://www.ismp.org.

U.S. Pharmacopeia, "USP Quality Review: Use Caution-Avoid Confusion," March 2001, No. 76. Available at: http://www.usp.org.

# SAFE WRITING

Health professionals and their support personnel frequently produce handwritten copies of information they see in print; therefore, such information is subjected to even greater possibilities for error or misinterpretation on the part of others. Thus, particular care must be given to how drug names and strengths are expressed when creating written health care documents.

The following are a few examples of safe writing rules suggested by the Institute for Safe Medication Practices, Inc.*

1. There should be a space between a number and its units as it is easier to read. There should be no periods after the abbreviations mg or mL.

   | Correct | Incorrect |
   |---------|-----------|
   | 10 mg   | 10mg      |
   | 100 mg  | 100mg     |

2. Never place a decimal and a zero after a whole number (2 mg is correct and 2.0 mg is incorrect). If the decimal point is not seen because it falls on a line or because individuals are working from copies where the decimal point is not seen, this causes a tenfold overdose.

3. Just the opposite is true for numbers less than one. Always place a zero before a naked decimal (0.5 mL is correct, .5 mL is incorrect).

4. Never abbreviate the word "unit." The handwritten U or u, looks like a 0 (zero), and may cause a tenfold overdose error to be made.

5. IU is not a safe abbreviation for international units. The handwritten IU looks like IV. Write out international units or use int. units.

6. Q.D. is not a safe abbreviation for once daily, as when the Q is followed by a sloppy dot, it looks like QID which means four times daily.

7. O.D. is not a safe abbreviation for once daily, as it is properly interpreted as meaning "right eye" and has caused liquid medications such as saturated solution of potassium iodide and Lugol's solution to be administered incorrectly. There is no safe abbreviation for once daily. It must be written out in full.

8. Do not use chemical names such as 6-mercaptopurine or 6-thioguanine, as 6-fold overdoses have been given when these were not recognized as chemical names. The proper names of these drugs are mercaptopurine or thioguanine.

9. Do not abbreviate drug names (5FC, 6MP, 5-ASA, MTX, HCTZ CPZ, PBZ, etc) as they are misinterpreted and cause error.

10. Do not use the apothecary system or symbols.

11. Do not abbreviate microgram as μg; instead use mcg as there is less likelihood of misinterpretation.

12. When writing an outpatient prescription, write a complete prescription. A complete prescription can prevent the prescriber, the pharmacist, and/or the patient from making a mistake and can eliminate the need for further clarification. The legible prescriptions should contain:

    a. patient's full name

    b. for pediatric or geriatric patients: their age (or weight where applicable)

*From "Safe Writing" by Davis NM, PharmD and Cohen MR, MS, Lecturers and Consultants for Safe Medication Practices, 1143 Wright Drive, Huntingdon Valley, PA 19006. Phone: (215) 947-7566.

c.  drug name, dosage form and strength; if a drug is new or rarely prescribed, print this information

d.  number or amount to be dispensed

e.  complete instructions for the patient, including the purpose of the medication

f.  when there are recognized contraindications for a prescribed drug, indicate to the pharmacist that you are aware of this fact (ie, when prescribing a potassium salt for a patient receiving an ACE inhibitor, write "K serum leveling being monitored")

# ALPHABETICAL LISTING OF DRUGS

**1370-999-397** *see* anagrelide *on page 52*

**A₁-PI** *see* alpha₁-proteinase inhibitor *on page 30*

**A200® Lice [US-OTC]** *see* permethrin *on page 635*

**A-200® Maximum Strength [US-OTC]** *see* pyrethrins and piperonyl butoxide *on page 699*

**A and D® Ointment [US-OTC]** *see* vitamin A and vitamin D *on page 849*

## abacavir (a BAK a veer)
**Synonyms** abacavir sulfate; ABC
**U.S./Canadian Brand Names** Ziagen® [US/Can]
**Therapeutic Category** Nucleoside Reverse Transcriptase Inhibitor (NRTI)
**Use** Treatment of HIV infections in combination with other antiretroviral agents
**Usual Dosage** Oral:
  Children: 3 months to 16 years: 8 mg/kg body weight twice daily (maximum: 300 mg twice daily) in combination with other antiretroviral agents
  Adults: 300 mg twice daily or 600 mg once daily in combination with other antiretroviral agents
**Dosage Forms**
  Solution, oral: 20 mg/mL (240 mL) [strawberry-banana flavor]
  Tablet: 300 mg

## abacavir and lamivudine (a BAK a veer & la MI vyoo deen)
**Synonyms** abacavir sulfate and lamivudine; lamivudine and abacavir
**U.S./Canadian Brand Names** Epzicom™ [US]
**Therapeutic Category** Antiretroviral Agent, Reverse Transcriptase Inhibitor (Nucleoside)
**Use** Treatment of HIV infections in combination with other antiretroviral agents
**Usual Dosage** Oral: Adults: HIV: One tablet (abacavir 600 mg and lamivudine 300 mg) once daily
**Dosage Forms** Tablet, film-coated: Abacavir 600 mg and lamivudine 300 mg

## abacavir, lamivudine, and zidovudine
(a BAK a veer, la MI vyoo deen, & zye DOE vyoo deen)
**Synonyms** 3TC, abacavir, and zidovudine; azidothymidine, abacavir, and lamivudine; AZT, abacavir, and lamivudine; compound S, abacavir, and lamivudine; lamivudine, abacavir, and zidovudine; ZDV, abacavir, and lamivudine; zidovudine, abacavir, and lamivudine
**U.S./Canadian Brand Names** Trizivir® [US]
**Therapeutic Category** Antiretroviral Agent, Nucleoside Reverse Transcriptase Inhibitor (NRTI)
**Use** Treatment of HIV infection (either alone or in combination with other antiretroviral agents) in patients whose regimen would otherwise contain the components of Trizivir®
**Usual Dosage** Oral: Adolescents and Adults: 1 tablet twice daily; **Note:** Not recommended for patients <40 kg
**Dosage Forms** Tablet [film coated]: Abacavir 300 mg, lamivudine 150 mg, and zidovudine 300 mg

**abacavir sulfate** *see* abacavir *on this page*

**abacavir sulfate and lamivudine** *see* abacavir and lamivudine *on this page*

## abarelix (a ba REL iks)
**Synonyms** PPI-149; R-3827
**Therapeutic Category** Gonadotropin Releasing Hormone Antagonist
**Use** Palliative treatment of advanced symptomatic prostate cancer; treatment is limited to men who are not candidates for LHRH therapy, refuse surgical castration, and have one or more of the following complications due to metastases or local encroachment: 1) risk of neurological compromise, 2) ureteral or bladder outlet obstruction, or 3) severe bone pain (persisting despite narcotic analgesia)
**Usual Dosage** I.M.: Male prostate cancer: 100 mg administered on days 1, 15, 29 (week 4), then every 4 weeks
**Dosage Forms** [DSC] = Discontinued product
  Injection, powder for reconstitution [preservative free]: 113 mg [provides 100 mg/2 mL depot suspension when reconstituted; packaged with diluent and syringe] [DSC]

## Abbokinase® *(Discontinued)*
**abbott-43818** *see* leuprolide acetate *on page 471*

**ABC** *see* abacavir *on previous page*

**ABCD** *see* amphotericin B cholesteryl sulfate complex *on page 48*

## abciximab (ab SIK si mab)
**Synonyms** 7E3; C7E3
**U.S./Canadian Brand Names** ReoPro® [US/Can]
**Therapeutic Category** Platelet Aggregation Inhibitor
**Use** Prevention of acute cardiac ischemic complications in patients at high risk for abrupt closure of the treated coronary vessel and patients at risk of restenosis; an adjunct with heparin to prevent cardiac ischemic complications in patients with unstable angina not responding to conventional therapy when a percutaneous coronary intervention is scheduled within 24 hours
**Usual Dosage** I.V.: 0.25 mg/kg bolus administered 10-60 minutes before the start of intervention followed by an infusion of 0.125 mcg/kg/minute (to a maximum of 10 mcg/minute) for 12 hours
Patients with unstable angina not responding to conventional medical therapy and who are planning to undergo percutaneous coronary intervention within 24 hours may be treated with abciximab 0.25 mg/kg intravenous bolus followed by an 18- to 24-hour intravenous infusion of 10 mcg/minute, concluding 1 hour after the percutaneous coronary intervention.
**Dosage Forms** Injection, solution: 2 mg/mL (5 mL)

**Abelcet**® **[US/Can]** *see* amphotericin B lipid complex *on page 49*

**Abenol**® **[Can]** *see* acetaminophen *on next page*

**Abilify**® **[US]** *see* aripiprazole *on page 70*

**ABLC** *see* amphotericin B lipid complex *on page 49*

**A/B Otic [US]** *see* antipyrine and benzocaine *on page 58*

**Abraxane**™ **[US]** *see* paclitaxel (protein bound) *on page 613*

**Abreva**® **[US-OTC]** *see* docosanol *on page 263*

**absorbable cotton** *see* cellulose, oxidized regenerated *on page 160*

**absorbable gelatin sponge** *see* gelatin (absorbable) *on page 368*

**Absorbine**® **Antifungal** *(Discontinued)* *see* tolnaftate *on page 809*

**Absorbine**® **Jock Itch** *(Discontinued)* *see* tolnaftate *on page 809*

**AC002993** *see* exenatide *on page 324*

**AC 2993** *see* exenatide *on page 324*

## acamprosate (a kam PROE sate)
**Synonyms** acamprosate calcium; calcium acetylhomotaurinate
**U.S./Canadian Brand Names** Campral® [US]
**Therapeutic Category** GABA Agonist/Glutamate Antagonist
**Use** Maintenance of alcohol abstinence
**Usual Dosage** Oral: Adults: Alcohol abstinence: 666 mg 3 times/day (a lower dose may be effective in some patients)
**Dosage Forms** Tablet, enteric coated, delayed release, as calcium: 333 mg [contains calcium 33 mg and sulfites]

**acamprosate calcium** *see* acamprosate *on this page*

## acarbose (AY car bose)
**Sound-Alike/Look-Alike Issues**
Precose® may be confused with PreCare®
**U.S./Canadian Brand Names** Prandase® [Can]; Precose® [US]
**Therapeutic Category** Antidiabetic Agent, Oral
**Use**
Monotherapy, as indicated as an adjunct to diet to lower blood glucose in patients with type 2 diabetes mellitus (noninsulin dependent, NIDDM) whose hyperglycemia cannot be managed on diet alone
Combination with a sulfonylurea, metformin, or insulin in patients with type 2 diabetes mellitus (noninsulin dependent, NIDDM) when diet plus acarbose do not result in adequate glycemic control. The effect of acarbose to enhance glycemic control is additive to that of other hypoglycemic agents when used in combination.
(Continued)

## acarbose *(Continued)*

**Usual Dosage** Oral:

Adults: Dosage must be individualized on the basis of effectiveness and tolerance while not exceeding the maximum recommended dose

**Initial dose:** 25 mg 3 times/day with the first bite of each main meal

**Maintenance dose:** Should be adjusted at 4- to 8-week intervals based on 1-hour postprandial glucose levels and tolerance. Dosage may be increased from 25 mg 3 times/day to 50 mg 3 times/day. Some patients may benefit from increasing the dose to 100 mg 3 times/day.
Maintenance dose ranges: 50-100 mg 3 times/day.

**Maximum dose:**
≤60 kg: 50 mg 3 times/day
>60 kg: 100 mg 3 times/day

**Patients receiving sulfonylureas:** Acarbose given in combination with a sulfonylurea will cause a further lowering of blood glucose and may increase the hypoglycemic potential of the sulfonylurea. If hypoglycemia occurs, appropriate adjustments in the dosage of these agents should be made.

**Dosage Forms** Tablet: 25 mg, 50 mg, 100 mg

**A-Caro-25**® **[US]** *see* beta-carotene *on page 101*

**Accolate**® **[US/Can]** *see* zafirlukast *on page 857*

**AccuHist**® **DM Pediatric Drops [US]** *see* brompheniramine, pseudoephedrine, and dextromethorphan *on page 116*

**AccuHist**® **PDX Drops [US]** *see* brompheniramine, pseudoephedrine, and dextromethorphan *on page 116*

**AccuHist**® **Pediatric** *(Discontinued) see* brompheniramine and pseudoephedrine *on page 115*

**AccuNeb**™ **[US]** *see* albuterol *on page 22*

**Accupril**® **[US/Can]** *see* quinapril *on page 704*

**Accuretic**® **[US/Can]** *see* quinapril and hydrochlorothiazide *on page 704*

**Accutane**® **[US/Can]** *see* isotretinoin *on page 452*

**Accuzyme**™ **[US]** *see* papain and urea *on page 618*

**ACE** *see* captopril *on page 139*

## acebutolol *(a se BYOO toe lole)*

**Sound-Alike/Look-Alike Issues**
Sectral® may be confused with Factrel®, Seconal®, Septra®

**Synonyms** acebutolol hydrochloride

**U.S./Canadian Brand Names** Apo-Acebutolol® [Can]; Gen-Acebutolol [Can]; Monitan® [Can]; Novo-Acebutolol [Can]; Nu-Acebutolol [Can]; Rhotral [Can]; Rhoxal-Acebutolol [Can]; Sectral® [US/Can]

**Therapeutic Category** Antiarrhythmic Agent, Class II; Beta-Adrenergic Blocker

**Use** Treatment of hypertension, ventricular arrhythmias, angina

**Usual Dosage** Oral: Adults:
Hypertension: 400-800 mg/day (larger doses may be divided); maximum: 1200 mg/day; usual dose range (JNC 7): 200-800 mg/day in 2 divided doses
Ventricular arrhythmias: Initial: 400 mg/day; maintenance: 600-1200 mg/day in divided doses

**Dosage Forms** Capsule, as hydrochloride: 200 mg, 400 mg

**acebutolol hydrochloride** *see* acebutolol *on this page*

**Aceon**® **[US]** *see* perindopril erbumine *on page 634*

**Acephen**® **[US-OTC]** *see* acetaminophen *on this page*

**Acetadote**® **[US]** *see* acetylcysteine *on page 15*

## acetaminophen *(a seet a MIN oh fen)*

**Sound-Alike/Look-Alike Issues**
Acephen® may be confused with AcipHex®
FeverALL® may be confused with Fiberall®
Tylenol® may be confused with atenolol, timolol, Tuinal®, Tylox®

**Synonyms** APAP; n-acetyl-p-aminophenol; paracetamol

**U.S./Canadian Brand Names** Abenol® [Can]; Acephen® [US-OTC]; Apo-Acetaminophen® [Can]; Aspirin Free Anacin® Maximum Strength [US-OTC]; Atasol® [Can]; Cetafen Extra® [US-OTC]; Cetafen® [US-OTC]; Comtrex® Sore Throat Maximum Strength [US-OTC]; ElixSure™ Fever/Pain [US-OTC]; FeverALL® [US-OTC]; Genapap® Children [US-OTC]; Genapap® Extra Strength [US-OTC]; Genapap® Infant [US-OTC]; Genapap® [US-OTC]; Genebs® Extra Strength [US-OTC]; Genebs® [US-OTC]; Mapap® Arthritis [US-OTC]; Mapap® Children's [US-OTC]; Mapap® Extra Strength [US-OTC]; Mapap® Infants [US-OTC]; Mapap® [US-OTC]; Novo-Gesic [Can]; Pediatrix [Can]; Redutemp® [US-OTC]; Silapap® Children's [US-OTC]; Silapap® Infants [US-OTC]; Tempra® [Can]; Tylenol® 8 Hour [US-OTC]; Tylenol® Arthritis Pain [US-OTC]; Tylenol® Children's [US-OTC]; Tylenol® Extra Strength [US-OTC]; Tylenol® Infants [US-OTC]; Tylenol® Junior Strength [US-OTC]; Tylenol® Sore Throat [US-OTC]; Tylenol® [US-OTC/Can]; Valorin Extra [US-OTC]; Valorin [US-OTC]

**Therapeutic Category** Analgesic, Nonnarcotic; Antipyretic

**Use** Treatment of mild to moderate pain and fever (antipyretic/analgesic); does not have antirheumatic or anti-inflammatory effects

**Usual Dosage** Oral, rectal:

Children <12 years: 10-15 mg/kg/dose every 4-6 hours as needed; do **not** exceed 5 doses (2.6 g) in 24 hours; alternatively, the following age-based doses may be used:

0-3 months: 40 mg
4-11 months: 80 mg
1-2 years: 120 mg
2-3 years: 160 mg
4-5 years: 240 mg
6-8 years: 320 mg
9-10 years: 400 mg
11 years: 480 mg

**Note:** Higher rectal doses have been studied for use in preoperative pain control in children. However, specific guidelines are not available and dosing may be product dependent. The safety and efficacy of alternating acetaminophen and ibuprofen dosing has not been established.

Adults: 325-650 mg every 4-6 hours or 1000 mg 3-4 times/day; do **not** exceed 4 g/day

**Dosage Forms** [DSC] = Discontinued product

Caplet (Cetafen Extra® Strength, Genapap® Extra Strength, Genebs® Extra Strength, Mapap® Extra Strength, Tylenol® Extra Strength): 500 mg

Caplet, extended release (Mapap® Arthritis, Tylenol® 8 Hour, Tylenol® Arthritis Pain): 650 mg

Capsule (Mapap® Extra Strength): 500 mg

Elixir: 160 mg/5 mL (120 mL, 480 mL, 3780 mL)

Mapap® Children's: 160 mg/5 mL (120 mL) [alcohol free; contains benzoic acid and sodium benzoate; cherry flavor]

Gelcap (Mapap® Extra Strength, Tylenol® Extra Strength): 500 mg

Geltab (Mapap® Extra Strength, Tylenol® Extra Strength): 500 mg

Geltab, extended release (Tylenol® 8 Hour): 650 mg

Liquid, oral: 500 mg/15 mL (240 mL)

Comtrex® Sore Throat Maximum Strength: 500 mg/15 mL (240 mL) [contains sodium benzoate; honey lemon flavor]

Genapap® Children: 160 mg/5 mL (120 mL) [contains sodium benzoate; cherry and grape flavors]

Silapap®: 160 mg/5 mL (120 mL, 240 mL, 480 mL) [sugar free; contains sodium benzoate; cherry flavor]

Tylenol® Extra Strength: 500 mg/15 mL (240 mL) [contains sodium benzoate; cherry flavor]

Tylenol® Sore Throat: 500 mg/15 mL (240 mL) [contains sodium benzoate; cherry and honey-lemon flavors]

Solution, oral drops: 80 mg/0.8 mL (15 mL) [droppers are marked at 0.4 mL (40 mg) and at 0.8 mL (80 mg)]

Genapap® Infant: 80 mg/0.8 mL (15 mL) [fruit flavor]

Silapap® Infant's: 80 mg/0.8 mL (15 mL, 30 mL) [contains sodium benzoate; cherry flavor]

Solution, oral: 160 mg/5 mL (120 mL, 480 mL)

Suppository, rectal: 120 mg, 325 mg, 650 mg

Acephen®: 120 mg, 325 mg, 650 mg

FeverALL®: 80 mg, 120 mg, 325 mg, 650 mg

Mapap®: 125 mg, 650 mg

Suspension, oral:

Mapap® Children's: 160 mg/5 mL (120 mL) [contains sodium benzoate; cherry flavor]

(Continued)

## acetaminophen (Continued)

Tylenol® Children's: 160 mg/5 mL (120 mL, 240 mL) [contains sodium benzoate; bubble gum yum, cherry blast, dye free cherry, grape splash, and very berry strawberry flavors]

Suspension, oral drops:

Mapap® Infants 80 mg/0.8 mL (15 mL, 30 mL) [contains sodium benzoate; cherry flavor]

Tylenol® Infants: 80 mg/0.8 mL (15 mL, 30 mL) [contains sodium benzoate; cherry, dye free cherry, and grape flavors]

Syrup, oral (ElixSure™ Fever/Pain): 160 mg/5 mL (120 mL) [bubble gum, cherry, and grape flavors]

Tablet: 325 mg, 500 mg

Aspirin Free Anacin® Extra Strength, Genapap® Extra Strength, Genebs® Extra Strength, Mapap® Extra Strength, Redutemp®, Tylenol® Extra Strength, Valorin Extra: 500 mg

Cetafen®, Genapap®, Genebs®, Mapap®, Tylenol®, Valorin: 325 mg

Tablet, chewable: 80 mg

Genapap® Children: 80 mg [contains phenylalanine 6 mg/tablet; fruit and grape flavors]

Mapap® Children's: 80 mg [contains phenylalanine 3 mg/tablet; bubble gum, fruit, and grape flavors]

Mapap® Junior Strength: 160 mg [contains phenylalanine 12 mg/tablet; grape flavor]

Tylenol® Children's: 80 mg [fruit and grape flavors contain phenylalanine 3 mg/tablet; bubble gum flavor contains phenylalanine 6 mg/tablet] [DSC]

Tylenol® Junior: 160 mg [contains phenylalanine 6 mg/tablet; fruit and grape flavors] [DSC]

Tablet, orally-disintegrating:

Tylenol® Children's Meltaways: 80 mg [bubble gum, grape, and watermelon flavors]

Tylenol® Junior Meltaways: 160 mg [bubble gum and grape flavors]

**acetaminophen and chlorpheniramine** *see* chlorpheniramine and acetaminophen *on page 171*

## acetaminophen and codeine (a seet a MIN oh fen & KOE deen)

**Sound-Alike/Look-Alike Issues**

Capital® may be confused with Capitrol®

Tylenol® may be confused with atenolol, timolol, Tuinal®, Tylox®

**Synonyms** codeine and acetaminophen

**U.S./Canadian Brand Names** Capital® and Codeine [US]; ratio-Emtec [Can]; ratio-Lenoltec [Can]; Triatec-30 [Can]; Triatec-8 Strong [Can]; Triatec-8 [Can]; Tylenol® Elixir with Codeine [Can]; Tylenol® No. 1 Forte [Can]; Tylenol® No. 1 [Can]; Tylenol® No. 2 with Codeine [Can]; Tylenol® No. 3 with Codeine [Can]; Tylenol® No. 4 with Codeine [Can]; Tylenol® With Codeine [US]

**Therapeutic Category** Analgesic, Narcotic

**Controlled Substance** C-III; C-V

**Use** Relief of mild to moderate pain

**Usual Dosage** Doses should be adjusted according to severity of pain and response of the patient. Adult doses ≥60 mg codeine fail to give commensurate relief of pain but merely prolong analgesia and are associated with an appreciably increased incidence of side effects. Oral:

Children: Analgesic:

Codeine: 0.5-1 mg codeine/kg/dose every 4-6 hours

Acetaminophen: 10-15 mg/kg/dose every 4 hours up to a maximum of 2.6 g/24 hours for children <12 years; **alternatively, the following can be used:**

3-6 years: 5 mL 3-4 times/day as needed of elixir

7-12 years: 10 mL 3-4 times/day as needed of elixir

>12 years: 15 mL every 4 hours as needed of elixir

Adults:

Antitussive: Based on codeine (15-30 mg/dose) every 4-6 hours (maximum: 360 mg/24 hours based on codeine component)

Analgesic: Based on codeine (30-60 mg/dose) every 4-6 hours (maximum: 4000 mg/24 hours based on acetaminophen component)

**Dosage Forms** [DSC] = Discontinued product; [CAN] = Canadian brand name

Caplet:

ratio-Lenoltec No. 1 [CAN], Tylenol No. 1 [CAN]: Acetaminophen 300 mg, codeine phosphate, 8 mg and caffeine 15 mg [not available in the U.S.]

Tylenol No. 1 Forte [CAN]: Acetaminophen 500 mg, codeine phosphate 8 mg, and caffeine 15 mg [not available in the U.S.]

Elixir, oral [C-V]: Acetaminophen 120 mg and codeine phosphate 12 mg per 5 mL (5 mL, 10 mL, 12.5 mL, 15 mL, 120 mL, 480 mL) [contains alcohol 7%]

Tylenol® with Codeine [DSC]: Acetaminophen 120 mg and codeine phosphate 12 mg per 5 mL (480 mL) [contains alcohol 7%; cherry flavor]

Tylenol Elixir with Codeine [CAN]: Acetaminophen 160 mg and codeine phosphate 8 mg per 5 mL (500 mL) [contains alcohol 7%, sucrose 31%; cherry flavor; not available in the U.S.]

Suspension, oral [C-V] (Capital® and Codeine): Acetaminophen 120 mg and codeine phosphate 12 mg per 5 mL (480 mL) [alcohol free; fruit punch flavor]

Tablet [C-III]: Acetaminophen 300 mg and codeine phosphate 15 mg; acetaminophen 300 mg and codeine phosphate 30 mg; acetaminophen 300 mg and codeine phosphate 60 mg

ratio-Emtec [CAN], Triatec-30 [CAN]: Acetaminophen 300 mg and codeine phosphate 30 mg [not available in the U.S.]

ratio-Lenoltec No. 1 [CAN]: Acetaminophen 300 mg, codeine phosphate 8 mg, and caffeine 15 mg [not available in the U.S.]

ratio-Lenoltec No. 2 [CAN], Tylenol No. 2 with Codeine [CAN]: Acetaminophen 300 mg, codeine phosphate 15 mg, and caffeine 15 mg [not available in the U.S.]

ratio-Lenoltec No. 3 [CAN], Tylenol No. 3 with Codeine [CAN]: Acetaminophen 300 mg, codeine phosphate 30 mg, and caffeine 15 mg [not available in the U.S.]

ratio-Lenoltec No. 4 [CAN], Tylenol No. 4 with Codeine [CAN]: Acetaminophen 300 mg and codeine phosphate 60 mg [not available in the U.S.]

Triatec-8 [CAN]: Acetaminophen 325 mg, codeine phosphate 8 mg, and caffeine 30 mg [not available in the U.S.]

Triatec-8 Strong [CAN]: Acetaminophen 500 mg, codeine phosphate 8 mg, and caffeine 30 mg [not available in the U.S.]

Tylenol® with Codeine No. 3: Acetaminophen 300 mg and codeine phosphate 30 mg [contains sodium metabisulfite]

Tylenol® with Codeine No. 4: Acetaminophen 300 mg and codeine phosphate 60 mg [contains sodium metabisulfite]

## acetaminophen and diphenhydramine (a seet a MIN oh fen & dye fen HYE dra meen)

**Sound-Alike/Look-Alike Issues**
Excedrin® may be confused with Dexatrim®, Dexedrine®
Percogesic® may be confused with paregoric, Percodan®
Tylenol® may be confused with atenolol, timolol, Tuinal®, Tylox®

**Synonyms** diphenhydramine and acetaminophen

**U.S./Canadian Brand Names** Excedrin® P.M. [US-OTC]; Goody's PM® Powder [US-OTC]; Legatrin PM® [US-OTC]; Percogesic® Extra Strength [US-OTC]; Tylenol® PM Extra Strength [US-OTC]; Tylenol® Severe Allergy [US-OTC]

**Therapeutic Category** Analgesic, Nonnarcotic

**Use** Aid in the relief of insomnia accompanied by minor pain

**Usual Dosage** Oral: Adults: 50 mg of diphenhydramine HCl (76 mg diphenhydramine citrate) at bedtime or as directed by physician; do not exceed recommended dosage; not for use in children <12 years of age

**Dosage Forms** [DSC] = Discontinued product
Caplet: Acetaminophen 500 mg and diphenhydramine hydrochloride 25 mg
Excedrin® P.M.: Acetaminophen 500 mg and diphenhydramine citrate 38 mg [contains benzoic acid]
Legatrin PM®: Acetaminophen 500 mg and diphenhydramine hydrochloride 50 mg
Percogesic® Extra Strength: Acetaminophen 500 mg and diphenhydramine hydrochloride 25 mg
Tylenol® PM: Acetaminophen 500 mg and diphenhydramine hydrochloride 25 mg [also available in vanilla caplets]
Tylenol® Severe Allergy: Acetaminophen 500 mg and diphenhydramine hydrochloride 12.5 mg
Gelcap (Tylenol® PM): Acetaminophen 500 mg and diphenhydramine hydrochloride 25 mg
Geltab: Acetaminophen 500 mg and diphenhydramine hydrochloride 25 mg
Excedrin® P.M.: Acetaminophen 500 mg and diphenhydramine citrate 38 mg [contains benzoic acid]
Tylenol® PM: Acetaminophen 500 mg and diphenhydramine hydrochloride 25 mg
Liquid (Tylenol® PM): Acetaminophen 500 mg and diphenhydramine hydrochloride 25 mg per 15 mL (240 mL) [contains sodium benzoate; vanilla flavor]
Powder for oral solution (Goody's PM® Powder): Acetaminophen 500 mg and diphenhydramine citrate 38 mg
Tablet: Acetaminophen 500 mg and diphenhydramine hydrochloride 25 mg
Excedrin® P.M.: Acetaminophen 500 mg and diphenhydramine citrate 38 mg [contains benzoic acid]

## acetaminophen and hydrocodone see hydrocodone and acetaminophen on page 411

## acetaminophen and oxycodone see oxycodone and acetaminophen on page 609

## acetaminophen and phenyltoloxamine (a seet a MIN oh fen & fen il to LOKS a meen)

**Sound-Alike/Look-Alike Issues**
Percogesic® may be confused with paregoric, Percodan®

**Synonyms** phenyltoloxamine and acetaminophen

**U.S./Canadian Brand Names** Genesec® [US-OTC]; Percogesic® [US-OTC]; Phenylgesic® [US-OTC]

**Therapeutic Category** Analgesic, Nonnarcotic

**Use** Relief of mild to moderate pain

**Usual Dosage** Oral:

Analgesic: Based on acetaminophen component:

Children: 10-15 mg/kg/dose every 4-6 hours as needed; do **not** exceed 5 doses/24 hours

Adults: 325-650 every 4-6 hours as needed; do **not** exceed 4 g/day

**Product labeling:** Percogesic®:

Children 6-12 years: 1 tablet every 4 hours; do **not** exceed 4 tablets/24 hours

Adults: 1-2 tablets every 4 hours; do **not** exceed 8 tablets/24 hours

**Dosage Forms** Tablet: Acetaminophen 325 mg and phenyltoloxamine citrate 30 mg

## acetaminophen and pseudoephedrine (a seet a MIN oh fen & soo doe e FED rin)

**Sound-Alike/Look-Alike Issues**
Ornex® may be confused with Orexin®, Orinase®

Sudafed® may be confused with Sufenta®

Tylenol® may be confused with atenolol, timolol, Tuinal®, Tylox®

**Synonyms** pseudoephedrine and acetaminophen

**U.S./Canadian Brand Names** Alka-Seltzer® Plus® Cold and Sinus Liqui-Gels [US-OTC]; Cetafen Cold® [US-OTC]; Contac® Cold and Sore Throat, Non Drowsy, Extra Strength [Can]; Dristan® N.D. [Can]; Dristan® N.D., Extra Strength [Can]; Genapap® Sinus Maximum Strength [US-OTC]; Mapap Sinus Maximum Strength [US-OTC]; Medi-Synal [US-OTC]; Ornex® Maximum Strength [US-OTC]; Ornex® [US-OTC]; Sinus-Relief® [US-OTC]; Sinutab® Non Drowsy [Can]; Sinutab® Sinus [US-OTC]; Sudafed® Head Cold and Sinus Extra Strength [Can]; Sudafed® Sinus and Cold [US-OTC]; Sudafed® Sinus Headache [US-OTC]; SudoGest Sinus [US-OTC]; Tylenol® Cold, Infants [US-OTC]; Tylenol® Decongestant [Can]; Tylenol® Sinus Day Non-Drowsy [US-OTC]; Tylenol® Sinus [Can]; Tylenol® Sinus, Children's [US-OTC]

**Therapeutic Category** Decongestant/Analgesic

**Use** Relief of mild to moderate pain; relief of congestion

**Usual Dosage** Oral:

Analgesic: Based on acetaminophen component:

Children: 10-15 mg/kg/dose every 4-6 hours as needed; do **not** exceed 5 doses in 24 hours

Adults: 325-650 mg every 4-6 hours as needed; do **not** exceed 4 g/day

Decongestant: Based on pseudoephedrine component:

Children:

2-6 years: 15 mg every 4 hours; do **not** exceed 90 mg/day

6-12 years: 30 mg every 4 hours; do **not** exceed 180 mg/day

Children >12 years and Adults: 60 mg every 4 hours; do **not** exceed 360 mg/day

**Product labeling:**

Alka-Seltzer Plus® Cold and Sinus:

Children 6-12 years: 1 dose with water every 4 hours (maximum: 4 doses/24 hours)

Adults: 2 doses with water every 4 hours (maximum: 4 doses/24 hours)

Children's Tylenol® Sinus: Children:

Liquid:

2-5 years (24-47 lb): 1 teaspoonful every 4-6 hours (maximum: 4 doses/24 hours)

6-11 years (48-95 lb): 2 teaspoonfuls every 4-6 hours (maximum: 4 doses/24 hours)

Tablet, chewable:

2-5 years (24-47 lb): 2 tablets every 4-6 hours (maximum: 4 doses/24 hours)

6-11 years (48-95 lb): 4 tablets every 4-6 hours (maximum: 4 doses/24 hours)

Sinutab® Sinus: Children >12 years and Adults: 2 doses every 6 hours (maximum: 8 doses/24 hours)

**Dosage Forms**

Caplet:

Ornex®: Acetaminophen 325 mg and pseudoephedrine hydrochloride 30 mg

Genapap™ Sinus Maximum Strength, Mapap Sinus Maximum Strength, Ornex® Maximum Strength, Sudafed® Sinus Headache, Tylenol® Sinus Day Non-Drowsy: Acetaminophen 500 mg and pseudoephedrine hydrochloride 30 mg

Capsule, liquid (Alka-Seltzer Plus® Cold and Sinus, Sudafed® Sinus and Cold): Acetaminophen 325 mg and pseudoephedrine hydrochloride 30 mg

Gelcap (Tylenol® Sinus Day Non-Drowsy): Acetaminophen 500 mg and pseudoephedrine hydrochloride 30 mg

Geltab (Mapap Sinus Maximum Strength, Tylenol® Sinus Day Non-Drowsy): Acetaminophen 500 mg and pseudoephedrine hydrochloride 30 mg

Liquid, oral drops (Infants Tylenol® Cold): Acetaminophen 80 mg/0.8 mL and pseudoephedrine 7.5 mg/0.8 mL [contains sodium benzoate; bubble gum flavor]

Suspension (Children's Tylenol® Sinus): Acetaminophen 160 mg and pseudoephedrine hydrochloride 15 mg/5 mL [contains sodium benzoate; fruit flavor]

Tablet:

Cetafen Cold®, Medi-Synal, Sinus-Relief: Acetaminophen 325 mg and pseudoephedrine hydrochloride 30 mg

Sinutab® Sinus, Sudafed® Sinus Headache, SudoGest Sinus: Acetaminophen 500 mg and pseudoephedrine hydrochloride 30 mg

# acetaminophen and tramadol (a seet a MIN oh fen & TRA ma dole)

**Synonyms** APAP and tramadol; tramadol hydrochloride and acetaminophen

**U.S./Canadian Brand Names** Tramacet [Can]; Ultracet™ [US]

**Therapeutic Category** Analgesic, Miscellaneous; Analgesic, Nonnarcotic

**Use** Short-term (≤5 days) management of acute pain

**Usual Dosage** Oral: Adults: Acute pain: Two tablets every 4-6 hours as needed for pain relief (maximum: 8 tablets/day); treatment should not exceed 5 days

**Dosage Forms** Tablet: Acetaminophen 325 mg and tramadol hydrochloride 37.5 mg

# acetaminophen, aspirin, and caffeine (a seet a MIN oh fen, AS pir in, & KAF een)

**Sound-Alike/Look-Alike Issues**

Excedrin® may be confused with Dexatrim®, Dexedrine®

**Synonyms** aspirin, acetaminophen, and caffeine; aspirin, caffeine, and acetaminophen; caffeine, acetaminophen, and aspirin; caffeine, aspirin, and acetaminophen

**U.S./Canadian Brand Names** Excedrin® Extra Strength [US-OTC]; Excedrin® Migraine [US-OTC]; Fem-Prin® [US-OTC]; Genaced™ [US-OTC]; Goody's® Extra Strength Headache Powder [US-OTC]; Goody's® Extra Strength Pain Relief [US-OTC]; Pain-Off [US-OTC]; Vanquish® Extra Strength Pain Reliever [US-OTC]

**Therapeutic Category** Analgesic, Nonnarcotic

**Use** Relief of mild to moderate pain; mild to moderate pain associated with migraine headache

**Usual Dosage** Oral: Adults:

Analgesic:

Based on **acetaminophen** component:

Mild to moderate pain: 325-650 mg every 4-6 hours as needed; do **not** exceed 4 g/day

Mild to moderate pain associated with migraine headache: 500 mg/dose (in combination with 500 mg aspirin and 130 mg caffeine) every 6 hours while symptoms persist; do not use for longer than 48 hours

Based on **aspirin** component:

Mild to moderate pain: 325-650 mg every 4-6 hours as needed; do **not** exceed 4 g/day

Mild to moderate pain associated with migraine headache: 500 mg/dose (in combination with 500 mg acetaminophen and 130 mg caffeine) every 6 hours; do not use for longer than 48 hours

**Product labeling:**

Excedrin® Extra Strength, Excedrin® Migraine: Children >12 years and Adults: 2 doses every 6 hours (maximum: 8 doses/24 hours)

**Note:** When used for migraine, do not use for longer than 48 hours

Goody's® Extra Strength Headache Powder: Children >12 years and Adults: 1 powder, placed on tongue or dissolved in water, every 4-6 hours (maximum: 4 powders/24 hours)

Goody's® Extra Strength Pain Relief Tablets: Children >12 years and Adults: 2 tablets every 4-6 hours (maximum: 8 tablets/24 hours)

Vanquish® Extra Strength Pain Reliever: Children >12 years and Adults: 2 tablets every 4 hours (maximum: 12 tablets/24 hours)

**Dosage Forms**

Caplet:

Excedrin® Extra Strength, Excedrin® Migraine: Acetaminophen 250 mg, aspirin 250 mg, and caffeine 65 mg

(Continued)

## acetaminophen, aspirin, and caffeine *(Continued)*

Vanquish® Extra Strength Pain Reliever: Acetaminophen 194 mg, aspirin 227 mg, and caffeine 33 mg

Geltab (Excedrin® Extra Strength, Excedrin® Migraine): Acetaminophen 250 mg, aspirin 250 mg, and caffeine 65 mg

Powder (Goody's® Extra Strength Headache Powder): Acetaminophen 260 mg, aspirin 520 mg, and caffeine 32.5 mg [contains lactose]

Tablet:

Excedrin® Extra Strength, Excedrin® Migraine, Genaced™, Pain-Off: Acetaminophen 250 mg, aspirin 250 mg, and caffeine 65 mg

Fem-Prin®: Acetaminophen 194.4 mg, aspirin 226.8 mg, and caffeine 32.4 mg

Goody's® Extra Strength Pain Relief: Acetaminophen 130 mg, aspirin 260 mg, and caffeine 16.25 mg

**acetaminophen, butalbital, and caffeine** *see* butalbital, acetaminophen, and caffeine *on* page 124

**acetaminophen, caffeine, hydrocodone, chlorpheniramine, and phenylephrine** *see* hydrocodone, chlorpheniramine, phenylephrine, acetaminophen, and caffeine *on page 414*

## acetaminophen, chlorpheniramine, and pseudoephedrine

(a seet a MIN oh fen, klor fen IR a meen, & soo doe e FED rin)

**Sound-Alike/Look-Alike Issues**

Thera-Flu® may be confused with Tamiflu®, Thera-Flur-N®

Tylenol® may be confused with atenolol, timolol, Tuinal®, Tylox®

**Synonyms** acetaminophen, pseudoephedrine, and chlorpheniramine; chlorpheniramine, acetaminophen, and pseudoephedrine; chlorpheniramine, pseudoephedrine, and acetaminophen; pseudoephedrine, acetaminophen, and chlorpheniramine; pseudoephedrine, chlorpheniramine, and acetaminophen

**U.S./Canadian Brand Names** Actifed® Cold and Sinus [US-OTC]; Alka-Seltzer® Plus® Cold Liqui-Gels [US-OTC]; Children's Tylenol® Plus Cold [US-OTC]; Comtrex® Maximum Strength Sinus and Nasal Decongestant [US-OTC]; Sinutab® Sinus & Allergy [Can]; Sinutab® Sinus Allergy Maximum Strength [US-OTC]; Thera-Flu® Cold and Sore Throat Night Time [US-OTC]; Tylenol® Allergy Sinus [US-OTC/Can]

**Therapeutic Category** Antihistamine/Decongestant/Analgesic

**Use** Temporary relief of sinus symptoms

**Usual Dosage** Oral:

Analgesic: Based on **acetaminophen** component:

Children: 10-15 mg/kg/dose every 4-6 hours as needed; do **not** exceed 5 doses in 24 hours

Adults: 325-650 mg every 4-6 hours as needed; do **not** exceed 4 g/day

Antihistamine: Based on **chlorpheniramine maleate** component:

Children:

2-6 years: 1 mg every 4-6 hours (maximum: 6 mg/24 hours)

6-12 years: 2 mg every 4-6 hours (maximum: 12 mg/24 hours)

Children >12 years and Adults: 4 mg every 4-6 hours (maximum: 24 mg/24 hours)

Decongestant: Based on **pseudoephedrine** component:

Children:

2-6 years: 15 mg every 4 hours (maximum: 90 mg/24 hours)

6-12 years: 30 mg every 4 hours (maximum: 180 mg/24 hours)

Children >12 years and Adults: 60 mg every 4 hours (maximum: 360 mg/24 hours)

**Product labeling:**

Alka-Seltzer Plus® Cold Medicine Liqui-Gels®:

Children 6-12 years: 1 softgel every 4 hours with water (maximum: 4 doses/24 hours)

Children >12 years and Adults: 2 softgels every 4 hours with water (maximum: 4 doses/24 hours)

Sinutab® Sinus Allergy Maximum Strength: Children >12 years and Adults: 2 tablets/caplets every 6 hours (maximum: 8 doses/24 hours)

Thera-Flu® Cold and Sore Throat Night Time: Children >12 years and Adults: 1 packet dissolved in hot water every 6 hours (maximum: 4 packets/24 hours)

**Dosage Forms** [DSC] = Discontinued product

Caplet: Acetaminophen 325 mg, chlorpheniramine maleate 2 mg, and pseudoephedrine hydrochloride 30 mg

Actifed® Cold and Sinus, Comtrex® Maximum Strength Sinus and Nasal Decongestant [DSC], Sinutab® Sinus Allergy Maximum Strength, Tylenol® Allergy Complete: Acetaminophen 500 mg, chlorpheniramine maleate 2 mg, and pseudoephedrine hydrochloride 30 mg

Kolephrin®: Acetaminophen 325 mg, chlorpheniramine maleate 2 mg, and pseudoephedrine hydrochloride 30 mg

Capsule, softgel (Alka-Seltzer® Plus Cold Liqui-Gels®): Acetaminophen 325 mg, chlorpheniramine maleate 2 mg, and pseudoephedrine hydrochloride 30 mg [contains potassium 25 mg]

Combination package: (Comtrex® Flu Therapy Day/Night):

Caplet [Daytime]: Acetaminophen 500 mg, and pseudoephedrine hydrochloride 30 mg

Caplet [Nighttime]: Acetaminophen 500 mg, chlorpheniramine maleate 2 mg, and pseudoephedrine hydrochloride 30 mg

Gelcap (Tylenol® Allergy Sinus): Acetaminophen 500 mg, chlorpheniramine maleate 2 mg, and pseudoephedrine hydrochloride 30 mg [DSC]

Geltab (Tylenol® Allergy Sinus): Acetaminophen 500 mg, chlorpheniramine maleate 2 mg, and pseudoephedrine hydrochloride 30 mg [DSC]

Liquid:

Comtrex® Flu Therapy Nighttime: Acetaminophen 100 mg, chlorpheniramine maleate 4 mg, and pseudoephedrine hydrochloride 60 mg per 30 mL (240 mL) [contains alcohol; cherry flavor]

Tylenol® Children's Plus Cold Nighttime: Acetaminophen 160 mg, chlorpheniramine maleate 1 mg, and pseudoephedrine hydrochloride 15 mg per 5 mL (120 mL) [contains sodium benzoate; grape flavor]

Powder for oral solution [packet] (Thera-Flu® Cold and Sore Throat Night Time): Acetaminophen 650 mg, chlorpheniramine maleate 4 mg, and pseudoephedrine hydrochloride 60 mg [contains phenylalanine 11 mg/packet; lemon flavor]

# acetaminophen, dextromethorphan, and pseudoephedrine

(a seet a MIN oh fen, deks troe meth OR fan, & soo doe e FED rin)

**Sound-Alike/Look-Alike Issues**

Sudafed® may be confused with Sufenta®

Thera-Flu® may be confused with Tamiflu®, Thera-Flur-N®

Tylenol® may be confused with atenolol, timolol, Tuinal®, Tylox®

**Synonyms** dextromethorphan, acetaminophen, and pseudoephedrine; pseudoephedrine, acetaminophen, and dextromethorphan; pseudoephedrine, dextromethorphan, and acetaminophen

**U.S./Canadian Brand Names** Alka Seltzer® Plus® Flu Liqui-Gels [US-OTC]; Comtrex® Non-Drowsy Cold and Cough Relief [US-OTC]; Contac® Complete [Can]; Contac® Cough, Cold and Flu Day & Night™ [Can]; Contac® Severe Cold and Flu/Non-Drowsy [US-OTC]; Infants' Tylenol® Cold Plus Cough Concentrated Drops [US-OTC]; Sudafed® Cold & Cough Extra Strength [Can]; Sudafed® Severe Cold [US-OTC]; Triaminic® Cough and Sore Throat Formula [US-OTC]; Tylenol® Cold Day Non-Drowsy [US-OTC]; Tylenol® Cold Daytime [Can]; Tylenol® Flu Non-Drowsy Maximum Strength [US-OTC]; Vicks® DayQuil® Multi-Symptom Cold and Flu [US-OTC]

**Therapeutic Category** Cold Preparation

**Use** Treatment of mild to moderate pain and fever; symptomatic relief of cough and congestion

**Usual Dosage** Oral:

Analgesic: Based on acetaminophen component:

Children: 10-15 mg/kg/dose every 4-6 hours as needed; do **not** exceed 5 doses/24 hours

Adults: 325-650 mg every 4-7 hours as needed; do **not** exceed 4 g/day

Cough suppressant: Based on dextromethorphan component:

Children 6-12 years: 15 mg every 6-8 hours; do **not** exceed 60 mg/24 hours

Children >12 years and Adults: 10-20 mg every 4-8 hours **or** 30 mg every 8 hours; do **not** exceed 120 mg/24 hours

Decongestant: Based on pseudoephedrine component:

Children:

2-6 years: 15 mg every 4 hours (maximum: 90 mg/24 hours)

6-12 years: 30 mg every 4 hours (maximum: 180 mg/24 hours)

Children >12 years and Adults: 60 mg every 4 hours (maximum: 360 mg/24 hours)

**Product labeling:**

Alka-Seltzer Plus® Cold and Flu Liqui-Gels®:

Children 6-12 years: 1 dose every 4 hours (maximum: 4 doses/24 hours)

Children >12 years and Adults: 2 dose every 4 hours (maximum: 4 doses/24 hours)

Infants' Tylenol® Cold Plus Cough Concentrated Drops: Children 2-3 years (24-55 lb): 2 dropperfuls every 4-6 hours (maximum: 4 doses/24 hours)

Sudafed® Severe Cold, Thera-Flu® Non-Drowsy Maximum Strength (gelcap), Tylenol® Flu Non-Drowsy Maximum Strength: Children >12 years and Adults: 2 doses every 6 hours (maximum: 8 doses/24 hours)

Tylenol® Cold Non-Drowsy:

Children 6-11 years: 1 dose every 6 hours (maximum: 4 doses/24 hours)

(Continued)

## acetaminophen, dextromethorphan, and pseudoephedrine *(Continued)*

Children ≥12 years and Adults: 2 doses every 6 hours (maximum: 8 doses/24 hours)

Thera-Flu® Non-Drowsy Maximum Strength: Children >12 years and Adults: 1 packet dissolved in hot water every 6 hours (maximum: 4 packets/24 hours)

**Dosage Forms** [DSC] = Discontinued product

Caplet:

Contac® Severe Cold and Flu/Non-Drowsy, Sudafed® Severe Cold, Tylenol® Cold Non-Drowsy: Acetaminophen 325 mg, dextromethorphan hydrobromide 15 mg, and pseudoephedrine hydrochloride 30 mg

Comtrex® Non-Drowsy Cold and Cough Relief: Acetaminophen 500 mg, dextromethorphan hydrobromide 15 mg, and pseudoephedrine hydrochloride 30 mg [contains benzoic acid]

Thera-Flu® Severe Cold Non-Drowsy: Acetaminophen 500 mg, dextromethorphan hydrobromide 15 mg, and pseudoephedrine hydrochloride 30 mg [contains lactose] [DSC]

Tylenol® Cold Day Non-Drowsy: Acetaminophen 325 mg dextromethorphan hydrobromide 15 mg, and pseudoephedrine hydrochloride 30 mg

Capsule, liquid:

Alka-Seltzer Plus® Flu Liqui-Gels®: Acetaminophen 325 mg, dextromethorphan hydrobromide 10 mg, and pseudoephedrine hydrochloride 30 mg

Vicks® DayQuil® Multi-Symptom Cold and Flu: Acetaminophen 250 mg, dextromethorphan hydrobromide 10 mg, and pseudoephedrine hydrochloride 30 mg

Gelcap:

Tylenol® Cold Day Non-Drowsy: Acetaminophen 325 mg dextromethorphan hydrobromide 15 mg, and pseudoephedrine hydrochloride 30 mg [contains benzyl alcohol]

Tylenol® Flu Non-Drowsy Maximum Strength: Acetaminophen 500 mg, dextromethorphan hydrobromide 15 mg, and pseudoephedrine hydrochloride 30 mg

Liquid:

Triaminic® Cough and Sore Throat Formula: Acetaminophen 160 mg, dextromethorphan hydrobromide 7.5 mg, and pseudoephedrine hydrochloride 15 mg per 5 mL (120 mL, 240 mL) [contains benzoic acid; grape flavor]

Vicks® DayQuil® Multi-Symptom Cold and Flu: Acetaminophen 325 mg, dextromethorphan hydrobromide 10 mg, and pseudoephedrine hydrochloride 30 mg per 15 mL (175 mL)

Powder for oral solution [packet] (Thera-Flu® Severe Cold Non-Drowsy): Acetaminophen 1000 mg, dextromethorphan hydrobromide 30 mg, and pseudoephedrine hydrochloride 60 mg [contains phenylalanine 17 mg/packet; lemon flavor] [DSC]

Suspension, oral drops (Infants' Tylenol® Cold Plus Cough Concentrated Drops): Acetaminophen 160 mg, dextromethorphan hydrobromide 5 mg, and pseudoephedrine hydrochloride 15 mg per 1.6 mL (15 mL) [1.6 mL = 2 dropperfuls] [cherry flavor]

**acetaminophen, dichloralphenazone, and isometheptene** *see* acetaminophen, isometheptene, and dichloralphenazone *on this page*

## acetaminophen, isometheptene, and dichloralphenazone

(a seet a MIN oh fen, eye soe me THEP teen, & dye KLOR al FEN a zone)

**Sound-Alike/Look-Alike Issues**

Midrin® may be confused with Mydfrin®

**Synonyms** acetaminophen, dichloralphenazone, and isometheptene; dichloralphenazone, acetaminophen, and isometheptene; dichloralphenazone, isometheptene, and acetaminophen; isometheptene, acetaminophen, and dichloralphenazone; isometheptene, dichloralphenazone, and acetaminophen

**U.S./Canadian Brand Names** Amidrine [US]; Duradrin® [US]; Midrin® [US]; Migrin-A [US]

**Therapeutic Category** Analgesic, Nonnarcotic

**Controlled Substance** C-IV

**Use** Relief of migraine and tension headache

**Usual Dosage** Oral: Adults:

Migraine headache: 2 capsules to start, followed by 1 capsule every hour until relief is obtained (maximum: 5 capsules/12 hours)

Tension headache: 1-2 capsules every 4 hours (maximum: 8 capsules/24 hours)

**Dosage Forms** Capsule: Acetaminophen 325 mg, isometheptene mucate 65 mg, dichloralphenazone 100 mg

**acetaminophen, pseudoephedrine, and chlorpheniramine** *see* acetaminophen, chlorpheniramine, and pseudoephedrine *on page 10*

**Acetasol**® **HC [US]** *see* acetic acid, propylene glycol diacetate, and hydrocortisone *on next page*

# acetazolamide (a set a ZOLE a mide)
### Sound-Alike/Look-Alike Issues
acetaZOLAMIDE may be confused with acetoHEXAMIDE
Diamox® Sequels® may be confused with Dobutrex®, Trimox®
### Tall-Man acetaZOLAMIDE
### U.S./Canadian Brand Names Apo-Acetazolamide® [Can]; Diamox® Sequels® [US]; Diamox® [Can]
### Therapeutic Category Anticonvulsant; Carbonic Anhydrase Inhibitor
### Use Treatment of glaucoma (chronic simple open-angle, secondary glaucoma, preoperatively in acute angle-closure); drug-induced edema or edema due to congestive heart failure (adjunctive therapy); centrencephalic epilepsies (immediate release dosage form); prevention or amelioration of symptoms associated with acute mountain sickness
### Usual Dosage Note: I.M. administration is not recommended because of pain secondary to the alkaline pH
Children:
Glaucoma:
Oral: 8-30 mg/kg/day or 300-900 mg/m$^2$/day divided every 8 hours
I.V.: 20-40 mg/kg/24 hours divided every 6 hours, not to exceed 1 g/day
Edema: Oral, I.V.: 5 mg/kg or 150 mg/m$^2$ once every day
Epilepsy: Oral: 8-30 mg/kg/day in 1-4 divided doses, not to exceed 1 g/day; sustained release capsule is not recommended for treatment of epilepsy
Adults:
Glaucoma:
Chronic simple (open-angle): Oral: 250 mg 1-4 times/day or 500 mg sustained release capsule twice daily
Secondary, acute (closed-angle): I.V.: 250-500 mg, may repeat in 2-4 hours to a maximum of 1 g/day
Edema: Oral, I.V.: 250-375 mg once daily
Epilepsy: Oral: 8-30 mg/kg/day in 1-4 divided doses; **sustained release capsule is not recommended for treatment of epilepsy**
Mountain sickness: Oral: 250 mg every 8-12 hours (or 500 mg extended release capsules every 12-24 hours)
Therapy should begin 24-48 hours before and continue during ascent and for at least 48 hours after arrival at the high altitude
**Note:** In situations of rapid ascent (such as rescue or military operations), 1000 mg/day is recommended.
### Dosage Forms
Capsule, sustained release (Diamox® Sequels®): 500 mg
Injection, powder for reconstitution: 500 mg
Tablet: 125 mg, 250 mg

# acetic acid (a SEE tik AS id)
### Sound-Alike/Look-Alike Issues
VoSol® may be confused with Vexol®
### Synonyms ethanoic acid
### U.S./Canadian Brand Names VoSol® [US]
### Therapeutic Category Antibacterial, Otic; Antibacterial, Topical
### Use Irrigation of the bladder; treatment of superficial bacterial infections of the external auditory canal
### Usual Dosage
Irrigation (note dosage of an irrigating solution depends on the capacity or surface area of the structure being irrigated):
For continuous irrigation of the urinary bladder with 0.25% acetic acid irrigation, the rate of administration will approximate the rate of urine flow; usually 500-1500 mL/24 hours
For periodic irrigation of an indwelling urinary catheter to maintain patency, about 50 mL of 0.25% acetic acid irrigation is required
Otic: Insert saturated wick; keep moist 24 hours; remove wick and instill 5 drops 3-4 times/day
### Dosage Forms
Solution for irrigation: 0.25% (250 mL, 500 mL, 1000 mL)
Solution, otic (VōSol®): 2% [in propylene glycol] (15 mL)

**acetic acid, hydrocortisone, and propylene glycol diacetate** *see* acetic acid, propylene glycol diacetate, and hydrocortisone *on this page*

## acetic acid, propylene glycol diacetate, and hydrocortisone
(a SEE tik AS id, PRO pa leen GLY kole dye AS e tate, & hye droe KOR ti sone)

**Synonyms** acetic acid, hydrocortisone, and propylene glycol diacetate; hydrocortisone, acetic acid, and propylene glycol diacetate; hydrocortisone, propylene glycol diacetate, and acetic acid; propylene glycol diacetate, acetic acid, and hydrocortisone; propylene glycol diacetate, hydrocortisone, and acetic acid

**U.S./Canadian Brand Names** Acetasol® HC [US]; VoSol® HC [US]

**Therapeutic Category** Antibiotic/Corticosteroid, Otic

**Use** Treatment of superficial infections of the external auditory canal caused by organisms susceptible to the action of the antimicrobial, complicated by swelling

**Usual Dosage** Adults: Otic: Instill 4 drops in ear(s) 3-4 times/day

**Dosage Forms** Solution, otic drops: Acetic acid 2%, propylene glycol diacetate 3%, and hydrocortisone 1% (10 mL)

## acetohexamide (a set oh HEKS a mide)
**Sound-Alike/Look-Alike Issues**
acetoHEXAMIDE may be confused with acetaZOLAMIDE
Dymelor® may be confused with Demerol®, Pamelor®

**Tall-Man** acetoHEXAMIDE

**Therapeutic Category** Antidiabetic Agent, Oral

**Use** Adjunct to diet for the management of mild to moderately severe, stable, type 2 diabetes mellitus (noninsulin dependent, NIDDM)

**Usual Dosage** Oral: Adults:
Initial: 250 mg/day; increase in increments of 250-500 mg daily at intervals of 5-7 days up to 1.5 g/day. Patients on ≤1 g/day can be controlled with once daily administration. Patients receiving 1.5 g/day usually benefit from twice daily administration before the morning and evening meals. Doses >1.5 g daily are not recommended.

**Dosage Forms** Tablet: 250 mg, 500 mg

## acetohydroxamic acid (a SEE toe hye droks am ik AS id)
**Sound-Alike/Look-Alike Issues**
Lithostat® may be confused with Lithobid®

**Synonyms** AHA

**U.S./Canadian Brand Names** Lithostat® [US/Can]

**Therapeutic Category** Urinary Tract Product

**Use** Adjunctive therapy in chronic urea-splitting urinary infection

**Usual Dosage** Oral:
Children: Initial: 10 mg/kg/day
Adults: 250 mg 3-4 times/day for a total daily dose of 10-15 mg/kg/day

**Dosage Forms** Tablet: 250 mg

**Acetoxyl® [Can]** *see* benzoyl peroxide *on page 98*

**acetoxymethylprogesterone** *see* medroxyprogesterone acetate *on page 507*

## acetylcholine (a se teel KOE leen)
**Sound-Alike/Look-Alike Issues**
acetylcholine may be confused with acetylcysteine

**Synonyms** acetylcholine chloride

**U.S./Canadian Brand Names** Miochol-E® [US/Can]

**Therapeutic Category** Cholinergic Agent

**Use** Produces complete miosis in cataract surgery, keratoplasty, iridectomy and other anterior segment surgery where rapid miosis is required

**Usual Dosage** Adults: Intraocular: 0.5-2 mL of 1% injection (5-20 mg) instilled into anterior chamber before or after securing one or more sutures

**Dosage Forms** Powder for intraocular solution, as chloride: 1:100 [10 mg/mL] (2 mL)

**acetylcholine chloride** *see* acetylcholine *on this page*

# acetylcysteine (a se teel SIS teen)

### Sound-Alike/Look-Alike Issues
acetylcysteine may be confused with acetylcholine

Mucomyst® may be confused with Mucinex®

**Synonyms** n-acetyl-L-cysteine; n-acetylcysteine; acetylcysteine sodium; mercapturic acid; NAC

**U.S./Canadian Brand Names** Acetadote® [US]; Mucomyst® [US/Can]; Parvolex® [Can]

**Therapeutic Category** Mucolytic Agent

**Use** Adjunctive mucolytic therapy in patients with abnormal or viscid mucous secretions in acute and chronic bronchopulmonary diseases; pulmonary complications of surgery and cystic fibrosis; diagnostic bronchial studies; antidote for acute acetaminophen toxicity

### Usual Dosage
Acetaminophen poisoning: Children and Adults:

Oral: 140 mg/kg; followed by 17 doses of 70 mg/kg every 4 hours; repeat dose if emesis occurs within 1 hour of administration; therapy should continue until all doses are administered even though the acetaminophen plasma level has dropped below the toxic range

I.V. (Acetadote®): Loading dose: 150 mg/kg over 15 minutes. Maintenance dose: 50 mg/kg infused over 4 hours followed by 100 mg/kg infused over 16 hours. **Note:** To avoid fluid overload in patients <40 kg and those requiring fluid restriction, decrease volume of $D_5W$ proportionally.

Adjuvant therapy in respiratory conditions: **Note:** Patients should receive an aerosolized bronchodilator 10-15 minutes prior to acetylcysteine.

Inhalation, nebulization (face mask, mouth piece, tracheostomy): Acetylcysteine 10% and 20% solution (Mucomyst®) (dilute 20% solution with sodium chloride or sterile water for inhalation); 10% solution may be used undiluted

Infants: 1-2 mL of 20% solution or 2-4 mL of 10% solution until nebulized given 3-4 times/day

Children and Adults: 3-5 mL of 20% solution or 6-10 mL of 10% solution until nebulized given 3-4 times/day; dosing range: 1-10 mL of 20% solution or 2-20 mL of 10% solution every 2-6 hours

Inhalation, nebulization (tent, croupette): Children and Adults: Dose must be individualized; may require up to 300 mL solution/treatment

Direct instillation: Adults:

Into tracheostomy: 1-2 mL of 10% to 20% solution every 1-4 hours

Through percutaneous intratracheal catheter: 1-2 mL of 20% or 2-4 mL of 10% solution every 1-4 hours via syringe attached to catheter

Diagnostic bronchogram: Nebulization or intratracheal: Adults: 1-2 mL of 20% solution or 2-4 mL of 10% solution administered 2-3 times prior to procedure

### Dosage Forms
Injection, solution (Acetadote®): 20% [200 mg/mL] (30 mL) [contains disodium edetate]

Solution, as sodium (Mucomyst®): 10% [100 mg/mL] (4 mL, 10 mL, 30 mL); 20% [200 mg/mL] (4 mL, 10 mL, 30 mL)

**acetylcysteine sodium** see acetylcysteine on this page

**acetylsalicylic acid** see aspirin on page 73

**Aches-N-Pain**® **(Discontinued)** see ibuprofen on page 427

**achromycin** see tetracycline on page 791

**aciclovir** see acyclovir on page 17

**acidulated phosphate fluoride** see fluoride on page 347

**Aci-jel**® **(Discontinued)** see acetic acid on page 13

**Acilac [Can]** see lactulose on page 464

**AcipHex**® **[US/Can]** see rabeprazole on page 706

# acitretin (a si TRE tin)

### Sound-Alike/Look-Alike Issues
Soriatane® may be confused with Loxitane®

**U.S./Canadian Brand Names** Soriatane® [US/Can]

**Therapeutic Category** Retinoid-like Compound

**Use** Treatment of severe psoriasis

**Usual Dosage** Oral: Adults: Individualization of dosage is required to achieve maximum therapeutic response while minimizing side effects

Initial therapy: Therapy should be initiated at 25-50 mg/day, given as a single dose with the main meal

(Continued)

## acitretin *(Continued)*

Maintenance doses of 25-50 mg/day may be given after initial response to treatment; the maintenance dose should be based on clinical efficacy and tolerability

**Dosage Forms** Capsule: 10 mg, 25 mg

**Aclasta**® **[Can]** *see* zoledronic acid *on page 863*

**Aclovate**® **[US]** *see* alclometasone *on page 24*

## acrivastine and pseudoephedrine (AK ri vas teen & soo doe e FED rin)

**Synonyms** pseudoephedrine and acrivastine

**U.S./Canadian Brand Names** Semprex®-D [US]

**Therapeutic Category** Antihistamine/Decongestant Combination

**Use** Temporary relief of nasal congestion, decongest sinus openings, running nose, itching of nose or throat, and itchy, watery eyes due to hay fever or other upper respiratory allergies

**Usual Dosage** Oral: Adults: 1 capsule 3-4 times/day

**Dosage Forms** Capsule: Acrivastine 8 mg and pseudoephedrine hydrochloride 60 mg

**ACT**® **[US-OTC]** *see* fluoride *on page 347*

**Act-D** *see* dactinomycin *on page 221*

**Actagen-C**® *(Discontinued) see* triprolidine, pseudoephedrine, and codeine *(Canada only) on page 827*

**Actagen**® **Syrup** *(Discontinued) see* triprolidine and pseudoephedrine *on page 827*

**Actagen**® **Tablet** *(Discontinued) see* triprolidine and pseudoephedrine *on page 827*

**Act-A-Med**® *(Discontinued) see* triprolidine and pseudoephedrine *on page 827*

**ACTH** *see* corticotropin *on page 208*

**ActHIB**® **[US/Can]** *see* Haemophilus B conjugate vaccine *on page 394*

**Acticin**® **[US]** *see* permethrin *on page 635*

**Actidose-Aqua**® **[US-OTC]** *see* charcoal *on page 165*

**Actidose**® **with Sorbitol [US-OTC]** *see* charcoal *on page 165*

**Actifed**® **[Can]** *see* triprolidine and pseudoephedrine *on page 827*

**Actifed**® **Allergy Tablet (Night)** *(Discontinued) see* diphenhydramine and pseudoephedrine *on page 256*

**Actifed**® **Cold and Allergy [US-OTC]** *see* triprolidine and pseudoephedrine *on page 827*

**Actifed**® **Cold and Sinus [US-OTC]** *see* acetaminophen, chlorpheniramine, and pseudoephedrine *on page 10*

**Actigall**® **[US]** *see* ursodiol *on page 836*

**Actimmune**® **[US/Can]** *see* interferon gamma-1b *on page 444*

**actinomycin** *see* dactinomycin *on page 221*

**actinomycin D** *see* dactinomycin *on page 221*

**actinomycin Cl** *see* dactinomycin *on page 221*

**Actiq**® **[US/Can]** *see* fentanyl *on page 332*

**Activase**® **[US]** *see* alteplase *on page 32*

**Activase**® **rt-PA [Can]** *see* alteplase *on page 32*

**activated carbon** *see* charcoal *on page 165*

**activated charcoal** *see* charcoal *on page 165*

**activated dimethicone** *see* simethicone *on page 748*

**activated ergosterol** *see* ergocalciferol *on page 292*

**activated methylpolysiloxane** *see* simethicone *on page 748*

**activated protein C, human, recombinant** *see* drotrecogin alfa *on page 274*

**Activella**® **[US]** *see* estradiol and norethindrone *on page 302*

**Actonel**® **[US/Can]** *see* risedronate *on page 724*

**Actos**® **[US/Can]** *see* pioglitazone *on page 649*

**ACU-dyne**® **[US-OTC]** *see* povidone-iodine *on page 668*

**Acular**® **[US/Can]** *see* ketorolac *on page 458*

**Acular LS**™ **[US/Can]** *see* ketorolac *on page 458*

**Acular**® **PF [US]** *see* ketorolac *on page 458*

**Acutrim**® **II, Maximum Strength** *(Discontinued)*

**Acutrim**® **16 Hours** *(Discontinued)*

**Acutrim**® **Late Day** *(Discontinued)*

**ACV** *see* acyclovir *on this page*

**acycloguanosine** *see* acyclovir *on this page*

# acyclovir (ay SYE kloe veer)

### Sound-Alike/Look-Alike Issues
Zovirax® may be confused with Zostrix®, Zyvox™

**Synonyms** aciclovir; ACV; acycloguanosine

**U.S./Canadian Brand Names** Apo-Acyclovir® [Can]; Gen-Acyclovir [Can]; Nu-Acyclovir [Can]; ratio-Acyclovir [Can]; Zovirax® [US/Can]

**Therapeutic Category** Antiviral Agent

**Use** Treatment of genital herpes simplex virus (HSV), herpes labialis (cold sores), herpes zoster (shingles), HSV encephalitis, neonatal HSV, mucocutaneous HSV, varicella-zoster (chickenpox)

**Usual Dosage Note:** Obese patients should be dosed using ideal body weight

**Genital HSV:**
I.V.: Children ≥12 years and Adults (immunocompetent): Initial episode, severe: 5 mg/kg every 8 hours for 5-7 days
Oral: Adults:
Initial episode: 200 mg every 4 hours while awake (5 times/day) for 10 days (per manufacturer's labeling); 400 mg 3 times/day for 5-10 days has also been reported
Recurrence: 200 mg every 4 hours while awake (5 times/day) for 5 days (per manufacturer's labeling; begin at earliest signs of disease); 400 mg 3 times/day for 5 days has also been reported
Chronic suppression: 400 mg twice daily or 200 mg 3-5 times/day, for up to 12 months followed by re-evaluation (per manufacturer's labeling); 400-1200 mg/day in 2-3 divided doses has also been reported
Topical: Adults (immunocompromised): Ointment: Initial episode: $1/2$" ribbon of ointment for a 4" square surface area every 3 hours (6 times/day) for 7 days

**Herpes labialis (cold sores):** Topical: Children ≥12 years and Adults: Cream: Apply 5 times/day for 4 days

**Herpes zoster (shingles):**
Oral: Adults (immunocompetent): 800 mg every 4 hours (5 times/day) for 7-10 days
I.V.:
Children <12 years (immunocompromised): 20 mg/kg/dose every 8 hours for 7 days
Children ≥12 years and Adults (immunocompromised): 10 mg/kg/dose or 500 mg/m$^2$/dose every 8 hours for 7 days

**HSV encephalitis:** I.V.:
Children 3 months to 12 years: 20 mg/kg/dose every 8 hours for 10 days (per manufacturer's labeling); dosing for 14-21 days also reported
Children ≥12 years and Adults: 10 mg/kg/dose every 8 hours for 10 days (per manufacturer's labeling); 10-15 mg/kg/dose every 8 hours for 14-21 days also reported

**Mucocutaneous HSV:**
I.V.:
Children <12 years (immunocompromised): 10 mg/kg/dose every 8 hours for 7 days
Children ≥12 years and Adults (immunocompromised): 5 mg/kg/dose every 8 hours for 7 days (per manufacturer's labeling); dosing for up to 14 days also reported
Topical: Ointment: Adults (nonlife-threatening, immunocompromised): $1/2$" ribbon of ointment for a 4" square surface area every 3 hours (6 times/day) for 7 days

**Neonatal HSV:** I.V.: Neonate: Birth to 3 months: 10 mg/kg/dose every 8 hours for 10 days (manufacturer's labeling); 15 mg/kg/dose or 20 mg/kg/dose every 8 hours for 14-21 days has also been reported
(Continued)

## acyclovir *(Continued)*

**Varicella-zoster (chickenpox):** Begin treatment within the first 24 hours of rash onset:
Oral:
Children ≥2 years and ≤40 kg (immunocompetent): 20 mg/kg/dose (up to 800 mg/dose) 4 times/day for 5 days
Children >40 kg and Adults (immunocompetent): 800 mg/dose 4 times a day for 5 days
**Dosage Forms**
Capsule: 200 mg
Cream, topical: 5% (2 g)
Injection, powder for reconstitution, as sodium: 500 mg, 1000 mg
Zovirax®: 500 mg
Injection, solution, as sodium [preservative free]: 25 mg/mL (20 mL, 40 mL); 50 mg/mL (10 mL, 20 mL)
Ointment, topical: 5% (15 g)
Suspension, oral: 200 mg/5 mL (480 mL) [banana flavor]
Tablet: 400 mg, 800 mg

**Aczone**™ **[US]** *see* dapsone *on page 224*

**Adacel**™ **[US/Can]** *see* diphtheria, tetanus toxoids, and acellular pertussis vaccine *on page 259*

**Adagen**® **[US/Can]** *see* pegademase (bovine) *on page 623*

**Adalat**® **XL**® **[Can]** *see* nifedipine *on page 575*

**Adalat**® **CC [US]** *see* nifedipine *on page 575*

**Adalat**® *(Discontinued) see* nifedipine *on page 575*

## adalimumab *(a da LIM yoo mab)*

**Sound-Alike/Look-Alike Issues**
Humira® may be confused with Humulin®
**Synonyms** antitumor necrosis factor apha (human); D2E7; human antitumor necrosis factor-alpha
**U.S./Canadian Brand Names** Humira® [US/Can]
**Therapeutic Category** Antirheumatic, Disease Modifying; Monoclonal Antibody
**Use** Treatment of active rheumatoid and active psoriatic arthritis (moderate to severe). **Note:** May be used alone or in combination with disease-modifying antirheumatic drugs (DMARDs)
**Usual Dosage** SubQ: Adults: Rheumatoid arthritis: 40 mg every other week; may be administered with other DMARDs; patients not taking methotrexate may increase dose to 40 mg/weekly
**Dosage Forms** Injection, solution [preservative free]: 40 mg/0.8 mL (1 mL) [prefilled glass syringe; packaged with alcohol preps; needle cover contains latex]

## adamantanamine hydrochloride *see* amantadine *on page 37*

## adapalene *(a DAP a leen)*

**U.S./Canadian Brand Names** Differin® [US/Can]
**Therapeutic Category** Acne Products
**Use** Treatment of acne vulgaris
**Usual Dosage** Topical: Children >12 years and Adults: Apply once daily at bedtime; therapeutic results should be noticed after 8-12 weeks of treatment
**Dosage Forms** [DSC] = Discontinued product
Cream, topical: 0.1% (15 g, 45 g)
Gel, topical: 0.1% (15 g, 45 g) [alcohol free]
Pledget, topical: 0.1% (60s) [DSC]
Solution, topical: 0.1% (30 mL) [DSC]

**Adderall**® **[US]** *see* dextroamphetamine and amphetamine *on page 237*

**Adderall XR**® **[US/Can]** *see* dextroamphetamine and amphetamine *on page 237*

## adefovir *(a DEF o veer)*

**Synonyms** adefovir dipivoxil
**U.S./Canadian Brand Names** Hepsera™ [US]
**Therapeutic Category** Antiretroviral Agent, Non-nucleoside Reverse Transcriptase Inhibitor (NNRTI)
**Use** Treatment of chronic hepatitis B with evidence of active viral replication (based on persistent elevation of ALT/AST or histologic evidence), including patients with lamivudine-resistant hepatitis B

Usual Dosage Oral: Adults: 10 mg once daily
Dosage Forms Tablet, as dipivoxil: 10 mg

**adefovir dipivoxil** *see* adefovir *on previous page*

**ADEKs [US-OTC]** *see* vitamins (multiple/pediatric) *on page 852*

**Adenocard® [US/Can]** *see* adenosine *on this page*

**Adenoscan® [US]** *see* adenosine *on this page*

# adenosine (a DEN oh seen)

Synonyms 9-beta-d-ribofuranosyladenine
U.S./Canadian Brand Names Adenocard® [US/Can]; Adenoscan® [US]
Therapeutic Category Antiarrhythmic Agent, Miscellaneous
Use
  Adenocard®: Treatment of paroxysmal supraventricular tachycardia (PSVT) including that associated with accessory bypass tracts (Wolff-Parkinson-White syndrome); when clinically advisable, appropriate vagal maneuvers should be attempted prior to adenosine administration; **not effective in atrial flutter, atrial fibrillation, or ventricular tachycardia**
  Adenoscan®: Pharmacologic stress agent used in myocardial perfusion thallium-201 scintigraphy
Usual Dosage
  Adenocard®: **Rapid I.V. push (over 1-2 seconds) via peripheral line:**
  Infants and Children:
  Manufacturer's recommendation:
    <50 kg: 0.05 to 0.1 mg/kg. If conversion of PSVT does not occur within 1-2 minutes, may increase dose by 0.05 to 0.1 mg/kg. May repeat until sinus rhythm is established or to a maximum single dose of 0.3 mg/kg or 12 mg. Follow each dose with normal saline flush.
    ≥50 kg: Refer to Adults dosing
  Pediatric advanced life support (PALS): Treatment of SVT: I.V., I.O.: 0.1 mg/kg; if not effective, administer 0.2 mg/kg of PSVT; medium dose required: 0.15 mg/kg; maximum single dose: 12 mg. Follow each dose with normal saline flush.
  Adults: 6 mg; if not effective within 1-2 minutes, 12 mg may be given; may repeat 12 mg bolus if needed
  Maximum single dose: 12 mg
  Follow each I.V. bolus of adenosine with normal saline flush
  **Note:** Preliminary results in adults suggest adenosine may be administered via a central line at lower doses (ie, initial adult dose: 3 mg).

  Adenoscan®: Stress testing: Continuous I.V. infusion via peripheral line: 140 mcg/kg/minute for 6 minutes using syringe or columetric infusion pump; total dose: 0.84 mg/kg. Thallium-201 is injected at midpoint (3 minutes) of infusion.
Dosage Forms
  Injection, solution [preservative free]: 3 mg/mL (2 mL)
  Adenocard®: 3 mg/mL (2 mL, 4 mL)
  Adenoscan®: 3 mg/mL (20 mL, 30 mL)

**ADH** *see* vasopressin *on page 842*

**Adipex-P® [US]** *see* phentermine *on page 639*

**Adlone® Injection *(Discontinued)*** *see* methylprednisolone *on page 531*

**Adoxa™ [US]** *see* doxycycline *on page 271*

**Adphen® *(Discontinued)***

**Adrenalin® [US/Can]** *see* epinephrine *on page 287*

**adrenaline** *see* epinephrine *on page 287*

**adrenocorticotropic hormone** *see* corticotropin *on page 208*

**adria** *see* doxorubicin *on page 270*

**Adriamycin® [Can]** *see* doxorubicin *on page 270*

**Adriamycin PFS® [US]** *see* doxorubicin *on page 270*

**Adriamycin RDF® [US]** *see* doxorubicin *on page 270*

**Adrucil® [US]** *see* fluorouracil *on page 349*

**adsorbent charcoal** *see* charcoal *on page 165*

**Adsorbocarpine**® **Ophthalmic** *(Discontinued)* *see* pilocarpine *on page 647*

**Adsorbonac**® *(Discontinued)* *see* sodium chloride *on page 752*

**Adsorbotear**® **Ophthalmic Solution** *(Discontinued)* *see* artificial tears *on page 71*

**Advair Diskus**® **[US/Can]** *see* fluticasone and salmeterol *on page 353*

**Advanced Formula Oxy**® **Sensitive Gel** *(Discontinued)* *see* benzoyl peroxide *on page 98*

**Advanced NatalCare**® **[US]** *see* vitamins (multiple/prenatal) *on page 852*

**Advantage-S**™ **[US-OTC]** *see* nonoxynol 9 *on page 580*

**Advate [US]** *see* antihemophilic factor (recombinant) *on page 57*

**Advicor**® **[US]** *see* niacin and lovastatin *on page 573*

**Advil**® **[US-OTC/Can]** *see* ibuprofen *on page 427*

**Advil**® **Children's [US-OTC]** *see* ibuprofen *on page 427*

**Advil**® **Cold, Children's [US-OTC]** *see* pseudoephedrine and ibuprofen *on page 694*

**Advil**® **Cold & Sinus [US-OTC/Can]** *see* pseudoephedrine and ibuprofen *on page 694*

**Advil**® **Infants' [US-OTC]** *see* ibuprofen *on page 427*

**Advil**® **Junior [US-OTC]** *see* ibuprofen *on page 427*

**Advil**® **Migraine [US-OTC]** *see* ibuprofen *on page 427*

**Aerius**® **[Can]** *see* desloratadine *on page 230*

**Aeroaid**® *(Discontinued)* *see* thimerosal *on page 797*

**AeroBid**® **[US]** *see* flunisolide *on page 344*

**AeroBid**®**-M [US]** *see* flunisolide *on page 344*

**AeroChamber**™ **[US]** *see* inhalation devices *on page 438*

**Aerodine**® *(Discontinued)* *see* povidone-iodine *on page 668*

**Afeditab**™ **CR [US]** *see* nifedipine *on page 575*

**A-Free Prenatal [US]** *see* vitamins (multiple/prenatal) *on page 852*

**Afrin**® **Children's Nose Drops** *(Discontinued)* *see* oxymetazoline *on page 610*

**Afrin**® **Extra Moisturizing [US-OTC]** *see* oxymetazoline *on page 610*

**Afrinol**® *(Discontinued)* *see* pseudoephedrine *on page 692*

**Afrin**® **Original [US-OTC]** *see* oxymetazoline *on page 610*

**Afrin**® **Saline Mist** *(Discontinued)* *see* sodium chloride *on page 752*

**Afrin**® **Severe Congestion [US-OTC]** *see* oxymetazoline *on page 610*

**Afrin**® **Sinus [US-OTC]** *see* oxymetazoline *on page 610*

**Aftate**® **Antifungal [US-OTC]** *see* tolnaftate *on page 809*

**AG** *see* aminoglutethimide *on page 40*

## agalsidase beta (aye GAL si days BAY ta)

Synonyms alpha-galactosidase-A (human, recombinant); r-h α-GAL
U.S./Canadian Brand Names Fabrazyme® [US/Can]
Therapeutic Category Enzyme
Use Replacement therapy for Fabry disease
Usual Dosage I.V.: Adults: 1 mg/kg every 2 weeks
Dosage Forms Injection, powder for reconstitution: 35 mg [contains mannitol 222 mg/vial; derived from Chinese hamster cells]

**Agenerase**® **[US/Can]** *see* amprenavir *on page 51*

**Aggrastat**® **[US/Can]** *see* tirofiban *on page 806*

**Aggrenox**® **[US/Can]** *see* aspirin and dipyridamole *on page 75*

**AgNO₃** *see* silver nitrate *on page 747*

**Agrylin**® **[US/Can]** *see* anagrelide *on page 52*

**AGT** *see* aminoglutethimide *on page 40*

**AHA** *see* acetohydroxamic acid *on page 14*

**AH-Chew® [US]** *see* chlorpheniramine, phenylephrine, and methscopolamine *on page 175*

**AH-Chew® II [US]** *see* chlorpheniramine, phenylephrine, and methscopolamine *on page 175*

**AHF (human)** *see* antihemophilic factor (human) *on page 55*

**AHF (porcine)** *see* antihemophilic factor (porcine) *on page 56*

**AHF (recombinant)** *see* antihemophilic factor (recombinant) *on page 57*

**A-hydroCort** *see* hydrocortisone (topical) *on page 417*

**Airet® (Discontinued)** *see* albuterol *on next page*

**Airomir [Can]** *see* albuterol *on next page*

**AKBeta® (Discontinued)** *see* levobunolol *on page 472*

**Ak-Chlor® Ophthalmic (Discontinued)** *see* chloramphenicol *on page 167*

**AK-Con™ [US]** *see* naphazoline *on page 561*

**AK-Dilate® [US]** *see* phenylephrine *on page 640*

**AK-Fluor [US]** *see* fluorescein sodium *on page 346*

**Ak-Homatropine® Ophthalmic (Discontinued)** *see* homatropine *on page 405*

**Akineton® [US/Can]** *see* biperiden *on page 107*

**AK-Mycin® (Discontinued)**

**AK-Nefrin® [US]** *see* phenylephrine *on page 640*

**Akne-Mycin® [US]** *see* erythromycin *on page 295*

**AK-Pentolate® (Discontinued)** *see* cyclopentolate *on page 214*

**AK-Poly-Bac® [US]** *see* bacitracin and polymyxin B *on page 86*

**AK-Pred® [US]** *see* prednisolone (ophthalmic) *on page 673*

**AK-Spore® H.C. Ophthalmic (Discontinued)** *see* bacitracin, neomycin, polymyxin B, and hydrocortisone *on page 87*

**AK-Spore® H.C. Otic (Discontinued)** *see* neomycin, polymyxin B, and hydrocortisone *on page 568*

**AK-Spore® Ophthalmic Ointment (Discontinued)** *see* bacitracin, neomycin, and polymyxin B *on page 87*

**AK-Taine® (Discontinued)** *see* proparacaine *on page 685*

**AKTob® [US]** *see* tobramycin *on page 807*

**AK-Tracin® (Discontinued)** *see* bacitracin *on page 86*

**AK-Trol® [US]** *see* neomycin, polymyxin B, and dexamethasone *on page 567*

**Akwa Tears® [US-OTC]** *see* artificial tears *on page 71*

**Alamag [US-OTC]** *see* aluminum hydroxide and magnesium hydroxide *on page 35*

**Alamag Plus [US-OTC]** *see* aluminum hydroxide, magnesium hydroxide, and simethicone *on page 35*

**Alamast® [US/Can]** *see* pemirolast *on page 626*

**Alavert™ [US-OTC]** *see* loratadine *on page 491*

**Alavert™ Allergy and Sinus [US-OTC]** *see* loratadine and pseudoephedrine *on page 491*

**Alazide® (Discontinued)** *see* hydrochlorothiazide and spironolactone *on page 410*

**Albalon® [US]** *see* naphazoline *on page 561*

**Albalon®-A Liquifilm [Can]** *see* naphazoline and antazoline *on page 561*

**Albalon®-A Ophthalmic (Discontinued)** *see* naphazoline and antazoline *on page 561*

## albendazole (al BEN da zole)
**U.S./Canadian Brand Names** Albenza® [US]
**Therapeutic Category** Anthelmintic
**Use** Treatment of parenchymal neurocysticercosis caused by *Taenia solium* and cystic hydatid disease of the liver, lung, and peritoneum caused by *Echinococcus granulosus*
(Continued)

## albendazole (Continued)

Usual Dosage Oral: Children and Adults:
Neurocysticercosis:
<60 kg: 15 mg/kg/day in 2 divided doses (maximum: 800 mg/day) for 8-30 days
≥60 kg: 400 mg twice daily for 8-30 days
**Note:** Give concurrent anticonvulsant and steroid therapy during first week.
Hydatid:
<60 kg: 15 mg/kg/day in 2 divided doses (maximum: 800 mg/day)
≥60 kg: 400 mg twice daily
**Note:** Administer dose for three 28-day cycles with a 14-day drug-free interval in between.
Dosage Forms Tablet: 200 mg

**Albenza® [US]** see albendazole on previous page

**Albert® Glyburide [Can]** see glyburide on page 378

**Albert® Pentoxifylline [Can]** see pentoxifylline on page 632

**Albert® Tiafen [Can]** see tiaprofenic acid (Canada only) on page 801

**Albumarc® [US]** see albumin on this page

## albumin (al BYOO min)
Sound-Alike/Look-Alike Issues
Albutein® may be confused with albuterol
Buminate® may be confused with bumetanide
Synonyms albumin (human); normal human serum albumin; normal serum albumin (human); salt poor albumin; SPA
U.S./Canadian Brand Names Albumarc® [US]; Albuminar® [US]; Albutein® [US]; Buminate® [US]; Plasbumin® [US]; Plasbumin®-25 [Can]; Plasbumin®-5 [Can]
Therapeutic Category Blood Product Derivative
Use Plasma volume expansion and maintenance of cardiac output in the treatment of certain types of shock or impending shock; may be useful for burn patients, ARDS, and cardiopulmonary bypass; other uses considered by some investigators (but not proven) are retroperitoneal surgery, peritonitis, and ascites; unless the condition responsible for hypoproteinemia can be corrected, albumin can provide only symptomatic relief or supportive treatment
Usual Dosage I.V.:
**5%** should be used in hypovolemic patients or intravascularly-depleted patients
**25%** should be used in patients in whom fluid and sodium intake must be minimized
**Dose depends on condition of patient:**
Children: Hypovolemia: 0.5-1 g/kg/dose (10-20 mL/kg/dose of albumin 5%); maximum dose: 6 g/kg/day
Adults: Usual dose: 25 g; initial dose may be repeated in 15-30 minutes if response is inadequate; no more than 250 g should be administered within 48 hours
Hypoproteinemia: 0.5-1 g/kg/dose; repeat every 1-2 days as calculated to replace ongoing losses
Hypovolemia: 0.5-1 g/kg/dose; repeat as needed; maximum dose: 6 g/kg/day
Dosage Forms
Injection, solution, human: 5% [50 mg/mL] (50 mL, 250 mL, 500 mL); 25% [250 mg/mL] (50 mL, 100 mL)
Albumarc®: 5% [50 mg/mL] (250 mL, 500 mL); 25% [250 mg/mL] (50 mL, 100 mL)
Albuminar®: 5% [50 mg/mL] (50 mL, 250 mL, 500 mL, 1000 mL); 25% [250 mg/mL] (20 mL, 50 mL, 100 mL)
Albutein®, Buminate®: 5% [50 mg/mL]: (250 mL, 500 mL); 25% [250 mg/mL] (20 mL, 50 mL, 100 mL)
Plasbumin®: 5% [50 mg/mL] (50 mL, 250 mL, 500 mL); 25% [250 mg/mL] (20 mL, 50 mL, 100 mL)

**Albuminar® [US]** see albumin on this page

**albumin (human)** see albumin on this page

**Albumisol® (Discontinued)** see albumin on this page

**Albunex® (Discontinued)** see albumin on this page

**Albutein® [US]** see albumin on this page

## albuterol (al BYOO ter ole)
Sound-Alike/Look-Alike Issues
albuterol may be confused with Albutein®, atenolol
Proventil® may be confused with Bentyl®, Prilosec® Prinivil®
salbutamol may be confused with salmeterol

Ventolin® may be confused with phentolamine, Benylin®, Vantin®
Volmax® may be confused with Flomax®

**Synonyms** albuterol sulfate; salbutamol

**U.S./Canadian Brand Names** AccuNeb™ [US]; Airomir [Can]; Alti-Salbutamol [Can]; Apo-Salvent® [Can]; Gen-Salbutamol [Can]; PMS-Salbutamol [Can]; Proventil® HFA [US]; Proventil® Repetabs® [US]; Proventil® [US]; ratio-Inspra-Sal [Can]; ratio-Salbutamol [Can]; Rhoxal-salbutamol [Can]; Salbu-2 [Can]; Salbu-4 [Can]; Ventolin® Diskus [Can]; Ventolin® HFA [US/Can]; Ventolin® [Can]; Ventrodisk [Can]; VoSpire ER™ [US]

**Therapeutic Category** Adrenergic Agonist Agent

**Use** Bronchodilator in reversible airway obstruction due to asthma or COPD; prevention of exercise-induced bronchospasm

**Usual Dosage**
Oral:
Children: Bronchospasm (treatment):
2-6 years: 0.1-0.2 mg/kg/dose 3 times/day; maximum dose not to exceed 12 mg/day (divided doses)
6-12 years: 2 mg/dose 3-4 times/day; maximum dose not to exceed 24 mg/day (divided doses)
Extended release: 4 mg every 12 hours; maximum dose not to exceed 24 mg/day (divided doses)
Children >12 years and Adults: Bronchospasm (treatment): 2-4 mg/dose 3-4 times/day; maximum dose not to exceed 32 mg/day (divided doses)
Extended release: 8 mg every 12 hours; maximum dose not to exceed 32 mg/day (divided doses). A 4 mg dose every 12 hours may be sufficient in some patients, such as adults of low body weight.
Inhalation: MDI 90 mcg/puff:
Children ≤12 years:
Bronchospasm (acute): 4-8 puffs every 20 minutes for 3 doses, then every 1-4 hours; spacer/holding-chamber device should be used
Exercise-induced bronchospasm (prophylaxis): 1-2 puffs 5 minutes prior to exercise
Children >12 years and Adults:
Bronchospasm (acute): 4-8 puffs every 20 minutes for up to 4 hours, then every 1-4 hours as needed
Exercise-induced bronchospasm (prophylaxis): 2 puffs 5-30 minutes prior to exercise
Children ≥4 years and Adults: Bronchospasm (chronic treatment): 1-2 inhalations every 4-6 hours; maximum: 12 inhalations/day
NIH guidelines: 2 puffs 3-4 times a day as needed; may double dose for mild exacerbations
Nebulization:
Children ≤12 years:
Bronchospasm (treatment): 0.05 mg/kg every 4-6 hours; minimum dose: 1.25 mg, maximum dose: 2.5 mg
2-12 years: AccuNeb™: 0.63 mg or 1.25 mg 3-4 times/day, as needed, delivered over 5-15 minutes
Children >40 kg, patients with more severe asthma, or children 11-12 years: May respond better with a 1.25 mg dose
Bronchospasm (acute): Solution 0.5%: 0.15 mg/kg (minimum dose: 2.5 mg) every 20 minutes for 3 doses, then 0.15-0.3 mg/kg (up to 10 mg) every 1-4 hours as needed; may also use 0.5 mg/kg/hour by continuous infusion. Continuous nebulized albuterol at 0.3 mg/kg/hour has been used safely in the treatment of severe status asthmaticus in children; continuous nebulized doses of 3 mg/kg/hour ± 2.2 mg/kg/hour in children whose mean age was 20.7 months resulted in no cardiac toxicity; the optimal dosage for continuous nebulization remains to be determined.
**Note:** Use of the 0.5% solution should be used for bronchospasm (acute or treatment) in children <15 kg. AccuNeb™ has not been studied for the treatment of acute bronchospasm; use of the 0.5% concentrated solution may be more appropriate.
Children >12 years and Adults:
Bronchospasm (treatment): 2.5 mg, diluted to a total of 3 mL, 3-4 times/day over 5-15 minutes
NIH guidelines: 1.25-5 mg every 4-8 hours
Bronchospasm (acute) in intensive care patients: 2.5-5 mg every 20 minutes for 3 doses, then 2.5-10 mg every 1-4 hours as needed, **or** 10-15 mg/hour continuously

**Dosage Forms** [DSC] = Discontinued product
Aerosol, oral (Proventil®): 90 mcg/dose (17 g) [200 doses]
Aerosol, oral, as sulfate [chlorofluorocarbon free]:
Proventil® HFA: 90 mcg/dose (6.7 g) [200 doses]
Ventolin® HFA: 90 mcg/dose (18 g) [200 doses]
Solution for oral inhalation, as sulfate: 0.083% (3 mL); 0.5% (20 mL)
AccuNeb™: 0.63 mg/3 mL (3 mL); 1.25 mg/3 mL (3 mL)
Proventil®: 0.083% (3 mL); 0.5% (20 mL)
Syrup, as sulfate: 2 mg/5 mL (480 mL)
(Continued)

## albuterol *(Continued)*

Tablet, as sulfate: 2 mg, 4 mg
Tablet, extended release, as sulfate:
Proventil® Repetabs®: 4 mg
Volmax® [DSC], VoSpire ER™: 4 mg, 8 mg

**albuterol and ipratropium** *see* ipratropium and albuterol *on page 446*

**albuterol sulfate** *see* albuterol *on page 22*

**Alcaine® [US/Can]** *see* proparacaine *on page 685*

**Alcalak [US-OTC]** *see* calcium carbonate *on page 130*

## alclometasone *(al kloe MET a sone)*

**Sound-Alike/Look-Alike Issues**
Aclovate® may be confused with Accolate®
**Synonyms** alclometasone dipropionate
**U.S./Canadian Brand Names** Aclovate® [US]
**Therapeutic Category** Corticosteroid, Topical
**Use** Treatment of inflammation of corticosteroid-responsive dermatosis (low potency topical corticosteroid)
**Usual Dosage** Topical: Apply a thin film to the affected area 2-3 times/day. Therapy should be discontinued when control is achieved; if no improvement is seen, reassessment of diagnosis may be necessary.
**Dosage Forms**
Cream, as dipropionate: 0.05% (15 g, 45 g, 60 g)
Ointment, as dipropionate: 0.05% (15 g, 45 g, 60 g)

**alclometasone dipropionate** *see* alclometasone *on this page*

**alcohol, absolute** *see* alcohol (ethyl) *on this page*

**alcohol, dehydrated** *see* alcohol (ethyl) *on this page*

## alcohol (ethyl) *(AL koe hol, ETH il)*

**Sound-Alike/Look-Alike Issues**
ethanol may be confused with Ethyol®, Ethamolin®
**Synonyms** alcohol, absolute; alcohol, dehydrated; ethanol; ethyl alcohol; EtOH
**U.S./Canadian Brand Names** Biobase-G™ [Can]; Biobase™ [Can]; Lavacol® [US-OTC]
**Therapeutic Category** Intravenous Nutritional Therapy; Pharmaceutical Aid
**Use** Topical anti-infective; pharmaceutical aid; therapeutic neurolysis (nerve or ganglion block); replenishment of fluid and carbohydrate calories
**Usual Dosage**
Oral: **Note:** Oral dosing is not recommended outside of a hospital setting: Initial dose: 600 mg/kg [equivalent to 1.8 mL/kg using a 43% solution]
Maintenance dose:
Nondrinker: 66 mg/kg/hour [equivalent to 0.2 mL/kg/hour using a 43% solution]
Chronic drinker: 154 mg/kg/hour [equivalent to 0.46 mL/kg/hour using a 43% solution]
Antiseptic: Children and Adults: Liquid denatured alcohol: Topical: Apply 1-3 times/day as needed
Therapeutic neurolysis (nerve or ganglion block): Adults: Dehydrated alcohol injection: Intraneural: Dosage variable depending upon the site of injection (eg, trigeminal neuralgia: 0.05-0.5 mL as a single injection per interspace vs subarachnoid injection: 0.5-1 mL as a single injection per interspace); single doses >1.5 mL are seldom required
Replenishment of fluid and carbohydrate calories: Adults: Dehydrated alcohol infusion: Alcohol 5% and dextrose 5%: 1-2 L/day by slow infusion
**Dosage Forms**
Infusion [in $D_5W$, dehydrated]: Alcohol 5% (1000 mL); alcohol 10% (1000 mL)
Injection, solution [dehydrated]: 98% (1 mL, 5 mL)
Liquid, topical [denatured] (Lavacol®): 70% (473 mL)

**Alcomicin® [Can]** *see* gentamicin *on page 372*

**Alconefrin® Nasal Solution *(Discontinued)*** *see* phenylephrine *on page 640*

**Aldactazide® [US]** *see* hydrochlorothiazide and spironolactone *on page 410*

**Aldactazide 25**® **[Can]** *see* hydrochlorothiazide and spironolactone *on page 410*

**Aldactazide 50**® **[Can]** *see* hydrochlorothiazide and spironolactone *on page 410*

**Aldactone**® **[US/Can]** *see* spironolactone *on page 764*

**Aldara**™ **[US/Can]** *see* imiquimod *on page 432*

## aldesleukin (al des LOO kin)

**Sound-Alike/Look-Alike Issues**
aldesleukin may be confused with oprelvekin
Proleukin® may be confused with oprelvekin
**Synonyms** epidermal thymocyte activating factor; ETAF; IL-2; interleukin-2; lymphocyte mitogenic factor; NSC-373364; T-cell growth factor; TCGF; thymocyte stimulating factor
**U.S./Canadian Brand Names** Proleukin® [US/Can]
**Therapeutic Category** Biological Response Modulator
**Use** Treatment of metastatic renal cell cancer, melanoma
**Usual Dosage** Refer to individual protocols.
I.V.:
Renal cell carcinoma: 600,000 int. units/kg every 8 hours for a maximum of 14 doses; repeat after 9 days for a total of 28 doses per course. Retreat if needed 7 weeks after previous course.
Melanoma:
Single-agent use: 600,000 int. units/kg every 8 hours for a maximum of 14 doses; repeat after 9 days for a total of 28 doses per course. Retreat if needed 7 weeks after previous course.
In combination with cytotoxic agents: 24 million int. units/m$^2$ days 12-16 and 19-23
SubQ:
Single-agent doses: 3-18 million int. units/day for 5 days each week, up to 6 weeks
In combination with interferon:
5 million int. units/m$^2$ 3 times/week
1.8 million int. units/m$^2$ twice daily 5 days/week for 6 weeks
**Dosage Forms** Injection, powder for reconstitution: 22 x 10$^6$ int. units [18 million int. units/mL = 1.1 mg/mL when reconstituted]

**Aldex**™ **[US]** *see* guaifenesin and phenylephrine *on page 387*

**Aldoclor**® *(Discontinued)*

**Aldomet**® *(Discontinued)* *see* methyldopa *on page 529*

**Aldoril**® **[US]** *see* methyldopa and hydrochlorothiazide *on page 529*

**Aldoril**® **D50** *(Discontinued)* *see* methyldopa and hydrochlorothiazide *on page 529*

**Aldroxicon I [US-OTC]** *see* aluminum hydroxide, magnesium hydroxide, and simethicone *on page 35*

**Aldroxicon II [US-OTC]** *see* aluminum hydroxide, magnesium hydroxide, and simethicone *on page 35*

**Aldurazyme**® **[US/Can]** *see* laronidase *on page 468*

## alefacept (a LE fa sept)

**Synonyms** B 9273; BG 9273; human LFA-3/IgG(1) fusion protein; LFA-3/IgG(1) fusion protein, human
**U.S./Canadian Brand Names** Amevive® [US/Can]
**Therapeutic Category** Monoclonal Antibody
**Use** Treatment of moderate to severe plaque psoriasis in adults who are candidates for systemic therapy or phototherapy
**Usual Dosage** Adults:
I.M.: 15 mg once weekly; usual duration of treatment: 12 weeks
I.V.: 7.5 mg once weekly; usual duration of treatment: 12 weeks
A second course of treatment may be initiated at least 12 weeks after completion of the initial course of treatment, provided CD4$^+$ T-lymphocyte counts are within the normal range.
**Note:** CD4$^+$ T-lymphocyte counts should be monitored before initiation of treatment and weekly during therapy. Dosing should be withheld if CD4$^+$ counts are <250 cells/µl, and dosing should be permanently discontinued if CD4$^+$ lymphocyte counts remain at <250 cell/µL for longer than 1 month.
**Dosage Forms** [DSC] = Discontinued product
Injection, powder for reconstitution: 7.5 mg [for I.V. administration; supplied with SWFI] [DSC]
Injection, powder for reconstitution: 15 mg [for I.M. administration; supplied with SWFI]

# alemtuzumab (ay lem TU zoo mab)

**Synonyms** campath-1H; DNA-derived humanized monoclonal antibody; humanized IgG1 anti-CD52 monoclonal antibody

**U.S./Canadian Brand Names** Campath® [US]

**Therapeutic Category** Antineoplastic Agent, Monoclonal Antibody

**Use** Treatment of B-cell chronic lymphocytic leukemia (B-CLL)

**Usual Dosage Note: Dose escalation is required;** usually accomplished in 3-7 days. Do not exceed single doses >30 mg or cumulative doses >90 mg/week.

I.V. infusion, SubQ: Adults: B-CLL:

Initial: 3 mg/day; increase to 10 mg/day, then to 30 mg/day as tolerated

Maintenance: 30 mg/day 3 times/week on alternate days for up to 12 weeks

**Dosage Forms** [DSC] = Discontinued product

Injection, solution [ampul]: 10 mg/mL (3 mL) [DSC]

Injection, solution [vial]: 30 mg/mL (1 mL)

# alendronate (a LEN droe nate)

**Sound-Alike/Look-Alike Issues**

Fosamax® may be confused with Flomax®

**Synonyms** alendronate sodium

**U.S./Canadian Brand Names** Apo-Alendronate® [Can]; Fosamax® [US/Can]; Novo-Alendronate [Can]

**Therapeutic Category** Bisphosphonate Derivative

**Use** Treatment and prevention of osteoporosis in postmenopausal females; treatment of osteoporosis in males; Paget's disease of the bone in patients who are symptomatic, at risk for future complications, or with alkaline phosphatase ≥2 times the upper limit of normal; treatment of glucocorticoid-induced osteoporosis in males and females with low bone mineral density who are receiving a daily dosage ≥7.5 mg of prednisone (or equivalent)

**Usual Dosage** Oral: Adults: **Note:** Patients treated with glucocorticoids and those with Paget's disease should receive adequate amounts of calcium and vitamin D.

**Osteoporosis in postmenopausal females:**

Prophylaxis: 5 mg once daily **or** 35 mg once weekly

Treatment: 10 mg once daily **or** 70 mg once weekly

**Osteoporosis in males:** 10 mg once daily **or** 70 mg once weekly

**Osteoporosis secondary to glucocorticoids in males and females:** Treatment: 5 mg once daily; a dose of 10 mg once daily should be used in postmenopausal females who are not receiving estrogen.

**Paget's disease of bone in males and females:** 40 mg once daily for 6 months

Retreatment: Relapses during the 12 months following therapy occurred in 9% of patients who responded to treatment. Specific retreatment data are not available. Retreatment with alendronate may be considered, following a 6-month post-treatment evaluation period, in patients who have relapsed based on increases in serum alkaline phosphatase, which should be measured periodically. Retreatment may also be considered in those who failed to normalize their serum alkaline phosphatase.

**Dosage Forms**

Solution, oral, as monosodium trihydrate: 70 mg/75 mL [contains parabens; raspberry flavor]

Tablet, as sodium: 5 mg, 10 mg, 35 mg, 40 mg, 70 mg

# alendronate and cholecalciferol (a LEN droe nate & kole e kal SI fer ole)

**Synonyms** alendronate sodium and cholecalciferol; cholecalciferol and alendronate; vitamin D3

**U.S./Canadian Brand Names** Fosamax Plus D™ [US]

**Therapeutic Category** Bisphosphonate Derivative; Vitamin D Analog

**Use** Treatment of osteoporosis in postmenopausal females; increase bone mass in males with osteoporosis

**Usual Dosage** Oral: Adults: One tablet once weekly

**Dosage Forms** Tablet: Alendronate 70 mg and cholecalciferol 2800 int. units

**alendronate sodium** see alendronate on this page

**alendronate sodium and cholecalciferol** see alendronate and cholecalciferol on this page

**Aler-Cap [US-OTC]** see diphenhydramine on page 254

**Aler-Dryl [US-OTC]** see diphenhydramine on page 254

**Aler-Tab [US-OTC]** see diphenhydramine on page 254

**Alertec**® **[Can]** *see* modafinil *on page 546*

**Alesse**® **[US/Can]** *see* ethinyl estradiol and levonorgestrel *on page 312*

**Aleve**® **[US-OTC]** *see* naproxen *on page 562*

**Alfenta**® **[US/Can]** *see* alfentanil *on this page*

## alfentanil (al FEN ta nil)

**Sound-Alike/Look-Alike Issues**
alfentanil may be confused with Anafranil®, fentanyl, remifentanil, sufentanil
Alfenta® may be confused with Sufenta®

**Synonyms** alfentanil hydrochloride

**U.S./Canadian Brand Names** Alfenta® [US/Can]

**Therapeutic Category** Analgesic, Narcotic; General Anesthetic

**Controlled Substance** C-II

**Use** Analgesic adjunct given by continuous infusion or in incremental doses in maintenance of anesthesia with barbiturate or $N_2O$ or a primary anesthetic agent for the induction of anesthesia in patients undergoing general surgery in which endotracheal intubation and mechanical ventilation are required

**Usual Dosage** Doses should be titrated to appropriate effects; wide range of doses is dependent upon desired degree of analgesia/anesthesia
Children <12 years: Dose not established
Adults: Dose should be based on ideal body weight.

**Dosage Forms** Injection, solution, as hydrochloride [preservative free]: 500 mcg/mL (2 mL, 5 mL, 10 mL, 20 mL)

**alfentanil hydrochloride** *see* alfentanil *on this page*

**Alferon**® **N [US/Can]** *see* interferon alfa-n3 *on page 443*

## alfuzosin (al FYOO zoe sin)

**Synonyms** alfuzosin hydrochloride

**U.S./Canadian Brand Names** Uroxatral™ [US]; Xatral [Can]

**Therapeutic Category** Alpha-Adrenergic Blocking Agent

**Use** Treatment of the functional symptoms of benign prostatic hyperplasia (BPH)

**Usual Dosage** Oral: Adults: 10 mg once daily

**Dosage Forms** Tablet, extended release, as hydrochloride: 10 mg

**alfuzosin hydrochloride** *see* alfuzosin *on this page*

## alglucerase (al GLOO ser ase)

**Sound-Alike/Look-Alike Issues**
Ceredase® may be confused with Cerezyme®

**Synonyms** glucocerebrosidase

**U.S./Canadian Brand Names** Ceredase® [US]

**Therapeutic Category** Enzyme

**Use** Replacement therapy for Gaucher disease (type 1)

**Usual Dosage** I.V.: Children and Adults: Initial: 30-60 units/kg every 2 weeks; dosing is individualized based on disease severity; average dose: 60 units/kg every 2 weeks. Range: 2.5 units/kg 3 times/week to 60 units/kg 1-4 times/week. Once patient response is well established, dose may be reduced every 3-6 months to determine maintenance therapy.

**Dosage Forms** Injection, solution [preservative free]: 10 units/mL (5 mL); 80 units/mL (5 mL) [contains human albumin 1%]

**Alimta**® **[US/Can]** *see* pemetrexed *on page 626*

**Alinia**® **[US]** *see* nitazoxanide *on page 576*

## alitretinoin (a li TRET i noyn)

**Sound-Alike/Look-Alike Issues**
Panretin® may be confused with pancreatin
(Continued)

## alitretinoin *(Continued)*

U.S./Canadian Brand Names Panretin® [US/Can]
Therapeutic Category Antineoplastic Agent, Miscellaneous; Retinoic Acid Derivative
Use Orphan drug: Topical treatment of cutaneous lesions in AIDS-related Kaposi's sarcoma
Usual Dosage Topical: Apply gel twice daily to cutaneous lesions
Dosage Forms Gel: 0.1% (60 g tube)

**Alka-Mints®** [US-OTC] *see* calcium carbonate *on page 130*

**Alka-Seltzer® Plus® Cold and Cough [US-OTC]** *see* chlorpheniramine, phenylephrine, and dextromethorphan *on page 174*

**Alka-Seltzer® Plus® Cold and Sinus Liqui-Gels [US-OTC]** *see* acetaminophen and pseudoephedrine *on page 8*

**Alka-Seltzer® Plus® Cold Liqui-Gels [US-OTC]** *see* acetaminophen, chlorpheniramine, and pseudoephedrine *on page 10*

**Alka-Seltzer® Plus® Flu Liqui-Gels [US-OTC]** *see* acetaminophen, dextromethorphan, and pseudoephedrine *on page 11*

**Alkeran®** [US/Can] *see* melphalan *on page 509*

**Allbee® C-800 [US-OTC]** *see* vitamin B complex combinations *on page 849*

**Allbee® C-800 + Iron [US-OTC]** *see* vitamin B complex combinations *on page 849*

**Allbee® with C [US-OTC]** *see* vitamin B complex combinations *on page 849*

**Allegra®** [US/Can] *see* fexofenadine *on page 337*

**Allegra® 60 mg Capsule *(Discontinued)*** *see* fexofenadine *on page 337*

**Allegra-D®** [Can] *see* fexofenadine and pseudoephedrine *on page 337*

**Allegra-D® 12 Hour [US]** *see* fexofenadine and pseudoephedrine *on page 337*

**Allegra-D® 24 Hour [US]** *see* fexofenadine and pseudoephedrine *on page 337*

**Aller-Chlor®** [US-OTC] *see* chlorpheniramine *on page 171*

**Allercon® Tablet *(Discontinued)*** *see* triprolidine and pseudoephedrine *on page 827*

**Allerdryl®** [Can] *see* diphenhydramine *on page 254*

**Allerest® 12 Hour Nasal Solution *(Discontinued)*** *see* oxymetazoline *on page 610*

**Allerest® Eye Drops *(Discontinued)*** *see* naphazoline *on page 561*

**Allerest® Maximum Strength Allergy and Hay Fever [US-OTC]** *see* chlorpheniramine and pseudoephedrine *on page 172*

**Allerfrim®** [US-OTC] *see* triprolidine and pseudoephedrine *on page 827*

**Allerfrin® Syrup *(Discontinued)*** *see* triprolidine and pseudoephedrine *on page 827*

**Allerfrin® Tablet *(Discontinued)*** *see* triprolidine and pseudoephedrine *on page 827*

**Allerfrin® with Codeine *(Discontinued)*** *see* triprolidine, pseudoephedrine, and codeine *(Canada only) on page 827*

**Allergen®** [US] *see* antipyrine and benzocaine *on page 58*

**AllerMax®** [US-OTC] *see* diphenhydramine *on page 254*

**Allernix [Can]** *see* diphenhydramine *on page 254*

**Allersol®** [US] *see* naphazoline *on page 561*

**Allfen-DM [US]** *see* guaifenesin and dextromethorphan *on page 385*

**Allfen Jr [US]** *see* guaifenesin *on page 383*

## allopurinol *(al oh PURE i nole)*

Sound-Alike/Look-Alike Issues
allopurinol may be confused with Apresoline
Zyloprim® may be confused with Xylo-Pfan®, ZORprin®
Synonyms allopurinol sodium
U.S./Canadian Brand Names Aloprim™ [US]; Apo-Allopurinol® [Can]; Novo-Purol [Can]; Zyloprim® [US/Can]

**Therapeutic Category** Xanthine Oxidase Inhibitor

**Use**

Oral: Prevention of attack of gouty arthritis and nephropathy; treatment of secondary hyperuricemia which may occur during treatment of tumors or leukemia; prevention of recurrent calcium oxalate calculi

I.V.: Treatment of elevated serum and urinary uric acid levels when oral therapy is not tolerated in patients with leukemia, lymphoma, and solid tumor malignancies who are receiving cancer chemotherapy

**Usual Dosage**

Oral: Doses >300 mg should be given in divided doses.

Children ≤10 years: Secondary hyperuricemia associated with chemotherapy: 10 mg/kg/day in 2-3 divided doses **or** 200-300 mg/m$^2$/day in 2-4 divided doses, maximum: 800 mg/24 hours

Alternative (manufacturer labeling): <6 years: 150 mg/day in 3 divided doses; 6-10 years: 300 mg/day in 2-3 divided doses

Children >10 years and Adults:

Secondary hyperuricemia associated with chemotherapy: 600-800 mg/day in 2-3 divided doses for prevention of acute uric acid nephropathy for 2-3 days starting 1-2 days before chemotherapy

Gout: Mild: 200-300 mg/day; Severe: 400-600 mg/day; to reduce the possibility of acute gouty attacks, initiate dose at 100 mg/day and increase weekly to recommended dosage.

Recurrent calcium oxalate stones: 200-300 mg/day in single or divided doses

I.V.: Hyperuricemia secondary to chemotherapy: Intravenous daily dose can be given as a single infusion or in equally divided doses at 6-, 8-, or 12-hour intervals. A fluid intake sufficient to yield a daily urinary output of at least 2 L in adults and the maintenance of a neutral or, preferably, slightly alkaline urine are desirable.

Children ≤10 years: Starting dose: 200 mg/m$^2$/day

Children >10 years and Adults: 200-400 mg/m$^2$/day (max: 600 mg/day)

**Dosage Forms**

Injection, powder for reconstitution, as sodium (Aloprim™): 500 mg

Tablet (Zyloprim®): 100 mg, 300 mg

**allopurinol sodium** *see* allopurinol *on previous page*

**all-*trans*-retinoic acid** *see* tretinoin (oral) *on page 817*

**Almacone® [US-OTC]** *see* aluminum hydroxide, magnesium hydroxide, and simethicone *on page 35*

**Almacone Double Strength® [US-OTC]** *see* aluminum hydroxide, magnesium hydroxide, and simethicone *on page 35*

**Almora® [US-OTC]** *see* magnesium gluconate *on page 498*

## almotriptan (al moh TRIP tan)

**Sound-Alike/Look-Alike Issues**

Axert™ may be confused with Antivert®

**Synonyms** almotriptan malate

**U.S./Canadian Brand Names** Axert™ [US/Can]

**Therapeutic Category** Serotonin 5-HT$_{1D}$ Receptor Agonist

**Use** Acute treatment of migraine with or without aura

**Usual Dosage** Oral: Adults: Migraine: Initial: 6.25-12.5 mg in a single dose; if the headache returns, repeat the dose after 2 hours; no more than 2 doses in 24-hour period

**Note:** If the first dose is ineffective, diagnosis needs to be re-evaluated. Safety of treating more than 4 migraines/month has not been established.

**Dosage Forms** Tablet, as malate: 6.25 mg, 12.5 mg

**almotriptan malate** *see* almotriptan *on this page*

**Alocril® [US/Can]** *see* nedocromil (ophthalmic) *on page 565*

**Aloe Vesta® 2-n-1 Antifungal [US-OTC]** *see* miconazole *on page 537*

**Alomide® [US/Can]** *see* lodoxamide tromethamine *on page 488*

**Alophen® [US-OTC]** *see* bisacodyl *on page 107*

**Aloprim™ [US]** *see* allopurinol *on previous page*

**Alor® 5/500 (Discontinued)** *see* hydrocodone and aspirin *on page 412*

**Alora® [US]** *see* estradiol *on page 299*

## alosetron (a LOE se tron)

**Sound-Alike/Look-Alike Issues**
Lotronex® may be confused with Lovenox®, Protonix®
**U.S./Canadian Brand Names** Lotronex® [US]
**Therapeutic Category** 5-HT$_3$ Receptor Antagonist
**Use** Treatment of women with severe diarrhea-predominant irritable bowel syndrome (IBS) who have failed to respond to conventional therapy
**Usual Dosage** Oral:
Children: Safety and efficacy have not been established.
Adults: Female: Initial: 0.5 mg twice daily for 4 weeks, with or without food; if tolerated, but response is inadequate, may be increased after 4 weeks to 1 mg twice daily. If response is inadequate after 4 weeks of 1 mg twice-daily dosing, discontinue treatment.
**Note:** Discontinue immediately if constipation or signs/symptoms of ischemic colitis occur. Do not reinitiate in patients who develop ischemic colitis.
**Dosage Forms** Tablet: 0.5 mg, 1 mg

**Aloxi™ [US]** *see* palonosetron *on page 614*
**alpha$_1$-antitrypsin** *see* alpha$_1$-proteinase inhibitor *on this page*
**alpha$_1$-PI** *see* alpha$_1$-proteinase inhibitor *on this page*

## alpha$_1$-proteinase inhibitor (al fa won PRO tee in ase in HI bi tor)

**Synonyms** A$_1$-PI; alpha$_1$-antitrypsin; alpha$_1$-PI; alpha$_1$-proteinase inhibitor, human; $\alpha_1$-PI
**U.S./Canadian Brand Names** Aralast™ [US]; Prolastin® [US/Can]; Zemaira™ [US]
**Therapeutic Category** Antitrypsin Deficiency Agent
**Use** Replacement therapy in congenital alpha$_1$-antitrypsin deficiency with clinical emphysema
**Usual Dosage** I.V.: Adults: 60 mg/kg once weekly
**Dosage Forms** Injection, powder for reconstitution [single-dose vial]:
Aralast™, Prolastin®: 500 mg, 1000 mg [packaged with diluent]
Zemaira™: 1000 mg [packaged with diluent]

**alpha$_1$-proteinase inhibitor, human** *see* alpha$_1$-proteinase inhibitor *on this page*
**alpha-galactosidase-A (human, recombinant)** *see* agalsidase beta *on page 20*
**Alphagan® [Can]** *see* brimonidine *on page 113*
**Alphagan® (Discontinued)** *see* brimonidine *on page 113*
**Alphagan® P [US]** *see* brimonidine *on page 113*
**Alphamul® (Discontinued)** *see* castor oil *on page 151*
**Alphanate® [US]** *see* antihemophilic factor (human) *on page 55*
**AlphaNine® SD [US]** *see* factor IX *on page 325*
**Alphaquin HP [US]** *see* hydroquinone *on page 420*

## alprazolam (al PRAY zoe lam)

**Sound-Alike/Look-Alike Issues**
alprazolam may be confused with alprostadil, lorazepam, triazolam
Xanax® may be confused with Lanoxin®, Tenex®, Tylox®, Xopenex®, Zantac®, Zyrtec®
**U.S./Canadian Brand Names** Alprazolam Intensol® [US]; Alti-Alprazolam [Can]; Apo-Alpraz® [Can]; Gen-Alprazolam [Can]; Niravam™ [US]; Novo-Alprazol [Can]; Nu-Alprax [Can]; Xanax TS™ [Can]; Xanax XR® [US]; Xanax® [US/Can]
**Therapeutic Category** Benzodiazepine
**Controlled Substance** C-IV
**Use** Treatment of anxiety disorder (GAD); panic disorder, with or without agoraphobia; anxiety associated with depression
**Usual Dosage** Oral: **Note:** Treatment >4 months should be re-evaluated to determine the patient's continued need for the drug
Adults:
Anxiety: Immediate release: Effective doses are 0.5-4 mg/day in divided doses; the manufacturer recommends starting at 0.25-0.5 mg 3 times/day; titrate dose upward; maximum: 4 mg/day
Anxiety associated with depression: Immediate release: Average dose required: 2.5-3 mg/day in divided doses

Panic disorder:

Immediate release: Initial: 0.5 mg 3 times/day; dose may be increased every 3-4 days in increments ≤1 mg/day; many patients obtain relief at 2 mg/day, as much as 10 mg/day may be required

Extended release: 0.5-1 mg once daily; may increase dose every 3-4 days in increments ≤1 mg/day (range: 3-6 mg/day)

Switching from immediate release to extended release: Patients may be switched to extended release tablets by taking the total daily dose of the immediate release tablets and giving it once daily using the extended release preparation.

Preoperative sedation: 0.5 mg in evening at bedtime and 0.5 mg 1 hour before procedure

**Dose reduction:** Abrupt discontinuation should be avoided. Daily dose may be decreased by 0.5 mg every 3 days, however, some patients may require a slower reduction. If withdrawal symptoms occur, resume previous dose and discontinue on a less rapid schedule.

### Dosage Forms

Solution, oral (Alprazolam Intensol®): 1 mg/mL (30 mL)

Tablet (Xanax®): 0.25 mg, 0.5 mg, 1 mg, 2 mg

Tablet, extended release (Xanax XR®): 0.5 mg, 1 mg, 2 mg, 3 mg

Tablet, orally-disintegrating (Niravam™): 0.25 mg, 0.5 mg, 1 mg, 2 mg [orange flavor]

## Alprazolam Intensol® [US] *see alprazolam on previous page*

# alprostadil (al PROS ta dill)

### Sound-Alike/Look-Alike Issues

alprostadil may be confused with alprazolam

**Synonyms** PGE$_1$; prostaglandin E$_1$

**U.S./Canadian Brand Names** Caverject® Impulse™ [US]; Caverject® [US/Can]; Edex® [US]; Muse® Pellet [Can]; Muse® [US]; Prostin VR Pediatric® [US]; Prostin® VR [Can]

**Therapeutic Category** Prostaglandin

### Use

Prostin VR Pediatric®: Temporary maintenance of patency of ductus arteriosus in neonates with ductal-dependent congenital heart disease until surgery can be performed. These defects include cyanotic (eg, pulmonary atresia, pulmonary stenosis, tricuspid atresia, Fallot's tetralogy, transposition of the great vessels) and acyanotic (eg, interruption of aortic arch, coarctation of aorta, hypoplastic left ventricle) heart disease

Caverject®: Treatment of erectile dysfunction of vasculogenic, psychogenic, or neurogenic etiology; adjunct in the diagnosis of erectile dysfunction

Edex®, Muse®: Treatment of erectile dysfunction of vasculogenic, psychogenic, or neurogenic etiology

### Usual Dosage

**Patent ductus arteriosus** (Prostin VR Pediatric®):

I.V. continuous infusion into a large vein, or alternatively through an umbilical artery catheter placed at the ductal opening: 0.05-0.1 mcg/kg/minute with therapeutic response, rate is reduced to lowest effective dosage; with unsatisfactory response, rate is increased gradually; maintenance: 0.01-0.4 mcg/kg/minute

PGE$_1$ is usually given at an infusion rate of 0.1 mcg/kg/minute, but it is often possible to reduce the dosage to $^1/_2$ or even $^1/_{10}$ without losing the therapeutic effect. The mixing schedule is as follows. Infusion rates deliver 0.1 mcg/kg/minute. **Note:** 500 mcg equals 1 ampul.

For a concentration of 2 mcg/mL, add 500 mcg to 250 mL; infuse at 0.05 mL/kg/minute (72 mL/kg/24 hours)

For a concentration of 5 mcg/mL, add 500 mcg to 100 mL; infuse at 0.02 mL/kg/minute (28.8 mL/kg/24 hours)

For a concentration of 10 mcg/mL, add 500 mcg to 50 mL; infuse at 0.01 mL/kg/minute (14.4 mL/kg/24 hours)

For a concentration of 20 mcg/mL, add 500 mcg to 25 mL; infuse at 0.005 mL/kg/minute (7.2 mL/kg/24 hours)

Therapeutic response is indicated by increased pH in those with acidosis or by an increase in oxygenation (PO$_2$) usually evident within 30 minutes

**Erectile dysfunction:**

Caverject®, Edex®: Intracavernous: Individualize dose by careful titration; doses >40 mcg (Edex®) or >60 mcg (Caverject®) are not recommended: Initial dose must be titrated in physicians office. Patient must stay in the physician's office until complete detumescence occurs; if there is no response, then the next higher dose may be given within 1 hour; if there is still no response, a 1-day interval before giving the next dose is recommended; increasing the dose or concentration in the treatment of impotence results in increasing pain and discomfort

(Continued)

# alprostadil (Continued)

Vasculogenic, psychogenic, or mixed etiology: Initiate dosage titration at 2.5 mcg, increasing by 2.5 mcg to a dose of 5 mcg and then in increments of 5-10 mcg depending on the erectile response until the dose produces an erection suitable for intercourse, not lasting >1 hour; if there is absolutely no response to initial 2.5 mcg dose, the second dose may be increased to 7.5 mcg, followed by increments of 5-10 mcg

Neurogenic etiology (eg, spinal cord injury): Initiate dosage titration at 1.25 mcg, increasing to a dose of 2.5 mcg and then 5 mcg; increase further in increments 5 mcg until the dose is reached that produces an erection suitable for intercourse, not lasting >1 hour

Maintenance: Once appropriate dose has been determined, patient may self-administer injections at a frequency of no more than 3 times/week with at least 24 hours between doses

Muse® Pellet: Intraurethral:

Initial: 125-250 mcg

Maintenance: Administer as needed to achieve an erection; duration of action is about 30-60 minutes; use only two systems per 24-hour period

**Dosage Forms** [DSC] = Discontinued product

Injection, powder for reconstitution:

Caverject®: 10 mcg, 20 mcg, 40 mcg [contains lactose; diluent contains benzyl alcohol]

Caverject® Impulse™: 10 mcg, 20 mcg [prefilled injection system; contains lactose; diluent contains benzyl alcohol]

Edex®: 10 mcg, 20 mcg, 40 mcg [contains lactose; diluent contains benzyl alcohol; also packaged in kits containing diluent, syringe, and alcohol swab]

Injection, solution: 500 mcg/mL (1 mL)

Caverject® [DSC]: 20 mcg/mL (2 mL)

Prostin VR Pediatric®: 500 mcg/mL (1 mL) [contains dehydrated alcohol]

Pellet, urethral (Muse®): 125 mcg, 250 mcg, 500 mcg, 1000 mcg

**Alrex® [US/Can]** see loteprednol on page 493

**AL-Rr® Oral (Discontinued)** see chlorpheniramine on page 171

**Altace® [US/Can]** see ramipril on page 710

**Altamist [US-OTC]** see sodium chloride on page 752

**Altarussin DM [US-OTC]** see guaifenesin and dextromethorphan on page 385

**Altaryl [US-OTC]** see diphenhydramine on page 254

# alteplase (AL te plase)

**Sound-Alike/Look-Alike Issues**

alteplase may be confused with Altace®

"tPA" abbreviation should not be used when writing orders for this medication; has been misread as TNKase (tenecteplase)

**Synonyms** alteplase, recombinant; alteplase, tissue plasminogen activator, recombinant; tPA

**U.S./Canadian Brand Names** Activase® rt-PA [Can]; Activase® [US]; Cathflo™ Activase® [US/Can]

**Therapeutic Category** Fibrinolytic Agent

**Use** Management of acute myocardial infarction for the lysis of thrombi in coronary arteries; management of acute massive pulmonary embolism (PE) in adults

Acute myocardial infarction (AMI): Chest pain ≥20 minutes, ≤12-24 hours; S-T elevation ≥0.1 mV in at least two ECG leads

Acute pulmonary embolism (APE): Age ≤75 years: Documented massive pulmonary embolism by pulmonary angiography or echocardiography or high probability lung scan with clinical shock

Cathflo™ Activase®: Restoration of central venous catheter function

**Usual Dosage**

I.V.:

Coronary artery thrombi: Front loading dose (weight-based):

Patients >67 kg: Total dose: 100 mg over 1.5 hours; infuse 15 mg over 1-2 minutes. Infuse 50 mg over 30 minutes. See "Note."

Patients ≤67 kg: Total dose: 1.25 mg/kg; infuse 15 mg I.V. bolus over 1-2 minutes, then infuse 0.75 mg/kg (not to exceed 50 mg) over next 30 minutes, followed by 0.5 mg/kg over next 60 minutes (not to exceed 35 mg). See "Note."

**Note:** Concurrently, begin heparin 60 units/kg bolus (maximum: 4000 units) followed by continuous infusion of 12 units/kg/hour (maximum: 1000 units/hour) and adjust to aPTT target of 1.5-2 times the upper limit of control. Infuse remaining 35 mg of alteplase over the next hour.

Acute pulmonary embolism: 100 mg over 2 hours.

Acute ischemic stroke: Doses should be given within the first 3 hours of the onset of symptoms; recommended total dose: 0.9 mg/kg (maximum dose should not exceed 90 mg) infused over 60 minutes.

Load with 0.09 mg/kg (10% of the 0.9 mg/kg dose) as an I.V. bolus over 1 minute, followed by 0.81 mg/kg (90% of the 0.9 mg/kg dose) as a continuous infusion over 60 minutes. Heparin should not be started for 24 hours or more after starting alteplase for stroke.

Intracatheter: Central venous catheter clearance: Cathflo™ Activase® 1 mg/mL:

Patients <30 kg: 110% of the internal lumen volume of the catheter, not to exceed 2 mg/2 mL; retain in catheter for 0.5-2 hours; may instill a second dose if catheter remains occluded

Patients ≥30 kg: 2 mg (2 mL); retain in catheter for 0.5-2 hours; may instill a second dose if catheter remains occluded

**Dosage Forms** Injection, powder for reconstitution, recombinant:

Activase®: 50 mg [29 million int. units]; 100 mg [58 million int. units]

Cathflo™ Activase®: 2 mg

**alteplase, recombinant** *see* alteplase *on previous page*

**alteplase, tissue plasminogen activator, recombinant** *see* alteplase *on previous page*

**ALternaGel® [US-OTC]** *see* aluminum hydroxide *on next page*

**Alti-Alprazolam [Can]** *see* alprazolam *on page 30*

**Alti-Amiodarone [Can]** *see* amiodarone *on page 41*

**Alti-Amoxi-Clav [Can]** *see* amoxicillin and clavulanate potassium *on page 47*

**Alti-Azathioprine [Can]** *see* azathioprine *on page 83*

**Alti-Captopril [Can]** *see* captopril *on page 139*

**Alti-Clindamycin [Can]** *see* clindamycin *on page 192*

**Alti-Clobazam [Can]** *see* clobazam *(Canada only) on page 194*

**Alti-Clonazepam [Can]** *see* clonazepam *on page 197*

**Alti-Desipramine [Can]** *see* desipramine *on page 230*

**Alti-Diltiazem CD [Can]** *see* diltiazem *on page 251*

**Alti-Divalproex [Can]** *see* valproic acid and derivatives *on page 837*

**Alti-Domperidone [Can]** *see* domperidone *(Canada only) on page 266*

**Alti-Doxazosin [Can]** *see* doxazosin *on page 268*

**Alti-Flunisolide [Can]** *see* flunisolide *on page 344*

**Alti-Fluoxetine [Can]** *see* fluoxetine *on page 349*

**Alti-Flurbiprofen [Can]** *see* flurbiprofen *on page 352*

**Alti-Fluvoxamine [Can]** *see* fluvoxamine *on page 356*

**Alti-Ipratropium [Can]** *see* ipratropium *on page 446*

**Alti-Metformin [Can]** *see* metformin *on page 519*

**Alti-Minocycline [Can]** *see* minocycline *on page 542*

**Alti-Moclobemide [Can]** *see* moclobemide *(Canada only) on page 546*

**Alti-MPA [Can]** *see* medroxyprogesterone acetate *on page 507*

**Alti-Nadolol [Can]** *see* nadolol *on page 556*

**Alti-Nortriptyline [Can]** *see* nortriptyline *on page 583*

**Alti-Ranitidine [Can]** *see* ranitidine hydrochloride *on page 710*

**Alti-Salbutamol [Can]** *see* albuterol *on page 22*

**Alti-Sotalol [Can]** *see* sotalol *on page 762*

**Alti-Sulfasalazine [Can]** *see* sulfasalazine *on page 774*

**Alti-Terazosin [Can]** *see* terazosin *on page 786*

**Alti-Ticlopidine [Can]** *see* ticlopidine *on page 802*

**Alti-Timolol [Can]** *see* timolol *on page 803*

**Alti-Trazodone [Can]** *see* trazodone *on page 817*

**Alti-Verapamil [Can]** *see* verapamil *on page 843*

**Alti-Zopiclone [Can]** *see* zopiclone *(Canada only) on page 864*

**Altocor™** *(Discontinued) see* lovastatin *on page 494*

**Altoprev™ [US]** *see* lovastatin *on page 494*

## altretamine (al TRET a meen)

**Synonyms** hexamethylmelamine; HEXM; HMM; HXM; NSC-13875
**U.S./Canadian Brand Names** Hexalen® [US/Can]
**Therapeutic Category** Antineoplastic Agent
**Use** Palliative treatment of persistent or recurrent ovarian cancer
**Usual Dosage** Refer to individual protocols. Oral:
  Adults: 4-12 mg/kg/day in 3-4 divided doses for 21-90 days
  Alternatively: 240-320 mg/m$^2$/day in 3-4 divided doses for 21 days, repeated every 6 weeks
  Alternatively: 260 mg/m$^2$/day for 14-21 days of a 28-day cycle in 4 divided doses
  Alternatively: 150 mg/m$^2$/day in 3-4 divided doses for 14 days of a 28-day cycle
**Dosage Forms** Gelcap: 50 mg [contains lactose]

**Alu-Cap®** *(Discontinued) see* aluminum hydroxide *on this page*

**Aludrox®** *(Discontinued) see* aluminum hydroxide and magnesium hydroxide *on next page*

## aluminum chloride hexahydrate (a LOO mi num KLOR ide heks a HYE drate)

**Sound-Alike/Look-Alike Issues**
  Drysol™ may be confused with Drisdol®
**U.S./Canadian Brand Names** Certain Dri® [US-OTC]; Drysol™ [US]; Xerac AC™ [US]
**Therapeutic Category** Topical Skin Product
**Use** Astringent in the management of hyperhidrosis
**Usual Dosage** Topical: Adults: Apply once daily at bedtime; once excessive sweating has stopped, may decrease to once or twice weekly, or as needed. Wash treated area in the morning.
**Dosage Forms**
  Solution, topical: 20% in SD alcohol 40 (35 mL, 37.5 mL, 60 mL) [contains ethyl alcohol]
  Certain Dri®: 12% (36 mL)
  Drysol™: 20% (35 mL, 37.5 mL, 60 mL) [contains ethyl alcohol 93%]
  Xerac AC™: 6.25% (35 mL, 60 mL) [contains ethyl alcohol 95%]

## aluminum hydroxide (a LOO mi num hye DROKS ide)

**U.S./Canadian Brand Names** ALternaGel® [US-OTC]; Amphojel® [Can]; Basaljel® [Can]; Dermagran® [US-OTC]
**Therapeutic Category** Antacid
**Use** Treatment of hyperacidity; hyperphosphatemia; temporary protection of minor cuts, scrapes, and burns
**Usual Dosage**
  Oral:
  Hyperphosphatemia:
    Children: 50-150 mg/kg/24 hours in divided doses every 4-6 hours, titrate dosage to maintain serum phosphorus within normal range
    Adults: Initial: 300-600 mg 3 times/day with meals
    Antacid: Adults: 600-1200 mg between meals and at bedtime
  Topical: Apply to affected area as needed; reapply at least every 12 hours
**Dosage Forms** [DSC] = Discontinued product
  Capsule (Alu-Cap®): 400 mg [DSC]
  Ointment (Dermagran®): 0.275% (5 g, 120 g)
  Suspension, oral: 320 mg/5 mL (473 mL)
  ALternaGel®: 600 mg/5 mL (360 mL)

## aluminum hydroxide and magnesium carbonate

(a LOO mi num hye DROKS ide & mag NEE zhum KAR bun nate)

**Synonyms** magnesium carbonate and aluminum hydroxide

**U.S./Canadian Brand Names** Gaviscon® Extra Strength [US-OTC]; Gaviscon® Liquid [US-OTC]

**Therapeutic Category** Antacid

**Use** Temporary relief of symptoms associated with gastric acidity

**Usual Dosage** Oral: Adults:

Liquid:

Gaviscon® Regular Strength: 15-30 mL 4 times/day after meals and at bedtime

Gaviscon® Extra Strength Relief: 15-30 mL 4 times/day after meals

Tablet (Gaviscon® Extra Strength Relief): Chew 2-4 tablets 4 times/day

**Dosage Forms**

Liquid:

Gaviscon®: Aluminum hydroxide 31.7 mg and magnesium carbonate 119.3 mg per 5 mL (355 mL) [contains sodium 0.57 mEq/5 mL]

Gaviscon® Extra Strength: Aluminum hydroxide 84.6 mg and magnesium carbonate 79.1 mg per 5 mL (355 mL) [contains sodium 0.9 mEq/5 mL]

Tablet, chewable (Gaviscon® Extra Strength): Aluminum hydroxide 160 mg and magnesium carbonate 105 mg [contains sodium 1.3 mEq/tablet]

## aluminum hydroxide and magnesium hydroxide

(a LOO mi num hye DROKS ide & mag NEE zhum hye DROK side)

**Sound-Alike/Look-Alike Issues**

Maalox® may be confused with Maox®, Monodox®

**Synonyms** magnesium hydroxide and aluminum hydroxide

**U.S./Canadian Brand Names** Alamag [US-OTC]; Diovol® Ex [Can]; Diovol® [Can]; Gelusil® Extra Strength [Can]; Mylanta™ [Can]; Rulox No. 1 [US]; Rulox [US]

**Therapeutic Category** Antacid

**Use** Antacid, hyperphosphatemia in renal failure

**Usual Dosage** Oral: 5-10 mL 4-6 times/day, between meals and at bedtime; may be used every hour for severe symptoms

**Dosage Forms** [DSC] = Discontinued product

Suspension (Alamag, Rulox): Aluminum hydroxide 225 mg and magnesium hydroxide 200 mg per 5 mL (360 mL)

Suspension, high potency (Maalox® TC) [DSC]: Aluminum hydroxide 600 mg and magnesium hydroxide 300 mg per 5 mL (360 mL)

Tablet, chewable:

Alamag: Aluminum hydroxide 300 mg and magnesium hydroxide 150 mg

Rulox No. 1: Aluminum hydroxide 200 mg and magnesium hydroxide 200 mg

## aluminum hydroxide, magnesium hydroxide, and simethicone

(a LOO mi num hye DROKS ide, mag NEE zhum hye DROKS ide, & sye METH i kone)

**Sound-Alike/Look-Alike Issues**

Maalox® may be confused with Maox®, Monodox®

Mylanta® may be confused with Mynatal®

**Synonyms** magnesium hydroxide, aluminum hydroxide, and simethicone; simethicone, aluminum hydroxide, and magnesium hydroxide

**U.S./Canadian Brand Names** Alamag Plus [US-OTC]; Aldroxicon I [US-OTC]; Aldroxicon II [US-OTC]; Almacone Double Strength® [US-OTC]; Almacone® [US-OTC]; Diovol Plus® [Can]; Gelusil® [US-OTC/Can]; Maalox® Max [US-OTC]; Maalox® [US-OTC]; Mi-Acid™ Maximum Strength [US-OTC]; Mi-Acid™ [US-OTC]; Mintox Extra Strength [US-OTC]; Mintox Plus [US-OTC]; Mylanta® Double Strength [Can]; Mylanta® Extra Strength [Can]; Mylanta® Liquid [US-OTC]; Mylanta® Maximum Strength Liquid [US-OTC]; Mylanta® Regular Strength [Can]

**Therapeutic Category** Antacid; Antiflatulent

**Use** Temporary relief of hyperacidity associated with gas; may also be used for indications associated with other antacids

**Usual Dosage** Oral: Adults: 10-20 mL or 2-4 tablets 4-6 times/day between meals and at bedtime; may be used every hour for severe symptoms

(Continued)

## aluminum hydroxide, magnesium hydroxide, and simethicone *(Continued)*

### Dosage Forms

Liquid: Aluminum hydroxide 200 mg, magnesium hydroxide 200 mg, and simethicone 20 mg per 5 mL (360 mL); aluminum hydroxide 400 mg, magnesium hydroxide 400 mg, and simethicone 40 mg per 5 mL (360 mL)

Aldroxicon I: Aluminum hydroxide 200 mg, magnesium hydroxide 200 mg, and simethicone 20 mg per 5 mL (30 mL)

Aldroxicon II: Aluminum hydroxide 400 mg, magnesium hydroxide 400 mg, and simethicone 40 mg per 5 mL (30 mL)

Almacone®: Aluminum hydroxide 200 mg, magnesium hydroxide 200 mg, and simethicone 20 mg per 5 mL (360 mL)

Almacone Double Strength®: Aluminum hydroxide 400 mg, magnesium hydroxide 400 mg, and simethicone 40 mg per 5 mL (360 mL)

Maalox®: Aluminum hydroxide 200 mg, magnesium hydroxide 200 mg, and simethicone 20 mg per 5 mL (360 mL, 770 mL) [lemon and mint flavors]

Maalox® Max: Aluminum hydroxide 400 mg, magnesium hydroxide 400 mg, and simethicone 40 mg per 5 mL (360 mL, 770 mL) [cherry, vanilla creme, and wild berry flavors]

Mi-Acid: Aluminum hydroxide 200 mg, magnesium hydroxide 200 mg, and simethicone 20 mg per 5 mL (360 mL)

Mi-Acid Maximum Strength: Aluminum hydroxide 400 mg, magnesium hydroxide 400 mg, and simethicone 40 mg per 5 mL (360 mL)

Mintox Extra Strength: Aluminum hydroxide 500 mg, magnesium hydroxide 450 mg, and simethicone 40 mg per 5 mL (360 mL) [lemon creme flavor]

Mylanta®: Aluminum hydroxide 200 mg, magnesium hydroxide 200 mg, and simethicone 20 mg per 5 mL (180 mL, 360 mL, 720 mL) [original, cherry, and mint flavors]

Mylanta® Maximum Strength: Aluminum hydroxide 400 mg, magnesium hydroxide 400 mg, and simethicone 40 mg per 5 mL (180 mL, 360 mL, 720 mL) [original, cherry, orange creme, and mint flavors]

Suspension (Alamag Plus): Aluminum hydroxide 225 mg, magnesium hydroxide 200 mg, and simethicone 25 mg per 5 mL (360 mL)

Tablet, chewable: Aluminum hydroxide 200 mg, magnesium hydroxide 200 mg, and simethicone 25 mg

Alamag Plus: Aluminum hydroxide 200 mg, magnesium hydroxide 200 mg, and simethicone 25 mg [cherry flavor]

Almacone®: Aluminum hydroxide 200 mg, magnesium hydroxide 200 mg, and simethicone 20 mg [peppermint flavor]

Gelusil®: Aluminum hydroxide 200 mg, magnesium hydroxide 200 mg, and simethicone 25 mg [peppermint flavor]

Mintox Plus: Aluminum hydroxide 200 mg, magnesium hydroxide 200 mg, and simethicone 25 mg

**Aluminum Sucrose Sulfate, Basic** *see* sucralfate *on page 769*

## aluminum sulfate and calcium acetate

(a LOO mi num SUL fate & KAL see um AS e tate)

**Synonyms** calcium acetate and aluminum sulfate

**U.S./Canadian Brand Names** Domeboro® [US-OTC]; Pedi-Boro® [US-OTC]

**Therapeutic Category** Topical Skin Product

**Use** Astringent wet dressing for relief of inflammatory conditions of the skin and to reduce weeping that may occur in dermatitis

**Usual Dosage** Topical: Soak affected area in the solution 2-4 times/day for 15-30 minutes or apply wet dressing soaked in the solution for more extended periods; rewet dressing with solution 2-4 times/day every 15-30 minutes

### Dosage Forms

Powder, for topical solution:

Domeboro®: Aluminum sulfate 1191 mg and calcium acetate 938 mg per packet (12s, 100s)

Pedi-Boro®: Aluminum sulfate 49% and calcium acetate 51% per packet (12s, 100s)

Tablet, effervescent, for topical solution (Domeboro®): Aluminum sulfate 878 mg and calcium acetate 604 mg

**Alupent® [US]** *see* metaproterenol *on page 518*

**Alupent® Inhalation Solution *(Discontinued)*** *see* metaproterenol *on page 518*

**Alu-Tab® *(Discontinued)*** *see* aluminum hydroxide *on page 34*

## amantadine (a MAN ta deen)

**Sound-Alike/Look-Alike Issues**
amantadine may be confused with ranitidine, rimantadine
Symmetrel® may be confused with Synthroid®

**Synonyms** adamantanamine hydrochloride; amantadine hydrochloride

**U.S./Canadian Brand Names** Endantadine® [Can]; PMS-Amantadine [Can]; Symmetrel® [US/Can]

**Therapeutic Category** Anti-Parkinson Agent; Antiviral Agent

**Use** Prophylaxis and treatment of influenza A viral infection; treatment of parkinsonism; treatment of drug-induced extrapyramidal symptoms

**Usual Dosage** Oral:
Children:
Influenza A treatment:
1-9 years: 5 mg/kg/day in 2 divided doses (manufacturers range: 4.4-8.8 mg/kg/day); maximum dose: 150 mg/day
≥10 years and <40 kg: 5 mg/kg/day; maximum dose: 150 mg/day
≥10 years and ≥40 kg: 100 mg twice daily
**Note:** Initiate within 24-48 hours after onset of symptoms; discontinue as soon as possible based on clinical response (generally within 3-5 days or within 24-48 hours after symptoms disappear)
Influenza A prophylaxis: Refer to "Influenza A treatment" dosing
**Note:** Continue treatment throughout the peak influenza activity in the community or throughout the entire influenza season in patients who cannot be vaccinated. Development of immunity following vaccination takes ~2 weeks; amantadine therapy should be considered for high-risk patients from the time of vaccination until immunity has developed. For children <9 years receiving influenza vaccine for the first time, amantadine prophylaxis should continue for 6 weeks (4 weeks after the first dose and 2 weeks after the second dose)
Adults:
Drug-induced extrapyramidal symptoms: 100 mg twice daily; may increase to 300-400 mg/day, if needed
Influenza A viral infection: 100 mg twice daily; initiate within 24-48 hours after onset of symptoms; discontinue as soon as possible based on clinical response (generally within 3-5 days or within 24-48 hours after symptoms disappear)
Influenza A prophylaxis: 100 mg twice daily
**Note:** Continue treatment throughout the peak influenza activity in the community or throughout the entire influenza season in patients who cannot be vaccinated. Development of immunity following vaccination takes ~2 weeks; amantadine therapy should be considered for high-risk patients from the time of vaccination until immunity has developed

**Dosage Forms** [DSC] = Discontinued product
Capsule, as hydrochloride: 100 mg
Syrup, as hydrochloride: 50 mg/5 mL (480 mL)
Symmetrel®: 50 mg/5 mL (480 mL) [raspberry flavor] [DSC]
Tablet, as hydrochloride (Symmetrel®): 100 mg

**amantadine hydrochloride** *see* amantadine *on this page*

**Amaphen® (Discontinued)**

**Amaryl® [US/Can]** *see* glimepiride *on page 375*

**Amatine® [Can]** *see* midodrine *on page 540*

## ambenonium (am be NOE nee um)

**Synonyms** ambenonium chloride

**U.S./Canadian Brand Names** Mytelase® [US/Can]

**Therapeutic Category** Cholinergic Agent

**Use** Treatment of myasthenia gravis

**Usual Dosage** Oral: Adults: 5-25 mg 3-4 times/day

**Dosage Forms** Caplet, as chloride [scored]: 10 mg [contains lactose and sucrose]

**ambenonium chloride** *see* ambenonium *on this page*

**Ambi 10® (Discontinued)** *see* benzoyl peroxide *on page 98*

**Ambien® [US]** *see* zolpidem *on page 863*

**Ambien CR™ [US]** *see* zolpidem *on page 863*

**Ambifed-G [US]** *see* guaifenesin and pseudoephedrine *on page 388*

**Ambifed-G DM [US]** *see* guaifenesin, pseudoephedrine, and dextromethorphan *on page 391*

**Ambi® Skin Tone *(Discontinued)*** *see* hydroquinone *on page 420*

**AmBisome® [US/Can]** *see* amphotericin B liposomal *on page 50*

## amcinonide (am SIN oh nide)
**U.S./Canadian Brand Names** Amcort® [Can]; Cyclocort® [US/Can]; ratio-Amcinonide [Can]
**Therapeutic Category** Corticosteroid, Topical
**Use** Relief of the inflammatory and pruritic manifestations of corticosteroid-responsive dermatoses (high potency corticosteroid)
**Usual Dosage** Topical: Adults: Apply in a thin film 2-3 times/day. Therapy should be discontinued when control is achieved; if no improvement is seen, reassessment of diagnosis may be necessary.
**Dosage Forms**
Cream: 0.1% (15 g, 30 g, 60 g) [contains benzyl alcohol]
Lotion: 0.1% (60 mL)
  Cyclocort®: 0.1% (20 mL, 60 mL) [contains benzyl alcohol]
Ointment: 0.1% (30 g, 60 g) [contains benzyl alcohol]
  Cyclocort®: 0.1% (15 g, 30 g, 60 g) [contains benzyl alcohol]

**Amcort® [Can]** *see* amcinonide *on this page*

**Amcort® Injection *(Discontinued)***

**Amen® *(Discontinued)***

**Amerge® [US/Can]** *see* naratriptan *on page 563*

**Americaine® [US-OTC]** *see* benzocaine *on page 95*

**Americaine® Anesthetic Lubricant *(Discontinued)*** *see* benzocaine *on page 95*

**Americaine® Hemorrhoidal [US-OTC]** *see* benzocaine *on page 95*

**A-methapred** *see* methylprednisolone *on page 531*

**amethocaine hydrochloride** *see* tetracaine *on page 791*

**amethopterin** *see* methotrexate *on page 524*

**Ametop™ [Can]** *see* tetracaine *on page 791*

**Amevive® [US/Can]** *see* alefacept *on page 25*

**amfepramone** *see* diethylpropion *on page 246*

**AMG 073** *see* cinacalcet *on page 183*

**Amibid DM [US]** *see* guaifenesin and dextromethorphan *on page 385*

**Amibid LA *(Discontinued)*** *see* guaifenesin *on page 383*

**Amicar® [US]** *see* aminocaproic acid *on page 40*

**Amidal [US]** *see* guaifenesin and phenylephrine *on page 387*

**Amidate® [US/Can]** *see* etomidate *on page 322*

**Amidrine [US]** *see* acetaminophen, isometheptene, and dichloralphenazone *on page 12*

## amifostine (am i FOS teen)
**Sound-Alike/Look-Alike Issues**
Ethyol® may be confused with ethanol
**Synonyms** ethiofos; gammaphos; WR-2721; YM-08310
**U.S./Canadian Brand Names** Ethyol® [US/Can]
**Therapeutic Category** Antidote
**Use** Reduce the incidence of moderate to severe xerostomia in patients undergoing postoperative radiation treatment for head and neck cancer, where the radiation port includes a substantial portion of the parotid glands. Reduce the cumulative renal toxicity associated with repeated administration of cisplatin in patients with advanced ovarian cancer or nonsmall cell lung cancer.
**Usual Dosage Note:** It is recommended that antiemetic medication including dexamethasone 20 mg I.V. and a serotonin 5-HT$_3$ receptor antagonist be administered prior to and in conjunction with amifostine.

Adults:

Cisplatin-induced renal toxicity, reduction: I.V.: 740-910 mg/m$^2$ once daily 30 minutes prior to cytotoxic therapy

**Note:** Doses >740 mg/m$^2$ are associated with a higher incidence of hypotension and may require interruption of therapy or dose modification for subsequent cycles. For 910 mg/m$^2$ doses, the manufacturer suggests the following blood pressure-based adjustment schedule:

The infusion of amifostine should be interrupted if the systolic blood pressure decreases significantly from baseline, as defined below:

Decrease of 20 mm Hg if baseline systolic blood pressure <100

Decrease of 25 mm Hg if baseline systolic blood pressure 100-119

Decrease of 30 mm Hg if baseline systolic blood pressure 120-139

Decrease of 40 mm Hg if baseline systolic blood pressure 140-179

Decrease of 50 mm Hg if baseline systolic blood pressure ≥180

If the blood pressure returns to normal within 5 minutes (assisted by fluid administration and postural management) and the patient is asymptomatic, the infusion may be restarted so that the full dose of amifostine may be administered. If the full dose of amifostine cannot be administered, the dose of amifostine for subsequent cycles should be 740 mg/m$^2$.

Xerostomia from head and neck cancer, reduction:

I.V.: 200mg/m$^2$/day during radiation therapy **or**

SubQ: 500 mg/day during radiation therapy

Dosage Forms Injection, powder for reconstitution: 500 mg

**Amigesic**® **[US/Can]** *see* salsalate *on page 738*

## amikacin (am i KAY sin)

Sound-Alike/Look-Alike Issues

amikacin may be confused with Amicar®, anakinra

Amikin® may be confused with Amicar®

Synonyms amikacin sulfate

U.S./Canadian Brand Names Amikin® [US/Can]

Therapeutic Category Aminoglycoside (Antibiotic)

Use Treatment of serious infections due to organisms resistant to gentamicin and tobramycin including *Pseudomonas*, *Proteus*, *Serratia*, and other gram-negative bacilli (bone infections, respiratory tract infections, endocarditis, and septicemia); documented infection of mycobacterial organisms susceptible to amikacin

Usual Dosage Individualization is critical because of the low therapeutic index

**Use of ideal body weight (IBW) for determining the mg/kg/dose appears to be more accurate than dosing on the basis of total body weight (TBW)**

In morbid obesity, dosage requirement may best be estimated using a dosing weight of IBW + 0.4 (TBW - IBW)

Initial and periodic peak and trough plasma drug levels should be determined, particularly in critically-ill patients with serious infections or in disease states known to significantly alter aminoglycoside pharmacokinetics (eg, cystic fibrosis, burns, or major surgery)

Infants, Children, and Adults: I.M., I.V.: 5-7.5 mg/kg/dose every 8 hours

Some clinicians suggest a daily dose of 15-20 mg/kg for all patients with normal renal function. This dose is at least as efficacious with similar, if not less, toxicity than conventional dosing.

Dosage Forms Injection, solution, as sulfate: 50 mg/mL (2 mL, 4 mL); 62.5 mg/mL (8 mL); 250 mg/mL (2 mL, 4 mL) [contains metabisulfite]

**amikacin sulfate** *see* amikacin *on this page*

**Amikin**® **[US/Can]** *see* amikacin *on this page*

## amiloride (a MIL oh ride)

Sound-Alike/Look-Alike Issues

amiloride may be confused with amiodarone, amlodipine, amrinone

Synonyms amiloride hydrochloride

U.S./Canadian Brand Names Apo-Amiloride® [Can]

Therapeutic Category Diuretic, Potassium Sparing

Use Counteracts potassium loss induced by other diuretics in the treatment of hypertension or edematous conditions including CHF, hepatic cirrhosis, and hypoaldosteronism; usually used in conjunction with more potent diuretics such as thiazides or loop diuretics

(Continued)

## amiloride *(Continued)*

**Usual Dosage** Oral:
Children: Although safety and efficacy in children have not been established by the FDA, a dosage of 0.625 mg/kg/day has been used in children weighing 6-20 kg.
Adults: 5-10 mg/day (up to 20 mg)
Hypertension (JNC 7): 5-10 mg/day in 1-2 divided doses
**Dosage Forms** Tablet, as hydrochloride: 5 mg

## amiloride and hydrochlorothiazide (a MIL oh ride & hye droe klor oh THYE a zide)

**Synonyms** hydrochlorothiazide and amiloride
**U.S./Canadian Brand Names** Apo-Amilzide® [Can]; Moduretic® [Can]; Novamilor [Can]; Nu-Amilzide [Can]
**Therapeutic Category** Diuretic, Combination
**Use** Potassium-sparing diuretic; antihypertensive
**Usual Dosage** Adults: Oral: Start with 1 tablet/day, then may be increased to 2 tablets/day if needed; usually given in a single dose
**Dosage Forms** Tablet: Amiloride hydrochloride 5 mg and hydrochlorothiazide 50 mg

**amiloride hydrochloride** *see* amiloride *on previous page*

**Aminate Fe-90 [US]** *see* vitamins (multiple/prenatal) *on page 852*

**2-amino-6-mercaptopurine** *see* thioguanine *on page 797*

**2-amino-6-trifluoromethoxy-benzothiazole** *see* riluzole *on page 723*

**aminobenzylpenicillin** *see* ampicillin *on page 50*

## aminocaproic acid (a mee noe ka PROE ik AS id)

**Sound-Alike/Look-Alike Issues**
Amicar® may be confused with amikacin, Amikin®
**Synonyms** epsilon aminocaproic acid
**U.S./Canadian Brand Names** Amicar® [US]
**Therapeutic Category** Hemostatic Agent
**Use** Treatment of excessive bleeding from fibrinolysis
**Usual Dosage** Acute bleeding syndrome: Adults: Oral, I.V.: 4-5 g during the first hour, followed by 1 g/hour for 8 hours or until bleeding controlled (maximum daily dose: 30 g)
**Dosage Forms**
Injection, solution: 250 mg/mL (20 mL) [contains benzyl alcohol]
Syrup: 1.25 g/5 mL (240 mL, 480 mL)
Amicar®: 1.25 g/5 mL (480 mL) [raspberry flavor]
Tablet [scored]: 500 mg, 1000 mg

**Amino-Cerv™ [US]** *see* urea *on page 834*

## aminoglutethimide (a mee noe gloo TETH i mide)

**Sound-Alike/Look-Alike Issues**
Cytadren® may be confused with cytarabine
**Synonyms** AG; AGT; BA-16038; elipten
**U.S./Canadian Brand Names** Cytadren® [US]
**Therapeutic Category** Antineoplastic Agent
**Use** Suppression of adrenal function in selected patients with Cushing's syndrome
**Usual Dosage** Oral: Adults: Adrenal suppression: 250 mg every 6 hours may be increased at 1- to 2-week intervals to a total of 2 g/day
**Dosage Forms** Tablet [scored]: 250 mg

## aminolevulinic acid (a MEE noh lev yoo lin ik AS id)

**Synonyms** aminolevulinic acid hydrochloride
**U.S./Canadian Brand Names** Levulan® Kerastick® [US]; Levulan® [Can]
**Therapeutic Category** Photosensitizing Agent, Topical; Porphyrin Agent, Topical
**Use** Treatment of minimally to moderately thick actinic keratoses (grade 1 or 2) of the face or scalp; to be used in conjunction with blue light illumination

**Usual Dosage** Adults: Topical: Apply to actinic keratoses (**not** perilesional skin) followed 14-18 hours later by blue light illumination. Application/treatment may be repeated at a treatment site after 8 weeks.

**Dosage Forms** Powder for topical solution: 20% (1s, 6s) [2-component system containing aminolevulinic acid hydrochloride 354 mg (powder) and diluent containing ethanol 48% (1.5 mL) packaged together in an applicator tube]

**aminolevulinic acid hydrochloride** *see* aminolevulinic acid *on previous page*

# aminophylline (am in OFF i lin)
**Sound-Alike/Look-Alike Issues**
  aminophylline may be confused with amitriptyline, ampicillin
**Synonyms** theophylline ethylenediamine
**U.S./Canadian Brand Names** Phyllocontin® [Can]; Phyllocontin®-350 [Can]
**Therapeutic Category** Theophylline Derivative
**Use** Bronchodilator in reversible airway obstruction due to asthma or COPD; increase diaphragmatic contractility
**Usual Dosage**
  Treatment of acute bronchospasm: I.V.:
    Loading dose (in patients not currently receiving aminophylline or theophylline): 6 mg/kg (based on aminophylline) administered I.V. over 20-30 minutes; administration rate should not exceed 25 mg/minute (aminophylline)
    Approximate I.V. maintenance dosages are based upon **continuous infusions**; bolus dosing (often used in children <6 months of age) may be determined by multiplying the hourly infusion rate by 24 hours and dividing by the desired number of doses/day
    6 weeks to 6 months: 0.5 mg/kg/hour
    6 months to 1 year: 0.6-0.7 mg/kg/hour
    1-9 years: 1 mg/kg/hour
    9-16 years and smokers: 0.8 mg/kg/hour
    Adults, nonsmoking: 0.5 mg/kg/hour
    Older patients and patients with cor pulmonale: 0.3 mg/kg/hour
    Patients with congestive heart failure: 0.1-0.2 mg/kg/hour
    Dosage should be adjusted according to serum level measurements during the first 12- to 24-hour period.
  Bronchodilator: Oral: Children ≥45 kg and Adults: Initial: 380 mg/day (equivalent to theophylline 300 mg/day) in divided doses every 6-8 hours; may increase dose after 3 days; maximum dose: 928 mg/day (equivalent to theophylline 800 mg/day)
**Dosage Forms** [DSC] = Discontinued product
  Injection, solution: 25 mg/mL (10 mL, 20 mL)
  Liquid, oral [DSC]: 105 mg/5 mL (500 mL) [apricot flavor]
  Tablet: 100 mg, 200 mg

**aminosalicylate sodium** *see* aminosalicylic acid *on this page*

# aminosalicylic acid (a mee noe sal i SIL ik AS id)
**Synonyms** 4-aminosalicylic acid; aminosalicylate sodium; para-aminosalicylate sodium; PAS; sodium PAS
**U.S./Canadian Brand Names** Paser® [US]
**Therapeutic Category** Nonsteroidal Antiinflammatory Drug (NSAID)
**Use** Adjunctive treatment of tuberculosis used in combination with other antitubercular agents
**Usual Dosage** Oral:
  Children: Tuberculosis: 200-300 mg/kg/day in 3-4 equally divided doses
  Adults: Tuberculosis: 150 mg/kg/day in 2-3 equally divided doses
**Dosage Forms** Granules: 4 g/packet (30s) [contains talc]

**4-aminosalicylic acid** *see* aminosalicylic acid *on this page*

**5-aminosalicylic acid** *see* mesalamine *on page 516*

**Aminoxin® [US-OTC]** *see* pyridoxine *on page 701*

# amiodarone (a MEE oh da rone)
**Sound-Alike/Look-Alike Issues**
  amiodarone may be confused with amiloride, amrinone
(Continued)

## amiodarone *(Continued)*

Cordarone® may be confused with Cardura®, Cordran®

**Synonyms** amiodarone hydrochloride

**U.S./Canadian Brand Names** Alti-Amiodarone [Can]; Apo-Amiodarone® [Can]; Cordarone® [US/Can]; Gen-Amiodarone [Can]; Novo-Amiodarone [Can]; Pacerone® [US]; Rhoxal-amiodarone [Can]

**Therapeutic Category** Antiarrhythmic Agent, Class III

**Use** Management of life-threatening recurrent ventricular fibrillation (VF) or hemodynamically-unstable ventricular tachycardia (VT) refractory to other antiarrythmic agents or in patients intolerant of other agents used for these conditions

**Usual Dosage Note:** Lower loading and maintenance doses are preferable in women and all patients with low body weight.

Oral: Adults: Ventricular arrhythmias: 800-1600 mg/day in 1-2 doses for 1-3 weeks, then when adequate arrhythmia control is achieved, decrease to 600-800 mg/day in 1-2 doses for 1 month; maintenance: 400 mg/day. Lower doses are recommended for supraventricular arrhythmias.

I.V.:
Children:
Pulseless VF or VT (PALS dosing): 5 mg/kg rapid I.V. bolus or I.O.
Perfusing tachycardias (PALS dosing): Loading dose: 5 mg/kg I.V. over 20-60 minutes or I.O.; may repeat up to maximum dose of 15 mg/kg/day
Adults:
Breakthrough VF or VT: 150 mg supplemental doses in 100 mL $D_5W$ over 10 minutes
Pulseless VF or VT: I.V. push: Initial: 300 mg in 20-30 mL NS or $D_5W$; if VF or VT recurs, supplemental dose of 150 mg followed by infusion of 1 mg/minute for 6 hours, then 0.5 mg/minute (maximum daily dose: 2.2 g)
Step 1: 150 mg (100 mL) over first 10 minutes (mix 3 mL in 100 mL $D_5W$)
Step 2: 360 mg (200 mL) over next 6 hours (mix 18 mL in 500 mL $D_5W$): 1 mg/minute
Step 3: 540 mg (300 mL) over next 18 hours: 0.5 mg/minute
**Note:** After the first 24 hours: 0.5 mg/minute utilizing concentration of 1-6 mg/mL
**Note:** When switching from I.V. to oral therapy, use the following as a guide:
<1-week I.V. infusion: 800-1600 mg/day
1- to 3-week I.V. infusion: 600-800 mg/day
>3-week I.V. infusion: 400 mg/day
**Recommendations for conversion to intravenous amiodarone after oral administration:** During long-term amiodarone therapy (ie, ≥4 months), the mean plasma-elimination half-life of the active metabolite of amiodarone is 61 days. Replacement therapy may not be necessary in such patients if oral therapy is discontinued for a period <2 weeks, since any changes in serum amiodarone concentrations during this period may **not** be clinically significant.

**Dosage Forms**
Injection, solution, as hydrochloride: 50 mg/mL (3 mL, 9 mL, 18 mL) [contains benzyl alcohol and polysorbate (Tween®) 80]
Cordarone®: 50 mg/mL (3 mL) [contains benzyl alcohol and polysorbate (Tween®) 80]
Tablet, as hydrochloride [scored]: 200 mg
Cordarone®: 200 mg
Pacerone®: 100 mg [not scored], 200 mg, 300 mg, 400 mg

**amiodarone hydrochloride** *see* amiodarone *on previous page*

**Amipaque® *(Discontinued)***

**Ami-Tex LA [US]** *see* guaifenesin and phenylephrine *on page 387*

**Ami-Tex PSE [US]** *see* guaifenesin and pseudoephedrine *on page 388*

**Amitone® [US-OTC]** *see* calcium carbonate *on page 130*

## amitriptyline *(a mee TRIP ti leen)*

**Sound-Alike/Look-Alike Issues**
amitriptyline may be confused with aminophylline, imipramine, nortriptyline
Elavil® may be confused with Aldoril®, Eldepryl®, enalapril, Equanil®, Mellaril®, Oruvail®, Plavix®

**Synonyms** amitriptyline hydrochloride

**U.S./Canadian Brand Names** Apo-Amitriptyline® [Can]; Levate® [Can]; Novo-Triptyn [Can]; PMS-Amitriptyline [Can]

**Therapeutic Category** Antidepressant, Tricyclic (Tertiary Amine)

**Use** Relief of symptoms of depression

**Usual Dosage**
Adolescents: Depressive disorders: Oral: Initial: 25-50 mg/day; may administer in divided doses; increase gradually to 100 mg/day in divided doses
Adults:
Depression:
Oral: 50-150 mg/day single dose at bedtime or in divided doses; dose may be gradually increased up to 300 mg/day
I.M.: 20-30 mg 4 times/day
**Dosage Forms** [DSC] = Discontinued product
Injection, as hydrochloride: 10 mg/mL (10 mL) [DSC]
Tablet, as hydrochloride: 10 mg, 25 mg, 50 mg, 75 mg, 100 mg, 150 mg

# amitriptyline and chlordiazepoxide (a mee TRIP ti leen & klor dye az e POKS ide)
**Synonyms** chlordiazepoxide and amitriptyline
**U.S./Canadian Brand Names** Limbitrol® DS [US]; Limbitrol® [US/Can]
**Therapeutic Category** Antidepressant, Tricyclic (Tertiary Amine)
**Controlled Substance** C-IV
**Use** Treatment of moderate to severe anxiety and/or agitation and depression
**Usual Dosage** Initial: 3-4 tablets in divided doses; this may be increased to 6 tablets/day as required; some patients respond to smaller doses and can be maintained on 2 tablets
**Dosage Forms** Tablet:
5-12.5 (Limbitrol®): Amitriptyline hydrochloride 12.5 mg and chlordiazepoxide 5 mg [contains lactose]
10-25 (Limbitrol® DS): Amitriptyline hydrochloride 25 mg and chlordiazepoxide 10 mg [contains lactose]

# amitriptyline and perphenazine (a mee TRIP ti leen & per FEN a zeen)
**Synonyms** perphenazine and amitriptyline
**U.S./Canadian Brand Names** Etrafon® [Can]; Triavil® [US]
**Therapeutic Category** Antidepressant/Phenothiazine
**Use** Treatment of patients with moderate to severe anxiety and depression
**Usual Dosage** Oral: 1 tablet 2-4 times/day
**Dosage Forms** Tablet:
2-10 (Triavil®): Amitriptyline hydrochloride 10 mg and perphenazine 2 mg
2-25 (Triavil®): Amitriptyline hydrochloride 25 mg and perphenazine 2 mg
4-10: Amitriptyline hydrochloride 10 mg and perphenazine 4 mg
4-25 (Triavil®): Amitriptyline hydrochloride 25 mg and perphenazine 4 mg
4-50: Amitriptyline hydrochloride 50 mg and perphenazine 4 mg

# amitriptyline hydrochloride see amitriptyline on previous page

# AMJ 9701 see palifermin on page 613

# AmLactin® [US-OTC] see lactic acid and ammonium hydroxide on page 462

# amlexanox (am LEKS an oks)
**U.S./Canadian Brand Names** Aphthasol® [US]
**Therapeutic Category** Antiinflammatory Agent, Locally Applied
**Use** Treatment of aphthous ulcers (ie, canker sores)
**Usual Dosage** Administer (0.5 cm - ¼") directly on ulcers 4 times/day following oral hygiene, after meals, and at bedtime
**Dosage Forms** Paste: 5% (5 g) [contains benzyl alcohol]

# amlodipine (am LOE di peen)
**Sound-Alike/Look-Alike Issues**
amlodipine may be confused with amiloride
Norvasc® may be confused with Navane®, Norvir®, Vascor®
**Synonyms** amlodipine besylate
**U.S./Canadian Brand Names** Norvasc® [US/Can]
**Therapeutic Category** Calcium Channel Blocker
**Use** Treatment of hypertension; treatment of symptomatic chronic stable angina, vasospastic (Prinzmetal's) angina (confirmed or suspected); prevention of hospitalization due to angina with documented CAD (limited to patients without heart failure or ejection fraction <40%)
(Continued)

## amlodipine *(Continued)*

**Usual Dosage** Oral:
Children 6-17 years: Hypertension: 2.5-5 mg once daily
Adults:
Hypertension: Initial dose: 5 mg once daily; maximum dose: 10 mg once daily. In general, titrate in 2.5 mg increments over 7-14 days. Usual dosage range (JNC 7): 2.5-10 mg once daily.
Angina: Usual dose: 5-10 mg
**Dosage Forms** Tablet: 2.5 mg, 5 mg, 10 mg

## amlodipine and atorvastatin (am LOW di peen & a TORE va sta tin)

**Synonyms** atorvastatin calcium and amlodipine besylate
**U.S./Canadian Brand Names** Caduet® [US]
**Therapeutic Category** Antilipemic Agent, HMG-CoA Reductase Inhibitor;  Calcium Channel Blocker
**Use** For use when treatment with both agents is appropriate:
Amlodipine is used for the treatment of hypertension and angina.
Atorvastatin is used with dietary therapy for the following:
Hyperlipidemias: To reduce elevations in total cholesterol, LDL-C, apolipoprotein B, and triglycerides in patients with primary hypercholesterolemia (elevations of 1 or more components are present in Fredrickson type IIa, IIb, III, and IV hyperlipidemias); treatment of homozygous familial hypercholesterolemia
Heterozygous familial hypercholesterolemia (HeFH): In adolescent patients (10-17 years of age, females >1 year postmenarche) with HeFH having LDL-C ≥190 mg/dL **or** LDL ≥160 mg/dL with positive family history of premature cardiovascular disease (CVD) or with 2 or more CVD risk factors in the adolescent patient
Primary prevention of CVD in high-risk patients
**Usual Dosage** Oral: Children 10-17 years (females >1 year postmenarche) and Adults: Treatment of hypertension/angina and hyperlipidemias: Dose is individualized, given once daily and substituted for each individual component. See individual agents. Maximum dose: Amlodipine 10 mg/day, atorvastatin 80 mg/day.
**Dosage Forms** Tablet:
2.5/10: Amlodipine 2.5 mg and atorvastatin 10 mg
2.5/20: Amlodipine 2.5 mg and atorvastatin 20 mg
2.5/40: Amlodipine 2.5 mg and atorvastatin 40 mg
5/10: Amlodipine 5 mg and atorvastatin 10 mg
5/20: Amlodipine 5 mg and atorvastatin 20 mg
5/40: Amlodipine 5 mg and atorvastatin 40 mg
5/80: Amlodipine 5 mg and atorvastatin 80 mg
10/10: Amlodipine 10 mg and atorvastatin 10 mg
10/20: Amlodipine 10 mg and atorvastatin 20 mg
10/40: Amlodipine 10 mg and atorvastatin 40 mg
10/80: Amlodipine 10 mg and atorvastatin 80 mg

## amlodipine and benazepril (am LOE di peen & ben AY ze pril)

**Synonyms** benazepril and amlodipine
**U.S./Canadian Brand Names** Lotrel® [US]
**Therapeutic Category** Antihypertensive Agent, Combination
**Use** Treatment of hypertension
**Usual Dosage** Oral: Adults: Dose is individualized, given once daily
**Dosage Forms** Capsule:
Amlodipine 2.5 mg and benazepril hydrochloride 10 mg
Amlodipine 5 mg and benazepril hydrochloride 10 mg
Amlodipine 5 mg and benazepril hydrochloride 20 mg
Amlodipine 10 mg and benazepril hydrochloride 20 mg

**amlodipine besylate** *see* amlodipine *on previous page*

**Ammens® Medicated Deodorant [US-OTC]** *see* zinc oxide *on page 861*

**ammonapse** *see* sodium phenylbutyrate *on page 756*

## ammonia spirit (aromatic) (a MOE nee ah SPEAR it, air oh MAT ik)
**Synonyms** smelling salts
**Therapeutic Category** Respiratory Stimulant
**Use** Respiratory and circulatory stimulant, treatment of fainting
**Usual Dosage** Used as "smelling salts" to treat or prevent fainting
**Dosage Forms** Solution for inhalation [ampul]: 1.7% to 2.1% (0.33 mL)

## ammonium chloride (a MOE nee um KLOR ide)
**Therapeutic Category** Electrolyte Supplement, Oral
**Use** Treatment of hypochloremic states or metabolic alkalosis
**Usual Dosage** Metabolic alkalosis: The following equations represent different methods of correction utilizing either the serum $HCO_3^-$, the serum chloride, or the base excess
   **Dosing of mEq $NH_4Cl$ via the chloride-deficit method (hypochloremia):**
   Dose of mEq $NH_4Cl$ = [0.2 L/kg x body weight (kg)] x [103 - observed serum chloride]; administer 50% of dose over 12 hours, then re-evaluate
   **Note:** 0.2 L/kg is the estimated chloride volume of distribution and 103 is the average normal serum chloride concentration (mEq/L)
   **Dosing of mEq $NH_4Cl$ via the bicarbonate-excess method (refractory hypochloremic metabolic alkalosis):**
   Dose of $NH_4Cl$ = [0.5 L/kg x body weight (kg)] x (observed serum $HCO_3^-$ - 24); administer 50% of dose over 12 hours, then re-evaluate
   **Note:** 0.5 L/kg is the estimated bicarbonate volume of distribution and 24 is the average normal serum bicarbonate concentration (mEq/L)
   These equations will yield different requirements of ammonium chloride
**Dosage Forms** Injection, solution: Ammonium 5 mEq/mL and chloride 5 mEq/mL (20 mL) [equivalent to ammonium chloride 267.5 mg/mL]

**ammonium lactate** *see* lactic acid and ammonium hydroxide *on page 462*

**Ammonul® [US]** *see* sodium phenylacetate and sodium benzoate *on page 755*

**Amnesteem™ [US]** *see* isotretinoin *on page 452*

## amobarbital (am oh BAR bi tal)
**Synonyms** amylobarbitone
**U.S./Canadian Brand Names** Amytal® [US/Can]
**Therapeutic Category** Barbiturate
**Controlled Substance** C-II
**Use** Hypnotic in short-term treatment of insomnia; reduce anxiety and provide sedation preoperatively
**Usual Dosage**
   Children:
   Sedative: I.M., I.V.: 6-12 years: Manufacturer's dosing range: 65- 500 mg
   Hypnotic: I.M.: 2-3 mg/kg (maximum: 500 mg)
   Adults:
   Hypnotic: I.M., I.V.: 65-200 mg at bedtime (maximum I.M. dose: 500 mg)
   Sedative: I.M., I.V.: 30-50 mg 2-3 times/day
**Dosage Forms** Injection, powder for reconstitution, as sodium: 500 mg

## amobarbital and secobarbital (am oh BAR bi tal & see koe BAR bi tal)
**Sound-Alike/Look-Alike Issues**
   Tuinal® may be confused with Luminal®, Tylenol®
**Synonyms** secobarbital and amobarbital
**Therapeutic Category** Barbiturate
**Controlled Substance** C-II
**Use** Short-term treatment of insomnia
**Usual Dosage** Adults: Oral: 1-2 capsules at bedtime
**Dosage Forms** Capsule: Amobarbital 50 mg and secobarbital 50 mg

**AMO Vitrax® *(Discontinued)*** *see* hyaluronate and derivatives *on page 406*

## amoxapine (a MOKS a peen)

**Sound-Alike/Look-Alike Issues**
amoxapine may be confused with amoxicillin, Amoxil®
Asendin may be confused with aspirin

**Therapeutic Category** Antidepressant, Tricyclic (Secondary Amine)

**Use** Treatment of depression, psychotic depression, depression accompanied by anxiety or agitation

**Usual Dosage** Oral:
Children: Not established in children <16 years of age.
Adolescents: Initial: 25-50 mg/day; increase gradually to 100 mg/day; may administer as divided doses or as a single dose at bedtime
Adults: Initial: 25 mg 2-3 times/day, if tolerated, dosage may be increased to 100 mg 2-3 times/day; may be given in a single bedtime dose when dosage <300 mg/day
Maximum daily dose:
Inpatient: 600 mg
Outpatient: 400 mg

**Dosage Forms** Tablet: 25 mg, 50 mg, 100 mg, 150 mg

## amoxicillin (a moks i SIL in)

**Sound-Alike/Look-Alike Issues**
amoxicillin may be confused with amoxapine, Amoxil®, Atarax®
Amoxil® may be confused with amoxapine, amoxicillin
Trimox® may be confused with Diamox®, Tylox®

**Synonyms** p-hydroxyampicillin; amoxicillin trihydrate; amoxycillin

**U.S./Canadian Brand Names** Amoxil® [US]; Apo-Amoxi® [Can]; DisperMox™ [US]; Gen-Amoxicillin [Can]; Lin-Amox [Can]; Moxilin® [US]; Novamoxin® [Can]; Nu-Amoxi [Can]; PMS-Amoxicillin [Can]; Trimox® [US]

**Therapeutic Category** Penicillin

**Use** Treatment of otitis media, sinusitis, and infections caused by susceptible organisms involving the respiratory tract, skin, and urinary tract; prophylaxis of bacterial endocarditis in patients undergoing surgical or dental procedures; as part of a multidrug regimen for *H. pylori* eradication

**Usual Dosage** Oral:
Children ≤3 months: 20-30 mg/kg/day divided every 12 hours
Children: >3 months and <40 kg: Dosing range: 20-50 mg/kg/day in divided doses every 8-12 hours
Ear, nose, throat, genitourinary tract, or skin/skin structure infections:
Mild to moderate: 25 mg/kg/day in divided doses every 12 hours **or** 20 mg/kg/day in divided doses every 8 hours
Severe: 45 mg/kg/day in divided doses every 12 hours **or** 40 mg/kg/day in divided doses every 8 hours
Acute otitis media: 80-90 mg/kg/day divided every 12 hours
Lower respiratory tract infections: 45 mg/kg/day in divided doses every 12 hours **or** 40 mg/kg/day in divided doses every 8 hours
Subacute bacterial endocarditis prophylaxis: 50 mg/kg 1 hour before procedure

Adults: Dosing range: 250-500 mg every 8 hours or 500-875 mg twice daily
Ear, nose, throat, genitourinary tract or skin/skin structure infections:
Mild to moderate: 500 mg every 12 hours **or** 250 mg every 8 hours
Severe: 875 mg every 12 hours **or** 500 mg every 8 hours
Lower respiratory tract infections: 875 mg every 12 hours **or** 500 mg every 8 hours
Endocarditis prophylaxis: 2 g 1 hour before procedure
*Helicobacter pylori* eradication: 1000 mg twice daily; requires combination therapy with at least one other antibiotic and an acid-suppressing agent (proton pump inhibitor or $H_2$ blocker)

**Dosage Forms** [DSC] = Discontinued product
Capsule, as trihydrate: 250 mg, 500 mg
Amoxil®: 250 mg [DSC], 500 mg
Moxilin®, Trimox®: 250 mg, 500 mg
Powder for oral suspension, as trihydrate: 125 mg/5 mL (80 mL, 100 mL, 150 mL); 200 mg/5 mL (50 mL, 75 mL, 100 mL); 250 mg/5 mL (80 mL, 100 mL, 150 mL); 400 mg/5 mL (50 mL, 75 mL, 100 mL)
Amoxil®: 125 mg/5 mL (150 mL) [contains sodium benzoate; strawberry flavor] [DSC]; 200 mg/5 mL (5 mL, 50 mL, 75 mL, 100 mL) [contains sodium benzoate; bubble gum flavor]; 250 mg/5 mL (100 mL, 150 mL) [contains sodium benzoate; bubble gum flavor]; 400 mg/5 mL (5 mL, 50 mL, 75 mL, 100 mL) [contains sodium benzoate; bubble gum flavor]
Moxilin®: 250 mg/5 mL (100 mL, 150 mL)

Trimox®: 125 mg/5 mL (80 mL, 100 mL, 150 mL); 250 mg/5 mL (80 mL, 100 mL, 150 mL) [contains sodium benzoate; raspberry-strawberry flavor]

Powder for oral suspension, as trihydrate [drops] (Amoxil®): 50 mg/mL (15 mL [DSC], 30 mL) [bubble gum flavor]

Tablet, as trihydrate [film coated] (Amoxil®): 500 mg, 875 mg

Tablet, chewable, as trihydrate: 125 mg, 200 mg, 250 mg, 400 mg

Amoxil®: 200 mg [contains phenylalanine 1.82 mg/tablet; cherry banana peppermint flavor]; 400 mg [contains phenylalanine 3.64 mg/tablet; cherry banana peppermint flavor]

Tablet, for oral suspension, as trihydrate (DisperMox™): 200 mg [contains phenylalanine 5.6 mg; strawberry flavor]; 400 mg [contains phenylalanine 5.6 mg; strawberry flavor]; 600 mg [contains phenylalanine 11.23 mg; strawberry flavor]

# amoxicillin and clavulanate potassium

(a moks i SIL in & klav yoo LAN ate poe TASS ee um)

### Sound-Alike/Look-Alike Issues

Augmentin® may be confused with Azulfidine®

**Synonyms** amoxicillin and clavulanic acid

### U.S./Canadian Brand Names
Alti-Amoxi-Clav [Can]; Apo-Amoxi-Clav® [Can]; Augmentin ES-600® [US]; Augmentin XR™ [US]; Augmentin® [US/Can]; Clavulin® [Can]; Novo-Clavamoxin [Can]; ratio-Aclavulanate [Can]

### Therapeutic Category   Penicillin

**Use** Treatment of otitis media, sinusitis, and infections caused by susceptible organisms involving the lower respiratory tract, skin and skin structure, and urinary tract; spectrum same as amoxicillin with additional coverage of beta-lactamase producing *B. catarrhalis*, *H. influenzae*, *N. gonorrhoeae*, and *S. aureus* (not MRSA). The expanded coverage of this combination makes it a useful alternative when amoxicillin resistance is present and patients cannot tolerate alternative treatments.

### Usual Dosage

Infants <3 months: 30 mg/kg/day divided every 12 hours using the 125 mg/5 mL suspension

Children ≥3 months and <40 kg:

Otitis media (Augmentin® ES-600): 90 mg/kg/day divided every 12 hours for 10 days in children with severe illness and when coverage for B-lactamase postitive *H. influenzae* and *M. catarrhalis* is needed.

Lower respiratory tract infections, severe infections, sinusitis: 45 mg/kg/day divided every 12 hours **or** 40 mg/kg/day divided every 8 hours

Less severe infections: 25 mg/kg/day divided every 12 hours or 20 mg/kg/day divided every 8 hours

Children >40 kg and Adults: 250-500 mg every 8 hours or 875 mg every 12 hours

Children ≥16 years and Adults:

Acute bacterial sinusitis: Extended release tablet: Two 1000 mg tablets every 12 hours for 10 days

Community-acquired pneumonia: Extended release tablet: Two 1000 mg tablets every 12 hours for 7-10 days

Hemodialysis: Moderately dialyzable (20% to 50%)

250-500 mg every 24 hours; administer dose during and after dialysis. Do not use extended release tablets.

Peritoneal dialysis: Moderately dialyzable (20% to 50%)

Amoxicillin: Administer 250 mg every 12 hours

Clavulanic acid: Dose for $Cl_{cr}$ <10 mL/minute

Continuous arteriovenous or venovenous hemofiltration effects:

Amoxicillin: ~50 mg of amoxicillin/L of filtrate is removed

Clavulanic acid: Dose for $Cl_{cr}$ <10 mL/minute

### Dosage Forms

Powder for oral suspension: 200: Amoxicillin 200 mg and clavulanate potassium 28.5 mg per 5 mL (100 mL) [contains phenylalanine]; 400: Amoxicillin 400 mg and clavulanate potassium 57 mg per 5 mL (100 mL) [contains phenylalanine]; 600: Amoxicillin 600 mg and clavulanic potassium 42.9 mg per 5 mL (75 mL, 125 mL, 200 mL) [contains phenylalanine]

Augmentin®:

125: Amoxicillin 125 mg and clavulanate potassium 31.25 mg per 5 mL (75 mL, 100 mL, 150 mL) [banana flavor]

200: Amoxicillin 200 mg and clavulanate potassium 28.5 mg per 5 mL (50 mL, 75 mL, 100 mL) [contains phenylalanine 7 mg/5 mL; orange-raspberry flavor]

250: Amoxicillin 250 mg and clavulanate potassium 62.5 mg per 5 mL (75 mL, 100 mL, 150 mL) [orange flavor]

(Continued)

## amoxicillin and clavulanate potassium *(Continued)*

400: Amoxicillin 400 mg and clavulanate potassium 57 mg per 5 mL (50 mL, 75 mL, 100 mL) [contains phenylalanine 7 mg/5 mL; orange-raspberry flavor]

Augmentin ES-600®: Amoxicillin 600 mg and clavulanic potassium 42.9 mg per 5 mL (75 mL, 125 mL, 200 mL) [contains phenylalanine 7 mg/5 mL; strawberry cream flavor]

Tablet: 500: Amoxicillin trihydrate 500 mg and clavulanate potassium 125 mg; 875: Amoxicillin trihydrate 875 mg and clavulanate potassium 125 mg

Augmentin®:

250: Amoxicillin trihydrate 250 mg and clavulanate potassium 125 mg

500: Amoxicillin trihydrate 500 mg and clavulanate potassium 125 mg

875: Amoxicillin trihydrate 875 mg and clavulanate potassium 125 mg

Tablet, chewable: 200: Amoxicillin trihydrate 200 mg and clavulanate potassium 28.5 mg [contains phenylalanine]; 400: Amoxicillin trihydrate 400 mg and clavulanate potassium 57 mg [contains phenylalanine]

Augmentin®:

125: Amoxicillin trihydrate 125 mg and clavulanate potassium 31.25 mg [lemon-lime flavor]

200: Amoxicillin trihydrate 200 mg and clavulanate potassium 28.5 mg [contains phenylalanine 2.1 mg/tablet; cherry-banana flavor]

250: Amoxicillin trihydrate 250 mg and clavulanate potassium 62.5 mg [lemon-lime flavor]

400: Amoxicillin trihydrate 400 mg and clavulanate potassium 57 mg [contains phenylalanine 4.2 mg/tablet; cherry-banana flavor]

Tablet, extended release (Augmentin XR™): Amoxicillin 1000 mg and clavulanic acid 62.5 mg [contains potassium 29.3 mg (1.27 mEq) and sodium 12.6 mg (0.32 mEq)

**amoxicillin and clavulanic acid** *see* amoxicillin and clavulanate potassium *on previous page*

**amoxicillin, lansoprazole, and clarithromycin** *see* lansoprazole, amoxicillin, and clarithromycin *on page 468*

**amoxicillin trihydrate** *see* amoxicillin *on page 46*

**Amoxil® [US]** *see* amoxicillin *on page 46*

**amoxycillin** *see* amoxicillin *on page 46*

**Amphadase™ [US]** *see* hyaluronidase *on page 407*

**amphetamine and dextroamphetamine** *see* dextroamphetamine and amphetamine *on page 237*

**Amphocin® [US]** *see* amphotericin B (conventional) *on next page*

**Amphojel® [Can]** *see* aluminum hydroxide *on page 34*

**Amphojel® *(Discontinued)*** *see* aluminum hydroxide *on page 34*

**Amphotec® [US/Can]** *see* amphotericin B cholesteryl sulfate complex *on this page*

## amphotericin B cholesteryl sulfate complex

(am foe TER i sin bee kole LES te ril SUL fate KOM plecks)

**Synonyms** ABCD; amphotericin B colloidal dispersion

**U.S./Canadian Brand Names** Amphotec® [US/Can]

**Therapeutic Category** Antifungal Agent

**Use** Treatment of invasive aspergillosis in patients who have failed amphotericin B deoxycholate treatment, or who have renal impairment or experience unacceptable toxicity which precludes treatment with amphotericin B deoxycholate in effective doses.

**Usual Dosage** Children and Adults: I.V.:

Premedication: For patients who experience chills, fever, hypotension, nausea, or other nonanaphylactic infusion-related immediate reactions, premedicate with the following drugs, 30-60 minutes prior to drug administration: a nonsteroidal (eg, ibuprofen, choline magnesium trisalicylate) with or without diphenhydramine; or acetaminophen with diphenhydramine; or hydrocortisone 50-100 mg. If the patient experiences rigors during the infusion, meperidine may be administered.

Range: 3-4 mg/kg/day (infusion of 1 mg/kg/hour); maximum: 7.5 mg/kg/day

**Dosage Forms** Injection, powder for reconstitution: 50 mg, 100 mg

**amphotericin B colloidal dispersion** *see* amphotericin B cholesteryl sulfate complex *on this page*

# amphotericin B (conventional) (am foe TER i sin bee con VEN sha nal)

**Synonyms** amphotericin B desoxycholate

**U.S./Canadian Brand Names** Amphocin® [US]; Fungizone® [Can]

**Therapeutic Category** Antifungal Agent

**Use** Treatment of severe systemic and central nervous system infections caused by susceptible fungi such as *Candida* species, *Histoplasma capsulatum*, *Cryptococcus neoformans*, *Aspergillus* species, *Blastomyces dermatitidis*, *Torulopsis glabrata*, and *Coccidioides immitis*; fungal peritonitis; irrigant for bladder fungal infections; used in fungal infection in patients with bone marrow transplantation, amebic meningoencephalitis, ocular aspergillosis (intraocular injection), candidal cystitis (bladder irrigation), chemoprophylaxis (low-dose I.V.), immunocompromised patients at risk of aspergillosis (intranasal/nebulized), refractory meningitis (intrathecal), coccidioidal arthritis (intra-articular/I.M.).

Low-dose amphotericin B has been administered after bone marrow transplantation to reduce the risk of invasive fungal disease.

## Usual Dosage

I.V.: Premedication: For patients who experience infusion-related immediate reactions, premedicate with the following drugs, 30-60 minutes prior to drug administration: NSAID (with or without diphenhydramine) **or** acetaminophen with diphenhydramine **or** hydrocortisone 50-100 mg. If the patient experiences rigors during the infusion, meperidine may be administered.

Infants and Children:

Test dose: I.V.: 0.1 mg/kg/dose to a maximum of 1 mg; infuse over 30-60 minutes. Many clinicians believe a test dose is unnecessary.

Maintenance dose: 0.25-1 mg/kg/day given once daily; infuse over 2-6 hours. Once therapy has been established, amphotericin B can be administered on an every-other-day basis at 1-1.5 mg/kg/dose; cumulative dose: 1.5-2 g over 6-10 week.

Adults:

Test dose: 1 mg infused over 20-30 minutes. Many clinicians believe a test dose is unnecessary.

Maintenance dose: Usual: 0.25-1.5 mg/kg/day; 1-1.5 mg/kg over 4-6 hours every other day may be given once therapy is established; aspergillosis, mucormycosis, rhinocerebral phycomycosis often require 1-1.5 mg/kg/day; do not exceed 1.5 mg/kg/day

Duration of therapy varies with nature of infection: Usual duration is 4-12 weeks or cumulative dose of 1-4 g

I.T.: Meningitis, coccidioidal or cryptococcal:

Children.: 25-100 mcg every 48-72 hours; increase to 500 mcg as tolerated

Adults: Initial: 25-300 mcg every 48-72 hours; increase to 500 mcg to 1 mg as tolerated; maximum total dose: 15 mg has been suggested

Bladder irrigation: Candidal cystitis: Irrigate with 50 mcg/mL solution instilled periodically or continuously for 5-10 days or until cultures are clear

**Dosage Forms** Injection, powder for reconstitution, as desoxycholate: 50 mg

# amphotericin B desoxycholate *see* amphotericin B (conventional) *on this page*

# amphotericin B lipid complex (am foe TER i sin bee LIP id KOM pleks)

**Synonyms** ABLC

**U.S./Canadian Brand Names** Abelcet® [US/Can]

**Therapeutic Category** Antifungal Agent

**Use** Treatment of aspergillosis or any type of progressive fungal infection in patients who are refractory to or intolerant of conventional amphotericin B therapy

**Usual Dosage** Children and Adults: I.V.:

Premedication: For patients who experience infusion-related immediate reactions, premedicate with the following drugs, 30-60 minutes prior to drug administration: a nonsteroidal anti-inflammatory agent ± diphenhydramine; or acetaminophen with diphenhydramine; or hydrocortisone 50-100 mg. If the patient experiences rigors during the infusion, meperidine may be administered.

Range: 2.5-5 mg/kg/day as a single infusion

**Dosage Forms** Injection, suspension [preservative free]: 5 mg/mL (20 mL)

## amphotericin B liposomal (am foe TER i sin bee lye po SO mal)

**Synonyms** L-AmB

**U.S./Canadian Brand Names** AmBisome® [US/Can]

**Therapeutic Category** Antifungal Agent, Systemic

**Use** Empirical therapy for presumed fungal infection in febrile, neutropenic patients. Treatment of patients with *Aspergillus* species, *Candida* species and/or *Cryptococcus* species infections refractory to amphotericin B desoxycholate, or in patients where renal impairment or unacceptable toxicity precludes the use of amphotericin B desoxycholate. Treatment of cryptococcal meningitis in HIV-infected patients. Treatment of visceral leishmaniasis.

**Usual Dosage** Children and Adults: I.V.:

**Note:** Premedication: For patients who experience chills, fever, hypotension, nausea, or other nonanaphylactic infusion-related immediate reactions, premedicate with the following drugs, 30-60 minutes prior to drug administration: a nonsteroidal (eg, ibuprofen, choline magnesium trisalicylate) with or without diphenhydramine; or acetaminophen with diphenhydramine; or hydrocortisone 50-100 mg. If the patient experiences rigors during the infusion, meperidine may be administered.

Empiric therapy: Recommended initial dose: 3 mg/kg/day

Systemic fungal infections (*Aspergillus*, *Candida*, *Cryptococcus*): Recommended initial dose of 3-5 mg/kg/day

Cryptococcal meningitis in HIV-infected patients: 6 mg/kg/day

Treatment of visceral leishmaniasis:

Immunocompetent patients: 3 mg/kg/day on days 1-5, and 3 mg/kg/day on days 14 and 21; a repeat course may be given in patients who do not achieve parasitic clearance

Immunocompromised patients: 4 mg/kg/day on days 1-5, and 4 mg/kg/day on days 10, 17, 24, 31, and 38

**Dosage Forms** Injection, powder for reconstitution: 50 mg

## ampicillin (am pi SIL in)

**Sound-Alike/Look-Alike Issues**

ampicillin may be confused with aminophylline

**Synonyms** aminobenzylpenicillin; ampicillin sodium; ampicillin trihydrate

**U.S./Canadian Brand Names** Apo-Ampi® [Can]; Novo-Ampicillin [Can]; Nu-Ampi [Can]; Principen® [US]

**Therapeutic Category** Penicillin

**Use** Treatment of susceptible bacterial infections (nonbeta-lactamase-producing organisms); susceptible bacterial infections caused by streptococci, pneumococci, nonpenicillinase-producing staphylococci, *Listeria*, meningococci; some strains of *H. influenzae*, *Salmonella*, *Shigella*, *E. coli*, *Enterobacter*, and *Klebsiella*

**Usual Dosage**

Infants and Children:

Mild-to-moderate infections:

I.M., I.V.: 100-150 mg/kg/day in divided doses every 6 hours (maximum: 2-4 g/day)

Oral: 50-100 mg/kg/day in doses divided every 6 hours (maximum: 2-4 g/day)

Severe infections/meningitis: I.M., I.V.: 200-400 mg/kg/day in divided doses every 6 hours (maximum: 6-12 g/day)

Endocarditis prophylaxis: I.M., I.V.:

Dental, oral, respiratory tract, or esophageal procedures: 50 mg/kg within 30 minutes prior to procedure in patients unable to take oral amoxicillin

Genitourinary and gastrointestinal tract (except esophageal) procedures:

High-risk patients: 50 mg/kg (maximum: 2 g) within 30 minutes prior to procedure, followed by ampicillin 25 mg/kg (or amoxicillin 25 mg/kg orally) 6 hours later; must be used in combination with gentamicin.

Moderate-risk patients: 50 mg/kg within 30 minutes prior to procedure

Adults:

Susceptible infections:

Oral: 250-500 mg every 6 hours

I.M., I.V.: 250-500 mg every 6 hours

Sepsis/meningitis: I.M., I.V.: 150-250 mg/kg/24 hours divided every 3-4 hours (range: 6-12 g/day)

Endocarditis prophylaxis: I.M., I.V.:

Dental, oral, respiratory tract, or esophageal procedures: 2 g within 30 minutes prior to procedure in patients unable to take oral amoxicillin

Genitourinary and gastrointestinal tract (except esophageal) procedures:

High-risk patients: 2 g within 30 minutes prior to procedure, followed by ampicillin 1 g (or amoxicillin 1 g orally) 6 hours later; must be used in combination with gentamicin

Moderate-risk patients: 2 g within 30 minutes prior to procedure

**Dosage Forms**

Capsule (Principen®): 250 mg, 500 mg

Injection, powder for reconstitution, as sodium: 125 mg, 250 mg, 500 mg, 1 g, 2 g, 10 g

Powder for oral suspension (Principen®): 125 mg/5 mL (100 mL, 200 mL); 250 mg/5 mL (100 mL, 200 mL)

## ampicillin and sulbactam (am pi SIL in & SUL bak tam)

**Synonyms** sulbactam and ampicillin

**U.S./Canadian Brand Names** Unasyn® [US/Can]

**Therapeutic Category** Penicillin

**Use** Treatment of susceptible bacterial infections involved with skin and skin structure, intra-abdominal infections, gynecological infections; spectrum is that of ampicillin plus organisms producing beta-lactamases such as *S. aureus*, *H. influenzae*, *E. coli*, *Klebsiella*, *Acinetobacter*, *Enterobacter*, and anaerobes

**Usual Dosage** Unasyn® (ampicillin/sulbactam) is a combination product. Dosage recommendations for Unasyn® are based on the ampicillin component.

Children ≥1 year: I.V.:

Mild-to-moderate infections: 100-150 mg ampicillin/kg/day (150-300 mg Unasyn®) divided every 6 hours; maximum: 8 g ampicillin/day (12 g Unasyn®)

Severe infections: 200-400 mg ampicillin/kg/day divided every 6 hours; maximum: 8 g ampicillin/day (12 g Unasyn®)

Adults: I.M., I.V.: 1-2 g ampicillin (1.5-3 g Unasyn®) every 6 hours; maximum: 8 g ampicillin/day (12 g Unasyn®)

**Dosage Forms**

Injection, powder for reconstitution: 3 g [ampicillin sodium 2 g and sulbactam sodium 1 g]; 15 g [ampicillin sodium 10 g and sulbactam sodium 5 g] [bulk package]

Unasyn®: 1.5 g [ampicillin sodium 1 g and sulbactam sodium 0.5 g]; 3 g [ampicillin sodium 2 g and sulbactam sodium 1 g]; 15 g [ampicillin sodium 10 g and sulbactam sodium 5 g] [bulk package]

## ampicillin sodium *see* ampicillin *on previous page*

## ampicillin trihydrate *see* ampicillin *on previous page*

## amprenavir (am PREN a veer)

**U.S./Canadian Brand Names** Agenerase® [US/Can]

**Therapeutic Category** Protease Inhibitor

**Use** Treatment of HIV infections in combination with at least two other antiretroviral agents; oral solution should only be used when capsules or other protease inhibitors are not therapeutic options

**Usual Dosage** Oral: **Note:** Capsule and oral solution are **not** interchangeable on a mg-per-mg basis.

Capsule:

Children 4-12 years **or** 13-16 years (<50 kg): 20 mg/kg twice daily or 15 mg/kg 3 times daily; maximum: 2400 mg/day

Children >13 years (≥50 kg) and Adults: 1200 mg twice daily

**Note:** Dosage adjustments for amprenavir when administered in combination therapy:

Efavirenz: Adjustments necessary for both agents:

Amprenavir 1200 mg 3 times/day (single protease inhibitor) **or**

Amprenavir 1200 mg twice daily plus ritonavir 200 mg twice daily

Ritonavir: Adjustments necessary for both agents:

Amprenavir 1200 mg plus ritonavir 200 mg once daily **or**

Amprenavir 600 mg plus ritonavir 100 mg twice daily

**Note:** Oral solution of ritonavir and amprenavir should not be coadministered.

Solution:

Children 4-12 years **or** 13-16 years (<50 kg): 22.5 mg/kg twice daily or 17 mg/kg 3 times daily; maximum: 2800 mg/day

Children >13 years (≥50 kg) and Adults: 1400 mg twice daily

**Dosage Forms** [DSC] = Discontinued product

Capsule: 50 mg, 150 mg [DSC]

(Continued)

## amprenavir (Continued)

Solution, oral [use only when there are no other options]: 15 mg/mL (240 mL) [contains propylene glycol 550 mg/mL and vitamin E 46 int. units/mL; grape-bubble gum-peppermint flavor]

**AMPT** see metyrosine on page 536

**amrinone lactate** see inamrinone on page 434

**Amvisc® (Discontinued)** see hyaluronate and derivatives on page 406

**Amvisc® Plus (Discontinued)** see hyaluronate and derivatives on page 406

## amyl nitrite (AM il NYE trite)

Synonyms isoamyl nitrite

Therapeutic Category Vasodilator

Use Coronary vasodilator in angina pectoris; adjunct in treatment of cyanide poisoning; produce changes in the intensity of heart murmurs

Usual Dosage Nasal inhalation:

Cyanide poisoning: Children and Adults: Inhale the vapor from a 0.3 mL crushed ampul every minute for 15-30 seconds until I.V. sodium nitrite infusion is available

Angina: Adults: 1-6 inhalations from 1 crushed ampul; may repeat in 3-5 minutes

Dosage Forms Vapor for inhalation [crushable glass perles]: 0.3 mL

**amyl nitrite, sodium thiosulfate, and sodium nitrite** see sodium nitrite, sodium thiosulfate, and amyl nitrite on page 755

**amylobarbitone** see amobarbital on page 45

**Amytal® [US/Can]** see amobarbital on page 45

**Anabolin® (Discontinued)** see nandrolone on page 560

**Anacin® PM Aspirin Free (Discontinued)** see acetaminophen and diphenhydramine on page 7

**Anadrol® [US]** see oxymetholone on page 611

**Anafranil® [US/Can]** see clomipramine on page 196

## anagrelide (an AG gre lide)

Synonyms 1370-999-397; 6,7-dichloro-1,5-dihydroimidazo [2,1b] quinazolin-2(3H)-one monohydrochloride; anagrelide hydrochloride; BL4162A

U.S./Canadian Brand Names Agrylin® [US/Can]; Rhoxal-Anagrelide [Can]

Therapeutic Category Platelet Reducing Agent

Use Treatment of essential thrombocythemia (ET) and thrombocythemia associated with chronic myelogenous leukemia (CML), polycythemia vera, and other myeloproliferative disorders

Usual Dosage Note: Maintain for ≥1 week, then adjust to the lowest effective dose to reduce and maintain platelet count <600,000/μL ideally to the normal range; the dose must not be increased by >0.5 mg/day in any 1 week; maximum dose: 10 mg/day or 2.5 mg/dose
Oral:
Children: Initial: 0.5 mg/day (range: 0.5 mg 1-4 times/day)
Adults: 0.5 mg 4 times/day or 1 mg twice daily

Dosage Forms Capsule: 0.5 mg, 1 mg

**anagrelide hydrochloride** see anagrelide on this page

## anakinra (an a KIN ra)

Sound-Alike/Look-Alike Issues
anakinra may be confused with amikacin

Synonyms IL-1Ra; interleukin-1 receptor antagonist

U.S./Canadian Brand Names Kineret® [US/Can]

Therapeutic Category Antirheumatic, Disease Modifying

Use Reduction of signs and symptoms of moderately- to severely-active rheumatoid arthritis in adult patients who have failed one or more disease-modifying antirheumatic drugs (DMARDs); may be used alone or in combination with DMARDs (other than tumor necrosis factor-blocking agents)

Usual Dosage Adults: SubQ: Rheumatoid arthritis: 100 mg once daily (administer at approximately the same time each day)

Dosage Forms Injection, solution [preservative free]: 100 mg/0.67 mL (1 mL) [prefilled syringe]

**Ana-Kit**® **[US]** *see* epinephrine and chlorpheniramine *on page 289*

**Analpram-HC**® **[US]** *see* pramoxine and hydrocortisone *on page 671*

**AnaMantle**® **HC [US]** *see* lidocaine and hydrocortisone *on page 482*

**Anamine**® **Syrup** *(Discontinued) see* chlorpheniramine and pseudoephedrine *on page 172*

**Anandron**® **[Can]** *see* nilutamide *on page 576*

**Anaplex**® **DM [US]** *see* brompheniramine, pseudoephedrine, and dextromethorphan *on page 116*

**Anaplex**® **Liquid** *(Discontinued) see* chlorpheniramine and pseudoephedrine *on page 172*

**Anaprox**® **[US/Can]** *see* naproxen *on page 562*

**Anaprox**® **DS [US/Can]** *see* naproxen *on page 562*

**Anaspaz**® **[US]** *see* hyoscyamine *on page 424*

**anastrozole** (an AS troe zole)
Synonyms ICI-D1033; ZD1033
U.S./Canadian Brand Names Arimidex® [US/Can]
Therapeutic Category Antineoplastic Agent
Use Treatment of locally-advanced or metastatic breast cancer (ER-positive or hormone receptor unknown) in postmenopausal women; treatment of advanced breast cancer in postmenopausal women with disease progression following tamoxifen therapy; adjuvant treatment of early ER-positive breast cancer in postmenopausal women
Usual Dosage Adults: Oral (refer to individual protocols): Breast cancer: 1 mg once daily
Dosage Forms Tablet: 1 mg

**Anatrast**® **[US]** *see* radiological/contrast media (ionic) *on page 707*

**Anatuss**® *(Discontinued)*

**Anbesol**® **[US-OTC]** *see* benzocaine *on page 95*

**Anbesol**® **Baby [US-OTC/Can]** *see* benzocaine *on page 95*

**Anbesol**® **Cold Sore Therapy [US-OTC]** *see* benzocaine *on page 95*

**Anbesol**® **Jr. [US-OTC]** *see* benzocaine *on page 95*

**Anbesol**® **Maximum Strength [US-OTC]** *see* benzocaine *on page 95*

**Ancef**® **[US]** *see* cefazolin *on page 153*

**Ancobon**® **[US/Can]** *see* flucytosine *on page 342*

**Andehist DM NR [US]** *see* brompheniramine, pseudoephedrine, and dextromethorphan *on page 116*

**Andehist DM NR Drops [US]** *see* carbinoxamine, pseudoephedrine, and dextromethorphan *on page 145*

**Andehist NR Drops [US]** *see* carbinoxamine and pseudoephedrine *on page 144*

**Andehist NR Syrup [US]** *see* brompheniramine and pseudoephedrine *on page 115*

**Andriol**® **[Can]** *see* testosterone *on page 788*

**Androcur**® **[Can]** *see* cyproterone *(Canada only) on page 218*

**Androcur**® **Depot [Can]** *see* cyproterone *(Canada only) on page 218*

**Androderm**® **[US/Can]** *see* testosterone *on page 788*

**AndroGel**® **[US/Can]** *see* testosterone *on page 788*

**Android**® **[US]** *see* methyltestosterone *on page 533*

**Andro-L.A.**® **Injection** *(Discontinued) see* testosterone *on page 788*

**Androlone**® *(Discontinued) see* nandrolone *on page 560*

**Androlone**®**-D** *(Discontinued) see* nandrolone *on page 560*

**Andropository [Can]** *see* testosterone *on page 788*

**Andropository**® **Injection** *(Discontinued) see* testosterone *on page 788*

**Anectine**® *(Discontinued) see* succinylcholine *on page 768*

**Anemagen™ OB [US]** *see* vitamins (multiple/prenatal) *on page 852*

**Anestacon® [US]** *see* lidocaine *on page 479*

**aneurine hydrochloride** *see* thiamine *on page 796*

**Anexate® [Can]** *see* flumazenil *on page 343*

**Anexsia® [US]** *see* hydrocodone and acetaminophen *on page 411*

**Angio Conray® [US]** *see* radiological/contrast media (ionic) *on page 707*

**Angiomax® [US/Can]** *see* bivalirudin *on page 109*

**Angiovist® [US]** *see* radiological/contrast media (ionic) *on page 707*

**Angiscein® [US]** *see* fluorescein sodium *on page 346*

## anisindione (an is in DY one)

**Therapeutic Category** Anticoagulant (Other)

**Use** Prophylaxis and treatment of venous thrombosis, pulmonary embolism, and thromboembolic disorders; atrial fibrillation with risk of embolism; adjunct in the prophylaxis of systemic embolism following myocardial infarction

**Usual Dosage** Oral: Adults:

Initial: 300 mg on first day, 200 mg on second day, 100 mg on third day

Maintenance dosage: Established by daily PT/INR determinations; range: 25-250 mg/day

**Note:** When discontinuing therapy, manufacturer recommends tapering dose over 3-4 weeks.

**Dosage Forms** Tablet: 50 mg

**Anodynos-DHC® *(Discontinued)*** *see* hydrocodone and acetaminophen *on page 411*

**Anolor 300 [US]** *see* butalbital, acetaminophen, and caffeine *on page 124*

**Anoquan® *(Discontinued)***

**Ansaid® [Can]** *see* flurbiprofen *on page 352*

**Ansaid® *(Discontinued)*** *see* flurbiprofen *on page 352*

**ansamycin** *see* rifabutin *on page 721*

**Antabuse® [US]** *see* disulfiram *on page 261*

**Antagon® [US/Can]** *see* ganirelix *on page 367*

**Antara™ [US]** *see* fenofibrate *on page 330*

**Antazoline-V® Ophthalmic *(Discontinued)*** *see* naphazoline and antazoline *on page 561*

**antazoline and naphazoline** *see* naphazoline and antazoline *on page 561*

**Anthra-Derm® *(Discontinued)*** *see* anthralin *on this page*

**Anthraforte® [Can]** *see* anthralin *on this page*

## anthralin (AN thra lin)

**Synonyms** dithranol

**U.S./Canadian Brand Names** Anthraforte® [Can]; Anthranol® [Can]; Anthrascalp® [Can]; Dritho-Scalp® [US]; Drithocreme® [US]; Micanol® [Can]; Psoriatec™ [US]

**Therapeutic Category** Keratolytic Agent

**Use** Treatment of psoriasis (quiescent or chronic psoriasis)

**Usual Dosage** Adults: Topical: Generally, apply once a day or as directed. The irritant potential of anthralin is directly related to the strength being used and each patient's individual tolerance. Always commence treatment using a short, daily contact time (5-10 minutes) for at least 1 week using the lowest strength possible. Contact time may be gradually increased (to 20-30 minutes) as tolerated.

Skin application: Apply sparingly only to psoriatic lesions and rub gently and carefully into the skin until absorbed. Avoid applying an excessive quantity which may cause unnecessary soiling and staining of the clothing or bed linen.

Scalp application: Comb hair to remove scalar debris, wet hair and, after suitably parting, rub cream well into the lesions, taking care to prevent the cream from spreading onto the forehead,

Remove by washing or showering; optimal period of contact will vary according to the strength used and the patient's response to treatment. Continue treatment until the skin is entirely clear (ie, when there is nothing to feel with the fingers and the texture is normal).

**Dosage Forms** Cream:

Drithocreme®, Psoriatec™: 1% (50 g)

Dritho-Scalp®: 0.5% (50 g)

**Anthranol**® **[Can]** *see* anthralin *on previous page*

**Anthrascalp**® **[Can]** *see* anthralin *on previous page*

## anthrax vaccine, adsorbed (AN thraks vak SEEN ad SORBED)
**Synonyms** AVA
**U.S./Canadian Brand Names** BioThrax™ [US]
**Therapeutic Category** Vaccine
**Use** Immunization against *Bacillus anthracis.* Recommended for individuals who may come in contact with animal products which come from anthrax endemic areas and may be contaminated with *Bacillus anthracis* spores; recommended for high-risk persons such as veterinarians and other handling potentially infected animals. Routine immunization for the general population is not recommended.

The Department of Defense is implementing an anthrax vaccination program against the biological warfare agent anthrax, which will be administered to all active duty and reserve personnel.
**Usual Dosage** SubQ:
Children <18 years: Safety and efficacy have not been established
Children ≥18 years and Adults:
Primary immunization: Three injections of 0.5 mL each given 2 weeks apart, followed by three additional injections given at 6-, 12-, and 18 months; it is not necessary to restart the series if a dose is not given on time; resume as soon as practical
Subsequent booster injections: 0.5 mL at 1-year intervals are recommended for immunity to be maintained
**Dosage Forms** Injection, suspension: 5 mL [vial stopper contains dry natural rubber]

**Antiben**® *(Discontinued)* *see* antipyrine and benzocaine *on page 58*

**AntibiOtic**® **Ear [US]** *see* neomycin, polymyxin B, and hydrocortisone *on page 568*

**anti-CD11a** *see* efalizumab *on page 280*

**anti-CD20 monoclonal antibody** *see* rituximab *on page 726*

**anti-CD20-murine monoclonal antibody I-131** *see* tositumomab and iodine I 131 tositumomab *on page 812*

**antidigoxin fab fragments, ovine** *see* digoxin immune Fab *on page 249*

**antidiuretic hormone** *see* vasopressin *on page 842*

## antihemophilic factor (human) (an tee hee moe FIL ik FAK tor HYU man)
**Synonyms** AHF (human); factor VIII (human)
**U.S./Canadian Brand Names** Alphanate® [US]; Hemofil® M [US/Can]; Humate-P® [US/Can]; Koāte®-DVI [US]; Monarc® M [US]; Monoclate-P® [US]
**Therapeutic Category** Blood Product Derivative
**Use** Management of hemophilia A for patients in whom a deficiency in factor VIII has been demonstrated; can be of significant therapeutic value in patients with acquired factor VIII inhibitors not exceeding 10 Bethesda units/mL
Humate-P®: In addition, indicated as treatment of spontaneous bleeding in patients with severe von Willebrand disease and in mild and moderate von Willebrand disease where desmopressin is known or suspected to be inadequate
**Orphan status:** Alphanate®: Management of von Willebrand disease
**Usual Dosage** Children and Adults: I.V.: Individualize dosage based on coagulation studies performed prior to treatment and at regular intervals during treatment; 1 AHF unit is the activity present in 1 mL of normal pooled human plasma; dosage should be adjusted to actual vial size currently stocked in the pharmacy. (General guidelines presented; consult individual product labeling for specific dosing recommendations.)
**Dosage based on desired factor VIII increase (%):**
To calculate dosage needed based on desired factor VIII increase (%):
Body weight (kg) x 0.5 int. units/kg x desired factor VIII increase (%) = int. units factor VIII required
For example:
50 kg x 0.5 int. units/kg x 30 (% increase) = 750 int. units factor VIII
(Continued)

# antihemophilic factor (human) *(Continued)*

## Dosage based on expected factor VIII increase (%):
It is also possible to calculate the **expected** % factor VIII increase:

(# int. units administered x 2%/int. units/kg) divided by body weight (kg) = expected % factor VIII increase

For example:

(1400 int. units x 2%/int. units/kg) divided by 70 kg = 40%

## General guidelines:
Minor Hemorrhage: Required peak postinfusion AHF level: 20% to 40% (10-20 int. units/kg), repeat dose every 12-24 hours for 1-3 days until bleeding is resolved or healing achieved; mild superficial or early hemorrhages may respond to a single dose

Moderate hemorrhage: Required peak postinfusion AHF level: 30% to 60% (15-30 int. units/kg): Infuse every 12-24 hours for ≥3 days until pain and disability are resolved

Alternatively, a loading dose to achieve 50% (25 int. units/kg) may be given, followed by 10-15 int. units/kg dose given every 8-12 hours; may be needed for >7 days

Severe/life-threatening hemorrhage: Required peak postinfusion AHF level: 60% to 100% (30-50 int. units/kg): Infuse every 8-24 hours until threat is resolved

Alternatively, a loading dose to achieve 80% to 100% (40-50 int. units/kg) may be given, followed by 20-25 int. units/kg dose given every 8-12 hours for ≥14 days

Minor surgery: Required peak postinfusion AHF level: 30% to 80% (15-40 int. units/kg): Highly dependent upon procedure and specific product recommendations; for some procedures, may be administered as a single infusion plus oral antifibrinolytic therapy within 1 hour; in other procedures, may repeat dose every 12-24 hours as needed

Major surgery: Required peak pre- and postsurgery AHF level: 80% to 100% (40-50 int. units/kg): Administer every 6-24 hours until healing is complete (10-14 days)

Prophylaxis: May also be given on a regular schedule to prevent bleeding

If bleeding is not controlled with adequate dose, test for presence of inhibitor. It may not be possible or practical to control bleeding if inhibitor titers >10 Bethesda units/mL; antihemophilic factor (porcine) may be considered as an alternative

## von Willebrand disease:
Treatment of hemorrhage in von Willebrand disease (Humate-P®): 1 int. units of factor VIII per kg of body weight would be expected to raise circulating vWF:RC of approximately 3.5-4 int. units/dL

Type 1, mild (if desmopressin is not appropriate): Major hemorrhage:

Loading dose: 40-60 int. units/kg

Maintenance dose: 40-50 int. units/kg every 8-12 hours for 3 days, keeping vWF:RC of nadir >50%; follow with 40-50 int. units/kg daily for up to 7 days

Type 1, moderate or severe:

Minor hemorrhage: 40-50 int. units/kg for 1-2 doses

Major hemorrhage:

Loading dose: 50-75 int. units/kg

Maintenance dose: 40-60 int. units/kg daily for up to 7 days

Types 2 and 3:

Minor hemorrhage: 40-50 int. units/kg for 1-2 doses

Major hemorrhage:

Loading dose: 60-80 int. units/kg

Maintenance dose: 40-60 int. units/kg every 8-12 hours for 3 days, keeping vWF:RC of nadir >50%; follow with 40-60 int. units/kg daily for up to 7 days

**Dosage Forms** Injection, human [single-dose vial]: Labeling on cartons and vials indicates number of int. units

# antihemophilic factor (porcine) (an tee hee moe FIL ik FAK ter POR seen)
**Synonyms** AHF (porcine); factor VIII (porcine)

**U.S./Canadian Brand Names** Hyate:C® [US]

**Therapeutic Category** Antihemophilic Agent

**Use** Management of hemophilia A in patients with antibodies to human factor VIII (consider use of human factor VIII in patients with antibody titer of <5 Bethesda units/mL); management of previously nonhemophilic patients with spontaneously-acquired inhibitors to human factor VIII, regardless of initial antihuman inhibitor titer

**Usual Dosage** Clinical response should be used to assess efficacy

Initial dose:

Antibody level to human factor VIII <50 Bethesda units/mL: 100-150 porcine units/kg (body weight) is recommended

Antibody level to human factor VIII >50 Bethesda units/mL: Activity of the antibody to antihemophilic (porcine) should be determined; **an antiporcine antibody level** >20 Bethesda units/mL indicates that the patient is unlikely to benefit from treatment; for lower titers, a dose of 100-150 porcine units/kg is recommended

The initial dose may also be calculated using the following method:

1. Determine patient's antibody titer against porcine factor VIII

2. Calculate average plasma volume:

(body weight kg) (average blood volume) (1 - hematocrit) = plasma volume

(body weight kg) (80 mL/kg) (1 - hematocrit) = plasma volume

**Note:** A hematocrit of 50% = 0.5 for the equation

3. Neutralizing dose:

(plasma volume mL) (antibody titer Bethesda units/mL) = neutralizing dose units

This is the predicted dose required to neutralize the circulating antibodies. An incremental dose must be added to the neutralizing dose in order to increase the plasma factor VIII to the desired level.

4. Incremental dose:

(desired plasma factor VIII level) (body weight) divided by 1.5 = incremental dose units

5. Total dose = neutralizing dose + incremental dose = total dose units

If a patient has previously been treated with Hyate:C®, this may provide a guide to his likely response and, therefore, assist in estimation of the preliminary dose

Subsequent doses: Following administration of the initial dose, if the recovery of factor VIII in the patient's plasma is not sufficient, another larger dose should be administered; if recovery after the second dose is still insufficient, a third and larger dose may prove effective. Once appropriate factor VIII levels are achieved, dosing can be repeated every 6-8 hours.

**Dosage Forms** Injection, powder for reconstitution: 400-700 porcine units [to be reconstituted with 20 mL SWFI]

# antihemophilic factor (recombinant) (an tee hee moe FIL ik FAK tor ree KOM be nant)

**Synonyms** AHF (recombinant); factor VIII (recombinant); rAHF

**U.S./Canadian Brand Names** Advate [US]; Helixate® FS [US/Can]; Kogenate® FS [US/Can]; Kogenate® [Can]; Recombinate™ [US/Can]; ReFacto® [US/Can]

**Therapeutic Category** Blood Product Derivative

**Use** Management of hemophilia A (classic hemophilia) for patients in whom a deficiency in factor VIII has been demonstrated; prevention and control of bleeding episodes; perioperative management of hemophilia A; can be of significant therapeutic value in patients with acquired factor VIII inhibitors not exceeding 10 Bethesda units/mL

**Usual Dosage** Children and Adults: I.V.: Individualize dosage based on coagulation studies performed prior to treatment and at regular intervals during treatment; 1 AHF unit is the activity present in 1 mL of normal pooled human plasma; dosage should be adjusted to actual vial size currently stocked in the pharmacy. (General guidelines presented; consult individual product labeling for specific dosing recommendations.)

**Dosage based on desired factor VIII increase (%):**

To calculate dosage needed based on desired factor VIII increase (%):

Body weight (kg) x 0.5 int. units/kg x desired factor VIII increase (%) = int. units factor VIII required

For example:

50 kg x 0.5 int. units/kg x 30 (% increase) = 750 int. units factor VIII

**Dosage based on expected factor VIII increase (%):**

It is also possible to calculate the **expected** % factor VIII increase:

(# int. units administered x 2%/int. units/kg) divided by body weight (kg) = expected % factor VIII increase

For example:

(1400 int. units x 2%/int. units/kg) divided by 70 kg = 40%

**General guidelines:**

Minor hemorrhage: Required peak postinfusion AHF level: 20% to 40% (10-20 int. units/kg); mild superficial or early hemorrhages may respond to a single dose; may repeat dose every 12-24 hours for 1-3 days until bleeding is resolved or healing achieved

Moderate hemorrhage/minor surgery: Required peak postinfusion AHF level: 30% to 60% (15-30 int. units/kg); repeat dose at 12-24 hours if needed; some products suggest continuing for ≥3 days until pain and disability are resolved

(Continued)

## antihemophilic factor (recombinant) *(Continued)*

Severe/life-threatening hemorrhage: Required peak postinfusion AHF level: Initial dose: 80% to 100% (40-50 int. units/kg); maintenance dose: 40% to 50% (20-25 int. units/kg) every 8-12 hours until threat is resolved

Major surgery: Required peak pre- and postsurgery AHF level: ~100% (50 int. units/kg) give first dose prior to surgery and repeat every 6-12 hours until healing complete (10-14 days)

Prophylaxis: May also be given on a regular schedule to prevent bleeding

If bleeding is not controlled with adequate dose, test for presence of inhibitor. It may not be possible or practical to control bleeding if inhibitor titers >10 Bethesda units/mL; antihemophilic factor (porcine) may be considered as an alternative

**Dosage Forms** Injection, powder for reconstitution, recombinant [preservative free]:

Advate: 250 int. units, 500 int. units, 1000 int. units, 1500 int. units [plasma/albumin free]

Helixate® FS, Kogenate® FS: 250 int. units, 500 int. units, 1000 int. units [contains sucrose 28 mg/vial]

Recombinate™: 250 int. units, 500 units, 1000 int. units [contains human albumin 12.5 mg/mL; packaging contains natural rubber latex]

ReFacto®: 250 int. units, 500 units, 1000 int. units, 2000 int. units [contains sucrose]

**Antihist-1**® *(Discontinued)* see clemastine *on page 191*

## anti-inhibitor coagulant complex (an tee-in HI bi tor coe AG yoo lant KOM pleks)

**Synonyms** coagulant complex inhibitor

**U.S./Canadian Brand Names** Autoplex® T [US]; Feiba VH® [US]; Feiba® VH Immuno [Can]

**Therapeutic Category** Hemophilic Agent

**Use** Patients with factor VIII inhibitors who are to undergo surgery or those who are bleeding

**Usual Dosage** Dosage range: 25-100 factor VIII correctional units per kg depending on the severity of hemorrhage

**Dosage Forms** Injection, powder for reconstitution:

Autoplex® T: Each bottle is labeled with correctional units of factor VIII [with heparin 2 units/mL; packaging contains natural rubber latex]

Feiba VH®: Each bottle is labeled with correctional units of factor VIII [heparin free; packaging contains natural rubber latex]

**Antilirium**® *(Discontinued)* see physostigmine *on page 646*

**Antiminth**® *(Discontinued)* see pyrantel pamoate *on page 698*

**Antiphlogistine Rub A-535 No Odour [Can]** see triethanolamine salicylate *on page 823*

## antipyrine and benzocaine (an tee PYE reen & BEN zoe kane)

**Sound-Alike/Look-Alike Issues**

Auralgan® may be confused with Ophthalgan®

**Synonyms** benzocaine and antipyrine

**U.S./Canadian Brand Names** A/B Otic [US]; Allergen® [US]; Auralgan® [Can]; Aurodex [US]; Auroto [US]

**Therapeutic Category** Otic Agent, Analgesic; Otic Agent, Ceruminolytic

**Use** Temporary relief of pain and reduction of swelling associated with acute congestive and serous otitis media, swimmer's ear, otitis externa; facilitates ear wax removal

**Usual Dosage** Otic: Fill ear canal; moisten cotton pledget, place in external ear, repeat every 1-2 hours until pain and congestion are relieved; for ear wax removal instill drops 3-4 times/day for 2-3 days

**Dosage Forms** Solution, otic: Antipyrine 5.4% and benzocaine 1.4% (15 mL)

**Antispas**® **Injection** *(Discontinued)* see dicyclomine *on page 245*

## antithrombin III (an tee THROM bin three)

**Synonyms** AT III; heparin cofactor I

**U.S./Canadian Brand Names** Thrombate III® [US/Can]

**Therapeutic Category** Blood Product Derivative

**Use** Treatment of hereditary antithrombin III deficiency in connection with surgical or obstetrical procedures; thromboembolism

**Usual Dosage** Adults:

Initial dose: Dosing is individualized based on pretherapy AT-III levels. The initial dose should raise antithrombin III levels (AT-III) to 120% and may be calculated based on the following formula:

Initial dosage (int. units) = [desired AT-III level % - baseline AT-III level %] x body weight (kg) divided by 1.4%/int. units/kg (eg, if a 70 kg adult patient had a baseline AT-III level of 57%, the initial dose would be (120% - 57%) x 70/1.4%/int. units/kg = 3150 int. units).

Maintenance dose: Subsequent dosing should be targeted to keep levels between 80% to 120% which may be achieved by administering 60% of the initial dose every 24 hours. Adjustments may be made by adjusting dose or interval. Maintain level within normal range for 2-8 days depending on type of surgery or procedure.

**Dosage Forms** Injection, powder for reconstitution [preservative free]: 500 int. units, 1000 int. units [contains heparin; packaged with diluent]

# antithymocyte globulin (equine) (an te THY moe site GLOB yu lin, E kwine)

**Sound-Alike/Look-Alike Issues**

Atgam® may be confused with Ativan®

**Synonyms** antithymocyte immunoglobulin; ATG; horse antihuman thymocyte gamma globulin; lymphocyte immune globulin

**U.S./Canadian Brand Names** Atgam® [US/Can]

**Therapeutic Category** Immunosuppressant Agent

**Use** Prevention and treatment of acute renal allograft rejection; treatment of moderate to severe aplastic anemia in patients not considered suitable candidates for bone marrow transplantation

**Usual Dosage** An intradermal skin test is recommended prior to administration of the initial dose of ATG; use 0.1 mL of a 1:1000 dilution of ATG in normal saline. A positive skin reaction consists of a wheal ≥10 mm in diameter. If a positive skin test occurs, the first infusion should be administered in a controlled environment with intensive life support immediately available. A systemic reaction precludes further administration of the drug. The absence of a reaction does **not** preclude the possibility of an immediate sensitivity reaction.

Premedication with diphenhydramine, hydrocortisone, and acetaminophen is recommended prior to first dose.

Children: I.V.:

Aplastic anemia protocol: 10-20 mg/kg/day for 8-14 days; then administer every other day for 7 more doses; addition doses may be given every other day for 21 total doses in 28 days

Renal allograft: 5-25 mg/kg/day

Adults: I.V.:

Aplastic anemia protocol: 10-20 mg/kg/day for 8-14 days, then administer every other day for 7 more doses, for a total of 21 doses in 28 days

Renal allograft:

Rejection prophylaxis: 15 mg/kg/day for 14 days followed by 14 days of alternative day therapy at the same dose; the first dose should be administered within 24 hours before or after transplantation

Rejection treatment: 10-15 mg/kg/day for 14 days, then administer every other day for 10-14 days up to 21 doses in 28 days

**Dosage Forms** Injection, solution: 50 mg/mL (5 mL)

# antithymocyte globulin (rabbit) (an te THY moe site GLOB yu lin (RAB bit)

**Synonyms** antithymocyte immunoglobulin; ATG

**U.S./Canadian Brand Names** Thymoglobulin® [US]

**Therapeutic Category** Immunosuppressant Agent

**Use** Treatment of renal transplant acute rejection in conjunction with concomitant immunosuppression

**Usual Dosage** I.V.: 1.5 mg/kg/day for 7-14 days

**Dosage adjustment for toxicity:**

WBC count 2000-3000 cells/mm$^3$ or platelet count 50,000-75,000 cells/mm$^3$: Reduce dose by 50%

WBC count <2000 cells/mm$^3$ or platelet count <50,000 cells/mm$^3$: Consider discontinuing treatment

**Dosage Forms** Injection, powder for reconstitution: 25 mg [packaged with diluent]

**antithymocyte immunoglobulin** see antithymocyte globulin (equine) on this page

**antitumor necrosis factor apha (human)** see adalimumab on page 18

**Anti-Tuss® Expectorant** *(Discontinued)* see guaifenesin on page 383

**anti-VEGF monoclonal antibody** see bevacizumab on page 105

# antivenin *(Crotalidae)* polyvalent (an tee VEN in (kroe TAL ih die) pol i VAY lent)

**Synonyms** crotaline antivenin, polyvalent; North and South American antisnake-bite serum; pit viper antivenin; snake (pit vipers) antivenin

**U.S./Canadian Brand Names** Antivenin Polyvalent [Equine] [US]; CroFab™ [Ovine] [US]

**Therapeutic Category** Antivenin

**Use** Neutralization of venoms of North and South American crotalids: Rattlesnake, copperhead, cottonmouth, tropical moccasins, fer-de-lance, bushmaster

**Usual Dosage** Children and Adults: Crotalid envenomation:

**Antivenin polyvalent (equine):** I.M., I.V.: Initial sensitivity test: 0.02-0.03 mL of a 1:10 dilution of normal horse serum or antivenin given intracutaneously; also give a control test using normal saline in the opposite extremity. A positive reaction occurs within 5-30 minutes. A negative reaction does not rule out the possibility of an immediate or delayed reaction with treatment.

Minimal envenomation: 20-40 mL (2-4 vials)

Moderate envenomation: 50-90 mL (5-9 vials)

Severe envenomation: 100-150 mL (10-15 vials) or more

**Note:** The entire initial dose of antivenin should be administered as soon as possible to be most effective (within 4 hours after the bite). I.V. is the preferred route of administration. When administered I.V., infuse the initial 5-10 mL dilution over 3-5 minutes while carefully observing the patient for signs and symptoms of sensitivity reactions. If no reaction occurs, continue infusion at a safe I.V. fluid delivery rate. Additional doses of antivenin are based on clinical response to the initial dose. If swelling continues to progress, symptoms increase in severity, hypotension occurs, or decrease in hematocrit appears, an additional 10-50 mL (1-5 vials) should be administered.

**Antivenin polyvalent (ovine):** I.V.: Minimal or moderate envenomation:

Initial dose: 4-6 vials, dependent upon patient response. Treatment should begin within 6 hours of snakebite; monitor for 1 hour following infusion. Repeat with an additional 4-6 vials if control is not achieved with initial dose. Continue to treat with 4- to 6-vial doses until complete arrest of local manifestations, coagulation tests, and systemic signs are normal. Administer I.V. over 60 minutes at a rate of 25-50 mL/hour for the first 10 minutes. If no allergic reaction is observed, increase rate to 250 mL/hour. Monitor closely

Maintenance dose: Once control is achieved, administer 2 vials every 6 hours for up to 18 hours; optimal dosing past 18 hours has not been established; however, treatment may be continued if deemed necessary based on the patients condition

**Dosage Forms** Injection, powder for reconstitution:

Antivenin polyvalent [equine]: Derived from *Crotalus adamanteus*, *C. atrox*, *C. durissus terrificus*, and *Bothrops atrox* snake venoms [equine origin; contains phenol and thimerosal; packaged with diluent]

CroFab™ [ovine]: Derived from *Crotalus adamanteus*, *C. atrox*, *C. scutulatus*, and *Agkistrodon piscivorus* snake venoms [ovine origin; contains thimerosal; manufactured with papain]

# antivenin *(Latrodectus mactans)* (an tee VEN in lak tro DUK tus MAK tans)

**Synonyms** black widow spider species antivenin (*Latrodectus mactans*)

**Therapeutic Category** Antivenin

**Use** Treatment of patients with symptoms of black widow spider bites

**Usual Dosage**

Skin test: Intradermal: Children and Adults: 0.02 mL of a 1:10 dilution in NS (also use a control solution of NS); evaluate in 10 minutes. Positive reaction is urticarial wheal surrounded by zone of erythema

Conjunctival test: Ophthalmic:

Children: Instill 1 drop of a 1:100 dilution into the conjunctival sac

Adults: Instill 1 drop of a 1:10 dilution into the conjunctival sac

**Note:** Itching of the eye and/or reddening of conjunctiva indicates a positive reaction, usually occurring within 10 minutes.

Desensitization: **Note:** In separate vials or syringes, prepare 1:10 and 1:100 dilutions of antivenin in NS.

SubQ: Inject 0.1, 0.2, and 0.5 mL of the 1:100 dilution at 15- to 30- minute intervals. Proceed with the next dose only if no reaction has occurred following the previous. Repeat procedure using the 1:10 dilution and then undiluted antivenin.

If a reaction occurs, apply tourniquet proximal to the injection site and administer epinephrine 1:1000. Wait at least 30 minutes, then administer another antivenin injection at the last dose which did not evoke a reaction.

If no reaction has occurred following 0.5 mL of undiluted antivenin, continue the dose at 15 minute intervals until entire dose has been administered.

Treatment of symptoms due to black widow spider bite: Administer only following the skin test or conjunctival test:
Children <12 years: I.V.: 2.5 mL
Children >12 years and Adults: I.M., I.V.: 2.5 mL
**Dosage Forms** Injection, powder for reconstitution: 6000 antivenin units [equine origin; contains thimerosal; packaged with diluent and normal horse serum for sensitivity testing]

# antivenin *(Micrurus fulvius)* (an tee VEN in mye KRU rus FUL vee us)
**Synonyms** North American coral snake antivenin
**Therapeutic Category** Antivenin
**Use** Neutralization of venoms of Eastern coral snake and Texas coral snake, but does **not** neutralize venom of Arizona or Sonoran coral snake
**Usual Dosage** I.V.: Children and Adults: 3-5 vials by slow injection (dependent on severity of signs/symptoms; some patients may need more than 10 vials)
**Dosage Forms** Injection, powder for reconstitution: Derived from *Micrurus fulvius* venom [equine origin; contains phenol and thimerosal; packaged with diluent]

**Antivenin Polyvalent [Equine] [US]** *see* antivenin *(Crotalidae)* polyvalent *on previous page*

**Antivert**® **[US]** *see* meclizine *on page 506*

**Antizol**® **[US]** *see* fomepizole *on page 358*

**Antrizine**® *(Discontinued)* *see* meclizine *on page 506*

**Anturane**® *(Discontinued)* *see* sulfinpyrazone *on page 775*

**Anucort-HC**® **[US]** *see* hydrocortisone (rectal) *on page 416*

**Anusol**®**-HC   [US]** *see* hydrocortisone (rectal) *on page 416*

**Anusol**® **HC-1 [US-OTC]** *see* hydrocortisone (rectal) *on page 416*

**Anusol**® **Ointment [US-OTC]** *see* pramoxine *on page 670*

**Anuzinc [Can]** *see* zinc sulfate *on page 861*

**Anxanil**® **Oral** *(Discontinued)* *see* hydroxyzine *on page 423*

**Anzemet**® **[US/Can]** *see* dolasetron *on page 265*

**Apacet**® *(Discontinued)* *see* acetaminophen *on page 4*

**APAP** *see* acetaminophen *on page 4*

**APAP and tramadol** *see* acetaminophen and tramadol *on page 9*

**Apaphen**® *(Discontinued)* *see* acetaminophen and phenyltoloxamine *on page 8*

**Apatate**® **[US-OTC]** *see* vitamin B complex combinations *on page 849*

**ApexiCon**™ **[US]** *see* diflorasone *on page 247*

**ApexiCon**™ **E [US]** *see* diflorasone *on page 247*

**Aphedrid**™ **[US-OTC]** *see* triprolidine and pseudoephedrine *on page 827*

**Aphrodyne**® **[US]** *see* yohimbine *on page 857*

**Aphthasol**® **[US]** *see* amlexanox *on page 43*

**Apidra**™ **[US]** *see* insulin preparations *on page 438*

**A.P.L.**® *(Discontinued)* *see* chorionic gonadotropin (human) *on page 181*

**Aplisol**® **[US]** *see* tuberculin tests *on page 830*

**Aplitest**® *(Discontinued)* *see* tuberculin tests *on page 830*

**aplonidine** *see* apraclonidine *on page 67*

**Apo-Acebutolol**® **[Can]** *see* acebutolol *on page 4*

**Apo-Acetaminophen**® **[Can]** *see* acetaminophen *on page 4*

**Apo-Acetazolamide**® **[Can]** *see* acetazolamide *on page 13*

**Apo-Acyclovir**® **[Can]** *see* acyclovir *on page 17*

**Apo-Alendronate**® **[Can]** *see* alendronate *on page 26*

**Apo-Allopurinol**® **[Can]** *see* allopurinol *on page 28*

**Apo-Alpraz**® **[Can]** *see* alprazolam *on page 30*

**Apo-Amiloride**® **[Can]** *see* amiloride *on page 39*

**Apo-Amilzide**® **[Can]** *see* amiloride and hydrochlorothiazide *on page 40*

**Apo-Amiodarone**® **[Can]** *see* amiodarone *on page 41*

**Apo-Amitriptyline**® **[Can]** *see* amitriptyline *on page 42*

**Apo-Amoxi**® **[Can]** *see* amoxicillin *on page 46*

**Apo-Amoxi-Clav**® **[Can]** *see* amoxicillin and clavulanate potassium *on page 47*

**Apo-Ampi**® **[Can]** *see* ampicillin *on page 50*

**Apo-Atenol**® **[Can]** *see* atenolol *on page 76*

**Apo-Azathioprine**® **[Can]** *see* azathioprine *on page 83*

**Apo-Baclofen**® **[Can]** *see* baclofen *on page 88*

**Apo-Beclomethasone**® **[Can]** *see* beclomethasone *on page 91*

**Apo-Benztropine**® **[Can]** *see* benztropine *on page 99*

**Apo-Benzydamine**® **[Can]** *see* benzydamine *(Canada only) on page 100*

**Apo-Bisacodyl**® **[Can]** *see* bisacodyl *on page 107*

**Apo-Bromazepam**® **[Can]** *see* bromazepam *(Canada only) on page 114*

**Apo-Bromocriptine**® **[Can]** *see* bromocriptine *on page 114*

**Apo-Buspirone**® **[Can]** *see* buspirone *on page 123*

**Apo-Butorphanol**® **[Can]** *see* butorphanol *on page 126*

**Apo-Cal**® **[Can]** *see* calcium carbonate *on page 130*

**Apo-Calcitonin**® **[Can]** *see* calcitonin *on page 129*

**Apo-Capto**® **[Can]** *see* captopril *on page 139*

**Apo-Carbamazepine**® **[Can]** *see* carbamazepine *on page 140*

**Apo-Carvedilol**® **[Can]** *see* carvedilol *on page 150*

**Apo-Cefaclor**® **[Can]** *see* cefaclor *on page 152*

**Apo-Cefadroxil**® **[Can]** *see* cefadroxil *on page 152*

**Apo-Cefuroxime**® **[Can]** *see* cefuroxime *on page 158*

**Apo-Cephalex**® **[Can]** *see* cephalexin *on page 161*

**Apo-Cetirizine**® **[Can]** *see* cetirizine *on page 162*

**Apo-Chlorax**® **[Can]** *see* clidinium and chlordiazepoxide *on page 191*

**Apo-Chlordiazepoxide**® **[Can]** *see* chlordiazepoxide *on page 167*

**Apo-Chlorhexadine**® **[Can]** *see* chlorhexidine gluconate *on page 168*

**Apo-Chlorpromazine**® **[Can]** *see* chlorpromazine *on page 178*

**Apo-Chlorpropamide**® **[Can]** *see* chlorpropamide *on page 179*

**Apo-Chlorthalidone**® **[Can]** *see* chlorthalidone *on page 179*

**Apo-Cimetidine**® **[Can]** *see* cimetidine *on page 183*

**Apo-Ciproflox**® **[Can]** *see* ciprofloxacin *on page 184*

**Apo-Citalopram**® **[Can]** *see* citalopram *on page 188*

**Apo-Clindamycin**® **[Can]** *see* clindamycin *on page 192*

**Apo-Clobazam**® **[Can]** *see* clobazam *(Canada only) on page 194*

**Apo-Clomipramine**® **[Can]** *see* clomipramine *on page 196*

**Apo-Clonazepam**® **[Can]** *see* clonazepam *on page 197*

**Apo-Clonidine**® **[Can]** *see* clonidine *on page 197*

**Apo-Clorazepate**® **[Can]** *see* clorazepate *on page 199*

**Apo-Cloxi**® **[Can]** *see* cloxacillin *on page 200*

**Apo-Clozapine**® **[Can]** *see* clozapine *on page 200*

**Apo-Cromolyn**® **[Can]** *see* cromolyn sodium *on page 211*

**Apo-Cyclobenzaprine**® **[Can]** *see* cyclobenzaprine *on page 213*

**Apo-Cyclosporine**® **[Can]** *see* cyclosporine *on page 215*

**Apo-Cyproterone**® **[Can]** *see* cyproterone *(Canada only) on page 218*

**Apo-Desipramine**® **[Can]** *see* desipramine *on page 230*

**Apo-Desmopressin**® **[Can]** *see* desmopressin acetate *on page 230*

**Apo-Dexamethasone**® **[Can]** *see* dexamethasone (systemic) *on page 233*

**Apo-Diazepam**® **[Can]** *see* diazepam *on page 241*

**Apo-Diclo**® **[Can]** *see* diclofenac *on page 243*

**Apo-Diclo Rapide**® **[Can]** *see* diclofenac *on page 243*

**Apo-Diclo SR**® **[Can]** *see* diclofenac *on page 243*

**Apo-Diflunisal**® **[Can]** *see* diflunisal *on page 247*

**Apo-Diltiaz**® **[Can]** *see* diltiazem *on page 251*

**Apo-Diltiaz CD**® **[Can]** *see* diltiazem *on page 251*

**Apo-Diltiaz SR**® **[Can]** *see* diltiazem *on page 251*

**Apo-Dimenhydrinate**® **[Can]** *see* dimenhydrinate *on page 252*

**Apo-Dipyridamole FC**® **[Can]** *see* dipyridamole *on page 260*

**Apo-Divalproex**® **[Can]** *see* valproic acid and derivatives *on page 837*

**Apo-Docusate-Calcium**® **[Can]** *see* docusate *on page 263*

**Apo-Docusate-Sodium**® **[Can]** *see* docusate *on page 263*

**Apo-Domperidone**® **[Can]** *see* domperidone *(Canada only) on page 266*

**Apo-Doxazosin**® **[Can]** *see* doxazosin *on page 268*

**Apo-Doxepin**® **[Can]** *see* doxepin *on page 269*

**Apo-Doxy**® **[Can]** *see* doxycycline *on page 271*

**Apo-Doxy Tabs**® **[Can]** *see* doxycycline *on page 271*

**Apo-Erythro Base**® **[Can]** *see* erythromycin *on page 295*

**Apo-Erythro E-C**® **[Can]** *see* erythromycin *on page 295*

**Apo-Erythro-ES**® **[Can]** *see* erythromycin *on page 295*

**Apo-Erythro-S**® **[Can]** *see* erythromycin *on page 295*

**Apo-Etodolac**® **[Can]** *see* etodolac *on page 321*

**Apo-Famotidine**® **[Can]** *see* famotidine *on page 327*

**Apo-Fenofibrate**® **[Can]** *see* fenofibrate *on page 330*

**Apo-Feno-Micro**® **[Can]** *see* fenofibrate *on page 330*

**Apo-Ferrous Gluconate**® **[Can]** *see* ferrous gluconate *on page 335*

**Apo-Ferrous Sulfate**® **[Can]** *see* ferrous sulfate *on page 335*

**Apo-Flavoxate**® **[Can]** *see* flavoxate *on page 339*

**Apo-Fluconazole**® **[Can]** *see* fluconazole *on page 341*

**Apo-Flunisolide**® **[Can]** *see* flunisolide *on page 344*

**Apo-Fluoxetine**® **[Can]** *see* fluoxetine *on page 349*

**Apo-Fluphenazine**® **[Can]** *see* fluphenazine *on page 351*

**Apo-Fluphenazine Decanoate**® **[Can]** *see* fluphenazine *on page 351*

**Apo-Flurazepam**® **[Can]** *see* flurazepam *on page 352*

**Apo-Flurbiprofen**® **[Can]** *see* flurbiprofen *on page 352*

**Apo-Flutamide**® **[Can]** *see* flutamide *on page 353*

**Apo-Fluvoxamine**® **[Can]** *see* fluvoxamine *on page 356*

**Apo-Folic**® **[Can]** *see* folic acid *on page 356*

**Apo-Furosemide**® **[Can]** *see* furosemide *on page 364*

**Apo-Gabapentin**® **[Can]** *see* gabapentin *on page 365*

**Apo-Gain**® **[Can]** *see* minoxidil *on page 543*

**Apo-Gemfibrozil**® **[Can]** *see* gemfibrozil *on page 370*

**Apo-Gliclazide**® **[Can]** *see* gliclazide *(Canada only) on page 375*

**Apo-Glyburide**® **[Can]** *see* glyburide *on page 378*

**Apo-Haloperidol**® **[Can]** *see* haloperidol *on page 396*

**Apo-Haloperidol LA**® **[Can]** *see* haloperidol *on page 396*

**Apo-Hydralazine**® **[Can]** *see* hydralazine *on page 408*

**Apo-Hydro**® **[Can]** *see* hydrochlorothiazide *on page 409*

**Apo-Hydroxyquine**® **[Can]** *see* hydroxychloroquine *on page 421*

**Apo-Hydroxyurea**® **[Can]** *see* hydroxyurea *on page 422*

**Apo-Hydroxyzine**® **[Can]** *see* hydroxyzine *on page 423*

**Apo-Ibuprofen**® **[Can]** *see* ibuprofen *on page 427*

**Apo-Imipramine**® **[Can]** *see* imipramine *on page 432*

**Apo-Indapamide**® **[Can]** *see* indapamide *on page 434*

**Apo-Indomethacin**® **[Can]** *see* indomethacin *on page 436*

**Apo-Ipravent**® **[Can]** *see* ipratropium *on page 446*

**Apo-ISDN**® **[Can]** *see* isosorbide dinitrate *on page 451*

**Apo-K**® **[Can]** *see* potassium chloride *on page 663*

**Apo-Keto**® **[Can]** *see* ketoprofen *on page 457*

**Apo-Ketoconazole**® **[Can]** *see* ketoconazole *on page 457*

**Apo-Keto-E**® **[Can]** *see* ketoprofen *on page 457*

**Apo-Ketorolac**® **[Can]** *see* ketorolac *on page 458*

**Apo-Ketorolac Injectable**® **[Can]** *see* ketorolac *on page 458*

**Apo-Keto SR**® **[Can]** *see* ketoprofen *on page 457*

**Apo-Ketotifen**® **[Can]** *see* ketotifen *on page 458*

**Apokyn**™ **[US]** *see* apomorphine *on next page*

**Apo-Labetalol**® **[Can]** *see* labetalol *on page 460*

**Apo-Lactulose**® **[Can]** *see* lactulose *on page 464*

**Apo-Lamotrigine**® **[Can]** *see* lamotrigine *on page 465*

**Apo-Leflunomide**® **[Can]** *see* leflunomide *on page 469*

**Apo-Levobunolol**® **[Can]** *see* levobunolol *on page 472*

**Apo-Levocarb**® **[Can]** *see* levodopa and carbidopa *on page 474*

**Apo-Lisinopril**® **[Can]** *see* lisinopril *on page 485*

**Apo-Lithium**® **[Can]** *see* lithium *on page 486*

**Apo-Loperamide**® **[Can]** *see* loperamide *on page 489*

**Apo-Loratadine**® **[Can]** *see* loratadine *on page 491*

**Apo-Lorazepam**® **[Can]** *see* lorazepam *on page 491*

**Apo-Lovastatin**® **[Can]** *see* lovastatin *on page 494*

**Apo-Loxapine**® **[Can]** *see* loxapine *on page 494*

**Apo-Medroxy**® **[Can]** *see* medroxyprogesterone acetate *on page 507*

**Apo-Mefenamic**® **[Can]** *see* mefenamic acid *on page 508*

**Apo-Mefloquine**® **[Can]** *see* mefloquine *on page 508*

**Apo-Megestrol**® **[Can]** *see* megestrol acetate *on page 508*

**Apo-Meloxicam**® **[Can]** *see* meloxicam *on page 509*

**Apo-Metformin**® **[Can]** *see* metformin *on page 519*

**Apo-Methazide**® **[Can]** *see* methyldopa and hydrochlorothiazide *on page 529*

**Apo-Methazolamide**® **[Can]** *see* methazolamide *on page 522*

**Apo-Methoprazine**® **[Can]** *see* methotrimeprazine *(Canada only) on page 526*

Otitis media:
  1-day regimen: 30 mg/kg as a single dose (maximum dose: 1500 mg)
  3-day regimen: 10 mg/kg once daily for 3 days (maximum: 500 mg/day)
  5-day regimen: 10 mg/kg on day 1 (maximum: 500 mg/day) followed by 5 mg/kg/day once daily on days 2-5 (maximum: 250 mg/day)
Children ≥2 years: Pharyngitis, tonsillitis: 12 mg/kg/day once daily for 5 days (maximum: 500 mg/day)
Adolescents ≥16 years and Adults:
  Community-acquired pneumonia: Extended release suspension (Zmax™): 2 g as a single dose
  Respiratory tract, skin and soft tissue infections: 500 mg on day 1 followed by 250 mg/day on days 2-5 (maximum: 500 mg/day)
  Alternative regimen: Bacterial exacerbation of COPD: 500 mg/day for a total of 3 days
  Bacterial sinusitis: 500 mg/day for a total of 3 days
  Extended release suspension (Zmax™): 2 g as a single dose
Urethritis/cervicitis:
  Due to *C. trachomatis*: 1 g as a single dose
  Due to *N. gonorrhoeae*: 2 g as a single dose
  Chancroid due to *H. ducreyi*: 1 g as a single dose
I.V.: Adults:
  Community-acquired pneumonia: 500 mg as a single dose for at least 2 days, follow I.V. therapy by the oral route with a single daily dose of 500 mg to complete a 7-10 day course of therapy
  Pelvic inflammatory disease (PID): 500 mg as a single dose for 1-2 days, follow I.V. therapy by the oral route with a single daily dose of 250 mg to complete a 7-day course of therapy

**Dosage Forms**

Injection, powder for reconstitution, as dihydrate: 500 mg [contains sodium 114 mg (4.96 mEq) per vial]
Microspheres for oral suspension, extended release, as dihydrate (Zmax™): 2 g [single-dose bottle; contains sodium 148 mg per bottle; cherry and banana flavor]
Powder for oral suspension, immediate release, as dihydrate: 100 mg/5 mL (15 mL) [contains sodium 3.7 mg/ 5 mL; cherry creme de vanilla and banana flavor]; 200 mg/5 mL (15 mL, 22.5 mL, 30 mL) [contains sodium 7.4 mg/5 mL; cherry creme de vanilla and banana flavor]; 1 g [single-dose packet; contains sodium 37 mg per packet; cherry creme de vanilla and banana flavor]
Tablet, as dihydrate: 250 mg, 500 mg, 600 mg [contains sodium 0.9 mg per 250 mg tablet, 1.8 mg per 500 mg tablet, 2.1 mg per 600 mg tablet]
Zithromax® TRI-PAK™ [unit-dose pack]: 500 mg (3s)
Zithromax® Z-PAK® [unit-dose pack]: 250 mg (6s)

**azithromycin dihydrate** *see* azithromycin *on previous page*

**Azmacort® [US/Can]** *see* triamcinolone (inhalation, oral) *on page 819*

**AZO-Gesic® [US-OTC]** *see* phenazopyridine *on page 636*

**Azopt® [US/Can]** *see* brinzolamide *on page 113*

**AZO-Standard® [US-OTC]** *see* phenazopyridine *on page 636*

**AZT™ [Can]** *see* zidovudine *on page 859*

**AZT, abacavir, and lamivudine** *see* abacavir, lamivudine, and zidovudine *on page 2*

**azthreonam** *see* aztreonam *on this page*

# aztreonam (AZ tree oh nam)

**Sound-Alike/Look-Alike Issues**
  aztreonam may be confused with azidothymidine
**Synonyms** azthreonam
**U.S./Canadian Brand Names** Azactam® [US/Can]
**Therapeutic Category** Antibiotic, Miscellaneous
**Use** Treatment of patients with urinary tract infections, lower respiratory tract infections, septicemia, skin/skin structure infections, intra-abdominal infections, and gynecological infections caused by susceptible gram-negative bacilli
**Usual Dosage**
Children >1 month: I.M., I.V.:
  Mild-to-moderate infections: 30 mg/kg every 8 hours
  Moderate-to-severe infections: 30 mg/kg every 6-8 hours; maximum: 120 mg/kg/day (8 g/day)
  Cystic fibrosis: 50 mg/kg/dose every 6-8 hours (ie, up to 200 mg/kg/day); maximum: 8 g/day
Adults:
  Urinary tract infection: I.M., I.V.: 500 mg to 1 g every 8-12 hours
(Continued)

## aztreonam *(Continued)*

Moderately-severe systemic infections: 1 g I.V. or I.M. or 2 g I.V. every 8-12 hours
Severe systemic or life-threatening infections (especially caused by *Pseudomonas aeruginosa*): I.V.: 2 g every 6-8 hours; maximum: 8 g/day

**Dosage Forms**
Infusion [premixed]: 1 g (50 mL); 2 g (50 mL)
Injection, powder for reconstitution: 500 mg, 1 g, 2 g

**Azulfidine®  [US]**  *see* sulfasalazine  *on page 774*

**Azulfidine® EN-tabs® [US]**  *see* sulfasalazine  *on page 774*

**B1**  *see* tositumomab and iodine I 131 tositumomab  *on page 812*

**B1 antibody**  *see* tositumomab and iodine I 131 tositumomab  *on page 812*

**B-D™ Glucose [US-OTC]**  *see* glucose (instant)  *on page 377*

**B2036-PEG**  *see* pegvisomant  *on page 625*

**B 9273**  *see* alefacept  *on page 25*

**BA-16038**  *see* aminoglutethimide  *on page 40*

**Babee® Cof Syrup [US-OTC]**  *see* dextromethorphan  *on page 238*

**BabyBIG® [US]**  *see* botulism immune globulin (intravenous-human)  *on page 112*

**BAC**  *see* benzalkonium chloride  *on page 95*

**Bacid® [US-OTC/Can]**  *see* Lactobacillus  *on page 462*

**Baciguent® [US-OTC/Can]**  *see* bacitracin  *on this page*

**BaciiM® [US]**  *see* bacitracin  *on this page*

**Baciject® [Can]**  *see* bacitracin  *on this page*

**bacillus calmette-Guérin (BCG) live**  *see* BCG vaccine  *on page 90*

## bacitracin  (bas i TRAY sin)

**Sound-Alike/Look-Alike Issues**
bacitracin may be confused with Bactrim®, Bactroban®
**U.S./Canadian Brand Names** Baciguent® [US-OTC/Can]; BaciiM® [US]; Baciject® [Can]
**Therapeutic Category** Antibiotic, Miscellaneous; Antibiotic, Ophthalmic; Antibiotic, Topical
**Use** Treatment of susceptible bacterial infections mainly; has activity against gram-positive bacilli; due to toxicity risks, systemic and irrigant uses of bacitracin should be limited to situations where less toxic alternatives would not be effective
**Usual Dosage Do not administer I.V.:**
Infants: I.M.:
≤2.5 kg: 900 units/kg/day in 2-3 divided doses
>2.5 kg: 1000 units/kg/day in 2-3 divided doses
Children: I.M.: 800-1200 units/kg/day divided every 8 hours
Adults: Oral: Antibiotic-associated colitis: 25,000 units 4 times/day for 7-10 days
Children and Adults:
Topical: Apply 1-5 times/day
Ophthalmic, ointment: Instill ¼" to ½" ribbon every 3-4 hours into conjunctival sac for acute infections, or 2-3 times/day for mild to moderate infections for 7-10 days
Irrigation, solution: 50-100 units/mL in normal saline, lactated Ringer's, or sterile water for irrigation; soak sponges in solution for topical compresses 1-5 times/day or as needed during surgical procedures
**Dosage Forms** [DSC] = Discontinued product
Injection, powder for reconstitution (BaciiM®): 50,000 units
Ointment, ophthalmic (AK-Tracin® [DSC]): 500 units/g (3.5 g)
Ointment, topical: 500 units/g (0.9 g, 15 g, 30 g, 120 g, 454 g)
Baciguent®: 500 units/g (15 g, 30 g)

## bacitracin and polymyxin B  (bas i TRAY sin & pol i MIKS in bee)

**Sound-Alike/Look-Alike Issues**
Betadine® may be confused with Betagan®, betaine

**Synonyms** polymyxin B and bacitracin

**U.S./Canadian Brand Names** AK-Poly-Bac® [US]; Betadine® First Aid Antibiotics + Moisturizer [US-OTC]; LID-Pack® [Can]; Optimyxin® [Can]; Polysporin® Ophthalmic [US]; Polysporin® Topical [US-OTC]

**Therapeutic Category** Antibiotic, Ophthalmic; Antibiotic, Topical

**Use** Treatment of superficial infections caused by susceptible organisms

**Usual Dosage** Children and Adults:

Ophthalmic ointment: Instill ½" ribbon in the affected eye(s) every 3-4 hours for acute infections or 2-3 times/day for mild to moderate infections for 7-10 days

Topical ointment/powder: Apply to affected area 1-4 times/day; may cover with sterile bandage if needed

**Dosage Forms**

Ointment, ophthalmic (AK-Poly-Bac®, Polysporin®): Bacitracin 500 units and polymyxin B sulfate 10,000 units per g (3.5 g)

Ointment, topical [OTC]: Bacitracin 500 units and polymyxin B sulfate 10,000 units per g in white petrolatum (15 g, 30 g)

Betadine® First Aid Antibiotics + Moisturizer: Bacitracin 500 units and polymyxin B sulfate 10,000 units per g (14 g)

Polysporin®: Bacitracin 500 units and polymyxin B sulfate 10,000 units per g (15 g, 30 g)

Powder, topical (Polysporin®): Bacitracin 500 units and polymyxin B sulfate 10,000 units per g (10 g)

# bacitracin, neomycin, and polymyxin B

(bas i TRAY sin, nee oh MYE sin, & pol i MIKS in bee)

**Synonyms** neomycin, bacitracin, and polymyxin B; polymyxin B, bacitracin, and neomycin; triple antibiotic

**U.S./Canadian Brand Names** Neosporin® Neo To Go® [US-OTC]; Neosporin® Ophthalmic Ointment [US/Can]; Neosporin® Topical [US-OTC]

**Therapeutic Category** Antibiotic, Ophthalmic; Antibiotic, Topical

**Use** Helps prevent infection in minor cuts, scrapes and burns; short-term treatment of superficial external ocular infections caused by susceptible organisms

**Usual Dosage** Children and Adults:

Ophthalmic: Ointment: Instill ½" into the conjunctival sac every 3-4 hours for 7-10 days for acute infections

Topical: Apply 1-3 times/day to infected area; may cover with sterile bandage as needed

**Dosage Forms**

Ointment, ophthalmic (Neosporin® [DSC]): Bacitracin 400 units, neomycin 3.5 mg, and polymyxin B 10,000 units per g (3.5 g)

Ointment, topical: Bacitracin 400 units, neomycin 3.5 mg, and polymyxin B 5000 units per g (0.9 g, 15 g, 30 g, 454 g)

Neosporin®: Bacitracin 400 units, neomycin 3.5 mg, and polymyxin B 5000 units per g (15 g, 30 g)

Neosporin® Neo To Go®: Bacitracin 400 units, neomycin 3.5 mg, and polymyxin B 5000 units per g (0.9 g)

# bacitracin, neomycin, polymyxin B, and hydrocortisone

(bas i TRAY sin, nee oh MYE sin, pol i MIKS in bee, & hye droe KOR ti sone)

**Synonyms** hydrocortisone, bacitracin, neomycin, and polymyxin B; neomycin, bacitracin, polymyxin B, and hydrocortisone; polymyxin B, bacitracin, neomycin, and hydrocortisone

**U.S./Canadian Brand Names** Cortisporin® Ointment [US]; Cortisporin® Topical Ointment [Can]

**Therapeutic Category** Antibiotic/Corticosteroid, Ophthalmic; Antibiotic/Corticosteroid, Topical

**Use** Prevention and treatment of susceptible inflammatory conditions where bacterial infection (or risk of infection) is present

**Usual Dosage** Children and Adults:

Ophthalmic: Ointment: Instill ½" ribbon to inside of lower lid every 3-4 hours until improvement occurs

Topical: Apply sparingly 2-4 times/day. Therapy should be discontinued when control is achieved; if no improvement is seen, reassessment of diagnosis may be necessary.

**Dosage Forms** [DSC] = Discontinued product

Ointment, ophthalmic (Cortisporin® [DSC]): Bacitracin 400 units, neomycin sulfate 3.5 mg, polymyxin B 10,000 units, and hydrocortisone 10 mg per g (3.5 g)

Ointment, topical (Cortisporin®): Bacitracin 400 units, neomycin 3.5 mg, polymyxin B 5000 units, and hydrocortisone 10 mg per g (15 g)

# baclofen (BAK loe fen)

**Sound-Alike/Look-Alike Issues**
baclofen may be confused with Bactroban®
Lioresal® may be confused with lisinopril, Loniten®, Lotensin®

**U.S./Canadian Brand Names** Apo-Baclofen® [Can]; Gen-Baclofen [Can]; Lioresal® [US/Can]; Liotec [Can]; Nu-Baclo [Can]; PMS-Baclofen [Can]

**Therapeutic Category** Skeletal Muscle Relaxant

**Use** Treatment of reversible spasticity associated with multiple sclerosis or spinal cord lesions
**Orphan drug:** Intrathecal: Treatment of intractable spasticity caused by spinal cord injury, multiple sclerosis, and other spinal disease (spinal ischemia or tumor, transverse myelitis, cervical spondylosis, degenerative myelopathy)

**Usual Dosage**
Oral (avoid abrupt withdrawal of drug):
Children:
2-7 years: Initial: 10-15 mg/24 hours divided every 8 hours; titrate dose every 3 days in increments of 5-15 mg/day to a maximum of 40 mg/day
≥8 years: Maximum: 60 mg/day in 3 divided doses
Adults: 5 mg 3 times/day, may increase 5 mg/dose every 3 days to a maximum of 80 mg/day
Hiccups: Adults: Usual effective dose: 10-20 mg 2-3 times/day
Intrathecal:
Test dose: 50-100 mcg, doses >50 mcg should be given in 25 mcg increments, separated by 24 hours. A screening dose of 25 mcg may be considered in very small patients. Patients not responding to screening dose of 100 mcg should not be considered for chronic infusion/implanted pump.
Maintenance: After positive response to test dose, a maintenance intrathecal infusion can be administered via an implanted intrathecal pump. Initial dose via pump: Infusion at a 24-hour rate dosed at twice the test dose. Avoid abrupt discontinuation.

**Dosage Forms**
Injection, solution, intrathecal [preservative free] (Lioresal®): 50 mcg/mL (1 mL); 500 mcg/mL (20 mL); 2000 mcg/mL (5 mL)
Tablet: 10 mg, 20 mg

**BactoShield® CHG [US-OTC]** *see* chlorhexidine gluconate *on page 168*

**BactoShield® (Discontinued)** *see* chlorhexidine gluconate *on page 168*

**Bactrim™ [US]** *see* sulfamethoxazole and trimethoprim *on page 773*

**Bactrim™ DS [US]** *see* sulfamethoxazole and trimethoprim *on page 773*

**Bactrim™ I.V. Infusion (Discontinued)** *see* sulfamethoxazole and trimethoprim *on page 773*

**Bactroban® [US/Can]** *see* mupirocin *on page 553*

**Bactroban® Nasal [US]** *see* mupirocin *on page 553*

**baking soda** *see* sodium bicarbonate *on page 752*

**BAL** *see* dimercaprol *on page 252*

**Balacet 325™ [US]** *see* propoxyphene and acetaminophen *on page 687*

# balanced salt solution (BAL anced salt soe LOO shun)

**U.S./Canadian Brand Names** AquaLase™ [US]; BSS Plus® [US/Can]; BSS® [US/Can]; Eye-Stream® [Can]

**Therapeutic Category** Ophthalmic Agent, Miscellaneous

**Use**
AquaLase™, BSS®: Intraocular or extraocular irrigating solution
BSS® Plus: Intraocular irrigating solution

**Usual Dosage** Adults: Ophthalmic irrigation: Based on standard for each surgical procedure

**Dosage Forms**
Solution, ophthalmic [irrigation; preservative free]: Sodium chloride 0.64%, potassium chloride 0.075%, calcium chloride 0.048%, magnesium chloride 0.03%, sodium acetate 0.39%, sodium citrate 0.17% (18 mL, 200 mL, 250 mL, 500 mL)
AquaLase™: Sodium chloride 0.64%, potassium chloride 0.075%, calcium chloride 0.048%, magnesium chloride 0.03%, sodium acetate 0.39%, sodium citrate 0.17% (90 mL)
BSS®: Sodium chloride 0.64%, potassium chloride 0.075%, calcium chloride 0.048%, magnesium chloride 0.03%, sodium acetate 0.39%, sodium citrate 0.17% (15 mL, 30 mL, 250 mL, 500 mL)

BSS Plus®: Sodium chloride 0.71%, potassium chloride 0.038%, calcium chloride 0.015%, magnesium chloride 0.02%, sodium phosphate 0.042%, sodium bicarbonate 0.21%, dextrose 0.092%, glutathione 0.018% (250 mL, 500 mL)

**Baldex**® *(Discontinued)*

**BAL in Oil**® [US] *see* dimercaprol *on page 252*

**Balmex**® [US-OTC] *see* zinc oxide *on page 861*

**Balminil Decongestant [Can]** *see* pseudoephedrine *on page 692*

**Balminil DM D [Can]** *see* pseudoephedrine and dextromethorphan *on page 693*

**Balminil DM + Decongestant + Expectorant [Can]** *see* guaifenesin, pseudoephedrine, and dextromethorphan *on page 391*

**Balminil DM E [Can]** *see* guaifenesin and dextromethorphan *on page 385*

**Balminil Expectorant [Can]** *see* guaifenesin *on page 383*

**Balnetar**® [Can] *see* coal tar, lanolin, and mineral oil *on page 202*

## balsalazide (bal SAL a zide)
**Sound-Alike/Look-Alike Issues**
Colazal® may be confused with Clozaril®
**Synonyms** balsalazide disodium
**U.S./Canadian Brand Names** Colazal® [US]
**Therapeutic Category** 5-Aminosalicylic Acid Derivative; Antiinflammatory Agent
**Use** Treatment of mild to moderate active ulcerative colitis
**Usual Dosage** Oral: Adults: 2.25 g (three 750 mg capsules) 3 times/day for 8-12 weeks
**Dosage Forms** Capsule: 750 mg

**balsalazide disodium** *see* balsalazide *on this page*

**balsam peru, trypsin, and castor oil** *see* trypsin, balsam peru, and castor oil *on page 830*

**Bancap HC**® [US] *see* hydrocodone and acetaminophen *on page 411*

**Band-Aid**® **Hurt-Free**™ **Antiseptic Wash [US-OTC]** *see* lidocaine *on page 479*

**Banophen**® [US-OTC] *see* diphenhydramine *on page 254*

**Banophen**® **Anti-Itch [US-OTC]** *see* diphenhydramine *on page 254*

**Banophen**® **Decongestant Capsule** *(Discontinued)* *see* diphenhydramine and pseudoephedrine *on page 256*

**Baraclude**™ [US] *see* entecavir *on page 286*

**Barbidonna**® *(Discontinued)* *see* hyoscyamine, atropine, scopolamine, and phenobarbital *on page 425*

**Barbita**® *(Discontinued)* *see* phenobarbital *on page 638*

**Barc**™ **Liquid** *(Discontinued)*

**Baricon**® [US] *see* radiological/contrast media (ionic) *on page 707*

**Baridium**® [US-OTC] *see* phenazopyridine *on page 636*

**barium sulfate** *see* radiological/contrast media (ionic) *on page 707*

**Barobag**® [US] *see* radiological/contrast media (ionic) *on page 707*

**Baro-CAT**® [US] *see* radiological/contrast media (ionic) *on page 707*

**Baroflave**® [US] *see* radiological/contrast media (ionic) *on page 707*

**Barosperse**® [US] *see* radiological/contrast media (ionic) *on page 707*

**Bar-Test**® [US] *see* radiological/contrast media (ionic) *on page 707*

**Basaljel**® [Can] *see* aluminum hydroxide *on page 34*

**base ointment** *see* zinc oxide *on page 861*

## basiliximab (ba si LIK si mab)
**U.S./Canadian Brand Names** Simulect® [US/Can]
**Therapeutic Category** Immunosuppressant Agent
**Use** Prophylaxis of acute organ rejection in renal transplantation
(Continued)

## basiliximab (Continued)

Usual Dosage Note: Patients previously administered basiliximab should only be re-exposed to a subsequent course of therapy with extreme caution.

I.V.:

Children <35 kg: Renal transplantation: 10 mg within 2 hours prior to transplant surgery, followed by a second 10 mg dose 4 days after transplantation; the second dose should be withheld if complications occur (including severe hypersensitivity reactions or graft loss)

Children ≥35 kg and Adults: Renal transplantation: 20 mg within 2 hours prior to transplant surgery, followed by a second 20 mg dose 4 days after transplantation; the second dose should be withheld if complications occur (including severe hypersensitivity reactions or graft loss)

Dosage Forms Injection, powder for reconstitution: 10 mg, 20 mg

**Bausch & Lomb® Computer Eye Drops [US-OTC]** see glycerin on page 379

**Baycol® (Discontinued)**

**Bayer® Aspirin [US-OTC]** see aspirin on page 73

**Bayer® Aspirin Extra Strength [US-OTC]** see aspirin on page 73

**Bayer® Aspirin Regimen Adult Low Strength [US-OTC]** see aspirin on page 73

**Bayer® Aspirin Regimen Children's [US-OTC]** see aspirin on page 73

**Bayer® Aspirin Regimen Regular Strength [US-OTC]** see aspirin on page 73

**Bayer® Extra Strength Arthritis Pain Regimen [US-OTC]** see aspirin on page 73

**Bayer® Plus Extra Strength [US-OTC]** see aspirin on page 73

**Bayer® Women's Aspirin Plus Calcium [US-OTC]** see aspirin on page 73

**BayGam® [US/Can]** see immune globulin (intramuscular) on page 432

**BayHep B® [US/Can]** see hepatitis B immune globulin on page 401

**BayRab® [US/Can]** see rabies immune globulin (human) on page 707

**BayRho-D® Full-Dose [US/Can]** see $Rh_o(D)$ immune globulin on page 717

**BayRho-D® Mini-Dose [US]** see $Rh_o(D)$ immune globulin on page 717

**BayTet™ [US/Can]** see tetanus immune globulin (human) on page 790

**Baza® Antifungal [US-OTC]** see miconazole on page 537

**Baza® Clear [US-OTC]** see vitamin A and vitamin D on page 849

**B-Caro-T™ [US]** see beta-carotene on page 101

**BCG, live** see BCG vaccine on this page

## BCG vaccine (bee see jee vak SEEN)

Synonyms bacillus calmette-Guérin (BCG) live; BCG, live

U.S./Canadian Brand Names ImmuCyst® [Can]; Oncotice™ [Can]; Pacis™ [Can]; TheraCys® [US]; TICE® BCG [US]

Therapeutic Category Biological Response Modulator

Use Immunization against tuberculosis and immunotherapy for cancer; treatment of bladder cancer

BCG vaccine is not routinely recommended for use in the U.S. for prevention of tuberculosis

BCG vaccine is strongly recommended for infants and children with negative tuberculin skin tests who:
- are at high risk of intimate and prolonged exposure to persistently untreated or ineffectively treated patients with infectious pulmonary tuberculosis
- cannot be removed from the source of exposure
- cannot be placed on long-term preventive therapy
- are continuously exposed with tuberculosis who have bacilli resistant to isoniazid and rifampin

BCG is also recommended for tuberculin-negative infants and children in groups in which the rate of new infections exceeds 1% per year and for whom the usual surveillance and treatment programs have been attempted but are not operationally feasible

Usual Dosage Children >1 month and Adults:

Immunization against tuberculosis (TICE® BCG): 0.2-0.3 mL percutaneous; initial lesion usually appears after 10-14 days consisting of small red papule at injection site and reaches maximum diameter of 3 mm in 4-6 weeks; conduct postvaccinal tuberculin test (ie, 5 TU of PPD) in 2-3 months; if test is negative, repeat vaccination

Immunotherapy for bladder cancer:
Intravesical treatment: Instill into bladder for 2 hours
TheraCys®: One dose instilled into bladder once weekly for 6 weeks followed by one treatment at 3, 6, 12, 18, and 24 months after initial treatment
TICE® BCG: One dose instilled into the bladder once weekly for 6 weeks followed by once monthly for 6-12 months
**Dosage Forms** Injection, powder for reconstitution, intravesical:
TheraCys®: 81 mg [with diluent]
TICE® BCG: 50 mg

**BCNU** *see* carmustine *on page 149*

**B complex combinations** *see* vitamin B complex combinations *on page 849*

**Bebulin® VH [US]** *see* factor IX complex (human) *on page 326*

## becaplermin (be KAP ler min)
**Sound-Alike/Look-Alike Issues**
Regranex® may be confused with Granulex®, Repronex®
**Synonyms** recombinant human platelet-derived growth factor B; rPDGF-BB
**U.S./Canadian Brand Names** Regranex® [US/Can]
**Therapeutic Category** Topical Skin Product
**Use** Debridement adjunct for the treatment of diabetic ulcers that occur on the lower limbs and feet
**Usual Dosage** Topical: Adults:
Diabetic ulcers: Apply appropriate amount of gel once daily with a cotton swab or similar tool, as a coating over the ulcer
The amount of becaplermin to be applied will vary depending on the size of the ulcer area. To calculate the length of gel applied to the ulcer, measure the greatest length of the ulcer by the greatest width of the ulcer in inches. Tube size will determine the formula used in the calculation. For a 15 or 7.5 g tube, multiply length x width x 0.6. For a 2 g tube, multiply length x width x 1.3.
**Note:** If the ulcer does not decrease in size by ~30% after 10 weeks of treatment or complete healing has not occurred in 20 weeks, continued treatment with becaplermin gel should be reassessed.
**Dosage Forms** Gel, topical: 0.01% (15 g)

## beclomethasone (be kloe METH a sone)
**Sound-Alike/Look-Alike Issues**
Vanceril® may be confused with Vancenase®
**Synonyms** beclomethasone dipropionate
**U.S./Canadian Brand Names** Apo-Beclomethasone® [Can]; Beconase® AQ [US]; Gen-Beclo [Can]; Nu-Beclomethasone [Can]; Propaderm® [Can]; QVAR® [US/Can]; Rivanase AQ [Can]; Vanceril® AEM [Can]
**Therapeutic Category** Adrenal Corticosteroid
**Use**
Oral inhalation: Maintenance and prophylactic treatment of asthma; includes those who require cortico-steroids and those who may benefit from a dose reduction/elimination of systemically administered corticosteroids. Not for relief of acute bronchospasm
Nasal aerosol: Symptomatic treatment of seasonal or perennial rhinitis and to prevent recurrence of nasal polyps following surgery
**Usual Dosage** Nasal inhalation and oral inhalation dosage forms are not to be used interchangeably
Aqueous inhalation, nasal (Beconase® AQ): Children ≥6 years and Adults: 1-2 inhalations each nostril twice daily; total dose 168-336 mcg/day
Intranasal (Beconase®):
Children 6-12 years: 1 inhalation in each nostril 3 times/day; total dose 252 mcg/day
Children ≥12 years and Adults: 1 inhalation in each nostril 2-4 times/day or 2 inhalations each nostril twice daily (total dose 168-336 mcg/day); usual maximum maintenance: 1 inhalation in each nostril 3 times/day (252 mcg/day)
Oral inhalation (doses should be titrated to the lowest effective dose once asthma is controlled) (QVAR®).
Children 5-11 years: Initial: 40 mcg twice daily; maximum dose: 80 mcg twice daily
Children ≥12 years and Adults:
Patients previously on bronchodilators only: Initial dose 40-80 mcg twice daily; maximum dose: 320 mcg twice day
(Continued)

# beclomethasone *(Continued)*

Patients previously on inhaled corticosteroids: Initial dose 40-160 mcg twice daily; maximum dose: 320 mcg twice daily

Oral cavity spray (dental use) (QVAR®): Children >12 years and Adults: Initial: 40-160 mcg twice daily; maximum dose: 320 mcg twice daily. Apply spray to back of oral cavity.

**Dosage Forms** [DSC] = Discontinued product

Aerosol for oral inhalation, as dipropionate (QVAR®): 40 mcg/inhalation [100 metered doses] (7.3 g); 80 mcg/inhalation [100 metered doses] (7.3 g)

Aerosol, intranasal, as dipropionate (Beconase® [DSC]): 42 mcg/inhalation: [80 metered doses] (6.7 g); [200 metered doses] (16.8 g)

Suspension, intranasal, aqueous, as dipropionate [spray] (Beconase® AQ): 42 mcg/inhalation [180 metered doses] (25 g)

**beclomethasone dipropionate** *see* beclomethasone *on previous page*

**Beclovent®** *(Discontinued)* *see* beclomethasone *on previous page*

**Beconase® AQ [US]** *see* beclomethasone *on previous page*

**Beconase®** *(Discontinued)* *see* beclomethasone *on previous page*

**Becotin® Pulvules®** *(Discontinued)*

**Beepen-VK®** *(Discontinued)* *see* penicillin V potassium *on page 627*

**behenyl alcohol** *see* docosanol *on page 263*

**Belix® Oral** *(Discontinued)* *see* diphenhydramine *on page 254*

**belladonna alkaloids with phenobarbital** *see* hyoscyamine, atropine, scopolamine, and phenobarbital *on page 425*

# belladonna and opium *(bel a DON a & OH pee um)*

**Synonyms** opium and belladonna

**U.S./Canadian Brand Names** B&O Supprettes® [US]

**Therapeutic Category** Analgesic, Narcotic

**Controlled Substance** C-II

**Use** Relief of moderate to severe pain associated with rectal or bladder tenesmus that may occur in postoperative states and neoplastic situations; pain associated with ureteral spasms not responsive to non-narcotic analgesics and to space intervals between injections of opiates

**Usual Dosage** Rectal: Adults: 1 suppository 1-2 times/day, up to 4 doses/day

**Dosage Forms** Suppository:

#15 A: Belladonna extract 16.2 mg and opium 30 mg

#16 A: Belladonna extract 16.2 mg and opium 60 mg

# belladonna, phenobarbital, and ergotamine tartrate

*(bel a DON a, fee noe BAR bi tal, & er GOT a meen)*

**Synonyms** belladonna, phenobarbital, and ergotamine tartrate; ergotamine tartrate, belladonna, and phenobarbital; phenobarbital, belladonna, and ergotamine tartrate

**U.S./Canadian Brand Names** Bel-Tabs [US]; Bellamine S [US]; Bellergal® Spacetabs® [Can]

**Therapeutic Category** Ergot Alkaloid and Derivative

**Use** Management and treatment of menopausal disorders, GI disorders, and recurrent throbbing headache

**Usual Dosage** Oral: 1 tablet each morning and evening

**Dosage Forms** Tablet: Belladonna alkaloids 0.2 mg, phenobarbital 40 mg, and ergotamine tartrate 0.6 mg

**Bellamine S [US]** *see* belladonna, phenobarbital, and ergotamine tartrate *on this page*

**Bellatal®** *(Discontinued)* *see* hyoscyamine, atropine, scopolamine, and phenobarbital *on page 425*

**Bellergal-S®** *(Discontinued)*

**Bellergal® Spacetabs® [Can]** *see* belladonna, phenobarbital, and ergotamine tartrate *on this page*

**Bel-Tabs [US]** *see* belladonna, phenobarbital, and ergotamine tartrate *on this page*

**Benadryl® [Can]** *see* diphenhydramine *on page 254*

**Benadryl**® **Allergy [US-OTC]** *see* diphenhydramine *on page 254*

**Benadryl**® **Allergy and Sinus Fastmelt**™ **[US-OTC]** *see* diphenhydramine and pseudoephedrine *on page 256*

**Benadryl**® **Allergy/Sinus [US-OTC]** *see* diphenhydramine and pseudoephedrine *on page 256*

**Benadryl**® **Children's Allergy [US-OTC]** *see* diphenhydramine *on page 254*

**Benadryl**® **Children's Allergy and Cold Fastmelt**™ **[US-OTC]** *see* diphenhydramine and pseudoephedrine *on page 256*

**Benadryl**® **Children's Allergy and Sinus [US-OTC]** *see* diphenhydramine and pseudoephedrine *on page 256*

**Benadryl**® **Children's Allergy Fastmelt**® **[US-OTC]** *see* diphenhydramine *on page 254*

**Benadryl**® **Dye-Free Allergy [US-OTC]** *see* diphenhydramine *on page 254*

**Benadryl**® **Injection [US]** *see* diphenhydramine *on page 254*

**Benadryl**® **Itch Stopping [US-OTC]** *see* diphenhydramine *on page 254*

**Benadryl**® **Itch Stopping Extra Strength [US-OTC]** *see* diphenhydramine *on page 254*

**Ben-Allergin-50**® **Injection *(Discontinued)*** *see* diphenhydramine *on page 254*

**Ben-Aqua**® ***(Discontinued)*** *see* benzoyl peroxide *on page 98*

## benazepril (ben AY ze pril)

**Sound-Alike/Look-Alike Issues**
benazepril may be confused with Benadryl®
Lotensin® may be confused with Lioresal®, Loniten®, lovastatin
**Synonyms** benazepril hydrochloride
**U.S./Canadian Brand Names** Lotensin® [US/Can]
**Therapeutic Category** Angiotensin-Converting Enzyme (ACE) Inhibitor
**Use** Treatment of hypertension, either alone or in combination with other antihypertensive agents
**Usual Dosage** Oral: Hypertension:
Children ≥6 years: Initial: 0.2 mg/kg/day as monotherapy; dosing range: 0.1-0.6 mg/kg/day (maximum dose: 40 mg/day)
Adults: Initial: 10 mg/day in patients not receiving a diuretic; 20-40 mg/day as a single dose or 2 divided doses; the need for twice-daily dosing should be assessed by monitoring peak (2-6 hours after dosing) and trough responses.
**Note:** Patients taking diuretics should have them discontinued 2-3 days prior to starting benazepril. If they cannot be discontinued, then initial dose should be 5 mg; restart after blood pressure is stabilized if needed.
**Dosage Forms** Tablet, as hydrochloride: 5 mg, 10 mg, 20 mg, 40 mg

**benazepril and amlodipine** *see* amlodipine and benazepril *on page 44*

## benazepril and hydrochlorothiazide (ben AY ze pril & hye droe klor oh THYE a zide)

**Synonyms** hydrochlorothiazide and benazepril
**U.S./Canadian Brand Names** Lotensin® HCT [US]
**Therapeutic Category** Antihypertensive Agent, Combination
**Use** Treatment of hypertension
**Usual Dosage** Dose is individualized
**Dosage Forms** Tablet:
5/6.25: Benazepril 5 mg and hydrochlorothiazide 6.25 mg
10/12.5: Benazepril 10 mg and hydrochlorothiazide 12.5 mg
20/12.5: Benazepril 20 mg and hydrochlorothiazide 12.5 mg
20/25: Benazepril 20 mg and hydrochlorothiazide 25 mg

**benazepril hydrochloride** *see* benazepril *on this page*

## bendroflumethiazide (ben droe floo meth EYE a zide)

**Therapeutic Category** Diuretic, Thiazide
**Use** Management of mild to moderate hypertension, edema associated with congestive heart failure, pregnancy, or nephrotic syndrome; reportedly does not alter serum electrolyte concentrations appreciably at recommended doses
(Continued)

# bendroflumethiazide *(Continued)*

**Usual Dosage** Oral:
Children: Initial: 0.1-0.4 mg/kg/day in 1-2 doses; maintenance dose: 0.05-0.1 mg/kg/day in 1-2 doses; maximum dose: 20 mg/day
Adults: 2.5-20 mg/day or twice daily in divided doses
**Dosage Forms** Tablet: 5 mg

**BeneFix®  [US/Can]** *see* factor IX *on page 325*

**Benemid®  *(Discontinued)*** *see* probenecid *on page 678*

**Benicar®  [US]** *see* olmesartan *on page 596*

**Benicar HCT®  [US]** *see* olmesartan and hydrochlorothiazide *on page 596*

**Benoquin®  [US]** *see* monobenzone *on page 548*

**Benoxyl®  [Can]** *see* benzoyl peroxide *on page 98*

# benserazide and levodopa *(Canada only)* (ben SER a zide & lee voe DOE pa)

**Synonyms** levodopa and benserazide
**U.S./Canadian Brand Names** Prolopa® [Can]
**Therapeutic Category** Anti-Parkinson Agent
**Use** Treatment of Parkinson disease (except drug-induced Parkinsonism)
**Usual Dosage** Oral: Adults: **Note:** Dosage expressed as levodopa/benserazide:
Initial: 100/25 mg 1-2 times/day, increase every 3-4 days until therapeutic effect; optimal dosage: 400/100 mg to 800/200 mg divided into 4-6 doses
**Note:** 200/50 mg used only when maintenance therapy is reached and not to exceed levodopa 1000-1200 mg/benserazide 250-300 mg per day
Patients previously on levodopa: Allow 12 hours or more to lapse between last dose of levodopa; start at 15% of previous levodopa dosage
**Note:** Dosages should be introduced gradually, individualized, and continued for 3-6 weeks before assessing benefit. Decrease dosage in patients with dystonia.
**Dosage Forms** Capsule:
50-12.5: Levodopa 50 mg and benserazide 12.5 mg
100-25: Levodopa 100 mg and benserazide 25 mg
200-50: Levodopa 200 mg and benserazide 50 mg

# bentoquatam (BEN toe kwa tam)

**Synonyms** quaternium-18 bentonite
**U.S./Canadian Brand Names** IvyBlock® [US-OTC]
**Therapeutic Category** Protectant, Topical
**Use** Skin protectant for the prevention of allergic contact dermatitis to poison oak, ivy, and sumac
**Usual Dosage** Children >6 years and Adults: Topical: Apply to skin 15 minutes prior to potential exposure to poison ivy, poison oak, or poison sumac, and reapply every 4 hours
**Dosage Forms** Lotion: 5% (120 mL) [contains benzyl alcohol]

**Bentyl®  [US]** *see* dicyclomine *on page 245*

**Bentyl®  Injection *(Discontinued)*** *see* dicyclomine *on page 245*

**Bentylol®  [Can]** *see* dicyclomine *on page 245*

**Benuryl™  [Can]** *see* probenecid *on page 678*

**Benylin®  3.3 mg-D-E [Can]** *see* guaifenesin, pseudoephedrine, and codeine *on page 391*

**Benylin®  D for Infants [Can]** *see* pseudoephedrine *on page 692*

**Benylin®  Adult [US-OTC]** *see* dextromethorphan *on page 238*

**Benylin®  Cough Syrup *(Discontinued)*** *see* diphenhydramine *on page 254*

**Benylin®  DM-D [Can]** *see* pseudoephedrine and dextromethorphan *on page 693*

**Benylin®  DM-D-E [Can]** *see* guaifenesin, pseudoephedrine, and dextromethorphan *on page 391*

**Benylin®  DM *(Discontinued)*** *see* dextromethorphan *on page 238*

**Benylin®  DM-E [Can]** *see* guaifenesin and dextromethorphan *on page 385*

**Benylin®  E Extra Strength [Can]** *see* guaifenesin *on page 383*

**Benylin® Expectorant [US-OTC]** *see* guaifenesin and dextromethorphan *on page 385*

**Benylin® Pediatric [US-OTC]** *see* dextromethorphan *on page 238*

**Benza® [US-OTC]** *see* benzalkonium chloride *on this page*

**Benzac® [US]** *see* benzoyl peroxide *on page 98*

**Benzac® AC [Can]** *see* benzoyl peroxide *on page 98*

**Benzac® AC Gel *(Discontinued)*** *see* benzoyl peroxide *on page 98*

**Benzac® AC Wash [US]** *see* benzoyl peroxide *on page 98*

**BenzaClin® [US/Can]** *see* clindamycin and benzoyl peroxide *on page 193*

**Benzac® W [US]** *see* benzoyl peroxide *on page 98*

**Benzac® W Gel [Can]** *see* benzoyl peroxide *on page 98*

**Benzac® W Gel *(Discontinued)*** *see* benzoyl peroxide *on page 98*

**Benzac® W Wash [Can]** *see* benzoyl peroxide *on page 98*

**Benzagel® [US]** *see* benzoyl peroxide *on page 98*

**Benzagel® Wash [US]** *see* benzoyl peroxide *on page 98*

## benzalkonium chloride (benz al KOE nee um KLOR ide)

**Sound-Alike/Look-Alike Issues**
Benza® may be confused with Benzac®
**Synonyms** BAC
**U.S./Canadian Brand Names** 3M™ Cavilon™ Skin Cleanser [US-OTC]; Benza® [US-OTC]; Hand-Clens® [US-OTC]; Zephiran® [US-OTC]
**Therapeutic Category** Antibacterial, Topical
**Use** Surface antiseptic and germicidal preservative
**Usual Dosage** Thoroughly rinse anionic detergents and soaps from the skin or other areas prior to use of solutions because they reduce the antibacterial activity of BAC. To protect metal instruments stored in BAC solution, add crushed Anti-Rust Tablets, 4 tablets/quart, to antiseptic solution, change solution at least once weekly. Not to be used for storage of aluminum or zinc instruments, instruments with lenses fastened by cement, lacquered catheters, or some synthetic rubber goods.
**Dosage Forms** [DSC] = Discontinued product
Solution, topical:
Benza®: 1:750 (60 mL, 240 mL, 480 mL, 3840 mL)
HandClens®: 0.13% (120 mL, 480 mL, 800 mL)
Ony-Clear [DSC]: 1% (30 mL)
Zephiran®: 1:750 (240 mL, 3840 mL) [aqueous]
Solution, topical spray (3M™ Cavilon™ Skin Cleanser): 0.11% (240 mL)

**Benzamycin® [US]** *see* erythromycin and benzoyl peroxide *on page 296*

**Benzamycin® Pak [US]** *see* erythromycin and benzoyl peroxide *on page 296*

**Benzashave® [US]** *see* benzoyl peroxide *on page 98*

**benzathine benzylpenicillin** *see* penicillin G benzathine *on page 628*

**benzathine penicillin G** *see* penicillin G benzathine *on page 628*

**Benzedrex® [US-OTC]** *see* propylhexedrine *on page 690*

**benzene hexachloride** *see* lindane *on page 483*

**benzhexol hydrochloride** *see* trihexyphenidyl *on page 824*

**benzmethyzin** *see* procarbazine *on page 680*

## benzocaine (BEN zoe kane)

**Sound-Alike/Look-Alike Issues**
Orabase®-B may be confused with Orinase®
**Synonyms** ethyl aminobenzoate
**U.S./Canadian Brand Names** Americaine® Hemorrhoidal [US-OTC]; Americaine® [US-OTC]; Anbesol® Baby [US-OTC/Can]; Anbesol® Cold Sore Therapy [US-OTC]; Anbesol® Jr. [US-OTC]; Anbesol® Maximum Strength [US-OTC]; Anbesol® [US-OTC]; Benzodent® [US-OTC]; Cepacol® Sore Throat [US-
(Continued)

# benzocaine *(Continued)*

OTC]; Chiggerex® [US-OTC]; Chiggertox® [US-OTC]; Cylex® [US-OTC]; Dent's Extra Strength Tooth-ache [US-OTC]; Dent's Maxi-Strength Toothache [US-OTC]; Dentapaine [US-OTC]; Dermoplast® Anti-bacterial [US-OTC]; Dermoplast® Pain Relieving [US-OTC]; Detane® [US-OTC]; Foille® [US-OTC]; HDA® Toothache [US-OTC]; Hurricaine® [US]; Ivy-Rid® [US-OTC]; Kanka® Soft Brush™ [US-OTC]; Lanacane® Maximum Strength [US-OTC]; Lanacane® [US-OTC]; Mycinettes® [US-OTC]; Orabase®-B with Benzocaine [US-OTC]; Orajel® Baby Teething Nighttime [US-OTC]; Orajel® Baby Teething [US-OTC]; Orajel® Denture Plus [US-OTC]; Orajel® Maximum Strength [US-OTC]; Orajel® Medicated Tooth-ache [US-OTC]; Orajel® Mouth Sore [US-OTC]; Orajel® Multi-Action Cold Sore [US-OTC]; Orajel® PM [US-OTC]; Orajel® Ultra Mouth Sore [US-OTC]; Orajel® [US-OTC]; Oticaine [US]; Otocaine™ [US]; Outgro® [US-OTC]; Red Cross™ Canker Sore [US-OTC]; Rid-A-Pain Dental Drops [US-OTC]; Skeeter Stik [US-OTC]; Solarcaine® [US-OTC]; Sting-Kill [US-OTC]; Thorets [US-OTC]; Trocaine® [US-OTC]; Zilactin® Baby [US-OTC/Can]; Zilactin®-B [US-OTC/Can]

**Therapeutic Category** Local Anesthetic

**Use** Temporary relief of pain associated with local anesthetic for pruritic dermatosis, pruritus, minor burns, acute congestive and serous otitis media, swimmer's ear, otitis externa, toothache, minor sore throat pain, canker sores, hemorrhoids, rectal fissures, anesthetic lubricant for passage of catheters and endoscopic tubes; nonprescription diet aid

**Usual Dosage** Children and Adults:

Mucous membranes: Dosage varies depending on area to be anesthetized and vascularity of tissues

Oral mouth/throat preparations: Refer to specific package labeling or as directed by physician. **Note:** Do not administer for >2 days or use in children <2 years of age, unless directed by physician.

Topical: Apply to affected area as needed

**Dosage Forms**

Aerosol, oral spray (Hurricaine®): 20% (60 mL) [dye free]; cherry flavor]

Aerosol, topical spray:

Americaine®: 20% (60 mL)

Dermoplast® Antibacterial: 20% (83 mL) [contains aloe vera, benzethonium chloride, menthol]

Dermoplast® Pain Relieving: 20% (83 mL) [contains menthol]

Foille®: 5% (97.5 mL) [contains chloroxylenol 0.63% and corn oil]

Ivy-Rid®: 5% (83 mL)

Lanacane® Maximum Strength: 20% (120 mL) [contains alcohol]

Solarcaine®: 20% (120 mL) [contains triclosan 0.13%, alcohol 35%]

Cream, oral:

Benzodent®: 20% (7.5 g, 30 g)

Orajel PM®: 20% (5.3 g)

Cream, topical:

Lanacane®: 6% (30 g, 60 g)

Lanacane® Maximum Strength: 20% (30 g)

Gel, oral:

Anbesol®: 10% (7.5 g) [cool mint flavor]

Anbesol® Baby: 7.5% (7.5 g) [contains benzoic acid; grape flavor]

Anbesol® Jr.: 10% (7 g) [contains benzyl alcohol; bubble gum flavor]

Anbesol® Maximum Strength: 20% (7.5 g, 10 g) [contains benzyl alcohol]

Dentapaine®: 20% (11 g) [contains clove oil]

HDA® Toothache: 6.5% (15 mL) [contains benzyl alcohol]

Hurricaine®: 20% (5 g) [dye free; wild cherry flavor]; (30 g) dye free; mint, pina colada, watermelon, and wild cherry flavors]

Kanka® Soft Brush™: 20% (2 mL) [packaged in applicator with brush tip]

Orabase® with Benzocaine®: 20% (7 g) [contains ethyl alcohol 48%; mild mint flavor]

Orajel®: 10% (7.5 g)

Orajel® Baby Teething: 7.5% (9.4 g) [cherry flavor]

Orajel® Baby Teething Nighttime: 10% (5.3 g)

Orajel® Denture Plus: 15% (9 g) [contains menthol 2%, ethyl alcohol 66.7%]

Orajel® Maximum Strength: 20% (5.3 g, 9.4 g)

Orajel® Mouth Sore: 20% (5.3 g, 9.4 g) [contains benzalkonium chloride 0.02%, zinc chloride 0.1%]

Orajel® Multi-Action Cold Sore: 20% (9.4 g) [contains allantoin 0.5%, camphor 3%, dimethicone 2%]

Orajel® Ultra Mouth Sore: 15% (9.4 g) [contains ethyl alcohol 66.7%, menthol 2%]

Zilactin®-B: 10% (7.5 g)

Zilactin® Baby: 10% (10 g) [alcohol free, dye free; grape flavor]

Gel, topical:

Americaine® Anesthetic Lubricant: 20% (2.5 g, 28 g) [contains 0.1% benzethonium chloride [DSC]

Detane®: 7.5% (15 g)
Gum [oral wax] (Dent's Extra Strength Toothache): 20% (1 g)
Liquid, oral:
 Anbesol®: 10% (9 mL) [cool mint flavor]
 Anbesol® Maximum Strength: 20% (9 mL) [contains benzyl alcohol]
 Hurricaine®: 20% (30 mL) [pina colada and wild cherry flavors]
 Orajel®: 10% (13 mL) [contains ethyl alcohol 44%, tartrazine]
 Orajel® Baby Teething: 7.5% (13 mL) [very berry flavor]
 Orajel® Maximum Strength: 20% (13 mL) [contains ethyl alcohol 44%, tartrazine]
Liquid, oral drop:
 Dent's Maxi-Strength Toothache: 20% (3.7 mL) [contains alcohol 74%]
 Rid-A-Pain Dental Drops: 6.3% (30 mL) [contains alcohol]
Liquid, topical:
 Chiggertox®: 2% (30 mL)
 Outgro®: 20% (9 mL)
 Skeeter Stik: 5% (14 mL) [contains menthol]
Lozenge: 6 mg (18s) [contains menthol]; 15 mg (10s)
 Cepacol® Sore Throat: 10 mg (18s) [contains cetylpyridinium, menthol; cherry, citrus, honey lemon, and menthol flavors]
 Cepacol® Sore Throat: 10 mg (16s) [sugar free; contains cetylpyridinium, menthol; cherry and menthol flavors]
 Cylex®: 15 mg [sugar free; contains cetylpyridinium chloride 5 mg; cherry flavor]
 Mycinettes®: 15 mg (12s) [sugar free; contains sodium 9 mg; cherry or regular flavor]
 Thorets: 18 mg (500s) [sugar free]
 Trocaine®: 10 mg (40s, 400s)
Ointment, oral:
 Anbesol® Cold Sore Therapy: 20% (7.1 g) [contains benzyl alcohol, aloe, camphor, menthol, vitamin E]
 Red Cross™ Canker Sore: 20% (7.5 g) [contains coconut oil]
Ointment, rectal (Americaine® Hemorrhoidal): 20% (30 g)
Ointment, topical:
 Chiggerex®: 2% (52 g) [contains aloe vera]
 Foille®: 5% (3.5 g, 14 g, 28 g) [contains chloroxylenol 0.1%, benzyl alcohol; corn oil base]
Pads, topical (Sting-Kill): 20% (8s) [contains menthol]
Paste, oral (Orabase® with Benzocaine): 20% (6 g)
Solution, otic drops (Oticaine, Otocaine™): 20% (15 mL)
Swabs, oral:
 Hurricaine®: 20% (6s, 100s) [dye free]
 Orajel® Baby Teething: 7.5% (12s) [berry flavor]
 Orajel® Medicated Mouth Sore, Orajel® Medicated Toothache: 20% (8s) [contains tartrazine]
 Zilactin®: 20% (8s)
Swabs, topical (Sting-Kill): 20% (5s) [contains menthol]

**benzocaine and antipyrine** *see* antipyrine and benzocaine *on page 58*

**benzocaine and cetylpyridinium chloride** *see* cetylpyridinium and benzocaine *on page 164*

# benzocaine, butyl aminobenzoate, tetracaine, and benzalkonium chloride

(BEN zoe kane, BYOO til a meen oh BENZ oh ate, TET ra kane, & benz al KOE nee um KLOR ide)
**Synonyms** tetracaine hydrochloride, benzocaine butyl aminobenzoate, and benzalkonium chloride
**U.S./Canadian Brand Names** Cetacaine® [US]
**Therapeutic Category** Local Anesthetic
**Use** Topical anesthetic to control pain or gagging
**Usual Dosage** Apply to affected area for approximately 1 second or less
**Dosage Forms**
 Aerosol, topical: Benzocaine 14%, butyl aminobenzoate 2%, tetracaine hydrochloride 2%, and benzalkonium chloride 0.5% (56 g) [also packaged in a kit with various sized cannulas]
 Gel, topical: Benzocaine 14%, butyl aminobenzoate 2%, tetracaine hydrochloride 2%, and benzalkonium chloride 0.5% (29 g)
 Liquid, topical: Benzocaine 14%, butyl aminobenzoate 2%, tetracaine hydrochloride 2%, and benzalkonium chloride 0.5% (56 mL)

**Benzocol®** *(Discontinued) see* benzocaine *on page 95*

**Benzodent®** [US-OTC] *see* benzocaine *on page 95*

# benzoin (BEN zoin)

**Synonyms** gum benjamin

**Therapeutic Category** Pharmaceutical Aid; Protectant, Topical

**Use** Protective application for irritations of the skin; sometimes used in boiling water as steam inhalants for their expectorant and their soothing action

**Usual Dosage** Apply 1-2 times/day

**Dosage Forms** [DSC] = Discontinued product

Tincture, USP: (15 mL, 60 mL, 120 mL, 480 mL, 4000 mL)

TinBen®: 120 mL [DSC]

Tincture, USP [spray]: 120 mL

# benzonatate (ben ZOE na tate)

**U.S./Canadian Brand Names** Tessalon® [US/Can]

**Therapeutic Category** Antitussive

**Use** Symptomatic relief of nonproductive cough

**Usual Dosage** Children >10 years and Adults: Oral: 100 mg 3 times/day or every 4 hours up to 600 mg/day

**Dosage Forms**

Capsule: 100 mg

Tessalon®: 100 mg, 200 mg

# benzoyl peroxide (BEN zoe il peer OKS ide)

**Sound-Alike/Look-Alike Issues**

Benoxyl® may be confused with Brevoxyl®, Peroxyl®

Benzac® may be confused with Benza®

Brevoxyl® may be confused with Benoxyl®

Fostex® may be confused with pHisoHex®

**U.S./Canadian Brand Names** Acetoxyl® [Can]; Benoxyl® [Can]; Benzac® AC Wash [US]; Benzac® AC [Can]; Benzac® AC [US]; Benzac® W Gel [Can]; Benzac® W Wash [Can]; Benzac® W Wash [US]; Benzac® W [US]; Benzac® [US]; Benzagel® Wash [US]; Benzagel® [US]; Benzashave® [US]; Brevoxyl® Cleansing [US]; Brevoxyl® Wash [US]; Brevoxyl® [US]; Clearplex [US-OTC]; Clinac™ BPO [US]; Del Aqua® [US]; Desquam-E™ [US]; Desquam-X® [US/Can]; Exact® Acne Medication [US-OTC]; Fostex® 10% BPO [US-OTC]; Loroxide® [US-OTC]; Neutrogena® Acne Mask [US-OTC]; Neutrogena® On The Spot® Acne Treatment [US-OTC]; Oxy 10® Balance Spot Treatment [US-OTC]; Oxy 10® Balanced Medicated Face Wash [US-OTC]; Oxyderm™ [Can]; Palmer's® Skin Success Acne [US-OTC]; PanOxyl® Aqua Gel [US]; PanOxyl® Bar [US-OTC]; PanOxyl® [US/Can]; PanOxyl®-AQ [US]; Seba-Gel™ [US]; Solugel® [Can]; Triaz® Cleanser [US]; Triaz® [US]; Zapzyt® [US-OTC]

**Therapeutic Category** Acne Products

**Use** Adjunctive treatment of mild to moderate acne vulgaris and acne rosacea

**Usual Dosage** Children and Adults:

Cleansers: Wash once or twice daily; control amount of drying or peeling by modifying dose frequency or concentration

Topical: Apply sparingly once daily; gradually increase to 2-3 times/day if needed. If excessive dryness or peeling occurs, reduce dose frequency or concentration; if excessive stinging or burning occurs, remove with mild soap and water; resume use the next day.

**Dosage Forms** [DSC] = Discontinued product

Cream, topical:

Benzashave®: 5% (120 g); 10% (120 g)

Exact® Acne Medication: 5% (18 g)

Neutrogena® Acne Mask: 5% (60 g)

Neutrogena® On The Spot® Acne Treatment: 2.5% (22.5 g)

Gel, topical: 2.5% (60 g); 5% (45 g, 60 g, 90 g); 10% (45 g, 60 g, 90 g)

Benzac® [alcohol based]: 5% (60 g); 10% (60 g) [contains alcohol 12%]

Benzac® AC [water based]: 5% (60 g); 10% (60 g)

Benzac® W [water based]: 2.5% (60 g); 5% (60 g); 10% (60 g)

Benzagel®: 5% (45 g); 10% (45 g)

Benzagel® Wash [water based]: 10% (60 g)

Brevoxyl®: 4% (43 g, 90 g); 8% (43 g, 90 g)

Clearplex: 5% (45 g); 10% (45 g)

Clinac™ BPO: 7% (45 g)

Desquam-E™ [water based]: 2.5% (42.5 g); 5% (42.5 g); 10% (42.5 g) [DSC] [emollient gel]

Desquam-X®: 5% (42.5 g, 90 g); 10% (42.5 g, 90 g)
Fostex® 10% BPO: 10% (45 g)
Oxy 10® Balance Spot Treatment: 5% (30 g); 10% (30 g)
PanOxyl® [alcohol based]: 5% (57 g, 113 g); 10% (57 g, 113 g)
PanOxyl® AQ [water based]: 2.5% (57 g, 113 g); 5% (57 g, 113 g); 10% (57 g, 113 g)
PanOxyl® Aqua Gel [water based]: 10% (42.5 g)
Seba-Gel™: 5% (60 g [DSC], 90 g); 10% (60 g [DSC], 90 g)
Triaz®: 3% (42.5 g); 6% (42.5 g); 10% (42.5 g)
Triaz® Cleanser: 3% (170 g, 340 g); 6% (170 g, 340 g); 10% (170 g, 340 g)
Zapzyt®: 10% (30 g)
Liquid, topical: 2.5% (240 mL); 5% (120 mL, 150 mL, 240 mL); 10% (150 mL, 240 mL)
Benzac® AC Wash [water based]: 5% (240 mL); 10% (240 mL)
Benzac® W Wash [water based]: 5% (240 mL)
Del-Aqua®: 5% (45 mL); 10% (45 mL)
Desquam-X®: 5% (150 mL)
Oxy-10® Balance Medicated Face Wash: 10% (240 mL)
Lotion, topical: 5% (30 mL); 10% (30 mL)
Brevoxyl® Cleansing: 4% (297 g); 8% (297 g) [in a lathering vehicle]
Brevoxyl® Wash: 4% (170 g); 8% (170 g) [in a lathering vehicle]
Fostex® 10% BPO: 10% (150 mL)
Loroxide®: 5.5% (26 mL)
Palmer's® Skin Success Acne: 10% (30 mL) [contains vitamin E and aloe]
Pad, topical (Triaz®): 3% (30s, 60s); 6% (30s, 60s); 9% (30s)
Soap, topical [bar]:
Desquam-X®: 10% (113 g) [DSC]
Fostex® 10% BPO: 10% (113 g)
PanOxyl® Bar: 5% (113 g); 10% (113 g)

**benzoyl peroxide and clindamycin** *see* clindamycin and benzoyl peroxide *on page 193*
**benzoyl peroxide and erythromycin** *see* erythromycin and benzoyl peroxide *on page 296*

# benzoyl peroxide and hydrocortisone
(BEN zoe il peer OKS ide & hye droe KOR ti sone)
**Synonyms** hydrocortisone and benzoyl peroxide
**U.S./Canadian Brand Names** Vanoxide-HC® [US/Can]
**Therapeutic Category** Acne Products
**Use** Treatment of acne vulgaris and oily skin
**Usual Dosage** Topical: Shake well; apply thin film 1-3 times/day, gently massage into skin
**Dosage Forms** Lotion: Benzoyl peroxide 5% and hydrocortisone acetate 0.5% (25 mL)

# benzphetamine (benz FET a meen)
**Synonyms** benzphetamine hydrochloride
**U.S./Canadian Brand Names** Didrex® [US/Can]
**Therapeutic Category** Anorexiant
**Controlled Substance** C-III
**Use** Short-term adjunct in exogenous obesity
**Usual Dosage** Adults: Oral: Dose should be individualized based on patient response: Initial: 25-50 mg once daily; titrate to 25-50 mg 1-3 times/day; once-daily dosing should be administered midmorning or midafternoon; maximum dose: 50 mg 3 times/day
**Dosage Forms** Tablet, as hydrochloride: 50 mg

**benzphetamine hydrochloride** *see* benzphetamine *on this page*

# benztropine (BENZ troe peen)
**Sound-Alike/Look-Alike Issues**
benztropine may be confused with bromocriptine
**Synonyms** benztropine mesylate
**U.S./Canadian Brand Names** Apo-Benztropine® [Can]; Cogentin® [US]
**Therapeutic Category** Anti-Parkinson Agent; Anticholinergic Agent
**Use** Adjunctive treatment of Parkinson disease; treatment of drug-induced extrapyramidal symptoms (except tardive dyskinesia)
*(Continued)*

# benztropine *(Continued)*

**Usual Dosage** Use in children ≤3 years of age should be reserved for life-threatening emergencies
Drug-induced extrapyramidal symptom: Oral, I.M., I.V.:
  Children >3 years: 0.02-0.05 mg/kg/dose 1-2 times/day
  Adults: 1-4 mg/dose 1-2 times/day
Acute dystonia: Adults: I.M., I.V.: 1-2 mg
Parkinsonism: Oral:
  Adults: 0.5-6 mg/day in 1-2 divided doses; if one dose is greater, administer at bedtime; titrate dose in
  0.5 mg increments at 5- to 6-day intervals
**Dosage Forms**
Injection, solution, as mesylate (Cogentin®): 1 mg/mL (2 mL)
Tablet, as mesylate: 0.5 mg, 1 mg, 2 mg

**benztropine mesylate** *see* benztropine *on previous page*

# benzydamine *(Canada only)* (ben ZID a meen)

**Synonyms** benzydamine hydrochloride
**U.S./Canadian Brand Names** Apo-Benzydamine® [Can]; Dom-Benzydamine [Can]; Novo-Benzyda-mine [Can]; PMS-Benzydamine [Can]; ratio-Benzydamine [Can]; Sun-Benz® [Can]; Tantum® [Can]
**Therapeutic Category** Analgesic, Topical
**Use** Symptomatic treatment of pain associated with acute pharyngitis; treatment of pain associated with radiation-induced oropharyngeal mucositis
**Usual Dosage** Oral rinse: Adults:
  Radiation-associated mucositis: 15 mL as a gargle or rinse 3-4 times/day; contact between the liquid and the oral mucosa should be maintained for at least 30 seconds, followed by expulsion from the mouth. Clinical studies maintained contact for ~2 minutes, up to 8 times/day. Patient should not swallow the liquid. Begin treatment 1 day prior to initiation of radiation therapy and continue daily during treatment. Continue oral rinse treatments after the completion of radiation therapy until desired result/healing is achieved.
  Acute pharyngitis: Gargle with 15 mL every 1½-3 hours until symptoms resolve. Patient should expel solution from mouth following use; solution should not be swallowed.
**Dosage Forms** Oral rinse, as hydrochloride: 0.15% (100 mL, 250 mL)

**benzydamine hydrochloride** *see* benzydamine *(Canada only) on this page*
**benzylpenicillin benzathine** *see* penicillin G benzathine *on page 628*
**benzylpenicillin potassium** *see* penicillin G (parenteral/aqueous) *on page 629*
**benzylpenicillin sodium** *see* penicillin G (parenteral/aqueous) *on page 629*

# benzylpenicilloyl-polylysine (BEN zil pen i SIL oyl pol i LIE seen)

**Synonyms** penicilloyl-polylysine; PPL
**Therapeutic Category** Diagnostic Agent
**Use** Adjunct in assessing the risk of administering penicillin (penicillin or benzylpenicillin) in adults with a history of clinical penicillin hypersensitivity
**Usual Dosage** PPL is administered by a scratch technique or by intradermal injection. For initial testing, PPL should always be applied via the scratch technique. **Do not administer intradermally to patients who have positive reactions to a scratch test.** PPL test alone does not identify those patients who react to a minor antigenic determinant and does not appear to predict reliably the occurrence of late reactions.
**Scratch test:** Use scratch technique with a 20-gauge needle to make 3-5 mm nonbleeding scratch on epidermis, apply a small drop of solution to scratch, rub in gently with applicator or toothpick. A positive reaction consists of a pale wheal surrounding the scratch site which develops within 10 minutes and ranges from 5-15 mm or more in diameter.
**Intradermal test:** Use intradermal test with a tuberculin syringe with a 26- to 30-gauge short bevel needle; a dose of 0.01-0.02 mL is injected intradermally. A control of 0.9% sodium chloride should be injected at least 1.5" from the PPL test site. Most skin responses to the intradermal test will develop within 5-15 minutes.
**Interpretation:**
(-) Negative: No reaction
(±) Ambiguous: Wheal only slightly larger than original bleb with or without erythematous flare and larger than control site

(+) Positive: Itching and marked increase in size of original bleb
Control site should be reactionless
**Dosage Forms** [DSC] = Discontinued product
Injection, solution: 6 x 10$^{-5}$ M (0.25 mL) [DSC]

# bepridil (BE pri dil)
**Sound-Alike/Look-Alike Issues**
bepridil may be confused with Prepidil®
Vascor® may be confused with Norvasc®
**Synonyms** bepridil hydrochloride
**U.S./Canadian Brand Names** Vascor® [Can]
**Therapeutic Category** Calcium Channel Blocker
**Use** Treatment of chronic stable angina; due to side effect profile, reserve for patients who have been intolerant of other antianginal therapy; bepridil may be used alone or in combination with nitrates or beta-blockers
**Usual Dosage** Adults: Oral: Initial: 200 mg/day, then adjust dose at 10-day intervals until optimal response is achieved; usual dose: 300 mg/day; maximum daily dose: 400 mg
**Dosage Forms** Tablet, as hydrochloride: 200 mg, 300 mg

**bepridil hydrochloride** see bepridil on this page

# beractant (ber AKT ant)
**Sound-Alike/Look-Alike Issues**
Survanta® may be confused with Sufenta®
**Synonyms** bovine lung surfactant; natural lung surfactant
**U.S./Canadian Brand Names** Survanta® [US/Can]
**Therapeutic Category** Lung Surfactant
**Use** Prevention and treatment of respiratory distress syndrome (RDS) in premature infants

Prophylactic therapy: Body weight <1250 g in infants at risk for developing or with evidence of surfactant deficiency (administer within 15 minutes of birth)
Rescue therapy: Treatment of infants with RDS confirmed by x-ray and requiring mechanical ventilation (administer as soon as possible - within 8 hours of age)
**Usual Dosage**
Prophylactic treatment: Administer 100 mg phospholipids (4 mL/kg) intratracheal as soon as possible; as many as 4 doses may be administered during the first 48 hours of life, no more frequently than 6 hours apart. The need for additional doses is determined by evidence of continuing respiratory distress; if the infant is still intubated and requiring at least 30% inspired oxygen to maintain a PaO$_2$ ≤80 torr.
Rescue treatment: Administer 100 mg phospholipids (4 mL/kg) as soon as the diagnosis of RDS is made; may repeat if needed, no more frequently than every 6 hours to a maximum of 4 doses
**Dosage Forms** Suspension for inhalation: 25 mg/mL (4 mL, 8 mL)

**Berocca® (Discontinued)**

**Berocca® Plus (Discontinued)**

**Berotec® [Can]** see fenoterol (Canada only) on page 331

**Berubigen® (Discontinued)** see cyanocobalamin on page 212

**Betacaine® [Can]** see lidocaine on page 479

# beta-carotene (BAY ta KARE oh teen)
**U.S./Canadian Brand Names** A-Caro-25® [US]; B-Caro-T™ [US]; Lumitene™ [US]
**Therapeutic Category** Vitamin, Fat Soluble
**Usual Dosage** Oral:
Children <14 years: 30-150 mg/day
Adults: 30-300 mg/day
**Dosage Forms**
Capsule: 10,000 int. units (6 mg); 25,000 int. units (15 mg)
A-Caro-25®, B-Caro-T™: 25,000 int. units (15 mg)
Lumitene™: 50,000 int. units (30 mg)
Tablet: 10,000 int. units

**Betachron® (Discontinued)** see propranolol on page 688

**Betaderm [Can]** *see* betamethasone (topical) *on next page*

**Betadine® [US-OTC/Can]** *see* povidone-iodine *on page 668*

**Betadine® First Aid Antibiotics + Moisturizer [US-OTC]** *see* bacitracin and polymyxin B *on page 86*

**Betadine® Ophthalmic [US]** *see* povidone-iodine *on page 668*

**9-beta-d-ribofuranosyladenine** *see* adenosine *on page 19*

**Betagan® [US/Can]** *see* levobunolol *on page 472*

**Beta-HC® [US]** *see* hydrocortisone (topical) *on page 417*

## betahistine *(Canada only)* (bay ta HISS teen)
**Synonyms** betahistine dihydrochloride
**U.S./Canadian Brand Names** Serc® [Can]
**Therapeutic Category** Antihistamine
**Use** Treatment of Ménière disease (to decrease episodes of vertigo)
**Usual Dosage** Oral: Adults: 8-16 mg 3 times/day; administration with meals is recommended
**Dosage Forms** Tablet, as dihydrochloride: 8 mg, 16 mg

**betahistine dihydrochloride** *see* betahistine *(Canada only)* *on this page*

## betaine anhydrous (BAY ta een an HY drus)
**Sound-Alike/Look-Alike Issues**
betaine may be confused with Betadine®
**U.S./Canadian Brand Names** Cystadane® [US/Can]
**Therapeutic Category** Homocystinuria Agent
**Use Orphan drug:** Treatment of homocystinuria to decrease elevated homocysteine blood levels; included within the category of homocystinuria are deficiencies or defects in cystathionine beta-synthase (CBS), 5,10-methylenetetrahydrofolate reductase (MTHFR), and cobalamin cofactor metabolism (CBL).
**Usual Dosage** Oral:
Children <3 years: Dosage may be started at 100 mg/kg/day and then increased weekly by 100 mg/kg increments
Children ≥3 years and Adults: 6 g/day administered in divided doses of 3 g twice daily. Dosages of up to 20 g/day have been necessary to control homocysteine levels in some patients.
Dosage in all patients can be gradually increased until plasma homocysteine is undetectable or present only in small amounts
**Dosage Forms** Powder for oral solution: 1 g/scoop (180 g) [1 scoop = 1.7 mL]

**Betaject™ [Can]** *see* betamethasone (systemic) *on next page*

**Betalene® Topical *(Discontinued)***

**Betalin® S *(Discontinued)*** *see* thiamine *on page 796*

**Betaloc® [Can]** *see* metoprolol *on page 534*

**Betaloc® Durules® [Can]** *see* metoprolol *on page 534*

## betamethasone and calcipotriol *(Canada only)*
(bay ta METH a sone & kal si POE try ole)
**Synonyms** calcipotriol and betamethasone dipropionate
**U.S./Canadian Brand Names** Dovobet® [Can]
**Therapeutic Category** Corticosteroid, Topical; Vitamin D Analog
**Use** Treatment of psoriasis vulgaris
**Usual Dosage** Topical: Adults: Psoriasis vulgaris: Apply to affected area once daily (maximum recommended dose: 100 g/week); treatment may be discontinued when response is noted. Treatment should generally be limited to 4 weeks.
**Dosage Forms** Cream: Calcipotriol 50 mcg and betamethasone 0.5 mg per gram (3 g, 30 g, 60 g, 100 g, 120 g)

## betamethasone and clotrimazole (bay ta METH a sone & kloe TRIM a zole)
**Sound-Alike/Look-Alike Issues**
Lotrisone® may be confused with Lotrimin®

**Synonyms** clotrimazole and betamethasone

**U.S./Canadian Brand Names** Lotriderm® [Can]; Lotrisone® [US]

**Therapeutic Category** Antifungal/Corticosteroid

**Use** Topical treatment of various dermal fungal infections (including tinea pedis, cruris, and corpora in patients ≥17 years of age)

**Usual Dosage** Topical:

Children <17 years: Do not use

Children ≥17 years and Adults:

Allergic or inflammatory diseases: Apply to affected area twice daily, morning and evening

Tinea corporis, tinea cruris: Massage into affected area twice daily, morning and evening; do not use for longer than 2 weeks; re-evaluate after 1 week if no clinical improvement; do not exceed 45 g cream/week or 45 mL lotion/week

Tinea pedis: Massage into affected area twice daily, morning and evening; do not use for longer than 4 weeks; re-evaluate after 2 weeks if no clinical improvement; do not exceed 45 g cream/week or 45 mL lotion/week

**Dosage Forms**

Cream: Betamethasone dipropionate 0.05% and clotrimazole 1% (15 g, 45 g) [contains benzyl alcohol]

Lotion: Betamethasone dipropionate 0.05% and clotrimazole 1% (30 mL) [contains benzyl alcohol]

**betamethasone dipropionate** *see* betamethasone (topical) *on this page*

**betamethasone dipropionate, augmented** *see* betamethasone (topical) *on this page*

**betamethasone sodium phosphate** *see* betamethasone (systemic) *on this page*

# betamethasone (systemic) (bay ta METH a sone sis TEM ik)

**Synonyms** betamethasone sodium phosphate; flubenisolone

**U.S./Canadian Brand Names** Betaject™ [Can]; Betnesol® [Can]; Betnovate® [Can]; Celestone® Soluspan® [US/Can]; Celestone® [US]; Maxivate® [US]; Prevex® B [Can]; Taro-Sone® [Can]

**Therapeutic Category** Adrenal Corticosteroid

**Use** Antiinflammatory; immunosuppressant agent; corticosteroid replacement

**Usual Dosage** Base dosage on severity of disease and patient response

Children: Use lowest dose listed as initial dose for adrenocortical insufficiency (physiologic replacement)

I.M.: 0.0175-0.125 mg base/kg/day divided every 6-12 hours **or** 0.5-7.5 mg base/m²/day divided every 6-12 hours

Oral: 0.0175-0.25 mg/kg/day divided every 6-8 hours **or** 0.5-7.5 mg/m²/day divided every 6-8 hours

Adolescents and Adults:

Oral: 2.4-4.8 mg/day in 2-4 doses; range: 0.6-7.2 mg/day

I.M.: Betamethasone sodium phosphate and betamethasone acetate: 0.6-9 mg/day (generally, $^1/_3$ to $^1/_2$ of oral dose) divided every 12-24 hours

Adults:

Intrabursal, intra-articular, intradermal: 0.25-2 mL

Intralesional: Rheumatoid arthritis/osteoarthritis:

Very large joints: 1-2 mL

Large joints: 1 mL

Medium joints: 0.5-1 mL

Small joints: 0.25-0.5 mL

**Dosage Forms Note:** Potency expressed as betamethasone base.

Injection, suspension (Celestone® Soluspan®): Betamethasone sodium phosphate 3 mg/mL and betamethasone acetate 3 mg/mL [6 mg/mL] (5 mL)

Syrup, as base (Celestone®): 0.6 mg/5 mL (118 mL)

# betamethasone (topical) (bay ta METH a sone TOP i kal)

**Sound-Alike/Look-Alike Issues**

Luxiq® may be confused with Lasix®

**Synonyms** betamethasone dipropionate, augmented; betamethasone dipropionate; betamethasone valerate; flubenisolone

**U.S./Canadian Brand Names** Beta-Val® [US]; Betaderm [Can]; Betnesol® [Can]; Betnovate® [Can]; Diprolene® AF [US]; Diprolene® Glycol [Can]; Diprolene® [US]; Diprosone® [Can]; Ectosone [Can]; Luxiq® [US]; Maxivate® [US]; Prevex® B [Can]; Taro-Sone® [Can]; Topilene® [Can]; Topisone® [Can]; Valisone® Scalp Lotion [Can]

(Continued)

## betamethasone (topical) *(Continued)*

**Therapeutic Category** Corticosteroid, Topical
**Use** Inflammatory dermatoses such as seborrheic or atopic dermatitis, neurodermatitis, anogenital pruritus, psoriasis, inflammatory phase of xerosis
**Usual Dosage** Topical:
≤12 years: Use is not recommended.
>12 years: Apply a thin film twice daily; use minimal amount for shortest period of time to avoid HPA axis suppression
Adolescents and Adults: Foam: Apply twice daily, once in the morning and once at night to scalp
Adults: Apply thin film 2-4 times/day. Therapy should be discontinued when control is achieved; if no improvement is seen, reassessment of diagnosis may be necessary.
**Dosage Forms** [DSC] = Discontinued product
**Note:** Potency expressed as betamethasone base.
Cream, topical, as dipropionate: 0.05% (15 g, 45 g)
 Maxivate®: 0.05% (45 g)
Cream, topical, as dipropionate augmented (Diprolene® AF): 0.05% (15 g, 50 g)
Cream, topical, as valerate (Beta-Val®): 0.1% (15 g, 45 g)
Foam, topical, as valerate (Luxiq®): 0.12% (50 g, 100 g, 150 g) [contains alcohol 60.4%]
Gel, topical, as dipropionate augmented (Diprolene® [DSC]): 0.05% (15 g, 50 g)
Lotion, topical, as dipropionate (Maxivate®): 0.05% (60 mL)
Lotion, topical, as dipropionate augmented (Diprolene®): 0.05% (30 mL, 60 mL)
Lotion, topical, as valerate (Beta-Val®): 0.1% (60 mL)
Ointment, topical, as dipropionate: 0.05% (15 g, 45 g)
 Maxivate®: 0.05% (45 g)
Ointment, topical, as dipropionate augmented (Diprolene®): 0.05% (15 g, 50 g)
Ointment, topical, as valerate: 0.1% (15 g, 45 g)

**betamethasone valerate** *see* betamethasone (topical) *on previous page*

**Betapace® [US]** *see* sotalol *on page 762*

**Betapace AF® [US/Can]** *see* sotalol *on page 762*

**Betasept® [US-OTC]** *see* chlorhexidine gluconate *on page 168*

**Betaseron® [US/Can]** *see* interferon beta-1b *on page 443*

**Betatar® [US-OTC]** *see* coal tar *on page 201*

**Beta-Val® [US]** *see* betamethasone (topical) *on previous page*

**Betaxin® [Can]** *see* thiamine *on page 796*

## betaxolol (be TAKS oh lol)

**Sound-Alike/Look-Alike Issues**
betaxolol may be confused with bethanechol, labetalol
**Synonyms** betaxolol hydrochloride
**U.S./Canadian Brand Names** Betoptic® S [US/Can]; Kerlone® [US]
**Therapeutic Category** Beta-Adrenergic Blocker
**Use** Treatment of chronic open-angle glaucoma and ocular hypertension; management of hypertension
**Usual Dosage** Adults:
Ophthalmic: Instill 1 drop twice daily.
Oral: 5-10 mg/day; may increase dose to 20 mg/day after 7-14 days if desired response is not achieved.
**Dosage Forms**
Solution, ophthalmic, as hydrochloride: 0.5% (5 mL, 10 mL, 15 mL) [contains benzalkonium chloride]
Suspension, ophthalmic, as hydrochloride (Betoptic® S): 0.25% (2.5 mL, 5 mL, 10 mL, 15 mL) [contains benzalkonium chloride]
Tablet, as hydrochloride (Kerlone®): 10 mg, 20 mg

**betaxolol hydrochloride** *see* betaxolol *on this page*

## bethanechol (be THAN e kole)

**Sound-Alike/Look-Alike Issues**
bethanechol may be confused with betaxolol

**Synonyms** bethanechol chloride

**U.S./Canadian Brand Names** Duvoid® [Can]; Myotonachol® [Can]; PMS-Bethanechol [Can]; Urecholine® [US]

**Therapeutic Category** Cholinergic Agent

**Use** Nonobstructive urinary retention and retention due to neurogenic bladder

**Usual Dosage** Oral: Adults:

Urinary retention, neurogenic bladder, and/or bladder atony:

Oral: Initial: 10-50 mg 2-4 times/day (some patients may require dosages of 50-100 mg 4 times/day). To determine effective dose, may initiate at a dose of 5-10 mg, with additional doses of 5-10 mg hourly until an effective cumulative dose is reached. Cholinergic effects at higher oral dosages may be cumulative.

SubQ: Initial: 2.575 mg, may repeat in 15-30 minutes (maximum cumulative initial dose: 10.3 mg); subsequent doses may be given 3-4 times daily as needed (some patients may require more frequent dosing at 2.5- to 3-hour intervals). Chronic neurogenic atony may require doses of 7.5-10 every 4 hours.

**Dosage Forms** Tablet, as chloride: 5 mg, 10 mg, 25 mg, 50 mg

**bethanechol chloride** *see* bethanechol *on previous page*

**Betimol® [US]** *see* timolol *on page 803*

**Betnesol® [Can]** *see* betamethasone (topical) *on page 103*

**Betnovate® [Can]** *see* betamethasone (topical) *on page 103*

**Betoptic® *(Discontinued)*** *see* betaxolol *on previous page*

**Betoptic® S [US/Can]** *see* betaxolol *on previous page*

**bevacizumab** (be vuh SIZ uh mab)

**Sound-Alike/Look-Alike Issues**

bevacizumab may be confused with cetuximab

**Synonyms** anti-VEGF monoclonal antibody; rhuMAb-VEGF

**U.S./Canadian Brand Names** Avastin™ [US]

**Therapeutic Category** Antineoplastic Agent, Monoclonal Antibody; Vaccine, Recombinant

**Use** Treatment of metastatic colorectal cancer (in combination with I.V. fluorouracil-based regimen)

**Usual Dosage** I.V.: Adults: Colorectal cancer: 5-10 mg/kg every 2 weeks

**Dosage Forms** Injection, solution [preservative free]: 25 mg/mL (4 mL, 16 mL)

**bexarotene** (beks AIR oh teen)

**U.S./Canadian Brand Names** Targretin® [US/Can]

**Therapeutic Category** Retinoic Acid Derivative; Vitamin A Derivative; Vitamin, Fat Soluble

**Use**

Oral: Treatment of cutaneous manifestations of cutaneous T-cell lymphoma in patients who are refractory to at least one prior systemic therapy

Topical: Treatment of cutaneous lesions in patients with refractory cutaneous T-cell lymphoma (stage 1A and 1B) or who have not tolerated other therapies

**Usual Dosage**

Oral: 300 mg/m²/day taken as a single daily dose. If there is no tumor response after 8 weeks and the initial dose was well tolerated, then an increase to 400 mg/m²/day can be made with careful monitoring. Maintain as long as the patient is deriving benefit.

If the initial dose is not tolerated, then it may be adjusted to 200 mg/m²/day, then to 100 mg/m²/day or temporarily suspended if necessary to manage toxicity

Topical: Apply once every other day for first week, then increase on a weekly basis to once daily, 2 times/day, 3 times/day, and finally 4 times/day, according to tolerance

**Dosage Forms**

Capsule: 75 mg

Gel: 1% (60 g)

**Bextra® [US]** *see* valdecoxib *on page 837*

**Bexxar® [US]** *see* tositumomab and iodine I 131 tositumomab *on page 812*

## bezafibrate *(Canada only)* (be za FYE brate)
**U.S./Canadian Brand Names** Bezalip® [Can]; PMS-Bezafibrate [Can]
**Therapeutic Category** Antihyperlipidemic Agent, Miscellaneous
**Use** Adjunct to diet and other therapeutic measures for treatment of type IIa and IIb mixed hyperlipidemia, to regulate lipid and apoprotein levels (reduce serum TG, LDL-cholesterol, and apolipoprotein B, increase HDL-cholesterol and apolipoprotein A); treatment of adult patients with high to very high triglyceride levels (Fredrickson classification type IV and V hyperlipidemias), who are at high risk of sequelae and complications from their dyslipidemia.
**Usual Dosage** Oral: Adults:
Immediate release: 200 mg 2-3 times/day; may reduce to 200 mg twice daily in patients with good response
Sustained release: 400 mg once daily
**Dosage Forms**
Tablet, immediate release: 200 mg
Tablet, sustained release: 400 mg

**Bezalip® [Can]** *see* bezafibrate *(Canada only) on this page*

**BG 9273** *see* alefacept *on page 25*

**BI-007** *see* paclitaxel (protein bound) *on page 613*

**Biavax® II *(Discontinued)***

**Biaxin® [US/Can]** *see* clarithromycin *on page 190*

**Biaxin® XL [US/Can]** *see* clarithromycin *on page 190*

## bicalutamide (bye ka LOO ta mide)
**Synonyms** CDX; ICI-176334
**U.S./Canadian Brand Names** Casodex® [US/Can]
**Therapeutic Category** Androgen
**Use** In combination therapy with LHRH agonist analogues in treatment of advanced prostatic carcinoma
**Usual Dosage** Adults: Oral: 50-150 mg/day
**Dosage Forms** Tablet: 50 mg

**Bicillin® L-A [US]** *see* penicillin G benzathine *on page 628*

**Bicillin® C-R [US]** *see* penicillin G benzathine and penicillin G procaine *on page 628*

**Bicillin® C-R 900/300 [US]** *see* penicillin G benzathine and penicillin G procaine *on page 628*

**BiCNu® [US/Can]** *see* carmustine *on page 149*

**BiDil® [US]** *see* isosorbide dinitrate and hydralazine *on page 451*

**BIG-IV** *see* botulism immune globulin (intravenous-human) *on page 112*

**Bilopaque® *(Discontinued)*** *see* radiological/contrast media (ionic) *on page 707*

**Biltricide® [US/Can]** *see* praziquantel *on page 672*

## bimatoprost (bi MAT oh prost)
**U.S./Canadian Brand Names** Lumigan® [US/Can]
**Therapeutic Category** Ophthalmic Agent, Miscellaneous
**Use** Reduction of intraocular pressure (IOP) in patients with open-angle glaucoma or ocular hypertension; should be used in patients who are intolerant of other IOP-lowering medications or failed treatment with another IOP-lowering medication
**Usual Dosage** Ophthalmic: Adult: Open-angle glaucoma or ocular hypertension: Instill 1 drop into affected eye(s) once daily in the evening; do not exceed once-daily dosing (may decrease IOP-lowering effect). If used with other topical ophthalmic agents, separate administration by at least 5 minutes.
**Dosage Forms** Solution, ophthalmic: 0.03% (2.5 mL, 5 mL, 7.5 mL) [contains benzalkonium chloride]

**Biobase™ [Can]** *see* alcohol (ethyl) *on page 24*

**Biobase-G™ [Can]** *see* alcohol (ethyl) *on page 24*

**Biocef® [US]** *see* cephalexin *on page 161*

**Bioclate® *(Discontinued)*** *see* antihemophilic factor (recombinant) *on page 57*

**Biodine® *(Discontinued)*** *see* povidone-iodine *on page 668*

**Biofed [US-OTC]** *see* pseudoephedrine *on page 692*

**Biolon**™ **[US]** *see* hyaluronate and derivatives *on page 406*

**Bion® Tears [US-OTC]** *see* artificial tears *on page 71*

**Biopatch®** *(Discontinued) see* chlorhexidine gluconate *on page 168*

**BioQuin® Durules**™ **[Can]** *see* quinidine *on page 705*

**Bio-Statin® [US]** *see* nystatin *on page 592*

**BioThrax**™ **[US]** *see* anthrax vaccine, adsorbed *on page 55*

**Biozyme-C®** *(Discontinued) see* collagenase *on page 206*

## biperiden (bye PER i den)

**Synonyms** biperiden hydrochloride; biperiden lactate
**U.S./Canadian Brand Names** Akineton® [US/Can]
**Therapeutic Category** Anti-Parkinson Agent; Anticholinergic Agent
**Use** Adjunct in the therapy of all forms of Parkinsonism; control of extrapyramidal symptoms secondary to antipsychotics
**Usual Dosage** Oral: Adults:
 Parkinsonism: 2 mg 3-4 times/day
 Extrapyramidal: 2 mg 1-3 times/day
**Dosage Forms** Tablet, as hydrochloride: 2 mg

**biperiden hydrochloride** *see* biperiden *on this page*

**biperiden lactate** *see* biperiden *on this page*

**Bisac-Evac**™ **[US-OTC]** *see* bisacodyl *on this page*

## bisacodyl (bis a KOE dil)

**Sound-Alike/Look-Alike Issues**
 Doxidan® may be confused with doxepin
 Modane® may be confused with Matulane®, Moban®
**U.S./Canadian Brand Names** Alophen® [US-OTC]; Apo-Bisacodyl® [Can]; Bisac-Evac™ [US-OTC]; Bisacodyl Uniserts® [US-OTC]; Carter's Little Pills® [Can]; Correctol® Tablets [US-OTC]; Doxidan® *(reformulation)* [US-OTC]; Dulcolax® [US-OTC/Can]; Femilax™ [US-OTC]; Fleet® Bisacodyl Enema [US-OTC]; Fleet® Stimulant Laxative [US-OTC]; Gentlax® [Can]; Modane Tablets® [US-OTC]; Veracolate [US-OTC]
**Therapeutic Category** Laxative
**Use** Treatment of constipation; colonic evacuation prior to procedures or examination
**Usual Dosage**
 Children:
 Oral: >6 years: 5-10 mg (0.3 mg/kg) at bedtime or before breakfast
 Rectal suppository:
  <2 years: 5 mg as a single dose
  >2 years: 10 mg
 Adults:
 Oral: 5-15 mg as single dose (up to 30 mg when complete evacuation of bowel is required)
 Rectal suppository: 10 mg as single dose
**Dosage Forms**
 Enema (Fleet® Bisacodyl Enema): 10 mg/30 mL (37 mL)
 Suppository, rectal (Bisac-Evac™, Bisacodyl Uniserts®; Dulcolax®): 10 mg
 Tablet, enteric coated (Alophen®; Bisac-Evac™, Correctol®, Dulcolax®, Femilax™, Fleet® Stimulant Laxative, Gentlax® [DSC], Modane®, Veracolate): 5 mg
 Tablet, delayed release (Doxidan®): 5 mg

**Bisacodyl Uniserts® [US-OTC]** *see* bisacodyl *on this page*

**bis-chloronitrosourea** *see* carmustine *on page 149*

## bismuth subgallate (BIZ muth sub GAL ate)

**Therapeutic Category** Gastrointestinal Agent, Miscellaneous
**Use** Symptomatic treatment of mild, nonspecific diarrhea
**Usual Dosage** Oral: 1-2 tablets 3 times/day with meals
**Dosage Forms** Tablet, chewable: 200 mg

## bismuth subsalicylate (BIZ muth sub sa LIS i late)

**Synonyms** pink bismuth

**U.S./Canadian Brand Names** Children's Kaopectate® (reformulation) [OTC]; Colo-Fresh™ [OTC]; Diotame® [OTC]; Kaopectate® Extra Strength [OTC]; Kaopectate® [OTC]; Pepto-Bismol® Maximum Strength [OTC]; Pepto-Bismol® [OTC]

**Therapeutic Category** Gastrointestinal Agent, Miscellaneous

**Use** Symptomatic treatment of mild, nonspecific diarrhea including traveler's diarrhea; chronic infantile diarrhea

**Usual Dosage** Oral:

Nonspecific diarrhea:

Children: Up to 8 doses/24 hours:

3-6 years: $\frac{1}{3}$ tablet or 5 mL every 30 minutes to 1 hour as needed

6-9 years: $\frac{2}{3}$ tablet or 10 mL every 30 minutes to 1 hour as needed

9-12 years: 1 tablet or 15 mL every 30 minutes to 1 hour as needed

Adults: 2 tablets or 30 mL every 30 minutes to 1 hour as needed up to 8 doses/24 hours

Prevention of traveler's diarrhea: 2.1 g/day or 2 tablets 4 times/day before meals and at bedtime

**Dosage Forms**

Liquid: 262 mg/15 mL (240 mL, 360 mL, 480 mL); 525 mg/15 mL (240 mL, 360 mL)

Children's Kaopectate®: 87 mg/5 mL (180 mL) [cherry flavor]

Diotame®: 262 mg/15 mL (30 mL)

Kaopectate®: 262 mg/15 mL (240 mL) [regular and peppermint flavor]

Kaopectate® Extra Strength: 525 mg/15 mL (240 mL) [peppermint flavor]

Pepto-Bismol®: 262 mg/15 mL (120 mL, 240 mL, 360 mL, 480 mL) [wintergreen flavor]

Pepto-Bismol® Maximum Strength: 525 mg/15 mL (120 mL, 240 mL, 360 mL) [wintergreen flavor]

Tablet, chewable (Diotame®, Pepto-Bismol®): 262 mg

## bismuth subsalicylate, metronidazole, and tetracycline

(BIZ muth sub sa LIS i late, me troe NI da zole, & tet ra SYE kleen)

**Synonyms** bismuth subsalicylate, tetracycline, and metronidazole; metronidazole, bismuth subsalicylate, and tetracycline; metronidazole, tetracycline, and bismuth subsalicylate; tetracycline, bismuth subsalicylate, and metronidazole; tetracycline, metronidazole, and bismuth subsalicylate

**U.S./Canadian Brand Names** Helidac® [US]

**Therapeutic Category** Antidiarrheal

**Use** In combination with an $H_2$ antagonist, as part of a multidrug regimen for *H. pylori* eradication to reduce the risk of duodenal ulcer recurrence

**Usual Dosage** Adults: Chew 2 bismuth subsalicylate 262.4 mg tablets, swallow 1 metronidazole 250 mg tablet, and swallow 1 tetracycline 500 mg capsule 4 times/day at meals and bedtime, plus an $H_2$ antagonist (at the appropriate dose) for 14 days; follow with 8 oz of water; the $H_2$ antagonist should be continued for a total of 28 days

**Dosage Forms** Combination package [each package contains 14 blister cards (2-week supply); each card contains the following]:

Capsule: Tetracycline hydrochloride: 500 mg (4)

Tablet: Bismuth subsalicylate [chewable]: 262.4 mg (8)

Tablet: Metronidazole: 250 mg (4)

**bismuth subsalicylate, tetracycline, and metronidazole** *see* bismuth subsalicylate, metronidazole, and tetracycline *on this page*

## bisoprolol (bis OH proe lol)

**Sound-Alike/Look-Alike Issues**

Zebeta® may be confused with DiaBeta®

**Synonyms** bisoprolol fumarate

**U.S./Canadian Brand Names** Monocor® [Can]; Zebeta® [US/Can]

**Therapeutic Category** Beta-Adrenergic Blocker

**Use** Treatment of hypertension, alone or in combination with other agents

**Usual Dosage** Oral:

Adults: 2.5-5 mg once daily, may be increased to 10 mg, and then up to 20 mg once daily, if necessary

Hypertension (JNC 7): 2.5-10 mg once daily
**Dosage Forms** Tablet, as fumarate: 5 mg, 10 mg

## bisoprolol and hydrochlorothiazide (bis OH proe lol & hye droe klor oh THYE a zide)
**Sound-Alike/Look-Alike Issues**
Ziac® may be confused with Tiazac®, Zerit®
**Synonyms** hydrochlorothiazide and bisoprolol
**U.S./Canadian Brand Names** Ziac® [US/Can]
**Therapeutic Category** Antihypertensive Agent, Combination
**Use** Treatment of hypertension
**Usual Dosage** Oral: Adults: Dose is individualized, given once daily
**Dosage Forms** Tablet:
2.5/6.25: Bisoprolol fumarate 2.5 mg and hydrochlorothiazide 6.25 mg
5/6.25: Bisoprolol fumarate 5 mg and hydrochlorothiazide 6.25 mg
10/6.25: Bisoprolol fumarate 10 mg and hydrochlorothiazide 6.25 mg

**bisoprolol fumarate** *see* bisoprolol *on previous page*

**bistropamide** *see* tropicamide *on page 829*

## bivalirudin (bye VAL i roo din)
**Synonyms** hirulog
**U.S./Canadian Brand Names** Angiomax® [US/Can]
**Therapeutic Category** Anticoagulant (Other)
**Use** Anticoagulant used in conjunction with aspirin for patients with unstable angina undergoing percutaneous transluminal coronary angioplasty (PTCA) or percutaneous coronary intervention (PCI) with provisional glycoprotein IIb/IIIa inhibitor
**Usual Dosage** I.V.: Adults: Anticoagulant in patients undergoing PTCA or PCI (treatment should be started just prior to procedure): Initial: Bolus: 0.75 mg/kg, followed by continuous infusion: 1.75 mg/kg/hour for the duration of procedure up to 4 hours post-procedure; determine ACT 5 minutes after bolus dose; may administer additional bolus of 0.3 mg/kg if necessary.
A glycoprotein IIb/IIIa inhibitor may be administered concomitantly during the procedure.
If needed, infusion may be continued beyond initial 4 hours at 0.2 mg/kg/hour for up to 20 hours.
**Dosage Forms** Injection, powder for reconstitution: 250 mg

**BL4162A** *see* anagrelide *on page 52*

**Black Draught Tablets [US-OTC]** *see* senna *on page 743*

**black widow spider species antivenin (*Latrodectus mactans*)** *see* antivenin *(Latrodectus mactans) on page 60*

**BlemErase® Lotion *(Discontinued)*** *see* benzoyl peroxide *on page 98*

**Blenoxane® [US/Can]** *see* bleomycin *on this page*

**bleo** *see* bleomycin *on this page*

## bleomycin (blee oh MYE sin)
**Sound-Alike/Look-Alike Issues**
bleomycin may be confused with Cleocin®
**Synonyms** bleo; bleomycin sulfate; BLM; NSC-125066
**U.S./Canadian Brand Names** Blenoxane® [US/Can]
**Therapeutic Category** Antineoplastic Agent
**Use** Treatment of squamous cell carcinoma, melanomas, sarcomas, testicular carcinoma, Hodgkin lymphoma, and non-Hodgkin lymphoma
**Orphan drug:** Sclerosing agent for malignant pleural effusion
**Usual Dosage** Maximum cumulative lifetime dose: 400 units; refer to individual protocols; 1 unit = 1 mg
May be administered I.M., I.V., SubQ, or intracavitary
Children and Adults:
Test dose for lymphoma patients: I.M., I.V., SubQ: Because of the possibility of an anaphylactoid reaction, ≤2 units of bleomycin for the first 2 doses; monitor vital signs every 15 minutes; wait a minimum of 1 hour before administering remainder of dose; if no acute reaction occurs, then the regular dosage schedule may be followed
(Continued)

# bleomycin *(Continued)*

**Single-agent therapy:**
I.M., I.V., SubQ: Squamous cell carcinoma, lymphoma, testicular carcinoma: 0.25-0.5 units/kg (10-20 units/m$^2$) 1-2 times/week
CIV: 15 units/m$^2$ over 24 hours daily for 4 days
Pleural sclerosing: 60 units as a single infusion. Dose may be repeated at intervals of several days if fluid continues to accumulate (mix in 50-100 mL of D$_5$W, NS, or SWFI); may add lidocaine 100-200 mg to reduce local discomfort.

**Dosage Forms** Injection, powder for reconstitution, as sulfate: 15 units, 30 units

**bleomycin sulfate** *see* bleomycin *on previous page*

**Bleph®-10 [US]** *see* sulfacetamide *on page 771*

**Blephamide® [US/Can]** *see* sulfacetamide and prednisolone *on page 771*

**Blis-To-Sol® [US-OTC]** *see* tolnaftate *on page 809*

**BLM** *see* bleomycin *on previous page*

**Blocadren® [US]** *see* timolol *on page 803*

**BMS-232632** *see* atazanavir *on page 76*

**BMS 337039** *see* aripiprazole *on page 70*

**Bonamine™ [Can]** *see* meclizine *on page 506*

**Bondronat® [Can]** *see* ibandronate *on page 426*

**Bonefos® [Can]** *see* clodronate disodium *(Canada only) on page 195*

**Bonine® [US-OTC/Can]** *see* meclizine *on page 506*

**Boniva® [US]** *see* ibandronate *on page 426*

**Bontril® [Can]** *see* phendimetrazine *on page 637*

**Bontril® PDM [US]** *see* phendimetrazine *on page 637*

**Bontril® Slow-Release [US]** *see* phendimetrazine *on page 637*

**Boostrix® [US]** *see* diphtheria, tetanus toxoids, and acellular pertussis vaccine *on page 259*

# boric acid *(BOR ik AS id)*

**Therapeutic Category** Pharmaceutical Aid
**Use**
Ophthalmic: Mild antiseptic used for inflamed eyelids
Otic: Prophylaxis of swimmer's ear
Topical ointment: Temporary relief of chapped, chafed, or dry skin, diaper rash, abrasions, minor burns, sunburn, insect bites, and other skin irritations
**Usual Dosage**
Ophthalmic: Apply to lower eyelid 1-2 times/day
Otic: Place 2-4 drops in ears
Topical: Apply as needed
**Dosage Forms**
Ointment:
Ophthalmic: 5% (3.5 g); 10% (3.5 g)
Topical: 5% (52.5 g); 10% (28 g)
Topical (Borofax®): 5% boric acid and lanolin (1$^3$/$_4$ oz)
Solution, otic: 2.75% with isopropyl alcohol (30 mL)

# bortezomib *(bore TEZ oh mib)*

**Synonyms** LDP-341; MLN341; PS-341
**U.S./Canadian Brand Names** Velcade™ [US/Can]
**Therapeutic Category** Proteasome Inhibitor
**Use** Treatment of multiple myeloma in patients who have had at least one prior therapy
**Usual Dosage** I.V.: Adults: Multiple myeloma: 1.3 mg/m$^2$ twice weekly for 2 weeks on days 1, 4, 8, 11, every 21 days. Consecutive doses should be separated by at least 72 hours.
**Dosage Forms** Injection, powder for reconstitution [preservative free]: 3.5 mg [contains mannitol 35 mg]

# bosentan (boe SEN tan)

**U.S./Canadian Brand Names** Tracleer® [US/Can]

**Therapeutic Category** Endothelin Antagonist

**Use** Treatment of pulmonary artery hypertension (PAH) in patients with World Health Organization (WHO) Class III or IV symptoms to improve exercise capacity and decrease the rate of clinical deterioration

**Usual Dosage** Oral: Adults: Initial: 62.5 mg twice daily for 4 weeks; increase to maintenance dose of 125 mg twice daily; adults <40 kg should be maintained at 62.5 mg twice daily

**Note:** When discontinuing treatment, consider a reduction in dosage to 62.5 mg twice daily for 3-7 days (to avoid clinical deterioration).

**Dosage Forms** Tablet: 62.5 mg, 125 mg

**B&O Supprettes® [US]** *see* belladonna and opium *on page 92*

**Botox® [US/Can]** *see* botulinum toxin type A *on this page*

**Botox® Cosmetic [US/Can]** *see* botulinum toxin type A *on this page*

# botulinum toxin type A (BOT yoo lin num TOKS in type aye)

**Synonyms** BTX-A

**U.S./Canadian Brand Names** Botox® Cosmetic [US/Can]; Botox® [US/Can]

**Therapeutic Category** Ophthalmic Agent, Toxin

**Use** Treatment of strabismus and blepharospasm associated with dystonia (including benign essential blepharospasm or VII nerve disorders in patients ≥12 years of age); cervical dystonia (spasmodic torticollis) in patients ≥16 years of age; temporary improvement in the appearance of lines/wrinkles of the face (moderate to severe glabellar lines associated with corrugator and/or procerus muscle activity) in adult patients ≤65 years of age; treatment of severe primary axillary hyperhidrosis in adults not adequately controlled with topical treatments

**Orphan drug:** Treatment of dynamic muscle contracture in pediatric cerebral palsy patients

**Usual Dosage**

Cervical dystonia: Children ≥16 years and Adults: I.M.: For dosing guidance, the mean dose is 236 units (25th to 75th percentile range 198-300 units) divided among the affected muscles in patients previously treated with botulinum toxin. Initial dose in previously untreated patients should be lower. Sequential dosing should be based on the patient's head and neck position, localization of pain, muscle hypertrophy, patient response, and previous adverse reactions. The total dose injected into the sternocleidomastoid muscles should be ≤100 units to decrease the occurrence of dysphagia.

Blepharospasm: Children ≥12 years and Adults: I.M.: Initial dose: 1.25-2.5 units injected into the medial and lateral pretarsal orbicularis oculi of the upper and lower lid; dose may be increased up to twice the previous dose if the response from the initial dose lasted ≤2 months; maximum dose per site: 5 units; cumulative dose in a 30-day period: ≤200 units. Tolerance may occur if treatments are given more often than every 3 months, but the effect is not usually permanent.

Strabismus: Children ≥12 years and Adults: I.M.:

Initial dose:

Vertical muscles and for horizontal strabismus <20 prism diopters: 1.25-2.5 units in any one muscle

Horizontal strabismus of 20-50 prism diopters: 2.5-5 units in any one muscle

Persistent VI nerve palsy >1 month: 1.5-2.5 units in the medial rectus muscle

Re-examine patients 7-14 days after each injection to assess the effect of that dose. Subsequent doses for patients experiencing incomplete paralysis of the target may be increased up to twice the previous administered dose. The maximum recommended dose as a single injection for any one muscle is 25 units. Do not administer subsequent injections until the effects of the previous dose are gone.

Primary axillary hyperhidrosis: Adults ≥18 years: Intradermal: 50 units/axilla. Injection area should be defined by standard staining techniques. Injections should be evenly distributed into multiple sites (10-15), administered in 0.1-0.2 mL aliquots, ~1-2 cm apart.

Reduction of glabellar lines: Adults ≤65 years: I.M.: An effective dose is determined by gross observation of the patient's ability to activate the superficial muscles injected. The location, size and use of muscles may vary markedly among individuals. Inject 0.1 mL dose into each of five sites, two in each corrugator muscle and one in the procerus muscle (total dose 0.5 mL).

**Dosage Forms** Injection, powder for reconstitution [preservative free]: *Clostridium botulinum* toxin type A 100 units [contains human albumin]

# botulinum toxin type B (BOT yoo lin num TOKS in type bee)

**U.S./Canadian Brand Names** Myobloc® [US]

**Therapeutic Category** Neuromuscular Blocker Agent, Toxin

**Use** Treatment of cervical dystonia (spasmodic torticollis)

**Usual Dosage**

Children: Not established in pediatric patients

Adults: Cervical dystonia: I.M.: Initial: 2500-5000 units divided among the affected muscles in patients **previously treated** with botulinum toxin; initial dose in **previously untreated** patients should be lower. Subsequent dosing should be optimized according to patient's response.

**Dosage Forms** Injection, solution [single-dose vial]: 5000 units/mL (0.5 mL, 1 mL, 2 mL) [contains albumin 0.05%]

# botulism immune globulin (intravenous-human)

(BOT yoo lism i MYUN GLOB you lin, in tra VEE nus, YU man)

**Synonyms** BIG-IV

**U.S./Canadian Brand Names** BabyBIG® [US]

**Therapeutic Category** Immune Globulin

**Use** Treatment of infant botulism caused by toxin type A or B

**Usual Dosage** I.V.: Children <1 year: Infant botulism: 1 mL/kg (50 mg/kg) as a single dose; infuse at 0.5 mL/kg/hour (25 mg/kg/hour) for the first 15 minutes; if well tolerated, may increase to 1 mL/kg/hour (50 mg/kg/hour)

**Dosage Forms** Injection, powder for reconstitution [preservative free]: ~100 mg [contains albumin 1% and sucrose 5%; packaged with SWFI]

**Boudreaux's**® **Butt Paste [US-OTC]** *see* zinc oxide *on page 861*

**bovine lung surfactant** *see* beractant *on page 101*

**Breathe Right**® **Saline [US-OTC]** *see* sodium chloride *on page 752*

**Breezee**® **Mist Antifungal *(Discontinued)*** *see* miconazole *on page 537*

**Breonesin**® ***(Discontinued)*** *see* guaifenesin *on page 383*

**Brethaire**® ***(Discontinued)*** *see* terbutaline *on page 787*

**Brethine**® **[US]** *see* terbutaline *on page 787*

# bretylium (bre TIL ee um)

**Sound-Alike/Look-Alike Issues**

bretylium may be confused with Brevibloc®

**Synonyms** bretylium tosylate

**Therapeutic Category** Antiarrhythmic Agent, Class III

**Use** Treatment of ventricular tachycardia and fibrillation; treatment of other serious ventricular arrhythmias resistant to lidocaine

**Usual Dosage Note:** Patients should undergo defibrillation/cardioversion before and after bretylium doses as necessary.

Children (**Note:** Not well established, although the following dosing has been suggested):

I.M.: 2-5 mg/kg as a single dose

I.V.: Acute ventricular fibrillation: Initial: 5 mg/kg, then attempt electrical defibrillation; repeat with 10 mg/kg if ventricular fibrillation persists at 15- to 30-minute intervals to maximum total of 30 mg/kg.

Maintenance dose: I.M., I.V.: 5 mg/kg every 6 hours

Adults:

Immediate life-threatening ventricular arrhythmias (ventricular fibrillation, unstable ventricular tachycardia): Initial dose: I.V.: 5 mg/kg (undiluted) over 1 minute; if arrhythmia persists, administer 10 mg/kg (undiluted) over 1 minute and repeat as necessary (usually at 15- to 30-minute intervals) up to a total dose of 30-35 mg/kg.

Other life-threatening ventricular arrhythmias:

Initial dose: I.M., I.V.: 5-10 mg/kg, may repeat every 1-2 hours if arrhythmia persists; administer I.V. dose (diluted) over 8-10 minutes.

Maintenance dose: I.M.: 5-10 mg/kg every 6-8 hours; I.V. (diluted): 5-10 mg/kg every 6 hours; I.V. infusion (diluted): 1-2 mg/minute (little experience with doses >40 mg/kg/day)

Example dilution: 2 g/250 mL $D_5W$ (infusion pump should be used for I.V. infusion administration)

Rate of I.V. infusion: 1-4 mg/minute

1 mg/minute = 7 mL/hour

2 mg/minute = 15 mL/hour
3 mg/minute = 22 mL/hour
4 mg/minute = 30 mL/hour
**Dosage Forms** [DSC] = Discontinued product
Injection, solution, as tosylate: 50 mg/mL (10 mL) [DSC]
Injection, solution, as tosylate [premixed in $D_5W$]: 2 mg/mL (250 mL); 4 mg/mL (250 mL) [DSC]

**bretylium tosylate** *see* bretylium *on previous page*

**Brevibloc**® **[US/Can]** *see* esmolol *on page 297*

**Brevicon**® **[US]** *see* ethinyl estradiol and norethindrone *on page 314*

**Brevicon**® **0.5/35 [Can]** *see* ethinyl estradiol and norethindrone *on page 314*

**Brevicon**® **1/35 [Can]** *see* ethinyl estradiol and norethindrone *on page 314*

**Brevital**® **[Can]** *see* methohexital *on page 524*

**Brevital**® **Sodium [US]** *see* methohexital *on page 524*

**Brevoxyl**® **[US]** *see* benzoyl peroxide *on page 98*

**Brevoxyl**® **Cleansing [US]** *see* benzoyl peroxide *on page 98*

**Brevoxyl**® **Wash [US]** *see* benzoyl peroxide *on page 98*

**Bricanyl**® *(Discontinued)* *see* terbutaline *on page 787*

**brimonidine** (bri MOE ni deen)
**Sound-Alike/Look-Alike Issues**
brimonidine may be confused with bromocriptine
**Synonyms** brimonidine tartrate
**U.S./Canadian Brand Names** Alphagan® P [US]; Alphagan® [Can]; PMS-Brimonidine Tartrate [Can]; ratio-Brimonidine [Can]
**Therapeutic Category** Alpha$_2$-Adrenergic Agonist Agent, Ophthalmic
**Use** Lowering of intraocular pressure (IOP) in patients with open-angle glaucoma or ocular hypertension
**Usual Dosage** Ophthalmic: Children ≥2 years of age and Adults: Glaucoma: Instill 1 drop in affected eye(s) 3 times/day (approximately every 8 hours)
**Dosage Forms**
Solution, ophthalmic, as tartrate: 0.2% (5 mL, 10 mL, 15 mL) [may contain benzalkonium chloride]
Alphagan® P: 0.1% (5 mL, 10 mL, 15 mL) [contains Purite® as preservative]; 0.15% (5 mL, 10 mL, 15 mL) [contains Purite® as preservative]

**brimonidine tartrate** *see* brimonidine *on this page*

**brinzolamide** (brin ZOH la mide)
**U.S./Canadian Brand Names** Azopt® [US/Can]
**Therapeutic Category** Carbonic Anhydrase Inhibitor
**Use** Lowers intraocular pressure in patients with ocular hypertension or open-angle glaucoma
**Usual Dosage** Ophthalmic: Adults: Instill 1 drop in affected eye(s) 3 times/day
**Dosage Forms** Suspension, ophthalmic: 1% (5 mL, 10 mL, 15 mL) [contains benzalkonium chloride]

**Brioschi**® **[US-OTC]** *see* sodium bicarbonate *on page 752*

**British anti-lewisite** *see* dimercaprol *on page 252*

**BRL 43694** *see* granisetron *on page 382*

**Brofed**® **[US]** *see* brompheniramine and pseudoephedrine *on page 115*

**Bromaline**® **[US-OTC]** *see* brompheniramine and pseudoephedrine *on page 115*

**Bromaline**® **DM [US-OTC]** *see* brompheniramine, pseudoephedrine, and dextromethorphan *on page 116*

**Bromarest**® *(Discontinued)* *see* brompheniramine *on page 115*

**Bromaxefed DM RF [US]** *see* brompheniramine, pseudoephedrine, and dextromethorphan *on page 116*

**Bromaxefed RF [US]** *see* brompheniramine and pseudoephedrine *on page 115*

# bromazepam *(Canada only)* (broe MA ze pam)
**U.S./Canadian Brand Names** Apo-Bromazepam® [Can]; Gen-Bromazepam [Can]; Lectopam® [Can]; Novo-Bromazepam [Can]; Nu-Bromazepam [Can]
**Therapeutic Category** Benzodiazepine; Sedative
**Use** Short-term, symptomatic treatment of anxiety
**Usual Dosage** Oral: Adults: Initial: 6-18 mg/day in equally divided doses; initial course of treatment should not last longer than 1 week; optimal dosage range: 6-30 mg/day
**Dosage Forms** Tablet: 1.5 mg, 3 mg, 6 mg

**Brombay**® *(Discontinued)* *see* brompheniramine *on next page*

**brometane DX** *see* brompheniramine, pseudoephedrine, and dextromethorphan *on page 116*

**Bromfed**® *(Discontinued)* *see* brompheniramine and pseudoephedrine *on next page*

**Bromfed-PD**® *(Discontinued)* *see* brompheniramine and pseudoephedrine *on next page*

# bromfenac (BROME fen ak)
**Synonyms** bromfenac sodium
**U.S./Canadian Brand Names** Xibrom™ [US]
**Therapeutic Category** Analgesic, Nonnarcotic; Nonsteroidal Antiinflammatory Drug (NSAID), Oral
**Use** Treatment of postoperative inflammation following cataract removal
**Usual Dosage** Ophthalmic: Adults: Instill 1 drop into affected eye(s) twice daily beginning 24 hours after surgery and continuing for 2 weeks postoperatively
**Dosage Forms** Solution, ophthalmic: 0.09% (5 mL) [contains benzoic acid and sodium sulfite]

**bromfenac sodium** *see* bromfenac *on this page*

**Bromfenex**® **[US]** *see* brompheniramine and pseudoephedrine *on next page*

**Bromfenex**® **PD [US]** *see* brompheniramine and pseudoephedrine *on next page*

**Bromhist-DM [US]** *see* brompheniramine, pseudoephedrine, and dextromethorphan *on page 116*

**Bromhist Pediatric [US]** *see* brompheniramine and pseudoephedrine *on next page*

# bromocriptine (broe moe KRIP teen)
**Sound-Alike/Look-Alike Issues**
bromocriptine may be confused with benztropine, brimonidine
Parlodel® may be confused with pindolol, Provera®
**Synonyms** bromocriptine mesylate
**U.S./Canadian Brand Names** Apo-Bromocriptine® [Can]; Parlodel® [US/Can]; PMS-Bromocriptine [Can]
**Therapeutic Category** Anti-Parkinson Agent; Ergot Alkaloid and Derivative
**Use**
Amenorrhea with or without galactorrhea; infertility or hypogonadism; prolactin-secreting adenomas; acromegaly; Parkinson's disease
**A previous indication for prevention of postpartum lactation was withdrawn voluntarily by Sandoz Pharmaceuticals Corporation.**
**Usual Dosage** Oral:
Children: Prolactin-secreting adenoma:
11-15 years (based on limited information): Initial: 1.25-2.5 mg daily; dosage may be increased as tolerated to achieve a therapeutic response (range 2.5-10 mg daily).
≥16 years: Refer to Adults dosing
Adults:
Parkinsonism: 1.25 mg 2 times/day, increased by 2.5 mg/day in 2- to 4-week intervals (usual dose range is 30-90 mg/day in 3 divided doses)
Neuroleptic malignant syndrome: 2.5-5 mg 3 times/day
Hyperprolactinemia: 2.5 mg 2-3 times/day
Acromegaly: Initial: 1.25-2.5 mg increasing as necessary every 3-7 days; usual dose: 20-30 mg/day
Prolactin-secreting adenomas: Initial: 1.25-2.5 mg/day; may be increased as tolerated every 2-7 days until optimal response (range: 2.5-15 mg/day)
**Dosage Forms**
Capsule, as mesylate: 5 mg
Tablet, as mesylate: 2.5 mg

**bromocriptine mesylate** *see* bromocriptine *on previous page*

**Bromphen®** *(Discontinued)* *see* brompheniramine *on this page*

# brompheniramine (brome fen IR a meen)

**Synonyms** parabromdylamine

**U.S./Canadian Brand Names** Colhist® Solution [US-OTC]; Dimetane® Extentabs® [US-OTC]; Dimetapp® Allergy Children's [US-OTC]; Dimetapp® Allergy [US-OTC]; Lodrane® 12 Hour [US-OTC]; ND-Stat® Solution [US-OTC]; Polytapp® Allergy Dye-Free Medication [US-OTC]

**Therapeutic Category** Antihistamine

**Use** Perennial and seasonal allergic rhinitis and other allergic symptoms including urticaria

**Usual Dosage**

Oral:

Children:

<6 years: 0.125 mg/kg/dose administered every 6 hours; maximum: 6-8 mg/day

6-12 years: 2-4 mg every 6-8 hours; maximum: 12-16 mg/day

Adults: 4 mg every 4-6 hours or 8 mg of sustained release form every 8-12 hours or 12 mg of sustained release every 12 hours; maximum: 24 mg/day

I.M., I.V., SubQ:

Children <12 years: 0.5 mg/kg/24 hours divided every 6-8 hours

Adults: 5-50 mg every 4-12 hours, maximum: 40 mg/24 hours

**Dosage Forms**

Capsule, as maleate: 4 mg

Elixir, as maleate: 2 mg/5 mL with 3% alcohol (120 mL)

Liquid, as maleate: 2 mg/5 mL (60 mL, 120 mL, 240 mL)

Solution, as maleate: 2 mg/5 mL (10 mL)

Tablet, as maleate: 4 mg

Tablet, sustained release, as maleate: 6 mg, 12 mg

# brompheniramine and pseudoephedrine (brome fen IR a meen & soo doe e FED rin)

**Sound-Alike/Look-Alike Issues**

Bromfed® may be confused with Bromphen®

**Synonyms** brompheniramine maleate and pseudoephedrine hydrochloride; brompheniramine maleate and pseudoephedrine sulfate; pseudoephedrine and brompheniramine

**U.S./Canadian Brand Names** Andehist NR Syrup [US]; Brofed® [US]; Bromaline® [US-OTC]; Bromaxefed RF [US]; Bromfenex® PD [US]; Bromfenex® [US]; Bromhist Pediatric [US]; Children's Dimetapp® Elixir Cold & Allergy [US-OTC]; Histex™ SR [US]; Lodrane® 12D [US]; Lodrane® LD [US]; Lodrane® [US]; Rondec® Syrup [US]; Touro™ Allergy [US]

**Therapeutic Category** Antihistamine/Decongestant Combination

**Use** Temporary relief of symptoms of seasonal and perennial allergic rhinitis, and vasomotor rhinitis, including nasal obstruction

**Usual Dosage** Oral:

Capsule, long acting:

Based on 60 mg pseudoephedrine:

Children 6-12 years: 1 capsule every 12 hours

Children ≥12 years and Adults: 1-2 capsules every 12 hours

Based on 120 mg pseudoephedrine: Children ≥12 years and Adults: 1 capsule every 12 hours

Liquid:

Based on brompheniramine 1 mg/pseudoephedrine 15 mg per 1 mL: Children:

1-3 months: 0.25 mL 4 times/day

3-6 months: 0.5 mL 4 times/day

6-12 months: 0.75 mL 4 times/day

12-24 months: 1 mL 4 times/day

Based on brompheniramine 1 mg/pseudoephedrine 15 mg per 5 mL: Children:

6-11 months (6-8 kg): 2.5 mL every 6-8 hours (maximum: 4 doses/24 hours)

12-23 months (8-10 kg): 3.75 mL every 6-8 hours (maximum: 4 doses/24 hours)

2-6 years: 5 mL every 6-8 hours (maximum: 4 doses/24 hours)

6-12 years: 10 mL every 6-8 hours (maximum: 4 doses/24 hours)

>12 years and Adults: 20 mg every 4 hours (maximum: 4 doses/24 hours)

Based on brompheniramine 4 mg/pseudoephedrine 30 mg:

Children 2-6 years: 2.5 mL 3 times/day

Children >6 years and Adults: 5 mL 3 times/day

(Continued)

# brompheniramine and pseudoephedrine *(Continued)*

Brompheniramine 4 mg/pseudoephedrine 45 mg per 5 mL:
  Children 2-6 years: 2.5 mL 4 times/day
  Children >6 years and Adults: 5 mL 4 times/day
Tablet, extended release: Based on pseudoephedrine 45 mg:
  Children 6-12 years: 1 tablet every 12 hours
  Children ≥12 years and Adults: 1-2 tablets every 12 hours

**Dosage Forms** [DSC] = Discontinued product

Capsule, extended release: Brompheniramine maleate 6 mg and pseudoephedrine hydrochloride 60 mg; Brompheniramine maleate 12 mg and pseudoephedrine hydrochloride 120 mg

Bromfed® [DSC], Bromfenex®: Brompheniramine maleate 12 mg and pseudoephedrine hydrochloride 120 mg

Bromfed-PD® [DSC], Bromfenex® PD, Lodrane® LD: Brompheniramine maleate 6 mg and pseudoephedrine hydrochloride 60 mg

Histex™ SR: Brompheniramine maleate 10 mg and pseudoephedrine hydrochloride 120 mg

Capsule, sustained release (Touro™ Allergy): Brompheniramine maleate 5.75 mg and pseudoephedrine hydrochloride 60 mg

Elixir: Brompheniramine maleate 1 mg and pseudoephedrine hydrochloride 15 mg per 5 mL (120 mL, 480 mL)

Children's Dimetapp® Elixir Cold & Allergy: Brompheniramine maleate 1 mg and pseudoephedrine hydrochloride 15 mg per 5 mL (240 mL) [alcohol free; contains sodium benzoate; grape flavor]

Liquid (Lodrane®): Brompheniramine maleate 4 mg and pseudoephedrine hydrochloride 60 mg per 5 mL (480 mL) [alcohol free, dye free, sugar free; cherry flavor]

Liquid, oral drops (AccuHist® Pediatric [DSC], Bromhist Pediatric): Brompheniramine maleate 1 mg and pseudoephedrine hydrochloride 15 mg per 1 mL (30 mL) [contains sodium benzoate; cherry flavor]

Solution (Bromaline®): Brompheniramine maleate 1 mg and pseudoephedrine hydrochloride 15 mg per 5 mL (120 mL, 480 mL) [alcohol free; contains sodium benzoate; grape flavor]

Syrup: Brompheniramine maleate 4 mg and pseudoephedrine sulfate 45 mg per 5 mL (120 mL, 480 mL)

Andehist NR: Brompheniramine maleate 4 mg and pseudoephedrine sulfate 45 mg per 5 mL (473 mL) [raspberry flavor]

Brofed®: Brompheniramine maleate 4 mg and pseudoephedrine hydrochloride 30 mg per 5 mL(480 mL) [mint flavor]

Bromaxefed RF: Brompheniramine maleate 4 mg and pseudoephedrine hydrochloride 45 mg per 5 mL (120 mL, 480 mL) [alcohol free; cherry flavor]

Rondec®: Brompheniramine maleate 4 mg and pseudoephedrine hydrochloride 45 mg per 5 mL (120 mL, 480 mL) [cherry flavor]

Tablet, extended release (Lodrane® 12D): Brompheniramine maleate 6 mg and pseudoephedrine hydrochloride 45 mg

# brompheniramine maleate and pseudoephedrine hydrochloride *see* brompheniramine and pseudoephedrine *on previous page*

# brompheniramine maleate and pseudoephedrine sulfate *see* brompheniramine and pseudoephedrine *on previous page*

# brompheniramine, pseudoephedrine, and dextromethorphan

(brome fen IR a meen, soo doe e FED rin, & deks troe meth OR fan)

**Synonyms** brometane DX; dextromethorphan, brompheniramine, and pseudoephedrine; pseudoephedrine, dextromethorphan, and brompheniramine

**U.S./Canadian Brand Names** AccuHist® DM Pediatric Drops [US]; AccuHist® PDX Drops [US]; Anaplex® DM [US]; Andehist DM NR [US]; Bromaline® DM [US-OTC]; Bromaxefed DM RF [US]; Bromhist-DM [US]; Brotapp-DM [US]; Carbofed DM [US]; Dimaphen DM [US-OTC]; Dimetapp® DM Children's Cold and Cough [US-OTC]; EndaCof-DM [US]; EndaCof-PD [US]; PediaHist DM [US]; Rondec®-DM Syrup [US]

**Therapeutic Category** Antihistamine; Cough Preparation; Decongestant

**Use** Relief of cough and upper respiratory symptoms (including nasal congestion) associated with allergy or the common cold

**Usual Dosage**

Children:
  1-3 months (AccuHist® DM, AccuHist® PDX, EndaCof-PD): 0.25 mL 4 times/day
  3-6 months (AccuHist® DM, AccuHist® PDX, EndaCof-PD): 0.5 mL 4 times/day
  6-12 months (AccuHist® DM, AccuHist® PDX, EndaCof-PD): 0.75 mL 4 times/day

12-24 months (AccuHist® DM, AccuHist® PDX, EndaCof-PD): 1 mL 4 times/day
2-6 years:
  Anaplex® DM, EndaCof-DM: 1.25 mL every 4-6 hours (maximum: 4 doses/24 hours)
  Rondec®-DM: 2.5 mL 4 times/day
6-12 years:
  Anaplex® DM, EndaCof-DM: 2.5 mL every 4-6 hours (maximum: 4 doses/24 hours)
  Bromaline® DM, Dimaphen DM, Dimetapp® DM Children's Cough and Cold: 10 mL every 4-6 hours (maximum: 4 doses/24 hours)
  Rondec®-DM: Refer to Adults dosing
Children ≥12 years and Adults:
  Anaplex® DM: 5 mL every 4-6 hours (maximum: 4 doses/24 hours)
  Bromaline® DM, Dimaphen DM, Dimetapp® DM Children's Cough and Cold: 20 mL every 4-6 hours (maximum: 4 doses/24 hours)
  Rondec®-DM: 5 mL 4 times/day

## Dosage Forms

Elixir:
  Bromaline® DM: Brompheniramine maleate 1 mg, pseudoephedrine hydrochloride 15 mg, and dextromethorphan hydrobromide 5 mg per 5 mL (120 mL, 480 mL) [alcohol free; contains sodium benzoate; grape flavor]
  Dimetapp® DM Children's Cold and Cough: Brompheniramine maleate 1 mg, pseudoephedrine hydrochloride 15 mg, and dextromethorphan hydrobromide 5 mg per 5 mL (120 mL, 240 mL, 360 mL) [alcohol free; contains sodium benzoate; grape flavor]
  Dimaphen DM: Brompheniramine maleate 1 mg, pseudoephedrine hydrochloride 15 mg, and dextromethorphan hydrobromide 5 mg per 5 mL (120 mL)
  Q-Tapp DM: Brompheniramine maleate 1 mg, pseudoephedrine hydrochloride 15 mg, and dextromethorphan hydrobromide 5 mg per 5 mL (120 mL) [grape flavor]
Liquid:
  Brotapp-DM: Brompheniramine maleate 1 mg, pseudoephedrine hydrochloride 15 mg, and dextromethorphan hydrobromide 5 mg per 5 mL (120 mL, 240 mL) [grape flavor]
  Bromophed DX: Brompheniramine maleate 2 mg, pseudoephedrine hydrochloride 30 mg, and dextromethorphan hydrobromide 10 mg per 5 mL (480 mL) [butterscotch flavor]
Solution, oral drops: Brompheniramine maleate 1 mg, pseudoephedrine hydrochloride 15 mg, and dextromethorphan hydrobromide 4 mg per 1 mL (30 mL); Brompheniramine maleate 1 mg, pseudoephedrine hydrochloride 12.5 mg, and dextromethorphan hydrobromide 3 mg per 1 mL (30 mL)
  AccuHist® DM Pediatric: Brompheniramine maleate 1 mg, pseudoephedrine hydrochloride 15 mg, and dextromethorphan hydrobromide 4 mg per 1 mL (30 mL) [contains sodium benzoate; grape flavor]
  AccuHist® PDX: Brompheniramine maleate 1 mg, pseudoephedrine hydrochloride 12.5 mg, and dextromethorphan hydrobromide 3 mg per 1 mL (30 mL) [alcohol free, sugar free; contains sodium benzoate; grape flavor]
  Bromhist DM: Brompheniramine maleate 1 mg, pseudoephedrine hydrochloride 15 mg, and dextromethorphan hydrobromide 4 mg per 1 mL (30 mL) [grape flavor]
  Bromhist PDX, EndaCof-PD: Brompheniramine maleate 1 mg, pseudoephedrine hydrochloride 12.5 mg, and dextromethorphan hydrobromide 3 mg per 1 mL (30 mL) [grape flavor]
  Histacol DM Pediatric: Brompheniramine maleate 1 mg, pseudoephedrine hydrochloride 15 mg, and dextromethorphan hydrobromide 4 mg per 1 mL (30 mL)
  PediaHist DM: Brompheniramine maleate 1 mg, pseudoephedrine hydrochloride 15 mg, and dextromethorphan hydrobromide 4 mg per 1 mL (30 mL) [grape flavor]
Syrup: Brompheniramine maleate 4 mg, pseudoephedrine hydrobromide 60 mg, and dextromethorphan hydrochloride 30 mg per 5 mL (480 mL)
  Anaplex® DM: Brompheniramine maleate 4 mg, pseudoephedrine hydrobromide 60 mg, and dextromethorphan hydrochloride 30 mg per 5 mL (480 mL) [alcohol free, dye free, sugar free; fruit flavor]
  Andehist DM NR: Brompheniramine maleate 4 mg, pseudoephedrine hydrobromide 45 mg, and dextromethorphan hydrochloride 15 mg per 5 mL (480 mL) [grape flavor]
  Bromatane DX, Brometane DX: Brompheniramine maleate 2 mg, pseudoephedrine hydrobromide 30 mg, and dextromethorphan hydrochloride 10 mg per 5 mL (480 mL)
  Bromaxefed DM RF: Brompheniramine maleate 4 mg, pseudoephedrine hydrobromide 45 mg, and dextromethorphan hydrochloride 15 mg per 5 mL (120 mL, 240 mL, 480 mL) [alcohol free; grape flavor]
  Bromphenex DM: Brompheniramine maleate 4 mg, pseudoephedrine hydrochloride 60 mg, and dextromethorphan hydrobromide 30 mg per 5 mL (480 mL)
  Carbofed DM: Brompheniramine maleate 4 mg, pseudoephedrine hydrobromide 45 mg, and dextromethorphan hydrochloride 15 mg per 5 mL (480 mL) [alcohol free, sugar free; grape flavor]
(Continued)

## brompheniramine, pseudoephedrine, and dextromethorphan *(Continued)*

Cardec DM: Brompheniramine maleate 4 mg, pseudoephedrine hydrobromide 45 mg, and dextromethorphan hydrochloride 15 mg per 5 mL (120 mL, 480 mL) [grape flavor]

EndaCof-DM: Brompheniramine maleate 4 mg, pseudoephedrine hydrochloride 60 mg, and dextromethorphan hydrobromide 30 mg per 5 mL (480 mL) [alcohol free, dye free, sugar free; fruit flavor]

Rondec®-DM: Brompheniramine maleate 4 mg, pseudoephedrine hydrobromide 45 mg, and dextromethorphan hydrochloride 15 mg per 5 mL (120 mL, 480 mL) [contains sodium benzoate; grape flavor]

Sildec-DM: Brompheniramine maleate 4 mg, pseudoephedrine hydrobromide 45 mg, and dextromethorphan hydrochloride 15 mg per 5 mL (480 mL) [grape flavor]

**Brompheril®** *(Discontinued)* see dexbrompheniramine and pseudoephedrine on page 234

**Bronchial®** *(Discontinued)* see theophylline and guaifenesin on page 795

**Bronchial Mist®** *(Discontinued)* see epinephrine on page 287

**Broncho Saline®** **[US-OTC]** see sodium chloride on page 752

**Bronitin® Mist** *(Discontinued)* see epinephrine on page 287

**Brontex®** **[US]** see guaifenesin and codeine on page 384

**Brotane®** *(Discontinued)* see brompheniramine on page 115

**Brotapp-DM [US]** see brompheniramine, pseudoephedrine, and dextromethorphan on page 116

**BSS®** **[US/Can]** see balanced salt solution on page 88

**BSS Plus®** **[US/Can]** see balanced salt solution on page 88

**BTX-A** see botulinum toxin type A on page 111

**B-type natriuretic peptide (human)** see nesiritide on page 570

**Bubbli-Pred™ [US]** see prednisolone (systemic) on page 674

## budesonide (byoo DES oh nide)

**U.S./Canadian Brand Names** Entocort® [Can]; Entocort™ EC [US]; Gen-Budesonide AQ [Can]; Pulmicort Respules® [US]; Pulmicort Turbuhaler® [US]; Pulmicort® [Can]; Rhinocort® Aqua® [US]; Rhinocort® Turbuhaler® [Can]

**Therapeutic Category** Adrenal Corticosteroid

**Use**

Intranasal: Children ≥6 years of age and Adults: Management of symptoms of seasonal or perennial rhinitis

Nebulization: Children 12 months to 8 years: Maintenance and prophylactic treatment of asthma

Oral capsule: Treatment of active Crohn disease (mild to moderate) involving the ileum and/or ascending colon; maintenance of remission (for up to 3 months) of Crohn disease (mild to moderate) involving the ileum and/or ascending colon

Oral inhalation: Maintenance and prophylactic treatment of asthma; includes patients who require corticosteroids and those who may benefit from systemic dose reduction/elimination

**Usual Dosage**

Nasal inhalation: (Rhinocort® Aqua®): Children ≥6 years and Adults: 64 mcg/day as a single 32 mcg spray in each nostril. Some patients who do not achieve adequate control may benefit from increased dosage. A reduced dosage may be effective after initial control is achieved.

Maximum dose: Children <12 years: 128 mcg/day; Adults: 256 mcg/day

Nebulization: Children 12 months to 8 years: Pulmicort Respules®: Titrate to lowest effective dose once patient is stable; start at 0.25 mg/day or use as follows:

Previous therapy of bronchodilators alone: 0.5 mg/day administered as a single dose or divided twice daily (maximum daily dose: 0.5 mg)

Previous therapy of inhaled corticosteroids: 0.5 mg/day administered as a single dose or divided twice daily (maximum daily dose: 1 mg)

Previous therapy of oral corticosteroids: 1 mg/day administered as a single dose or divided twice daily (maximum daily dose: 1 mg)

Oral inhalation:

Children ≥6 years:

Previous therapy of bronchodilators alone: 200 mcg twice initially which may be increased up to 400 mcg twice daily

Previous therapy of inhaled corticosteroids: 200 mcg twice initially which may be increased up to 400 mcg twice daily

Previous therapy of oral corticosteroids: The highest recommended dose in children is 400 mcg twice daily

Adults:

Previous therapy of bronchodilators alone: 200-400 mcg twice initially which may be increased up to 400 mcg twice daily

Previous therapy of inhaled corticosteroids: 200-400 mcg twice initially which may be increased up to 800 mcg twice daily

Previous therapy of oral corticosteroids: 400-800 mcg twice daily which may be increased up to 800 mcg twice daily

NIH Guidelines (NIH, 1997) (give in divided doses twice daily):

Children:

"Low" dose: 100-200 mcg/day

"Medium" dose: 200-400 mcg/day (1-2 inhalations/day)

"High" dose: >400 mcg/day (>2 inhalation/day)

Adults:

"Low" dose: 200-400 mcg/day (1-2 inhalations/day)

"Medium" dose: 400-600 mcg/day (2-3 inhalations/day)

"High" dose: >600 mcg/day (>3 inhalation/day)

Oral: Adults: Crohn disease (active): 9 mg once daily in the morning for up to 8 weeks; recurring episodes may be treated with a repeat 8-week course of treatment

**Note:** Patients receiving CYP3A4 inhibitors should be monitored closely for signs and symptoms of hypercorticism; dosage reduction may be required. If switching from oral prednisolone, prednisolone dosage should be tapered while budesonide (Entocort™ EC) treatment is initiated.

Maintenance of remission: Following treatment of active disease (control of symptoms with CDAI <150), treatment may be continued at a dosage of 6 mg once daily for up to 3 months. If symptom control is maintained for 3 months, tapering of the dosage to complete cessation is recommended. Continued dosing beyond 3 months has not been demonstrated to result in substantial benefit.

**Dosage Forms**

Capsule, enteric coated (Entocort™ EC): 3 mg

Powder for oral inhalation (Pulmicort Turbuhaler®): 200 mcg/inhalation (104 g) [delivers ~160 mcg/inhalation; 200 metered doses]

Additional dosage strengths available in Canada: 100 mcg/inhalation, 400 mcg/inhalation

Suspension, nasal spray (Rhinocort® Aqua®): 32 mcg/inhalation (8.6 g) [120 metered doses]

Suspension for oral inhalation (Pulmicort Respules®): 0.25 mg/2 mL (30s), 0.5 mg/2 mL (30s)

**budesonide and eformoterol** *see* budesonide and formoterol *(Canada only)* on this page

# budesonide and formoterol *(Canada only)* (byoo DES oh nide & for MOH te rol)

**Synonyms** budesonide and eformoterol; eformoterol and budesonide; formoterol fumarate dehydrate and budesonide

**U.S./Canadian Brand Names** Symbicort® [Can]

**Therapeutic Category** Beta$_2$-Adrenergic Agonist Agent; Corticosteroid, Inhalant (Oral)

**Use** Treatment of asthma in patients ≥12 years of age where combination therapy is indicated

**Usual Dosage** Oral inhalation: Children ≥12 years and Adults: 1-2 inhalations once or twice daily

Maximum long-term maintenance dose: 4 inhalations/day; in periods of worsening asthma, this may be temporarily increased to 4 inhalations twice daily

Manufacturer's recommendation: Initial: Symbicort® 200 once or twice daily to establish symptom control. Following the establishment of response/symptom control: Titrate to the lowest dosage possible to maintain control (may substitute Symbicort® 100).

**Dosage Forms** Powder for oral inhalation:

Symbicort® 100 Turbuhaler®: Budesonide 100 mcg and formoterol dehydrate 6 mcg per inhalation (available in 60 or 120 metered doses) [delivers ~80 mcg budesonide and 4.5 mcg formoterol per inhalation; contains lactose]

Symbicort® 200 Turbuhaler®: Budesonide 200 mcg and formoterol dehydrate 6 mcg per inhalation (available in 60 or 120 metered doses) [delivers ~160 mcg budesonide and 4.5 mcg formoterol per inhalation; contains lactose]

**buffered aspirin and pravastatin sodium** *see* aspirin and pravastatin *on page 75*

**Bufferin® [US-OTC]** *see* aspirin *on page 73*

**Bufferin® Extra Strength [US-OTC]** *see* aspirin *on page 73*

**Buffinol [US-OTC]** *see* aspirin *on page 73*

**Buffinol Extra [US-OTC]** *see* aspirin *on page 73*

# bumetanide (byoo MET a nide)

**Sound-Alike/Look-Alike Issues**
bumetanide may be confused with Buminate®
Bumex® may be confused with Brevibloc®, Buprenex®, Permax®

**U.S./Canadian Brand Names** Bumex® [US/Can]; Burinex® [Can]

**Therapeutic Category** Diuretic, Loop

**Use** Management of edema secondary to congestive heart failure or hepatic or renal disease including nephrotic syndrome; may be used alone or in combination with antihypertensives in the treatment of hypertension; can be used in furosemide-allergic patients

**Usual Dosage**
Oral, I.M., I.V.:
Neonates: 0.01-0.05 mg/kg/dose every 24-48 hours
Infants and Children: 0.015-0.1 mg/kg/dose every 6-24 hours (maximum dose: 10 mg/day)
Adults:
Edema:
Oral: 0.5-2 mg/dose (maximum dose: 10 mg/day) 1-2 times/day
I.M., I.V.: 0.5-1 mg/dose; may repeat in 2-3 hours for up to 2 doses if needed (maximum dose: 10 mg/day)
Continuous I.V. infusion: 0.9-1 mg/hour
Hypertension: Oral: 0.5 mg daily (maximum dose: 5 mg/day); usual dosage range (JNC 7): 0.5-2 mg/day in 2 divided doses

**Dosage Forms**
Injection, solution: 0.25 mg/mL (2 mL, 4 mL, 10 mL) [contains benzyl alcohol]
Tablet (Bumex®): 0.5 mg, 1 mg, 2 mg

**Bumex® [US/Can]** *see* bumetanide *on this page*

**Bumex® Injection (Discontinued)** *see* bumetanide *on this page*

**Buminate® [US]** *see* albumin *on page 22*

**Buphenyl® [US]** *see* sodium phenylbutyrate *on page 756*

# bupivacaine (byoo PIV a kane)

**Sound-Alike/Look-Alike Issues**
bupivacaine may be confused with mepivacaine, ropivacaine
Marcaine® may be confused with Narcan®

**Synonyms** bupivacaine hydrochloride

**U.S./Canadian Brand Names** Marcaine® Spinal [US]; Marcaine® [US/Can]; Sensorcaine® [US/Can]; Sensorcaine®-MPF [US]

**Therapeutic Category** Local Anesthetic

**Use** Local anesthetic (injectable) for peripheral nerve block, infiltration, sympathetic block, caudal or epidural block, retrobulbar block

**Usual Dosage** Dose varies with procedure, depth of anesthesia, vascularity of tissues, duration of anesthesia and condition of patient. Some formulations contain metabisulfites (in epinephrine-containing injection); do not use solutions containing preservatives for caudal or epidural block.
Local anesthesia: Infiltration: 0.25% infiltrated locally; maximum: 175 mg
Caudal block (with or without epinephrine, preservative free):
Children: 1-3.7 mg/kg
Adults: 15-30 mL of 0.25% or 0.5%
Epidural block (other than caudal block - with or without epinephrine, preservative free):
Administer in 3-5 mL increments, allowing sufficient time to detect toxic manifestations of inadvertent I.V. or I.T. administration:
Children: 1.25 mg/kg/dose
Adults: 10-20 mL of 0.25% or 0.5%
Surgical procedures requiring a high degree of muscle relaxation and prolonged effects **only**: 10-20 mL of 0.75% (**Note:** Not to be used in obstetrical cases)
Maxillary and mandibular infiltration and nerve block: 9 mg (1.8 mL) of 0.5% (with epinephrine) per injection site; a second dose may be administered if necessary to produce adequate anesthesia after allowing up to 10 minutes for onset, up to a maximum of 90 mg per dental appointment

Obstetrical anesthesia: Incremental dose: 3-5 mL of 0.5% (not exceeding 50-100 mg in any dosing interval); allow sufficient time to detect toxic manifestations or inadvertent I.V. or I.T. injection

Peripheral nerve block: 5 mL of 0.25 or 0.5%; maximum: 400 mg/day

Sympathetic nerve block: 20-50 mL of 0.25%

Retrobulbar anesthesia: 2-4 mL of 0.75%

Spinal anesthesia: Solution of 0.75% bupivacaine in 8.25% dextrose is used:

Lower extremity and perineal procedures: 1 mL

Lower abdominal procedures: 1.6 mL

Obstetrical:

Normal vaginal delivery: 0.8 mL (higher doses may be required in some patients)

Cesarean section: 1-1.4 mL

## Dosage Forms

Injection, solution, as hydrochloride [preservative free]: 0.25% [2.5 mg/mL] (10 mL, 20 mL, 30 mL, 50 mL); 0.5% [5 mg/mL] (10 mL, 20 mL, 30 mL); 0.75% [7.5 mg/mL] (10 mL, 20 mL, 30 mL)

Marcaine®: 0.25% [2.5 mg/mL] (10 mL, 30 mL, 50 mL); 0.5% [5 mg/mL] (10 mL, 30 mL); 0.75% [7.5 mg/mL] (10 mL, 30 mL)

Marcaine® Spinal: 0.75% [7.5 mg/mL] (2 mL) [in dextrose 8.25%]

Sensorcaine®-MPF: 0.25% [2.5 mg/mL] (10 mL, 30 mL); 0.5% [5 mg/mL] (10 mL, 30 mL); 0.75% [7.5 mg/mL] (10 mL, 30 mL)

Injection, solution, as hydrochloride (Marcaine®, Sensorcaine®): 0.25% [2.5 mg/mL] (50 mL); 0.5% [5 mg/mL] (50 mL) [contains methylparaben]

Injection, solution, with epinephrine 1:200,000, as hydrochloride [preservative free]: 0.25% [2.5 mg/mL] (10 mL, 30 mL); 0.5 % [5 mg/mL] (30 mL)

Marcaine®: 0.25% [2.5 mg/mL] (10 mL, 30 mL); 0.5% [5 mg/mL] (3 mL, 10 mL, 30 mL); 0.75% [7.5 mg/mL] (30 mL) [contains sodium metabisulfite]

Sensorcaine®-MPF: 0.25% [2.5 mg/mL] (10 mL, 30 mL); 0.5% [5 mg/mL] (10 mL, 30 mL); 0.75% [7.5 mg/mL] (30 mL) [contains sodium metabisulfite]

Injection, solution, with epinephrine 1:200,000, as hydrochloride [with preservative] (Marcaine®, Sensorcaine®): 0.25% [2.5 mg/mL] (50 mL); 0.5% [5 mg/mL] (50 mL) [contains methylparaben and sodium metabisulfite]

**bupivacaine hydrochloride** *see* bupivacaine *on previous page*

**Buprenex® [US/Can]** *see* buprenorphine *on this page*

# buprenorphine (byoo pre NOR feen)

## Sound-Alike/Look-Alike Issues

Buprenex® may be confused with Brevibloc®, Bumex®

**Synonyms** buprenorphine hydrochloride

**U.S./Canadian Brand Names** Buprenex® [US/Can]; Subutex® [US/Can]

**Therapeutic Category** Analgesic, Narcotic

**Controlled Substance** Injection: C-V; Tablet: C-III

## Use

Injection: Management of moderate to severe pain

Tablet: Treatment of opioid dependence

## Usual Dosage Long-term use is not recommended

**Note:** These are guidelines and do not represent the maximum doses that may be required in all patients. Doses should be titrated to pain relief/prevention. In high-risk patients (eg, elderly, debilitated, presence of respiratory disease) and/or concurrent CNS depressant use, reduce dose by one-half. Buprenorphine has an analgesic ceiling.

Acute pain (moderate to severe):

Children 2-12 years: I.M., slow I.V.: 2-6 mcg/kg every 4-6 hours

Children ≥13 years and Adults:

I.M.: Initial: Opiate-naive: 0.3 mg every 6-8 hours as needed; initial dose (up to 0.3 mg) may be repeated once in 30-60 minutes after the initial dose if needed; usual dosage range: 0.15-0.6 mg every 4-8 hours as needed

Slow I.V.: Initial: Opiate-naive: 0.3 mg every 6-8 hours as needed; initial dose (up to 0.3 mg) may be repeated once in 30-60 minutes after the initial dose if needed

Sublingual: Children ≥16 years and Adults: Opioid dependence:

Induction: Range: 12-16 mg/day (doses during an induction study used 8 mg on day 1, followed by 16 mg on day 2; induction continued over 3-4 days). Treatment should begin at least 4 hours after last use of heroin or short-acting opioid, preferably when first signs of withdrawal appear. Titrating dose to (Continued)

# buprenorphine *(Continued)*

clinical effectiveness should be done as rapidly as possible to prevent undue withdrawal symptoms and patient drop-out during the induction period.

Maintenance: Target dose: 16 mg/day; range: 4-24 mg/day; patients should be switched to the buprenorphine/naloxone combination product for maintenance and unsupervised therapy

**Dosage Forms**
Injection, solution (Buprenex®): 0.3 mg/mL (1 mL)
Tablet, sublingual (Subutex®): 2 mg, 8 mg
Additional dosage strength available in Canada: 0.4 mg

# buprenorphine and naloxone *(byoo pre NOR feen & nal OKS one)*

**Synonyms** buprenorphine hydrochloride and naloxone hydrochloride dihydrate; naloxone and buprenorphine; naloxone hydrochloride dihydrate and buprenorphine hydrochloride

**U.S./Canadian Brand Names** Suboxone® [US]

**Therapeutic Category** Analgesic, Narcotic

**Controlled Substance** C-III

**Use** Treatment of opioid dependence

**Usual Dosage** Sublingual: Children ≥16 years and Adults: Opioid dependence: **Note:** This combination product is not recommended for use during the induction period; initial treatment should begin using buprenorphine oral tablets. Patients should be switched to the combination product for maintenance and unsupervised therapy.

Maintenance: Target dose (based on buprenorphine content): 16 mg/day; range: 4-24 mg/day

**Dosage Forms** Tablet, sublingual: Buprenorphine 2 mg and naloxone 0.5 mg; buprenorphine 8 mg and naloxone 2 mg [lemon-lime flavor]

**buprenorphine hydrochloride** *see* buprenorphine *on previous page*

**buprenorphine hydrochloride and naloxone hydrochloride dihydrate** *see* buprenorphine and naloxone *on this page*

# bupropion *(byoo PROE pee on)*

**Sound-Alike/Look-Alike Issues**
buPROPion may be confused with busPIRone
Wellbutrin SR® may be confused with Wellbutrin XL™
Wellbutrin XL™ may be confused with Wellbutrin SR®
Zyban® may be confused with Zagam®

**Tall-Man** buPROPion

**U.S./Canadian Brand Names** Novo-Bupropion SR [Can]; Wellbutrin SR® [US]; Wellbutrin XL™ [US]; Wellbutrin® [US/Can]; Zyban® [US/Can]

**Therapeutic Category** Antidepressant, Aminoketone

**Use** Treatment of depression; adjunct in smoking cessation

**Usual Dosage** Oral: Adults:
Depression:
Immediate release: 100 mg 3 times/day; begin at 100 mg twice daily; may increase to a maximum dose of 450 mg/day
Sustained release: Initial: 150 mg/day in the morning; may increase to 150 mg twice daily by day 4 if tolerated; target dose: 300 mg/day given as 150 mg twice daily; maximum dose: 400 mg/day given as 200 mg twice daily
Extended release: Initial: 150 mg/day in the morning; may increase as early as day 4 of dosing to 300 mg/day; maximum dose: 450 mg/day
Smoking cessation (Zyban®): Initiate with 150 mg once daily for 3 days; increase to 150 mg twice daily; treatment should continue for 7-12 weeks

**Dosage Forms**
Tablet, as hydrochloride (Wellbutrin®): 75 mg, 100 mg
Tablet, extended release, as hydrochloride (Wellbutrin XL™): 150 mg, 300 mg
Tablet, sustained release, as hydrochloride: 100 mg, 150 mg [equivalent to Wellbutrin® SR], 150 mg [equivalent to Zyban®]
Wellbutrin® SR: 100 mg, 150 mg, 200 mg
Zyban®: 150 mg

**Burinex® [Can]** *see* bumetanide *on page 120*

**Burnamycin [US-OTC]** *see* lidocaine *on page 479*

**Burn Jel [US-OTC]** *see* lidocaine *on page 479*

**Burn-O-Jel [US-OTC]** *see* lidocaine *on page 479*

**Buscopan® [Can]** *see* scopolamine derivatives *on page 740*

## buserelin acetate *(Canada only)* (BYOO se rel in AS e tate)

**Therapeutic Category** Luteinizing Hormone-Releasing Hormone Analog

**Use** For the palliative treatment of patients with hormone-dependent advanced carcinoma of the prostate gland (Stage D). Buserelin is also indicated for the treatment of endometriosis in patients who do not require surgery as primary therapy. The duration of treatment is usually 6 months and should not exceed 9 months. Experience with buserelin for the management of endometriosis has been limited to women 18 years of age and older.

**Usual Dosage** Buserelin should be administered at approximately equal time intervals to ensure that the desired therapeutic effect is maintained.

Prostatic Cancer: Initial Treatment: For the first 7 days of treatment give buserelin 500 mcg (0.5 mL) every 8 hours by SubQ injection. For patient comfort, vary the injection site.

Maintenance Treatment: Depending upon patient preference, or physician recommendation, maintenance treatment may be by daily SubQ injection or by intranasal administration 3 times daily. During maintenance dosing by the SubQ route, the buserelin dose is 200 mcg (0.2 mL) daily. For patient comfort, vary the site of injection.

During maintenance dosing by the intranasal administration route, the buserelin dose is 400 mcg (200 mcg into each nostril) 3 times daily using the metered-dose pump (nebulizer) provided. Each pump action delivers 100 mcg buserelin acetate or 0.1mL solution.

Endometriosis: The dose of buserelin in patients with endometriosis is 400 mcg (200 mcg into each nostril) 3 times daily using the metered-dose pump (nebulizer) provided. Each pump action delivers 100 mcg or 0.1 mL solution. The treatment duration is usually 6 months and should not exceed 9 months.

**Dosage Forms** Injection, depot: 6.6 mg [2 month]; 9.9 mg [3 month]

**BuSpar® [US/Can]** *see* buspirone *on this page*

**Buspirex [Can]** *see* buspirone *on this page*

## buspirone (byoo SPYE rone)

**Sound-Alike/Look-Alike Issues**

busPIRone may be confused with buPROPion

**Synonyms** buspirone hydrochloride

**Tall-Man** busPIRone

**U.S./Canadian Brand Names** Apo-Buspirone® [Can]; BuSpar® [US/Can]; Buspirex [Can]; Gen-Buspirone [Can]; Lin-Buspirone [Can]; Novo-Buspirone [Can]; Nu-Buspirone [Can]; PMS-Buspirone [Can]

**Therapeutic Category** Antianxiety Agent

**Use** Management of generalized anxiety disorder (GAD)

**Usual Dosage** Oral: Generalized anxiety disorder:

Children and Adolescents: Initial: 5 mg daily; increase in increments of 5 mg/day at weekly intervals as needed, to a maximum dose of 60 mg/day divided into 2-3 doses

Adults: 15 mg/day (7.5 mg twice daily); may increase in increments of 5 mg/day every 2-4 days to a maximum of 60 mg/day; target dose for most people is 30 mg/day (15 mg twice daily)

**Dosage Forms**

Tablet, as hydrochloride: 5 mg, 7.5 mg, 10 mg, 15 mg, 30 mg

BuSpar®: 5 mg, 10 mg, 15 mg, 30 mg

**buspirone hydrochloride** *see* buspirone *on this page*

## busulfan (byoo SUL fan)

**Sound-Alike/Look-Alike Issues**

busulfan may be confused with Butalan®

Myleran® may be confused with melphalan, Mylicon®

**U.S./Canadian Brand Names** Busultex® [US/Can]; Myleran® [US/Can]

**Therapeutic Category** Antineoplastic Agent

**Use**

Oral: Chronic myelogenous leukemia; conditioning regimens for bone marrow transplantation
(Continued)

# busulfan *(Continued)*

I.V.: Combination therapy with cyclophosphamide as a conditioning regimen prior to allogeneic hemato-poietic progenitor cell transplantation for chronic myelogenous leukemia

**Usual Dosage** Busulfan should be based on adjusted ideal body weight because actual body weight, ideal body weight, or other factors can produce significant differences in busulfan clearance among lean, normal, and obese patients; refer to individual protocols

Children:

For remission induction of CML: Oral: 0.06-0.12 mg/kg/day **OR** 1.8-4.6 mg/m$^2$/day; titrate dosage to maintain leukocyte count above 40,000/mm$^3$; reduce dosage by 50% if the leukocyte count reaches 30,000-40,000/mm$^3$; discontinue drug if counts fall to ≤20,000/mm$^3$

BMT marrow-ablative conditioning regimen:

Oral: 1 mg/kg/dose (ideal body weight) every 6 hours for 16 doses

I.V.:

≤12 kg: 1.1 mg/kg/dose (ideal body weight) every 6 hours for 16 doses

>12 kg: 0.8 mg/kg/dose (ideal body weight) every 6 hours for 16 doses

Adjust dose to desired AUC [1125 μmol(min)] using the following formula:

Adjusted dose (mg) = Actual dose (mg) x [target AUC μmol(min) / actual AUC μmol(min)]

Adults:

For remission induction of CML: Oral: 4-8 mg/day (may be as high as 12 mg/day); Maintenance doses: Controversial, range from 1-4 mg/day to 2 mg/week; treatment is continued until WBC reaches 10,000-20,000 cells/mm$^3$ at which time drug is discontinued; when WBC reaches 50,000/mm$^3$, maintenance dose is resumed

BMT marrow-ablative conditioning regimen:

Oral: 1 mg/kg/dose (ideal body weight) every 6 hours for 16 doses

I.V.: 0.8 mg/kg (ideal body weight or actual body weight, whichever is lower) every 6 hours for 4 days (a total of 16 doses)

I.V. dosing in morbidly obese patients: Dosing should be based on adjusted ideal body weight (AIBW) which should be calculated as ideal body weight (IBW) + 0.25 times (actual weight minus ideal body weight)

AIBW = IBW + 0.25 x (AW - IBW)

**Dosage Forms**

Injection, solution (Busulfex®): 6 mg/mL (10 mL)

Tablet (Myleran®): 2 mg

**Busulfex® [US/Can]** *see* busulfan *on previous page*

# butabarbital sodium *(byoo ta BAR bi tal SOW dee um)*

**Sound-Alike/Look-Alike Issues**

butabarbital may be confused with butalbital

**U.S./Canadian Brand Names** Butisol Sodium® [US]

**Therapeutic Category** Barbiturate

**Controlled Substance** C-III

**Use** Sedative; hypnotic

**Usual Dosage** Oral:

Children: Preoperative sedation: 2-6 mg/kg/dose (maximum: 100 mg)

Adults:

Sedative: 15-30 mg 3-4 times/day

Hypnotic: 50-100 mg

Preop: 50-100 mg 1-1½ hours before surgery

**Dosage Forms**

Elixir, as sodium: 30 mg/5 mL (480 mL) [contains alcohol 7% and tartrazine]

Tablet, as sodium: 30 mg, 50 mg [contains tartrazine]

**Butalan® *(Discontinued)***

# butalbital, acetaminophen, and caffeine

*(byoo TAL bi tal, a seet a MIN oh fen, & KAF een)*

**Sound-Alike/Look-Alike Issues**

Fioricet® may be confused with Fiorinal®, Lorcet®

Repan® may be confused with Riopan®

Synonyms acetaminophen, butalbital, and caffeine

U.S./Canadian Brand Names Anolor 300 [US]; Dolgic® LQ [US]; Dolgic® Plus [US]; Esgic-Plus™ [US]; Esgic® [US]; Fioricet® [US]; Medigesic® [US]; Repan® [US]; Zebutal™ [US]

Therapeutic Category Barbiturate/Analgesic

Use Relief of the symptomatic complex of tension or muscle contraction headache

Usual Dosage Adults: Oral: 1-2 tablets or capsules (or 15-30 mL elixir) every 4 hours; not to exceed 6 tablets or capsules (or 180 mL elixir) daily

Dosage Forms
Capsule:
Anolor 300, Esgic®, Medigesic®: Butalbital 50 mg, caffeine 40 mg, and acetaminophen 325 mg
Dolgic® Plus: Butalbital 50 mg, caffeine 40 mg, and acetaminophen 750 mg
Esgic-Plus™, Zebutal™: Butalbital 50 mg, caffeine 40 mg, and acetaminophen 500 mg
Elixir (Dolgic® LQ): Butalbital 50 mg, caffeine 40 mg, and acetaminophen 325 mg per 15 mL (480 mL) [contains alcohol 7%; fruit flavor]
Tablet: Butalbital 50 mg, caffeine 40 mg, and acetaminophen 325 mg; butalbital 50 mg, caffeine 40 mg, and acetaminophen 500 mg
Esgic®, Fioricet®, Repan®: Butalbital 50 mg, caffeine 40 mg, and acetaminophen 325 mg

## butalbital, aspirin, and caffeine (byoo TAL bi tal, AS pir in, & KAF een)

Sound-Alike/Look-Alike Issues
Fiorinal® may be confused with Fioricet®, Florical®, Florinef®

Synonyms aspirin, caffeine, and butalbital; butalbital compound

U.S./Canadian Brand Names Fiorinal® [US/Can]

Therapeutic Category Barbiturate/Analgesic

Controlled Substance C-III

Use Relief of the symptomatic complex of tension or muscle contraction headache

Usual Dosage Oral: Adults: 1-2 tablets or capsules every 4 hours; not to exceed 6/day

Dosage Forms Capsule: Butalbital 50 mg, caffeine 40 mg, and aspirin 325 mg

## butalbital, aspirin, caffeine, and codeine
(byoo TAL bi tal, AS pir in, KAF een, & KOE deen)

Sound-Alike/Look-Alike Issues
Fiorinal® may be confused with Fioricet®, Florical®, Florinef®
Phrenilin® may be confused with Phenergan®, Trinalin®

Synonyms butalbital compound and codeine; codeine and butalbital compound; codeine, butalbital, aspirin, and caffeine

U.S./Canadian Brand Names Fiorinal® With Codeine [US]; Fiorinal®-C 1/2 [Can]; Fiorinal®-C 1/4 [Can]; Phrenilin® With Caffeine and Codeine [US]; Tecnal C 1/2 [Can]; Tecnal C 1/4 [Can]

Therapeutic Category Analgesic, Narcotic; Barbiturate

Controlled Substance C-III

Use Mild to moderate pain when sedation is needed

Usual Dosage Adults: Oral: 1-2 capsules every 4 hours as needed for pain; up to 6/day

Dosage Forms
Capsule: Butalbital 50 mg, caffeine 40 mg, aspirin 325 mg, and codeine phosphate 30 mg
Fioricet® with Codeine: Butalbital 50 mg, caffeine 40 mg, acetaminophen 325 mg, and codeine phosphate 30 mg [may contain benzyl alcohol]
Phrenilin® with Caffeine and Codeine: Butalbital 50 mg, caffeine 40 mg, acetaminophen 325 mg, and codeine phosphate 30 mg [contains benzyl alcohol and lactose]

**butalbital compound** see butalbital, aspirin, and caffeine on this page

**butalbital compound and codeine** see butalbital, aspirin, caffeine, and codeine on this page

## butenafine (byoo TEN a feen)

Sound-Alike/Look-Alike Issues
lotrimin may be confused with Lotrisone®, Otrivin®

Synonyms butenafine hydrochloride

U.S./Canadian Brand Names Lotrimin® Ultra™ [US-OTC]; Mentax® [US]

Therapeutic Category Antifungal Agent

Use Topical treatment of tinea pedis (athlete's foot), tinea cruris (jock itch), tinea corporis (ringworm), and tinea versicolor
(Continued)

125

# butenafine (Continued)

**Usual Dosage** Children >12 years and Adults: Topical:
Tinea corporis, tinea cruris, or tinea versicolor: Apply once daily for 2 weeks to affected area and surrounding skin
Tinea pedis: Apply once daily for 4 weeks or twice daily for 7 days to affected area and surrounding skin (7-day regimen may have lower efficacy)
**Dosage Forms** Cream, as hydrochloride:
Lotrimin® Ultra™: 1% (12 g, 24 g) [contains benzyl alcohol and sodium benzoate]
Mentax®: 1% (15 g, 30 g) [contains benzyl alcohol and sodium benzoate]

**butenafine hydrochloride** see butenafine on previous page

**Buticaps® (Discontinued)**

**Butisol Sodium® [US]** see butabarbital sodium on page 124

# butoconazole (byoo toe KOE na zole)
**Sound-Alike/Look-Alike Issues**
Mycelex® may be confused with Myoflex®
**Synonyms** butoconazole nitrate
**U.S./Canadian Brand Names** Femstat® One [Can]; Gynazole-1® [US/Can]; Mycelex®-3 [US-OTC]
**Therapeutic Category** Antifungal Agent
**Use** Local treatment of vulvovaginal candidiasis
**Usual Dosage** Adults: Female:
Femstat®-3 [OTC]: Insert 1 applicatorful (~5 g) intravaginally at bedtime for 3 consecutive days
Gynazole-1®: Insert 1 applicatorful (~5 g) intravaginally as a single dose; treatment may need to be extended for up to 6 days in pregnant women (use in pregnancy during 2nd or 3rd trimester only)
**Dosage Forms** Cream, vaginal, as nitrate:
Mycelex®-3: 2% (5 g) [prefilled applicator], (20 g) [with disposable applicator]
Gynazole-1®: 2% (5 g) [prefilled applicator]

**butoconazole nitrate** see butoconazole on this page

# butorphanol (byoo TOR fa nole)
**Sound-Alike/Look-Alike Issues**
Stadol® may be confused with Haldol®, sotalol
**Synonyms** butorphanol tartrate
**U.S./Canadian Brand Names** Apo-Butorphanol® [Can]; PMS-Butorphanol [Can]; Stadol® [US]
**Therapeutic Category** Analgesic, Narcotic
**Controlled Substance** C-IV
**Use**
Parenteral: Management of moderate to severe pain; preoperative medication; supplement to balanced anesthesia; management of pain during labor
Nasal spray: Management of moderate to severe pain, including migraine headache pain
**Usual Dosage Note:** These are guidelines and do not represent the maximum doses that may be required in all patients. Doses should be titrated to pain relief/prevention. Butorphanol has an analgesic ceiling.
Adults:
**Parenteral:**
Acute pain (moderate to severe):
I.M.: Initial: 2 mg, may repeat every 3-4 hours as needed; usual range: 1-4 mg every 3-4 hours as needed
I.V.: Initial: 1 mg, may repeat every 3-4 hours as needed; usual range: 0.5-2 mg every 3-4 hours as needed
Preoperative medication: I.M.: 2 mg 60-90 minutes before surgery
Supplement to balanced anesthesia: I.V.: 2 mg shortly before induction and/or an incremental dose of 0.5-1 mg (up to 0.06 mg/kg), depending on previously administered sedative, analgesic, and hypnotic medications
Pain during labor (fetus >37 weeks gestation and no signs of fetal distress):
I.M., I.V.: 1-2 mg; may repeat in 4 hours
**Note:** Alternative analgesia should be used for pain associated with delivery or if delivery is anticipated within 4 hours

**Nasal spray:**
Moderate to severe pain (including migraine headache pain): Initial: 1 spray (~1 mg per spray) in 1 nostril; if adequate pain relief is not achieved within 60-90 minutes, an additional 1 spray in 1 nostril may be given; may repeat initial dose sequence in 3-4 hours after the last dose as needed

Alternatively, an initial dose of 2 mg (1 spray in each nostril) may be used in patients who will be able to remain recumbent (in the event drowsiness or dizziness occurs); additional 2 mg doses should not be given for 3-4 hours

**Note:** In some clinical trials, an initial dose of 2 mg (as 2 doses 1 hour apart or 2 mg initially - 1 spray in each nostril) has been used, followed by 1 mg in 1 hour; side effects were greater at these dosages

Dosage Forms [DSC] Discontinued product
Injection, solution, as tartrate [preservative free] (Stadol®): 1 mg/mL (1 mL); 2 mg/mL (1 mL, 2 mL)
Injection, solution, as tartrate [with preservative] (Stadol®): 2 mg/mL (10 mL)
Solution, intranasal spray, as tartrate: 10 mg/mL (2.5 mL) [14-15 doses]
Stadol® NS [DSC]: 10 mg/mL (2.5 mL)

**butorphanol tartrate** *see* butorphanol *on previous page*

**B vitamin combinations** *see* vitamin B complex combinations *on page 849*

**BW-430C** *see* lamotrigine *on page 465*

**BW524W91** *see* emtricitabine *on page 282*

**Byclomine® Injection *(Discontinued)*** *see* dicyclomine *on page 245*

**Bydramine® Cough Syrup *(Discontinued)*** *see* diphenhydramine *on page 254*

**Byetta™ [US]** *see* exenatide *on page 324*

**C2B8** *see* rituximab *on page 726*

**C2B8 monoclonal antibody** *see* rituximab *on page 726*

**C7E3** *see* abciximab *on page 3*

**C8-CCK** *see* sincalide *on page 749*

**311C90** *see* zolmitriptan *on page 863*

**C225** *see* cetuximab *on page 163*

**C-500-GR™ [US-OTC]** *see* ascorbic acid *on page 71*

## cabergoline (ca BER goe leen)

U.S./Canadian Brand Names Dostinex® [US/Can]
Therapeutic Category Ergot-like Derivative
Use Treatment of hyperprolactinemic disorders, either idiopathic or due to pituitary adenomas
Usual Dosage Oral: Initial dose: 0.25 mg twice weekly; the dose may be increased by 0.25 mg twice weekly up to a maximum of 1 mg twice weekly according to the patient's serum prolactin level. Dosage increases should not occur more rapidly than every 4 weeks. Once a normal serum prolactin level is maintained for 6 months, the dose may be discontinued and prolactin levels monitored to determine if cabergoline is still required. The durability of efficacy beyond 24 months of therapy has not been established.
Dosage Forms Tablet: 0.5 mg

**Ca-DTPA** *see* diethylene triamine penta-acetic acid *on page 246*

**Caduet® [US]** *see* amlodipine and atorvastatin *on page 44*

**Caelyx® [Can]** *see* doxorubicin (liposomal) *on page 271*

**Cafatine-PB® *(Discontinued)*** *see* ergotamine *on page 294*

**Cafcit® [US/Can]** *see* caffeine (citrated) *on next page*

**Cafetrate® *(Discontinued)*** *see* ergotamine *on page 294*

**caffeine, acetaminophen, and aspirin** *see* acetaminophen, aspirin, and caffeine *on page 9*

## caffeine and sodium benzoate (KAF een & SOW dee um BEN zoe ate)

Synonyms sodium benzoate and caffeine
Therapeutic Category Diuretic, Miscellaneous
Use Emergency stimulant in acute circulatory failure; as a diuretic; and to relieve spinal puncture headache
(Continued)

## caffeine and sodium benzoate *(Continued)*

**Usual Dosage**
Children: I.M., I.V., S.C.: 8 mg/kg every 4 hours as needed
Adults: I.M., I.V.: 500 mg, maximum single dose: 1 g

**Dosage Forms** Injection, solution: Caffeine 121 mg and sodium benzoate 129 mg per mL (2 mL); caffeine 125 mg and sodium benzoate 125 mg per mL (2 mL)

**caffeine, aspirin, and acetaminophen** *see* acetaminophen, aspirin, and caffeine *on page 9*

## caffeine (citrated) (KAF een SIT rated)
**U.S./Canadian Brand Names** Cafcit® [US/Can]
**Therapeutic Category** Respiratory Stimulant; Stimulant
**Use** Central nervous system stimulant; used in the treatment of apnea of prematurity (28 to <33 weeks gestational age). Has several advantages over theophylline in the treatment of neonatal apnea, its half-life is about 3 times as long, allowing once daily dosing, drug levels do not need to be drawn at peak and trough; has a wider therapeutic window, allowing more room between an effective concentration and toxicity.
**Usual Dosage** Apnea of prematurity: Neonates:
Loading dose (usually administered I.V.): 10-20 mg/kg as caffeine citrate (5-10 mg/kg as caffeine base). If theophylline has been administered to the patient within the previous 3 days, a full or modified loading dose (50% to 75% of a loading dose) may be given (caffeine is a significant metabolite of theophylline in the newborn).
Maintenance dose: Oral, I.V.: 5 mg/kg/day as caffeine citrate (2.5 mg/kg/day as caffeine base) once daily starting 24 hours after the loading dose. Maintenance dose is adjusted based on patient's response (efficacy and adverse effects), and serum caffeine concentrations.
**Dosage Forms**
Injection: 20 mg/mL as caffeine citrate [equivalent to 10 mg/mL caffeine base] (3 mL)
Solution, oral: 20 mg/mL as caffeine citrate [equivalent to 10 mg/mL caffeine base] (3 mL)

**caffeine, hydrocodone, chlorpheniramine, phenylephrine, and acetaminophen** *see* hydrocodone, chlorpheniramine, phenylephrine, acetaminophen, and caffeine *on page 414*

**caffeine, orphenadrine, and aspirin** *see* orphenadrine, aspirin, and caffeine *on page 603*

**caffeine, propoxyphene, and aspirin** *see* propoxyphene, aspirin, and caffeine *on page 688*

**Caladryl® Clear [US-OTC]** *see* pramoxine *on page 670*

**CalaMycin® Cool and Clear [US-OTC]** *see* pramoxine *on page 670*

**Calan® [US/Can]** *see* verapamil *on page 843*

**Calan® SR [US]** *see* verapamil *on page 843*

**Calcarb 600 [US-OTC]** *see* calcium carbonate *on page 130*

**Calcibind® [US/Can]** *see* cellulose sodium phosphate *on page 160*

**Calci-Chew® [US-OTC]** *see* calcium carbonate *on page 130*

**Calciday-667® *(Discontinued)*** *see* calcium carbonate *on page 130*

**Calciferol™ [US]** *see* ergocalciferol *on page 292*

**Calcijex® [US/Can]** *see* calcitriol *on next page*

**Calcimar® [Can]** *see* calcitonin *on next page*

**Calcimar® *(Discontinued)*** *see* calcitonin *on next page*

**Calci-Mix® [US-OTC]** *see* calcium carbonate *on page 130*

## calcipotriene (kal si POE try een)
**U.S./Canadian Brand Names** Dovonex® [US]
**Therapeutic Category** Antipsoriatic Agent
**Use** Treatment of plaque psoriasis
**Usual Dosage** Topical: Adults: Apply in a thin film to the affected skin twice daily and rub in gently and completely
**Dosage Forms**
Cream: 0.005% (60 g, 120 g)
Ointment: 0.005% (60 g, 120 g)
Solution, topical: 0.005% (60 mL)

**calcipotriol and betamethasone dipropionate** *see* betamethasone and calcipotriol *(Canada only) on page 102*

**Calcite-500 [Can]** *see* calcium carbonate *on next page*

# calcitonin (kal si TOE nin)
### Sound-Alike/Look-Alike Issues
calcitonin may be confused with calcitriol
Miacalcin® may be confused with Micatin®
**Synonyms** calcitonin (salmon)
**U.S./Canadian Brand Names** Apo-Calcitonin® [Can]; Calcimar® [Can]; Caltine® [Can]; Miacalcin® NS [Can]; Miacalcin® [US]
**Therapeutic Category** Polypeptide Hormone
**Use** Calcitonin (salmon): Treatment of Paget's disease of bone (osteitis deformans); adjunctive therapy for hypercalcemia; postmenopausal osteoporosis
**Usual Dosage** Salmon calcitonin:
Children: Dosage not established
Adults:
Paget's disease: I.M., SubQ: Initial: 100 units/day; maintenance: 50 units/day or 50-100 units every 1-3 days
Hypercalcemia: I.M., SubQ: Initial: 4 units/kg every 12 hours; may increase up to 8 units/kg every 12 hours to a maximum of every 6 hours
Osteogenesis imperfecta: I.M., SubQ: 2 units/kg 3 times/week
Postmenopausal osteoporosis:
I.M., SubQ: 100 units/day
Intranasal: 200 units (1 spray)/day
### Dosage Forms
Injection, solution, calcitonin-salmon: (Miacalcin®): 200 int. units/mL (2 mL)
Solution, nasal spray, calcitonin-salmon:
Fortical®: 200 int. units/0.09 mL (3.7 mL) [rDNA origin; contains benzyl alcohol; delivers 30 doses, 200 units/actuation]
Miacalcin®: 200 int. units/0.09 mL (3.7 mL) [contains benzalkonium chloride; delivers 30 doses, 200 units/actuation]

**calcitonin (salmon)** *see* calcitonin *on this page*

**Cal-Citrate® 250 [US-OTC]** *see* calcium citrate *on page 133*

# calcitriol (kal si TRYE ole)
### Sound-Alike/Look-Alike Issues
calcitriol may be confused with calcifediol, Calciferol®, calcitonin
**Synonyms** 1,25 dihydroxycholecalciferol
**U.S./Canadian Brand Names** Calcijex® [US/Can]; Rocaltrol® [US/Can]
**Therapeutic Category** Vitamin D Analog
**Use** Management of hypocalcemia in patients on chronic renal dialysis; management of secondary hyperparathyroidism in moderate-to-severe chronic renal failure; management of hypocalcemia in hypoparathyroidism and pseudohypoparathyroidism
**Usual Dosage** Individualize dosage to maintain calcium levels of 9-10 mg/dL
Renal failure:
Children:
Oral: 0.25-2 mcg/day have been used (with hemodialysis); 0.014-0.041 mcg/kg/day (not receiving hemodialysis); increases should be made at 4- to 8-week intervals
I.V.: 0.01-0.05 mcg/kg 3 times/week if undergoing hemodialysis
Adults:
Oral: 0.25 mcg/day or every other day (may require 0.5-1 mcg/day); increases should be made at 4- to 8-week intervals
I.V.: 0.5 mcg/day 3 times/week (may require from 0.5-3 mcg/day given 3 times/week) if undergoing hemodialysis
Hypoparathyroidism/pseudohypoparathyroidism: Oral (evaluate dosage at 2- to 4-week intervals):
Children:
<1 year: 0.04-0.08 mcg/kg once daily
(Continued)

## calcitriol *(Continued)*

1-5 years: 0.25-0.75 mcg once daily
Children >6 years and Adults: 0.5-2 mcg once daily
Vitamin D-dependent rickets: Children and Adults: Oral: 1 mcg once daily
Vitamin D-resistant rickets (familial hypophosphatemia): Children and Adults: Oral: Initial: 0.015-0.02
mcg/kg once daily; maintenance: 0.03-0.06 mcg/kg once daily; maximum dose: 2 mcg once daily
Hypocalcemia in premature infants: Oral: 1 mcg once daily for 5 days
Hypocalcemic tetany in premature infants: I.V.: 0.05 mcg/kg once daily for 5-12 days

**Dosage Forms**
Capsule (Rocaltrol®): 0.25 mcg, 0.5 mcg [each strength contains coconut oil]
Injection, solution: 1 mcg/mL (1 mL); 2 mcg/mL (2 mL)
Calcijex®: 1 mcg/mL (1 mL)
Solution, oral (Rocaltrol®): 1 mcg/mL (15 mL) [contains palm seed oil]

## calcium acetate (KAL see um AS e tate)

**Sound-Alike/Look-Alike Issues**
PhosLo® may be confused with Phos-Flur®, ProSom™

**U.S./Canadian Brand Names** PhosLo® [US]

**Therapeutic Category** Electrolyte Supplement, Oral

**Use**
Oral: Control of hyperphosphatemia in end-stage renal failure; does not promote aluminum absorption
I.V.: Calcium supplementation in parenteral nutrition therapy

**Usual Dosage**
**Dietary Reference Intake:**
0-6 months: 210 mg/day
7-12 months: 270 mg/day
1-3 years: 500 mg/day
4-8 years: 800 mg/day
Adults, Male/Female:
 9-18 years: 1300 mg/day
 19-50 years: 1000 mg/day
 ≥51 years: 1200 mg/day
Female: Pregnancy: Same as for Adults, Male/Female
Female: Lactating: Same as for Adults, Male/Female

Oral: Adults, on dialysis: Initial: 1334 mg with each meal, can be increased gradually to bring the serum
phosphate value <6 mg/dL as long as hypercalcemia does not develop (usual dose: 2001-2868 mg
calcium acetate with each meal); do not give additional calcium supplements
I.V.: Dose is dependent on the requirements of the individual patient; in central venous total parental
nutrition (TPN), calcium is administered at a concentration of 5 mEq (10 mL)/L of TPN solution; the
additive maintenance dose in neonatal TPN is 0.5 mEq calcium/kg/day (1.0 mL/kg/day)
Neonates: 70-200 mg/kg/day
Infants and Children: 70-150 mg/kg/day
Adolescents: 18-35 mg/kg/day

**Dosage Forms** [DSC] = Discontinued product. **Note:** Elemental calcium listed in brackets:
Gelcap (PhosLo®): 667 mg [169 mg]
Injection, solution: 0.5 mEq/mL (10 mL, 50 mL, 100 mL)
Tablet (PhosLo®): 667 mg [169 mg] [DSC]

**calcium acetate and aluminum sulfate** *see* aluminum sulfate and calcium acetate *on
page 36*

**calcium acetylhomotaurinate** *see* acamprosate *on page 3*

## calcium carbonate (KAL see um KAR bun ate)

**Sound-Alike/Look-Alike Issues**
Florical® may be confused with Fiorinal®
Mylanta® may be confused with Mynatal®
Nephro-Calci® may be confused with Nephrocaps®
Os-Cal® may be confused with Asacol®

**U.S./Canadian Brand Names** Alcalak [US-OTC]; Alka-Mints® [US-OTC]; Amitone® [US-OTC]; Apo-
Cal® [Can]; Cal-Gest [US-OTC]; Cal-Mint [US-OTC]; Calcarb 600 [US-OTC]; Calci-Chew® [US-OTC];
Calci-Mix® [US-OTC]; Calcite-500 [Can]; Caltrate® 600 [US-OTC]; Caltrate® Select [Can]; Caltrate®

[Can]; Chooz® [US-OTC]; Florical® [US-OTC]; Mylanta® Children's [US-OTC]; Nephro-Calci® [US-OTC]; Os-Cal® 500 [US-OTC]; Os-Cal® [Can]; Oysco 500 [US-OTC]; Oyst-Cal 500 [US-OTC]; Titralac™ Extra Strength [US-OTC]; Titralac™ [US-OTC]; Tums® 500 [US-OTC]; Tums® E-X [US-OTC]; Tums® Extra Strength Sugar Free [US-OTC]; Tums® Smooth Dissolve [US-OTC]; Tums® Ultra [US-OTC]; Tums® [US-OTC]

**Therapeutic Category** Antacid; Electrolyte Supplement, Oral

**Use** As an antacid, and treatment and prevention of calcium deficiency or hyperphosphatemia (eg, osteoporosis, osteomalacia, mild/moderate renal insufficiency, hypoparathyroidism, postmenopausal osteoporosis, rickets); has been used to bind phosphate

**Usual Dosage** Oral (dosage is in terms of **elemental** calcium):

**Dietary Reference Intake:**
0-6 months: 210 mg/day
7-12 months: 270 mg/day
1-3 years: 500 mg/day
4-8 years: 800 mg/day
Adults, Male/Female:
 9-18 years: 1300 mg/day
 19-50 years: 1000 mg/day
 ≥51 years: 1200 mg/day
Female: Pregnancy: Same as for Adults, Male/Female
Female: Lactating: Same as for Adults, Male/Female

Hypocalcemia (dose depends on clinical condition and serum calcium level): Dose expressed in mg of **elemental calcium**
Neonates: 50-150 mg/kg/day in 4-6 divided doses; not to exceed 1 g/day
Children: 45-65 mg/kg/day in 4 divided doses
Adults: 1-2 g or more/day in 3-4 divided doses
Adults:
Dietary supplementation: 500 mg to 2 g divided 2-4 times/day
Antacid: Dosage based on acid-neutralizing capacity of specific product; generally, 1-2 tablets or 5-10 mL every 2 hours; maximum: 7000 mg calcium carbonate per 24 hours; specific product labeling should be consulted
Adults >51 years: Osteoporosis: 1200 mg/day

**Dosage Forms**
Capsule:
Calci-Mix®: 1250 mg [equivalent to elemental calcium 500 mg]
Florical®: 364 mg [equivalent to elemental calcium 145.6 mg; contains sodium fluoride 8.3 mg]
Powder: 1600 mg/teaspoonful (960 g)
Suspension, oral: 1250 mg/5 mL (5 mL, 500 mL) [equivalent to elemental calcium 500 mg/5 mL; mint flavor]
Tablet: 1250 mg [equivalent to elemental calcium 500 mg]; 1500 mg [equivalent to elemental calcium 600 mg]
Calcarb 600, Caltrate® 600, Nephro-Calci®: 1500 mg [equivalent to elemental calcium 600 mg]
Florical®: 364 mg [equivalent to elemental calcium 145.6 mg; contains sodium fluoride 8.3 mg]
Os-Cal® 500, Oysco 500, Oyst-Cal 500: 1250 mg [equivalent to elemental calcium 500 mg]
Tablet, chewable: 500 mg [equivalent to elemental calcium 200 mg]; 650 mg [equivalent to elemental calcium 260 mg]; 750 mg [equivalent to elemental calcium 300 mg]
Alcalak: 420 mg [equivalent to elemental calcium 168 mg]
Alka-Mints®: 850 mg [equivalent to elemental calcium 340 mg; assorted and spearmint flavors]
Amitone®: 420 mg [equivalent to elemental calcium 168 mg; spearmint flavor]
Cal-Gest: 500 mg [equivalent to elemental calcium 200 mg]
Calci-Chew®: 1250 mg [equivalent to elemental calcium 500 mg; cherry, lemon, and orange flavors]
Cal-Mint: 650 mg [equivalent to elemental calcium 260 mg; mint flavor]
Chooz®: 500 mg [equivalent to elemental calcium 200 mg; contains phenylalanine]
Mylanta® Children's: 400 mg [equivalent to elemental calcium 160 mg; bubble gum flavor]
Os-Cal® 500: 1250 mg [equivalent to elemental calcium 500 mg; Bavarian cream flavor]
Titralac™: 420 mg [equivalent to elemental calcium 168 mg; sugar free; mint flavor]
Titralac™ Extra Strength: 750 mg [equivalent to elemental calcium 300 mg; sugar free; mint flavor]
Tums®: 500 mg [equivalent to elemental calcium 200 mg; assorted fruit (contains tartrazine) and peppermint flavors]
Tums® E-X: 750 mg [equivalent to elemental calcium 300 mg; assorted fruit (contains tartrazine), fresh blend, tropical assorted fruit, wintergreen (contains tartrazine), and assorted berry flavors]
(Continued)

# calcium carbonate *(Continued)*

Tums® Extra Strength Sugar Free: 750 mg [equivalent to elemental calcium 300 mg; sugar free; contains phenylalanine <1 mg/tablet; orange cream flavor]

Tums® Smooth Dissolve: 750 mg [equivalent to elemental calcium 300 mg; assorted fruit (contains tartrazine) and peppermint flavors]

Tums® Ultra®: 1000 mg [equivalent to elemental calcium 400 mg; assorted mint, assorted berry, and tropical assorted berry (contains tartrazine) flavors]

## calcium carbonate and magnesium hydroxide

(KAL see um KAR bun ate & mag NEE zhum hye DROKS ide)

**Sound-Alike/Look-Alike Issues**
Mylanta® may be confused with Mynatal®

**Synonyms** magnesium hydroxide and calcium carbonate

**U.S./Canadian Brand Names** Mi-Acid™ Double Strength [US-OTC]; Mylanta® Gelcaps® [US-OTC]; Mylanta® Supreme [US-OTC]; Mylanta® Ultra [US-OTC]; Rolaids® Extra Strength [US-OTC]; Rolaids® [US-OTC]

**Therapeutic Category** Antacid

**Use** Hyperacidity

**Usual Dosage** Adults: Oral: 2-4 tablets between meals, at bedtime, or as directed by healthcare provider

**Dosage Forms**
Gelcap (Mylanta® Gelcaps®): Calcium carbonate 550 mg and magnesium hydroxide 125 mg

Liquid (Mylanta® Supreme): Calcium carbonate 400 mg and magnesium hydroxide 135 mg per 5 mL (360 mL, 720 mL) [cherry flavor]

Tablet, chewable:
Mi-Acid™ Double Strength: Calcium carbonate 700 mg and magnesium hydroxide 300 mg

Mylanta® Ultra: Calcium carbonate 700 mg and magnesium hydroxide 300 mg [cherry créme and cool mint flavors]

Rolaids®: Calcium carbonate 550 mg and magnesium hydroxide 110 mg [sodium free; contains elemental calcium 220 mg and elemental magnesium 45 mg; original (peppermint), cherry, and spearmint flavors]

Rolaids® Extra Strength: Calcium carbonate 675 mg and magnesium hydroxide 135 mg [sodium free; contains elemental calcium 271 mg and elemental magnesium 56 mg, fruit flavor contains tartrazine; cool strawberry, fresh mint, fruit, and tropical fruit punch flavors]

## calcium carbonate and simethicone (KAL see um KAR bun ate & sye METH i kone)

**Synonyms** simethicone and calcium carbonate

**U.S./Canadian Brand Names** Gas Ban™ [US-OTC]; Titralac® Plus [US-OTC]

**Therapeutic Category** Antacid; Antiflatulent

**Use** Relief of acid indigestion, heartburn

**Usual Dosage** Oral (OTC labeling): Adults: Two tablets every 2-3 hours as needed (maximum: 19 tablets/24 hours)

**Dosage Forms** Tablet, chewable:
Gas Ban™: Calcium carbonate 300 mg and simethicone 40 mg

Titralac® Plus: Calcium carbonate 420 mg and simethicone 21 mg [equivalent to elemental calcium 168 mg; sugar free; spearmint flavor]

## calcium carbonate, magnesium hydroxide, and famotidine *see* famotidine, calcium carbonate, and magnesium hydroxide *on page 328*

## calcium chloride (KAL see um KLOR ide)

**Therapeutic Category** Electrolyte Supplement, Oral

**Use** Cardiac resuscitation when epinephrine fails to improve myocardial contractions, cardiac disturbances of hyperkalemia, hypocalcemia, or calcium channel blocking agent toxicity; emergent treatment of hypocalcemic tetany, treatment of hypermagnesemia

**Usual Dosage Note:** Per gram of each salt, calcium chloride contains 3 times the amount of elemental calcium as compared to calcium gluconate. Dosages are expressed in terms of the calcium chloride salt based on a solution concentration of 100 mg/mL (10%) containing 1.4 mEq (27.3 mg)/mL elemental calcium).

Cardiac arrest in the presence of hyperkalemia or hypocalcemia, magnesium toxicity, or calcium antagonist toxicity: I.V.:
Infants and Children: 20 mg/kg; may repeat in 10 minutes if necessary

Adolescents and Adults: 2-4 mg/kg, repeated every 10 minutes if necessary

Hypocalcemia: I.V.:

Children (manufacturer's recommendation): 2.7-5 mg/kg/dose every 4-6 hours

Alternative pediatric dosing: Infants and Children: 10-20 mg/kg/dose, repeat every 4-6 hours if needed

Adults: 500 mg to 1 g/dose repeated every 4-6 hours if needed

Hypocalcemic tetany: I.V.:

Neonates: Divided doses totaling approximately 170 mg/kg/24 hours

Infants and Children: 10 mg/kg over 5-10 minutes; may repeat after 6-8 hours or follow with an infusion with a maximum dose of 200 mg/kg/day; alternatively, higher doses of 35-50 mg/kg/dose repeated every 6-8 hours have been used

Adults: 1 g over 10-30 minutes; may repeat after 6 hours

Hypocalcemia secondary to citrated blood transfusion: I.V.: **Note:** Routine administration of calcium, in the absence of signs/symptoms of hypocalcemia, is generally not recommended. A number of recommendations have been published seeking to address potential hypocalcemia during massive transfusion of citrated blood; however, many practitioners recommend replacement only as guided by clinical evidence of hypocalcemia and/or serial monitoring of ionized calcium.

Neonates, Infants, and Children: Give 32 mg (0.45 mEq elemental calcium) for each 100 mL citrated blood infused

Adults: 200-500 mg per 500 mL of citrated blood (infused into another vein)

**Dosage Forms** Injection, solution [preservative free]: 10% [100 mg/mL] (10 mL) [equivalent to elemental calcium 27.2 mg/mL, calcium 1.36 mEq/mL]

## calcium citrate (KAL see um SIT rate)

**Sound-Alike/Look-Alike Issues**

Citracal® may be confused with Citrucel®

**U.S./Canadian Brand Names** Cal-Citrate® 250 [US-OTC]; Citracal® [US-OTC]; Osteocit® [Can]

**Therapeutic Category** Electrolyte Supplement, Oral

**Use** Antacid; treatment and prevention of calcium deficiency or hyperphosphatemia (eg, osteoporosis, osteomalacia, mild/moderate renal insufficiency, hypoparathyroidism, postmenopausal osteoporosis, rickets)

**Usual Dosage** Oral: Dosage is in terms of **elemental** calcium

**Dietary Reference Intake:**

0-6 months: 210 mg/day

7-12 months: 270 mg/day

1-3 years: 500 mg/day

4-8 years: 800 mg/day

Adults, Male/Female:

9-18 years: 1300 mg/day

19-50 years: 1000 mg/day

≥51 years: 1200 mg/day

Female: Pregnancy: Same as for Adults, Male/Female

Female: Lactating: Same as for Adults, Male/Female

Dietary supplement: Usual dose: 500 mg to 2 g 2-4 times/day

**Dosage Forms**

Granules: 760 mg/teaspoonful (480 g)

Tablet: Elemental calcium 200 mg, 250 mg

Cal-Citrate®: Elemental calcium 250 mg

Citracal®: 950 mg [equivalent to elemental calcium 200 mg]

## calcium disodium edetate see edetate calcium disodium on page 278

## Calcium Disodium Versenate® [US] see edetate calcium disodium on page 278

## calcium EDTA see edetate calcium disodium on page 278

## calcium glubionate (KAL see um gloo BYE oh nate)

**Sound-Alike/Look-Alike Issues**

calcium glubionate may be confused with calcium gluconate

**Therapeutic Category** Electrolyte Supplement, Oral

**Use** Adjunct in treatment and prevention of postmenopausal osteoporosis; treatment and prevention of calcium depletion or hyperphosphatemia (eg, osteoporosis, osteomalacia, mild/moderate renal insufficiency, hypoparathyroidism, rickets)

**Usual Dosage** Dosage is in terms of **elemental** calcium

(Continued)

# calcium glubionate *(Continued)*

**Dietary Reference Intake:**
0-6 months: 210 mg/day
7-12 months: 270 mg/day
1-3 years: 500 mg/day
4-8 years: 800 mg/day
Adults, Male/Female:
 9-18 years: 1300 mg/day
 19-50 years: 1000 mg/day
 ≥51 years: 1200 mg/day
Female: Pregnancy: Same as for Adults, Male/Female
Female: Lactating: Same as for Adults, Male/Female

Syrup is a hyperosmolar solution; dosage is in terms of calcium glubionate, elemental calcium is in parentheses
Neonatal hypocalcemia: 1200 mg (77 mg $Ca^{++}$)/kg/day in 4-6 divided doses
 Maintenance: Infants and Children: 600-2000 mg (38-128 mg $Ca^{++}$)/kg/day in 4 divided doses up to a maximum of 9 g (575 mg $Ca^{++}$)/day
 Adults: 6-18 g (~0.5-1 g $Ca^{++}$)/day in divided doses
**Dosage Forms** Syrup: 1.8 g/5 mL (480 mL) [equivalent to elemental calcium 115 mg/5 mL]

# calcium gluconate (KAL see um GLOO koe nate)

**Sound-Alike/Look-Alike Issues**
 calcium gluconate may be confused with calcium glubionate
**Therapeutic Category** Electrolyte Supplement, Oral
**Use** Treatment and prevention of hypocalcemia; treatment of tetany, cardiac disturbances of hyperkalemia, cardiac resuscitation when epinephrine fails to improve myocardial contractions, hypocalcemia, or calcium channel blocker toxicity; calcium supplementation
**Usual Dosage**
**Dietary Reference Intake (expressed as elemental calcium):**
0-6 months: 210 mg/day
7-12 months: 270 mg/day
1-3 years: 500 mg/day
4-8 years: 800 mg/day
9-18 years: 1300 mg/day
Adults, Male/Female:
 19-50 years: 1000 mg/day
 ≥51 years: 1200 mg/day
Female: Pregnancy: Same as for Adults, Male/Female
Female: Lactating: Same as for Adults, Male/Female

**Dosage note:** The following dosages are expressed in terms of the calcium gluconate salt based on a solution concentration of 100 mg/mL (10%) containing 0.465 mEq (9.3 mg)/mL elemental calcium):
Hypocalcemia: I.V.:
 Neonates: 200-800 mg/kg/day as a continuous infusion or in 4 divided doses (maximum: 1 g/dose)
 Infants and Children: 200-500 mg/kg/day as a continuous infusion or in 4 divided doses (maximum: 2-3 g/dose)
 Adults: 2-15 g/24 hours as a continuous infusion or in divided doses
Hypocalcemia: Oral:
 Children: 200-500 mg/kg/day divided every 6 hours
 Adults: 500 mg to 2 g 2-4 times/day
Osteoporosis/bone loss: Oral: 1000-1500 mg in divided doses/day
Hypocalcemia secondary to citrated blood infusion: I.V.: **Note:** Routine administration of calcium, in the absence of signs/symptoms of hypocalcemia, is generally not recommended. A number of recommendations have been published seeking to address potential hypocalcemia during massive transfusion of citrated blood; however, many practitioners recommend replacement only as guided by clinical evidence of hypocalcemia and/or serial monitoring of ionized calcium.
 Neonates, Infants, and Children: Give 98 mg (0.45 mEq **elemental** calcium) for each 100 mL citrated blood infused
 Adults: 500 mg to 1 g per 500 mL of citrated blood (infused into another vein). Single doses up to 2 g have also been recommended.

Hypocalcemic tetany: I.V.:
Neonates, Infants and Children: 100-200 mg/kg/dose over 5-10 minutes; may repeat every 6-8 hours **or** follow with an infusion of 500 mg/kg/day
Adults: 1-3 g may be administered until therapeutic response occurs
Calcium antagonist toxicity, magnesium intoxication, or cardiac arrest in the presence of hyperkalemia or hypocalcemia: I.V.:
Infants and Children: 60-100 mg/kg/dose (maximum: 3 g/dose)
Adults: 500-800 mg/dose (maximum: 3 g/dose)
Maintenance electrolyte requirements for total parenteral nutrition: I.V.: Daily requirements: Adults: 1.7-3.4 g/1000 kcal/24 hours

**Dosage Forms**
Injection, solution [preservative free]: 10% [100 mg/mL] (10 mL, 50 mL, 100 mL, 200 mL) [equivalent to elemental calcium 9 mg/mL; calcium 0.46 mEq/mL]
Powder: 347 mg/tablespoonful (480 g)
Tablet: 500 mg [equivalent to elemental calcium 45 mg]; 650 mg [equivalent to elemental calcium 58.5 mg]; 975 mg [equivalent to elemental calcium 87.75 mg]

## calcium lactate (KAL see um LAK tate)

**Therapeutic Category** Electrolyte Supplement, Oral
**Use** Adjunct in prevention of postmenopausal osteoporosis; treatment and prevention of calcium depletion
**Usual Dosage** Oral (in terms of calcium lactate):
**Dietary Reference Intake (in terms of elemental calcium):**
0-6 months: 210 mg/day
7-12 months: 270 mg/day
1-3 years: 500 mg/day
4-8 years: 800 mg/day
Adults, Male/Female:
9-18 years: 1300 mg/day
19-50 years: 1000 mg/day
≥51 years: 1200 mg/day
Female: Pregnancy: Same as Adults, Male/Female
Female: Lactating: Same as Adults, Male/Female
Children: 500 mg/kg/day divided every 6-8 hours; maximum daily dose: 9 g
Adults: 1.5-3 g divided every 8 hours
**Dosage Forms** Tablet: 650 mg [equivalent to elemental calcium 84.5 mg]

**calcium leucovorin** *see* leucovorin *on page 470*

**calcium pantothenate** *see* pantothenic acid *on page 618*

## calcium phosphate (tribasic) (KAL see um FOS fate tri BAY sik)

**Synonyms** tricalcium phosphate
**U.S./Canadian Brand Names** Posture® [US-OTC]
**Therapeutic Category** Electrolyte Supplement, Oral
**Use** Adjunct in prevention of postmenopausal osteoporosis; treatment and prevention of calcium depletion
**Usual Dosage** Oral (dosage is in terms of **elemental** calcium):
**Dietary Reference Intake:**
0-6 months: 210 mg/day
7-12 months: 270 mg/day
1-3 years: 500 mg/day
4-8 years: 800 mg/day
Adults, Male/Female:
9-18 years: 1300 mg/day
19-50 years: 1000 mg/day
≥51 years: 1200 mg/day
Female: Pregnancy: Same as for Adults, Male/Female
Female: Lactating: Same as for Adults, Male/Female
Prevention of osteoporosis:
Children: 45-65 mg/kg/day
Adults: 1-2 g/day
**Dosage Forms** Tablet: 1565.2 mg [equivalent to elemental calcium 600 mg; sugar free]

**Caldecort**® **[US-OTC]** *see* hydrocortisone (topical) *on page 417*

**calfactant** (kaf AKT ant)
**U.S./Canadian Brand Names** Infasurf® [US]
**Therapeutic Category** Lung Surfactant
**Use** Prevention of respiratory distress syndrome (RDS) in premature infants at high risk for RDS and for the treatment ("rescue") of premature infants who develop RDS

Prophylaxis: Therapy at birth with calfactant is indicated for premature infants <29 weeks of gestational age at significant risk for RDS. Should be administered as soon as possible, preferably within 30 minutes after birth.

Treatment: For infants ≤72 hours of age with RDS (confirmed by clinical and radiologic findings) and requiring endotracheal intubation.

**Usual Dosage** Intratracheal administration **only**: Each dose is 3 mL/kg body weight at birth; should be administered every 12 hours for a total of up to 3 doses

**Dosage Forms** Suspension, intratracheal [preservative free]: 35 mg/mL (6 mL)

**Cal-Gest [US-OTC]** *see* calcium carbonate *on page 130*

**Callergy Clear [US-OTC]** *see* pramoxine *on page 670*

**Calm-X**® **Oral** *(Discontinued)* *see* dimenhydrinate *on page 252*

**Cal-Mint [US-OTC]** *see* calcium carbonate *on page 130*

**Calmylin with Codeine [Can]** *see* guaifenesin, pseudoephedrine, and codeine *on page 391*

**Cal-Nate**™ **[US]** *see* vitamins (multiple/prenatal) *on page 852*

**Calphron**® *(Discontinued)* *see* calcium acetate *on page 130*

**Cal-Plus**® *(Discontinued)* *see* calcium carbonate *on page 130*

**Caltine**® **[Can]** *see* calcitonin *on page 129*

**Caltrate**® **[Can]** *see* calcium carbonate *on page 130*

**Caltrate**® **600 [US-OTC]** *see* calcium carbonate *on page 130*

**Caltrate**® **Jr.** *(Discontinued)* *see* calcium carbonate *on page 130*

**Caltrate**® **Select [Can]** *see* calcium carbonate *on page 130*

**Camila**™ **[US]** *see* norethindrone *on page 582*

**Campath**® **[US]** *see* alemtuzumab *on page 26*

**campath-1H** *see* alemtuzumab *on page 26*

**Campho-Phenique**® **[US-OTC]** *see* camphor and phenol *on this page*

**camphor and phenol** (KAM for & FEE nole)
**Synonyms** phenol and camphor
**U.S./Canadian Brand Names** Campho-Phenique® [US-OTC]
**Therapeutic Category** Topical Skin Product
**Use** Relief of pain and itching associated with minor burns, sunburn, minor cuts, insect bites, minor skin irritation; temporary relief of pain from cold sores
**Usual Dosage** Topical: Adults: Relief of pain/itching: Apply 1-3 times/day
**Dosage Forms**
Gel, topical: Camphor 10.8% and phenol 4.7% (7 g, 15 g)
Liquid, topical: Camphor 10.8% and phenol 4.7% (45 mL)
Campho-Phenique®: Camphor 10.8% and phenol 4.7% (22.5 mL, 45 mL)

**camphor, menthol, and phenol** (KAM for, MEN thol, & FEE nole)
**Therapeutic Category** Topical Skin Product
**Use** Relief of dry, itching skin
**Usual Dosage** Topical: Apply as needed for dry skin
**Dosage Forms** Lotion, topical: Camphor 0.5%, menthol 0.5%, and phenol 0.5% in emollient base (240 mL)

**Campral**® **[US]** *see* acamprosate *on page 3*

**Camptosar**® **[US/Can]** *see* irinotecan *on page 447*

**camptothecin-11** *see* irinotecan *on page 447*

**Canasa**™ **[US]** *see* mesalamine *on page 516*

**Cancidas**® **[US/Can]** *see* caspofungin *on page 151*

## candesartan (kan de SAR tan)

**Synonyms** candesartan cilexetil

**U.S./Canadian Brand Names** Atacand® [US/Can]

**Therapeutic Category** Angiotensin II Receptor Antagonist

**Use** Alone or in combination with other antihypertensive agents in treating essential hypertension; treatment of heart failure (NYHA class II-IV)

**Usual Dosage** Adults: Oral:

Hypertension: Usual dose is 4-32 mg once daily; dosage must be individualized. Blood pressure response is dose-related over the range of 2-32 mg. The usual recommended starting dose of 16 mg once daily when it is used as monotherapy in patients who are not volume depleted. It can be administered once or twice daily with total daily doses ranging from 8-32 mg. Larger doses do not appear to have a greater effect and there is relatively little experience with such doses.

Congestive heart failure: Initial: 4 mg once daily; double the dose at 2-week intervals, as tolerated; target dose: 32 mg

**Note:** In selected cases, concurrent therapy with an ACE inhibitor may provide additional benefit.

**Dosage Forms** Tablet, as cilexetil: 4 mg, 8 mg, 16 mg, 32 mg

## candesartan and hydrochlorothiazide (kan de SAR tan & hye droe klor oh THYE a zide)

**Synonyms** candesartan cilexetil and hydrochlorothiazide

**U.S./Canadian Brand Names** Atacand HCT™ [US]; Atacand® Plus [Can]

**Therapeutic Category** Antihypertensive Agent, Combination

**Use** Treatment of hypertension; combination product should not be used for initial therapy

**Usual Dosage** Oral: Adults: Replacement therapy: Combination product can be substituted for individual agents; maximum therapeutic effect would be expected within 4 weeks

Usual dosage range:

Candesartan: 8-32 mg/day, given once daily or twice daily in divided doses

Hydrochlorothiazide: 12.5-50 mg once daily

**Dosage Forms** Tablet:

16-12.5: Candesartan 16 mg and hydrochlorothiazide 12.5 mg

32-12.5: Candesartan 32 mg and hydrochlorothiazide 12.5 mg

**candesartan cilexetil** *see* candesartan *on this page*

**candesartan cilexetil and hydrochlorothiazide** *see* candesartan and hydrochlorothiazide *on this page*

## *Candida albicans (Monilia)* (KAN dee da AL bi kans mo NIL ya)

**Synonyms** *Monilia* skin test

**U.S./Canadian Brand Names** Candin® [US]

**Therapeutic Category** Diagnostic Agent

**Use** Screen for detection of nonresponsiveness to antigens in immunocompromised individuals

**Usual Dosage** Intradermal: 0.1 mL, examine reaction site in 24-48 hours; induration of ≥5 mm in diameter is a positive reaction

**Dosage Forms** Injection, solution: 0.1 mL/dose (1 mL)

**Candin**® **[US]** *see Candida albicans (Monilia) on this page*

**Candistatin**® **[Can]** *see* nystatin *on page 592*

**Canesten**® **Topical [Can]** *see* clotrimazole *on page 199*

**Canesten**® **Vaginal [Can]** *see* clotrimazole *on page 199*

**Cankaid**® **[US-OTC]** *see* carbamide peroxide *on page 141*

**Cantil**® **[Can]** *see* mepenzolate *on page 512*

**Cantil**® ***(Discontinued)*** *see* mepenzolate *on page 512*

**Capastat® Sulfate [US]** *see capreomycin on this page*

## capecitabine (ka pe SITE a been)
**U.S./Canadian Brand Names** Xeloda® [US/Can]
**Therapeutic Category** Antineoplastic Agent, Antimetabolite
**Use** Treatment of metastatic colorectal cancer; adjuvant therapy of Dukes C colon cancer; treatment of metastatic breast cancer
**Usual Dosage** Oral:
 Adults: 2500 mg/m$^2$/day in 2 divided doses (~12 hours apart) at the end of a meal for 2 weeks followed by a 1- or 2-week rest period
 Adjuvant therapy of Dukes C colon cancer: Recommended for a total of 24 weeks (8 cycles of 2 weeks of drug administration and 1 week rest period.
**Dosage Forms** Tablet: 150 mg, 500 mg

**Capex™ [US/Can]** *see fluocinolone on page 344*

**Capital® and Codeine [US]** *see acetaminophen and codeine on page 6*

**Capitrol® [US/Can]** *see chloroxine on page 171*

**Capoten® [US/Can]** *see captopril on next page*

**Capozide® [US/Can]** *see captopril and hydrochlorothiazide on next page*

## capreomycin (kap ree oh MYE sin)
**Sound-Alike/Look-Alike Issues**
 Capastat® may be confused with Cepastat®
**Synonyms** capreomycin sulfate
**U.S./Canadian Brand Names** Capastat® Sulfate [US]
**Therapeutic Category** Antibiotic, Miscellaneous
**Use** Treatment of tuberculosis in conjunction with at least one other antituberculosis agent
**Usual Dosage** I.M., I.V.:
 Infants and Children: 15-30 mg/kg/day, up to 1 g/day maximum
 Adults: 1 g/day (not to exceed 20 mg/kg/day) for 60-120 days, followed by 1 g 2-3 times/week
**Dosage Forms** Injection, powder for reconstitution, as sulfate: 1 g

**capreomycin sulfate** *see capreomycin on this page*

**Capsagel® [US-OTC]** *see capsaicin on this page*

## capsaicin (kap SAY sin)
**Sound-Alike/Look-Alike Issues**
 Zostrix® may be confused with Zestril®, Zovirax®
**U.S./Canadian Brand Names** ArthriCare® for Women Extra Moisturizing [US-OTC]; ArthriCare® for Women Multi-Action [US-OTC]; ArthriCare® for Women Silky Dry [US-OTC]; ArthriCare® for Women Ultra Strength [US-OTC]; Capsagel® [US-OTC]; Capzasin-HP® [US-OTC]; Capzasin-P® [US-OTC]; Zostrix® [US-OTC/Can]; Zostrix®-HP [US-OTC/Can]
**Therapeutic Category** Analgesic, Topical
**Use** Topical treatment of pain associated with postherpetic neuralgia, rheumatoid arthritis, osteoarthritis, diabetic neuropathy; postsurgical pain
**Usual Dosage** Children ≥2 years and Adults: Topical: Apply to affected area at least 3-4 times/day; application frequency less than 3-4 times/day prevents the total depletion, inhibition of synthesis, and transport of substance P resulting in decreased clinical efficacy and increased local discomfort
**Dosage Forms** [DSC] = Discontinued product
 Cream, topical: 0.025% (60 g); 0.075% (60 g)
 ArthriCare® for Women Multi-Action: 0.025% (42 g) [contains menthol]
 ArthriCare® for Women Silky Dry: 0.025% (42 g)
 ArthriCare® for Women Ultra Strength: 0.075% (42 g) [contains benzalkonium chloride and menthol]
 Capzasin-P®: 0.025% (45 g)
 Capzasin-HP®: 0.075% (45 g)
 Zostrix®: 0.025% (60 g)
 Zostrix®-HP: 0.075% (60 g)
 Gel, topical (Capsagel®): 0.025% (60 g); 0.05% (60 g); 0.075% (30 g)
 Lotion, topical (ArthriCare® for Women Extra Moisturizing): 0.025% (120 mL, 240 mL)
 Patch, topical (TheraPatch® Warm): 0.09% (6s) [DSC]
 Stick (Zostrix®-HP): 0.075% (21 g) [DSC]

## captopril (KAP toe pril)

**Sound-Alike/Look-Alike Issues**
captopril may be confused with Capitrol®, carvedilol

**Synonyms** ACE

**U.S./Canadian Brand Names** Alti-Captopril [Can]; Apo-Capto® [Can]; Capoten® [US/Can]; Gen-Captopril [Can]; Novo-Captopril [Can]; Nu-Capto [Can]; PMS-Captopril [Can]

**Therapeutic Category** Angiotensin-Converting Enzyme (ACE) Inhibitor

**Use** Management of hypertension; treatment of congestive heart failure, left ventricular dysfunction after myocardial infarction, diabetic nephropathy

**Usual Dosage Note:** Dosage must be titrated according to patient's response; use lowest effective dose.
Oral:
Infants: Initial: 0.15-0.3 mg/kg/dose; titrate dose upward to maximum of 6 mg/kg/day in 1-4 divided doses; usual required dose: 2.5-6 mg/kg/day
Children: Initial: 0.5 mg/kg/dose; titrate upward to maximum of 6 mg/kg/day in 2-4 divided doses
Older Children: Initial: 6.25-12.5 mg/dose every 12-24 hours; titrate upward to maximum of 6 mg/kg/day
Adolescents: Initial: 12.5-25 mg/dose given every 8-12 hours; increase by 25 mg/dose to maximum of 450 mg/day
Adults:
Acute hypertension (urgency/emergency): 12.5-25 mg, may repeat as needed (may be given sublingually, but no therapeutic advantage demonstrated)
Hypertension:
Initial dose: 12.5-25 mg 2-3 times/day; may increase by 12.5-25 mg/dose at 1- to 2-week intervals up to 50 mg 3 times/day; maximum dose: 150 mg 3 times/day; add diuretic before further dosage increases
Usual dose range (JNC 7): 25-100 mg/day in 2 divided doses
Congestive heart failure:
Initial dose: 6.25-12.5 mg 3 times/day in conjunction with cardiac glycoside and diuretic therapy; initial dose depends upon patient's fluid/electrolyte status
Target dose: 50 mg 3 times/day
Maximum dose: 150 mg 3 times/day
LVD after MI: Initial dose: 6.25 mg followed by 12.5 mg 3 times/day; then increase to 25 mg 3 times/day during next several days and then over next several weeks to target dose of 50 mg 3 times/day
Diabetic nephropathy: 25 mg 3 times/day; other antihypertensives often given concurrently

**Dosage Forms** Tablet: 12.5 mg, 25 mg, 50 mg, 100 mg

## captopril and hydrochlorothiazide (KAP toe pril & hye droe klor oh THYE a zide)

**Synonyms** hydrochlorothiazide and captopril

**U.S./Canadian Brand Names** Capozide® [US/Can]

**Therapeutic Category** Antihypertensive Agent, Combination

**Use** Management of hypertension and treatment of congestive heart failure

**Usual Dosage** Oral: Adults: Hypertension, CHF: May be substituted for previously titrated dosages of the individual components; alternatively, may initiate as follows:
Initial: Single tablet (captopril 25 mg/hydrochlorothiazide 15 mg) taken once daily; daily dose of captopril should not exceed 150 mg; daily dose of hydrochlorothiazide should not exceed 50 mg

**Dosage Forms** Tablet:
25/15: Captopril 25 mg and hydrochlorothiazide 15 mg
25/25: Captopril 25 mg and hydrochlorothiazide 25 mg
50/15: Captopril 50 mg and hydrochlorothiazide 15 mg
50/25: Captopril 50 mg and hydrochlorothiazide 25 mg

**Capzasin-HP® [US-OTC]** see capsaicin on previous page

**Capzasin-P® [US-OTC]** see capsaicin on previous page

**Carac™ [US]** see fluorouracil on page 349

**Carafate® [US]** see sucralfate on page 769

**Carapres® [Can]** see clonidine on page 197

# carbachol (KAR ba kole)

**Sound-Alike/Look-Alike Issues**
Isopto® Carbachol may be confused with Isopto® Carpine
**Synonyms** carbacholine; carbamylcholine chloride
**U.S./Canadian Brand Names** Isopto® Carbachol [US/Can]; Miostat® [US/Can]
**Therapeutic Category** Cholinergic Agent
**Use** Lowers intraocular pressure in the treatment of glaucoma; cause miosis during surgery
**Usual Dosage** Adults:
Ophthalmic: Instill 1-2 drops up to 3 times/day
Intraocular: 0.5 mL instilled into anterior chamber before or after securing sutures
**Dosage Forms** [DSC] = Discontinued product
Solution, intraocular (Carbastat® [DSC], Miostat®): 0.01% (1.5 mL)
Solution, ophthalmic (Isopto® Carbachol): 1.5% (15 mL); 3% (30 mL) [contains benzalkonium chloride]

**carbacholine** *see* carbachol *on this page*

# carbamazepine (kar ba MAZ e peen)

**Sound-Alike/Look-Alike Issues**
Carbatrol® may be confused with Cartrol®
Epitol® may be confused with Epinal®
Tegretol® may be confused with Mebaral®, Tegrin®, Toradol®, Trental®
**Synonyms** CBZ; SPD417
**U.S./Canadian Brand Names** Apo-Carbamazepine® [Can]; Carbatrol® [US]; Epitol® [US]; Equetro™ [US]; Gen-Carbamazepine CR [Can]; Novo-Carbamaz [Can]; Nu-Carbamazepine [Can]; PMS-Carbamazepine [Can]; Taro-Carbamazepine Chewable [Can]; Tegretol® [US/Can]; Tegretol®-XR [US]
**Therapeutic Category** Anticonvulsant
**Use**
Carbatrol®, Tegretol®, Tegretol®-XR: Partial seizures with complex symptomatology (psychomotor, temporal lobe), generalized tonic-clonic seizures (grand mal), mixed seizure patterns, trigeminal neuralgia
Equetro™: Acute manic and mixed episodes associated with bipolar 1 disorder
**Usual Dosage** Dosage must be adjusted according to patient's response and serum concentrations. Administer tablets (chewable or conventional) in 2-3 divided doses daily and suspension in 4 divided doses daily. Oral:
**Epilepsy:**
Children:
<6 years: Initial: 10-20 mg/kg/day divided twice or 3 times daily as tablets or 4 times/day as suspension; increase dose every week until optimal response and therapeutic levels are achieved
Maintenance dose: Divide into 3-4 doses daily (tablets or suspension); maximum recommended dose: 35 mg/kg/day
6-12 years: Initial: 100 mg twice daily (tablets or extended release tablets) or 50 mg of suspension 4 times/day (200 mg/day); increase by up to 100 mg/day at weekly intervals using a twice daily regimen of extended release tablets or 3-4 times daily regimen of other formulations until optimal response and therapeutic levels are achieved
Maintenance: Usual: 400-800 mg/day; maximum recommended dose: 1000 mg/day
**Note:** Children <12 years who receive ≥400 mg/day of carbamazepine may be converted to extended release capsules (Carbatrol®) using the same total daily dosage divided twice daily
Children >12 years and Adults: Initial: 200 mg twice daily (tablets, extended release tablets, or extended release capsules) or 100 mg of suspension 4 times/day (400 mg daily); increase by up to 200 mg/day at weekly intervals using a twice daily regimen of extended release tablets or capsules, or a 3-4 times/day regimen of other formulations until optimal response and therapeutic levels are achieved; usual dose: 800-1200 mg/day
Maximum recommended doses:
Children 12-15 years: 1000 mg/day
Children >15 years: 1200 mg/day
Adults: 1600 mg/day; however, some patients have required up to 1.6-2.4 g/day

**Trigeminal or glossopharyngeal neuralgia:** Adults: Initial: 100 mg twice daily with food, gradually increasing in increments of 100 mg twice daily as needed
Maintenance: Usual: 400-800 mg daily in 2 divided doses; maximum dose: 1200 mg/day

**Bipolar disorder (Equetro™):** Adults: Initial: 400 mg/day in divided doses, twice daily; may adjust by 200 mg daily increments; maximum dose: 1600 mg/day

Dosage Forms
Capsule, extended release (Carbatrol®, Equetro™): 100 mg, 200 mg, 300 mg
Suspension, oral: 100 mg/5 mL (10 mL, 450 mL)
 Tegretol®: 100 mg/5 mL (450 mL) [citrus vanilla flavor]
Tablet (Epitol®, Tegretol®): 200 mg
Tablet, chewable (Tegretol®): 100 mg
Tablet, extended release (Tegretol®-XR): 100 mg, 200 mg, 400 mg

**carbamide** *see* urea *on page 834*

# carbamide peroxide (KAR ba mide per OKS ide)

Synonyms urea peroxide
U.S./Canadian Brand Names Cankaid® [US-OTC]; Debrox® [US-OTC]; Dent's Ear Wax [US-OTC]; E•R•O [US-OTC]; Gly-Oxide® [US-OTC]; Murine® Ear Wax Removal System [US-OTC]; Orajel® Perioseptic® Spot Treatment [US-OTC]
Therapeutic Category Antiinfective Agent, Oral; Otic Agent, Ceruminolytic
Use Relief of minor inflammation of gums, oral mucosal surfaces and lips including canker sores and dental irritation; emulsify and disperse ear wax
Usual Dosage Children and Adults:
Oral: Inflammation/dental irritation: Solution (should not be used for >7 days): Oral preparation should not be used in children <2 years of age; apply several drops undiluted on affected area 4 times/day after meals and at bedtime; expectorate after 2-3 minutes **or** place 10 drops onto tongue, mix with saliva, swish for several minutes, expectorate
Otic:
Children <12 years: Tilt head sideways and individualize the dose according to patient size; 3 drops (range: 1-5 drops) twice daily for up to 4 days, tip of applicator should not enter ear canal; keep drops in ear for several minutes by keeping head tilted and placing cotton in ear
Children ≥12 years and Adults: Tilt head sideways and instill 5-10 drops twice daily up to 4 days, tip of applicator should not enter ear canal; keep drops in ear for several minutes by keeping head tilted and placing cotton in ear
Dosage Forms
Solution, oral: 10% (60 mL)
Cankaid®: 10% (22 mL) [in anhydrous glycerol]
Gly-Oxide®: 10% (15 mL, 60 mL) [contains glycerin]
Orajel® Perioseptic® Spot Treatment: 15% (13.3 mL) [contains anhydrous glycerin]
Solution, otic: 6.5% (15 mL)
Debrox®: 6.5% (15 mL, 30 mL) [contains propylene glycol]
Dent's Ear Wax: 6.5% (3.7 mL) [contains glycerin]
E•R•O: 6.5% (15 mL)
Murine® Ear Wax Removal System: 6.5% (15 mL) [contains alcohol 6.3% and glycerin]

**carbamylcholine chloride** *see* carbachol *on previous page*

**Carbaphen 12® [US]** *see* carbetapentane, phenylephrine, and chlorpheniramine *on next page*

**Carbaphen 12 Ped® [US]** *see* carbetapentane, phenylephrine, and chlorpheniramine *on next page*

**Carbastat® (Discontinued)** *see* carbachol *on previous page*

**Carbatrol® [US]** *see* carbamazepine *on previous page*

**Carbaxefed DM RF [US]** *see* carbinoxamine, pseudoephedrine, and dextromethorphan *on page 145*

**Carbaxefed RF [US]** *see* carbinoxamine and pseudoephedrine *on page 144*

# carbenicillin (kar ben i SIL in)

Synonyms carbenicillin indanyl sodium; carindacillin
U.S./Canadian Brand Names Geocillin® [US]
Therapeutic Category Penicillin
Use Treatment of serious urinary tract infections and prostatitis caused by susceptible gram-negative aerobic bacilli
Usual Dosage Oral:
Children: 30-50 mg/kg/day divided every 6 hours; maximum dose: 2-3 g/day
Adults: 1-2 tablets every 6 hours for urinary tract infections or 2 tablets every 6 hours for prostatitis
Dosage Forms Tablet [film coated]: 382 mg [contains sodium 23 mg/tablet]

**carbenicillin indanyl sodium** *see* carbenicillin *on previous page*

# carbetapentane and chlorpheniramine (kar bay ta PEN tane & klor fen IR a meen)

**Synonyms** carbetapentane tannate and chlorpheniramine tannate; chlorpheniramine and carbetapentane

**U.S./Canadian Brand Names** Tannate 12 S [US]; Tannic-12 S [US]; Tannic-12 [US]; Tannihist-12 RF [US]; Tussi-12 S™ [US]; Tussi-12® [US]; Tussizone-12 RF™ [US]

**Therapeutic Category** Antihistamine/Antitussive

**Use** Symptomatic relief of cough associated with upper respiratory tract conditions, such as the common cold, bronchitis, bronchial asthma

**Usual Dosage** Oral:

Children: Based on carbetapentane 30 mg and chlorpheniramine 4 mg per 5 mL suspension:

2-6 years: 2.5-5 mL every 12 hours

>6 years: 5-10 mL every 12 hours

Adults: Based on carbetapentane 60 mg and chlorpheniramine 5 mg per tablet: 1-2 tablets every 12 hours

**Dosage Forms**

Suspension:

Tannate 12 S: Carbetapentane tannate 30 mg and chlorpheniramine tannate 4 mg per 5 mL (120 mL, 480 mL)

Tannic-12 S: Carbetapentane tannate 30 mg and chlorpheniramine tannate 4 mg per 5 mL (120 mL) [contains benzoic acid; strawberry flavor]

Tannihist-12 RF: Carbetapentane tannate 30 mg and chlorpheniramine tannate 4 mg per 5 mL (120 mL, 480 mL) [strawberry-black currant flavor]

Tussi-12 S™: Carbetapentane tannate 30 mg and chlorpheniramine tannate 4 mg per 5 mL (120 mL) [contains benzoic acid and tartrazine; strawberry-currant flavor]

Tussizone-12 RF™: Carbetapentane tannate 30 mg and chlorpheniramine tannate 4 mg per 5 mL (120 mL, 480 mL) [contains benzoic acid and tartrazine; strawberry-black currant flavor]

Tablet (Tannic-12, Tussi-12®, Tussizone-12 RF™): Carbetapentane tannate 60 mg and chlorpheniramine tannate 5 mg

# carbetapentane and pseudoephedrine (kar bay ta PEN tane & soo doe e FED rin)

**Synonyms** carbetapentane tannate and pseudoephedrine tannate; pseudoephedrine and carbetapentane

**U.S./Canadian Brand Names** Respi-Tann™ [US]

**Therapeutic Category** Antitussive/Decongestant

**Use** Relief of cough and congestion due to the common cold, influenza, sinusitis, or bronchitis

**Usual Dosage** Relief of cough and congestion: Oral:

Children:

2-6 years: ½ tablet or 2.5 mL suspension every 12 hours (maximum 4 doses/24 hours)

6-12 years: 1 tablet or 5 mL suspension every 12 hours (maximum: 4 doses/24 hours)

>12 years: Refer to Adults dosing

Adults: 2 tablets or 10 mL suspension every 12 hours (maximum: 4 doses/24 hours)

**Dosage Forms**

Suspension: Carbetapentane tannate 25 mg and pseudoephedrine tannate 75 mg per 5 mL (480 mL) [dye free; contains sodium benzoate; cherry flavor]

Tablet, chewable: Carbetapentane tannate 25 mg and pseudoephedrine tannate 75 mg [dye free; cherry flavor]

**carbetapentane, ephedrine, phenylephrine, and chlorpheniramine** *see* chlorpheniramine, ephedrine, phenylephrine, and carbetapentane *on page 173*

# carbetapentane, phenylephrine, and chlorpheniramine
(kar bay ta PEN tane, fen il EF rin, & klor fen IR a meen)

**Synonyms** chlorpheniramine, carbetapentane, and phenylephrine; phenylephrine, chlorpheniramine, and carbetapentane

**U.S./Canadian Brand Names** Carbaphen 12 Ped® [US]; Carbaphen 12® [US]; XiraTuss [US]

**Therapeutic Category** Antihistamine/Decongestant/Antitussive; Antitussive; Sympathomimetic

**Use** Symptomatic relief of cough, nasal congestion, and discharge associated with the common cold, bronchial asthma, acute and chronic bronchitis, and other respiratory tract conditions

**Usual Dosage** Oral: Relief of cough, congestion:

Children 2-6 years:

Carbaphen 12 Ped®: 1-2 mL every 12 hours

XiraTuss suspension: 2.5-5 mL every 12 hours

Children 6-12 years:

Carbaphen 12 Ped®: 2-4 mL every 12 hours

XiraTuss suspension: 5-10 mL every 12 hours

Children >12 years and Adults:

Carbaphen 12®: 5-10 mL every 12 hours

XiraTuss tablet: 1-2 tablets every 12 hours

**Dosage Forms**

Suspension:

Carbaphen 12®: Carbetapentane tannate 60 mg, phenylephrine tannate 20 mg, and chlorpheniramine tannate 8 mg per 5 mL (480 mL) [contains benzoic acid, phenylalanine 1 mg/5 mL; alcohol free, sugar free; blueberry-banana flavor]

Carbaphen 12 Ped®: Carbetapentane tannate 15 mg, phenylephrine tannate 2.5 mg, and chlorpheniramine tannate 2 mg per mL (60 mL) [contains benzoic acid, phenylalanine 1.6 mg/mL; alcohol free, sugar free; blueberry-banana flavor]

XiraTuss: Carbetapentane tannate 30 mg, phenylephrine tannate 12.5 mg, and chlorpheniramine tannate 4 mg per 5 mL (120 mL) [strawberry flavor]

Tablet (XiraTuss): Carbetapentane tannate 60 mg, phenylephrine tannate 10 mg, and chlorpheniramine tannate 5 mg

**carbetapentane tannate and chlorpheniramine tannate** *see* carbetapentane and chlorpheniramine *on previous page*

**carbetapentane tannate and pseudoephedrine tannate** *see* carbetapentane and pseudoephedrine *on previous page*

## carbetocin *(Canada only)* (kar BE toe sin)

**U.S./Canadian Brand Names** Duratocin™ [Can]

**Therapeutic Category** Uteronic Agent

**Use** For the prevention of uterine atony and postpartum hemorrhage following elective cesarean section under epidural or spinal anesthesia.

**Usual Dosage** A single I.V. dose of 100 mcg (1 mL) is administered by bolus injection, over 1 minute, only when delivery of the infant has been completed by cesarean section under epidural anesthetic. Carbetocin can be administered either before or after delivery of the placenta

**Dosage Forms** Injection: 1 mcg/mL (1 mL)

## carbidopa (kar bi DOE pa)

**U.S./Canadian Brand Names** Lodosyn® [US]

**Therapeutic Category** Anti-Parkinson Agent; Dopaminergic Agent (Anti-Parkinson)

**Use** Given with levodopa in the treatment of parkinsonism to enable a lower dosage of levodopa to be used and a more rapid response to be obtained and to decrease side-effects; for details of administration and dosage, see Levodopa; has no effect without levodopa

**Usual Dosage** Oral: Adults: 70-100 mg/day; maximum daily dose: 200 mg

**Dosage Forms** Tablet: 25 mg

**carbidopa and levodopa** *see* levodopa and carbidopa *on page 474*

**carbidopa, levodopa, and entacapone** *see* levodopa, carbidopa, and entacapone *on page 475*

**Carbihist [US]** *see* carbinoxamine *on next page*

# carbinoxamine (kar bi NOKS a meen)

**Synonyms** carbinoxamine maleate; carbinoxamine tannate

**U.S./Canadian Brand Names** Carbihist [US]; Carbinoxamine PD [US]; Carboxine [US]; Histex™ CT [US]; Histex™ I/E [US]; Histex™ PD [US]; Histex™ PD-12 [US]; Palgic [US]; Pediatex™ 12 [US]; Pediatex™ [US]

**Therapeutic Category** Antihistamine

**Use** Seasonal and perennial allergic rhinitis; urticaria

**Usual Dosage** Oral: Allergic rhinitis/urticaria:

Children:

1-3 months (Pediatex™): 0.4 mg (1.25 mL) every 4-6 hours

3-9 months:

Histex™ PD: 1 mg (1.25 mL) 4 times/day

Pediatex™: 0.9-1.3 mg (2.5-3.75 mL) every 4-6 hours

9-18 months:

Histex™ PD: 1-2 mg (1.25-2.5 mL) 4 times/day

Histex™ PD-12: 1.25 mL every 12 hours

Pediatex™: 1.3-1.75 mg (3.75-5 mL) every 4-6 hours

18 months to 6 years:

Histex™ PD, Palgic: 2 mg (2.5 mL) 4 times/day

Histex™ PD-12: 2.5 mL every 12 hours

Pediatex™: 1.75 mg (5 mL) every 4-6 hours

2-6 years (Pediatex™ 12): 2.5-5 mL every 12 hours

6-12 years:

Histex™ CT: One-half tablet every 12 hours

Histex™ PD, Histex™ PD-12, Palgic, Pediatex™: Refer to Adults dosing

Pediatex™ 12: 5-10 mL every 12 hours

≥12 years: Refer to Adults dosing

Adults:

Histex™ CT, Histex™ I/E: One capsule or tablet every 12 hours; maximum: 2 doses/24 hours

Histex™ PD, Palgic: 4 mg (5 mL) 4 times/day

Histex™ PD-12: 5 mL every 12 hours

Pediatex™: 3.5 mg (10 mL) every 4-6 hours

Pediatex™ 12: 10-20 mL every 12 hours

**Dosage Forms** [DSC] = Discontinued product

Capsule, variable release (Histex™ I/E): Carbinoxamine maleate 2 mg [immediate release] and carbinoxamine maleate 8 mg [extended release]

Liquid, as maleate:

Carbihist: 4 mg/5 mL (120 mL) [cotton candy flavor]

Carbinoxamine PD: 4 mg/5 mL (480 mL) [bubble gum flavor]

Carboxine: 1.75 mg/5 mL (480 mL) [bubble gum flavor]

Histex™ PD: 4 mg/5 mL (480 mL) [alcohol free, dye free, sugar free; bubble gum flavor]

Pediatex™: 1.75 mg/5 mL (480 mL) [alcohol free, dye free, sugar free; cotton candy flavor]

Solution, as maleate (Palgic): 4 mg/5 mL (120 mL [DSC], 480 mL) [bubble gum flavor]

Suspension, as tannate (Pediatex™ 12): Carbinoxamine 3.6 mg per 5 mL (480 mL) [contains sodium benzoate; candy apple flavor]

Suspension, variable release (Histex™ PD-12): Carbinoxamine maleate 2 mg [immediate release] and carbinoxamine tannate 6 mg [extended release] per 5 mL (120 mL, 480 mL) [alcohol free, dye free, sugar free; contains sodium benzoate; bubble gum flavor]

Tablet, as maleate [scored] (Palgic): 4 mg

Tablet, timed release, as maleate (Histex™ CT): 8 mg

# carbinoxamine and pseudoephedrine (kar bi NOKS a meen & soo doe e FED rin)

**Synonyms** pseudoephedrine and carbinoxamine

**U.S./Canadian Brand Names** Andehist NR Drops [US]; Carbaxefed RF [US]; Carboxine-PSE [US]; Hydro-Tussin™-CBX [US]; Palgic®-D [US]; Palgic®-DS [US]; Pediatex™-D [US]; Rondec-TR® [US]; Rondec® Drops [US]; Rondec® Tablets [US]; Sildec [US]

**Therapeutic Category** Antihistamine/Decongestant Combination

**Use** Seasonal and perennial allergic rhinitis; vasomotor rhinitis

**Usual Dosage** Oral:
Children:
Drops (Andehist NR, Carbaxefed RF, Rondec®, Sildec):
1-3 months: 0.25 mL 4 times/day
3-6 months: 0.5 mL 4 times/day
6-12 months: 0.75 mL 4 times/day
12-24 months: 1 mL 4 times/day
Liquid (Pediatex™-D):
1-3 months: 1.25 mL up to 4 times/day
3-6 months: 2.5 mL up to 4 times/day
6-9 months: 3.75 mL up to 4 times/day
9-18 months: 3.75-5 mL up to 4 times/day
18 months to 6 years: 5 mL 3-4 times/day
>6 years: Refer to Adults dosing
Syrup (Hydro-Tussin™-CBX, Palgic®-DS):
1-3 months: 1.25 mL up to 4 times/day
3-6 months: 2.5 mL up to 4 times/day
6-9 months: 3.75 mL up to 4 times/day
9-18 months: 3.75-5 mL up to 4 times/day
18 months to 6 years: 5 mL 3-4 times/day
>6 years: Refer to Adults dosing
Tablet (Rondec®): ≥6 years: Refer to Adults dosing
Tablet, timed release:
6-12 years (Palgic®-D): One-half tablet every 12 hours
≥12 years (Palgic®-D, Rondec-TR®): Refer to Adults dosing
Adults:
Liquid (Pediatex™-D): 10 mL 4 times/day
Syrup (Hydro-Tussin™-CBX, Palgic®-DS): 10 mL 4 times/day
Tablet (Rondec®): 1 tablet 4 times a day
Tablet, timed release (Palgic®-D, Rondec-TR®): 1 tablet every 12 hours

**Dosage Forms**
Liquid (Pediatex™-D): Carbinoxamine maleate 2 mg and pseudoephedrine hydrochloride 20 mg per 5 mL (480 mL) [alcohol free, dye free, sugar free; cotton candy flavor]
Solution, oral drops:
Andehist NR: Carbinoxamine maleate 1 mg and pseudoephedrine hydrochloride 15 mg per mL (30 mL) [alcohol and sugar free; raspberry flavor]
Carbaxefed RF, Rondec®: Carbinoxamine maleate 1 mg and pseudoephedrine hydrochloride 15 mg per mL (30 mL) [alcohol free; contains sodium benzoate; cherry flavor]
Sildec: Carbinoxamine maleate 1 mg and pseudoephedrine hydrochloride 15 mg per mL (30 mL) [raspberry flavor]
Solution: Carbinoxamine maleate 2 mg and pseudoephedrine hydrochloride 25 mg per 5 mL (480 mL)
Carboxine-PSE: Carbinoxamine maleate 2 mg and pseudoephedrine hydrochloride 20 mg per 5 mL (480 mL) [peach flavor]
Syrup: Carbinoxamine maleate 2 mg and pseudoephedrine hydrochloride 25 mg per 5 mL (480 mL)
Hydro-Tussin™-CBX, Palgic®-DS: Carbinoxamine maleate 2 mg and pseudoephedrine hydrochloride 25 mg per 5 mL (480 mL) [alcohol, dye, and sugar free; strawberry/pineapple flavor]
Tablet (Rondec®): Carbinoxamine maleate 4 mg and pseudoephedrine hydrochloride 60 mg
Tablet, timed release:
Palgic®-D: Carbinoxamine maleate 8 mg and pseudoephedrine hydrochloride 80 mg [dye free]
Rondec-TR®: Carbinoxamine maleate 8 mg and pseudoephedrine hydrochloride 120 mg

**carbinoxamine, dextromethorphan, and pseudoephedrine** *see* carbinoxamine, pseudoephedrine, and dextromethorphan *on this page*

**carbinoxamine maleate** *see* carbinoxamine *on previous page*

**Carbinoxamine PD [US]** *see* carbinoxamine *on previous page*

# carbinoxamine, pseudoephedrine, and dextromethorphan
(kar bi NOKS a meen, soo doe e FED rin, & deks troe meth OR fan)
**Sound-Alike/Look-Alike Issues**
Tussafed® may be confused with Tussafin®
(Continued)

## carbinoxamine, pseudoephedrine, and dextromethorphan *(Continued)*

**Synonyms** carbinoxamine, dextromethorphan, and pseudoephedrine; dextromethorphan, carbinoxamine, and pseudoephedrine; dextromethorphan, pseudoephedrine, and carbinoxamine; pseudoephedrine, carbinoxamine, and dextromethorphan; pseudoephedrine, dextromethorphan, and carbinoxamine

**U.S./Canadian Brand Names** Andehist DM NR Drops [US]; Carbaxefed DM RF [US]; Decahist-DM [US]; Pediatex™-DM [US]; Rondec®-DM Drops [US]; Sildec-DM [US]; Tussafed® [US]

**Therapeutic Category** Antihistamine/Decongestant/Antitussive

**Use** Relief of coughs and upper respiratory symptoms, including nasal congestion, associated with allergy or the common cold

**Usual Dosage** Oral:

Drops (Rondec®-DM): Infants and Children:
1-3 months: 1/4 mL 4 times/day
3-6 months: 1/2 mL 4 times/day
6-12 months: 3/4 mL 4 times/day
12-24 months: 1 mL 4 times/day
Liquid (Pediatex™-DM):
Children 18 months to 6 years: 2.5 mL 4 times/day
Children 6-12 years: 5 mL 4 times/day
Children ≥12 years and Adults: 10 mL 4 times/day
Syrup (Tussafed®):
Children 18 months to 6 years: 2.5 mL 4 times/day
Children >6 years and Adults: 5 mL 4 times/day

**Dosage Forms**

Liquid:
Decahist-DM: Carbinoxamine maleate 2 mg, pseudoephedrine hydrochloride 15 mg and dextromethorphan hydrobromide 15 mg per 5 mL (480 mL) [peach flavor]
Pediatex™ DM: Carbinoxamine maleate 2 mg, pseudoephedrine hydrochloride 15 mg and dextromethorphan hydrobromide 15 mg per 5 mL (480 mL) [alcohol free, dye free, sugar free; cotton candy flavor]
Liquid, oral drops: Carbinoxamine maleate 1 mg, pseudoephedrine hydrochloride 15 mg and dextromethorphan hydrobromide 4 mg per mL (30 mL)
Andehist DM NR: Carbinoxamine maleate 1 mg, pseudoephedrine hydrochloride 15 mg and dextromethorphan hydrobromide 4 mg per mL (30 mL) [alcohol and sugar free; grape flavor]
Carbaxefed DM RF: Carbinoxamine maleate 1 mg, pseudoephedrine hydrochloride 15 mg and dextromethorphan hydrobromide 4 mg per mL (30 mL) [alcohol free; grape flavor]
Rondec®-DM: Carbinoxamine maleate 1 mg, pseudoephedrine hydrochloride 15 mg and dextromethorphan hydrobromide 4 mg per mL (30 mL) [alcohol free; contains sodium benzoate; grape flavor]
Sildec-DM: Carbinoxamine maleate 1 mg, pseudoephedrine hydrochloride 15 mg and dextromethorphan hydrobromide 4 mg per mL (30 mL)
Syrup, oral (Tussafed®): Carbinoxamine maleate 4 mg, pseudoephedrine hydrochloride 60 mg, and dextromethorphan hydrobromide 15 mg per 5 mL (480 mL) [alcohol and sugar free]

**carbinoxamine, pseudoephedrine, and hydrocodone** *see* hydrocodone, carbinoxamine, and pseudoephedrine *on page 414*

**carbinoxamine tannate** *see* carbinoxamine *on page 144*

**Carbiset® Tablet *(Discontinued)*** *see* carbinoxamine and pseudoephedrine *on page 144*

**Carbiset-TR® Tablet *(Discontinued)*** *see* carbinoxamine and pseudoephedrine *on page 144*

**Carbocaine® [US/Can]** *see* mepivacaine *on page 514*

**Carbodec® Syrup *(Discontinued)*** *see* carbinoxamine and pseudoephedrine *on page 144*

**Carbodec® Tablet *(Discontinued)*** *see* carbinoxamine and pseudoephedrine *on page 144*

**Carbodec® TR Tablet *(Discontinued)*** *see* carbinoxamine and pseudoephedrine *on page 144*

**Carbofed DM [US]** *see* brompheniramine, pseudoephedrine, and dextromethorphan *on page 116*

## carbol-fuchsin solution (kar bol-FOOK sin soe LOO shun)

**Synonyms** Castellani Paint
**U.S./Canadian Brand Names** Castellani Paint Modified [US]
**Therapeutic Category** Antifungal Agent
**Use** Treatment of superficial mycotic infections
**Usual Dosage** Topical: Apply to affected area 2-4 times/day

Dosage Forms Solution, topical: Phenol 1.5%, alcohol 13%, basic fuchsin, resorcinol, acetone (30 mL, 480 mL)

**carbolic acid** *see* phenol *on page 638*

**Carbolith™ [Can]** *see* lithium *on page 486*

# carboplatin (KAR boe pla tin)

**Sound-Alike/Look-Alike Issues**
carboplatin may be confused with cisplatin
Paraplatin® may be confused with Platinol®

**Synonyms** CBDCA

**U.S./Canadian Brand Names** Paraplatin-AQ [Can]; Paraplatin® [US]

**Therapeutic Category** Antineoplastic Agent

**Use** Treatment of ovarian cancer

**Usual Dosage** Refer to individual protocols: **Note:** Doses are usually determined by the AUC using the Calvert formula

IVPB, I.V. infusion, intraperitoneal:
Children:
Solid tumor: 300-600 mg/m$^2$ once every 4 weeks
Brain tumor: 175 mg/m$^2$ weekly for 4 weeks every 6 weeks, with a 2-week recovery period between courses
Adults:
Ovarian cancer: 300-360 mg/m$^2$ I.V. every 3-4 weeks
Autologous BMT: I.V.: 1600 mg/m$^2$ (total dose) divided over 4 days

**Dosage Forms**
Injection, powder for reconstitution: 50 mg, 150 mg, 450 mg
Injection, solution: 10 mg/mL (5 mL, 15 mL, 45 mL, 60 mL)

# carbopol 940 *(Canada only)* (KAR boe pol nine forty)

**U.S./Canadian Brand Names** Lacrinorm [Can]

**Therapeutic Category** Ophthalmic Agent, Miscellaneous

**Use** Artificial tear

**Usual Dosage** Ophthalmic: Use as needed for dry eyes

**Dosage Forms** Gel, ophthalmic: 20 mg (10 g)

**carboprost** *see* carboprost tromethamine *on this page*

# carboprost tromethamine (KAR boe prost tro METH a meen)

**Synonyms** carboprost

**U.S./Canadian Brand Names** Hemabate® [US/Can]

**Therapeutic Category** Prostaglandin

**Use** Termination of pregnancy and refractory postpartum uterine bleeding

**Usual Dosage** I.M.: Adults:
Abortion: Initial: 250 mcg, then 250 mcg at 1$^1$/$_2$-hour to 3$^1$/$_2$-hour intervals depending on uterine response; a 500 mcg dose may be given if uterine response is not adequate after several 250 mcg doses; do not exceed 12 mg total dose or continuous administration for >2 days
Refractory postpartum uterine bleeding: Initial: 250 mcg; may repeat at 15- to 90-minute intervals to a total dose of 2 mg
Bladder irrigation for hemorrhagic cystitis (refer to individual protocols): [0.4-1.0 mg/dL as solution] 50 mL instilled into bladder 4 times/day for 1 hour

**Dosage Forms** Injection, solution: Carboprost 250 mcg and tromethamine 83 mcg per mL (1 mL) [contains benzyl alcohol]

**carbose D** *see* carboxymethylcellulose *on next page*

**Carboxine [US]** *see* carbinoxamine *on page 144*

**Carboxine-PSE [US]** *see* carbinoxamine and pseudoephedrine *on page 144*

## carboxymethylcellulose (kar boks ee meth il SEL yoo lose)
**Synonyms** carbose D; carboxymethylcellulose sodium
**U.S./Canadian Brand Names** Celluvisc™ [Can]; Refresh Liquigel™ [US-OTC]; Refresh Plus® [US-OTC/Can]; Refresh Tears® [US-OTC/Can]; Tears Again® Gel Drops™ [US-OTC]; Tears Again® Night and Day™ [US-OTC]; Theratears® [US]
**Therapeutic Category** Ophthalmic Agent, Miscellaneous
**Use** Artificial tear substitute
**Usual Dosage** Ophthalmic: Adults: Instill 1-2 drops into eye(s) 3-4 times/day
**Dosage Forms**
  Gel, ophthalmic, as sodium (Tears Again® Night and Day™): 1.5% (3.5 g)
  Solution ophthalmic, as sodium:
    Refresh Liquigel™: 1% (15 mL) [liquid gel formulation]
    Refresh Plus®: 0.5% (0.4 mL) [preservative free; available in packages of 30 or 50]
    Refresh Tears®: 0.5% (15 mL)
    Tears Again® Gel Drops™: 0.7% (15 mL)
    Theratears®: 0.25% (0.6 mL [preservative free], 15 mL)

**carboxymethylcellulose sodium** *see* carboxymethylcellulose *on this page*

**Cardene® [US]** *see* nicardipine *on page 573*

**Cardene® I.V. [US]** *see* nicardipine *on page 573*

**Cardene® SR [US]** *see* nicardipine *on page 573*

**Cardilate® (Discontinued)**

**Cardio-Green® (Discontinued)** *see* indocyanine green *on page 435*

**Cardioquin® (Discontinued)** *see* quinidine *on page 705*

**Cardizem® [US/Can]** *see* diltiazem *on page 251*

**Cardizem® CD [US/Can]** *see* diltiazem *on page 251*

**Cardizem® Injection (Discontinued)** *see* diltiazem *on page 251*

**Cardizem® LA [US]** *see* diltiazem *on page 251*

**Cardizem® SR [Can]** *see* diltiazem *on page 251*

**Cardizem® SR (Discontinued)** *see* diltiazem *on page 251*

**Cardura® [US]** *see* doxazosin *on page 268*

**Cardura-1™ [Can]** *see* doxazosin *on page 268*

**Cardura-2™ [Can]** *see* doxazosin *on page 268*

**Cardura-4™ [Can]** *see* doxazosin *on page 268*

**CareNate™ 600 [US]** *see* vitamins (multiple/prenatal) *on page 852*

**Carimune™ (Discontinued)** *see* immune globulin (intravenous) *on page 433*

**Carimune™ NF [US]** *see* immune globulin (intravenous) *on page 433*

**carindacillin** *see* carbenicillin *on page 141*

**carisoprodate** *see* carisoprodol *on this page*

## carisoprodol (kar eye soe PROE dole)
**Synonyms** carisoprodate; isobamate
**U.S./Canadian Brand Names** Soma® [US/Can]
**Therapeutic Category** Skeletal Muscle Relaxant
**Use** Skeletal muscle relaxant
**Usual Dosage** Oral: Adults: 350 mg 3-4 times/day; take last dose at bedtime; compound: 1-2 tablets 4 times/day
**Dosage Forms** Tablet: 350 mg

## carisoprodol and aspirin (kar eye soe PROE dole & AS pir in)
**Synonyms** aspirin and carisoprodol
**U.S./Canadian Brand Names** Soma® Compound [US]
**Therapeutic Category** Skeletal Muscle Relaxant
**Use** Skeletal muscle relaxant

Usual Dosage Oral: Adults: 1-2 tablets 4 times/day
Dosage Forms Tablet: Carisoprodol 200 mg and aspirin 325 mg

## carisoprodol, aspirin, and codeine (kar eye soe PROE dole, AS pir in, and KOE deen)
Synonyms aspirin, carisoprodol, and codeine; codeine, aspirin, and carisoprodol
U.S./Canadian Brand Names Soma® Compound w/Codeine [US]
Therapeutic Category Skeletal Muscle Relaxant
Controlled Substance C-III
Use Skeletal muscle relaxant
Usual Dosage Oral: Adults: 1 or 2 tablets 4 times/day
Dosage Forms Tablet: Carisoprodol 200 mg, aspirin 325 mg, and codeine phosphate 16 mg

**Carmol® 10 [US-OTC]** see urea on page 834

**Carmol® 20 [US-OTC]** see urea on page 834

**Carmol® 40 [US]** see urea on page 834

**Carmol® Deep Cleaning [US]** see urea on page 834

**Carmol-HC® [US]** see urea and hydrocortisone on page 835

**Carmol® Scalp [US]** see sulfacetamide on page 771

## carmustine (kar MUS teen)
Sound-Alike/Look-Alike Issues
carmustine may be confused with lomustine
Synonyms BCNU; bis-chloronitrosourea; carmustinum; NSC-409962; WR-139021
U.S./Canadian Brand Names BiCNu® [US/Can]; Gliadel® [US]
Therapeutic Category Antineoplastic Agent
Use
Injection: Treatment of brain tumors (glioblastoma, brainstem glioma, medulloblastoma, astrocytoma, ependymoma, and metastatic brain tumors), multiple myeloma, Hodgkin disease, non-Hodgkin lymphomas, melanoma, lung cancer, colon cancer
Wafer (implant): Adjunct to surgery in patients with recurrent glioblastoma multiforme; adjunct to surgery and radiation in patients with high-grade malignant glioma
Usual Dosage
I.V. (refer to individual protocols):
Children: 200-250 mg/m$^2$ every 4-6 weeks as a single dose
Adults: Usual dosage (per manufacturer labeling): 150-200 mg/m$^2$ every 6 weeks as a single dose or divided into daily injections on 2 successive days
**Alternative regimens:**
75-120 mg/m$^2$ days 1 and 2 every 6-8 weeks **or**
50-80 mg/m$^2$ days 1,2,3 every 6-8 weeks
Primary brain cancer:
150-200 mg/m$^2$ every 6-8 weeks as a single dose **or**
75-120 mg/m$^2$ days 1 and 2 every 6-8 weeks **or**
20-65 mg/m$^2$ every 4-6 weeks **or**
0.5-1 mg/kg every 4-6 weeks **or**
40-80 mg/m$^2$/day for 3 days every 6-8 weeks
Autologous BMT: ALL OF THE FOLLOWING DOSES ARE FATAL WITHOUT BMT
Combination therapy: Up to 300-900 mg/m$^2$
Single-agent therapy: Up to 1200 mg/m$^2$ (fatal necrosis is associated with doses >2 g/m$^2$)
Implantation (wafer): Adults: Recurrent glioblastoma multiforme, malignant glioma: Up to 8 wafers may be placed in the resection cavity (total dose 62.6 mg); should the size and shape not accommodate 8 wafers, the maximum number of wafers allowed should be placed
Dosage Forms
Injection, powder for reconstitution (BiCNu®): 100 mg [packaged with 3 mL of absolute alcohol as diluent]
Wafer (Gliadel®): 7.7 mg (8s)

**carmustinum** see carmustine on this page

**Carnation Instant Breakfast® [US-OTC]** see nutritional formula, enteral/oral on page 591

**Carnitor® [US/Can]** see levocarnitine on page 474

**Carrington Antifungal [US-OTC]** *see* miconazole *on page 537*

## carteolol (KAR tee oh lole)

**Sound-Alike/Look-Alike Issues**

carteolol may be confused with carvedilol

Cartrol® may be confused with Carbatrol®

Ocupress® may be confused with Ocufen®

**Synonyms** carteolol hydrochloride

**U.S./Canadian Brand Names** Cartrol® [US/Can]; Ocupress® Ophthalmic [Can]

**Therapeutic Category** Beta-Adrenergic Blocker

**Use** Management of hypertension; treatment of chronic open-angle glaucoma and intraocular hypertension

**Usual Dosage** Adults:

Oral: 2.5 mg as a single daily dose, with a maintenance dose normally 2.5-5 mg once daily; doses >10 mg do not increase response and may in fact decrease effect.

Ophthalmic: Instill 1 drop in affected eye(s) twice daily.

**Dosage Forms** [DSC] = Discontinued product

Solution, ophthalmic, as hydrochloride: 1% (5 mL, 10 mL, 15 mL) [contains benzalkonium chloride]

Ocupress® [DSC]: 1% (5 mL, 10 mL, 15 mL) [contains benzalkonium chloride]

Tablet, as hydrochloride (Cartrol®): 2.5 mg, 5 mg

**carteolol hydrochloride** *see* carteolol *on this page*

**Carter's Little Pills® [Can]** *see* bisacodyl *on page 107*

**Carter's Little Pills® (Discontinued)** *see* bisacodyl *on page 107*

**Cartia XT™ [US]** *see* diltiazem *on page 251*

**Cartrol® [US/Can]** *see* carteolol *on this page*

## carvedilol (KAR ve dil ole)

**Sound-Alike/Look-Alike Issues**

carvedilol may be confused with captopril, carteolol

**U.S./Canadian Brand Names** Apo-Carvedilol® [Can]; Coreg® [US/Can]; Novo-Carvedilol [Can]; PMS-Carvedilol [Can]; ratio-Carvedilol [Can]

**Therapeutic Category** Beta-Adrenergic Blocker

**Use** Mild to severe heart failure of ischemic or cardiomyopathic origin (usually in addition to standardized therapy); left ventricular dysfunction following myocardial infarction (MI); management of hypertension

**Usual Dosage** Oral: Adults: Reduce dosage if heart rate drops to <55 beats/minute.

Hypertension: 6.25 mg twice daily; if tolerated, dose should be maintained for 1-2 weeks, then increased to 12.5 mg twice daily. Dosage may be increased to a maximum of 25 mg twice daily after 1-2 weeks. Maximum dose: 50 mg/day

Congestive heart failure: 3.125 mg twice daily for 2 weeks; if this dose is tolerated, may increase to 6.25 mg twice daily. Double the dose every 2 weeks to the highest dose tolerated by patient. (Prior to initiating therapy, other heart failure medications should be stabilized and fluid retention minimized.)

Maximum recommended dose:

Mild to moderate heart failure:

<85 kg: 25 mg twice daily

>85 kg: 50 mg twice daily

Severe heart failure: 25 mg twice daily

Left ventricular dysfunction following MI: Initial 3.125-6.25 mg twice daily; increase dosage incrementally (ie, from 6.25 to 12.5 mg twice daily) at intervals of 3-10 days, based on tolerance, to a target dose of 25 mg twice daily. **Note:** Should be initiated only after patient is hemodynamically stable and fluid retention has been minimized.

**Dosage Forms** Tablet: 3.125 mg, 6.25 mg, 12.5 mg, 25 mg

**Casodex® [US/Can]** *see* bicalutamide *on page 106*

## caspofungin (kas poe FUN jin)

**Synonyms** caspofungin acetate

**U.S./Canadian Brand Names** Cancidas® [US/Can]

**Therapeutic Category** Antifungal Agent, Systemic

**Use** Treatment of invasive *Aspergillus* infections in patients who are refractory or intolerant of other therapy; treatment of candidemia and other *Candida* infections (intra-abdominal abscesses, esophageal, peritonitis, pleural space); empirical treatment for presumed fungal infections in febrile neutropenic patient

**Usual Dosage** I.V.:

Children: Safety and efficacy in pediatric patients have not been established

Adults: **Note:** Duration of caspofungin treatment should be determined by patient status and clinical response. Empiric therapy should be given until neutropenia resolves. In patients with positive cultures, treatment should continue until 14 days after last positive culture. In neutropenic patients, treatment should be given at least 7 days after both signs and symptoms of infection **and** neutropenia resolve.

Empiric therapy: Initial dose: 70 mg on day 1; subsequent dosing: 50 mg/day; may increase up to 70 mg/day if tolerated, but clinical response is inadequate

Invasive *Aspergillus*, candidiasis: Initial dose: 70 mg on day 1; subsequent dosing: 50 mg/day

Esophageal candidiasis: 50 mg/day; **Note:** The majority of patients studied for this indication also had oropharyngeal involvement.

Concomitant use of an enzyme inducer:

Patients receiving rifampin: 70 mg caspofungin daily

Patients receiving carbamazepine, dexamethasone, efavirenz, nevirapine, **or** phenytoin (and possibly other enzyme inducers) may require an increased daily dose of caspofungin (70 mg/day).

**Dosage Forms** Injection, powder for reconstitution, as acetate: 50 mg [contains sucrose 39 mg], 70 mg [contains sucrose 54 mg]

**caspofungin acetate** *see* caspofungin *on this page*

**Castellani Paint** *see* carbol-fuchsin solution *on page 146*

**Castellani Paint Modified [US]** *see* carbol-fuchsin solution *on page 146*

## castor oil (KAS tor oyl)

**Synonyms** oleum ricini

**U.S./Canadian Brand Names** Purge® [US-OTC]

**Therapeutic Category** Laxative

**Use** Preparation for rectal or bowel examination or surgery; rarely used to relieve constipation; also applied to skin as emollient and protectant

**Usual Dosage** Oral: Oil:

Children 2-11 years: 5-15 mL as a single dose

Children ≥12 years and Adults: 15-60 mL as a single dose

**Dosage Forms** [DSC] = Discontinued product

Emulsion, oral (Emulsoil® [DSC]): 95% (60 mL)

Oil, oral: 100% (60 mL, 120 mL, 480 mL, 3840 mL)

Purge®: 95% (30 mL, 60 mL) [lemon flavor]

**castor oil, trypsin, and balsam peru** *see* trypsin, balsam peru, and castor oil *on page 830*

**Cataflam® [US/Can]** *see* diclofenac *on page 243*

**Catapres® [US]** *see* clonidine *on page 197*

**Catapres-TTS® [US]** *see* clonidine *on page 197*

**Cathflo™ Activase® [US/Can]** *see* alteplase *on page 32*

**Caverject® [US/Can]** *see* alprostadil *on page 31*

**Caverject® Impulse™ [US]** *see* alprostadil *on page 31*

**CB-1348** *see* chlorambucil *on page 166*

**CBDCA** *see* carboplatin *on page 147*

**CBZ** *see* carbamazepine *on page 140*

**CCNU** *see* lomustine *on page 488*

**C-Crystals® *(Discontinued)*** *see* ascorbic acid *on page 71*

**2-CdA** *see* cladribine *on page 189*

**CDDP** *see* cisplatin *on page 187*

**CDX** *see* bicalutamide *on page 106*

**Cebid**® *(Discontinued)* *see* ascorbic acid *on page 71*

**Ceclor**® **[Can]** *see* cefaclor *on this page*

**Cecon**® **[US-OTC]** *see* ascorbic acid *on page 71*

**Cedax**® **[US]** *see* ceftibuten *on page 157*

**Cedocard**®**-SR [Can]** *see* isosorbide dinitrate *on page 451*

**CEE** *see* estrogens (conjugated/equine) *on page 304*

**CeeNU**® **[US/Can]** *see* lomustine *on page 488*

**Ceepryn**® *(Discontinued)* *see* cetylpyridinium *on page 164*

## cefaclor (SEF a klor)

**Sound-Alike/Look-Alike Issues**
cefaclor may be confused with cephalexin

**U.S./Canadian Brand Names** Apo-Cefaclor® [Can]; Ceclor® [Can]; Novo-Cefaclor [Can]; Nu-Cefaclor [Can]; PMS-Cefaclor [Can]; Raniclor™ [US]

**Therapeutic Category** Cephalosporin (Second Generation)

**Use** Treatment of susceptible bacterial infections including otitis media, lower respiratory tract infections, acute exacerbations of chronic bronchitis, pharyngitis and tonsillitis, urinary tract infections, skin and skin structure infections

**Usual Dosage** Oral:
Children >1 month: Dosing range: 20-40 mg/kg/day divided every 8-12 hours; maximum dose: 1 g/day
Otitis media: 40 mg/kg/day divided every 12 hours
Pharyngitis: 20 mg/kg/day divided every 12 hours
Adults: Dosing range: 250-500 mg every 8 hours

**Dosage Forms**
Capsule: 250 mg, 500 mg
Powder for oral suspension: 125 mg/5 mL (75 mL, 150 mL); 187 mg/5 mL (50 mL, 100 mL); 250 mg/5 mL (75 mL, 150 mL); 375 mg/5 mL (50 mL, 100 mL)
Tablet, chewable (Raniclor™): 125 mg [contains phenylalanine 2.8 mg; fruity flavor], 187 mg [contains phenylalanine 4.2 mg; fruity flavor], 250 mg [contains phenylalanine 5.6 mg; fruity flavor], 375 mg [contains phenylalanine 8.4 mg; fruity flavor]

## cefadroxil (sef a DROKS il)

**Synonyms** cefadroxil monohydrate

**U.S./Canadian Brand Names** Apo-Cefadroxil® [Can]; Duricef® [US/Can]; Novo-Cefadroxil [Can]

**Therapeutic Category** Cephalosporin (First Generation)

**Use** Treatment of susceptible bacterial infections, including those caused by group A beta-hemolytic *Streptococcus*; prophylaxis against bacterial endocarditis in patients who are allergic to penicillin and undergoing surgical or dental procedures

**Usual Dosage** Oral:
Children: 30 mg/kg/day divided twice daily up to a maximum of 2 g/day
Adults: 1-2 g/day in 2 divided doses
Prophylaxis against bacterial endocarditis:
Children: 50 mg/kg 1 hour prior to the procedure
Adults: 2 g 1 hour prior to the procedure

**Dosage Forms**
Capsule, as monohydrate: 500 mg
Powder for oral suspension, as monohydrate: 250 mg/5 mL (50 mL, 100 mL); 500 mg/5 mL (75 mL, 100 mL) [contains sodium benzoate; orange-pineapple flavor]
Tablet, as monohydrate: 1 g

**cefadroxil monohydrate** *see* cefadroxil *on this page*

**Cefadyl**® *(Discontinued)*

**Cefanex**® *(Discontinued)* *see* cephalexin *on page 161*

## cefazolin (sef A zoe lin)

**Sound-Alike/Look-Alike Issues**
cefazolin may be confused with cefprozil, cephalexin, cephalothin
Kefzol® may be confused with Cefzil®

**Synonyms** cefazolin sodium

**U.S./Canadian Brand Names** Ancef® [US]

**Therapeutic Category** Cephalosporin (First Generation)

**Use** Treatment of respiratory tract, skin and skin structure, genital, urinary tract, biliary tract, bone and joint infections, and septicemia due to susceptible gram-positive cocci (except enterococcus); some gram-negative bacilli including *E. coli*, *Proteus*, and *Klebsiella* may be susceptible; perioperative prophylaxis

**Usual Dosage** I.M., I.V.:
Children >1 month: 25-100 mg/kg/day divided every 6-8 hours; maximum: 6 g/day
Adults: 250 mg to 2 g every 6-12 (usually 8) hours, depending on severity of infection; maximum dose: 12 g/day

**Dosage Forms** [DSC] = Discontinued product
Infusion [premixed in $D_5W$]: 500 mg (50 mL); 1 g (50 mL)
Injection, powder for reconstitution: 500 mg, 1 g, 10 g, 20 g
Ancef®: 1 g; 10 g [DSC]

**cefazolin sodium** *see* cefazolin *on this page*

## cefdinir (SEF di ner)

**Synonyms** CFDN

**U.S./Canadian Brand Names** Omnicef® [US/Can]

**Therapeutic Category** Cephalosporin (Third Generation)

**Use** Treatment of community-acquired pneumonia, acute exacerbations of chronic bronchitis, acute bacterial otitis media, acute maxillary sinusitis, pharyngitis/tonsillitis, and uncomplicated skin and skin structure infections.

**Usual Dosage** Oral:
Children 6 months to 12 years:
Acute bacterial otitis media, pharyngitis/tonsillitis: 7 mg/kg/dose twice daily for 5-10 days **or** 14 mg/kg/dose once daily for 10 days (maximum: 600 mg/day)
Acute maxillary sinusitis: 7 mg/kg/dose twice daily **or** 14 mg/kg/dose once daily for 10 days (maximum: 600 mg/day)
Uncomplicated skin and skin structure infections: 7 mg/kg/dose twice daily for 10 days (maximum: 600 mg/day)
Adolescents and Adults:
Community-acquired pneumonia, uncomplicated skin and skin structure infections: 300 mg twice daily for 10 days
Acute exacerbations of chronic bronchitis, pharyngitis/tonsillitis: 300 mg twice daily for 5-10 days **or** 600 mg once daily for 10 days
Acute maxillary sinusitis: 300 mg twice daily **or** 600 mg once daily for 10 days

**Dosage Forms**
Capsule: 300 mg
Powder for oral suspension: 125 mg/5 mL (60 mL, 100 mL) [contains sodium benzoate and sucrose 2.86 g/5 mL; strawberry flavor]; 250 mg/5 mL (60 mL, 100 mL) [contains sodium benzoate and sucrose 2.86 g/5 mL; strawberry flavor]

## cefditoren (sef de TOR en)

**Synonyms** cefditoren pivoxil

**U.S./Canadian Brand Names** Spectracef™ [US]

**Therapeutic Category** Antibiotic, Cephalosporin

**Use** Treatment of acute bacterial exacerbation of chronic bronchitis or community-acquired pneumonia (due to susceptible organisms including *Haemophilus influenzae*, *Haemophilus parainfluenzae*, *Streptococcus pneumoniae*-penicillin susceptible only, *Moraxella catarrhalis*); pharyngitis or tonsillitis (*Streptococcus pyogenes*); and uncomplicated skin and skin-structure infections (*Staphylococcus aureus* - not MRSA, *Streptococcus pyogenes*)

**Usual Dosage** Oral: Children ≥12 years and Adults:
Acute bacterial exacerbation of chronic bronchitis: 400 mg twice daily for 10 days
Community-acquired pneumonia: 400 mg twice daily for 14 days
(Continued)

## cefditoren *(Continued)*

Pharyngitis, tonsillitis, uncomplicated skin and skin structure infections: 200 mg twice daily for 10 days

**Dosage Forms** Tablet, as pivoxil: 200 mg [equivalent to cefditoren; contains sodium caseinate]

**cefditoren pivoxil** *see* cefditoren *on previous page*

## cefepime (SEF e pim)

**Synonyms** cefepime hydrochloride

**U.S./Canadian Brand Names** Maxipime® [US/Can]

**Therapeutic Category** Cephalosporin (Fourth Generation)

**Use** Treatment of uncomplicated and complicated urinary tract infections, including pyelonephritis caused by typical urinary tract pathogens; monotherapy for febrile neutropenia; uncomplicated skin and skin structure infections caused by *Streptococcus pyogenes*; moderate to severe pneumonia caused by pneumococcus, *Pseudomonas aeruginosa*, and other gram-negative organisms; complicated intra-abdominal infections (in combination with metronidazole). Also active against methicillin-susceptible staphylococci, *Enterobacter* sp, and many other gram-negative bacilli.

Children 2 months to 16 years: Empiric therapy of febrile neutropenia patients, uncomplicated skin/soft tissue infections, pneumonia, and uncomplicated/complicated urinary tract infections.

**Usual Dosage**

Children:

Febrile neutropenia: I.V.: 50 mg/kg every 8 hours for 7-10 days

Uncomplicated skin/soft tissue infections, pneumonia, and complicated/uncomplicated UTI: I.V.: 50 mg/kg twice daily

Adults:

Most infections: I.V.: 1-2 g every 12 hours for 7-10 days; higher doses or more frequent administration may be required in pseudomonal infections

Urinary tract infections, mild to moderate: I.M., I.V.: 500-1000 mg every 12 hours

Monotherapy for febrile neutropenic patients: I.V.: 2 g every 8 hours for 7 days or until the neutropenia resolves

**Dosage Forms** Injection, powder for reconstitution, as hydrochloride: 500 mg, 1 g, 2 g

**cefepime hydrochloride** *see* cefepime *on this page*

## cefixime (sef IKS eem)

**Sound-Alike/Look-Alike Issues**

Suprax® may be confused with Sporanox®, Surbex®

**U.S./Canadian Brand Names** Suprax® [US/Can]

**Therapeutic Category** Cephalosporin (Third Generation)

**Use** Treatment of urinary tract infections, otitis media, respiratory infections due to susceptible organisms including *S. pneumoniae* and *S. pyogenes*, *H. influenzae* and many Enterobacteriaceae; uncomplicated cervical/urethral gonorrhea due to *N. gonorrhoeae*

**Usual Dosage** Oral:

Children ≥6 months: 8 mg/kg/day divided every 12-24 hours

Children >50 kg or >12 years and Adults: 400 mg/day divided every 12-24 hours

Uncomplicated cervical/urethral gonorrhea due to *N. gonorrhoeae*: 400 mg as a single dose

For *S. pyogenes* infections, treat for 10 days

**Dosage Forms** Powder for oral suspension: 100 mg/5 mL (50 mL, 75 mL, 100 mL) [contains sodium benzoate; strawberry flavor]

**Cefizox® [US/Can]** *see* ceftizoxime *on page 157*

**Cefotan® [US/Can]** *see* cefotetan *on next page*

## cefotaxime (sef oh TAKS eem)

**Sound-Alike/Look-Alike Issues**

cefotaxime may be confused with cefoxitin, ceftizoxime, cefuroxime

**Synonyms** cefotaxime sodium

**U.S./Canadian Brand Names** Claforan® [US/Can]

**Therapeutic Category** Cephalosporin (Third Generation)

**Use** Treatment of susceptible infection in respiratory tract, skin and skin structure, bone and joint, urinary tract, gynecologic as well as septicemia, and documented or suspected meningitis. Active against most gram-negative bacilli (not *Pseudomonas*) and gram-positive cocci (not enterococcus). Active against many penicillin-resistant pneumococci.

**Usual Dosage**
Infants and Children 1 month to 12 years: I.M., I.V.: <50 kg: 50-180 mg/kg/day in divided doses every 4-6 hours
Meningitis: 200 mg/kg/day in divided doses every 6 hours
Children >12 years and Adults:
Uncomplicated infections: I.M., I.V.: 1 g every 12 hours
Moderate/severe infections: I.M., I.V.: 1-2 g every 8 hours
Infections commonly needing higher doses (eg, septicemia): I.V.: 2 g every 6-8 hours
Life-threatening infections: I.V.: 2 g every 4 hours
Preop: I.M., I.V.: 1 g 30-90 minutes before surgery
C-section: 1 g as soon as the umbilical cord is clamped, then 1 g I.M., I.V. at 6- and 12-hour intervals

**Dosage Forms**
Infusion, as sodium [premixed in $D_5W$]: 1 g (50 mL); 2 g (50 mL)
Injection, powder for reconstitution, as sodium: 500 mg, 1 g, 2 g, 10 g, 20 g
Claforan®: 500 mg, 1 g, 2 g, 10 g [contains sodium 50.5 mg (2.2 mEq) per cefotaxime 1 g]

**cefotaxime sodium** *see* cefotaxime *on previous page*

# cefotetan (SEF oh tee tan)
**Sound-Alike/Look-Alike Issues**
cefotetan may be confused with cefoxitin, Ceftin®
Cefotan® may be confused with Ceftin®
**Synonyms** cefotetan disodium
**U.S./Canadian Brand Names** Cefotan® [US/Can]
**Therapeutic Category** Cephalosporin (Second Generation)
**Use** Surgical prophylaxis; intra-abdominal infections and other mixed infections; respiratory tract, skin and skin structure, bone and joint, urinary tract and gynecologic as well as septicemia; active against gram-negative enteric bacilli including *E. coli*, *Klebsiella*, and *Proteus*; less active against staphylococci and streptococci than first generation cephalosporins, but active against anaerobes including *Bacteroides fragilis*
**Usual Dosage**
Adolescents and Adults: I.V.: Pelvic inflammatory disease: 2 g every 12 hours; used in combination with doxycycline
Adults: I.M., I.V.: 1-6 g/day in divided doses every 12 hours; usual dose: 1-2 g every 12 hours for 5-10 days; 1-2 g may be given every 24 hours for urinary tract infection
Preoperative prophylaxis: I.M., I.V.: 1-2 g 30-60 minutes prior to surgery; when used for cesarean section, dose should be given as soon as umbilical cord is clamped
**Dosage Forms** [DSC] = Discontinued product
Infusion [premixed iso-osmotic solution]: 1 g (50 mL); 2 g (50 mL) [contains sodium 80 mg/g (3.5 mEq/g)]
Injection, powder for reconstitution: 1 g, 2 g [contains sodium 80 mg/g (3.5 mEq/g)] [DSC]

**cefotetan disodium** *see* cefotetan *on this page*

# cefoxitin (se FOKS i tin)
**Sound-Alike/Look-Alike Issues**
cefoxitin may be confused with cefotaxime, cefotetan, Cytoxan®
Mefoxin® may be confused with Lanoxin®
**Synonyms** cefoxitin sodium
**U.S./Canadian Brand Names** Mefoxin® [US]
**Therapeutic Category** Cephalosporin (Second Generation)
**Use** Less active against staphylococci and streptococci than first generation cephalosporins, but active against anaerobes including *Bacteroides fragilis*; active against gram-negative enteric bacilli including *E. coli*, *Klebsiella*, and *Proteus*; used predominantly for respiratory tract, skin and skin structure, bone and joint, urinary tract and gynecologic as well as septicemia; surgical prophylaxis; intra-abdominal infections and other mixed infections; indicated for bacterial *Eikenella corrodens* infections
**Usual Dosage**
Infants >3 months and Children: I.M., I.V.:
Mild to moderate infection: 80-100 mg/kg/day in divided doses every 4-6 hours
Severe infection: 100-160 mg/kg/day in divided doses every 4-6 hours; maximum dose: 12 g/day
(Continued)

## cefoxitin *(Continued)*

Perioperative prophylaxis: 30-40 mg/kg 30-60 minutes prior to surgery followed by 30-40 mg/kg/dose every 6 hours for no more than 24 hours after surgery depending on the procedure

Adolescents and Adults: I.M., I.V.: Perioperative prophylaxis: 1-2 g 30-60 minutes prior to surgery followed by 1-2 g every 6-8 hours for no more than 24 hours after surgery depending on the procedure

Adults: I.M., I.V.: 1-2 g every 6-8 hours (I.M. injection is painful); up to 12 g/day

Pelvic inflammatory disease:

Inpatients: I.V.: 2 g every 6 hours **plus** doxycycline 100 mg I.V. or 100 mg orally every 12 hours until improved, followed by doxycycline 100 mg orally twice daily to complete 14 days

Outpatients: I.M.: 2 g **plus** probenecid 1 g orally as a single dose, followed by doxycycline 100 mg orally twice daily for 14 days

**Dosage Forms**

Infusion, as sodium [premixed iso-osmotic solution]: 1 g (50 mL); 2 g (50 mL) [contains sodium 53.8 mg/g (2.3 mEq/g)]

Injection, powder for reconstitution, as sodium: 1 g, 2 g, 10 g [contains sodium 53.8 mg/g (2.3 mEq/g)]

**cefoxitin sodium** *see* cefoxitin *on previous page*

## cefpodoxime *(sef pode OKS eem)*

**Sound-Alike/Look-Alike Issues**

Vantin® may be confused with Ventolin®

**Synonyms** cefpodoxime proxetil

**U.S./Canadian Brand Names** Vantin® [US/Can]

**Therapeutic Category** Cephalosporin (Second Generation)

**Use** Treatment of susceptible acute, community-acquired pneumonia caused by *S. pneumoniae* or nonbeta-lactamase producing *H. influenzae*; acute uncomplicated gonorrhea caused by *N. gonorrhoeae*; uncomplicated skin and skin structure infections caused by *S. aureus* or *S. pyogenes*; acute otitis media caused by *S. pneumoniae, H. influenzae*, or *M. catarrhalis*; pharyngitis or tonsillitis; and uncomplicated urinary tract infections caused by *E. coli, Klebsiella*, and *Proteus*

**Usual Dosage** Oral:

Children 2 months to 12 years:

Acute otitis media: 10 mg/kg/day divided every 12 hours (400 mg/day) for 5 days (maximum: 200 mg/dose)

Acute maxillary sinusitis: 10 mg/kg/day divided every 12 hours for 10 days (maximum: 200 mg/dose)

Pharyngitis/tonsillitis: 10 mg/kg/day in 2 divided doses for 5-10 days (maximum: 100 mg/dose)

Children ≥12 years and Adults:

Acute community-acquired pneumonia and bacterial exacerbations of chronic bronchitis: 200 mg every 12 hours for 14 days and 10 days, respectively

Acute maxillary sinusitis: 200 mg every 12 hours for 10 days

Skin and skin structure: 400 mg every 12 hours for 7-14 days

Uncomplicated gonorrhea (male and female) and rectal gonococcal infections (female): 200 mg as a single dose

Pharyngitis/tonsillitis: 100 mg every 12 hours for 5-10 days

Uncomplicated urinary tract infection: 100 mg every 12 hours for 7 days

**Dosage Forms**

Granules for oral suspension: 50 mg/5 mL (50 mL, 75 mL, 100 mL); 100 mg/5 mL (50 mL, 75 mL, 100 mL) [contains sodium benzoate; lemon creme flavor]

Tablet [film coated]: 100 mg, 200 mg

**cefpodoxime proxetil** *see* cefpodoxime *on this page*

## cefprozil *(sef PROE zil)*

**Sound-Alike/Look-Alike Issues**

cefprozil may be confused with cefazolin, cefuroxime

Cefzil® may be confused with Cefol®, Ceftin®, Kefzol®

**U.S./Canadian Brand Names** Cefzil® [US/Can]

**Therapeutic Category** Cephalosporin (Second Generation)

**Use** Treatment of otitis media and infections involving the respiratory tract and skin and skin structure; active against methicillin-sensitive staphylococci, many streptococci, and various gram-negative bacilli including *E. coli*, some *Klebsiella, P. mirabilis, H. influenzae*, and *Moraxella*.

**Usual Dosage** Oral:

Infants and Children >6 months to 12 years: Otitis media: 15 mg/kg every 12 hours for 10 days

Pharyngitis/tonsillitis:

Children 2-12 years: 7.5 -15 mg/kg/day divided every 12 hours for 10 days (administer for >10 days if due to *S. pyogenes*); maximum: 1 g/day

Children >13 years and Adults: 500 mg every 24 hours for 10 days

Uncomplicated skin and skin structure infections:

Children 2-12 years: 20 mg/kg every 24 hours for 10 days; maximum: 1 g/day

Children >13 years and Adults: 250 mg every 12 hours, or 500 mg every 12-24 hours for 10 days

Secondary bacterial infection of acute bronchitis or acute bacterial exacerbation of chronic bronchitis: 500 mg every 12 hours for 10 days

**Dosage Forms**

Powder for oral suspension, as anhydrous: 125 mg/5 mL (50 mL, 75 mL, 100 mL); 250 mg/5 mL (50 mL, 75 mL, 100 mL) [contains phenylalanine 28 mg/5 mL and sodium benzoate; bubble gum flavor]

Tablet, as anhydrous: 250 mg, 500 mg

## ceftazidime (SEF tay zi deem)

**Sound-Alike/Look-Alike Issues**

ceftazidime may be confused with ceftizoxime

Ceptaz® may be confused with Septra®

Tazicef® may be confused with Tazidime®

Tazidime® may be confused with Tazicef®

**U.S./Canadian Brand Names** Fortaz® [US/Can]; Tazicef® [US]

**Therapeutic Category** Cephalosporin (Third Generation)

**Use** Treatment of documented susceptible *Pseudomonas aeruginosa* infection and infections due to other susceptible aerobic gram-negative organisms; empiric therapy of a febrile, granulocytopenic patient

**Usual Dosage**

Infants and Children 1 month to 12 years: I.V.: 30-50 mg/kg/dose every 8 hours; maximum dose: 6 g/day

Adults: I.M., I.V.: 500 mg to 2 g every 8-12 hours

Urinary tract infections: 250-500 mg every 12 hours

**Dosage Forms** [DSC] = Discontinued product

Infusion, as sodium [premixed iso-osmotic solution] (Fortaz®): 1 g (50 mL); 2 g (50 mL)

Injection, powder for reconstitution:

Ceptaz® [DSC]: 10 g [L-arginine formulation]

Fortaz®: 500 mg, 1 g, 2 g, 6 g [contains sodium carbonate]

Tazicef®: 1 g, 2 g, 6 g [contains sodium carbonate]

## ceftibuten (sef TYE byoo ten)

**U.S./Canadian Brand Names** Cedax® [US]

**Therapeutic Category** Cephalosporin (Third Generation)

**Use** Oral cephalosporin for treatment of bronchitis, otitis media, and pharyngitis/tonsillitis due to *H. influenzae* and *M. catarrhalis*, both beta-lactamase-producing and nonproducing strains, as well as *S. pneumoniae* (weak) and *S. pyogenes*

**Usual Dosage** Oral:

Children <12 years: 9 mg/kg/day for 10 days; maximum daily dose: 400 mg

Children ≥12 years and Adults: 400 mg once daily for 10 days; maximum: 400 mg

**Dosage Forms**

Capsule: 400 mg

Powder for oral suspension: 90 mg/5 mL (30 mL, 60 mL, 120 mL) [contains sodium benzoate; cherry flavor]

**Ceftin® [US/Can]** see cefuroxime *on next page*

**Ceftin® Tablet 125 mg *(Discontinued)*** see cefuroxime *on next page*

## ceftizoxime (sef ti ZOKS eem)

**Sound-Alike/Look-Alike Issues**

ceftizoxime may be confused with cefotaxime, ceftazidime, cefuroxime

(Continued)

## ceftizoxime *(Continued)*

**Synonyms** ceftizoxime sodium

**U.S./Canadian Brand Names** Cefizox® [US/Can]

**Therapeutic Category** Cephalosporin (Third Generation)

**Use** Treatment of susceptible bacterial infection, mainly respiratory tract, skin and skin structure, bone and joint, urinary tract and gynecologic, as well as septicemia; active against many gram-negative bacilli (not *Pseudomonas*), some gram-positive cocci (not *Enterococcus*), and some anaerobes

**Usual Dosage** I.M., I.V.:

Children ≥6 months: 150-200 mg/kg/day divided every 6-8 hours (maximum of 12 g/24 hours)

Adults: 1-2 g every 8-12 hours, up to 2 g every 4 hours or 4 g every 8 hours for life-threatening infections

**Dosage Forms**

Infusion [premixed iso-osmotic solution]: 1 g (50 mL); 2 g (50 mL)

Injection, powder for reconstitution: 1 g, 2 g, 10 g

**ceftizoxime sodium** *see ceftizoxime on previous page*

## ceftriaxone *(sef trye AKS one)*

**Sound-Alike/Look-Alike Issues**

Rocephin® may be confused with Roferon®

**Synonyms** ceftriaxone sodium

**U.S./Canadian Brand Names** Rocephin® [US/Can]

**Therapeutic Category** Cephalosporin (Third Generation)

**Use** Treatment of lower respiratory tract infections, acute bacterial otitis media, skin and skin structure infections, bone and joint infections, intra-abdominal and urinary tract infections, pelvic inflammatory disease (PID), uncomplicated gonorrhea, bacterial septicemia, and meningitis; used in surgical prophylaxis

**Usual Dosage**

Infants and Children:

Usual dose: I.M., I.V.:

Mild-to-moderate infections: 50-75 mg/kg/day in 1-2 divided doses every 12-24 hours (maximum: 2 g/day); continue until at least 2 days after signs and symptoms of infection have resolved

Serious infections: 80-100 mg/kg/day in 1-2 divided doses (maximum: 4 g/day)

Gonococcal infection, uncomplicated: I.M.: 125 mg in a single dose

Meningitis: I.M., I.V.:

Uncomplicated: Loading dose of 100 mg/kg (maximum: 4 g), followed by 100 mg/kg/day divided every 12-24 hours (maximum: 4 g/day); usual duration of treatment is 7-14 days

Gonococcal, complicated:

<45 kg: 50 mg/kg/day given every 12 hours (maximum: 2 g/day); usual duration of treatment is 10-14 days

>45 kg: I.V.: 1-2 g every 12 hours; usual duration of treatment is 10-14 days

Otitis media: I.M., I.V.:

Acute: 50 mg/kg in a single dose (maximum: 1 g)

Adults: Usual dose: I.M., I.V.: 1-2 g every 12-24 hours, depending on the type and severity of infection

Gonococcal infection, uncomplicated: I.M.: 125-250 mg in a single dose

PID: I.M.: 250 mg in a single dose

Surgical prophylaxis: I.V.: 1 g 30 minutes to 2 hours before surgery

**Dosage Forms Note:** Contains sodium 83 mg (3.6 mEq) per ceftriaxone 1 g

Infusion [premixed in dextrose]: 1 g (50 mL); 2 g (50 mL)

Injection, powder for reconstitution: 250 mg, 500 mg, 1 g, 2 g, 10 g

**ceftriaxone sodium** *see ceftriaxone on this page*

## cefuroxime *(se fyoor OKS eem)*

**Sound-Alike/Look-Alike Issues**

cefuroxime may be confused with cefotaxime, cefprozil, ceftizoxime, deferoxamine

Ceftin® may be confused with Cefotan®, cefotetan, Cefzil®, Cipro®

Zinacef® may be confused with Zithromax®

**Synonyms** cefuroxime axetil; cefuroxime sodium

**U.S./Canadian Brand Names** Apo-Cefuroxime® [Can]; Ceftin® [US/Can]; ratio-Cefuroxime [Can]; Zinacef® [US/Can]

**Therapeutic Category** Cephalosporin (Second Generation)

**Use** Treatment of infections caused by staphylococci, group B streptococci, *H. influenzae* (type A and B), *E. coli*, *Enterobacter*, *Salmonella*, and *Klebsiella*; treatment of susceptible infections of the lower respiratory tract, otitis media, urinary tract, skin and soft tissue, bone and joint, sepsis and gonorrhea

**Usual Dosage Note:** Cefuroxime axetil film-coated tablets and oral suspension are not bioequivalent and are not substitutable on a mg/mg basis

Children ≥3 months to 12 years:

Pharyngitis, tonsillitis: Oral:

Suspension: 20 mg/kg/day (maximum: 500 mg/day) in 2 divided doses for 10 days

Tablet: 125 mg every 12 hours for 10 days

Acute otitis media, impetigo: Oral:

Suspension: 30 mg/kg/day (maximum: 1 g/day) in 2 divided doses for 10 days

Tablet: 250 mg twice daily for 10 days

I.M., I.V.: 75-150 mg/kg/day divided every 8 hours; maximum dose: 6 g/day

Meningitis: Not recommended (doses of 200-240 mg/kg/day divided every 6-8 hours have been used); maximum dose: 9 g/day

Acute bacterial maxillary sinusitis:

Suspension: 30 mg/kg/day in 2 divided doses for 10 days; maximum dose: 1 g/day

Tablet: 250 mg twice daily for 10 days

Children ≥13 years and Adults:

Oral: 250-500 mg twice daily for 10 days (5 days in selected patients with acute bronchitis)

Uncomplicated urinary tract infection: 125-250 mg every 12 hours for 7-10 days

Uncomplicated gonorrhea: 1 g as a single dose

Early Lyme disease: 500 mg twice daily for 20 days

I.M., I.V.: 750 mg to 1.5 g/dose every 8 hours or 100-150 mg/kg/day in divided doses every 6-8 hours; maximum: 6 g/24 hours

**Dosage Forms**

Infusion, as sodium [premixed] (Zinacef®): 750 mg (50 mL); 1.5 g (50 mL) [contains sodium 4.8 mEq (111 mg) per 750 mg]

Injection, powder for reconstitution, as sodium (Zinacef®): 750 mg, 1.5 g, 7.5 g [contains sodium 4.8 mEq (111 mg) per 750 mg]

Powder for oral suspension, as axetil (Ceftin®): 125 mg/5 mL (100 mL) [contains phenylalanine 11.8 mg/5 mL; tutti-frutti flavor]; 250 mg/5 mL (50 mL, 100 mL) [contains phenylalanine 25.2 mg/5 mL; tutti-frutti flavor]

Tablet, as axetil (Ceftin®): 250 mg, 500 mg

**cefuroxime axetil** *see* cefuroxime *on previous page*

**cefuroxime sodium** *see* cefuroxime *on previous page*

**Cefzil® [US/Can]** *see* cefprozil *on page 156*

**Celebrex® [US/Can]** *see* celecoxib *on this page*

**celecoxib** (se le KOKS ib)

**Sound-Alike/Look-Alike Issues**

Celebrex® may be confused with Celexa™, cerebra, Cerebyx®

**U.S./Canadian Brand Names** Celebrex® [US/Can]

**Therapeutic Category** Nonsteroidal Antiinflammatory Drug (NSAID), COX-2 Selective

**Use** Relief of the signs and symptoms of osteoarthritis, ankylosing spondylitis, and rheumatoid arthritis; management of acute pain; treatment of primary dysmenorrhea; decreasing intestinal polyps in familial adenomatous polyposis (FAP). **Note:** The Notice of Compliance for the use of celecoxib in FAP has been suspended by Health Canada.

**Usual Dosage** Adults: Oral:

Acute pain or primary dysmenorrhea: Initial dose: 400 mg, followed by an additional 200 mg if needed on day 1; maintenance dose: 200 mg twice daily as needed

Ankylosing spondylitis: 200 mg/day as a single dose or in divided doses twice daily; if no effect after 6 weeks, may increase to 400 mg/day. If no response following 6 weeks of treatment with 400 mg/day, consider discontinuation and alternative treatment.

Familial adenomatous polyposis: 400 mg twice daily

Osteoarthritis: 200 mg/day as a single dose or in divided dose twice daily

Rheumatoid arthritis: 100-200 mg twice daily

**Dosage Forms** Capsule: 100 mg, 200 mg, 400 mg

Celestone® [US] *see* betamethasone (systemic) *on page 103*

Celestone® Soluspan® [US/Can] *see* betamethasone (systemic) *on page 103*

Celexa™ [US/Can] *see* citalopram *on page 188*

CellCept® [US/Can] *see* mycophenolate *on page 554*

Cellugel® [US] *see* hydroxypropyl methylcellulose *on page 422*

## cellulose, oxidized regenerated (SEL yoo lose, OKS i dyzed re JEN er aye ted)

Sound-Alike/Look-Alike Issues

Surgicel® may be confused with Serentil®

Synonyms absorbable cotton; oxidized regenerated cellulose

Therapeutic Category Hemostatic Agent

Use Hemostatic; temporary packing for the control of capillary, venous, or small arterial hemorrhage

Usual Dosage Minimal amounts of the fabric strip are laid on the bleeding site or held firmly against the tissues until hemostasis occurs; remove excess material

Dosage Forms

Fabric, fibrous (Surgicel® Fibrillar):
1" x 2" (10s)
2" x 4" (10s)
4" x 4" (10s)

Fabric, knitted (Surgicel® NuKnit):
1" x 1" (24s)
1" x 3½" (10s)
3" x 4" (24s)
6" x 9" (10s)

Fabric, sheer weave (Surgicel®):
½" x 2" (24s)
2" x 3" (24s)
2" x 14" (24s)
4" x 8" (24s)

## cellulose sodium phosphate (sel yoo lose SOW dee um FOS fate)

Synonyms CSP; sodium cellulose phosphate

U.S./Canadian Brand Names Calcibind® [US/Can]

Therapeutic Category Urinary Tract Product

Use Adjunct to dietary restriction to reduce renal calculi formation in absorptive hypercalciuria type I

Usual Dosage Adults: Oral: 5 g 3 times/day with meals; decrease dose to 5 g with main meal and 2.5 g with each of two other meals when urinary calcium declines to <150 mg/day

Dosage Forms Powder: 2.5 g/scoop (45 g)

Celluvisc™ [Can] *see* carboxymethylcellulose *on page 148*

Celontin® [US/Can] *see* methsuximide *on page 528*

Cena-K® *(Discontinued) see* potassium chloride *on page 663*

Cenestin® [US] *see* estrogens (conjugated A/synthetic) *on page 303*

Centany™ [US] *see* mupirocin *on page 553*

Centrum® [US-OTC] *see* vitamins (multiple/oral) *on page 852*

Centrum® Kids Jimmy Neutron® Complete [US-OTC] *see* vitamins (multiple/pediatric) *on page 852*

Centrum® Kids Jimmy Neutron® Extra C [US-OTC] *see* vitamins (multiple/pediatric) *on page 852*

Centrum® Kids Rugrats™ Complete [US-OTC] *see* vitamins (multiple/pediatric) *on page 852*

Centrum® Kids Rugrats™ Extra C [US-OTC] *see* vitamins (multiple/pediatric) *on page 852*

Centrum® Kids Rugrats™ Extra Calcium [US-OTC] *see* vitamins (multiple/pediatric) *on page 852*

Centrum® Performance™ [US-OTC] *see* vitamins (multiple/oral) *on page 852*

Centrum® Silver® [US-OTC] *see* vitamins (multiple/oral) *on page 852*

Cepacol® [Can] *see* cetylpyridinium and benzocaine *on page 164*

**Cepacol® Antibacterial Mouthwash [US-OTC]** *see* cetylpyridinium *on page 164*

**Cepacol® Antibacterial Mouthwash Gold [US-OTC]** *see* cetylpyridinium *on page 164*

**Cepacol® Dual Action Maximum Strength [US-OTC]** *see* dyclonine *on page 277*

**Cepacol® Sore Throat [US-OTC]** *see* benzocaine *on page 95*

**Cepastat® [US-OTC]** *see* phenol *on page 638*

**Cepastat® Extra Strength [US-OTC]** *see* phenol *on page 638*

## cephalexin (sef a LEKS in)

**Sound-Alike/Look-Alike Issues**
cephalexin may be confused with cefaclor, cefazolin, cephalothin, ciprofloxacin

**Synonyms** cephalexin monohydrate

**U.S./Canadian Brand Names** Apo-Cephalex® [Can]; Biocef® [US]; Keflex® [US]; Keftab® [Can]; Novo-Lexin [Can]; Nu-Cephalex [Can]; Panixine DisperDose™ [US]

**Therapeutic Category** Cephalosporin (First Generation)

**Use** Treatment of susceptible bacterial infections including respiratory tract infections, otitis media, skin and skin structure infections, bone infections and genitourinary tract infections, including acute prostatitis; alternative therapy for acute bacterial endocarditis prophylaxis

**Usual Dosage** Oral:
Children >1 year: Dosing range: 25-50 mg/kg/day every 6-8 hours; more severe infections: 50-100 mg/kg/day in divided doses every 6-8 hours; maximum: 4 g/24 hours
Otitis media: 75-100 mg/kg/day in 4 divided doses
Streptococcal pharyngitis, skin and skin structure infections: 25-50 mg/kg/day divided every 12 hours
Uncomplicated cystitis: Children >15 years: Refer to Adults dosing
Prophylaxis of bacterial endocarditis (dental, oral, respiratory tract, or esophageal procedures): 50 mg/kg 1 hour prior to procedure (maximum: 2 g)
Adults: Dosing range: 250-1000 mg every 6 hours; maximum: 4 g/day
Streptococcal pharyngitis, skin and skin structure infections: 500 mg every 12 hours
Uncomplicated cystitis: 500 mg every 12 hours for 7-14 days
Prophylaxis of bacterial endocarditis (dental, oral, respiratory tract, or esophageal procedures): 2 g 1 hour prior to procedure

**Dosage Forms**
Capsule: 250 mg, 500 mg
Biocef®: 500 mg
Keflex®: 250 mg, 500 mg
Powder for oral suspension: 125 mg/5 mL (100 mL, 200 mL); 250 mg/5 mL (100 mL, 200 mL)
Biocef®: 125 mg/5 mL (100 mL); 250 mg/5 mL (100 mL)
Keflex®: 125 mg/5 mL (100 mL, 200 mL); 250 mg/5 mL (100 mL, 200 mL)
Tablet, for oral suspension (Panixine DisperDose™): 125 mg [contains phenylalanine 2.8 mg; peppermint flavor], 250 mg [contains phenylalanine 5.6 mg; peppermint flavor]

**cephalexin monohydrate** *see* cephalexin *on this page*

## cephalothin (sef A loe thin)

**Sound-Alike/Look-Alike Issues**
cephalothin may be confused with cefazolin, cephalexin

**Synonyms** cephalothin sodium

**Therapeutic Category** Cephalosporin (First Generation)

**Use** Treatment of infections when caused by susceptible strains in respiratory, genitourinary, gastrointestinal, skin and soft tissue, bone and joint infections; septicemia; treatment of susceptible gram-positive bacilli and cocci (never enterococcus); some gram-negative bacilli including *E. coli*, *Proteus*, and *Klebsiella* may be susceptible

**Usual Dosage** I.V.:
Neonates:
Postnatal age <7 days:
<2000 g: 20 mg every 12 hours
>2000 g: 20 mg every 8 hours
Postnatal age >7 days:
<2000 g: 20 mg every 8 hours
>2000 g: 20 mg every 6 hours
Children: 75-125 mg/kg/day divided every 4-6 hours; maximum dose: 10 g in a 24-hour period
(Continued)

# cephalothin *(Continued)*

Adults: 500 mg to 2 g every 4-6 hours
Dosage Forms [DSC] = Discontinued product
Infusion, as sodium [frozen]: 1 g (50 mL); 2 g (50 mL) [DSC]

**cephalothin sodium** *see* cephalothin *on previous page*

# cephradine (SEF ra deen)
Sound-Alike/Look-Alike Issues
cephradine may be confused with cephapirin
Velosef® may be confused with Vasosulf®
U.S./Canadian Brand Names Velosef® [US]
Therapeutic Category Cephalosporin (First Generation)
Use Treatment of infections when caused by susceptible strains in respiratory, genitourinary, gastrointestinal, skin and soft tissue, bone and joint infections; treatment of susceptible gram-positive bacilli and cocci (never enterococcus); some gram-negative bacilli including *E. coli*, *Proteus*, and *Klebsiella* may be susceptible
Usual Dosage Oral:
Children ≥9 months: Usual dose: 25-50 mg/kg/day in divided doses every 6 hours
Otitis media: 75-100 mg/kg/day in divided doses every 6 or 12 hours (maximum: 4 g/day)
Adults: 250-500 mg every 6-12 hours
Dosage Forms [DSC] = Discontinued product
Capsule: 250 mg, 500 mg [DSC]
Powder for oral suspension: 250 mg/5 mL (100 mL) [fruit flavor]

**Cephulac® *(Discontinued)*** *see* lactulose *on page 464*

**Ceptaz® *(Discontinued)*** *see* ceftazidime *on page 157*

**Cerebyx® [US/Can]** *see* fosphenytoin *on page 361*

**Ceredase® [US]** *see* alglucerase *on page 27*

**Cerezyme® [US/Can]** *see* imiglucerase *on page 431*

**Certain Dri® [US-OTC]** *see* aluminum chloride hexahydrate *on page 34*

**Cerubidine® [US/Can]** *see* daunorubicin hydrochloride *on page 225*

**Cerumenex® [Can]** *see* triethanolamine polypeptide oleate-condensate *on page 822*

**Cerumenex® *(Discontinued)*** *see* triethanolamine polypeptide oleate-condensate *on page 822*

**Cervidil® [US/Can]** *see* dinoprostone *on page 253*

**C.E.S.** *see* estrogens (conjugated/equine) *on page 304*

**Cetacaine® [US]** *see* benzocaine, butyl aminobenzoate, tetracaine, and benzalkonium chloride *on page 97*

**Cetacort® [US]** *see* hydrocortisone (topical) *on page 417*

**Cetafen® [US-OTC]** *see* acetaminophen *on page 4*

**Cetafen Cold® [US-OTC]** *see* acetaminophen and pseudoephedrine *on page 8*

**Cetafen Extra® [US-OTC]** *see* acetaminophen *on page 4*

**Cetamide™ [Can]** *see* sulfacetamide *on page 771*

**Ceta-Plus® [US]** *see* hydrocodone and acetaminophen *on page 411*

**Cetapred® Ophthalmic *(Discontinued)*** *see* sulfacetamide and prednisolone *on page 771*

# cetirizine (se TI ra zeen)
Sound-Alike/Look-Alike Issues
Zyrtec® may be confused with Serax®, Xanax®, Zantac®, Zyprexa®
Synonyms cetirizine hydrochloride; P-071; UCB-P071
U.S./Canadian Brand Names Apo-Cetirizine® [Can]; Reactine™ [Can]; Zyrtec® [US]
Therapeutic Category Antihistamine
Use Perennial and seasonal allergic rhinitis and other allergic symptoms including urticaria; chronic idiopathic urticaria

**Usual Dosage** Oral:
Children:

6-12 months: Chronic urticaria, perennial allergic rhinitis: 2.5 mg once daily

12 months to <2 years: Chronic urticaria, perennial allergic rhinitis: 2.5 mg once daily; may increase to 2.5 mg every 12 hours if needed

2-5 years: Chronic urticaria, perennial or seasonal allergic rhinitis: Initial: 2.5 mg once daily; may be increased to 2.5 mg every 12 hours **or** 5 mg once daily

Children ≥6 years and Adults: Chronic urticaria, perennial or seasonal allergic rhinitis: 5-10 mg once daily, depending upon symptom severity

**Dosage Forms**

Syrup, as hydrochloride: 5 mg/5 mL (120 mL, 480 mL) [banana-grape flavor]

Tablet, as hydrochloride: 5 mg, 10 mg

Tablet, chewable, as hydrochloride: 5 mg, 10 mg [grape flavor]

## cetirizine and pseudoephedrine (se TI ra zeen & soo doe e FED rin)

**Sound-Alike/Look-Alike Issues**

Zyrtec® may be confused with Serax®, Xanax®, Zantac®, Zyprexa®

**Synonyms** cetirizine hydrochloride and pseudoephedrine hydrochloride; pseudoephedrine hydrochloride and cetirizine hydrochloride

**U.S./Canadian Brand Names** Reactine® Allergy and Sinus [Can]; Zyrtec-D 12 Hour™ [US]

**Therapeutic Category** Antihistamine/Decongestant Combination

**Use** Treatment of symptoms of seasonal or perennial allergic rhinitis

**Usual Dosage** Oral: Children ≥12 years and Adults: Seasonal/perennial allergic rhinitis: 1 tablet twice daily

**Dosage Forms** Tablet, extended release: Cetirizine hydrochloride 5 mg and pseudoephedrine hydrochloride 120 mg

## cetirizine hydrochloride *see* cetirizine *on previous page*

## cetirizine hydrochloride and pseudoephedrine hydrochloride *see* cetirizine and pseudoephedrine *on this page*

## cetrorelix (set roe REL iks)

**Synonyms** cetrorelix acetate

**U.S./Canadian Brand Names** Cetrotide® [US/Can]

**Therapeutic Category** Antigonadotropic Agent

**Use** Inhibits premature luteinizing hormone (LH) surges in women undergoing controlled ovarian stimulation

**Usual Dosage** SubQ: Adults: Female: Used in conjunction with controlled ovarian stimulation therapy using gonadotropins (FSH, HMG):

Single-dose regimen: 3 mg given when serum estradiol levels show appropriate stimulation response, usually stimulation day 7 (range days 5-9). If hCG is not administered within 4 days, continue cetrorelix at 0.25 mg/day until hCG is administered

Multiple-dose regimen: 0.25 mg morning or evening of stimulation day 5, or morning of stimulation day 6; continue until hCG is administered.

**Dosage Forms** Injection, powder for reconstitution: 0.25 mg, 3 mg [supplied with SWFI in prefilled syringe]

## cetrorelix acetate *see* cetrorelix *on this page*

## Cetrotide® [US/Can] *see* cetrorelix *on this page*

## cetuximab (se TUK see mab)

**Sound-Alike/Look-Alike Issues**

cetuximab may be confused with bevacizumab

**Synonyms** C225; IMC-C225

**U.S./Canadian Brand Names** Erbitux™ [US]

**Therapeutic Category** Antineoplastic Agent, Monoclonal Antibody; Epidermal Growth Factor Receptor (EGFR) Inhibitor

**Use** Treatment of epidermal growth factor receptor (EGFR) expressing, metastatic colorectal carcinoma; may be used in combination with irinotecan in patients who are refractory to irinotecan-based chemotherapy or as a single agent in patients who are intolerant to irinotecan-based chemotherapy. (Continued)

# cetuximab *(Continued)*

**Usual Dosage** I.V.: Adults: Colorectal cancer:
Initial loading dose: 400 mg/m$^2$ infused over 120 minutes
Maintenance dose: 250 mg/m$^2$ infused over 60 minutes
**Dosage Forms** Injection, solution [preservative free]: 2 mg/mL (50 mL)

# cetylpyridinium *(SEE til peer i DI nee um)*

**Synonyms** cetylpyridinium chloride; CPC
**U.S./Canadian Brand Names** Cepacol® Antibacterial Mouthwash Gold [US-OTC]; Cepacol® Antibacterial Mouthwash [US-OTC]; DiabetAid Gingivitis Mouth Rinse [US-OTC]
**Therapeutic Category** Local Anesthetic
**Use** Antiseptic to aid in the prevention and reduction of plaque and gingivitis, and to freshen breath
**Usual Dosage** Children ≥6 years and Adults: Oral (OTC labeling): Rinse or gargle to freshen mouth; may be used before or after brushing
**Dosage Forms** Liquid, as chloride, oral [mouthwash/gargle]:
Cepacol® Antibacterial Mouthwash Gold: 0.05% (120 mL, 360 mL, 720 mL, 960 mL) [contains alcohol 14% and tartrazine; original flavor]
Cepacol® Antibacterial Mouthwash: 0.05% (120 mL, 360 mL, 720 mL, 960 mL) [contains alcohol 14% and tartrazine; mint flavor]
DiabetAid Gingivitis Mouth Rinse: 0.1% (480 mL) [sugar free]

# cetylpyridinium and benzocaine *(SEE til peer i DI nee um & BEN zoe kane)*

**Synonyms** benzocaine and cetylpyridinium chloride; cetylpyridinium chloride and benzocaine
**U.S./Canadian Brand Names** Cepacol® [Can]; Kank-A® [Can]
**Therapeutic Category** Local Anesthetic
**Use** Symptomatic relief of sore throat
**Usual Dosage** Antiseptic/anesthetic: Oral: Dissolve in mouth as needed for sore throat

**cetylpyridinium chloride** *see* cetylpyridinium *on this page*

**cetylpyridinium chloride and benzocaine** *see* cetylpyridinium and benzocaine *on this page*

**Cevalin® *(Discontinued)*** *see* ascorbic acid *on page 71*

**Cevi-Bid® [US-OTC]** *see* ascorbic acid *on page 71*

# cevimeline *(se vi ME leen)*

**Sound-Alike/Look-Alike Issues**
Evoxac® may be confused with Eurax®
**Synonyms** cevimeline hydrochloride
**U.S./Canadian Brand Names** Evoxac® [US/Can]
**Therapeutic Category** Cholinergic Agent
**Use** Treatment of symptoms of dry mouth in patients with Sjögren syndrome
**Usual Dosage** Adults: Oral: 30 mg 3 times/day
**Dosage Forms** Capsule, as hydrochloride: 30 mg

**cevimeline hydrochloride** *see* cevimeline *on this page*

**CFDN** *see* cefdinir *on page 153*

**CG** *see* chorionic gonadotropin (human) *on page 181*

**CGP-42446** *see* zoledronic acid *on page 863*

**CGP 57148B** *see* imatinib *on page 430*

**C-Gram [US-OTC]** *see* ascorbic acid *on page 71*

**Charcadole® [Can]** *see* charcoal *on next page*

**Charcadole®, Aqueous [Can]** *see* charcoal *on next page*

**Charcadole® TFS [Can]** *see* charcoal *on next page*

**Char-Caps [US-OTC]** *see* charcoal *on next page*

**CharcoAid® *(Discontinued)*** *see* charcoal *on next page*

**CharcoAid G® *(Discontinued)*** *see* charcoal *on next page*

# charcoal (CHAR kole)

**Sound-Alike/Look-Alike Issues**
Actidose® may be confused with Actos®

**Synonyms** activated carbon; activated charcoal; adsorbent charcoal; liquid antidote; medicinal carbon; medicinal charcoal

**U.S./Canadian Brand Names** Actidose-Aqua® [US-OTC]; Actidose® with Sorbitol [US-OTC]; Char-Caps [US-OTC]; Charcadole® TFS [Can]; Charcadole® [Can]; Charcadole®, Aqueous [Can]; Charcoal Plus® DS [US-OTC]; Charcocaps® [US-OTC]; EZ-Char™ [US-OTC]; Kerr Insta-Char® [US-OTC]

**Therapeutic Category** Antidote

**Use** Emergency treatment in poisoning by drugs and chemicals; aids the elimination of certain drugs and improves decontamination of excessive ingestions of sustained-release products or in the presence of bezoars; repetitive doses have proven useful to enhance the elimination of certain drugs (eg, theophylline, phenobarbital, and aspirin); repetitive doses for gastric dialysis in uremia to adsorb various waste products; dietary supplement (digestive aid)

**Usual Dosage** Oral:
Acute poisoning: **Note:** ~10 g of activated charcoal for each 1 g of toxin is considered adequate; this may require multiple doses. If sorbitol is also used, sorbitol dose should not exceed 1.5 g/kg. When using multiple doses of charcoal, sorbitol should be given with every other dose (not to exceed 2 doses/day).
Children: 1 g/kg as a single dose; if multiple doses are needed, additional doses can be given as 0.25 g/kg every hour or equivalent (ie, 0.5 g/kg every 2 hours) **or**
>1 year-12 years: 25-50 g as a single dose; smaller doses (10-25 g) may be used in children 1-5 years due to smaller gut lumen capacity
Children >12 years and Adults: 25-100 g as a single dose; if multiple doses are needed, additional doses may be given as 12.5 g/hour or equivalent (ie, 25 g every 2 hours)
Dietary supplement: Adult: 500-520 mg after meals; may repeat in 2 hours if needed (maximum 10 g/day)

**Dosage Forms** [DSC] = Discontinued product
Capsule, activated (Char-Caps, Charcocaps®): 260 mg
Granules, activated (CharcoAid G®): 15 g (120 mL) [DSC]
Liquid, activated:
Actidose-Aqua®: 15 g (72 mL); 25 g (120 mL); 50 g (240 mL)
Kerr Insta-Char®: 25 g (120 mL) [cherry flavor]; 50 g (240 mL) [unflavored or cherry flavor]
Liquid, activated [with sorbitol]:
Actidose® with Sorbitol: 25 g (120 mL); 50 g (240 mL)
Kerr Insta-Char®: 25 g (120 mL); 50 g (240 mL) [cherry flavor]
Pellets, activated (EZ-Char™): 25 g
Powder for suspension, activated: 30 g, 240 g
Tablets, activated (Charcoal Plus® DS): 250 mg

**Children's Kaopectate®** *(Discontinued)* see attapulgite *on page 81*

**Children's Kaopectate®** **(reformulation) [OTC]** see bismuth subsalicylate *on page 108*

**Children's Tylenol®** **Plus Cold [US-OTC]** see acetaminophen, chlorpheniramine, and pseudoephedrine *on page 10*

**children's vitamins** see vitamins (multiple/pediatric) *on page 852*

**Chirocaine® [Can]** see levobupivacaine *on page 473*

**Chirocaine®** *(Discontinued)* see levobupivacaine *on page 473*

**Chlo-Amine® Oral** *(Discontinued)* see chlorpheniramine *on page 171*

**Chlorafed® Liquid** *(Discontinued)* see chlorpheniramine and pseudoephedrine *on page 172*

**chloral** see chloral hydrate *on this page*

## chloral hydrate (KLOR al HYE drate)

**Synonyms** chloral; hydrated chloral; trichloroacetaldehyde monohydrate

**U.S./Canadian Brand Names** Aquachloral® Supprettes® [US]; PMS-Chloral Hydrate [Can]; Somnote™ [US]

**Therapeutic Category** Hypnotic, Nonbarbiturate

**Controlled Substance** C-IV

**Use** Short-term sedative and hypnotic (<2 weeks), sedative/hypnotic for diagnostic procedures; sedative prior to EEG evaluations

**Usual Dosage**
Children:
Sedation or anxiety: Oral, rectal: 5-15 mg/kg/dose every 8 hours (maximum: 500 mg/dose)
Prior to EEG: Oral, rectal: 20-25 mg/kg/dose, 30-60 minutes prior to EEG; may repeat in 30 minutes to maximum of 100 mg/kg or 2 g total
Hypnotic: Oral, rectal: 20-40 mg/kg/dose up to a maximum of 50 mg/kg/24 hours or 1 g/dose or 2 g/24 hours
Conscious sedation: Oral: 50-75 mg/kg/dose 30-60 minutes prior to procedure; may repeat 30 minutes after initial dose if needed, to a total maximum dose of 120 mg/kg or 1 g total
Adults: Oral, rectal:
Sedation, anxiety: 250 mg 3 times/day
Hypnotic: 500-1000 mg at bedtime or 30 minutes prior to procedure, not to exceed 2 g/24 hours

**Dosage Forms**
Capsule (Somnote™): 500 mg
Suppository, rectal (Aquachloral® Supprettes®): 325 mg [contains tartrazine], 650 mg
Syrup: 500 mg/5 mL (480 mL) [contains sodium benzoate]

## chlorambucil (klor AM byoo sil)

**Sound-Alike/Look-Alike Issues**
chlorambucil may be confused with Chloromycetin®
Leukeran® may be confused with Alkeran®, leucovorin, Leukine®

**Synonyms** CB-1348; chlorambucilum; chloraminophene; chlorbutinum; NSC-3088; WR-139013

**U.S./Canadian Brand Names** Leukeran® [US/Can]

**Therapeutic Category** Antineoplastic Agent

**Use** Management of chronic lymphocytic leukemia, Hodgkin and non-Hodgkin lymphoma; breast and ovarian carcinoma; Waldenström macroglobulinemia, testicular carcinoma, thrombocythemia, choriocarcinoma

**Usual Dosage** Oral (refer to individual protocols):
Children:
General short courses: 0.1-0.2 mg/kg/day **or** 4.5 mg/m$^2$/day for 3-6 weeks for remission induction (usual: 4-10 mg/day); maintenance therapy: 0.03-0.1 mg/kg/day (usual: 2-4 mg/day)
Nephrotic syndrome: 0.1-0.2 mg/kg/day every day for 5-15 weeks with low-dose prednisone
Chronic lymphocytic leukemia (CLL):
Biweekly regimen: Initial: 0.4 mg/kg/dose every 2 weeks; increase dose by 0.1 mg/kg every 2 weeks until a response occurs and/or myelosuppression occurs
Monthly regimen: Initial: 0.4 mg/kg, increase dose by 0.2 mg/kg every 4 weeks until a response occurs and/or myelosuppression occurs
Malignant lymphomas:
Non-Hodgkin's lymphoma: 0.1 mg/kg/day

Hodgkin's lymphoma: 0.2 mg/kg/day
Adults: 0.1-0.2 mg/kg/day **or**
3-6 mg/m$^2$/day for 3-6 weeks, then adjust dose on basis of blood counts **or**
0.4 mg/kg and increased by 0.1 mg/kg biweekly or monthly **or**
14 mg/m$^2$/day for 5 days, repeated every 21-28 days
**Dosage Forms** Tablet [film coated]: 2 mg

**chlorambucilum** *see* chlorambucil *on previous page*

**chloraminophene** *see* chlorambucil *on previous page*

# chloramphenicol (klor am FEN i kole)
**Sound-Alike/Look-Alike Issues**
Chloromycetin® may be confused with chlorambucil, Chlor-Trimeton®
**U.S./Canadian Brand Names** Chloromycetin® Sodium Succinate [US]; Chloromycetin® [Can]; Diochloram® [Can]; Pentamycetin® [Can]
**Therapeutic Category** Antibiotic, Miscellaneous; Antibiotic, Ophthalmic; Antibiotic, Otic
**Use** Treatment of serious infections due to organisms resistant to other less toxic antibiotics or when its penetrability into the site of infection is clinically superior to other antibiotics to which the organism is sensitive, useful in infections caused by *Bacteroides*, *H. influenzae*, *Neisseria meningitidis*, *Salmonella*, and *Rickettsia*; active against many vancomycin-resistant enterococci
**Usual Dosage**
Meningitis: I.V.: Infants >30 days and Children: 50-100 mg/kg/day divided every 6 hours
Other infections: I.V.:
Infants >30 days and Children: 50-75 mg/kg/day divided every 6 hours; maximum daily dose: 4 g/day
Adults: 50-100 mg/kg/day in divided doses every 6 hours; maximum daily dose: 4 g/day
**Dosage Forms** Injection, powder for reconstitution: 1 g [contains sodium ~52 mg/g (2.25 mEq/g)]

**ChloraPrep® [US-OTC]** *see* chlorhexidine gluconate *on next page*

**Chloraseptic® Gargle [US-OTC]** *see* phenol *on page 638*

**Chloraseptic® Mouth Pain Spray [US-OTC]** *see* phenol *on page 638*

**Chloraseptic® Rinse [US-OTC]** *see* phenol *on page 638*

**Chloraseptic® Spray [US-OTC]** *see* phenol *on page 638*

**Chloraseptic® Spray for Kids [US-OTC]** *see* phenol *on page 638*

**Chlorate® Oral *(Discontinued)*** *see* chlorpheniramine *on page 171*

**chlorbutinum** *see* chlorambucil *on previous page*

# chlordiazepoxide (klor dye az e POKS ide)
**Sound-Alike/Look-Alike Issues**
Librium® may be confused with Librax®
**Synonyms** methaminodiazepoxide hydrochloride
**U.S./Canadian Brand Names** Apo-Chlordiazepoxide® [Can]; Librium® [US]
**Therapeutic Category** Benzodiazepine
**Controlled Substance** C-IV
**Use** Management of anxiety disorder or for the short-term relief of symptoms of anxiety; withdrawal symptoms of acute alcoholism; preoperative apprehension and anxiety
**Usual Dosage**
Children:
<6 years: Not recommended
>6 years: Anxiety: Oral, I.M.: 0.5 mg/kg/24 hours divided every 6-8 hours
Adults:
Anxiety:
Oral: 15-100 mg divided 3-4 times/day
I.M., I.V.: Initial: 50-100 mg followed by 25-50 mg 3-4 times/day as needed
Preoperative anxiety: I.M.: 50-100 mg prior to surgery
Ethanol withdrawal symptoms: Oral, I.V.: 50-100 mg to start, dose may be repeated in 2-4 hours as necessary to a maximum of 300 mg/24 hours
**Note:** Up to 300 mg may be given I.M. or I.V. during a 6-hour period, but not more than this in any 24-hour period.
(Continued)

# chlordiazepoxide *(Continued)*

## Dosage Forms
Capsule, as hydrochloride: 5 mg, 10 mg, 25 mg
Injection, powder for reconstitution, as hydrochloride: 100 mg [diluent contains benzyl alcohol, polysorbate 80, and propylene glycol]

**chlordiazepoxide and amitriptyline** *see* amitriptyline and chlordiazepoxide *on page 43*

**chlordiazepoxide and clidinium** *see* clidinium and chlordiazepoxide *on page 191*

**chlorethazine** *see* mechlorethamine *on page 505*

**chlorethazine mustard** *see* mechlorethamine *on page 505*

# chlorhexidine gluconate (klor HEKS i deen GLOO koe nate)

## Sound-Alike/Look-Alike Issues
Peridex® may be confused with Precedex™

## Synonyms CHG

## U.S./Canadian Brand Names Apo-Chlorhexidine® [Can]; Avagard™ [US-OTC]; BactoShield® CHG [US-OTC]; Betasept® [US-OTC]; ChloraPrep® [US-OTC]; Dyna-Hex® [US-OTC]; Hibiclens® [US-OTC]; Hibidil® 1:2000 [Can]; Hibistat® [US-OTC]; Operand® Chlorhexidine Gluconate [US-OTC]; ORO-Clense [Can]; Peridex® [US]; PerioChip® [US]; PerioGard® [US]

## Therapeutic Category Antibiotic, Oral Rinse; Antibiotic, Topical

## Use Skin cleanser for surgical scrub, cleanser for skin wounds, preoperative skin preparation, germicidal hand rinse, and as antibacterial dental rinse. Chlorhexidine is active against gram-positive and gram-negative organisms, facultative anaerobes, aerobes, and yeast.

**Orphan drug:** Peridex®: Oral mucositis with cytoreductive therapy when used for patients undergoing bone marrow transplant

## Usual Dosage Adults:
**Oral rinse (Peridex®, PerioGard®):**
Floss and brush teeth, completely rinse toothpaste from mouth and swish 15 mL (one capful) undiluted oral rinse around in mouth for 30 seconds, then expectorate. Caution patient not to swallow the medicine and instruct not to eat for 2-3 hours after treatment. (Cap on bottle measures 15 mL.)

Treatment of gingivitis: Oral prophylaxis: Swish for 30 seconds with 15 mL chlorhexidine, then expectorate; repeat twice daily (morning and evening). Patient should have a re-evaluation followed by a dental prophylaxis every 6 months.

**Periodontal chip:** One chip is inserted into a periodontal pocket with a probing pocket depth ≥5 mm. Up to 8 chips may be inserted in a single visit. Treatment is recommended every 3 months in pockets with a remaining depth ≥5 mm. If dislodgment occurs 7 days or more after placement, the subject is considered to have had the full course of treatment. If dislodgment occurs within 48 hours, a new chip should be inserted. The chip biodegrades completely and does not need to be removed. Patients should avoid dental floss at the site of PerioChip® insertion for 10 days after placement because flossing might dislodge the chip.

Insertion of periodontal chip: Pocket should be isolated and surrounding area dried prior to chip insertion. The chip should be grasped using forceps with the rounded edges away from the forceps. The chip should be inserted into the periodontal pocket to its maximum depth. It may be maneuvered into position using the tips of the forceps or a flat instrument.

Cleanser:
Surgical scrub: Scrub 3 minutes and rinse thoroughly, wash for an additional 3 minutes

Hand sanitizer (Avagard™): Dispense 1 pumpful in palm of one hand; dip fingertips of opposite hand into solution and work it under nails. Spread remainder evenly over hand and just above elbow, covering all surfaces. Repeat on other hand. Dispense another pumpful in each hand and reapply to each hand up to the wrist. Allow to dry before gloving.

Hand wash: Wash for 15 seconds and rinse
Hand rinse: Rub 15 seconds and rinse

## Dosage Forms
Chip, for periodontal pocket insertion (PerioChip®): 2.5 mg
Liquid, topical [surgical scrub]:
Avagard™: 1% (500 mL) [contains ethyl alcohol and moisturizers]
BactoShield® CHG: 2% (120 mL, 480 mL, 750 mL, 1000 mL, 3800 mL); 4% (120 mL, 480 mL, 750 mL, 1000 mL, 3800 mL) [contains isopropyl alcohol]
Betasept®: 4% (120 mL, 240 mL, 480 mL, 960 mL, 3840 mL) [contains isopropyl alcohol]

ChloraPrep®: 2% (0.67 mL, 1.5 mL, 3 mL, 10.5 mL) [contains isopropyl alcohol 70%; prefilled applicator]

Dyna-Hex®: 2% (120 mL, 960 mL, 3840 mL); 4% (120 mL, 960 mL, 3840 mL)

Hibiclens®: 4% (15 mL, 120 mL, 240 mL, 480 mL, 960 mL, 3840 mL) [contains isopropyl alcohol]

Operand® Chlorhexidine Gluconate: 2% (120 mL); 4% (120 mL, 240 mL, 480 mL, 960 mL, 3840 mL) [contains isopropyl alcohol]

Liquid, oral rinse: 0.12% (480 mL)

Peridex®: 0.12% (480 mL) [contains alcohol 11.6%]

PerioGard®: 0.12% (480 mL) [contains alcohol 11.6%; mint flavor]

Pad [prep pad] (Hibistat®): 0.5% (50s) [contains isopropyl alcohol]

Sponge/Brush (BactoShield® CHG): 4% per sponge/brush [contains isopropyl alcohol]

**chlormeprazine** *see* prochlorperazine *on page 680*

**Chlor-Mes-D [US]** *see* chlorpheniramine, phenylephrine, and methscopolamine *on page 175*

**2-chlorodeoxyadenosine** *see* cladribine *on page 189*

**chloroethane** *see* ethyl chloride *on page 320*

**Chloromag® [US]** *see* magnesium chloride *on page 497*

**Chloromycetin® [Can]** *see* chloramphenicol *on page 167*

**Chloromycetin® Sodium Succinate [US]** *see* chloramphenicol *on page 167*

## chlorophyll (KLOR oh fil)

**Synonyms** chlorophyllin

**U.S./Canadian Brand Names** Nullo® [US-OTC]

**Therapeutic Category** Gastrointestinal Agent, Miscellaneous

**Use** Control fecal odors in colostomy or ileostomy

**Usual Dosage**

Oral: Children >12 years and Adults: 100-200 mg/day in divided doses; may increase to 300 mg/day if odor is not controlled (maximum: 300 mg/day)

Ostomy: Tablet: May also place 1-2 tablets in empty pouch each time it is reused or changed.

**Dosage Forms** [DSC] = Discontinued product

Caplet: Chlorophyllin copper complex 100 mg

Tablet: Chlorophyllin copper complex 33.3 mg [DSC]

**chlorophyllin** *see* chlorophyll *on this page*

## chloroprocaine (klor oh PROE kane)

**Sound-Alike/Look-Alike Issues**

Nesacaine® may be confused with Neptazane®

**Synonyms** chloroprocaine hydrochloride

**U.S./Canadian Brand Names** Nesacaine® [US]; Nesacaine®-CE [Can]; Nesacaine®-MPF [US]

**Therapeutic Category** Local Anesthetic

**Use** Infiltration anesthesia and peripheral and epidural anesthesia

**Usual Dosage** Dosage varies with anesthetic procedure, the area to be anesthetized, the vascularity of the tissues, depth of anesthesia required, degree of muscle relaxation required, and duration of anesthesia; range.

Children >3 years (normally developed): Maximum dose (without epinephrine): 11 mg/kg; for infiltration, concentrations of 0.5% to 1% are recommended; for nerve block, concentrations of 1% to 1.5% are recommended

Adults:

Maximum single dose (without epinephrine): 11 mg/kg; maximum dose: 800 mg

Maximum single dose (with epinephrine): 14 mg/kg; maximum dose: 1000 mg

Infiltration and peripheral nerve block:

Mandibular: 2%: 2-3 mL; total dose 40-60 mg

Infraorbital: 2%: 0.5-1 mL; total dose 10-20 mg

Brachial plexus: 2%; 30-40 mL; total dose 600-800 mg

DIgItal (without epinephrine): 1%; 3-4 mL; total dose: 30-40 mg

Pudendal: 2%; 10 mL each side; total dose: 400 mg

Paracervical: 1%; 3 mL per each of four sites

Caudal block: Preservative-free: 2% or 3%: 15-25 mL; may repeat at 40-60 minute intervals

(Continued)

# chloroprocaine *(Continued)*

Lumbar epidural block: Preservative-free: 2% or 3%: 2-2.5 mL per segment; usual total volume: 15-25 mL; may repeat with doses that are 2-6 mL less than initial dose every 40-50 minutes.

**Dosage Forms**

Injection, solution, as hydrochloride (Nesacaine®): 1% (30 mL); 2% (30 mL) [contains disodium EDTA and methylparaben]

Injection, solution, as hydrochloride (Nesacaine®-MPF) [preservative free]: 2% (20 mL); 3% (20 mL)

**chloroprocaine hydrochloride** *see* chloroprocaine *on previous page*

**Chloroptic® Ophthalmic Solution *(Discontinued)*** *see* chloramphenicol *on page 167*

**Chloroptic® SOP *(Discontinued)*** *see* chloramphenicol *on page 167*

# chloroquine phosphate (KLOR oh kwin FOS fate)

**U.S./Canadian Brand Names** Aralen® [US/Can]; Novo-Chloroquine [Can]

**Therapeutic Category** Aminoquinoline (Antimalarial)

**Use** Suppression or chemoprophylaxis of malaria; treatment of uncomplicated or mild to moderate malaria; extraintestinal amebiasis

**Usual Dosage** Oral:

Suppression or prophylaxis of malaria:

Children: Administer 5 mg base/kg/week on the same day each week (not to exceed 300 mg base/dose); begin 1-2 weeks prior to exposure; continue for 4-6 weeks after leaving endemic area; if suppressive therapy is not begun prior to exposure, double the initial loading dose to 10 mg base/kg and administer in 2 divided doses 6 hours apart, followed by the usual dosage regimen

Adults: 500 mg/week (300 mg base) on the same day each week; begin 1-2 weeks prior to exposure; continue for 4-6 weeks after leaving endemic area; if suppressive therapy is not begun prior to exposure, double the initial loading dose to 1 g (600 mg base) and administer in 2 divided doses 6 hours apart, followed by the usual dosage regimen

Acute attack:

Children: 10 mg/kg (base) on day 1, followed by 5 mg/kg (base) 6 hours later and 5 mg/kg (base) on days 2 and 3

Adults: 1 g (600 mg base) on day 1, followed by 500 mg (300 mg base) 6 hours later, followed by 500 mg (300 mg base) on days 2 and 3

Extraintestinal amebiasis:

Children: 10 mg/kg (base) once daily for 2-3 weeks (up to 300 mg base/day)

Adults: 1 g/day (600 mg base) for 2 days followed by 500 mg/day (300 mg base) for at least 2-3 weeks

**Dosage Forms**

Tablet, as phosphate: 250 mg [equivalent to 150 mg base]; 500 mg [equivalent to 300 mg base]

Aralen®: 500 mg [equivalent to 300 mg base]

# chlorothiazide (klor oh THYE a zide)

**U.S./Canadian Brand Names** Diuril® [US/Can]

**Therapeutic Category** Diuretic, Thiazide

**Use** Management of mild to moderate hypertension; adjunctive treatment of edema

**Usual Dosage Note:** The manufacturer states that I.V. and oral dosing are equivalent. Some clinicians may use lower I.V. doses, however, because of chlorothiazide's poor oral absorption. I.V. dosing in infants and children has not been well established.

Infants <6 months: Oral: 20-40 mg/kg/day in 2 divided doses (maximum dose: 375 mg/day)

Infants >6 months and Children: Oral: 10-20 mg/kg/day in 2 divided doses (maximum dose: 375 mg/day in children <2 years or 1 g/day in children 2-12 years)

Adults:

Hypertension: Oral: 500 mg to 2 g/day divided in 1-2 doses (manufacturer labeling); doses of 125-500 mg/day have also been recommended

Edema: Oral, I.V.: 500 mg to 1 g once or twice daily. Intermittent treatment (ie, therapy on alternate days) may be appropriate for some patients.

**Dosage Forms**

Injection, powder for reconstitution, as sodium: 500 mg

Suspension, oral: 250 mg/5 mL (237 mL) [contains alcohol 0.5% and benzoic acid]

Tablet: 250 mg, 500 mg

# chloroxine (klor OKS een)

**Sound-Alike/Look-Alike Issues**
Capitrol® may be confused with Capital®, captopril
**U.S./Canadian Brand Names** Capitrol® [US/Can]
**Therapeutic Category** Antiseborrheic Agent, Topical
**Use** Treatment of dandruff or seborrheic dermatitis of the scalp
**Usual Dosage** Use twice weekly, massage into wet scalp, avoid contact with eyes, lather should remain on the scalp for approximately 3 minutes, then rinsed; application should be repeated and the scalp rinsed thoroughly
**Dosage Forms** [DSC] = Discontinued product
Shampoo, topical: 2% (110 g) [contains benzyl alcohol] [DSC]

**Chlorphed®** *(Discontinued)* *see* brompheniramine *on page 115*

**Chlorphed®-LA Nasal Solution** *(Discontinued)* *see* oxymetazoline *on page 610*

**Chlorphen [US-OTC]** *see* chlorpheniramine *on this page*

# chlorpheniramine (klor fen IR a meen)

**Sound-Alike/Look-Alike Issues**
Chlor-Trimeton® may be confused with Chloromycetin®
**Synonyms** chlorpheniramine maleate; CTM
**U.S./Canadian Brand Names** Aller-Chlor® [US-OTC]; Chlor-Trimeton® [US-OTC]; Chlor-Tripolon® [Can]; Chlorphen [US-OTC]; Diabetic Tussin® Allergy Relief [US-OTC]; Novo-Pheniram [Can]; Teldrin® HBP [US-OTC]
**Therapeutic Category** Antihistamine
**Use** Perennial and seasonal allergic rhinitis and other allergic symptoms including urticaria
**Usual Dosage**
Children: Oral: 0.35 mg/kg/day in divided doses every 4-6 hours
2-6 years: 1 mg every 4-6 hours, not to exceed 6 mg in 24 hours
6-12 years: 2 mg every 4-6 hours, not to exceed 12 mg/day or sustained release 8 mg at bedtime
Children >12 years and Adults: Oral: 4 mg every 4-6 hours, not to exceed 24 mg/day or sustained release 8-12 mg every 8-12 hours, not to exceed 24 mg/day
**Dosage Forms**
Syrup, as maleate:
Aller-Chlor®: 2 mg/5 mL (120 mL) [contains alcohol 5%]
Diabetic Tussin® Allergy Relief: 2 mg/5 mL (120 mL) [alcohol free, dye free, sugar free]
Tablet, as maleate (Aller-Chlor®, Chlor-Trimeton®, Chlorphen, Teldrin® HBP): 4 mg
Tablet, extended release, as maleate (Chlor-Trimeton®): 12 mg

**chlorpheniramine, acetaminophen, and pseudoephedrine** *see* acetaminophen, chlorpheniramine, and pseudoephedrine *on page 10*

# chlorpheniramine and acetaminophen (klor fen IR a meen & a seet a MIN oh fen)

**Synonyms** acetaminophen and chlorpheniramine
**U.S./Canadian Brand Names** Coricidin HBP® Cold and Flu [US-OTC]
**Therapeutic Category** Antihistamine/Analgesic
**Use** Symptomatic relief of congestion, headache, aches and pains of colds and flu
**Usual Dosage** Adults: Oral: 2 tablets every 4 hours
**Dosage Forms** Tablet: Chlorpheniramine maleate 2 mg and acetaminophen 325 mg

**chlorpheniramine and carbetapentane** *see* carbetapentane and chlorpheniramine *on page 142*

**chlorpheniramine and hydrocodone** *see* hydrocodone and chlorpheniramine *on page 412*

# chlorpheniramine and phenylephrine (klor fen IR a meen & fen il EF rin)

**Sound-Alike/Look-Alike Issues**
Rynatan® may be confused with Rynatuss®
**Synonyms** chlorpheniramine maleate and phenylephrine hydrochloride; chlorpheniramine tannate and phenylephrine tannate; phenylephrine and chlorpheniramine
**U.S./Canadian Brand Names** Dallergy-JR® [US]; Ed A-Hist® [US]; Rynatan® Pediatric Suspension [US]; Rynatan® [US]
(Continued)

## chlorpheniramine and phenylephrine *(Continued)*

**Therapeutic Category** Antihistamine/Decongestant Combination

**Use** Temporary relief of nasal congestion and eustachian tube congestion as well as runny nose, sneezing, itching of nose or throat, itchy and watery eyes

**Usual Dosage** General dosing guidelines; consult specific product labeling. Antihistamine/decongestant:
Oral:
Children:
2-6 years: Chlorpheniramine tannate 4.5 mg and phenylephrine tannate 5 mg per 5 mL: 2.5-5 mL every 12 hours
6-12 years:
Chlorpheniramine maleate 4 mg and phenylephrine hydrochloride 20 mg every 12 hours **or**
Chlorpheniramine tannate 4.5 mg and phenylephrine tannate 5 mg per 5 mL: 5-10 mL every 12 hours
≥12 years: Chlorpheniramine maleate 8 mg and phenylephrine hydrochloride 40 mg every 12 hours
Adults:
Chlorpheniramine maleate 8 mg and phenylephrine hydrochloride 40 mg every 12 hours **or**
Chlorpheniramine tannate 9 mg and phenylephrine tannate 25 mg every 12 hours

**Dosage Forms** [DSC] = Discontinued product
Caplet, prolonged release (Ed A-Hist®): Chlorpheniramine maleate 8 mg and phenylephrine hydrochloride 20 mg
Capsule, extended release (Dallergy-JR®): Chlorpheniramine maleate 4 mg and phenylephrine hydrochloride 20 mg
Liquid (Ed A-Hist®): Chlorpheniramine maleate 4 mg and phenylephrine hydrochloride 10 mg per 5 mL (480 mL) [sugar free; grape flavor]
Suspension, oral (Rynatan® Pediatric Suspension): Chlorpheniramine tannate 4.5 mg and phenylephrine tannate 5 mg per 5 mL (480 mL) [contains benzoic acid and tartrazine; strawberry flavor]
Tablet:
Histatab® Plus: Chlorpheniramine maleate 2 mg and phenylephrine hydrochloride 5 mg [DSC]
Rynatan®: Chlorpheniramine tannate 9 mg and phenylephrine tannate 25 mg

## chlorpheniramine and pseudoephedrine (klor fen IR a meen & soo doe e FED rin)

**Sound-Alike/Look-Alike Issues**
Allerest® may be confused with Sinarest®
Chlor-Trimeton® may be confused with Chloromycetin®
Sudafed® may be confused with Sufenta®

**Synonyms** chlorpheniramine maleate and pseudoephedrine hydrochloride; chlorpheniramine tannate and pseudoephedrine tannate; pseudoephedrine and chlorpheniramine

**U.S./Canadian Brand Names** A.R.M® [US-OTC]; Allerest® Maximum Strength Allergy and Hay Fever [US-OTC]; C-Phed Tannate [US]; Chlor-Trimeton® Allergy D [US-OTC]; Deconamine® SR [US]; Deconamine® [US]; Histade™ [US]; Histex™ [US]; Kronofed-A® [US]; Kronofed-A®-Jr [US]; LoHist-D [US]; PediaCare® Cold and Allergy [US-OTC]; Rescon-Jr. [US]; Sudafed® Sinus & Allergy [US-OTC]; Sudal® 12 [US]; Triaminic® Cold and Allergy [US-OTC/Can]

**Therapeutic Category** Antihistamine/Decongestant Combination

**Use** Relief of nasal congestion associated with the common cold, hay fever, and other allergies, sinusitis, eustachian tube blockage, and vasomotor and allergic rhinitis

**Usual Dosage** General dosing guidelines; consult specific product labeling. Rhinitis/decongestant: Oral:
Children:
2-6 years:
Chlorpheniramine maleate 1 mg and pseudoephedrine hydrochloride 15 mg every 4-6 hours
Tanafed®: Chlorpheniramine tannate 4.5 mg and pseudoephedrine tannate 75 mg: 2.5-5 mL every 12 hours (maximum: 10 mL/24 hours)
6-12 years:
Chlorpheniramine maleate 2 mg and pseudoephedrine hydrochloride 30 mg every 4-6 hours (immediate release products)
Rescon-Jr: Chlorpheniramine maleate 4 mg and pseudoephedrine hydrochloride 60 mg every 12 hours
Tanafed®: Chlorpheniramine tannate 4.5 mg and pseudoephedrine tannate 75 mg: 5-10 mL every 12 hours (maximum: 20 mL/24 hours)
Children ≥12 years and Adults:
Chlorpheniramine maleate 4 mg and pseudoephedrine hydrochloride 60 mg every 4-6 hours (immediate release products)

Deconamine® SR, Kronofed-A®: Chlorpheniramine maleate 8 mg and pseudoephedrine hydrochloride 120 mg every 12 hours

Tanafed®: Chlorpheniramine tannate 4.5 mg and pseudoephedrine tannate 75 mg: 10-20 mL every 12 hours (maximum: 40 mL/24 hours)

**Dosage Forms** [DSC] = Discontinued product

Caplet (A.R.M.®): Chlorpheniramine maleate 4 mg and pseudoephedrine hydrochloride 60 mg

Capsule, extended release: Chlorpheniramine maleate 8 mg and pseudoephedrine hydrochloride 120 mg

Histade™: Chlorpheniramine maleate 12 mg and pseudoephedrine hydrochloride 120 mg

Capsule, sustained release:

Deconamine® SR, Kronofed-A®: Chlorpheniramine maleate 8 mg and pseudoephedrine hydrochloride 120 mg

Kronofed-A®-Jr, Rescon-Jr: Chlorpheniramine maleate 4 mg and pseudoephedrine hydrochloride 60 mg

Liquid:

Histex™: Chlorpheniramine maleate 2 mg and pseudoephedrine sulfate 30 mg per 5 mL (480 mL) [peach flavor]

PediaCare® Cold and Allergy: Chlorpheniramine maleate 1 mg and pseudoephedrine sulfate 15 mg per 5 mL (120 mL) [alcohol free; contains sodium benzoate; bubble gum flavor]

Triaminic® Cold and Allergy: Chlorpheniramine maleate 1 mg and pseudoephedrine sulfate 15 mg per 5 mL (120 mL) [contains benzoic acid; orange flavor]

Suspension: Chlorpheniramine tannate 4.5 mg and pseudoephedrine tannate 75 mg per 5 mL (120 mL, 480 mL)

C-Phed Tannate: Chlorpheniramine tannate 4.5 mg and pseudoephedrine tannate 75 mg per 5 mL (120 mL, 480 mL) [alcohol free; strawberry-banana flavor]

Tanafed®: Chlorpheniramine tannate 4.5 mg and pseudoephedrine tannate 75 mg per 5 mL (120 mL, 480 mL) [contains sodium benzoate; strawberry-banana flavor] [DSC]

Suspension, sustained release (Sudal®12): Chlorpheniramine maleate 6 mg and pseudoephedrine hydrochloride 30 mg per 5 mL (480 mL)

Syrup: Chlorpheniramine maleate 2 mg and pseudoephedrine hydrochloride 30 mg per 5 mL (480 mL)

Deconamine®: Chlorpheniramine maleate 2 mg and pseudoephedrine sulfate 30 mg per 5 mL (480 mL) [alcohol free, dye free; contains sodium benzoate; grape flavor]

LoHist-D: Chlorpheniramine maleate 2 mg and pseudoephedrine hydrochloride 30 mg per 5 mL (480 mL) [alcohol free, dye free; peach flavor]

Tablet: Chlorpheniramine maleate 4 mg and pseudoephedrine hydrochloride 60 mg

Allerest® Maximum Strength Allergy and Hay Fever: Chlorpheniramine maleate 2 mg and pseudoephedrine hydrochloride 30 mg

Chlor-Trimeton® Allergy D, Sudafed® Sinus & Allergy: Chlorpheniramine maleate 4 mg and pseudoephedrine hydrochloride 60 mg

Deconamine®: Chlorpheniramine maleate 4 mg and pseudoephedrine hydrochloride 60 mg [dye free]

Tablet, chewable: Chlorpheniramine maleate 2 mg and pseudoephedrine sulfate 15 mg

Triaminic® Cold and Allergy: Chlorpheniramine maleate 1 mg and pseudoephedrine sulfate 15 mg [contains coconut oil; phenylalanine 17.6 mg/tablet, sodium 5 mg/tablet; orange flavor]

**chlorpheniramine, carbetapentane, and phenylephrine** *see* carbetapentane, phenylephrine, and chlorpheniramine *on page 142*

# chlorpheniramine, ephedrine, phenylephrine, and carbetapentane
(klor fen IR a meen, e FED rin, fen il EF rin, & kar bay ta PEN tane)

**Sound-Alike/Look-Alike Issues**
Rynatuss® may be confused with Rynatan®

**Synonyms** carbetapentane, ephedrine, phenylephrine, and chlorpheniramine; ephedrine, chlorpheniramine, phenylephrine, and carbetapentane; phenylephrine, ephedrine, chlorpheniramine, and carbetapentane

**U.S./Canadian Brand Names** Rynatuss® Pediatric [US]; Rynatuss® [US]; Tetra Tannate Pediatric [US]

**Therapeutic Category** Antihistamine/Decongestant/Antitussive

**Use** Symptomatic relief of cough with a decongestant and an antihistamine

**Usual Dosage** Oral:

Children:
<2 years: Titrate dose individually
2-6 years: 2.5-5 mL every 12 hours
>6 years: 5-10 mL every 12 hours

(Continued)

## chlorpheniramine, ephedrine, phenylephrine, and carbetapentane
*(Continued)*
Adults: 1-2 tablets every 12 hours

**Dosage Forms**
Suspension (Rynatuss® Pediatric, Tetra Tannate Pediatric): Carbetapentane tannate 30 mg, ephedrine tannate 5 mg, phenylephrine tannate 5 mg, and chlorpheniramine tannate 4 mg per 5 mL (240 mL, 480 mL) [contains tartrazine and benzoic acid; strawberry flavor]
Tablet (Rynatuss®): Carbetapentane tannate 60 mg, ephedrine tannate 10 mg, phenylephrine tannate 10 mg, and chlorpheniramine tannate 5 mg

**chlorpheniramine, hydrocodone, phenylephrine, acetaminophen, and caffeine** *see* hydrocodone, chlorpheniramine, phenylephrine, acetaminophen, and caffeine *on page 414*

**chlorpheniramine maleate** *see* chlorpheniramine *on page 171*

**chlorpheniramine maleate and phenylephrine hydrochloride** *see* chlorpheniramine and phenylephrine *on page 171*

**chlorpheniramine maleate and pseudoephedrine hydrochloride** *see* chlorpheniramine and pseudoephedrine *on page 172*

**chlorpheniramine maleate, pseudoephedrine hydrochloride, and dextromethorphan hydrobromide** *see* chlorpheniramine, pseudoephedrine, and dextromethorphan *on page 177*

## chlorpheniramine, phenylephrine, and dextromethorphan
(klor fen IR a meen, fen il EF rin, & deks troe meth OR fan)
**Synonyms** dextromethorphan, chlorpheniramine, and phenylephrine; phenylephrine, chlorpheniramine, and dextromethorphan
**U.S./Canadian Brand Names** Alka-Seltzer® Plus® Cold and Cough [US-OTC]; Coldtuss DR [US]; Corfen DM [US]; De-Chlor DM [US]; De-Chlor DR [US]; Dex PC [US]; Tri-Vent™ DPC [US]
**Therapeutic Category** Antihistamine/Decongestant/Antitussive
**Use** Temporary relief of cough and upper respiratory symptoms associated with allergies or the common cold
**Usual Dosage** Oral: Relief of cough and cold symptoms:
Children:
2-6 years (Tri-Vent™ DPC): 2.5 mL every 6 hours (maximum: 10 mL/24 hours)
6-12 years (Tri-Vent™ DPC): 5 mL every 6 hours (maximum: 20 mL/24 hours)
Children ≥12 years and Adults:
Alka-Seltzer Plus® Cold and Cough: 2 tablets dissolved in water every 4 hours (maximum: 8 tablets/24 hours)
Tri-Vent™ DPC: 10 mL every 6 hours (maximum: 40 mL/24 hours)
**Dosage Forms**
Liquid: Chlorpheniramine maleate 4 mg, phenylephrine hydrochloride 10 mg, and dextromethorphan hydrobromide 15 mg per 5 mL (480 mL)
Corfen DM: Chlorpheniramine maleate 4 mg, phenylephrine hydrochloride 10 mg, and dextromethorphan hydrobromide 15 mg per 5 mL (480 mL) [grape flavor]
De-Chlor DM: Chlorpheniramine maleate 2 mg, phenylephrine hydrochloride 10 mg, and dextromethorphan hydrobromide 15 mg per 5 mL (480 mL) [strawberry flavor]
De-Chlor DR: Chlorpheniramine maleate 2 mg, phenylephrine hydrochloride 6 mg, and dextromethorphan hydrobromide 15 mg per 5 mL (480 mL) [strawberry flavor]
Syrup: Chlorpheniramine maleate 2 mg, phenylephrine hydrochloride 10 mg, and dextromethorphan hydrobromide 15 mg per 5 mL (480 mL)
Coldtuss DR: Chlorpheniramine maleate 4 mg, phenylephrine hydrochloride 6 mg, and dextromethorphan hydrobromide 15 mg per 5 mL (480 mL) [strawberry flavor]
Dex PC: Chlorpheniramine maleate 2 mg, phenylephrine hydrochloride 6 mg, and dextromethorphan hydrobromide 15 mg per 5 mL (480 mL) [strawberry flavor]
Tri-Vent™ DPC: Chlorpheniramine maleate 2 mg, phenylephrine hydrochloride 6 mg, and dextromethorphan hydrobromide 15 mg per 5 mL (480 mL) [alcohol free; contains sodium benzoate; strawberry flavor]
Tablet, effervescent (Alka-Seltzer Plus® Cold and Cough): Chlorpheniramine maleate 2 mg, phenylephrine hydrochloride 5 mg, and dextromethorphan hydrobromide 10 mg [contains phenylalanine 11 mg/tablet and sodium 504 mg/tablet]

**chlorpheniramine, phenylephrine, and hydrocodone** *see* phenylephrine, hydrocodone, and
chlorpheniramine *on page 643*

# chlorpheniramine, phenylephrine, and methscopolamine
(klor fen IR a meen, fen il EF rin, & meth skoe POL a meen)

**Synonyms** methscopolamine, chlorpheniramine, and phenylephrine; phenylephrine, chlorpheniramine,
and methscopolamine

**U.S./Canadian Brand Names** AH-Chew® II [US]; AH-Chew® [US]; Chlor-Mes-D [US]; Dallergy® [US];
Dehistine [US]; Drize®-R [US]; Extendryl JR [US]; Extendryl SR [US]; Extendryl [US]; Hista-Vent® DA
[US]; PCM Allergy [US]; PCM [US]

**Therapeutic Category** Antihistamine/Decongestant/Anticholinergic

**Use** Treatment of upper respiratory symptoms such as respiratory congestion, allergic rhinitis, vasomotor
rhinitis, sinusitis, and allergic skin reactions of urticaria and angioedema

**Usual Dosage**

Children 6-11 years: Relief of respiratory symptoms: Oral:

Extendryl chewable tablet: One tablet every 4 hours; do not exceed 4 doses in 24 hours

Dallergy®: One-half caplet every 12 hours

Extendryl JR: One capsule every 12 hours

Extendryl syrup: 2.5-5 mL, may repeat up to every 4 hours depending on age and body weight

Children ≥12 years and Adults: Relief of respiratory symptoms: Oral: **Note:** If disturbances in urination
occur in patients without renal impairment, medication should be discontinued for 1-2 days and should
then be restarted at a lower dose

Dallergy®, Extendryl SR: One capsule every 12 hours

Extendryl: 1-2 chewable tablets every 4 hours

Extendryl syrup: 5-10 mL every 3-4 hours (4 times/day)

**Dosage Forms** [DSC] = Discontinued product

Caplet, extended release (Dallergy®): Chlorpheniramine maleate 12 mg, phenylephrine hydrochloride
20 mg, and methscopolamine nitrate 2.5 mg

Capsule, extended release:

Extendryl JR: Chlorpheniramine maleate 4 mg, phenylephrine hydrochloride 10 mg, and methscopolamine nitrate 1.25 mg

Extendryl SR: Chlorpheniramine maleate 8 mg, phenylephrine hydrochloride 20 mg, and methscopolamine nitrate 2.5 mg

Liquid (Chlor-Mes-D): Chlorpheniramine maleate 2 mg, phenylephrine hydrochloride 10 mg, and methscopolamine nitrate 0.625 mg per 5 mL (480 mL)

Syrup:

Dallergy®: Chlorpheniramine maleate 2 mg, phenylephrine hydrochloride 10 mg, and methscopolamine
nitrate 0.625 mg per 5 mL (480 mL)

Dehistine: Chlorpheniramine maleate 2 mg, phenylephrine hydrochloride 10 mg, and methscopolamine
nitrate 1.25 mg per 5 mL (480 mL) [root beer flavor]

Extendryl: Chlorpheniramine maleate 2 mg, phenylephrine hydrochloride 10 mg, and methscopolamine
nitrate 1.25 mg per 5 mL (480 mL) [contains sodium benzoate; root beer flavor]

Tablet:

Dallergy®: Chlorpheniramine maleate 4 mg, phenylephrine hydrochloride 10 mg, and methscopolamine
nitrate 1.25 mg [scored]

Vanex Forte™-D [DSC]: Chlorpheniramine maleate 8 mg, phenylephrine hydrochloride 20 mg, and
methscopolamine nitrate 2.5 mg [dye free; scored]

Tablet, chewable:

AH-Chew®: Chlorpheniramine maleate 2 mg, phenylephrine hydrochloride 10 mg, and methscopolamine nitrate 1.25 mg [grape flavor]

AH-Chew II: Chlorpheniramine maleate 2 mg, phenylephrine hydrochloride 15 mg, and methscopolamine nitrate 1.25 mg [grape flavor]

Extendryl: Chlorpheniramine maleate 2 mg, phenylephrine hydrochloride 10 mg, and methscopolamine
nitrate 1.25 mg [root beer flavor]

PCM: Chlorpheniramine maleate 2 mg, phenylephrine hydrochloride 10 mg, and methscopolamine
nitrate 1.25 mg

Tablet, extended release: Chlorpheniramine maleate 8 mg, phenylephrine hydrochloride 20 mg, and
methscopolamine nitrate 2.5 mg

Drize®-R: Chlorpheniramine maleate 8 mg, phenylephrine hydrochloride 20 mg, and methscopolamine
nitrate 2.5 mg [dye free; scored]

Hista-Vent® DA: Chlorpheniramine maleate 8 mg, phenylephrine hydrochloride 20 mg, and methscopolamine nitrate 2.5 mg [scored]

(Continued)

## chlorpheniramine, phenylephrine, and methscopolamine *(Continued)*

PCM Allergy: Chlorpheniramine maleate 12 mg, phenylephrine hydrochloride 20 mg, and methscopolamine nitrate 2.5 mg

## chlorpheniramine, phenylephrine, and phenyltoloxamine

(klor fen IR a meen, fen il EF rin, & fen il tole LOKS a meen)

**Synonyms** phenylephrine, chlorpheniramine, and phenyltoloxamine; phenyltoloxamine, chlorpheniramine, and phenylephrine

**U.S./Canadian Brand Names** Comhist® [US]; Nalex®-A [US]

**Therapeutic Category** Antihistamine/Decongestant Combination

**Use** Symptomatic relief of rhinitis and nasal congestion due to colds or allergy

**Usual Dosage** Oral:
Children:
  2-6 years: Nalex®-A liquid: 1.25-2.5 mL every 4-6 hours
  6-12 years:
    Nalex®-A liquid: 5 mL every 4-6 hours
    Nalex®-A tablet: ½ tablet 2-3 times/day
  Children >12 years and Adults:
    Nalex®-A liquid: 10 mL every 4-6 hours
    Nalex®-A tablet: 1 tablet 2-3 times/day

**Dosage Forms**
Liquid (Nalex®-A): Chlorpheniramine maleate 2.5 mg, phenylephrine hydrochloride 5 mg, and phenyltoloxamine citrate 7.5 mg per 5 mL (480 mL) [alcohol free, sugar free; cotton candy flavor]
Tablet: (Comhist®): Chlorpheniramine maleate 2 mg, phenylephrine hydrochloride 10 mg, and phenyltoloxamine citrate 25 mg
Tablet, prolonged release (Nalex®-A): Chlorpheniramine maleate 4 mg, phenylephrine hydrochloride 20 mg, and phenyltoloxamine citrate 40 mg

## chlorpheniramine, phenylephrine, codeine, and potassium iodide

(klor fen IR a meen, fen il EF rin, KOE deen, & poe TASS ee um EYE oh dide)

**Synonyms** codeine, chlorpheniramine, phenylephrine, and potassium iodide; phenylephrine, chlorpheniramine, codeine, and potassium iodide; potassium iodide, chlorpheniramine, phenylephrine, and codeine

**Therapeutic Category** Antihistamine/Decongestant/Antitussive

**Controlled Substance** C-V

**Use** Symptomatic relief of rhinitis, nasal congestion and cough due to colds or allergy

**Usual Dosage** Children 6 months to 12 years: 1.25-10 mL every 4-6 hours

**Dosage Forms** Syrup: Chlorpheniramine maleate 0.75 mg, phenylephrine hydrochloride 2.5 mg, codeine phosphate 5 mg, and potassium iodide 75 mg per 5 mL (480 mL) [contains alcohol 5% and sodium benzoate; raspberry flavor] [DSC]

**chlorpheniramine, pseudoephedrine, and acetaminophen** *see* acetaminophen, chlorpheniramine, and pseudoephedrine *on page 10*

## chlorpheniramine, pseudoephedrine, and codeine

(klor fen IR a meen, soo doe e FED rin, & KOE deen)

**Synonyms** codeine, chlorpheniramine, and pseudoephedrine; pseudoephedrine, chlorpheniramine, and codeine

**U.S./Canadian Brand Names** Dihistine® DH [US]

**Therapeutic Category** Antihistamine/Decongestant/Antitussive

**Controlled Substance** C-V

**Use** Temporary relief of cough associated with minor throat or bronchial irritation or nasal congestion due to common cold, allergic rhinitis, or sinusitis

**Usual Dosage** Oral:
Children:
  25-50 lb: 1.25-2.50 mL every 4-6 hours, up to 4 doses in 24-hour period
  50-90 lb: 2.5-5 mL every 4-6 hours, up to 4 doses in 24-hour period
Adults: 10 mL every 4-6 hours, up to 4 doses in 24-hour period

**Dosage Forms**
Elixir: Chlorpheniramine maleate 2 mg, pseudoephedrine hydrochloride 30 mg, and codeine phosphate 10 mg per 5 mL (120 mL, 480 mL)
Dihistine® DH: Chlorpheniramine maleate 2 mg, pseudoephedrine hydrochloride 30 mg, and codeine phosphate 10 mg per 5 mL (120 mL, 480 mL) [contains alcohol; grape flavor]

## chlorpheniramine, pseudoephedrine, and dextromethorphan
(klor fen IR a meen, soo doe e FED rin, & deks troe meth OR fan)

**Synonyms** chlorpheniramine maleate, pseudoephedrine hydrochloride, and dextromethorphan hydrobromide; chlorpheniramine tannate, pseudoephedrine tannate, and dextromethorphan tannate; dexchlorpheniramine tannate, pseudoephedrine tannate, and dextromethorphan tannate; dextromethorphan, chlorpheniramine, and pseudoephedrine; pseudoephedrine, chlorpheniramine, and dextromethorphan

**U.S./Canadian Brand Names** Kidkare Cough and Cold [US-OTC]; PediaCare® Multi-Symptom Cold [US-OTC]; PediaCare® NightRest Cough and Cold [US-OTC]; Rescon DM [US-OTC]; Robitussin® Pediatric Night Relief [US-OTC]; Tanafed DMX™ [US]; Triaminic® Cold and Cough [US-OTC]; Triaminic® Night Time Cough and Cold [US-OTC]; Vicks® Children's NyQuil® [US-OTC]; Vicks® Pediatric 44®m [US-OTC]

**Therapeutic Category** Antihistamine/Decongestant/Antitussive

**Use** Temporarily relieves nasal congestion, runny nose, cough, and sneezing due to the common cold, hay fever, or allergic rhinitis

**Usual Dosage** General dosing guidelines; consult specific product labeling. Relief of cold symptoms: Oral:
Children:
2-6 years: Dexchlorpheniramine tannate 2.5 mg, pseudoephedrine tannate 75 mg, and dextromethorphan tannate 25 mg (Tanafed DMX™): 2.5-5 mL every 12 hours (maximum: 10 mL/24 hours)
6-12 years:
Chlorpheniramine maleate 1 mg, pseudoephedrine 15 mg, and dextromethorphan hydrobromide 7.5 mg per 5 mL: 10 mL every 6 hours
Chlorpheniramine maleate 1 mg, pseudoephedrine 15 mg, and dextromethorphan hydrobromide 5 mg per tablet or 5 mL: 2 tablets or 10 mL every 4-6 hours (maximum: 4 doses/24 hours)
Chlorpheniramine maleate 2 mg, pseudoephedrine 30 mg, and dextromethorphan hydrobromide 10 mg per tablet or 5 mL (Rescon DM): 5 mL every 4-6 hours (maximum: 4 doses/24 hours)
Dexchlorpheniramine tannate 2.5 mg, pseudoephedrine tannate 75 mg, and dextromethorphan tannate 25 mg (Tanafed DMX™): 5-10 mL every 12 hours (maximum: 20 mL/24 hours)
>12 years: Refer to Adults dosing
Adults:
Chlorpheniramine maleate 1 mg, pseudoephedrine 15 mg, and dextromethorphan hydrobromide 7.5 mg per 5 mL: 20 mL every 6 hours
Chlorpheniramine maleate 2 mg, pseudoephedrine 30 mg, and dextromethorphan hydrobromide 10 mg per tablet or 5 mL (Rescon DM): 10 mL every 4-6 hours (maximum: 4 doses/24 hours)
Dexchlorpheniramine tannate 2.5 mg, pseudoephedrine tannate 75 mg, and dextromethorphan tannate 25 mg (Tanafed DMX™): 10-20 mL every 12 hours (maximum: 40 mL/24 hours)

**Dosage Forms**
Liquid: Chlorpheniramine maleate 1 mg, pseudoephedrine hydrochloride 15 mg, and dextromethorphan hydrobromide 5 mg per 5 mL (120 mL, 480 mL)
Kidkare Cough and Cold: Chlorpheniramine maleate 1 mg, pseudoephedrine hydrochloride 15 mg, and dextromethorphan hydrobromide 5 mg per 5 mL (120 mL)
PediaCare® Multi-Symptom Cold: Chlorpheniramine maleate 1 mg, pseudoephedrine hydrochloride 15 mg, and dextromethorphan hydrobromide 5 mg per 5 mL (120 mL) [contains sodium benzoate; cherry flavor]
PediaCare® NightRest Cough and Cold: Chlorpheniramine maleate 1 mg, pseudoephedrine hydrochloride 15 mg, and dextromethorphan hydrobromide 7.5 mg per 5 mL (120 mL) [contains sodium benzoate; cherry flavor]
Rescon DM: Chlorpheniramine maleate 2 mg, pseudoephedrine hydrochloride 30 mg, and dextromethorphan hydrobromide 10 mg per 5 mL (120 mL, 480 mL) [dye free; cherry flavor]
Triaminic® Cold and Cough: Chlorpheniramine maleate 1 mg, pseudoephedrine hydrochloride 15 mg, and dextromethorphan hydrobromide 5 mg per 5 mL (120 mL)[contains sodium 10 mg/5 mL and benzoic acid; cherry flavor]
Triaminic® Night Time Cough and Cold: Chlorpheniramine maleate 1 mg, pseudoephedrine hydrochloride 15 mg, and dextromethorphan hydrobromide 7.5 mg per 5 mL (120 mL) [contains sodium 7.5 mg/5 mL and benzoic acid;  grape flavor]
(Continued)

## chlorpheniramine, pseudoephedrine, and dextromethorphan *(Continued)*

Vicks® Pediatric 44®m: Chlorpheniramine maleate 2 mg, pseudoephedrine hydrochloride 30 mg, and dextromethorphan hydrobromide 15 mg per 15 mL (120 mL) [contains sodium 30 mg/15 mL and sodium benzoate; cherry flavor]

Vicks® Children's NyQuil®: Chlorpheniramine maleate 2 mg, pseudoephedrine hydrochloride 30 mg, and dextromethorphan hydrobromide 15 mg per 15 mL (120 mL) [contains sodium 71 mg/15 mL; cherry flavor]

Suspension (Tanafed DMX™): Dexchlorpheniramine tannate 2.5 mg, pseudoephedrine tannate 75 mg, and dextromethorphan tannate 25 mg (120 mL, 480 mL) [contains sodium benzoate; cotton candy flavor]

Syrup (Robitussin® Pediatric Night Relief): Chlorpheniramine maleate 1 mg, pseudoephedrine hydrochloride 15 mg, and dextromethorphan hydrobromide 7.5 mg per 5 mL (120 mL) [contains sodium benzoate; fruit punch flavor]

Tablet, chewable (PediaCare® Multi-Symptom Cold): Chlorpheniramine maleate 1 mg, pseudoephedrine hydrochloride 15 mg, and dextromethorphan hydrobromide 5 mg [contains phenylalanine 8.4 mg/tablet; cherry flavor]

**chlorpheniramine, pseudoephedrine, and hydrocodone** *see* pseudoephedrine, hydrocodone, and chlorpheniramine *on page 695*

**chlorpheniramine tannate and phenylephrine tannate** *see* chlorpheniramine and phenylephrine *on page 171*

**chlorpheniramine tannate and pseudoephedrine tannate** *see* chlorpheniramine and pseudoephedrine *on page 172*

**chlorpheniramine tannate, pseudoephedrine tannate, and dextromethorphan tannate** *see* chlorpheniramine, pseudoephedrine, and dextromethorphan *on previous page*

**Chlor-Pro® Injection *(Discontinued)*** *see* chlorpheniramine *on page 171*

## chlorpromazine (klor PROE ma zeen)

**Sound-Alike/Look-Alike Issues**

chlorproMAZINE may be confused with chlorproPAMIDE, clomiPRAMINE, prochlorperazine, promethazine

Thorazine® may be confused with thiamine, thioridazine

**Synonyms** chlorpromazine hydrochloride; CPZ

**Tall-Man** chlorproMAZINE

**U.S./Canadian Brand Names** Apo-Chlorpromazine® [Can]; Largactil® [Can]; Novo-Chlorpromazine [Can]

**Therapeutic Category** Phenothiazine Derivative

**Use** Control of mania; treatment of schizophrenia; control of nausea and vomiting; relief of restlessness and apprehension before surgery; acute intermittent porphyria; adjunct in the treatment of tetanus; intractable hiccups; combativeness and/or explosive hyperexcitable behavior in children 1-12 years of age and in short-term treatment of hyperactive children

**Usual Dosage**

Children ≥6 months:

Schizophrenia/psychoses:

Oral: 0.5-1 mg/kg/dose every 4-6 hours; older children may require 200 mg/day or higher

I.M., I.V.: 0.5-1 mg/kg/dose every 6-8 hours

<5 years (22.7 kg): Maximum: 40 mg/day

5-12 years (22.7-45.5 kg): Maximum: 75 mg/day

Nausea and vomiting:

Oral: 0.5-1 mg/kg/dose every 4-6 hours as needed

I.M., I.V.: 0.5-1 mg/kg/dose every 6-8 hours

<5 years (22.7 kg): Maximum: 40 mg/day

5-12 years (22.7-45.5 kg): Maximum: 75 mg/day

Adults:

Schizophrenia/psychoses:

Oral: Range: 30-2000 mg/day in 1-4 divided doses, initiate at lower doses and titrate as needed; usual dose: 400-600 mg/day; some patients may require 1-2 g/day

I.M., I.V.: Initial: 25 mg, may repeat (25-50 mg) in 1-4 hours, gradually increase to a maximum of 400 mg/dose every 4-6 hours until patient is controlled; usual dose: 300-800 mg/day

Intractable hiccups: Oral, I.M.: 25-50 mg 3-4 times/day

Nausea and vomiting:
Oral: 10-25 mg every 4-6 hours
I.M., I.V.: 25-50 mg every 4-6 hours
**Dosage Forms**
Injection, solution, as hydrochloride: 25 mg/mL (10 mL) [contains benzyl alcohol, sodium bisulfite, and sodium sulfite]
Tablet, as hydrochloride: 10 mg, 25 mg, 50 mg, 100 mg, 200 mg

**chlorpromazine hydrochloride** *see* chlorpromazine *on previous page*

# chlorpropamide (klor PROE pa mide)

**Sound-Alike/Look-Alike Issues**
chlorproPAMIDE may be confused with chlorproMAZINE
Diabinese® may be confused with DiaBeta®, Dialume®
**Tall-Man** chlorpro**PAMIDE**
**U.S./Canadian Brand Names** Apo-Chlorpropamide® [Can]; Diabinese® [US]; Novo-Propamide [Can]
**Therapeutic Category** Antidiabetic Agent, Oral
**Use** Management of blood sugar in type 2 diabetes mellitus (noninsulin dependent, NIDDM)
**Usual Dosage** Oral: The dosage of chlorpropamide is variable and should be individualized based upon the patient's response
Initial dose: Adults: 250 mg/day in mild to moderate diabetes in middle-aged, stable diabetic
Subsequent dosages may be increased or decreased by 50-125 mg/day at 3- to 5-day intervals
Maintenance dose: 100-250 mg/day; severe diabetics may require 500 mg/day; avoid doses >750 mg/day
**Dosage Forms** Tablet: 100 mg, 250 mg

# chlorthalidone (klor THAL i done)

**U.S./Canadian Brand Names** Apo-Chlorthalidone® [Can]; Thalitone® [US]
**Therapeutic Category** Diuretic, Miscellaneous
**Use** Management of mild to moderate hypertension when used alone or in combination with other agents; treatment of edema associated with congestive heart failure or nephrotic syndrome. Recent studies have found chlorthalidone effective in the treatment of isolated systolic hypertension in the elderly.
**Usual Dosage** Oral:
Children (nonapproved): 2 mg/kg/dose 3 times/week or 1-2 mg/kg/day
Adults: 25-100 mg/day or 100 mg 3 times/week; usual dosage range (JNC 7): 12.5-25 mg/day
**Dosage Forms**
Tablet: 25 mg, 50 mg, 100 mg
Thalitone®: 15 mg

**chlorthalidone and atenolol** *see* atenolol and chlorthalidone *on page 77*

**chlorthalidone and clonidine** *see* clonidine and chlorthalidone *on page 198*

**Chlor-Trimeton® [US-OTC]** *see* chlorpheniramine *on page 171*

**Chlor-Trimeton® Allergy D [US-OTC]** *see* chlorpheniramine and pseudoephedrine *on page 172*

**Chlor-Trimeton® Syrup *(Discontinued)*** *see* chlorpheniramine *on page 171*

**Chlor-Tripolon® [Can]** *see* chlorpheniramine *on page 171*

**Chlor-Tripolon ND® [Can]** *see* loratadine and pseudoephedrine *on page 491*

# chlorzoxazone (klor ZOKS a zone)

**Sound-Alike/Look-Alike Issues**
Parafon Forte® may be confused with Fam-Pren Forte
**U.S./Canadian Brand Names** Parafon Forte® [Can]; Strifon Forte® [Can]
**Therapeutic Category** Skeletal Muscle Relaxant
**Use** Symptomatic treatment of muscle spasm and pain associated with acute musculoskeletal conditions
**Usual Dosage** Oral:
Children: 20 mg/kg/day or 600 mg/m$^2$/day in 3-4 divided doses
Adults: 250-500 mg 3-4 times/day up to 750 mg 3-4 times/day
**Dosage Forms**
Caplet (Parafon Forte® DSC): 500 mg
Tablet: 250 mg, 500 mg

**Cholebrine**® **[US]** *see* radiological/contrast media (ionic) *on page 707*

**cholecalciferol** (kole e kal SI fer ole)
Synonyms $D_3$
**U.S./Canadian Brand Names** D-Vi-Sol® [Can]; Delta-D® [US]
**Therapeutic Category** Vitamin D Analog
**Use** Dietary supplement, treatment of vitamin D deficiency, or prophylaxis of deficiency
**Usual Dosage** Adults: Oral: 400-1000 units/day
**Dosage Forms**
  Tablet: 1000 int. units
  Delta-D®: 400 int. units

**cholecalciferol and alendronate** *see* alendronate and cholecalciferol *on page 26*

**cholera vaccine (all products)** *(Discontinued)*

**cholestyramine resin** (koe LES teer a meen REZ in)
**U.S./Canadian Brand Names** Novo-Cholamine Light [Can]; Novo-Cholamine [Can]; PMS-Cholestyramine [Can]; Prevalite® [US]; Questran® Light Sugar Free [Can]; Questran® Light [US]; Questran® [US/Can]
**Therapeutic Category** Bile Acid Sequestrant
**Use** Adjunct in the management of primary hypercholesterolemia; pruritus associated with elevated levels of bile acids; diarrhea associated with excess fecal bile acids; binding toxicologic agents; pseudomembraneous colitis
**Usual Dosage** Oral (dosages are expressed in terms of anhydrous resin):
  Children: 240 mg/kg/day in 3 divided doses; need to titrate dose depending on indication
  Adults: 4 g 1-2 times/day to a maximum of 24 g/day and 6 doses/day
**Dosage Forms**
  Powder for oral suspension: 4 g of resin/5.7 g of powder (5.7 g packets, 240 g can) [light formulation]; 4 g of resin/9 g of powder (9 g packets, 378 g can)
    Prevalite®: 4 g of resin/5.5 g of powder (5.5 g packets, 231 g can) [contains phenylalanine 14.1 mg/5.5 g; orange flavor]
    Questran®: 4 g of resin/9 g of powder (9 g packets, 378 g can)
    Questran® Light: 4 g of resin/5 g of powder (5 g packets, 210 g can) [contains phenylalanine 16.8 g/5 g]

**choline magnesium trisalicylate** (KOE leen mag NEE zhum trye sa LIS i late)
Synonyms tricosal
**Therapeutic Category** Analgesic, Nonnarcotic; Nonsteroidal Antiinflammatory Drug (NSAID)
**Use** Management of osteoarthritis, rheumatoid arthritis, and other arthritis; acute painful shoulder
**Usual Dosage** Oral (based on total salicylate content):
  Children <37 kg: 50 mg/kg/day given in 2 divided doses; 2250 mg/day for heavier children
  Adults: 500 mg to 1.5 g 2-3 times/day **or** 3 g at bedtime; usual maintenance dose: 1-4.5 g/day
**Dosage Forms**
  Liquid: 500 mg/5 mL (240 mL) [choline salicylate 293 mg and magnesium salicylate 362 mg per 5 mL; cherry cordial flavor]
  Tablet: 500 mg [choline salicylate 293 mg and magnesium salicylate 362 mg]; 750 mg [choline salicylate 440 mg and magnesium salicylate 544 mg]; 1000 mg [choline salicylate 587 mg and magnesium salicylate 725 mg]

**Cholografin**® **Meglumine [US]** *see* radiological/contrast media (ionic) *on page 707*

**chondroitin sulfate and sodium hyaluronate**
  (kon DROY tin SUL fate & SOW de um hye al yoor ON ate)
Synonyms sodium hyaluronate-chrondroitin sulfate
**U.S./Canadian Brand Names** Viscoat® [US]
**Therapeutic Category** Ophthalmic Agent, Viscoelastic
**Use** Surgical aid in anterior segment procedures, protects corneal endothelium and coats intraocular lens thus protecting it

**Usual Dosage** Carefully introduce (using a 27-gauge needle or cannula) into anterior chamber after thoroughly cleaning the chamber with a balanced salt solution

**Dosage Forms** Solution, ophthalmic: Sodium chondroitin 4% and sodium hyaluronate 3% (0.5 mL)

**Chooz® [US-OTC]** *see* calcium carbonate *on page 130*

**choriogonadotropin alfa** *see* chorionic gonadotropin (recombinant) *on this page*

## chorionic gonadotropin (human) (kor ee ON ik goe NAD oh troe pin, HYU man)

**Synonyms** CG; hCG

**U.S./Canadian Brand Names** Humegon® [Can]; Novarel™ [US]; Pregnyl® [US/Can]; Profasi® HP [Can]

**Therapeutic Category** Gonadotropin

**Use** Induces ovulation and pregnancy in anovulatory, infertile females; treatment of hypogonadotropic hypogonadism, prepubertal cryptorchidism; spermatogenesis induction with follitropin alfa or follitropin beta

**Usual Dosage** I.M.:

Children:

Prepubertal cryptorchidism: 1000-2000 units/m²/dose 3 times/week for 3 weeks **or** 4000 units 3 times/week for 3 weeks **or** 5000 units every second day for 4 injections **or** 500 units 3 times/week for 4-6 weeks

Hypogonadotropic hypogonadism: 500-1000 units 3 times/week for 3 weeks, followed by the same dose twice weekly for 3 weeks **or** 1000-2000 units 3 times/week **or** 4000 units 3 times/week for 6-9 months; reduce dosage to 2000 units 3 times/week for additional 3 months

Adults:

Induction of ovulation: Female: 5000-10,000 units one day following last dose of menotropins

Spermatogenesis induction: Male: Initial: 1500 int. units twice weekly to normalize serum testosterone levels. If no response in 8 weeks, increase dose to 3000 int. units twice weekly. After normalization of testosterone levels, combine with follitropin beta (Follistim®). Continue hCG at same dose used to normalize testosterone levels. Treatment response was noted at up to 12 months.

**Dosage Forms**

Injection, powder for reconstitution: 10,000 units [packaged with diluent; diluent contains benzyl alcohol and mannitol]

Novarel™: 10,000 units [packaged with diluent; diluent contains benzyl alcohol and mannitol]

Pregnyl®: 10,000 units [packaged with diluent; diluent contains benzyl alcohol]

## chorionic gonadotropin (recombinant)

(kor ee ON ik goe NAD oh troe pin ree KOM be nant)

**Synonyms** choriogonadotropin alfa; r-hCG

**U.S./Canadian Brand Names** Ovidrel® [US/Can]

**Therapeutic Category** Gonadotropin; Ovulation Stimulator

**Use** As part of an assisted reproductive technology (ART) program, induces ovulation in infertile females who have been pretreated with follicle stimulating hormones (FSH); induces ovulation and pregnancy in infertile females when the cause of infertility is functional

**Usual Dosage** SubQ: Adults: Female: Assisted reproductive technologies (ART) and ovulation induction: 250 mcg given 1 day following the last dose of follicle stimulating agent. Use only after adequate follicular development has been determined. Hold treatment when there is an excessive ovarian response.

**Dosage Forms** [DSC] = Discontinued product

Injection, powder for reconstitution: 285 mcg [packaged with 1 mL SWFI; delivers 250 mcg r-hCG following reconstitution] [DSC]

Injection, solution: 257.5 mcg/0.515 mL (0.515 mL) [prefilled syringe; delivers 250 mcg r-hCG/0.5 mL]

**Choron® *(Discontinued)*** *see* chorionic gonadotropin (human) *on this page*

**Chromagen® OB [US]** *see* vitamins (multiple/prenatal) *on page 852*

**chromium** *see* trace metals *on page 813*

**Chronovera® [Can]** *see* verapamil *on page 843*

**Chronulac® *(Discontinued)*** *see* lactulose *on page 464*

**Cialis® [US/Can]** *see* tadalafil *on page 779*

**Cibacalcin® *(Discontinued)*** *see* calcitonin *on page 129*

# ciclopirox (sye kloe PEER oks)

**Sound-Alike/Look-Alike Issues**
Loprox® may be confused with Lonox®

**Synonyms** ciclopirox olamine

**U.S./Canadian Brand Names** Loprox® [US/Can]; Penlac® [US/Can]

**Therapeutic Category** Antifungal Agent

**Use**
Cream/suspension: Treatment of tinea pedis (athlete's foot), tinea cruris (jock itch), tinea corporis (ringworm), cutaneous candidiasis, and tinea versicolor (pityriasis)

Gel: Treatment of tinea pedis (athlete's foot), tinea corporis (ringworm); seborrheic dermatitis of the scalp

Lacquer (solution): Topical treatment of mild-to-moderate onychomycosis of the fingernails and toenails due to *Trichophyton rubrum* (not involving the lunula) and the immediately-adjacent skin

Shampoo: Treatment of seborrheic dermatitis of the scalp

**Usual Dosage** Topical:
Children >10 years and Adults: Tinea pedis, tinea cruris, tinea corporis, cutaneous candidiasis, and tinea versicolor: Cream/suspension: Apply twice daily, gently massage into affected areas; if no improvement after 4 weeks of treatment, re-evaluate the diagnosis

Children >16 years and Adults:
Tinea pedis, tinea corporis, seborrheic dermatitis of the scalp: Gel: Apply twice daily, gently massage into affected areas and surrounding skin; if no improvement after 4 weeks of treatment, re-evaluate diagnosis

Seborrheic dermatitis of the scalp: Shampoo: Apply to wet hair, lather, and leave in place ~3 minute; rinse. Repeat twice weekly for 4 weeks; allow a minimum of 3 days between applications

Onychomycosis of the fingernails and toenails: Children ≥12 years and Adults: Lacquer (solution): Apply to adjacent skin and affected nails daily (as a part of a comprehensive management program for onychomycosis). Remove with alcohol every 7 days

**Dosage Forms**
Cream, as olamine (Loprox®): 0.77% (15 g, 30 g, 90 g)
Gel (Loprox®): 0.77% (30 g, 45 g, 100 g)
Shampoo (Loprox®): 1% (120 mL)
Solution, topical [nail lacquer] (Penlac®): 8% (6.6 mL)
Suspension, topical, as olamine (Loprox®): 0.77% (30 mL, 60 mL)

**ciclopirox olamine** *see ciclopirox on this page*

**Cidecin** *see daptomycin on page 224*

# cidofovir (si DOF o veer)

**U.S./Canadian Brand Names** Vistide® [US]

**Therapeutic Category** Antiviral Agent

**Use** Treatment of cytomegalovirus (CMV) retinitis in patients with acquired immunodeficiency syndrome (AIDS). **Note:** Should be administered with probenecid.

**Usual Dosage** Adults:
Induction: 5 mg/kg I.V. over 1 hour once weekly for 2 consecutive weeks
Maintenance: 5 mg/kg over 1 hour once every other week
**Note: Administer with probenecid 2 g orally 3 hours prior to each cidofovir dose and 1 g at 2 hours and 8 hours after completion of the infusion (total: 4 g)**
Hydrate with 1 L of 0.9% NS I.V. prior to cidofovir infusion; a second liter may be administered over a 1- to 3-hour period immediately following infusion, if tolerated

**Dosage Forms** Injection, solution [preservative free]: 75 mg/mL (5 mL)

# cilazapril *(Canada only)* (sye LAY za pril)

**Synonyms** cilazapril monohydrate

**U.S./Canadian Brand Names** Inhibace® [Can]; Novo-Cilazapril [Can]

**Therapeutic Category** Angiotensin-Converting Enzyme (ACE) Inhibitor

**Use** Management of hypertension; treatment of congestive heart failure

**Usual Dosage** Oral:
Hypertension: 2.5-5 mg once daily (maximum dose: 10 mg/day)
Congestive heart failure: Initial: 0.5 mg once daily; if tolerated, after 5 days increase to 1 mg/day (lowest maintenance dose); may increase to maximum of 2.5 mg once daily

**Dosage Forms** Tablet: 1 mg, 2.5 mg, 5 mg

**cilazapril monohydrate** *see* cilazapril *(Canada only)* *on previous page*

# cilostazol (sil OH sta zol)

**Sound-Alike/Look-Alike Issues**
Pletal® may be confused with Plendil®

**Synonyms** OPC-13013

**U.S./Canadian Brand Names** Pletal® [US/Can]

**Therapeutic Category** Platelet Aggregation Inhibitor

**Use** Symptomatic management of peripheral vascular disease, primarily intermittent claudication

**Usual Dosage** Adults: Oral: 100 mg twice daily taken at least one-half hour before or 2 hours after breakfast and dinner; dosage should be reduced to 50 mg twice daily during concurrent therapy with inhibitors of CYP3A4 or CYP2C19

**Dosage Forms** Tablet: 50 mg, 100 mg

**Ciloxan® [US/Can]** *see* ciprofloxacin *on next page*

# cimetidine (sye MET i deen)

**Sound-Alike/Look-Alike Issues**
clmetldlne may be confused wlth slmethlcone

**U.S./Canadian Brand Names** Apo-Cimetidine® [Can]; Gen-Cimetidine [Can]; Novo-Cimetidine [Can]; Nu-Cimet [Can]; PMS-Cimetidine [Can]; Tagamet® HB 200 [US-OTC]; Tagamet® HB [Can]; Tagamet® [US]

**Therapeutic Category** Histamine $H_2$ Antagonist

**Use** Short-term treatment of active duodenal ulcers and benign gastric ulcers; long-term prophylaxis of duodenal ulcer; gastric hypersecretory states; gastroesophageal reflux; prevention of upper GI bleeding in critically-ill patients; labeled for OTC use for prevention or relief of heartburn, acid indigestion, or sour stomach

**Usual Dosage**
Children: Oral, I.M., I.V.: 20-40 mg/kg/day in divided doses every 6 hours

Children ≥12 years and Adults: Oral: Heartburn, acid indigestion, sour stomach (OTC labeling): 200 mg up to twice daily; may take 30 minutes prior to eating foods or beverages expected to cause heartburn or indigestion

Adults:
Short-term treatment of active ulcers:
 Oral: 300 mg 4 times/day or 800 mg at bedtime or 400 mg twice daily for up to 8 weeks
 I.M., I.V.: 300 mg every 6 hours or 37.5 mg/hour by continuous infusion; I.V. dosage should be adjusted to maintain an intragastric pH ≥5
Patients with an active bleed: Administer cimetidine as a continuous infusion (see above)
Duodenal ulcer prophylaxis: Oral: 400-800 mg at bedtime
Gastric hypersecretory conditions: Oral, I.M., I.V.: 300-600 mg every 6 hours; dosage not to exceed 2.4 g/day

**Dosage Forms**
Infusion, as hydrochloride [premixed in NS]: 300 mg (50 mL)
Injection, solution, as hydrochloride: 150 mg/mL (2 mL, 8 mL) [8 mL size contains benzyl alcohol]
Liquid, oral, as hydrochloride: 300 mg/5 mL (240 mL, 480 mL) [contains alcohol 2.8%; mint-peach flavor]
Tablet: 200 mg [OTC], 300 mg, 400 mg, 800 mg
 Tagamet®: 300 mg, 400 mg
 Tagamet® HB 200: 200 mg

# cinacalcet (sin a KAL cet)

**Synonyms** AMG 073; cinacalcet hydrochloride

**U.S./Canadian Brand Names** Sensipar™ [US]

**Therapeutic Category** Calcimimetic

**Use** Treatment of secondary hyperparathyroidism in dialysis patients; treatment of hypercalcemia in patients with parathyroid carcinoma

**Usual Dosage** Oral: Adults: **Do not titrate dose more frequently than every 2-4 weeks.**
Secondary hyperparathyroidism: Initial: 30 mg once daily (maximum daily dose: 180 mg); increase dose incrementally (60 mg, 90 mg, 120 mg, 180 mg once daily) as necessary to maintain iPTH level between 150-300 pg/mL.
(Continued)

# cinacalcet *(Continued)*

Parathyroid carcinoma: Initial: 30 mg twice daily (maximum daily dose: 360 mg daily as 90 mg 4 times/day); increase dose incrementally (60 mg twice daily, 90 mg twice daily, 90 mg 4 times/day) as necessary to normalize serum calcium levels.

**Dosage Forms** Tablet [film coated]: 30 mg, 60 mg, 90 mg

**cinacalcet hydrochloride** *see* cinacalcet *on previous page*

**Cipralex® [Can]** *see* escitalopram *on page 297*

**Cipro® [US/Can]** *see* ciprofloxacin *on this page*

**Cipro® XL [Can]** *see* ciprofloxacin *on this page*

**Ciprodex® [US/Can]** *see* ciprofloxacin and dexamethasone *on page 186*

# ciprofloxacin *(sip roe FLOKS a sin)*

**Sound-Alike/Look-Alike Issues**

ciprofloxacin may be confused with cephalexin

Ciloxan® may be confused with cinoxacin, Cytoxan®

Cipro® may be confused with Ceftin®

**Synonyms** ciprofloxacin hydrochloride

**U.S./Canadian Brand Names** Apo-Ciproflox® [Can]; Ciloxan® [US/Can]; Cipro® XL [Can]; Cipro® XR [US]; Cipro® [US/Can]; CO Ciprofloxacin [Can]; Gen-Ciprofloxacin [Can]; Novo-Ciprofloxacin [Can]; PMS-Ciprofloxacin [Can]; Proquin® XR [US]; ratio-Ciprofloxacin [Can]; Rhoxal-ciprofloxacin [Can]

**Therapeutic Category** Antibiotic, Ophthalmic; Quinolone

**Use**

Children: Complicated urinary tract infections and pyelonephritis due to *E. coli*. **Note:** Although effective, ciprofloxacin is not the drug of first choice in children.

Children and adults: To reduce incidence or progression of disease following exposure to aerolized *Bacillus anthracis*. Ophthalmologically, for superficial ocular infections (corneal ulcers, conjunctivitis) due to susceptible strains

Adults: Treatment of the following infections when caused by susceptible bacteria: Urinary tract infections; acute uncomplicated cystitis in females; chronic bacterial prostatitis; lower respiratory tract infections (including acute exacerbations of chronic bronchitis); acute sinusitis; skin and skin structure infections; bone and joint infections; complicated intra-abdominal infections (in combination with metronidazole); infectious diarrhea; typhoid fever due to *Salmonella typhi* (eradication of chronic typhoid carrier state has not been proven); uncomplicated cervical and urethra gonorrhea (due to *N. gonorrhoeae*); nosocomial pneumonia; empirical therapy for febrile neutropenic patients (in combination with piperacillin)

**Usual Dosage Note:** Extended release tablets and immediate release formulations are not interchangeable. Unless otherwise specified, oral dosing reflects the use of immediate release formulations.

Children:

Oral:

Complicated urinary tract infection or pyelonephritis: Children 1-17 years: 20-30 mg/kg/day in 2 divided doses (every 12 hours) for 10-21 days; maximum: 1.5 g/day

Anthrax:

Inhalational (postexposure prophylaxis): 15 mg/kg/dose every 12 hours for 60 days; maximum: 500 mg/dose

Cutaneous (treatment, CDC guidelines): 10-15 mg/kg every 12 hours for 60 days (maximum: 1 g/day); amoxicillin 80 mg/kg/day divided every 8 hours is an option for completion of treatment after clinical improvement. **Note:** In the presence of systemic involvement, extensive edema, lesions on head/neck, refer to I.V. dosing for treatment of inhalational/gastrointestinal/oropharyngeal anthrax

I.V.:

Complicated urinary tract infection or pyelonephritis: Children 1-17 years: 6-10 mg/kg every 8 hours for 10-21 days (maximum: 400 mg/dose)

Anthrax:

Inhalational (postexposure prophylaxis): 10 mg/kg/dose every 12 hours for 60 days; do **not** exceed 400 mg/dose (800 mg/day)

Inhalational/gastrointestinal/oropharyngeal (treatment, CDC guidelines): Initial: 10-15 mg/kg every 12 hours for 60 days (maximum: 500 mg/dose); switch to oral therapy when clinically appropriate; refer to Adults dosing for notes on combined therapy and duration

Adults: Oral:
Urinary tract infection:
  Acute uncomplicated: Immediate release formulation: 250 mg every 12 hours for 3 days
  Acute uncomplicated pyelonephritis: Extended release formulation (Cipro® XR): 1000 mg every 24 hours for 7-14 days
  Uncomplicated/acute cystitis: Extended release formulation (Cipro® XR, Proquin® XR): 500 mg every 24 hours for 3 days
  Mild/moderate: Immediate release formulation: 250 mg every 12 hours for 7-14 days
  Severe/complicated:
    Immediate release formulation: 500 mg every 12 hours for 7-14 days
    Extended release formulation (Cipro® XR): 1000 mg every 24 hours for 7-14 days
Lower respiratory tract, skin/skin structure infections: 500-750 mg twice daily for 7-14 days depending on severity and susceptibility
Bone/joint infections: 500-750 mg twice daily for 4-6 weeks, depending on severity and susceptibility
Infectious diarrhea: 500 mg every 12 hours for 5-7 days
Intra-abdominal (in combination with metronidazole): 500 mg every 12 hours for 7-14 days
Typhoid fever: 500 mg every 12 hours for 10 days
Urethral/cervical gonococcal infections: 250-500 mg as a single dose (CDC recommends concomitant doxycycline or azithromycin due to developing resistance; avoid use in Asian or Western Pacific travelers)
Disseminated gonococcal infection (CDC guidelines): 500 mg twice daily to complete 7 days of therapy (initial treatment with ceftriaxone 1 g I.M./I.V. daily for 24-48 hours after improvement begins)
Chancroid (CDC guidelines): 500 mg twice daily for 3 days
Sinusitis (acute): 500 mg every 12 hours for 10 days
Chronic bacterial prostatitis: 500 mg every 12 hours for 28 days
Anthrax:
  Inhalational (postexposure prophylaxis): 500 mg every 12 hours for 60 days
  Cutaneous (treatment, CDC guidelines): Immediate release formulation: 500 mg every 12 hours for 60 days. **Note:** In the presence of systemic involvement, extensive edema, lesions on head/neck, refer to I.V. dosing for treatment of inhalational/gastrointestinal/oropharyngeal anthrax
Adults: I.V.:
Bone/joint infections:
  Mild to moderate: 400 mg every 12 hours for 4-6 weeks
  Severe or complicated: 400 mg every 8 hours for 4-6 weeks
Lower respiratory tract, skin/skin structure infections:
  Mild to moderate: 400 mg every 12 hours for 7-14 days
  Severe or complicated: 400 mg every 8 hours for 7-14 days
Nosocomial pneumonia (mild to moderate to severe): 400 mg every 8 hours for 10-14 days
Prostatitis (chronic, bacterial): 400 mg every 12 hours for 28 days
Sinusitis (acute): 400 mg every 12 hours for 10 days
Urinary tract infection:
  Mild to moderate: 200 mg every 12 hours for 7-14 days
  Severe or complicated: 400 mg every 12 hours for 7-14 days
Febrile neutropenia (with piperacillin): 400 mg every 8 hours for 7-14 days
Intra-abdominal infection (with metronidazole): 400 mg every 12 hours for 7-14 days
Anthrax:
  Inhalational (postexposure prophylaxis): 400 mg every 12 hours for 60 days
  Inhalational/gastrointestinal/oropharyngeal (treatment, CDC guidelines): 400 mg every 12 hours. **Note:** Initial treatment should include two or more agents predicted to be effective (per CDC recommendations). Agents suggested for use in conjunction with ciprofloxacin or doxycycline include rifampin, vancomycin, imipenem, penicillin, ampicillin, chloramphenicol, clindamycin, and clarithromycin. May switch to oral antimicrobial therapy when clinically appropriate. Continue combined therapy for 60 days.

Ophthalmic:
Solution: Children >1 year and Adults:
  Bacterial conjunctivitis: Instill 1-2 drops in eye(s) every 2 hours while awake for 2 days and 1-2 drops every 4 hours while awake for the next 5 days
  Corneal ulcer: Instill 2 drops into affected eye every 15 minutes for the first 6 hours, then 2 drops into the affected eye every 30 minutes for the remainder of the first day. On day 2, instill 2 drops into the affected eye hourly. On days 3-14, instill 2 drops into affected eye every 4 hours. Treatment may continue after day 14 if re-epithelialization has not occurred.
(Continued)

## ciprofloxacin *(Continued)*

Ointment: Children >2 years and Adults: Bacterial conjunctivitis: Apply a ½" ribbon into the conjunctival sac 3 times/day for the first 2 days, followed by a ½" ribbon applied twice daily for the next 5 days

**Dosage Forms** [DSC] = Discontinued product

Infusion, [premixed in D₅W] (Cipro®): 200 mg (100 mL); 400 mg (200 mL) [latex free]

Injection, solution (Cipro®): 10 mg/mL (20 mL, 40 mL, 120 mL [DSC])

Microcapsules for oral suspension (Cipro®): 250 mg/5 mL (100 mL); 500 mg/5 mL (100 mL) [strawberry flavor]

Ointment, ophthalmic, as hydrochloride (Ciloxan®): 3.33 mg/g [0.3% base] (3.5 g)

Solution, ophthalmic, as hydrochloride (Ciloxan®): 3.5 mg/mL [0.3% base] (2.5 mL, 5 mL, 10 mL) [contains benzalkonium chloride]

Tablet: 250 mg, 500 mg, 750 mg

Cipro®: 100 mg, 250 mg, 500 mg, 750 mg

Tablet, extended release:

Cipro® XR: 500 mg [equivalent to ciprofloxacin hydrochloride 287.5 mg and ciprofloxacin base 212.6 mg]; 1000 mg [equivalent to ciprofloxacin hydrochloride 574.9 mg and ciprofloxacin base 425.2 mg]

Proquin® XR: 500 mg

## ciprofloxacin and dexamethasone *(sip roe FLOKS a sin & deks a METH a sone)*

**Synonyms** ciprofloxacin hydrochloride and dexamethasone; dexamethasone and ciprofloxacin

**U.S./Canadian Brand Names** Ciprodex® [US/Can]

**Therapeutic Category** Antibiotic/Corticosteroid, Otic

**Use** Treatment of acute otitis media in pediatric patients with tympanostomy tubes or acute otitis externa in children and adults

**Usual Dosage** Otic:

Children: Acute otitis media in patients with tympanostomy tubes or acute otitis externa: Instill 4 drops into affected ear(s) twice daily for 7 days

Adults: Acute otitis externa: Instill 4 drops into affected ear(s) twice daily for 7 days

**Dosage Forms** Suspension, otic: Ciprofloxacin 0.3% and dexamethasone 0.1% (7.5 mL) [contains benzalkonium chloride]

## ciprofloxacin and hydrocortisone *(sip roe FLOKS a sin & hye droe KOR ti sone)*

**Synonyms** hydrocortisone and ciprofloxacin

**U.S./Canadian Brand Names** Cipro® HC [US/Can]

**Therapeutic Category** Antibiotic/Corticosteroid, Otic

**Use** Treatment of acute otitis externa, sometimes known as "swimmer's ear"

**Usual Dosage** Children >1 year of age and Adults: Otic: The recommended dosage for all patients is three drops of the suspension in the affected ear twice daily for seven day; twice-daily dosing schedule is more convenient for patients than that of existing treatments with hydrocortisone, which are typically administered three or four times a day; a twice-daily dosage schedule may be especially helpful for parents and caregivers of young children

**Dosage Forms** Suspension, otic: Ciprofloxacin hydrochloride 0.2% and hydrocortisone 1% (10 mL) [contains benzyl alcohol]

**ciprofloxacin hydrochloride** *see ciprofloxacin on page 184*

**ciprofloxacin hydrochloride and dexamethasone** *see ciprofloxacin and dexamethasone on this page*

**Cipro® HC [US/Can]** *see ciprofloxacin and hydrocortisone on this page*

**Cipro® XR [US]** *see ciprofloxacin on page 184*

## cisapride *(SIS a pride)*

**Sound-Alike/Look-Alike Issues**

Propulsid® may be confused with propranolol

**U.S./Canadian Brand Names** Propulsid® [US]

**Therapeutic Category** Gastrointestinal Agent, Prokinetic

**Use** Treatment of nocturnal symptoms of gastroesophageal reflux disease (GERD); has demonstrated effectiveness for gastroparesis, refractory constipation, and nonulcer dyspepsia

**Usual Dosage** Oral:

Children: 0.15-0.3 mg/kg/dose 3-4 times/day; maximum: 10 mg/dose

Adults: Initial: 10 mg 4 times/day at least 15 minutes before meals and at bedtime; in some patients the dosage will need to be increased to 20 mg to obtain a satisfactory result

# cisatracurium (sis a tra KYOO ree um)
## Sound-Alike/Look-Alike Issues
Nimbex® may be confused with Revex®
## Synonyms cisatracurium besylate
## U.S./Canadian Brand Names Nimbex® [US/Can]
## Therapeutic Category Skeletal Muscle Relaxant
## Use Adjunct to general anesthesia to facilitate endotracheal intubation and to relax skeletal muscles during surgery; to facilitate mechanical ventilation in ICU patients; does not relieve pain or produce sedation
## Usual Dosage I.V. (not to be used I.M.):
**Operating room administration:**
Children 2-12 years: Intubating doses: 0.1 mg over 5-15 seconds during either halothane or opioid anesthesia. (**Note:** When given during stable opioid/nitrous oxide/oxygen anesthesia, 0.1 mg/kg produces maximum neuromuscular block in an average of 2.8 minutes and clinically effective block for 28 minutes.)
Adults: Intubating doses: 0.15-0.2 mg/kg as component of propofol/nitrous oxide/oxygen induction-intubation technique. (**Note:** May produce generally good or excellent conditions for tracheal intubation in 1.5-2 minutes with clinically effective duration of action during propofol anesthesia of 55-61 minutes.); initial dose after succinylcholine for intubation: 0.1 mg/kg; maintenance dose: 0.03 mg/kg 40-60 minutes after initial dose, then at ~20-minute intervals based on clinical criteria
Children ≥2 years and Adults: Continuous infusion: After an initial bolus, a diluted solution can be given by continuous infusion for maintenance of neuromuscular blockade during extended surgery; adjust the rate of administration according to the patient's response as determined by peripheral nerve stimulation. An initial infusion rate of 3 mcg/kg/minute may be required to rapidly counteract the spontaneous recovery of neuromuscular function; thereafter, a rate of 1-2 mcg/kg/minute should be adequate to maintain continuous neuromuscular block in the 89% to 99% range in most pediatric and adult patients. Consider reduction of the infusion rate by 30% to 40% when administering during stable isoflurane, enflurane, sevoflurane, or desflurane anesthesia. Spontaneous recovery from neuromuscular blockade following discontinuation of infusion of cisatracurium may be expected to proceed at a rate comparable to that following single bolus administration.
**Intensive care unit administration:** Follow the principles for infusion in the operating room. At initial signs of recovery from bolus dose, begin the infusion at a dose of 3 mcg/kg/minute and adjust rates accordingly; dosage ranges of 0.5-10 mcg/kg/minute have been reported. If patient is allowed to recover from neuromuscular blockade, readministration of a bolus dose may be necessary to quickly re-establish neuromuscular block prior to reinstituting the infusion.
## Dosage Forms
Injection, solution: 2 mg/mL (5 mL); 10 mg/mL (20 mL)
Injection, solution: 2 mg/mL (10 mL) [contains benzyl alcohol]

**cisatracurium besylate** *see* cisatracurium *on this page*

# cisplatin (SIS pla tin)
## Sound-Alike/Look-Alike Issues
cisplatin may be confused with carboplatin
Platinol®-AQ may be confused with Paraplatin®, Patanol®, Plaquenil®
## Synonyms CDDP
## Therapeutic Category Antineoplastic Agent
## Use Treatment of head and neck, breast, testicular, and ovarian cancer; Hodgkin and non-Hodgkin lymphoma; neuroblastoma; sarcomas, bladder, gastric, lung, esophageal, cervical, and prostate cancer; myeloma, melanoma, mesothelioma, small cell lung cancer, and osteosarcoma
## Usual Dosage
Children: Various dosage schedules range from 30-100 mg/m$^2$ once every 2-3 weeks; may also dose similar to adult dosing
Recurrent brain tumors: 60 mg/m$^2$ once daily for 2 consecutive days every 3-4 weeks
Adults:
Advanced bladder cancer: 50-70 mg/m$^2$ every 3-4 weeks
Head and neck cancer: 100-120 mg/m$^2$ every 3-4 weeks
Malignant pleural mesothelioma (in combination with pemetrexed): 75 mg/m$^2$ on day 1 of each 21-day cycle; see pemetrexed monograph for additional details
(Continued)

## cisplatin (Continued)

Metastatic ovarian cancer: 75-100 mg/m$^2$ every 3 weeks

Intraperitoneal: Cisplatin has been administered intraperitoneal with systemic sodium thiosulfate for ovarian cancer; doses up to 90-270 mg/m$^2$ have been administered and retained for 4 hours before draining

Testicular cancer: 10-20 mg/m$^2$/day for 5 days repeated every 3-4 weeks

**Dosage Forms** [DSC] = Discontinued product

Injection, solution: 1 mg/mL (50 mL, 100 mL, 200 mL)

Platinol®-AQ: 1 mg/mL (50 mL, 100 mL) [DSC]

**13-*cis*-retinoic acid** *see* isotretinoin *on page 452*

## citalopram (sye TAL oh pram)

**Sound-Alike/Look-Alike Issues**

Celexa™ may be confused with Celebrex®, Cerebra®, Cerebyx®, Zyprexa®

**Synonyms** citalopram hydrobromide; nitalapram

**U.S./Canadian Brand Names** Apo-Citalopram® [Can]; Celexa™ [US/Can]; CO Citalopram [Can]; Gen-Citalopram [Can]; Novo-Citalopram [Can]; PMS-Citalopram [Can]; ratio-Citalopram [Can]; Rhoxal-citalopram [Can]

**Therapeutic Category** Antidepressant

**Use** Treatment of depression

**Usual Dosage** Oral: Adults: Depression: Initial: 20 mg/day, generally with an increase to 40 mg/day; doses of more than 40 mg are not usually necessary. Should a dose increase be necessary, it should occur in 20 mg increments at intervals of no less than 1 week. Maximum dose: 60 mg/day

**Dosage Forms**

Solution, oral: 10 mg/5 mL (240 mL) [alcohol free, sugar free; peppermint flavor]

Tablet: 10 mg, 20 mg, 40 mg

**citalopram hydrobromide** *see* citalopram *on this page*

**Citanest® Plain [US/Can]** *see* prilocaine *on page 677*

**Citracal® [US-OTC]** *see* calcium citrate *on page 133*

**Citracal® Prenatal Rx [US]** *see* vitamins (multiple/prenatal) *on page 852*

**citrate of magnesia** *see* magnesium citrate *on page 498*

**citric acid and d-gluconic acid irrigant** *see* citric acid, magnesium carbonate, and glucono-delta-lactone *on this page*

**citric acid and potassium citrate** *see* potassium citrate and citric acid *on page 665*

**citric acid bladder mixture** *see* citric acid, magnesium carbonate, and glucono-delta-lactone *on this page*

## citric acid, magnesium carbonate, and glucono-delta-lactone

(SI trik AS id, mag NEE see um KAR bo nate, and GLOO kon o DEL ta LAK tone)

**Sound-Alike/Look-Alike Issues**

Renacidin® may be confused with Remicade®

**Synonyms** citric acid and d-gluconic acid irrigant; citric acid bladder mixture; citric acid, magnesium hydroxycarbonate, D-gluconic acid, magnesium acid citrate, and calcium carbonate; hemiacidrin

**U.S./Canadian Brand Names** Renacidin® [US]

**Therapeutic Category** Irrigating Solution

**Use** Prevention of formation of calcifications of indwelling urinary tract catheters; treatment of renal and bladder calculi of the apatite or struvite type

**Usual Dosage** Adults:

Dissolution or prevention of calcifications: Irrigation (indwelling urethral catheters): 30-60 mL 2-3 times/day by means of a rubber syringe

Renal calculi: Irrigation: Infuse NS at 60 mL/hour and increase until pain, elevated pressure, or maximum flow rate of 120 mL/hour is reached. Begin flow of solution at maximum rate achieved with NS.

Bladder calculi: 30 mL instilled through urinary catheter; clamp for 30-60 minutes, then release and drain; repeat 4-6 times/day

**Dosage Forms** Solution, irrigation: Citric acid 6.602 g, magnesium carbonate 3.177 g, glucono-delta-lactone 0.198 g per 100 mL (500 mL) [contains benzoic acid]

**citric acid, magnesium hydroxycarbonate, D-gluconic acid, magnesium acid citrate, and calcium carbonate** *see* citric acid, magnesium carbonate, and glucono-delta-lactone *on previous page*

## citric acid, sodium citrate, and potassium citrate
(SIT rik AS id, SOW dee um SIT rate, & poe TASS ee um SIT rate)

**Synonyms** potassium citrate, citric acid, and sodium citrate; sodium citrate, citric acid, and potassium citrate

**U.S./Canadian Brand Names** Cytra-3 [US]; Polycitra® [US]; Polycitra®-LC [US]

**Therapeutic Category** Alkalinizing Agent

**Use** Conditions where long-term maintenance of an alkaline urine is desirable as in control and dissolution of uric acid and cystine calculi of the urinary tract

**Usual Dosage** Oral:
Children: 5-15 mL diluted in water after meals and at bedtime
Adults: 15-30 mL diluted in water after meals and at bedtime

**Dosage Forms Note:** Equivalent to potassium 1 mEq/mL, sodium 1 mEq/mL, and bicarbonate 2 mEq/mL
Solution, oral:
Cytra-3: Citric acid 334 mg, sodium citrate 500 mg, and potassium citrate 550 mg per 5 mL (480 mL) [alcohol free, sugar free; contains sodium benzoate; raspberry flavor]
Polycitra®-LC: Citric acid 334 mg, sodium citrate 500 mg, and potassium citrate 550 mg per 5 mL (480 mL) [alcohol free, sugar free]
Syrup, oral (Polycitra®): Citric acid 334 mg, sodium citrate 500 mg, and potassium citrate 550 mg per 5 mL (480 mL) [alcohol free]

**Citro-Mag® [Can]** *see* magnesium citrate *on page 498*

**Citrotein® [US-OTC]** *see* nutritional formula, enteral/oral *on page 591*

**citrovorum factor** *see* leucovorin *on page 470*

**Citrucel® [US-OTC]** *see* methylcellulose *on page 529*

**CL-118,532** *see* triptorelin *on page 828*

**Cl-719** *see* gemfibrozil *on page 370*

**CL-825** *see* pentostatin *on page 632*

**CL-184116** *see* porfimer *on page 661*

## cladribine (KLA dri been)
**Sound-Alike/Look-Alike Issues**
Leustatin® may be confused with lovastatin

**Synonyms** 2-CdA; 2-chlorodeoxyadenosine

**U.S./Canadian Brand Names** Leustatin® [US/Can]

**Therapeutic Category** Antineoplastic Agent

**Use** Treatment of hairy cell leukemia, chronic lymphocytic leukemia (CLL), chronic myelogenous leukemia (CML)

**Usual Dosage** I.V.: Refer to individual protocols.
Pediatrics: Acute leukemias: 6.2-7.5 mg/m$^2$/day continuous infusion for days 1-5; maximum tolerated dose was 8.9 mg/m$^2$/day.
Adults:
Hairy cell leukemia: Continuous infusion:
0.09-0.1 mg/kg/day days 1-7; may be repeated every 28-35 days **or**
3.4 mg/m$^2$/day SubQ days 1-7
Chronic lymphocytic leukemia: Continuous infusion:
0.1 mg/kg/day days 1-7 **or**
0.028-0.14 mg/kg/day as a 2-hour infusion days 1-5
Chronic myelogenous leukemia: 15 mg/m$^2$/day as a 1-hour infusion days 1-5; if no response increase dose to 20 mg/m$^2$/day in the second course.

**Dosage Forms** Injection, solution [preservative free]: 1 mg/mL (10 mL)

**Claforan® [US/Can]** *see* cefotaxime *on page 154*

**Claravis™ [US]** *see* isotretinoin *on page 452*

**Clarinex® [US]** *see* desloratadine *on page 230*

**Claripel**™ **[US]** *see* hydroquinone *on page 420*

# clarithromycin (kla RITH roe mye sin)
## Sound-Alike/Look-Alike Issues
clarithromycin may be confused with erythromycin

**U.S./Canadian Brand Names** Biaxin® XL [US/Can]; Biaxin® [US/Can]; ratio-Clarithromycin [Can]

**Therapeutic Category** Macrolide (Antibiotic)

## Use
Children:

Pharyngitis/tonsillitis, acute maxillary sinusitis, uncomplicated skin/skin structure infections, and mycobacterial infections due to the above organisms

Acute otitis media (*H. influenzae, M. catarrhalis,* or *S. pneumoniae*)

Prevention of disseminated mycobacterial infections due to MAC disease in patients with advanced HIV infection

Adults:

Pharyngitis/tonsillitis due to susceptible *S. pyogenes*

Acute maxillary sinusitis and acute exacerbation of chronic bronchitis due to susceptible *H. influenzae, M. catarrhalis,* or *S. pneumoniae*

Pneumonia due to susceptible *H. influenzae, Mycoplasma pneumoniae, S. pneumoniae,* or *Chlamydia pneumoniae* (TWAR)

Uncomplicated skin/skin structure infections due to susceptible *S. aureus, S. pyogenes*

Disseminated mycobacterial infections due to *M. avium* or *M. intracellulare*

Prevention of disseminated mycobacterial infections due to *M. avium* complex (MAC) disease (eg, patients with advanced HIV infection)

Duodenal ulcer disease due to *H. pylori* in regimens with other drugs including amoxicillin and lansoprazole or omeprazole, ranitidine bismuth citrate, bismuth subsalicylate, tetracycline, and/or an $H_2$ antagonist

Alternate antibiotic for prophylaxis of bacterial endocarditis in patients who are allergic to penicillin and undergoing surgical or dental procedures

## Usual Dosage Oral:
Children ≥6 months: 15 mg/kg/day divided every 12 hours for 10 days

Mycobacterial infection (prevention and treatment): 7.5 mg/kg twice daily, up to 500 mg twice daily

Prophylaxis of bacterial endocarditis: 15 mg/kg 1 hour before procedure (maximum dose: 500 mg)

Adults:

Usual dose: 250-500 mg every 12 hours **or** 1000 mg (two 500 mg extended release tablets) once daily for 7-14 days

Upper respiratory tract: 250-500 mg every 12 hours for 10-14 days

Pharyngitis/tonsillitis: 250 mg every 12 hours for 10 days

Acute maxillary sinusitis: 500 mg every 12 hours **or** 1000 mg (two 500 mg extended release tablets) once daily for 14 days

Lower respiratory tract: 250-500 mg every 12 hours for 7-14 days

Acute exacerbation of chronic bronchitis due to:

*M. catarrhalis* and *S. pneumoniae*: 250 mg every 12 hours **or** 1000 mg (two 500 mg extended release tablets) once daily for 7-14 days

*H. influenzae*: 500 mg every 12 hours for 7-14 days

Pneumonia due to:

*C. pneumoniae, M. pneumoniae,* and *S. pneumoniae*: 250 mg every 12 hours for 7-14 days **or** 1000 mg (two 500 mg extended release tablets) once daily for 7 days

*H. influenzae*: 250 mg every 12 hours for 7 days **or** 1000 mg (two 500 mg extended release tablets) once daily for 7 days

Mycobacterial infection (prevention and treatment): 500 mg twice daily (use with other antimycobacterial drugs, eg, ethambutol, clofazimine, or rifampin)

Prophylaxis of bacterial endocarditis: 500 mg 1 hour prior to procedure

Uncomplicated skin and skin structure: 250 mg every 12 hours for 7-14 days

*Helicobacter pylori*: Combination regimen with bismuth subsalicylate, tetracycline, clarithromycin, and an $H_2$-receptor antagonist; or combination of omeprazole and clarithromycin; 250 mg twice daily to 500 mg 3 times/day

## Dosage Forms
Granules for oral suspension (Biaxin®): 125 mg/5 mL (50 mL, 100 mL); 250 mg/5 mL (50 mL, 100 mL) [fruit punch flavor]

Tablet [film coated] (Biaxin®): 250 mg, 500 mg

Tablet, extended release [film coated] (Biaxin® XL): 500 mg

**clarithromycin, lansoprazole, and amoxicillin** *see* lansoprazole, amoxicillin, and clarithromycin *on page 468*

**Claritin**® **[US-OTC/Can]** *see* loratadine *on page 491*

**Claritin-D**® **12-Hour [US-OTC]** *see* loratadine and pseudoephedrine *on page 491*

**Claritin-D**® **24-Hour [US-OTC]** *see* loratadine and pseudoephedrine *on page 491*

**Claritin**® **Allergic Decongestant [Can]** *see* oxymetazoline *on page 610*

**Claritin**® **Extra [Can]** *see* loratadine and pseudoephedrine *on page 491*

**Claritin**® **Hives Relief [US-OTC]** *see* loratadine *on page 491*

**Claritin**® **Kids [Can]** *see* loratadine *on page 491*

**Claritin**® **Liberator [Can]** *see* loratadine and pseudoephedrine *on page 491*

**Clavulin**® **[Can]** *see* amoxicillin and clavulanate potassium *on page 47*

**Clear Away**® **Disc** *(Discontinued)* *see* salicylic acid *on page 734*

**Clear By Design**® **Gel** *(Discontinued)* *see* benzoyl peroxide *on page 98*

**Clear Eyes**® **ACR [US-OTC]** *see* naphazoline *on page 561*

**Clear Eyes**® **Extra Relief [US-OTC]** *see* naphazoline *on page 561*

**Clearplex [US-OTC]** *see* benzoyl peroxide *on page 98*

**Clearsil**® **Maximum Strength** *(Discontinued)* *see* benzoyl peroxide *on page 98*

**Clear Tussin**® **30** *(Discontinued)* *see* guaifenesin and dextromethorphan *on page 385*

## clemastine (KLEM as teen)

Synonyms clemastine fumarate
U.S./Canadian Brand Names Dayhist® Allergy [US-OTC]; Tavist® Allergy [US-OTC]
Therapeutic Category Antihistamine
Use Perennial and seasonal allergic rhinitis and other allergic symptoms including urticaria
Usual Dosage Oral:
Infants and Children <6 years: 0.05 mg/kg/day as **clemastine base** or 0.335-0.67 mg/day clemastine fumarate (0.25-0.5 mg base/day) divided into 2 or 3 doses; maximum daily dosage: 1.34 mg (1 mg base)
Children 6-12 years: 0.67-1.34 mg clemastine fumarate (0.5-1 mg base) twice daily; do not exceed 4.02 mg/day (3 mg/day base)
Children ≥12 years and Adults:
1.34 mg clemastine fumarate (1 mg base) twice daily to 2.68 mg (2 mg base) 3 times/day; do not exceed 8.04 mg/day (6 mg base)
OTC labeling: 1.34 mg clemastine fumarate (1 mg base) twice daily; do not exceed 2 mg base/24 hours
Dosage Forms
Syrup, as fumarate [prescription formulation]: 0.67 mg/5 mL (120 mL) [0.5 mg base/5 mL; contains alcohol 5.5%; citrus flavor]
Tablet, as fumarate: 1.34 mg [1 mg base; OTC], 2.68 mg [2 mg base; prescription formulation]
Dayhist® Allergy, Tavist® Allergy: 1.34 mg [1 mg base]

**clemastine fumarate** *see* clemastine *on this page*

**Clenia**™ **[US]** *see* sulfur and sulfacetamide *on page 776*

**Cleocin**® **[US]** *see* clindamycin *on next page*

**Cleocin HCl**® **[US]** *see* clindamycin *on next page*

**Cleocin Pediatric**® **[US]** *see* clindamycin *on next page*

**Cleocin Phosphate**® **[US]** *see* clindamycin *on next page*

**Cleocin T**® **[US]** *see* clindamycin *on next page*

## clidinium and chlordiazepoxide (kli DI nee um & klor dye az e POKS ide)

Sound-Alike/Look-Alike Issues
Librax® may be confused with Librium®
(Continued)

# clidinium and chlordiazepoxide *(Continued)*

**Synonyms** chlordiazepoxide and clidinium
**U.S./Canadian Brand Names** Apo-Chlorax® [Can]; Librax® [Can]
**Therapeutic Category** Anticholinergic Agent
**Use** Adjunct treatment of peptic ulcer; treatment of irritable bowel syndrome
**Usual Dosage** Oral: 1-2 capsules 3-4 times/day, before meals or food and at bedtime
**Dosage Forms** Capsule: Clidinium bromide 2.5 mg and chlordiazepoxide hydrochloride 5 mg

**Climara® [US/Can]** *see* estradiol *on page 299*

**ClimaraPro™ [US]** *see* estradiol and levonorgestrel *on page 301*

**Clinac™ BPO [US]** *see* benzoyl peroxide *on page 98*

**Clindagel® [US]** *see* clindamycin *on this page*

**ClindaMax™ [US]** *see* clindamycin *on this page*

## clindamycin (klin da MYE sin)

**Sound-Alike/Look-Alike Issues**
Cleocin® may be confused with bleomycin, Clinoril®, Lincocin®
**Synonyms** clindamycin hydrochloride; clindamycin palmitate; clindamycin phosphate
**U.S./Canadian Brand Names** Alti-Clindamycin [Can]; Apo-Clindamycin® [Can]; Cleocin HCl® [US]; Cleocin Pediatric® [US]; Cleocin Phosphate® [US]; Cleocin T® [US]; Cleocin® [US]; Clindagel® [US]; ClindaMax™ [US]; Clindesse™ [US]; Clindets® [US]; Clindoxyl® [Can]; Dalacin® C [Can]; Dalacin® T [Can]; Dalacin® Vaginal [Can]; Evoclin™ [US]; Novo-Clindamycin [Can]
**Therapeutic Category** Acne Products; Antibiotic, Miscellaneous
**Use** Treatment against aerobic and anaerobic streptococci (except enterococci), most staphylococci, *Bacteroides* sp and *Actinomyces*; bacterial vaginosis (vaginal cream, vaginal suppository); pelvic inflammatory disease (I.V.); topically in treatment of severe acne; vaginally for *Gardnerella vaginalis*
**Usual Dosage**
Infants and Children:
 Oral: 8-20 mg/kg/day as hydrochloride; 8-25 mg/kg/day as palmitate in 3-4 divided doses; minimum dose of palmitate: 37.5 mg 3 times/day
 I.M., I.V.:
 <1 month: 15-20 mg/kg/day
 >1 month: 20-40 mg/kg/day in 3-4 divided doses
Children ≥12 years and Adults: Topical:
 Gel, pledget, lotion, solution: Apply a thin film twice daily
 Foam (Evoclin™): Apply once daily
Adults:
 Oral: 150-450 mg/dose every 6-8 hours; maximum dose: 1.8 g/day
 I.M., I.V.: 1.2-1.8 g/day in 2-4 divided doses; maximum dose: 4.8 g/day
 Pelvic inflammatory disease: I.V.: 900 mg every 8 hours with gentamicin 2 mg/kg, then 1.5 mg/kg every 8 hours; continue after discharge with doxycycline 100 mg twice daily to complete 14 days of total therapy
 Bacterial vaginosis: Intravaginal:
 Suppositories: Insert one ovule (100 mg clindamycin) daily into vagina at bedtime for 3 days
 Cream:
  Cleocin®: One full applicator inserted intravaginally once daily before bedtime for 3 or 7 consecutive days in nonpregnant patients or for 7 consecutive days in pregnant patients
  Clindesse™: One full applicator inserted intravaginally as a single dose at anytime during the day in nonpregnant patients
**Dosage Forms Note:** Strength is expressed as base
Capsule, as hydrochloride: 150 mg, 300 mg
 Cleocin HCl®: 75 mg [contains tartrazine], 150 mg [contains tartrazine], 300 mg
Cream, vaginal, as phosphate:
 Cleocin®: 2% (40 g) [contains benzyl alcohol and mineral oil; packaged with 7 disposable applicators]
 Clindesse™: 2% (5 g) [contains mineral oil; prefilled single disposable applicator]
Foam, topical, as phosphate (Evoclin™): 1% (50 g, 100 g) [contains ethanol 58%]
Gel, topical, as phosphate: 1% [10 mg/g] (30 g, 60 g)
 Cleocin T®: 1% [10 mg/g] (30 g, 60 g)
 Clindagel®: 1% [10 mg/g] (40 mL, 75 mL)
 ClindaMax™: 1% (30 g, 60 g)

Granules for oral solution, as palmitate (Cleocin Pediatric®): 75 mg/5 mL (100 mL) [cherry flavor]

Infusion, as phosphate [premixed in D$_5$W] (Cleocin Phosphate®): 300 mg (50 mL); 600 mg (50 mL); 900 mg (50 mL)

Injection, solution, as phosphate (Cleocin Phosphate®): 150 mg/mL (2 mL, 4 mL, 6 mL, 60 mL) [contains benzyl alcohol and disodium edetate 0.5 mg]

Lotion, as phosphate (Cleocin T®, ClindaMax™): 1% [10 mg/mL] (60 mL)

Pledgets, topical: 1% (60s) [contains alcohol]

Clindets®: 1% (69s) [contains isopropyl alcohol 52%]

Cleocin T®: 1% (60s) [contains isopropyl alcohol 50%]

Solution, topical, as phosphate (Cleocin T®): 1% [10 mg/mL] (30 mL, 60 mL) [contains isopropyl alcohol 50%]

Suppository (ovule), vaginal, as phosphate (Cleocin®): 100 mg (3s) [contains oleaginous base; single reusable applicator]

## clindamycin and benzoyl peroxide (klin da MYE sin & BEN zoe il peer OKS ide)

**Synonyms** benzoyl peroxide and clindamycin; clindamycin phosphate and benzoyl peroxide

**U.S./Canadian Brand Names** BenzaClin® [US/Can]; Duac™ [US]

**Therapeutic Category** Topical Skin Product; Topical Skin Product, Acne

**Use** Topical treatment of acne vulgaris

**Usual Dosage** Topical: Children ≥12 years and Adults: Apply to affected areas after skin has been cleansed and dried

BenzaClin®: Acne: Apply twice daily (morning and evening)

Duac™: Inflammatory acne: Apply once daily in the evening

**Dosage Forms** Gel, topical:

BenzaClin®: Clindamycin phosphate 1% and benzoyl peroxide 5% (25 g, 50 g)

Duac™: Clindamycin phosphate 1% and benzoyl peroxide 5% (45 g)

**clindamycin hydrochloride** *see* clindamycin *on previous page*

**clindamycin palmitate** *see* clindamycin *on previous page*

**clindamycin phosphate** *see* clindamycin *on previous page*

**clindamycin phosphate and benzoyl peroxide** *see* clindamycin and benzoyl peroxide *on this page*

**Clindesse™ [US]** *see* clindamycin *on previous page*

**Clindets® [US]** *see* clindamycin *on previous page*

**Clindex® *(Discontinued)*** *see* clidinium and chlordiazepoxide *on page 191*

**Clindoxyl® [Can]** *see* clindamycin *on previous page*

**Clinoril® [US]** *see* sulindac *on page 776*

## clioquinol (klye oh KWIN ole)

**Synonyms** iodochlorhydroxyquin

**Therapeutic Category** Antifungal Agent

**Use** Treatment of tinea pedis, tinea cruris, and skin infections caused by dermatophytic fungi (ringworm)

**Usual Dosage** Children and Adults: Topical: Apply 2-4 times/day; do not use for >7 days

**Dosage Forms**

Cream: 3% (30 g)

Ointment, topical: 3% (30 g)

## clioquinol (all products) *(Discontinued)*

## clioquinol and flumethasone *(Canada only)* (klye ok KWIN ole & floo METH a sone)

**Synonyms** flumethasone and clioquinol; iodochlorhydroxyquin and flumethasone

**U.S./Canadian Brand Names** Locacorten® Vioform® [Can]

**Therapeutic Category** Antibiotic, Topical; Corticosteroid, Topical

**Use** Treatment of corticosteroid-responsive dermatoses complicated by infection with bacterial and/or fungal agents

**Usual Dosage** Children >2 years and Adults:

Otic solution (drops): Instill 2-3 drops into affected ear(s) 2 times/day; generally limit duration to 10 days

Topical: Apply in a thin layer to affected area 2-3 times/day; generally limit duration to 7 days

(Continued)

# clioquinol and flumethasone *(Canada only)* *(Continued)*

**Dosage Forms**
Cream, topical: Clioquinol 3% and flumethasone pivalate 0.02% (15 g, 50 g)
Solution, otic: Clioquinol 1% and flumethasone pivalate 0.02% (10 mL)

# clobazam *(Canada only)* (KLOE ba zam)

**U.S./Canadian Brand Names** Alti-Clobazam [Can]; Apo-Clobazam® [Can]; Frisium® [Can]; Novo-Clobazam [Can]; PMS-Clobazam [Can]
**Therapeutic Category** Anticonvulsant; Antidepressant
**Use** Adjunctive treatment of epilepsy
**Usual Dosage** Oral:
Children:
<2 years: Initial 0.5-1 mg/kg/day
2-16 years: Initial: 5 mg/day; may be increased (no more frequently than every 5 days) to a maximum of 40 mg/day
Adults: Initial: 5-15 mg/day; dosage may be gradually adjusted (based on tolerance and seizure control) to a maximum of 80 mg/day
**Note:** Daily doses of up to 30 mg may be taken as a single dose at bedtime; higher doses should be divided.
**Dosage Forms** Tablet: 10 mg

# clobetasol (kloe BAY ta sol)

**Synonyms** clobetasol propionate
**U.S./Canadian Brand Names** Clobevate® [US]; Clobex® [US/Can]; Cormax® [US]; Dermovate® [Can]; Embeline™ E [US]; Embeline™ [US]; Gen-Clobetasol [Can]; Novo-Clobetasol [Can]; Olux® [US]; Temovate E® [US]; Temovate® [US]
**Therapeutic Category** Corticosteroid, Topical
**Use** Short-term relief of inflammation of moderate to severe corticosteroid-responsive dermatoses (very high potency topical corticosteroid)
**Usual Dosage** Topical: Discontinue when control achieved; if improvement not seen within 2 weeks, reassessment of diagnosis may be necessary.
Children <12 years: Use is not recommended
Children ≥12 years and Adults:
Oral mucosal inflammation (dental use): Apply twice daily for up to 2 weeks (maximum dose: 50 g/week); discontinue application when control is achieved; if no improvement is seen, reassessment of diagnosis may be necessary
Steroid-responsive dermatoses:
Cream, emollient cream, gel, lotion, ointment: Apply twice daily for up to 2 weeks (maximum dose: 50 g/week)
Foam, solution: Apply to affected scalp twice daily for up to 2 weeks (maximum dose: 50 g/week or 50 mL/week)
Mild to moderate plaque-type psoriasis of nonscalp areas: Foam: Apply to affected area twice daily for up to 2 weeks (maximum dose: 50 g/week); do not apply to face or intertriginous areas
Children ≥16 years and Adults: Moderate to severe plaque-type psoriasis: Emollient cream, lotion: Apply twice daily for up to 2 weeks, has been used for up to 4 weeks when application is <10% of body surface area; use with caution (maximum dose: 50 g/week)
**Dosage Forms** [DSC] = Discontinued product
Cream, as propionate: 0.05% (15 g, 30 g, 45 g, 60 g)
Cormax®: 0.05% (15 g [DSC], 30 g, 45 g [DSC])
Embeline™, Temovate®: 0.05% (15 g, 30 g, 45 g, 60 g)
Cream, as propionate [in emollient base]: 0.05% (15 g, 30 g, 60 g)
Embeline™ E, Temovate E®: 0.05% (15 g, 30 g, 60 g)
Foam, topical, as propionate [for scalp application] (Olux®): 0.05% (50 g, 100 g) [contains ethanol 60%]
Gel, as propionate (Clobevate®, Embeline™; Temovate®): 0.05% (15 g, 30 g, 60 g)
Lotion, as propionate (Clobex®): 0.05% (30 mL, 59 mL)
Ointment, as propionate: 0.05% (15 g, 30 g, 45 g, 60 g)
Cormax®: 0.05% (15 g, 45 g)
Embeline™, Temovate®: 0.05% (15 g, 30 g, 45 g, 60 g)
Solution, topical, as propionate [for scalp application] (Cormax®, Embeline™, Temovate®): 0.05% (25 mL, 50 mL) [contains isopropyl alcohol 40%]

**clobetasol propionate** *see* clobetasol *on previous page*

**Clobevate® [US]** *see* clobetasol *on previous page*

**Clobex® [US/Can]** *see* clobetasol *on previous page*

## clocortolone (kloe KOR toe lone)
**Sound-Alike/Look-Alike Issues**
Cloderm® may be confused with Clocort®
**Synonyms** clocortolone pivalate
**U.S./Canadian Brand Names** Cloderm® [US/Can]
**Therapeutic Category** Corticosteroid, Topical
**Use** Inflammation of corticosteroid-responsive dermatoses (intermediate-potency topical corticosteroid)
**Usual Dosage** Adults: Apply sparingly and gently; rub into affected area from 1-4 times/day. Therapy should be discontinued when control is achieved; if no improvement is seen, reassessment of diagnosis may be necessary.
**Dosage Forms** Cream, as pivalate: 0.1% (15 g, 45 g, 90 g)

**clocortolone pivalate** *see* clocortolone *on this page*

**Clocream® [US-OTC]** *see* vitamin A and vitamin D *on page 849*

**Cloderm® [US/Can]** *see* clocortolone *on this page*

**clodronate disodium** *see* clodronate disodium *(Canada only) on this page*

## clodronate disodium *(Canada only)* (KLOE droh nate)
**Synonyms** clodronate disodium
**U.S./Canadian Brand Names** Bonefos® [Can]; Ostac® [Can]
**Therapeutic Category** Bisphosphonate Derivative
**Use** Management of hypercalcemia of malignancy
**Usual Dosage**
I.V.:
Multiple infusions: 300 mg/day; should not be prolonged beyond 10 days.
Single infusion: 1500 mg as a single dose
Oral: Recommended daily maintenance dose following I.V. therapy: Range: 1600 mg (4 capsules) to 2400 mg (6 capsules) given in single or 2 divided doses; maximum recommended daily dose: 3200 mg (8 capsules). Should be taken at least 1 hour before or after food, because food may decrease the amount of clodronate absorbed by the body.
**Dosage Forms**
Injection, as disodium: 30 mg/mL (10 mL); 60 mg/mL (5 mL)
Capsule, as disodium: 400 mg

## clofarabine (klo FARE a been)
**Synonyms** Clofarex; NSC606869
**U.S./Canadian Brand Names** Clolar™ [US]
**Therapeutic Category** Antineoplastic Agent, Antimetabolite (Purine Antagonist)
**Use** Treatment of relapsed or refractory acute lymphoblastic leukemia
**Usual Dosage** I.V.: Children 1-21 years: ALL: 52 mg/m² over 2 hours once daily for 5 consecutive days; repeat every 2-6 weeks following recovery or return to baseline organ function
**Dosage Forms** Injection, solution [preservative free]: 1 mg/mL (20 mL)

**Clofarex** *see* clofarabine *on this page*

## clofazimine (kloe FA zi meen)
**Sound-Alike/Look-Alike Issues**
clofazimine may be confused with clonazepam, clozapine
**Synonyms** clofazimine palmitate
**U.S./Canadian Brand Names** Lamprene® [Can]
**Therapeutic Category** Leprostatic Agent
**Use** Treatment of lepromatous leprosy including dapsone-resistant leprosy and lepromatous leprosy with erythema nodosum leprosum; multibacillary leprosy
**Usual Dosage** Oral:
Children: Leprosy: 1 mg/kg/day every 24 hours in combination with dapsone and rifampin
(Continued)

## clofazimine (Continued)

Adults:

Dapsone-resistant leprosy: 100 mg/day in combination with one or more antileprosy drugs for 3 years; then alone 100 mg/day

Dapsone-sensitive multibacillary leprosy: 100 mg/day in combination with two or more antileprosy drugs for at least 2 years and continue until negative skin smears are obtained, then institute single drug therapy with appropriate agent

Erythema nodosum leprosum: 100-200 mg/day for up to 3 months or longer then taper dose to 100 mg/day when possible

**Dosage Forms** [DSC] = Discontinued product

Capsule: 50 mg [DSC]

**clofazimine palmitate** *see* clofazimine *on previous page*

**Clolar™ [US]** *see* clofarabine *on previous page*

**Clomid® [US/Can]** *see* clomiphene *on this page*

## clomiphene (KLOE mi feen)

**Sound-Alike/Look-Alike Issues**

clomiPHENE may be confused with clomiPRAMINE, clonidine

Clomid® may be confused with clonidine

Serophene® may be confused with Sarafem™

**Synonyms** clomiphene citrate

**Tall-Man** clomiPHENE

**U.S./Canadian Brand Names** Clomid® [US/Can]; Milophene® [Can]; Serophene® [US/Can]

**Therapeutic Category** Ovulation Stimulator

**Use** Treatment of ovulatory failure in patients desiring pregnancy

**Usual Dosage** Adults: Oral:

Male (infertility): 25 mg/day for 25 days with 5 days rest, or 100 mg every Monday, Wednesday, Friday

Female (ovulatory failure): 50 mg/day for 5 days (first course); start the regimen on or about the fifth day of cycle. The dose should be increased only in those patients who do not ovulate in response to cyclic 50 mg Clomid®. A low dosage or duration of treatment course is particularly recommended if unusual sensitivity to pituitary gonadotropin is suspected, such as in patients with polycystic ovary syndrome.

If ovulation does not appear to occur after the first course of therapy, a second course of 100 mg/day (two 50 mg tablets given as a single daily dose) for 5 days should be given. This course may be started as early as 30 days after the previous one after precautions are taken to exclude the presence of pregnancy. Increasing the dosage or duration of therapy beyond 100 mg/day for 5 days is not recommended. The majority of patients who are going to ovulate will do so after the first course of therapy. If ovulation does not occur after 3 courses of therapy, further treatment is not recommended and the patient should be reevaluated. If 3 ovulatory responses occur, but pregnancy has not been achieved, further treatment is not recommended. If menses does not occur after an ovulatory response, the patient should be reevaluated. Long-term cyclic therapy is not recommended beyond a total of about 6 cycles.

**Dosage Forms** Tablet, as citrate: 50 mg

**clomiphene citrate** *see* clomiphene *on this page*

## clomipramine (kloe MI pra meen)

**Sound-Alike/Look-Alike Issues**

clomiPRAMINE may be confused with chlorproMAZINE, clomiPHENE, desipramine, Norpramin®

Anafranil® may be confused with alfentanil, enalapril, nafarelin

**Synonyms** clomipramine hydrochloride

**Tall-Man** clomiPRAMINE

**U.S./Canadian Brand Names** Anafranil® [US/Can]; Apo-Clomipramine® [Can]; CO Clomipramine [Can]; Gen-Clomipramine [Can]

**Therapeutic Category** Antidepressant, Tricyclic (Tertiary Amine)

**Use** Treatment of obsessive-compulsive disorder (OCD)

**Usual Dosage** Oral: Initial:

Children:

<10 years: Safety and efficacy have not been established.

≥10 years: OCD: 25 mg/day; gradually increase, as tolerated, to a maximum of 3 mg/kg/day or 200 mg/day (whichever is smaller)

Adults: OCD: 25 mg/day and gradually increase, as tolerated, to 100 mg/day the first 2 weeks, may then be increased to a total of 250 mg/day maximum

**Dosage Forms** Capsule, as hydrochloride: 25 mg, 50 mg, 75 mg

## clomipramine hydrochloride *see* clomipramine *on previous page*

## Clonapam [Can] *see* clonazepam *on this page*

# clonazepam (kloe NA ze pam)

**Sound-Alike/Look-Alike Issues**

clonazepam may be confused with clofazimine, clonidine, clorazepate, Klonopin®, lorazepam

Klonopin® may be confused with clonazepam, clonidine

**U.S./Canadian Brand Names** Alti-Clonazepam [Can]; Apo-Clonazepam® [Can]; Clonapam [Can]; Gen-Clonazepam [Can]; Klonopin® [US/Can]; Novo-Clonazepam [Can]; Nu-Clonazepam [Can]; PMS-Clonazepam [Can]; Rho-Clonazepam [Can]; Rivotril® [Can]

**Therapeutic Category** Benzodiazepine

**Controlled Substance** C-IV

**Use** Alone or as an adjunct in the treatment of petit mal variant (Lennox-Gastaut), akinetic, and myoclonic seizures; petit mal (absence) seizures unresponsive to succimides; panic disorder with or without agoraphobla

**Usual Dosage** Oral:

Children <10 years or 30 kg: Seizure disorders:

Initial daily dose: 0.01-0.03 mg/kg/day (maximum: 0.05 mg/kg/day) given in 2-3 divided doses; increase by no more than 0.5 mg every third day until seizures are controlled or adverse effects seen

Usual maintenance dose: 0.1-0.2 mg/kg/day divided 3 times/day, not to exceed 0.2 mg/kg/day

Adults:

Burning mouth syndrome (dental use): 0.25-3 mg/day in 2 divided doses, in morning and evening

Seizure disorders:

Initial daily dose not to exceed 1.5 mg given in 3 divided doses; may increase by 0.5-1 mg every third day until seizures are controlled or adverse effects seen (maximum: 20 mg/day)

Usual maintenance dose: 0.05-0.2 mg/kg; do not exceed 20 mg/day

Panic disorder: 0.25 mg twice daily; increase in increments of 0.125-0.25 mg twice daily every 3 days; target dose: 1 mg/day (maximum: 4 mg/day)

Discontinuation of treatment: To discontinue, treatment should be withdrawn gradually. Decrease dose by 0.125 mg twice daily every 3 days until medication is completely withdrawn.

**Dosage Forms**

Tablet: 0.5 mg, 1 mg, 2 mg

Tablet, orally-disintegrating [wafer]: 0.125 mg, 0.25 mg, 0.5 mg, 1 mg, 2 mg

# clonidine (KLON i deen)

**Sound-Alike/Look-Alike Issues**

clonidine may be confused with Clomid®, clomiPHENE, clonazepam, clozapine, Klonopin™, Loniten®, quinidine

Catapres® may be confused with Cataflam®, Cetapred®, Combipres®

**Synonyms** clonidine hydrochloride

**U.S./Canadian Brand Names** Apo-Clonidine® [Can]; Carapres® [Can]; Catapres-TTS® [US]; Catapres® [US]; Dixarit® [Can]; Duraclon™ [US]; Novo-Clonidine [Can]; Nu-Clonidine [Can]

**Therapeutic Category** Alpha-Adrenergic Agonist

**Use** Management of mild to moderate hypertension; either used alone or in combination with other antihypertensives

**Orphan drug:** Duraclon™: For continuous epidural administration as adjunctive therapy with intraspinal opiates for treatment of cancer pain in patients tolerant to or unresponsive to intraspinal opiates

**Usual Dosage**

Children:

Oral:

Hypertension: Initial: 5-10 mcg/kg/day in divided doses every 8-12 hours; increase gradually at 5- to 7-day intervals to 25 mcg/kg/day in divided doses every 6 hours; maximum: 0.9 mg/day

Clonidine tolerance test (test of growth hormone release from pituitary): 0.15 mg/m2 or 4 mcg/kg as single dose

Epidural infusion: Pain management: Reserved for patients with severe intractable pain, unresponsive to other analgesics or epidural or spinal opiates: Initial: 0.5 mcg/kg/hour; adjust with caution, based on clinical effect

(Continued)

# clonidine *(Continued)*

Adults:
Oral:
Acute hypertension (urgency): Initial 0.1-0.2 mg; may be followed by additional doses of 0.1 mg every hour, if necessary, to a maximum total dose of 0.6 mg.
Hypertension: Initial dose: 0.1 mg twice daily (maximum recommended dose: 2.4 mg/day); usual dose range (JNC 7): 0.1-0.8 mg/day in 2 divided doses
Nicotine withdrawal symptoms: 0.1 mg twice daily to maximum of 0.4 mg/day for 3-4 weeks
Transdermal: Hypertension: Apply once every 7 days; for initial therapy start with 0.1 mg and increase by 0.1 mg at 1- to 2-week intervals (dosages >0.6 mg do not improve efficacy); usual dose range (JNC 7): 0.1-0.3 mg once weekly
Epidural infusion: Pain management: Starting dose: 30 mcg/hour; titrate as required for relief of pain or presence of side effects; minimal experience with doses >40 mcg/hour; should be considered an adjunct to intraspinal opiate therapy

**Dosage Forms**
Injection, epidural solution, as hydrochloride [preservative free] (Duraclon™): 100 mcg/mL (10 mL); 500 mcg/mL (10 mL)
Patch, transdermal [once-weekly patch]:
Catapres-TTS®-1: 0.1 mg/24 hours (4s)
Catapres-TTS®-2: 0.2 mg/24 hours (4s)
Catapres-TTS®-3: 0.3 mg/24 hours (4s)
Tablet, as hydrochloride (Catapres®): 0.1 mg, 0.2 mg, 0.3 mg

# clonidine and chlorthalidone (KLON i deen & klor THAL i done)

**Sound-Alike/Look-Alike Issues**
Combipres® may be confused with Catapres®
**Synonyms** chlorthalidone and clonidine
**U.S./Canadian Brand Names** Clorpres® [US]
**Therapeutic Category** Antihypertensive Agent, Combination
**Use** Management of mild to moderate hypertension
**Usual Dosage** Oral: 1 tablet 1-2 times/day; maximum: 0.6 mg clonidine and 30 mg chlorthalidone
**Dosage Forms** Tablet:
0.1: Clonidine hydrochloride 0.1 mg and chlorthalidone 15 mg
0.2: Clonidine hydrochloride 0.2 mg and chlorthalidone 15 mg
0.3: Clonidine hydrochloride 0.3 mg and chlorthalidone 15 mg

**clonidine hydrochloride** *see* clonidine *on previous page*

# clopidogrel (kloh PID oh grel)

**Sound-Alike/Look-Alike Issues**
Plavix® may be confused with Elavil®, Paxil®
**Synonyms** clopidogrel bisulfate
**U.S./Canadian Brand Names** Plavix® [US/Can]
**Therapeutic Category** Antiplatelet Agent
**Use** Reduce atherosclerotic events (myocardial infarction, stroke, vascular deaths) in patients with atherosclerosis documented by recent myocardial infarction (MI), recent stroke, or established peripheral arterial disease; acute coronary syndrome (unstable angina or non-Q-wave MI) managed medically or through PCI (with or without stent)
**Usual Dosage** Oral: Adults:
Recent MI, recent stroke, or established arterial disease: 75 mg once daily
Acute coronary syndrome: Initial: 300 mg loading dose, followed by 75 mg once daily (in combination with aspirin 75-325 mg once daily). **Note:** A loading dose of 600 mg has been used in some investigations; limited research exists comparing the two doses.
**Dosage Forms** Tablet [film coated]: 75 mg

**clopidogrel bisulfate** *see* clopidogrel *on this page*

**Clopixol® [Can]** *see* zuclopenthixol *(Canada only) on page 864*

**Clopixol-Acuphase® [Can]** *see* zuclopenthixol *(Canada only) on page 864*

**Clopixol® Depot [Can]** *see* zuclopenthixol *(Canada only) on page 864*

**Clopra®** *(Discontinued)*

## clorazepate (klor AZ e pate)

**Sound-Alike/Look-Alike Issues**
clorazepate may be confused with clofibrate, clonazepam
**Synonyms** clorazepate dipotassium; Tranxene T-Tab®
**U.S./Canadian Brand Names** Apo-Clorazepate® [Can]; Novo-Clopate [Can]; T-Tab® [US]; Tranxene® SD™ [US]; Tranxene® SD™-Half Strength [US]; Tranxene® [US]
**Therapeutic Category** Anticonvulsant; Benzodiazepine
**Controlled Substance** C-IV
**Use** Treatment of generalized anxiety disorder; management of ethanol withdrawal; adjunct anticonvulsant in management of partial seizures
**Usual Dosage** Oral:
Children 9-12 years: Anticonvulsant: Initial: 3.75-7.5 mg/dose twice daily; increase dose by 3.75 mg at weekly intervals, not to exceed 60 mg/day in 2-3 divided doses
Children >12 years and Adults: Anticonvulsant: Initial: Up to 7.5 mg/dose 2-3 times/day; increase dose by 7.5 mg at weekly intervals, not to exceed 90 mg/day
Adults:
Anxiety:
Regular release tablets (Tranxene® T-Tab®): 7.5-15 mg 2-4 times/day
Sustained release (Tranxene® SD): 11.25 or 22.5 mg once daily at bedtime
Ethanol withdrawal: Initial: 30 mg, then 15 mg 2-4 times/day on first day; maximum daily dose: 90 mg; gradually decrease dose over subsequent days
**Dosage Forms**
Tablet, as dipotassium: 3.75 mg, 7.5 mg, 15 mg
Tranxene® SD™: 22.5 mg [once daily]
Tranxene® SD™-Half Strength: 11.25 mg [once daily]
Tranxene® T-Tab®: 3.75 mg, 7.5 mg, 15 mg

**clorazepate dipotassium** see clorazepate on this page

**Clorpactin® WCS-90 [US-OTC]** see oxychlorosene on page 608

**Clorpres® [US]** see clonidine and chlorthalidone on previous page

**Clotrimaderm [Can]** see clotrimazole on this page

## clotrimazole (kloe TRIM a zole)

**Sound-Alike/Look-Alike Issues**
clotrimazole may be confused with co-trimoxazole
Lotrimin® may be confused with Lotrisone®, Otrivin®
Mycelex® may be confused with Myoflex®
**U.S./Canadian Brand Names** Canesten® Topical [Can]; Canesten® Vaginal [Can]; Clotrimaderm [Can]; Cruex® Cream [US-OTC]; Gyne-Lotrimin® 3 [US-OTC]; Lotrimin® AF Athlete's Foot Cream [US-OTC]; Lotrimin® AF Athlete's Foot Solution [US-OTC]; Lotrimin® AF Jock Itch Cream [US-OTC]; Mycelex® Twin Pack [US-OTC]; Mycelex® [US]; Mycelex®-7 [US-OTC]; Trivagizole-3® [Can]
**Therapeutic Category** Antifungal Agent
**Use** Treatment of susceptible fungal infections, including oropharyngeal candidiasis, dermatophytoses, superficial mycoses, and cutaneous candidiasis, as well as vulvovaginal candidiasis; limited data suggest that clotrimazole troches may be effective for prophylaxis against oropharyngeal candidiasis in neutropenic patients
**Usual Dosage**
Children >3 years and Adults:
Oral:
Prophylaxis: 10 mg troche dissolved 3 times/day for the duration of chemotherapy or until steroids are reduced to maintenance levels
Treatment: 10 mg troche dissolved slowly 5 times/day for 14 consecutive days
Topical (cream, solution): Apply twice daily; if no improvement occurs after 4 weeks of therapy, re-evaluate diagnosis
Children >12 years and Adults:
Vaginal:
Cream:
1%: Insert 1 applicatorful vaginal cream daily (preferably at bedtime) for 7 consecutive days
2%: Insert 1 applicatorful vaginal cream daily (preferably at bedtime) for 3 consecutive days
Tablet: Insert 100 mg/day for 7 days or 500 mg single dose
(Continued)

## clotrimazole *(Continued)*

Topical (cream, solution): Apply to affected area twice daily (morning and evening) for 7 consecutive days

**Dosage Forms**
Combination pack (Mycelex®-7): Vaginal tablet 100 mg (7s) and vaginal cream 1% (7 g)
Cream, topical: 1% (15 g, 30 g, 45 g)
  Cruex®: 1% (15 g)
  Lotrimin® AF Athlete's Foot: 1% (12 g, 24 g)
  Lotrimin® AF Jock Itch: 1% (12 g)
Cream, vaginal: 2% (21 g)
  Mycelex®-7: 1% (45 g)
Solution, topical: 1% (10 mL, 30 mL)
  Lotrimin® AF Athlete's Foot: 1% (10 mL)
Tablet, vaginal (Gyne-Lotrimin® 3): 200 mg (3s)
Troche (Mycelex®): 10 mg

**clotrimazole and betamethasone** *see* betamethasone and clotrimazole *on page 102*

## cloxacillin (kloks a SIL in)

**Synonyms** cloxacillin sodium
**U.S./Canadian Brand Names** Apo-Cloxi® [Can]; Novo-Cloxin [Can]; Nu-Cloxi [Can]; Riva-Cloxacillin [Can]
**Therapeutic Category** Penicillin
**Use** Treatment of susceptible bacterial infections, notably penicillinase-producing staphylococci causing respiratory tract, skin and skin structure, bone and joint, urinary tract infections
**Usual Dosage** Oral:
Children >1 month (<20 kg): 50-100 mg/kg/day in divided doses every 6 hours; up to a maximum of 4 g/day
Children (>20 kg) and Adults: 250-500 mg every 6 hours
**Dosage Forms**
Capsule, as sodium: 250 mg, 500 mg
Powder for oral suspension, as sodium: 125 mg/5 mL (100 mL, 200 mL)

**cloxacillin sodium** *see* cloxacillin *on this page*

**Cloxapen® *(Discontinued)*** *see* cloxacillin *on this page*

## clozapine (KLOE za peen)

**Sound-Alike/Look-Alike Issues**
clozapine may be confused with clofazimine, clonidine
Clozaril® may be confused with Clinoril®, Colazal®
**U.S./Canadian Brand Names** Apo-Clozapine® [Can]; Clozaril® [US/Can]; FazaClo® [US]; Gen-Clozapine [Can]
**Therapeutic Category** Antipsychotic Agent, Dibenzodiazepine
**Use** Treatment-refractory schizophrenia; to reduce risk of recurrent suicidal behavior in schizophrenia or schizoaffective disorder
**Usual Dosage** Oral: Adults:
Schizophrenia: Initial: 12.5 mg once or twice daily; increased, as tolerated, in increments of 25-50 mg/day to a target dose of 300-450 mg/day after 2-4 weeks, may require doses as high as 600-900 mg/day
Reduce risk of suicidal behavior: Initial: 12.5 mg once or twice daily; increased, as tolerated, in increments of 25-50 mg/day to a target dose of 300-450 mg/day after 2-4 weeks; median dose is ~300 mg/day (range: 12.5-900 mg)

**Termination of therapy**: If dosing is interrupted for ≥48 hours, therapy must be reinitiated at 12.5-25 mg/day; may be increased more rapidly than with initial titration, unless cardiopulmonary arrest occurred during initial titration.
In the event of planned termination of clozapine, gradual reduction in dose over a 1- to 2-week period is recommended. If conditions warrant abrupt discontinuation (leukopenia), monitor patient for psychosis and cholinergic rebound (headache, nausea, vomiting, diarrhea).
Patients discontinued on clozapine therapy due to WBC <2000/mm$^3$ or ANC <1000/mm$^3$ should not be restarted on clozapine.
**Dosage Forms**
Tablet: 12.5 mg, 25 mg, 100 mg

Clozaril®: 25 mg, 100 mg
Tablet, orally-disintegrating (FazaClo®): 25 mg [contains phenylalanine 1.75 mg; mint flavor], 100 mg [contains phenylalanine 6.96 mg; mint flavor]

**Clozaril® [US/Can]** see clozapine on previous page

**Clysodrast® (Discontinued)** see bisacodyl on page 107

**CMV-IGIV** see cytomegalovirus immune globulin (intravenous-human) on page 219

**CoActifed® [Can]** see triprolidine, pseudoephedrine, and codeine (Canada only) on page 827

**coagulant complex inhibitor** see anti-inhibitor coagulant complex on page 58

**coagulation factor VIIa** see factor VIIa (recombinant) on page 325

## coal tar (KOLE tar)

### Sound-Alike/Look-Alike Issues
Pentrax® may be confused with Permax®
Tegrin® may be confused with Tegretol®

**Synonyms** crude coal tar; LCD; pix carbonis

**U.S./Canadian Brand Names** Balnetar® [US-OTC/Can]; Betatar® [US-OTC]; Cutar® [US-OTC]; DHS™ Tar [US-OTC]; DHS™ Targel [US-OTC]; Doak® Tar [US-OTC]; Estar® [US-OTC/Can]; Exorex® [US]; Ionil T® Plus [US-OTC]; Ionil T® [US-OTC]; MG 217® Medicated Tar [US-OTC]; MG 217® [US-OTC]; Neutrogena® T/Gel Extra Strength [US-OTC]; Neutrogena® T/Gel [US-OTC]; Oxipor® VHC [US-OTC]; Pentrax® [US-OTC]; Polytar® [US-OTC]; PsoriGel® [US-OTC]; Reme-t™ [US-OTC]; Targel® [Can]; Tegrin® [US-OTC]; Zetar® [US-OTC]

**Therapeutic Category** Antipsoriatic Agent; Antiseborrheic Agent, Topical

**Use** Topically for controlling dandruff, seborrheic dermatitis, or psoriasis

**Usual Dosage** Topical:
Bath: Add appropriate amount to bath water; soak 5-20 minutes, then pat dry; use once daily to 3 days
Shampoo: Rub shampoo onto wet hair and scalp, rinse thoroughly; repeat; leave on 5 minutes; rinse thoroughly; apply twice weekly for the first 2 weeks then once weekly or more often if needed
Soap: Use on affected areas in place of regular soap. Work into a lather using warm water; massage into skin; rinse.
Skin: Apply to the affected area 1-4 times/day; decrease frequency to 2-3 times/week once condition has been controlled
Scalp psoriasis: Tar oil bath or coal tar solution may be painted sparingly to the lesions 3-12 hours before each shampoo
Psoriasis of the body, arms, legs: Apply at bedtime; if thick scales are present, use product with salicylic acid and apply several times during the day

**Dosage Forms**
Emulsion, topical (Cutar®): Coal tar solution 7.5% (180 mL, 3840 mL)
Gel, shampoo:
Betatar®: Coal tar solution 5% (240 mL) [green apple scent]
DHS™ Targel: Coal tar solution 2.9% (240 mL) [equivalent to 0.5% coal tar]
Gel, topical:
Estar®: Coal tar 5% (90 g)
PsoriGel®: Coal tar solution 7.5% (120 g)
Lotion, topical:
Doak® Tar: Coal tar distillate 5% (240 mL) [equivalent to coal tar 2%]
Exorex®: Coal tar 1% (240 mL)
MG 217®: Coal tar solution 5% (120 mL) [equivalent to 1% coal tar; contains jojoba]
Oxipor® VHC: Coal tar solution 25% (60 mL, 120 mL)
Oil, topical:
Balnetar®: Water-dispersible emollient tar 2.5%, lanolin fraction, and mineral oil (225 mL) [for use in bath]
Doak® Tar: Coal tar distillate 2% (240 mL) [equivalent to coal tar 0.8%; for use in bath]
Ointment, topical (MG 217®): Coal tar solution 10% (107 g, 430 g) [equivalent to 2% coal tar]
Shampoo:
DHS™ Tar: Coal tar solution 2.9% (120 mL, 240 mL, 480 mL) [equivalent to 0.5% coal tar]
Doak® Tar: Coal tar distillate 3% (240 mL) [equivalent to coal tar 1.2%]
Ionil T®: Coal tar 1% (240 mL, 480 mL, 960 mL)
Ionil T® Plus: Coal tar 2% (240 mL) [with conditioner]
MG 217® Medicated Tar: Coal tar solution 15% (120 mL, 240 mL, 480 mL) [equivalent to 3% coal tar]
(Continued)

## coal tar *(Continued)*

Neutrogena® T/Gel: Coal tar extract 2% (132 mL, 480 mL) [coal tar 0.5%]
Neutrogena® T/Gel Extra Strength: Coal tar extract 4% (132 mL) [coal tar 1%]
Pentrax®: Coal tar 5% (240 mL)
Polytar®: Coal tar 0.5% (177 mL, 355 mL)
Reme-t™: Coal tar distillate 5% (236 mL)
Tegrin®: Coal tar solution 7% (210 mL) [equivalent to 1% coal tar; available with or without conditioner]
Zetar®: Coal tar 1% (180 mL)
Soap (Polytar®): Coal tar 0.5% (113 g)

## coal tar and salicylic acid (KOLE tar & sal i SIL ik AS id)

**Synonyms** salicylic acid and coal tar
**U.S./Canadian Brand Names** Sebcur/T® [Can]; Tarsum® [US-OTC]; X-Seb T® Pearl [US-OTC]; X-Seb T® Plus [US-OTC]
**Therapeutic Category** Antipsoriatic Agent; Antiseborrheic Agent, Topical
**Use** Seborrheal dermatitis, dandruff, psoriasis
**Usual Dosage** Psoriasis: Scalp:
Gel: Apply directly to plaques; may leave in place for up to 1 hour. Apply water and work into a lather; rinse.
Shampoo: Apply to wet hair; massage into scalp; rinse.
**Dosage Forms**
Gel [shampoo] (Tarsum®): Coal tar solution 10% [equivalent to coal tar 2%] and salicylic acid (120 mL, 240 mL)
Shampoo, topical:
X-Seb T® Pearl: Coal tar solution 10% [equivalent to coal tar 2%] and salicylic acid (120 mL, 240 mL)
X-Seb T® Plus: Coal tar solution 10% [equivalent to coal tar 2%] and salicylic acid (120 mL, 240 mL) [conditioning shampoo]

## coal tar, lanolin, and mineral oil (KOLE tar, LAN oh lin, & MIN er al oyl)

**Synonyms** coal tar, mineral oil, and lanolin; lanolin, coal tar, and mineral oil; lanolin, mineral oil, and coal tar; mineral oil, coal tar, and lanolin; mineral oil, lanolin, and coal tar
**U.S./Canadian Brand Names** Balnetar® [Can]
**Therapeutic Category** Antipsoriatic Agent; Antiseborrheic Agent, Topical
**Use** Treatment of psoriasis, seborrheal dermatitis, atopic dermatitis, eczematoid dermatitis
**Usual Dosage** Add to bath water, soak for 5-20 minutes then pat dry
**Dosage Forms** Oil, bath: Water-dispersible emollient tar 2.5%, lanolin fraction, and mineral oil (225 mL)

**coal tar, mineral oil, and lanolin** *see* coal tar, lanolin, and mineral oil *on this page*

**Cobex® *(Discontinued)*** *see* cyanocobalamin *on page 212*

## cocaine (koe KANE)

**Synonyms** cocaine hydrochloride
**Therapeutic Category** Local Anesthetic
**Controlled Substance** C-II
**Use** Topical anesthesia for mucous membranes
**Usual Dosage** Topical application (ear, nose, throat, bronchoscopy): Dosage depends on the area to be anesthetized, tissue vascularity, technique of anesthesia, and individual patient tolerance; the lowest dose necessary to produce adequate anesthesia should be used; concentrations of 1% to 10% are used (not to exceed 1 mg/kg). Use reduced dosages for children, elderly, or debilitated patients.
**Dosage Forms**
Powder, as hydrochloride: 1 g, 5 g, 25 g
Solution, topical, as hydrochloride: 4% [40 mg/mL] (4 mL, 10 mL); 10% [100 mg/mL] (4 mL, 10 mL)

**cocaine hydrochloride** *see* cocaine *on this page*

**CO Ciprofloxacin [Can]** *see* ciprofloxacin *on page 184*

**CO Citalopram [Can]** *see* citalopram *on page 188*

**CO Clomipramine [Can]** *see* clomipramine *on page 196*

**Codal-DM [US-OTC]** *see* phenylephrine, pyrilamine, and dextromethorphan *on page 644*

**Codamine® *(Discontinued)***

**Codamine® Pediatric** *(Discontinued)*

**Codehist® DH** *(Discontinued)* *see* chlorpheniramine, pseudoephedrine, and codeine *on page 176*

# codeine (KOE deen)

**Sound-Alike/Look-Alike Issues**
codeine may be confused with Cardene®, Cophene®, Cordran®, iodine, Lodine®

**Synonyms** codeine phosphate; codeine sulfate; methylmorphine

**U.S./Canadian Brand Names** Codeine Contin® [Can]

**Therapeutic Category** Analgesic, Narcotic; Antitussive

**Controlled Substance** C-II

**Use** Treatment of mild to moderate pain; antitussive in lower doses; dextromethorphan has equivalent antitussive activity but has much lower toxicity in accidental overdose

**Usual Dosage Note:** These are guidelines and do not represent the maximum doses that may be required in all patients. Doses should be titrated to pain relief/prevention. Doses >1.5 mg/kg body weight are not recommended.

Analgesic:

Children: Oral, I.M., SubQ: 0.5-1 mg/kg/dose every 4-6 hours as needed; maximum: 60 mg/dose

Adults:

Oral: 30 mg every 4-6 hours as needed; patients with prior opiate exposure may require higher initial doses. Usual range: 15-120 mg every 4-6 hours as needed

Oral, controlled release formulation (Codeine Contin®, not available in U.S.): 50-300 mg every 12 hours. **Note:** A patient's codeine requirement should be established using prompt release formulations; conversion to long acting products may be considered when chronic, continuous treatment is required. Higher dosages should be reserved for use only in opioid-tolerant patients.

I.M., SubQ: 30 mg every 4-6 hours as needed; patients with prior opiate exposure may require higher initial doses. Usual range: 15-120 mg every 4-6 hours as needed; more frequent dosing may be needed

Antitussive: Oral (for nonproductive cough):

Children: 1-1.5 mg/kg/day in divided doses every 4-6 hours as needed: Alternative dose according to age:

2-6 years: 2.5-5 mg every 4-6 hours as needed; maximum: 30 mg/day

6-12 years: 5-10 mg every 4-6 hours as needed; maximum: 60 mg/day

Adults: 10-20 mg/dose every 4-6 hours as needed; maximum: 120 mg/day

**Dosage Forms**

Injection, as phosphate: 15 mg/mL (2 mL); 30 mg/mL (2 mL) [contains sodium metabisulfite]

Solution, oral, as phosphate: 15 mg/5 mL (5 mL, 500 mL) [strawberry flavor]

Tablet, controlled release (Codeine Contin®) [not available in U.S.]: 50 mg, 100 mg, 150 mg, 200 mg

Tablet, as phosphate: 30 mg, 60 mg

Tablet, as sulfate: 15 mg, 30 mg, 60 mg

**codeine and acetaminophen** *see* acetaminophen and codeine *on page 6*

**codeine and aspirin** *see* aspirin and codeine *on page 74*

**codeine and butalbital compound** *see* butalbital, aspirin, caffeine, and codeine *on page 125*

**codeine and guaifenesin** *see* guaifenesin and codeine *on page 384*

**codeine and promethazine** *see* promethazine and codeine *on page 683*

**codeine, aspirin, and carisoprodol** *see* carisoprodol, aspirin, and codeine *on page 149*

**codeine, butalbital, aspirin, and caffeine** *see* butalbital, aspirin, caffeine, and codeine *on page 125*

**codeine, chlorpheniramine, and pseudoephedrine** *see* chlorpheniramine, pseudoephedrine, and codeine *on page 176*

**codeine, chlorpheniramine, phenylephrine, and potassium iodide** *see* chlorpheniramine, phenylephrine, codeine, and potassium iodide *on page 176*

**Codeine Contin® [Can]** *see* codeine *on this page*

**codeine, guaifenesin, and pseudoephedrine** *see* guaifenesin, pseudoephedrine, and codeine *on page 391*

**codeine phosphate** *see* codeine *on this page*

**codeine, promethazine, and phenylephrine** *see* promethazine, phenylephrine, and codeine *on page 684*

**codeine, pseudoephedrine, and triprolidine** *see* triprolidine, pseudoephedrine, and codeine *(Canada only) on page 827*

**codeine sulfate** *see* codeine *on previous page*

**codeine, triprolidine, and pseudoephedrine** *see* triprolidine, pseudoephedrine, and codeine *(Canada only) on page 827*

**Codiclear® DH [US]** *see* hydrocodone and guaifenesin *on page 412*

**Codimal® DM [US-OTC]** *see* phenylephrine, pyrilamine, and dextromethorphan *on page 644*

**Codituss DM [US-OTC]** *see* phenylephrine, pyrilamine, and dextromethorphan *on page 644*

**cod liver oil** *see* vitamin A and vitamin D *on page 849*

**CO Fluoxetine [Can]** *see* fluoxetine *on page 349*

**Cogentin® [US]** *see* benztropine *on page 99*

**Co-Gesic® [US]** *see* hydrocodone and acetaminophen *on page 411*

**Cognex® [US]** *see* tacrine *on page 778*

**Colace® [US-OTC/Can]** *see* docusate *on page 263*

**Colace® Adult/Children Suppositories [US-OTC]** *see* glycerin *on page 379*

**Colace® Infant/Children Suppositories [US-OTC]** *see* glycerin *on page 379*

**Colax-C® [Can]** *see* docusate *on page 263*

**Colazal® [US]** *see* balsalazide *on page 89*

**ColBenemid® *(Discontinued)*** *see* colchicine and probenecid *on this page*

## colchicine (KOL chi seen)

**Therapeutic Category** Antigout Agent

**Use** Treatment of acute gouty arthritis attacks and prevention of recurrences of such attacks

**Usual Dosage**

Gouty arthritis: Adults:

Prophylaxis of acute attacks: Oral: 0.6 mg twice daily; initial and/or subsequent dosage may be decreased (ie, 0.6 mg once daily) in patients at risk of toxicity or in those who are intolerant (including weakness, loose stools, or diarrhea); range: 0.6 mg every other day to 0.6 mg 3 times/day

Acute attacks:

Oral: Initial: 0.6-1.2 mg, followed by 0.6 every 1-2 hours; some clinicians recommend a maximum of 3 doses; more aggressive approaches have recommended a maximum dose of up to 6 mg. Wait at least 3 days before initiating another course of therapy

I.V.: Initial: 1-2 mg, then 0.5 mg every 6 hours until response, not to exceed total dose of 4 mg. If pain recurs, it may be necessary to administer additional daily doses. The amount of colchicine administered intravenously in an acute treatment period (generally ~1 week) should not exceed a total dose of 4 mg. Do not administer more colchicine by any route for at least 7 days after a full course of I.V. therapy.

**Note:** Many experts would avoid use because of potential for serious, life-threatening complications. Should not be administered to patients with renal insufficiency, hepatobiliary obstruction, patients >70 years of age, or recent oral colchicine use. Should be reserved for hospitalized patients who are under the care of a physician experienced in the use of intravenous colchicine.

Surgery: Gouty arthritis, prophylaxis of recurrent attacks: Adults: Oral: 0.6 mg/day or every other day; patients who are to undergo surgical procedures may receive 0.6 mg 3 times/day for 3 days before and 3 days after surgery

**Dosage Forms**

Injection, solution: 0.5 mg/mL (2 mL)

Tablet: 0.6 mg

## colchicine and probenecid (KOL chi seen & proe BEN e sid)

**Synonyms** probenecid and colchicine

**Therapeutic Category** Antigout Agent

**Use** Treatment of chronic gouty arthritis when complicated by frequent, recurrent acute attacks of gout

**Usual Dosage** Adults: Oral: 1 tablet daily for 1 week, then 1 tablet twice daily thereafter

**Dosage Forms** Tablet: Colchicine 0.5 mg and probenecid 0.5 g

**Coldcough HC [US]** *see* pseudoephedrine, hydrocodone, and chlorpheniramine *on page 695*

**Coldlac-LA® *(Discontinued)***

**Coldloc® *(Discontinued)***

**Coldtuss DR [US]** *see* chlorpheniramine, phenylephrine, and dextromethorphan *on page 174*

## colesevelam (koh le SEV a lam)

**U.S./Canadian Brand Names** WelChol® [US/Can]

**Therapeutic Category** Antihyperlipidemic Agent, Miscellaneous; Bile Acid Sequestrant

**Use** Adjunctive therapy to diet and exercise in the management of elevated LDL in primary hypercholesterolemia (Fredrickson type IIa) when used alone or in combination with an HMG-CoA reductase inhibitor

**Usual Dosage** Adult: Oral:

Monotherapy: 3 tablets twice daily with meals or 6 tablets once daily with a meal; maximum dose: 7 tablets/day

Combination therapy with an HMG-CoA reductase inhibitor: 4-6 tablets daily; maximum dose: 6 tablets/day

**Dosage Forms** Tablet, as hydrochloride [film coated]: 625 mg

**Colestid® [US/Can]** *see* colestipol *on this page*

## colestipol (koe LES ti pole)

**Synonyms** colestipol hydrochloride

**U.S./Canadian Brand Names** Colestid® [US/Can]

**Therapeutic Category** Antihyperlipidemic Agent, Miscellaneous

**Use** Adjunct in management of primary hypercholesterolemia; regression of arteriolosclerosis; relief of pruritus associated with elevated levels of bile acids; possibly used to decrease plasma half-life of digoxin in toxicity

**Usual Dosage** Adults: Oral:

Granules: 5-30 g/day given once or in divided doses 2-4 times/day; initial dose: 5 g 1-2 times/day; increase by 5 g at 1- to 2-month intervals

Tablets: 2-16 g/day; initial dose: 2 g 1-2 times/day; increase by 2 g at 1- to 2-month intervals

**Dosage Forms**

Granules, as hydrochloride:

5 g/7.5 g packet (30s, 90s) [unflavored]

5 g/7.5 g (300 g, 500 g) [unflavored]

5 g/7.5 g packet (60s) [contains phenylalanine 18.2 mg/7.5 g; orange flavor]

5 g/7.5 g (450 g) [contains phenylalanine 18.2 mg/7.5 g; orange flavor]

Tablet, as hydrochloride: 1 g

**colestipol hydrochloride** *see* colestipol *on this page*

**Colhist® Solution [US-OTC]** *see* brompheniramine *on page 115*

## colistimethate (koe lis ti METH ate)

**Synonyms** colistimethate sodium

**U.S./Canadian Brand Names** Coly-Mycin® M [US/Can]

**Therapeutic Category** Antibiotic, Miscellaneous

**Use** Treatment of infections due to sensitive strains of certain gram-negative bacilli which are resistant to other antibacterials or in patients allergic to other antibacterials

**Usual Dosage** Children and Adults:

I.M., I.V.: 2.5-5 mg/kg/day in 2-4 divided doses

Inhalation: 50-75 mg in NS (3-4 mL total) via nebulizer 2-3 times/day

**Dosage Forms** Injection, powder for reconstitution: 150 mg

**colistimethate sodium** *see* colistimethate *on this page*

**colistin, neomycin, hydrocortisone, and thonzonium** *see* neomycin, colistin, hydrocortisone, and thonzonium *on page 567*

**collagen** *see* collagen hemostat *on next page*

**collagen absorbable hemostat** *see* collagen hemostat *on next page*

## collagenase (KOL la je nase)
**U.S./Canadian Brand Names** Santyl® [US]
**Therapeutic Category** Enzyme
**Use** Promotes debridement of necrotic tissue in dermal ulcers and severe burns
  **Orphan drug:** Injection: Treatment of Peyronie's disease; treatment of Dupytren's disease
**Usual Dosage** Topical: Apply once daily (or more frequently if the dressing becomes soiled)
**Dosage Forms** Ointment: 250 units/g (15 g, 30 g)

## collagen hemostat (KOL la jen HEE moe stat)
**Sound-Alike/Look-Alike Issues**
  Avitene® may be confused with Ativan®
**Synonyms** collagen absorbable hemostat; collagen; MCH; microfibrillar collagen hemostat
**U.S./Canadian Brand Names** Avitene® Flour [US]; Avitene® Ultrafoam [US]; Avitene® UltraWrap™ [US]; Avitene® [US]; EndoAvitene® [US]; Helistat® [US]; Helitene® [US]; Instat™ MCH [US]; Instat™ [US]; SyringeAvitene™ [US]
**Therapeutic Category** Hemostatic Agent
**Use** Adjunct to hemostasis when control of bleeding by ligature is ineffective or impractical
**Usual Dosage** Apply dry directly to source of bleeding; remove excess material after ~10-15 minutes
**Dosage Forms**
  Pad (Instat™) [bovine derived]: 1 inch x 2 inch (24s); 3 inch x 4 inch (24s)
  Powder:
  Avitene® Flour [microfibrillar product, bovine derived]: 0.5 g, 1 g, 5 g
  Helitene® [bovine derived]: 0.5 g, 1 g
  Instat™ MCH [microfibrillar product, bovine derived]: 0.5 g, 1 g
  SyringeAvitene™ [microfibrillar product, bovine derived, prefilled syringe]: 1 g
  Sheet:
  Avitene® [microfibrillar product, bovine derived, nonwoven web]: 35 mm x 35 mm (1s); 70 mm x 35 mm (6s, 12s); 70 mm x 70 mm (6s, 12s)
  EndoAvitene® [microfibrillar product, bovine derived, preloaded applicator]: 5 mm diameter (6s); 10 mm diameter (6s)
  Sponge:
  Avitene® Ultrafoam [microfibrillar product, bovine derived]: 2 cm x 6.25 cm x 7 mm (12s); 8 cm x 6.25 cm x 1 cm (6s); 8 cm x 12.5 cm x 1 cm (6s); 8 cm x 12.5 cm x 3 mm (6s)
  Avitene® UltraWrap™ [microfibrillar product, bovine derived]: 8 cm x 12.5 cm (6s)
  Helistat® [bovine derived]: 0.5 inch x 1 inch x 7 mm (18s) [packaged as 3 strips of 6 sponges]; 3 inch x 4 inch x 5 inch (10s)

## collagen implants (KOL a jen im PLANTS)
**U.S./Canadian Brand Names** Soft Plug® [US]
**Therapeutic Category** Ophthalmic Agent, Miscellaneous
**Use** Relief of dry eyes; enhance the effect of ocular medications
**Usual Dosage** Implants inserted by physician
**Dosage Forms**
  Implant, ophthalmic [bovine collagen]: 0.2 mm, 0.3 mm, 0.4 mm, 0.5 mm, 0.6 mm
  Soft Plug®: 0.2 mm, 0.3 mm, 0.4 mm

**Colo-Fresh™ [OTC]** *see* bismuth subsalicylate *on page 108*

**CO Lovastatin [Can]** *see* lovastatin *on page 494*

**Coly-Mycin® M [US/Can]** *see* colistimethate *on previous page*

**Coly-Mycin® S [US]** *see* neomycin, colistin, hydrocortisone, and thonzonium *on page 567*

**Colyte® [US/Can]** *see* polyethylene glycol-electrolyte solution *on page 658*

**Combantrin™ [Can]** *see* pyrantel pamoate *on page 698*

**CombiPatch® [US]** *see* estradiol and norethindrone *on page 302*

**Combipres® (Discontinued)** *see* clonidine and chlorthalidone *on page 198*

**Combivent® [US/Can]** *see* ipratropium and albuterol *on page 446*

**Combivir® [US/Can]** *see* zidovudine and lamivudine *on page 860*

**CO Meloxicam [Can]** *see* meloxicam *on page 509*

Comfort® Ophthalmic *(Discontinued)* see naphazoline on page 561

Comfort® Tears Solution *(Discontinued)* see artificial tears on page 71

Comhist® [US] see chlorpheniramine, phenylephrine, and phenyltoloxamine on page 176

Commit™ [US-OTC] see nicotine on page 574

Compazine® [Can] see prochlorperazine on page 680

Compazine® *(Discontinued)* see prochlorperazine on page 680

compound E see cortisone acetate on page 209

compound F see hydrocortisone (systemic) on page 416

compound S see zidovudine on page 859

compound S, abacavir, and lamivudine see abacavir, lamivudine, and zidovudine on page 2

Compound W® [US-OTC] see salicylic acid on page 734

Compound W® One Step Wart Remover [US-OTC] see salicylic acid on page 734

Compoz® Nighttime Sleep Aid [US-OTC] see diphenhydramine on page 254

Compro™ [US] see prochlorperazine on page 680

Comtan® [US/Can] see entacapone on page 286

Comtrex® Maximum Strength Sinus and Nasal Decongestant [US-OTC] see acetaminophen, chlorpheniramine, and pseudoephedrine on page 10

Comtrex® Non-Drowsy Cold and Cough Relief [US-OTC] see acetaminophen, dextromethorphan, and pseudoephedrine on page 11

Comtrex® Sore Throat Maximum Strength [US-OTC] see acetaminophen on page 4

Comvax® [US] see Haemophilus B conjugate and hepatitis B vaccine on page 394

Conceptrol® [US-OTC] see nonoxynol 9 on page 580

Concerta® [US/Can] see methylphenidate on page 530

Condyline™ [Can] see podofilox on page 656

Condylox® [US] see podofilox on page 656

Conex® *(Discontinued)*

Congess® Jr *(Discontinued)* see guaifenesin and pseudoephedrine on page 388

Congess® Sr *(Discontinued)* see guaifenesin and pseudoephedrine on page 388

Congestac® [US-OTC] see guaifenesin and pseudoephedrine on page 388

conjugated estrogen and methyltestosterone see estrogens (esterified) and methyltestosterone on page 306

Conray® [US] see radiological/contrast media (ionic) on page 707

Constulose® [US] see lactulose on page 464

Contac® Cold 12 Hour Relief Non Drowsy [Can] see pseudoephedrine on page 692

Contac® Cold 12 Hour Relief Non-Drowsy *(Discontinued)* see pseudoephedrine on page 692

Contac® Cold and Sore Throat, Non Drowsy, Extra Strength [Can] see acetaminophen and pseudoephedrine on page 8

Contac® Cold-Chest Congestion, Non Drowsy, Regular Strength [Can] see guaifenesin and pseudoephedrine on page 388

Contac® Complete [Can] see acetaminophen, dextromethorphan, and pseudoephedrine on page 11

Contac® Cough, Cold and Flu Day & Night™ [Can] see acetaminophen, dextromethorphan, and pseudoephedrine on page 11

Contac® Cough Formula Liquid *(Discontinued)* see guaifenesin and dextromethorphan on page 385

Contac® Severe Cold and Flu/Non-Drowsy [US-OTC] see acetaminophen, dextromethorphan, and pseudoephedrine on page 11

Contact® Cold [US-OTC] see pseudoephedrine on page 692

**Control**® *(Discontinued)*

**Contuss**® *(Discontinued)*

**Contuss**® **XT** *(Discontinued)*

**CO Paroxetine [Can]** *see* paroxetine *on page 620*

**Copaxone**® **[US/Can]** *see* glatiramer acetate *on page 374*

**Copegus**® **[US]** *see* ribavirin *on page 720*

**Cophene-B**® *(Discontinued) see* brompheniramine *on page 115*

**Cophene XP**® *(Discontinued) see* hydrocodone, pseudoephedrine, and guaifenesin *on page 415*

**copolymer-1** *see* glatiramer acetate *on page 374*

**copper** *see* trace metals *on page 813*

**CO Pravastatin [Can]** *see* pravastatin *on page 671*

**Co-Pyronil**® **2 Pulvules**® *(Discontinued) see* chlorpheniramine and pseudoephedrine *on page 172*

**CO Ranitidine [Can]** *see* ranitidine hydrochloride *on page 710*

**Cordarone**® **[US/Can]** *see* amiodarone *on page 41*

**Cordran**® **[US/Can]** *see* flurandrenolide *on page 351*

**Cordran**® **SP [US]** *see* flurandrenolide *on page 351*

**Cordron-HC [US]** *see* pseudoephedrine, hydrocodone, and chlorpheniramine *on page 695*

**Coreg**® **[US/Can]** *see* carvedilol *on page 150*

**Corfen DM [US]** *see* chlorpheniramine, phenylephrine, and dextromethorphan *on page 174*

**Corgard**® **[US/Can]** *see* nadolol *on page 556*

**Coricidin HBP**® **Chest Congestion and Cough [US-OTC]** *see* guaifenesin and dextromethorphan *on page 385*

**Coricidin HBP**® **Cold and Flu [US-OTC]** *see* chlorpheniramine and acetaminophen *on page 171*

**Corlopam**® **[US/Can]** *see* fenoldopam *on page 331*

**Cormax**® **[US]** *see* clobetasol *on page 194*

**Coronex**® **[Can]** *see* isosorbide dinitrate *on page 451*

**Correctol**® **Tablets [US-OTC]** *see* bisacodyl *on page 107*

**Cortaid**® **Intensive Therapy [US-OTC]** *see* hydrocortisone (topical) *on page 417*

**Cortaid**® **Maximum Strength [US-OTC]** *see* hydrocortisone (topical) *on page 417*

**Cortaid**® **Sensitive Skin [US-OTC]** *see* hydrocortisone (topical) *on page 417*

**Cortamed**® **[Can]** *see* hydrocortisone (topical) *on page 417*

**Cortatrigen**® **Otic** *(Discontinued) see* neomycin, polymyxin B, and hydrocortisone *on page 568*

**Cortef**® **[US/Can]** *see* hydrocortisone (systemic) *on page 416*

**Cortenema**® **[Can]** *see* hydrocortisone (rectal) *on page 416*

**Corticool**® **[US-OTC]** *see* hydrocortisone (topical) *on page 417*

**corticotropin** (kor ti koe TROE pin)

Synonyms ACTH; adrenocorticotropic hormone; corticotropin, repository

U.S./Canadian Brand Names H.P. Acthar® Gel [US]

Therapeutic Category Adrenal Corticosteroid

Use Acute exacerbations of multiple sclerosis; diagnostic aid in adrenocortical insufficiency, severe muscle weakness in myasthenia gravis

Cosyntropin is preferred over corticotropin for diagnostic test of adrenocortical insufficiency (cosyntropin is less allergenic and test is shorter in duration)

**Usual Dosage**
Children:
Anti-inflammatory/immunosuppressant: I.M.: 0.8 units/kg/day or 25 units/m²/day divided every 12-24 hours

Infantile spasms: Various regimens have been used. Some neurologists recommend low-dose ACTH (5-40 units/day) for short periods (1-6 weeks), while others recommend larger doses of ACTH (40-160 units/day) for long periods of treatment (3-12 months). Well designed comparative dosing studies are needed. Example of low dose regimen:

Initial: I.M.: 20 units/day for 2 weeks, if patient responds, taper and discontinue; if patient does not respond, increase dose to 30 units/day for 4 weeks then taper and discontinue

I.M. usual dose: 20-40 units/day or 5-8 units/kg/day in 1-2 divided doses; range: 5-160 units/day

Oral prednisone (2 mg/kg/day) was as effective as I.M. ACTH gel (20 units/day) in controlling infantile spasms

Adults: Acute exacerbation of multiple sclerosis: I.M.: 80-120 units/day for 2-3 weeks
Repository injection: I.M., SubQ: 40-80 units every 24-72 hours

**Dosage Forms** Injection, gelatin: 80 units/mL (5 mL)

**corticotropin, repository** *see* corticotropin *on previous page*

**Cortifoam**® **[US/Can]** *see* hydrocortisone (rectal) *on page 416*

**Cortimyxin**® **[Can]** *see* neomycin, polymyxin B, and hydrocortisone *on page 568*

**cortisol** *see* hydrocortisone (systemic) *on page 416*

## cortisone acetate (KOR ti sone AS e tate)

**Sound-Alike/Look-Alike Issues**
cortisone may be confused with Cortizone®

**Synonyms** compound E

**Therapeutic Category** Adrenal Corticosteroid

**Use** Management of adrenocortical insufficiency

**Usual Dosage** If possible, administer glucocorticoids before 9 AM to minimize adrenocortical suppression; dosing depends upon the condition being treated and the response of the patient; **Note:** Supplemental doses may be warranted during times of stress in the course of withdrawing therapy
Children:
Anti-inflammatory or immunosuppressive: Oral: 2.5-10 mg/kg/day **or** 20-300 mg/m²/day in divided doses every 6-8 hours

Physiologic replacement: Oral: 0.5-0.75 mg/kg/day **or** 20-25 mg/m²/day in divided doses every 8 hours
Adults:
Anti-inflammatory or immunosuppressive: Oral: 25-300 mg/day in divided doses every 12-24 hours
Physiologic replacement: Oral: 25-35 mg/day

**Dosage Forms** Tablet, as acetate: 25 mg

**Cortisporin**® **Cream [US]** *see* neomycin, polymyxin B, and hydrocortisone *on page 568*

**Cortisporin**® **Ointment [US]** *see* bacitracin, neomycin, polymyxin B, and hydrocortisone *on page 87*

**Cortisporin**® **Ophthalmic [US]** *see* neomycin, polymyxin B, and hydrocortisone *on page 568*

**Cortisporin**® **Otic [US/Can]** *see* neomycin, polymyxin B, and hydrocortisone *on page 568*

**Cortisporin**®**-TC [US]** *see* neomycin, colistin, hydrocortisone, and thonzonium *on page 567*

**Cortisporin**® **Topical Cream *(Discontinued)*** *see* neomycin, polymyxin B, and hydrocortisone *on page 568*

**Cortisporin**® **Topical Ointment [Can]** *see* bacitracin, neomycin, polymyxin B, and hydrocortisone *on page 87*

**Cortizone**®**-10 Maximum Strength [US-OTC]** *see* hydrocortisone (topical) *on page 417*

**Cortizone**®**-10 Plus Maximum Strength [US-OTC]** *see* hydrocortisone (topical) *on page 417*

**Cortizone**®**-10 Quick Shot [US-OTC]** *see* hydrocortisone (topical) *on page 417*

**Cortone**® *(Discontinued)*

**Cortrosyn**® **[US/Can]** *see* cosyntropin *on next page*

**Corvert**® **[US]** *see* ibutilide *on page 429*

**Coryphen**® **Codeine [Can]** *see* aspirin and codeine *on page 74*

**CO Simvastatin [Can]** *see* simvastatin *on page 748*

**Cosmegen® [US/Can]** *see* dactinomycin *on page 221*

**Cosopt® [US/Can]** *see* dorzolamide and timolol *on page 267*

**cosyntropin** (koe sin TROE pin)
    **Sound-Alike/Look-Alike Issues**
      Cortrosyn® may be confused with Cotazym®
    **Synonyms** synacthen; tetracosactide
    **U.S./Canadian Brand Names** Cortrosyn® [US/Can]
    **Therapeutic Category** Diagnostic Agent
    **Use** Diagnostic test to differentiate primary adrenal from secondary (pituitary) adrenocortical insufficiency
    **Usual Dosage** Adrenocortical insufficiency: I.M., I.V. (over 2 minutes): Peak plasma cortisol concentrations usually occur 45-60 minutes after cosyntropin administration
      Children <2 years: 0.125 mg
      Children >2 years and Adults: 0.25-0.75 mg
      When greater cortisol stimulation is needed, an I.V. infusion may be used:
        Children >2 years and Adults: 0.25 mg administered at 0.04 mg/hour over 6 hours
    **Dosage Forms** Injection, powder for reconstitution: 0.25 mg

**Cotazym® [Can]** *see* pancrelipase *on page 615*

**Cotazym® (Discontinued)** *see* pancrelipase *on page 615*

**Cotazym-S® (Discontinued)** *see* pancrelipase *on page 615*

**CO Temazepam [Can]** *see* temazepam *on page 784*

**Cotrim® (Discontinued)**

**Cotrim® DS (Discontinued)**

**co-trimoxazole** *see* sulfamethoxazole and trimethoprim *on page 773*

**Coughtuss [US]** *see* phenylephrine, hydrocodone, and chlorpheniramine *on page 643*

**Coumadin® [US/Can]** *see* warfarin *on page 854*

**Covan® [Can]** *see* triprolidine, pseudoephedrine, and codeine *(Canada only) on page 827*

**Covera® [Can]** *see* verapamil *on page 843*

**Covera-HS® [US]** *see* verapamil *on page 843*

**Coversyl® [Can]** *see* perindopril erbumine *on page 634*

**Coversyl® Plus [Can]** *see* perindopril and indapamide *(Canada only) on page 634*

**co-vidarabine** *see* pentostatin *on page 632*

**coviracil** *see* emtricitabine *on page 282*

**Cozaar® [US/Can]** *see* losartan *on page 492*

**CP358774** *see* erlotinib *on page 294*

**CPC** *see* cetylpyridinium *on page 164*

**C-Phed Tannate [US]** *see* chlorpheniramine and pseudoephedrine *on page 172*

**CPM** *see* cyclophosphamide *on page 214*

**CPT-11** *see* irinotecan *on page 447*

**CPZ** *see* chlorpromazine *on page 178*

**Crantex ER [US]** *see* guaifenesin and phenylephrine *on page 387*

**Crantex LA [US]** *see* guaifenesin and phenylephrine *on page 387*

**Creomulsion® Cough [US-OTC]** *see* dextromethorphan *on page 238*

**Creomulsion® for Children [US-OTC]** *see* dextromethorphan *on page 238*

**Creon® [US]** *see* pancrelipase *on page 615*

**Creon® 5 [Can]** *see* pancrelipase *on page 615*

**Creon® 10 [Can]** *see* pancrelipase *on page 615*

**Creon® 20 [Can]** *see* pancrelipase *on page 615*

**Creon® 25 [Can]** *see* pancrelipase *on page 615*

**Creo-Terpin**® **[US-OTC]** *see* dextromethorphan *on page 238*

**Crestor**® **[US/Can]** *see* rosuvastatin *on page 732*

**Cresylate**® **[US]** *see* m-cresyl acetate *on page 504*

**Crinone**® **[US/Can]** *see* progesterone *on page 682*

**Critic-Aid Skin Care**® **[US-OTC]** *see* zinc oxide *on page 861*

**Criticare HN**® **[US-OTC]** *see* nutritional formula, enteral/oral *on page 591*

**Crixivan**® **[US/Can]** *see* indinavir *on page 435*

**CroFab**™ **[Ovine] [US]** *see* antivenin *(Crotalidae)* polyvalent *on page 60*

**Crolom**® **[US]** *see* cromolyn sodium *on this page*

**cromoglycic acid** *see* cromolyn sodium *on this page*

## cromolyn sodium (KROE moe lin SOW dee um)

**Sound-Alike/Look-Alike Issues**
Intal® may be confused with Endal®
NasalCrom® may be confused with Nasacort®, Nasalide®

**Synonyms** cromoglycic acid; disodium cromoglycate; DSCG

**U.S./Canadian Brand Names** Apo-Cromolyn® [Can]; Crolom® [US]; Gastrocrom® [US]; Intal® [US/Can]; Nalcrom® [Can]; NasalCrom® [US-OTC]; Nu-Cromolyn [Can]; Opticrom® [US/Can]

**Therapeutic Category** Mast Cell Stabilizer

**Use**
Inhalation: May be used as an adjunct in the prophylaxis of allergic disorders, including asthma; prevention of exercise-induced bronchospasm
Nasal: Prevention and treatment of seasonal and perennial allergic rhinitis
Oral: Systemic mastocytosis
Ophthalmic: Treatment of vernal keratoconjunctivitis, vernal conjunctivitis, and vernal keratitis

**Usual Dosage**

**Oral:**
Systemic mastocytosis:
Children 2-12 years: 100 mg 4 times/day; not to exceed 40 mg/kg/day; given $1/2$ hour prior to meals and at bedtime
Children >12 years and Adults: 200 mg 4 times/day; given $1/2$ hour prior to meals and at bedtime; if control of symptoms is not seen within 2-3 weeks, dose may be increased to a maximum 40 mg/kg/day

**Inhalation:**
For chronic control of asthma, taper frequency to the lowest effective dose (ie, 4 times/day to 3 times/day to twice daily):
Nebulization solution: Children >2 years and Adults: Initial: 20 mg 4 times/day; usual dose: 20 mg 3-4 times/day
Metered spray:
Children 5-12 years: Initial: 2 inhalations 4 times/day; usual dose: 1-2 inhalations 3-4 times/day
Children ≥12 years and Adults: Initial: 2 inhalations 4 times/day; usual dose: 2-4 inhalations 3-4 times/day
Prevention of allergen- or exercise-induced bronchospasm: Administer 10-15 minutes prior to exercise or allergen exposure but no longer than 1 hour before:
Nebulization solution: Children >2 years and Adults: Single dose of 20 mg
Metered spray: Children >5 years and Adults: Single dose of 2 inhalations

**Ophthalmic:** Children >4 years and Adults: 1-2 drops in each eye 4-6 times/day

**Nasal:** Allergic rhinitis (treatment and prophylaxis): Children ≥2 years and Adults: 1 spray into each nostril 3-4 times/day; may be increased to 6 times/day (symptomatic relief may require 2-4 weeks)

**Dosage Forms**
Aerosol, for oral inhalation, as sodium (Intal®): 800 mcg/inhalation (8.1 g) [112 metered inhalations; 56 doses], (14.2 g) [200 metered inhalations; 100 doses]
Solution for nebulization, as sodium (Intal®): 20 mg/2 mL (60s, 120s)
Solution, intranasal spray, as sodium (NasalCrom®): 40 mg/mL (13 mL, 26 mL) [5.2 mg/inhalation; contains benzalkonium chloride]
Solution, ophthalmic, as sodium (Crolom®, Opticrom®): 4% (10 mL) [contains benzalkonium chloride]
Solution, oral, as sodium (Gastrocrom®): 100 mg/5 mL (96s)

**Crosseal**™ **[US]** *see* fibrin sealant kit *on page 337*

**crotaline antivenin, polyvalent** *see* antivenin *(Crotalidae)* polyvalent *on page 60*

**crotamiton** (kroe TAM i tonn)
**Sound-Alike/Look-Alike Issues**
Eurax® may be confused with Efudex®, Eulexin®, Evoxac™, Serax®, Urex®
**U.S./Canadian Brand Names** Eurax® [US]
**Therapeutic Category** Scabicides/Pediculicides
**Use** Treatment of scabies (*Sarcoptes scabiei*) and symptomatic treatment of pruritus
**Usual Dosage** Topical:
Scabicide: Children and Adults: Wash thoroughly and scrub away loose scales, then towel dry; apply a thin layer and massage drug onto skin of the entire body from the neck to the toes (with special attention to skin folds, creases, and interdigital spaces). Repeat application in 24 hours. Take a cleansing bath 48 hours after the final application. Treatment may be repeated after 7-10 days if live mites are still present.
Pruritus: Massage into affected areas until medication is completely absorbed; repeat as necessary
**Dosage Forms**
Cream: 10% (60 g)
Lotion: 10% (60 mL, 480 mL)

**crude coal tar** *see* coal tar *on page 201*

**Cruex® Cream [US-OTC]** *see* clotrimazole *on page 199*

**Cryselle™ [US]** *see* ethinyl estradiol and norgestrel *on page 318*

**crystalline penicillin** *see* penicillin G (parenteral/aqueous) *on page 629*

**Crystamine® *(Discontinued)*** *see* cyanocobalamin *on this page*

**Crysti 1000® *(Discontinued)*** *see* cyanocobalamin *on this page*

**CsA** *see* cyclosporine *on page 215*

**CSP** *see* cellulose sodium phosphate *on page 160*

**CTM** *see* chlorpheniramine *on page 171*

**CTX** *see* cyclophosphamide *on page 214*

**Cubicin™ [US]** *see* daptomycin *on page 224*

**Culturelle® [US-OTC]** *see* Lactobacillus *on page 462*

**Cuprimine® [US/Can]** *see* penicillamine *on page 627*

**Curasore [US-OTC]** *see* pramoxine *on page 670*

**Curosurf® [US/Can]** *see* poractant alfa *on page 661*

**Cutar® [US-OTC]** *see* coal tar *on page 201*

**Cutivate® [US]** *see* fluticasone (topical) *on page 355*

**CyA** *see* cyclosporine *on page 215*

**cyanide antidote kit** *see* sodium nitrite, sodium thiosulfate, and amyl nitrite *on page 755*

**Cyanide Antidote Package [US]** *see* sodium nitrite, sodium thiosulfate, and amyl nitrite *on page 755*

**cyanocobalamin** (sye an oh koe BAL a min)
**Synonyms** vitamin $B_{12}$
**U.S./Canadian Brand Names** Nascobal® [US]; Twelve Resin-K [US]
**Therapeutic Category** Vitamin, Water Soluble
**Use** Treatment of pernicious anemia; vitamin $B_{12}$ deficiency due to malabsorption diseases, inadequaste secretion of intrinisic factor, and inadequate utilization of $B_{12}$ (eg, during neoplastic treatment); increased $B_{12}$ requirements due to pregnancy, thyrotoxicosis, hemorrhage, malignancy, liver or kidney disease
**Usual Dosage**
Recommended daily allowance (RDA):
Children: 0.9-2.4 mcg/day
Adults: 2.4 mcg/day
Pregnancy: 2.6 mcg/day
Lactation: 2.8 mcg/day

Vitamin B$_{12}$ deficiency:

Intranasal: 500 mcg in one nostril once weekly

Oral: 250 mcg/day

I.M., deep SubQ:

Children (dosage not well established): 0.2 mcg/kg for 2 days, followed by 1000 mcg/day for 2-7 days, followed by 100 mcg/week for one month; for malabsorptive causes of B$_{12}$ deficiency, monthly maintenance doses of 100 mcg have been recommended **or** as an alternative 100 mcg/day for 10-15 days, then once or twice weekly for several months

Adults: Initial: 30 mcg/day for 5-10 days; maintenance: 100-200 mcg/month

Pernicious anemia: I.M., deep SubQ (administer concomitantly with folic acid if needed, 1 mg/day for 1 month):

Children: 30-50 mcg/day for 2 or more weeks (to a total dose of 1000-5000 mcg), then follow with 100 mcg/month as maintenance dosage

Adults: 100 mcg/day for 6-7 days; if improvement, administer same dose on alternate days for 7 doses, then every 3-4 days for 2-3 weeks; once hematologic values have returned to normal, maintenance dosage: 100 mcg/month. **Note:** Alternative dosing of 1000 mcg/day for 5 days (followed by 500-1000 mcg/month) has been used.

Hematologic remission (without evidence of nervous system involvement):

Intranasal gel: 500 mcg in one nostril once weekly

Oral: 1000-2000 mcg/day

I.M., SubQ: 100-1000 mcg/month

Schilling test: I.M.: 1000 mcg

**Dosage Forms**

Gel, intranasal (Nascobal®): 500 mcg/0.1 mL (2.3 mL) [contains benzalkonium chloride; delivers 8 doses]

Injection, solution: 1000 mcg/mL (1 mL, 10 mL, 30 mL) [may contain benzyl alcohol and/or aluminum]

Lozenge [OTC]: 100 mcg, 250 mcg, 500 mcg

Solution, intranasal spray (Nascobal®): 500 mcg/0.1 mL actuation (2.3 mL) [contains benzalkonium chloride; delivers 8 doses]

Tablet [OTC]: 50 mcg, 100 mcg, 250 mcg, 500 mcg, 1000 mcg, 5000 mcg

Twelve Resin-K: 1000 mcg [may be used as oral, sublingual, or buccal]

Tablet, extended release [OTC]: 1500 mcg

Tablet, sublingual [OTC]: 2500 mcg

**cyanocobalamin, folic acid, and pyridoxine** *see* folic acid, cyanocobalamin, and pyridoxine *on page 357*

**Cyanoject**® *(Discontinued)* *see* cyanocobalamin *on previous page*

# cyclandelate (sye KLAN de late)

**Therapeutic Category** Vasodilator, Peripheral

**Use** Considered as "possibly effective" for adjunctive therapy in peripheral vascular disease and possibly senility due to cerebrovascular disease or multi-infarct dementia; migraine prophylaxis, vertigo, tinnitus, and visual disturbances secondary to cerebrovascular insufficiency and diabetic peripheral polyneuropathy

**Usual Dosage** Oral: Adults: Initial: 1.2-1.6 g/day in divided doses before meals and at bedtime until response; maintenance therapy: 400-800 mg/day in 2-4 divided doses; decrease dose by 200 mg decrements to achieve minimal maintenance dose; improvement can usually be seen over weeks of therapy and prolonged use; short courses of therapy are usually ineffective and not recommended

**Dosage Forms** Capsule: 200 mg, 400 mg

**Cyclen**® **[Can]** *see* ethinyl estradiol and norgestimate *on page 317*

**Cyclessa**® **[US]** *see* ethinyl estradiol and desogestrel *on page 309*

# cyclobenzaprine (sye kloe BEN za preen)

**Sound-Alike/Look-Alike Issues**

cyclobenzaprine may be confused with cycloSERINE, cyproheptadine

Flexeril® may be confused with Floxin®

**Synonyms** cyclobenzaprine hydrochloride

**U.S./Canadian Brand Names** Apo-Cyclobenzaprine® [Can]; Flexeril® [US/Can]; Flexitec [Can]; Gen-Cyclobenzaprine [Can]; Novo-Cycloprine [Can]; Nu-Cyclobenzaprine [Can]

(Continued)

## cyclobenzaprine *(Continued)*

**Therapeutic Category** Skeletal Muscle Relaxant
**Use** Treatment of muscle spasm associated with acute painful musculoskeletal conditions
**Usual Dosage** Oral: **Note:** Do not use longer than 2-3 weeks
Adults: Initial: 5 mg 3 times/day; may increase to 10 mg 3 times/day if needed
**Dosage Forms**
Tablet, as hydrochloride: 10 mg
Flexeril®: 5 mg, 10 mg [film coated]

**cyclobenzaprine hydrochloride** *see* cyclobenzaprine *on previous page*

**Cyclocort® [US/Can]** *see* amcinonide *on page 38*

**Cyclogyl® [US/Can]** *see* cyclopentolate *on this page*

**Cyclomen® [Can]** *see* danazol *on page 222*

**Cyclomydril® [US]** *see* cyclopentolate and phenylephrine *on this page*

## cyclopentolate *(sye kloe PEN toe late)*

**Synonyms** cyclopentolate hydrochloride
**U.S./Canadian Brand Names** Cyclogyl® [US/Can]; Cylate® [US]; Diopentolate® [Can]
**Therapeutic Category** Anticholinergic Agent
**Use** Diagnostic procedures requiring mydriasis and cycloplegia
**Usual Dosage** Ophthalmic:
Neonates and Infants: **Note:** Cyclopentolate and phenylephrine combination formulation is the preferred agent for use in neonates and infants due to lower cyclopentolate concentration and reduced risk for systemic reactions
Children: Instill 1 drop of 0.5%, 1%, or 2% in eye followed by 1 drop of 0.5% or 1% in 5 minutes, if necessary
Adults: Instill 1 drop of 1% followed by another drop in 5 minutes; 2% solution in heavily pigmented iris
**Dosage Forms** [DSC] = Discontinued product
Solution, ophthalmic, as hydrochloride: 1% (2 mL, 15 mL)
AK-Pentolate® [DSC], Cylate®: 1% (2 mL, 15 mL) [contains benzalkonium chloride]
Cyclogyl®: 0.5% (15 mL); 1% (2 mL, 5 mL, 15 mL); 2% (2 mL, 5 mL, 15 mL) [contains benzalkonium chloride]

## cyclopentolate and phenylephrine *(sye kloe PEN toe late & fen il EF rin)*

**Synonyms** phenylephrine and cyclopentolate
**U.S./Canadian Brand Names** Cyclomydril® [US]
**Therapeutic Category** Anticholinergic/Adrenergic Agonist
**Use** Induce mydriasis greater than that produced with cyclopentolate HCl alone
**Usual Dosage** Ophthalmic: Neonates, Infants, Children, and Adults: Instill 1 drop into the eye every 5-10 minutes, for up to 3 doses, approximately 40-50 minutes before the examination
**Dosage Forms** Solution, ophthalmic: Cyclopentolate hydrochloride 0.2% and phenylephrine hydrochloride 1% (2 mL, 5 mL) [contains benzalkonium chloride]

**cyclopentolate hydrochloride** *see* cyclopentolate *on this page*

## cyclophosphamide *(sye kloe FOS fa mide)*

**Sound-Alike/Look-Alike Issues**
cyclophosphamide may be confused with cycloSPORINE, ifosfamide
Cytoxan® may be confused with cefoxitin, Centoxin®, Ciloxan®, cytarabine, CytoGam®, Cytosar®, Cytosar-U®, Cytotec®
**Synonyms** CPM; CTX; CYT; NSC-26271
**U.S./Canadian Brand Names** Cytoxan® [US/Can]; Procytox® [Can]
**Therapeutic Category** Antineoplastic Agent
**Use**
**Oncologic:** Treatment of Hodgkin and non-Hodgkin lymphoma, Burkitt lymphoma, chronic lymphocytic leukemia (CLL), chronic myelocytic leukemia (CML), acute myelocytic leukemia (AML), acute lymphocytic leukemia (ALL), mycosis fungoides, multiple myeloma, neuroblastoma, retinoblastoma, rhabdomyosarcoma, Ewing sarcoma; breast, testicular, endometrial, ovarian, and lung cancers, and in conditioning regimens for bone marrow transplantation

**Nononcologic:** Prophylaxis of rejection for kidney, heart, liver, and bone marrow transplants, severe rheumatoid disorders, nephrotic syndrome, Wegener granulomatosis, idiopathic pulmonary hemosideroses, myasthenia gravis, multiple sclerosis, systemic lupus erythematosus, lupus nephritis, autoimmune hemolytic anemia, idiopathic thrombocytic purpura (ITP), macroglobulinemia, and antibody-induced pure red cell aplasia

**Usual Dosage** Refer to individual protocols

Patients who are heavily pretreated with cytotoxic radiation or chemotherapy, or who have compromised bone marrow function may require a 33% to 50% reduction in initial dose.

Children:

SLE: I.V.: 500-750 mg/m$^2$ every month; maximum dose: 1 g/m$^2$

JRA/vasculitis: I.V.: 10 mg/kg every 2 weeks

Children and Adults:

Oral: 50-100 mg/m$^2$/day as continuous therapy or 400-1000 mg/m$^2$ in divided doses over 4-5 days as intermittent therapy

I.V.:

Single doses: 400-1800 mg/m$^2$ (30-50 mg/kg) per treatment course (1-5 days) which can be repeated at 2-4 week intervals

Continuous daily doses: 60-120 mg/m$^2$ (1-2.5 mg/kg) per day

Autologous BMT: IVPB: 50 mg/kg/dose x 4 days or 60 mg/kg/dose for 2 days; total dose is usually divided over 2-4 days

Nephrotic syndrome: Oral: 2-3 mg/kg/day every day for up to 12 weeks when corticosteroids are unsuccessful

**Dosage Forms**

Injection, powder for reconstitution (Cytoxan®): 500 mg, 1 g, 2 g [contains mannitol 75 mg per cyclophosphamide 100 mg]

Tablet (Cytoxan®): 25 mg, 50 mg

# cycloserine (sye kloe SER een)

**Sound-Alike/Look-Alike Issues**

cycloSERINE may be confused with cyclobenzaprine, cycloSPORINE

**Tall-Man** cyclo**SERINE**

**U.S./Canadian Brand Names** Seromycin® [US]

**Therapeutic Category** Antibiotic, Miscellaneous

**Use** Adjunctive treatment in pulmonary or extrapulmonary tuberculosis

**Usual Dosage** Some of the neurotoxic effects may be relieved or prevented by the concomitant administration of pyridoxine

Tuberculosis: Oral:

Children: 10-20 mg/kg/day in 2 divided doses up to 1000 mg/day for 18-24 months

Adults: Initial: 250 mg every 12 hours for 14 days, then administer 500 mg to 1 g/day in 2 divided doses for 18-24 months (maximum daily dose: 1 g)

**Dosage Forms** Capsule: 250 mg

# cyclosporin A see cyclosporine on this page

# cyclosporine (SYE kloe spor een)

**Sound-Alike/Look-Alike Issues**

cycloSPORINE may be confused with cyclophosphamide, Cyklokapron®, cycloSERINE

Gengraf® may be confused with Prograf®

Neoral® may be confused with Neurontin®, Nizoral®

Sandimmune® may be confused with Sandostatin®

**Synonyms** CsA; CyA; cyclosporin A

**Tall-Man** cyclo**SPORINE**

**U.S./Canadian Brand Names** Apo-Cyclosporine® [Can]; Gengraf® [US]; Neoral® [US/Can]; Restasis™ [US]; Rhoxal-cyclosporine [Can]; Sandimmune® I.V. [Can]; Sandimmune® [US]

**Therapeutic Category** Immunosuppressant Agent

**Use** Prophylaxis of organ rejection in kidney, liver, and heart transplants, has been used with azathioprine and/or corticosteroids; severe, active rheumatoid arthritis (RA) not responsive to methotrexate alone; severe, recalcitrant plaque psoriasis in nonimmunocompromised adults unresponsive to or unable to tolerate other systemic therapy

(Continued)

## cyclosporine *(Continued)*

Ophthalmic emulsion (Restasis™): Increase tear production when suppressed tear production is presumed to be due to keratoconjunctivitis sicca-associated ocular inflammation (in patients not already using topical anti-inflammatory drugs or punctal plugs)

Usual Dosage Note: Neoral® and Sandimmune® are not bioequivalent and cannot be used interchangeably

Children: Transplant: Refer to adult dosing; children may require, and are able to tolerate, larger doses than adults.

Adults:

**Newly-transplanted patients:** Adjunct therapy with corticosteroids is recommended. Initial dose should be given 4-12 hours prior to transplant or may be given postoperatively; adjust initial dose to achieve desired plasma concentration

Oral: Dose is dependent upon type of transplant and formulation:

Cyclosporine (modified):

Renal: $9 \pm 3$ mg/kg/day, divided twice daily

Liver: $8 \pm 4$ mg/kg/day, divided twice daily

Heart: $7 \pm 3$ mg/kg/day, divided twice daily

Cyclosporine (non-modified): Initial dose: 15 mg/kg/day as a single dose (range 14-18 mg/kg); lower doses of 10-14 mg/kg/day have been used for renal transplants. Continue initial dose daily for 1-2 weeks; taper by 5% per week to a maintenance dose of 5-10 mg/kg/day; some renal transplant patients may be dosed as low as 3 mg/kg/day

**Note:** When using the non-modified formulation, cyclosporine levels may increase in liver transplant patients when the T-tube is closed; dose may need decreased

I.V.: Cyclosporine (non-modified): Manufacturer's labeling: Initial dose: 5-6 mg/kg/day as a single dose ($\frac{1}{3}$ the oral dose), infused over 2-6 hours; use should be limited to patients unable to take capsules or oral solution; patients should be switched to an oral dosage form as soon as possible

**Note:** Many transplant centers administer cyclosporine as "divided dose" infusions (in 2-3 doses/day) or as a continuous (24-hour) infusion; dosages range from 3-7.5 mg/kg/day. Specific institutional protocols should be consulted.

**Conversion to cyclosporine (modified) from cyclosporine (non-modified):** Start with daily dose previously used and adjust to obtain preconversion cyclosporine trough concentration. Plasma concentrations should be monitored every 4-7 days and dose adjusted as necessary, until desired trough level is obtained. When transferring patients with previously poor absorption of cyclosporine (non-modified), monitor trough levels at least twice weekly (especially if initial dose exceeds 10 mg/kg/day); high plasma levels are likely to occur.

**Rheumatoid arthritis:** Oral: Cyclosporine (modified): Initial dose: 2.5 mg/kg/day, divided twice daily; salicylates, NSAIDs, and oral glucocorticoids may be continued; dose may be increased by 0.5-0.75 mg/kg/day if insufficient response is seen after 8 weeks of treatment; additional dosage increases may be made again at 12 weeks (maximum dose: 4 mg/kg/day). Discontinue if no benefit is seen by 16 weeks of therapy.

**Note:** Increase the frequency of blood pressure monitoring after each alteration in dosage of cyclosporine. Cyclosporine dosage should be decreased by 25% to 50% in patients with no history of hypertension who develop sustained hypertension during therapy and, if hypertension persists, treatment with cyclosporine should be discontinued.

**Psoriasis:** Oral: Cyclosporine (modified): Initial dose: 2.5 mg/kg/day, divided twice daily; dose may be increased by 0.5 mg/kg/day if insufficient response is seen after 4 weeks of treatment. Additional dosage increases may be made every 2 weeks if needed (maximum dose: 4 mg/kg/day). Discontinue if no benefit is seen by 6 weeks of therapy. Once patients are adequately controlled, the dose should be decreased to the lowest effective dose. Doses lower than 2.5 mg/kg/day may be effective. Treatment longer than 1 year is not recommended.

**Note:** Increase the frequency of blood pressure monitoring after each alteration in dosage of cyclosporine. Cyclosporine dosage should be decreased by 25% to 50% in patients with no history of hypertension who develop sustained hypertension during therapy and, if hypertension persists, treatment with cyclosporine should be discontinued.

**Focal segmental glomerulosclerosis:** Initial: 3 mg/kg/day divided every 12 hours

**Autoimmune diseases:** 1-3 mg/kg/day

**Keratoconjunctivitis sicca**: Ophthalmic: Children ≥16 years and Adults: Instill 1 drop in each eye every 12 hours

### Dosage Forms

Capsule, soft gel, modified: 25 mg, 100 mg [contains castor oil, ethanol]

Gengraf®: 25 mg, 100 mg [contains ethanol, castor oil, propylene glycol]

Neoral®: 25 mg, 100 mg [contains dehydrated ethanol, corn oil, castor oil, propylene glycol]
Capsule, soft gel, non-modified (Sandimmune®): 25 mg, 100 mg [contains dehydrated ethanol, corn oil]
Emulsion, ophthalmic [preservative free, single-use vial] (Restasis™): 0.05% (0.4 mL) [contains glycerin, castor oil, polysorbate 80, carbomer 1342; 32 vials/box]
Injection, solution, non-modified (Sandimmune®): 50 mg/mL (5 mL) [contains Cremophor® EL (polyoxyethylated castor oil), ethanol]
Solution, oral, modified:
  Gengraf®: 100 mg/mL (50 mL) [contains castor oil, propylene glycol]
  Neoral®: 100 mg/mL (50 mL) [contains dehydrated ethanol, corn oil, castor oil, propylene glycol]
Solution, oral, non-modified (Sandimmune®): 100 mg/mL (50 mL) [contains olive oil, ethanol]

**Cycofed® Pediatric** *(Discontinued)* *see* guaifenesin, pseudoephedrine, and codeine *on page 391*

**Cyklokapron® [US/Can]** *see* tranexamic acid *on page 815*

**Cylate® [US]** *see* cyclopentolate *on page 214*

**Cylert®** *(Discontinued)* *see* pemoline *on page 626*

**Cylex® [US-OTC]** *see* benzocaine *on page 95*

**Cymbalta® [US]** *see* duloxetine *on page 275*

**Cyomin®** *(Discontinued)* *see* cyanocobalamin *on page 212*

## cyproheptadine (si proe HEP ta deen)
**Sound-Alike/Look-Alike Issues**
  cyproheptadine may be confused with cyclobenzaprine
  Periactin® may be confused with Perative®, Percodan®, Persantine®
**Synonyms** cyproheptadine hydrochloride
**Therapeutic Category** Antihistamine
**Use** Perennial and seasonal allergic rhinitis and other allergic symptoms including urticaria
**Usual Dosage** Oral:
  Children:
  Allergic conditions: 0.25 mg/kg/day or 8 mg/m$^2$/day in 2-3 divided doses **or**
    2-6 years: 2 mg every 8-12 hours (not to exceed 12 mg/day)
    7-14 years: 4 mg every 8-12 hours (not to exceed 16 mg/day)
  Migraine headaches: 4 mg 2-3 times/day
  Children ≥12 years and Adults: Spasticity associated with spinal cord damage: 4 mg at bedtime; increase by a 4 mg dose every 3-4 days; average daily dose: 16 mg in divided doses; not to exceed 36 mg/day
  Children >13 years and Adults: Appetite stimulation (anorexia nervosa): 2 mg 4 times/day; may be increased gradually over a 3-week period to 8 mg 4 times/day
  Adults:
  Allergic conditions: 4-20 mg/day divided every 8 hours (not to exceed 0.5 mg/kg/day)
  Cluster headaches: 4 mg 4 times/day
  Migraine headaches: 4-8 mg 3 times/day
**Dosage Forms**
  Syrup, as hydrochloride: 2 mg/5 mL (473 mL) [contains alcohol 5%; mint flavor]
  Tablet, as hydrochloride: 4 mg

**cyproheptadine hydrochloride** *see* cyproheptadine *on this page*

**cyproterone acetate** *see* cyproterone *(Canada only)* *on next page*

# cyproterone and ethinyl estradiol *(Canada only)*
(sye PROE ter one & ETH in il es tra DYE ole)
**Synonyms** ethinyl estradiol and cyproterone acetate
**U.S./Canadian Brand Names** Diane-35 [Can]
**Therapeutic Category** Acne Products; Estrogen and Androgen Combination
**Use** Treatment of females with severe acne, unresponsive to other therapies, with associated symptoms of androgenization (including mild hirsutism or seborrhea). **Should not be used solely for contraception;** however, will provide reliable contraception if taken as recommended for approved indications.
**Usual Dosage** Oral: Adults: Female: Acne: One tablet daily for 21 days, followed by 7 days off; first cycle should begin on the first day of menstrual flow. Discontinue therapy 3-4 cycles after symptoms have resolved.
**Dosage Forms** Tablet: Cyproterone acetate 2 mg and ethinyl estradiol 0.35 mg [orange tablets] (21s)

# cyproterone *(Canada only)* (sye PROE ter one)
**Synonyms** cyproterone acetate
**U.S./Canadian Brand Names** Androcur® Depot [Can]; Androcur® [Can]; Apo-Cyproterone® [Can]; Gen-Cyproterone [Can]
**Therapeutic Category** Antiandrogen;  Progestin
**Use** Palliative treatment of advanced prostate carcinoma
**Usual Dosage** Adults: Males: Prostatic carcinoma (palliative treatment):
Oral: 200-300 mg/day in 2-3 divided doses; following orchiectomy, reduce dose to 100-200 mg/day; should be taken with meals
I.M. (depot): 300 mg (3 mL) once weekly; reduce dose in orchiectomized patients to 300 mg every 2 weeks
**Dosage Forms**
Injection, solution, as acetate (Androcur® Depot): 100 mg/mL (3 mL) [contains benzyl benzoate and castor oil]
Tablet, as acetate (Androcur®): 50 mg

**Cystadane® [US/Can]** *see* betaine anhydrous *on page 102*

**Cystagon® [US]** *see* cysteamine *on this page*

# cysteamine (sis TEE a meen)
**Synonyms** cysteamine bitartrate
**U.S./Canadian Brand Names** Cystagon® [US]
**Therapeutic Category**  Urinary Tract Product
**Use Orphan drug:** Treatment of nephropathic cystinosis
**Usual Dosage** Oral: Initiate therapy with $1/4$ to $1/6$ of maintenance dose; titrate slowly upward over 4-6 weeks. **Note:** Dosage may be increased if cystine levels are <1 nmol/$1/2$ cystine/mg protein, although intolerance and incidence of adverse events may be increased.
Children <12 years: Maintenance: 1.3 g/m$^2$/day or 60 mg/kg/day divided into 4 doses (maximum dose: 1.95 g/m$^2$/day or 90 mg/kg/day)
Children >12 years and Adults (>110 lb): 2 g/day in 4 divided doses; maximum dose: 1.95 g/m$^2$/day or 90 mg/kg/day
**Dosage Forms** Capsule: 50 mg, 150 mg

**cysteamine bitartrate** *see* cysteamine *on this page*

# cysteine (SIS te een)
**Synonyms** cysteine hydrochloride
**Therapeutic Category**  Nutritional Supplement
**Use** Supplement to crystalline amino acid solutions, in particular the specialized pediatric formulas (eg, Aminosyn® PF, TrophAmine®) to meet the intravenous amino acid nutritional requirements of infants receiving parenteral nutrition (PN)
**Usual Dosage** Neonates and Infants: I.V.: Added as a fixed ratio to crystalline amino acid solution: 40 mg cysteine per g of amino acids; dosage will vary with the daily amino acid dosage (eg, 0.5-2.5 g/kg/day amino acids would result in 20-100 mg/kg/day cysteine); individual doses of cysteine of 0.8-1 mmol/kg/day have also been added directly to the daily PN solution; the duration of treatment relates to the need for PN; patients on chronic PN therapy have received cysteine until 6 months of age and in some cases until 2 years of age
**Dosage Forms** Injection, solution, as hydrochloride: 50 mg/mL (10 mL, 50 mL)

**cysteine hydrochloride** *see* cysteine *on this page*

**Cystistat® [Can]** *see* hyaluronate and derivatives *on page 406*

**Cystografin® [US]** *see* radiological/contrast media (ionic) *on page 707*

**Cystospaz® [US/Can]** *see* hyoscyamine *on page 424*

**Cystospaz-M® *(Discontinued)*** *see* hyoscyamine *on page 424*

**CYT** *see* cyclophosphamide *on page 214*

**Cytadren® [US]** *see* aminoglutethimide *on page 40*

## cytarabine (sye TARE a been)

### Sound-Alike/Look-Alike Issues

cytarabine may be confused with Cytadren®, Cytosar®, Cytoxan®, vidarabine

Cytosar-U® may be confused with cytarabine, Cytovene®, Cytoxan®, Neosar®

**Synonyms** ara-C; arabinosylcytosine; cytarabine hydrochloride; cytosine arabinosine hydrochloride; NSC-63878

**U.S./Canadian Brand Names** Cytosar-U® [US]; Cytosar® [Can]

**Therapeutic Category** Antineoplastic Agent

**Use** Cytarabine is one of the most active agents in leukemia; also active against lymphoma, meningeal leukemia, and meningeal lymphoma; has little use in the treatment of solid tumors

**Usual Dosage** I.V. bolus, IVPB, and CIV doses of cytarabine are very different. Bolus doses are relatively well tolerated since the drug is rapidly metabolized; but are associated with greater neurotoxicity. Continuous infusion uniformly results in myelosuppression. Refer to individual protocols. Children and Adults:

Remission induction:

I.V.: 100-200 mg/m$^2$/day for 5-10 days; a second course, beginning 2-4 weeks after the initial therapy, may be required in some patients.

I.T.: 5-75 mg/m$^2$ every 2-7 days until CNS findings normalize; or age-based dosing:

<1 year: 20 mg

1-2 years: 30 mg

2-3 years: 50 mg

>3 years: 75 mg

Remission maintenance:

I.V.: 70-200 mg/m$^2$/day for 2-5 days at monthly intervals

I.M., SubQ: 1-1.5 mg/kg single dose for maintenance at 1- to 4-week intervals

**High-dose therapies:**

Doses as high as 1-3 g/m$^2$ have been used for refractory or secondary leukemias or refractory non-Hodgkin's lymphoma.

Doses of 1-3 g/m$^2$ every 12 hours for up to 12 doses have been used

Bone marrow transplant: 1.5 g/m$^2$ continuous infusion over 48 hours

### Dosage Forms

Injection, powder for reconstitution: 100 mg, 500 mg, 1 g, 2 g

Injection, solution: 20 mg/mL (5 mL, 25 mL, 50 mL); 100 mg/mL (20 mL)

**cytarabine hydrochloride** *see* cytarabine *on this page*

## cytarabine (liposomal) (sye TARE a been lip po SOE mal)

### Sound-Alike/Look-Alike Issues

cytarabine may be confused with Cytadren®, Cytosar®, Cytoxan®, vidarabine

DepoCyt™ may be confused with Depoject®

**U.S./Canadian Brand Names** DepoCyt™ [US/Can]

**Therapeutic Category** Antineoplastic Agent, Antimetabolite (Purine)

**Use** Treatment of neoplastic (lymphomatous) meningitis

**Usual Dosage** Adults:

Induction: 50 mg intrathecally every 14 days for a total of 2 doses (weeks 1 and 3)

Consolidation: 50 mg intrathecally every 14 days for 3 doses (weeks 5, 7, and 9), followed by an additional dose at week 13

Maintenance: 50 mg intrathecally every 28 days for 4 doses (weeks 17, 21, 25, and 29)

If drug-related neurotoxicity develops, the dose should be reduced to 25 mg. If toxicity persists, treatment with liposomal cytarabine should be discontinued.

**Note:** Patients should be started on dexamethasone 4 mg twice daily (oral or I.V.) for 5 days, beginning on the day of liposomal cytarabine injection

**Dosage Forms** Injection, suspension: 10 mg/mL (5 mL) [preservative free]

**CytoGam® [US]** *see* cytomegalovirus immune globulin (intravenous-human) *on this page*

## cytomegalovirus immune globulin (intravenous-human)

(sye toe meg a low VYE rus i MYUN GLOB yoo lin in tra VEE nus HYU man)

### Sound-Alike/Look-Alike Issues

CytoGam® may be confused with Cytoxan®, Gamimune® N

(Continued)

## cytomegalovirus immune globulin (intravenous-human) *(Continued)*

**Synonyms** CMV-IGIV

**U.S./Canadian Brand Names** CytoGam® [US]

**Therapeutic Category** Immune Globulin

**Use** Prophylaxis of cytomegalovirus (CMV) disease associated with kidney, lung, liver, pancreas, and heart transplants; concomitant use with ganciclovir should be considered in organ transplants (other than kidney) from CMV seropositive donors to CMV seronegative recipients

**Usual Dosage** I.V.: Adults:

Kidney transplant:

Initial dose (within 72 hours of transplant): 150 mg/kg/dose

2-, 4-, 6-, and 8 weeks after transplant: 100 mg/kg/dose

12 and 16 weeks after transplant: 50 mg/kg/dose

Liver, lung, pancreas, or heart transplant:

Initial dose (within 72 hours of transplant): 150 mg/kg/dose

2-, 4-, 6-, and 8 weeks after transplant: 150 mg/kg/dose

12 and 16 weeks after transplant: 100 mg/kg/dose

Severe CMV pneumonia: Various regimens have been used, including 400 mg/kg CMV-IGIV in combination with ganciclovir on days 1, 2, 7, or 8, followed by 200 mg/kg CMV-IGIV on days 14 and 21

**Dosage Forms** Injection, solution [preservative free]: 50 mg ± 10 mg/mL (50 mL) [contains human albumin and sucrose]

**Cytomel® [US/Can]** *see* liothyronine *on page 484*

**Cytosar® [Can]** *see* cytarabine *on previous page*

**Cytosar-U® [US]** *see* cytarabine *on previous page*

**cytosine arabinosine hydrochloride** *see* cytarabine *on previous page*

**Cytotec® [US]** *see* misoprostol *on page 544*

**Cytovene® [US/Can]** *see* ganciclovir *on page 366*

**Cytoxan® [US/Can]** *see* cyclophosphamide *on page 214*

**Cytra-3 [US]** *see* citric acid, sodium citrate, and potassium citrate *on page 189*

**Cytra-K [US]** *see* potassium citrate and citric acid *on page 665*

**Cytuss HC [US]** *see* phenylephrine, hydrocodone, and chlorpheniramine *on page 643*

**D2E7** *see* adalimumab *on page 18*

**D₃** *see* cholecalciferol *on page 180*

**D-3-mercaptovaline** *see* penicillamine *on page 627*

**d4T** *see* stavudine *on page 765*

## dacarbazine *(da KAR ba zeen)*

**Sound-Alike/Look-Alike Issues**

dacarbazine may be confused with Dicarbosil®, procarbazine

**Synonyms** DIC; dimethyl triazeno imidazole carboxamide; DTIC; imidazole carboxamide dimethyl-triazene; imidazole carboxamide; WR-139007

**U.S./Canadian Brand Names** DTIC-Dome® [US]; DTIC® [Can]

**Therapeutic Category** Antineoplastic Agent

**Use** Treatment of malignant melanoma, Hodgkin disease, soft-tissue sarcomas, fibrosarcomas, rhabdomyosarcoma, islet cell carcinoma, medullary carcinoma of the thyroid, and neuroblastoma

**Usual Dosage** Refer to individual protocols. Some dosage regimens include:

Intra-arterial: 50-400 mg/m² for 5-10 days

I.V.:

Hodgkin disease, ABVD: 375 mg/m² days 1 and 15 every 4 weeks **or** 100 mg/m²/day for 5 days

Metastatic melanoma (alone or in combination with other agents): 150-250 mg/m² days 1-5 every 3-4 weeks

Metastatic melanoma: 850 mg/m² every 3 weeks

**High dose:** Bone marrow/blood cell transplantation: I.V.: 1-3 g/m²; maximum dose as a single agent: 3.38 g/m²; generally combined with other high-dose chemotherapeutic drugs

**Dosage Forms**

Injection, powder for reconstitution: 100 mg, 200 mg, 500 mg

DTIC-Dome®: 200 mg

## daclizumab (dac KLYE zue mab)
**U.S./Canadian Brand Names** Zenapax® [US/Can]
**Therapeutic Category** Immunosuppressant Agent
**Use** Part of an immunosuppressive regimen (including cyclosporine and corticosteroids) for the prophylaxis of acute organ rejection in patients receiving renal transplant
**Usual Dosage** Daclizumab is used adjunctively with other immunosuppressants (eg, cyclosporine, corticosteroids, mycophenolate mofetil, and azathioprine): I.V.:
Children: Use same weight-based dose as adults
Adults: Immunoprophylaxis against acute renal allograft rejection: 1 mg/kg infused over 15 minutes within 24 hours before transplantation (day 0), then every 14 days for 4 additional doses
**Dosage Forms** Injection, solution [preservative free]: 5 mg/mL (5 mL)

**Dacodyl® *(Discontinued)*** see bisacodyl *on page 107*

**DACT** see dactinomycin *on this page*

## dactinomycin (dak ti noe MYE sin)
**Sound-Alike/Look-Alike Issues**
dactinomycin may be confused with DAUNOrubicin
actinomycin may be confused with Achromycin
**Synonyms** Act-D; ACT; actinomycin Cl; actinomycin D; actinomycin; DACT; NSC-3053
**U.S./Canadian Brand Names** Cosmegen® [US/Can]
**Therapeutic Category** Antineoplastic Agent
**Use** Treatment of testicular tumors, melanoma, choriocarcinoma, Wilms tumor, neuroblastoma, retinoblastoma, rhabdomyosarcoma, uterine sarcomas, Ewing sarcoma, Kaposi sarcoma, sarcoma botryoides, and soft tissue sarcoma
**Usual Dosage** Refer to individual protocols: I.V.:
**Note: Medication orders for dactinomycin are commonly written in MICROgrams (eg, 150 mcg) although many regimens list the dose in MILLIgrams (eg, mg/kg or mg/m$^2$).** One-time doses for >1000 mcg, or multiple-day doses for >500 mcg/day are not common. Some practitioners recommend calculation of the dosage for obese or edematous patients on the basis of body surface area in an effort to relate dosage to lean body mass.
Children >6 months: 15 mcg/kg/day **or** 400-600 mcg/m$^2$/day for 5 days every 3-6 weeks
Adults: 2.5 mg/m$^2$ in divided doses over 1 week, repeated every 2 weeks **or**
0.75-2 mg/m$^2$ every 1-4 weeks **or**
400-600 mcg/m$^2$/day for 5 days, repeated every 3-6 weeks
**Dosage Forms** Injection, powder for reconstitution: 0.5 mg [contains mannitol 20 mg]

**DAD** see mitoxantrone *on page 545*

**Dairyaid® [Can]** see lactase *on page 461*

**Dakin's Solution [US]** see sodium hypochlorite solution *on page 754*

**Dakrina® Ophthalmic Solution *(Discontinued)*** see artificial tears *on page 71*

**Dalacin® C [Can]** see clindamycin *on page 192*

**Dalacin® T [Can]** see clindamycin *on page 192*

**Dalacin® Vaginal [Can]** see clindamycin *on page 192*

**Dallergy® [US]** see chlorpheniramine, phenylephrine, and methscopolamine *on page 175*

**Dallergy-D® Syrup *(Discontinued)*** see chlorpheniramine and phenylephrine *on page 171*

**Dallergy-JR® [US]** see chlorpheniramine and phenylephrine *on page 171*

**Dalmane® [US]** see flurazepam *on page 352*

***d*-alpha tocopherol** see vitamin E *on page 850*

## dalteparin (dal TE pa rin)
**U.S./Canadian Brand Names** Fragmin® [US/Can]
**Therapeutic Category** Anticoagulant (Other)
**Use** Prevention of deep vein thrombosis which may lead to pulmonary embolism, in patients requiring abdominal surgery who are at risk for thromboembolism complications (eg, patients >40 years of age, obesity, patients with malignancy, history of deep vein thrombosis or pulmonary embolism, and surgical procedures requiring general anesthesia and lasting >30 minutes); prevention of DVT in patients
(Continued)

## dalteparin *(Continued)*

undergoing hip-replacement surgery; patients immobile during an acute illness; acute treatment of unstable angina or non-Q-wave myocardial infarction; prevention of ischemic complications in patients on concurrent aspirin therapy

**Usual Dosage** Adults: SubQ:

Abdominal surgery:

Low-to-moderate DVT risk: 2500 int. units 1-2 hours prior to surgery, then once daily for 5-10 days postoperatively

High DVT risk: 5000 int. units 1-2 hours prior to surgery and then once daily for 5-10 days postoperatively

Patients undergoing total hip surgery: **Note:** Three treatment options are currently available. Dose is given for 5-10 days, although up to 14 days of treatment have been tolerated in clinical trials:

Postoperative start:

Initial: 2500 int. units 4-8 hours* after surgery

Maintenance: 5000 int. units once daily; start at least 6 hours after postsurgical dose

Preoperative (starting day of surgery):

Initial: 2500 int. units within 2 hours before surgery

Adjustment: 2500 int. units 4-8 hours* after surgery

Maintenance: 5000 int. units once daily; start at least 6 hours after postsurgical dose

Preoperative (starting evening prior to surgery):

Initial: 5000 int. units 10-14 hours before surgery

Adjustment: 5000 int. units 4-8 hours* after surgery

Maintenance: 5000 int. units once daily, allowing 24 hours between doses.

**\*Dose may be delayed if hemostasis is not yet achieved.**

Unstable angina or non-Q-wave myocardial infarction: 120 int. units/kg body weight (maximum dose: 10,000 int. units) every 12 hours for 5-8 days with concurrent aspirin therapy. Discontinue dalteparin once patient is clinically stable.

Immobility during acute illness: 5000 int. units once daily

**Dosage Forms**

Injection, solution [multidose vial]: Antifactor Xa 10,000 int. units per 1 mL (9.5 mL) [contains benzyl alcohol]; antifactor Xa 25,000 units per 1 mL (3.8 mL) [contains benzyl alcohol]

Injection, solution [preservative free; prefilled syringe]: Antifactor Xa 2500 int. units per 0.2 mL (0.2 mL); antifactor Xa 5000 int. units per 0.2 mL (0.2 mL); antifactor Xa 7500 int. units per 0.3 mL (0.3 mL); antifactor Xa 10,000 int. units per 1 mL (1 mL)

**Damason-P® [US]** *see* hydrocodone and aspirin *on page 412*

## danaparoid (da NAP a roid)

**Synonyms** danaparoid sodium

**U.S./Canadian Brand Names** Orgaran® [Can]

**Therapeutic Category** Anticoagulant (Other)

**Use** Prevention of postoperative deep vein thrombosis following elective hip replacement surgery

**Usual Dosage** SubQ:

Children: Safety and effectiveness have not been established.

Adults: Prevention of DVT following hip replacement: 750 anti-Xa units twice daily; beginning 1-4 hours before surgery and then not sooner than 2 hours after surgery and every 12 hours until the risk of DVT has diminished. The average duration of therapy is 7-10 days.

**Dosage Forms** Injection, solution, as sodium 750 anti-Xa units/0.6 mL (0.6 mL) [prefilled syringe or ampul; contains sodium sulfite]

**danaparoid sodium** *see* danaparoid *on this page*

## danazol (DA na zole)

**Sound-Alike/Look-Alike Issues**

danazol may be confused with Dantrium®

Danocrine® may be confused with Dacriose®

**U.S./Canadian Brand Names** Cyclomen® [Can]; Danocrine® [Can]

**Therapeutic Category** Androgen

**Use** Treatment of endometriosis, fibrocystic breast disease, and hereditary angioedema

**Usual Dosage** Adults: Oral:

Female: Endometriosis: Initial: 200-400 mg/day in 2 divided doses for mild disease; individualize dosage. Usual maintenance dose: 800 mg/day in 2 divided doses to achieve amenorrhea and rapid response to painful symptoms. Continue therapy uninterrupted for 3-6 months (up to 9 months).

Female: Fibrocystic breast disease: Range: 100-400 mg/day in 2 divided doses

Male/Female: Hereditary angioedema: Initial: 200 mg 2-3 times/day; after favorable response, decrease the dosage by 50% or less at intervals of 1-3 months or longer if the frequency of attacks dictates. If an attack occurs, increase the dosage by up to 200 mg/day.

**Dosage Forms** [DSC] = Discontinued product

Capsule: 50 mg, 100 mg, 200 mg

Danocrine®: 50 mg, 100 mg, 200 mg [DSC]

**Danocrine® [Can]** *see danazol on previous page*

**Danocrine® (Discontinued)** *see danazol on previous page*

**Dantrium® [US/Can]** *see dantrolene on this page*

# dantrolene (DAN troe leen)

**Sound-Alike/Look-Alike Issues**

Dantrium® may be confused with danazol, Daraprim®

**Synonyms** dantrolene sodium

**U.S./Canadian Brand Names** Dantrium® [US/Can]

**Therapeutic Category** Skeletal Muscle Relaxant

**Use** Treatment of spasticity associated with spinal cord injury, stroke, cerebral palsy, or multiple sclerosis; treatment of malignant hyperthermia

**Usual Dosage**

Spasticity: Oral:

Children: Initial: 0.5 mg/kg/dose twice daily, increase frequency to 3-4 times/day at 4- to 7-day intervals, then increase dose by 0.5 mg/kg to a maximum of 3 mg/kg/dose 2-4 times/day up to 400 mg/day

Adults: 25 mg/day to start, increase frequency to 2-4 times/day, then increase dose by 25 mg every 4-7 days to a maximum of 100 mg 2-4 times/day or 400 mg/day

Malignant hyperthermia: Children and Adults:

Preoperative prophylaxis:

Oral: 4-8 mg/kg/day in 4 divided doses, begin 1-2 days prior to surgery with last dose 3-4 hours prior to surgery

I.V.: 2.5 mg/kg ~1¼ hours prior to anesthesia and infused over 1 hour with additional doses as needed and individualized

Crisis: I.V.: 2.5 mg/kg; may repeat dose up to cumulative dose of 10 mg/kg; if physiologic and metabolic abnormalities reappear, repeat regimen

Postcrisis follow-up: Oral: 4-8 mg/kg/day in 4 divided doses for 1-3 days; I.V. dantrolene may be used when oral therapy is not practical; individualize dosage beginning with 1 mg/kg or more as the clinical situation dictates

**Dosage Forms**

Capsule, as sodium: 25 mg, 50 mg, 100 mg

Injection, powder for reconstitution, as sodium: 20 mg [contains mannitol 3 g]

**dantrolene sodium** *see dantrolene on this page*

**dapcin** *see daptomycin on next page*

# dapiprazole (DA pi pray zole)

**Synonyms** dapiprazole hydrochloride

**U.S./Canadian Brand Names** Rēv-Eyes™ [US]

**Therapeutic Category** Alpha-Adrenergic Blocking Agent

**Use** Reverse dilation due to drugs (adrenergic or parasympathomimetic) after eye exams

**Usual Dosage** Adults: Ophthalmic: Instill 2 drops followed 5 minutes later by an additional 2 drops into the conjunctiva of each eye; should not be used more frequently than once a week in the same patient

**Dosage Forms** Powder, ophthalmic, as hydrochloride: 25 mg [contains benzalkonium chloride; 0.5% solution when mixed with supplied diluent]

**dapiprazole hydrochloride** *see dapiprazole on this page*

## dapsone (DAP sone)

**Sound-Alike/Look-Alike Issues**
dapsone may be confused with Diprosone®

**Synonyms** diaminodiphenylsulfone

**U.S./Canadian Brand Names** Aczone™ [US]

**Therapeutic Category** Sulfone

**Use** Treatment of leprosy and dermatitis herpetiformis (infections caused by *Mycobacterium leprae*); treatment of acne vulgaris

**Usual Dosage** Oral:
Leprosy:
Children: 1-2 mg/kg/24 hours, up to a maximum of 100 mg/day
Adults: 50-100 mg/day for 3-10 years
Dermatitis herpetiformis: Adults: Start at 50 mg/day, increase to 300 mg/day, or higher to achieve full control, reduce dosage to minimum level as soon as possible
Topical: Acne vulgaris: Children ≥12 years and Adults: Apply pea-sized amount twice daily

**Dosage Forms**
Gel, topical (Aczone™): 5% (30 g)
Tablet: 25 mg, 100 mg

**Daptacel® [US]** *see* diphtheria, tetanus toxoids, and acellular pertussis vaccine *on page 259*

## daptomycin (DAP toe mye sin)

**Synonyms** Cidecin; dapcin; LY146032

**U.S./Canadian Brand Names** Cubicin™ [US]

**Therapeutic Category** Antibiotic, Cyclic Lipopeptide

**Use** Treatment of complicated skin and skin structure infections caused by susceptible aerobic Gram-positive organisms

**Usual Dosage** I.V.: Adults: Skin and soft tissue: 4 mg/kg once daily for 7-14 days

**Dosage Forms** Injection, powder for reconstitution: 250 mg, 500 mg

**Daranide® [US/Can]** *see* dichlorphenamide *on page 243*

**Daraprim® [US/Can]** *see* pyrimethamine *on page 701*

## darbepoetin alfa (dar be POE e tin AL fa)

**Sound-Alike/Look-Alike Issues**
darbepoetin alfa may be confused with epoetin alfa

**Synonyms** erythropoiesis stimulating protein

**U.S./Canadian Brand Names** Aranesp® [US/Can]

**Therapeutic Category** Colony-Stimulating Factor; Growth Factor; Recombinant Human Erythropoietin

**Use** Treatment of anemia associated with chronic renal failure (CRF), including patients on dialysis (ESRD) and patients not on dialysis; anemia associated with chemotherapy for nonmyeloid malignancies

**Usual Dosage** Adults:
Anemia associated with CRF: I.V., SubQ: Initial: 0.45 mcg/kg once weekly; titrate to response; some patients may respond to doses given once every 2 weeks
Anemia associated with chemotherapy: SubQ: Initial: 2.25 mcg/kg once weekly; with inadequate response: 4.5 mcg/kg once weekly
Treatment goals: **Note:** Titration may be required to limit rises of Hgb to <1 g/dL over any 2-week interval and to reach a Hgb concentration not to exceed 12 g/dL.
Inadequate response: Increase dose; refer to individual dosing regimens for adjustment when Hgb increase <1 g/dL after 4-6 weeks
Excessive response: Hold dose and/or decrease dose by 25%
Decrease dose by 25% when Hgb increases >1 g/dL in any 2-week period **or** Hgb increases and approaches 12 g/dL in any 2-week period
Hold dose, then decrease dose by 25% when Hgb increases despite previous dose decrease (hold until Hgb decreases) **or** when Hgb ≥13g/dL (hold until Hgb ≤12 g/dL)

**Dosage Forms**
Injection, solution, with human albumin 2.5 mg/mL [preservative free, single-dose vial]: 25 mcg/mL (1 mL); 40 mcg/mL (1 mL); 60 mcg/mL (1 mL); 100 mcg/mL (1 mL); 150 mcg/0.75 mL (0.75 mL); 200 mcg/mL (1 mL); 300 mcg/mL (1 mL)

Injection, solution, with human albumin 2.5 mg/mL [preservative free, prefilled syringe]: 25 mcg/0.42 mL (0.42 mL); 40 mcg/0.4 mL (0.4 mL); 60 mcg/0.3 mL (0.3 mL); 100 mcg/0.5 mL (0.5 mL); 200 mcg/0.4 mL (0.4 mL); 300 mcg/0.6 mL (0.6 mL); 500 mcg/mL (1 mL)

## darifenacin (dar i FEN a sin)

**Synonyms** darifenacin hydrobromide; UK-88,525
**U.S./Canadian Brand Names** Enablex® [US]
**Therapeutic Category** Anticholinergic Agent
**Use** Management of symptoms of bladder overactivity (urge incontinence, urgency, and frequency)
**Usual Dosage** Oral: Adults: Initial: 7.5 mg once daily. If response is not adequate after a minimum of 2 weeks, dosage may be increased to 15 mg once daily. Dosage should not be increased in patients with hepatic impairment or in those receiving potent inhibitors of CYP3A4.
**Dosage Forms** Tablet, extended release: 7.5 mg, 15 mg

**darifenacin hydrobromide** *see* darifenacin *on this page*

**Darvocet A500™ [US]** *see* propoxyphene and acetaminophen *on page 687*

**Darvocet-N® 50 [US/Can]** *see* propoxyphene and acetaminophen *on page 687*

**Darvocet-N® 100 [US/Can]** *see* propoxyphene and acetaminophen *on page 687*

**Darvon® [US]** *see* propoxyphene *on page 687*

**Darvon® Compound [US]** *see* propoxyphene, aspirin, and caffeine *on page 688*

**Darvon-N® [US/Can]** *see* propoxyphene *on page 687*

**daunomycin** *see* daunorubicin hydrochloride *on this page*

## daunorubicin citrate (liposomal) (daw noe ROO bi sin SI trate lip po SOE mal)

**Sound-Alike/Look-Alike Issues**
Sound-alike/look-alike issues:
DAUNOrubicin may be confused with dactinomycin, DOXOrubicin, epirubicin, idarubicin
liposomal formulations (DaunoXome®) may be confused with conventional formulations (Adriamycin PFS®, Adriamycin RDF®, Cerubidine®, Rubex®)
**Tall-Man DAUNO**rubicin citrate (liposomal)
**U.S./Canadian Brand Names** DaunoXome® [US]
**Therapeutic Category** Antineoplastic Agent
**Use** First-line cytotoxic therapy for advanced HIV-associated Kaposi sarcoma
**Usual Dosage** Refer to individual protocols. Adults: I.V.:
20-40 mg/m$^2$ every 2 weeks
100 mg/m$^2$ every 3 weeks
**Dosage Forms** Injection, solution [preservative free]: 2 mg/mL (25 mL) [contains sucrose 2125 mg/25 mL]

## daunorubicin hydrochloride (daw noe ROO bi sin hye droe KLOR ide)

**Sound-Alike/Look-Alike Issues**
Sound-alike/look-alike issues:
DAUNOrubicin may be confused with dactinomycin, DOXOrubicin, epirubicin, idarubicin
conventional formulations (Cerubidine®) may be confused with liposomal formulations (DaunoXome®, Doxil®)
**Synonyms** daunomycin; DNR; NSC-82151; rubidomycin hydrochloride
**Tall-Man DAUNO**rubicin hydrochloride
**U.S./Canadian Brand Names** Cerubidine® [US/Can]
**Therapeutic Category** Antineoplastic Agent
**Use** Treatment of acute lymphocytic (ALL) and nonlymphocytic (ANLL) leukemias
**Usual Dosage** I.V. (refer to individual protocols):
Children:
ALL combination therapy: Remission induction: 25-45 mg/m$^2$ on day 1 every week for 4 cycles **or** 30-45 mg/m$^2$/day for 3 days
AML combination therapy: Induction: I.V. continuous infusion: 30-60 mg/m$^2$/day on days 1-3 of cycle
**Note:** In children <2 years or <0.5 m$^2$, daunorubicin should be based on weight - mg/kg: 1 mg/kg per protocol with frequency dependent on regimen employed
*Cumulative dose should not exceed 300 mg/m$^2$ in children >2 years; maximum cumulative doses for younger children are unknown.*
(Continued)

## daunorubicin hydrochloride *(Continued)*

Adults:

Range: 30-60 mg/m$^2$/day for 3-5 days, repeat dose in 3-4 weeks

AML: Single agent induction: 60 mg/m$^2$/day for 3 days; repeat every 3-4 weeks

AML: Combination therapy induction: 45 mg/m$^2$/day for 3 days of the first course of induction therapy; subsequent courses: Every day for 2 days

ALL combination therapy: 45 mg/m$^2$/day for 3 days

*Cumulative dose should not exceed 400-600 mg/m$^2$*

**Dosage Forms**

Injection, powder for reconstitution: 20 mg, 50 mg

Cerubidine®: 20 mg

Injection, solution: 5 mg/mL (4 mL, 10 mL)

**DaunoXome® [US]** *see* daunorubicin citrate (liposomal) *on previous page*

**1-Day™ [US-OTC]** *see* tioconazole *on page 805*

**Dayhist® Allergy [US-OTC]** *see* clemastine *on page 191*

**Daypro® [US/Can]** *see* oxaprozin *on page 605*

**Dayto Himbin®** *(Discontinued)* *see* yohimbine *on page 857*

**DC 240® Softgel®** *(Discontinued)* *see* docusate *on page 263*

**dCF** *see* pentostatin *on page 632*

**DDAVP® [US/Can]** *see* desmopressin acetate *on page 230*

**ddC** *see* zalcitabine *on page 857*

**ddI** *see* didanosine *on page 245*

**1-deamino-8-D-arginine vasopressin** *see* desmopressin acetate *on page 230*

**Debrox® [US-OTC]** *see* carbamide peroxide *on page 141*

**Decadron® [US]** *see* dexamethasone (ophthalmic) *on page 232*

**Decadron® Phosphate** *(Discontinued)* *see* dexamethasone (systemic) *on page 233*

**Deca-Durabolin® [Can]** *see* nandrolone *on page 560*

**Deca-Durabolin®** *(Discontinued)* *see* nandrolone *on page 560*

**Decahist-DM [US]** *see* carbinoxamine, pseudoephedrine, and dextromethorphan *on page 145*

**Decavac™ [US]** *see* diphtheria and tetanus toxoid *on page 257*

**De-Chlor DM [US]** *see* chlorpheniramine, phenylephrine, and dextromethorphan *on page 174*

**De-Chlor DR [US]** *see* chlorpheniramine, phenylephrine, and dextromethorphan *on page 174*

**De-Chlor HC [US]** *see* phenylephrine, hydrocodone, and chlorpheniramine *on page 643*

**De-Chlor HD [US]** *see* phenylephrine, hydrocodone, and chlorpheniramine *on page 643*

**Declomycin® [US/Can]** *see* demeclocycline *on page 228*

**Deconamine® [US]** *see* chlorpheniramine and pseudoephedrine *on page 172*

**Deconamine® SR [US]** *see* chlorpheniramine and pseudoephedrine *on page 172*

**Deconsal® II [US]** *see* guaifenesin and phenylephrine *on page 387*

**Defen-LA®** *(Discontinued)* *see* guaifenesin and pseudoephedrine *on page 388*

## deferoxamine *(de fer OKS a meen)*

**Sound-Alike/Look-Alike Issues**

deferoxamine may be confused with cefuroxime

Desferal® may be confused with desflurane, Dexferrum®, Disophrol®

**Synonyms** deferoxamine mesylate

**U.S./Canadian Brand Names** Desferal® [US/Can]; PMS-Deferoxamine [Can]

**Therapeutic Category** Antidote

**Use** Acute iron intoxication or when clinical signs of significant iron toxicity exist; chronic iron overload secondary to multiple transfusions

## Usual Dosage

Acute iron toxicity: **Note:** I.V. route is used when severe toxicity is evidenced by systemic symptoms (coma, shock, metabolic acidosis, or severe gastrointestinal bleeding) or potentially severe intoxications (serum iron level >500 mcg/dL). When severe symptoms are not present, the I.M. route may be preferred (per manufacturer); however, the use of deferoxamine in situations where the serum iron concentration is <500 mcg/dL or when severe toxicity is not evident is a subject of some clinical debate.

Children:
  I.M.: 90 mg/kg/dose every 8 hours (maximum: 6 g/24 hours)
  I.V.: 15 mg/kg/hour (maximum: 6 g/24 hours)
Adults: I.M., I.V.: Initial: 1000 mg, may be followed by 500 mg every 4 hours for up to 2 doses; subsequent doses of 500 mg have been administered every 4-12 hours
  Maximum recommended dose: 6 g/day (per manufacturer, however, higher doses have been administered)

Chronic iron overload:
  Children: SubQ: 20-40 mg/kg/day over 8-12 hours (maximum: 1000-2000 mg/day)
  Adults:
  I.M., I.V.: 500-1000 mg/day I.M.; in addition, 2000 mg should be given I.V. with each unit of blood transfused (administer separately from blood); maximum: 6 g/day
  SubQ: 1-2 g every day over 8-24 hours

**Dosage Forms** Injection, powder for reconstitution, as mesylate: 500 mg, 2 g

**deferoxamine mesylate** *see* deferoxamine *on previous page*

**Deficol**® *(Discontinued)* *see* bisacodyl *on page 107*

**Definity**® **[US/Can]** *see* perflutren lipid microspheres *on page 633*

**Degest**® **2 Ophthalmic** *(Discontinued)* *see* naphazoline *on page 561*

**Dehistine [US]** *see* chlorpheniramine, phenylephrine, and methscopolamine *on page 175*

**Dehydral**® **[Can]** *see* methenamine *on page 522*

**dehydrobenzperidol** *see* droperidol *on page 274*

**Del Aqua**® **[US]** *see* benzoyl peroxide *on page 98*

**Delatest**® **Injection** *(Discontinued)* *see* testosterone *on page 788*

**Delatestryl**® **[US/Can]** *see* testosterone *on page 788*

## delavirdine (de la VIR deen)

**Synonyms** U-90152S
**U.S./Canadian Brand Names** Rescriptor® [US/Can]
**Therapeutic Category** Antiviral Agent
**Use** Treatment of HIV-1 infection in combination with at least two additional antiretroviral agents
**Usual Dosage** Adolescents ≥16 years and Adults: Oral: 400 mg 3 times/day
**Dosage Forms** Tablet, as mesylate: 100 mg, 200 mg

**Delestrogen**® **[US]** *see* estradiol *on page 299*

**Delfen**® **[US-OTC]** *see* nonoxynol 9 *on page 580*

**Del-Mycin**® **Topical** *(Discontinued)*

**Delsym**® **[US-OTC]** *see* dextromethorphan *on page 238*

**delta-9-tetrahydro-cannabinol** *see* dronabinol *on page 274*

**delta-9 THC** *see* dronabinol *on page 274*

**Delta-D**® **[US]** *see* cholecalciferol *on page 180*

**Delta-Cortef**® *(Discontinued)*

**deltacortisone** *see* prednisone *on page 674*

**deltadehydrocortisone** *see* prednisone *on page 674*

**deltahydrocortisone** *see* prednisolone (systemic) *on page 674*

**Delta-Tritex**® **Topical** *(Discontinued)*

**Del-Vi-A**® *(Discontinued)* *see* vitamin A *on page 848*

**Demadex**® **[US]** *see* torsemide *on page 812*

## demeclocycline (dem e kloe SYE kleen)
**Synonyms** demeclocycline hydrochloride; demethylchlortetracycline
**U.S./Canadian Brand Names** Declomycin® [US/Can]
**Therapeutic Category** Tetracycline Derivative
**Use** Treatment of susceptible bacterial infections (acne, gonorrhea, pertussis and urinary tract infections) caused by both gram-negative and gram-positive organisms
**Usual Dosage** Oral:
Children ≥8 years: 8-12 mg/kg/day divided every 6-12 hours
Adults: 150 mg 4 times/day or 300 mg twice daily
**Dosage Forms** Tablet, as hydrochloride: 150 mg, 300 mg

**demeclocycline hydrochloride** *see* demeclocycline *on this page*

**Demerol® [US/Can]** *see* meperidine *on page 512*

**4-demethoxydaunorubicin** *see* idarubicin *on page 429*

**demethylchlortetracycline** *see* demeclocycline *on this page*

**Demser® [US/Can]** *see* metyrosine *on page 536*

**Demulen® [US]** *see* ethinyl estradiol and ethynodiol diacetate *on page 310*

**Demulen® 30 [Can]** *see* ethinyl estradiol and ethynodiol diacetate *on page 310*

**Denavir® [US]** *see* penciclovir *on page 627*

## denileukin diftitox (de ni LOO kin DIF ti toks)
**U.S./Canadian Brand Names** ONTAK® [US]
**Therapeutic Category** Antineoplastic Agent, Miscellaneous
**Use** Treatment of persistent or recurrent cutaneous T-cell lymphoma whose malignant cells express the CD25 component of the IL-2 receptor
**Usual Dosage** Adults: I.V.: A treatment cycle consists of 9 or 18 mcg/kg/day for 5 consecutive days administered every 21 days. The optimal duration of therapy has not been determined. Only 2% of patients who failed to demonstrate a response (at least a 25% decrease in tumor burden) prior to the fourth cycle responded to subsequent treatment.
**Dosage Forms** Injection, solution [frozen]: 150 mcg/mL (2 mL)

**Dentapaine [US-OTC]** *see* benzocaine *on page 95*

**Dent's Ear Wax [US-OTC]** *see* carbamide peroxide *on page 141*

**Dent's Extra Strength Toothache [US-OTC]** *see* benzocaine *on page 95*

**Dent's Maxi-Strength Toothache [US-OTC]** *see* benzocaine *on page 95*

**deoxycoformycin** *see* pentostatin *on page 632*

**2'-deoxycoformycin** *see* pentostatin *on page 632*

**Depacon® [US]** *see* valproic acid and derivatives *on page 837*

**Depade® [US]** *see* naltrexone *on page 560*

**Depakene® [US/Can]** *see* valproic acid and derivatives *on page 837*

**Depakote® Delayed Release [US]** *see* valproic acid and derivatives *on page 837*

**Depakote® ER [US]** *see* valproic acid and derivatives *on page 837*

**Depakote® Sprinkle® [US]** *see* valproic acid and derivatives *on page 837*

**depAndro® Injection *(Discontinued)*** *see* testosterone *on page 788*

**Depen® [US/Can]** *see* penicillamine *on page 627*

**depGynogen® Injection *(Discontinued)*** *see* estradiol *on page 299*

**depMedalone® Injection *(Discontinued)*** *see* methylprednisolone *on page 531*

**DepoCyt™ [US/Can]** *see* cytarabine (liposomal) *on page 219*

**DepoDur™ [US]** *see* morphine sulfate *on page 549*

**Depo®-Estradiol [US/Can]** *see* estradiol *on page 299*

**Depoject® Injection *(Discontinued)*** *see* methylprednisolone *on page 531*

**Depo-Medrol® [US/Can]** *see* methylprednisolone *on page 531*

**Deponit® Patch *(Discontinued)*** see nitroglycerin *on page 578*

**Depo-Prevera® [Can]** see medroxyprogesterone acetate *on page 507*

**Depo-Provera® [US]** see medroxyprogesterone acetate *on page 507*

**Depo-Provera® Contraceptive [US]** see medroxyprogesterone acetate *on page 507*

**depo-subQ provera 104™ [US]** see medroxyprogesterone acetate *on page 507*

**Depotest® 100 [Can]** see testosterone *on page 788*

**Depotest® Injection *(Discontinued)*** see testosterone *on page 788*

**Depo®-Testosterone [US]** see testosterone *on page 788*

**deprenyl** see selegiline *on page 742*

## dequalinium *(Canada only)* (de kwal LI ne um)

**Therapeutic Category** Antibacterial, Topical; Antifungal Agent, Topical
**Use** Treatment of mouth and throat infections
**Usual Dosage** Adults:
Lozenge: One lozenge sucked slowly every 2-3 hours
Oral paint: Apply freely to infected area, every 2-3 hours, or as directed by physician
**Dosage Forms**
Lozenge, as chloride: 0.25 mg (20s)
Oral paint, as chloride: 0.5% (25 mL)

**Dermaflex® Gel *(Discontinued)*** see lidocaine *on page 479*

**DermaFungal [US-OTC]** see miconazole *on page 537*

**Dermagran® [US-OTC]** see aluminum hydroxide *on page 34*

**Dermagran® AF [US-OTC]** see miconazole *on page 537*

**Dermamycin® [US-OTC]** see diphenhydramine *on page 254*

**Dermarest Dricort® [US-OTC]** see hydrocortisone (topical) *on page 417*

**Dermarest® Insect Bite [US-OTC]** see diphenhydramine *on page 254*

**Dermarest® Plus [US-OTC]** see diphenhydramine *on page 254*

**Dermarest® Skin Correction Cream Plus [US-OTC]** see hydroquinone *on page 420*

**Derma-Smoothe/FS® [US/Can]** see fluocinolone *on page 344*

**Dermatop® [US/Can]** see prednicarbate *on page 673*

**Dermatophytin-O *(Discontinued)***

**Dermazene® [US]** see iodoquinol and hydrocortisone *on page 445*

**Dermazole [Can]** see miconazole *on page 537*

**Dermoplast® Antibacterial [US-OTC]** see benzocaine *on page 95*

**Dermoplast® Pain Relieving [US-OTC]** see benzocaine *on page 95*

**Dermovate® [Can]** see clobetasol *on page 194*

**Dermtex® HC [US-OTC]** see hydrocortisone (topical) *on page 417*

**deserpidine and methyclothiazide** see methyclothiazide and deserpidine *on page 528*

**Desferal® [US/Can]** see deferoxamine *on page 226*

## desflurane (DES flure ane)

**Sound-Alike/Look-Alike Issues**
desflurane may be confused with Desferal®
**U.S./Canadian Brand Names** Suprane® [US/Can]
**Therapeutic Category** General Anesthetic
**Use** Maintenance of general anesthesia
**Usual Dosage**
Children: Maintenance: Surgical levels of anesthesia range between 5.2% to 10%
Adults: The minimum alveolar concentration (MAC), the concentration at which 50% of patients do not respond to surgical incision, ranges from 6.0% (45 years of age) to 7.3% (25 years of age). The concentration at which amnesia and loss of awareness occur (MAC - awake) is 2.4%. Surgical levels of anesthesia are achieved with concentrations between 2.5% to 8.5%.
(Continued)

## desflurane *(Continued)*

**Note:** Because of the higher vapor pressure of desflurane, its vaporizer is heated in order to deliver a constant concentration

**Dosage Forms** Liquid, for inhalation: 240 mL

**desiccated thyroid** *see* thyroid *on page 800*

## desipramine (des IP ra meen)

**Sound-Alike/Look-Alike Issues**

desipramine may be confused with clomiPRAMINE, deserpidine, diphenhydrAMINE, disopyramide, imipramine, nortriptyline

Norpramin® may be confused with clomiPRAMINE, imipramine, Norpace®, nortriptyline, Tenormin®

**Synonyms** desipramine hydrochloride; desmethylimipramine hydrochloride

**U.S./Canadian Brand Names** Alti-Desipramine [Can]; Apo-Desipramine® [Can]; Norpramin® [US/Can]; Nu-Desipramine [Can]; PMS-Desipramine [Can]

**Therapeutic Category** Antidepressant, Tricyclic (Secondary Amine)

**Use** Treatment of depression

**Usual Dosage** Oral (dose is generally administered at bedtime):

Adolescents: Depression: Initial: 25-50 mg/day; gradually increase to 100 mg/day in single or divided doses (maximum: 150 mg/day)

Adults: Depression: Initial: 75 mg/day in divided doses; increase gradually to 150-200 mg/day in divided or single dose (maximum: 300 mg/day)

**Dosage Forms** Tablet, as hydrochloride: 10 mg, 25 mg, 50 mg, 75 mg, 100 mg, 150 mg

**desipramine hydrochloride** *see* desipramine *on this page*

**Desitin® [US-OTC]** *see* zinc oxide *on page 861*

**Desitin® Creamy [US-OTC]** *see* zinc oxide *on page 861*

## desloratadine (des lor AT a deen)

**U.S./Canadian Brand Names** Aerius® [Can]; Clarinex® [US]

**Therapeutic Category** Antihistamine, Nonsedating

**Use** Relief of nasal and non-nasal symptoms of seasonal allergic rhinitis (SAR) and perennial allergic rhinitis (PAR); treatment of chronic idiopathic urticaria (CIU)

**Usual Dosage** Oral:

Children:

6-11 months: 1 mg once daily

12 months to 5 years: 1.25 mg once daily

6-11 years: 2.5 mg once daily

Children ≥12 years and Adults: 5 mg once daily

**Dosage Forms**

Syrup (Clarinex®): 0.5 mg/mL (120 mL, 480 mL) [bubble gum flavor]

Tablet (Clarinex®): 5 mg

Tablet, orally-disintegrating (Clarinex® RediTabs®): 2.5 mg [contains phenylalanine 1.28 mg/tablet; tutti-frutti flavor]; 5 mg [contains phenylalanine 2.55 mg/tablet; tutti-frutti flavor]

**desmethylimipramine hydrochloride** *see* desipramine *on this page*

## desmopressin acetate (des moe PRES in AS e tate)

**Synonyms** 1-deamino-8-D-arginine vasopressin

**U.S./Canadian Brand Names** Apo-Desmopressin® [Can]; DDAVP® [US/Can]; Minirin® [Can]; Octostim® [Can]; Stimate™ [US]

**Therapeutic Category** Vasopressin Analog, Synthetic

**Use** Treatment of diabetes insipidus; control of bleeding in hemophilia A, and mild-to-moderate classic von Willebrand disease (type I); primary nocturnal enuresis

**Usual Dosage**

Children:

Diabetes insipidus:

Intranasal (using 100 mcg/mL nasal solution): 3 months to 12 years: Initial: 5 mcg/day (0.05 mL/day) divided 1-2 times/day; range: 5-30 mcg/day (0.05-0.3 mL/day) divided 1-2 times/day; adjust morning and evening doses separately for an adequate diurnal rhythm of water turnover; doses <10 mcg should be administered using the rhinal tube system

Oral: ≥4 years: Initial: 0.05 mg twice daily; total daily dose should be increased or decreased as needed to obtain adequate antidiuresis (range: 0.1-1.2 mg divided 2-3 times/day)

Hemophilia A and von Willebrand disease (type I):

I.V.: >3 months: 0.3 mcg/kg by slow infusion; may repeat dose if needed; begin 30 minutes before procedure

Intranasal: ≥11 months: Refer to adult dosing.

Nocturnal enuresis:

Intranasal (using 100 mcg/mL nasal solution): ≥6 years: Initial: 20 mcg (0.2 mL) at bedtime; range: 10-40 mcg; it is recommended that $1/_2$ of the dose be given in each nostril

Oral: 0.2 mg at bedtime; dose may be titrated up to 0.6 mg to achieve desired response. Patients previously on intranasal therapy can begin oral tablets 24 hours after the last intranasal dose.

Children ≥12 years and Adults:

Diabetes insipidus:

I.V., SubQ: 2-4 mcg/day (0.5-1 mL) in 2 divided doses or $1/_{10}$ of the maintenance intranasal dose

Intranasal (using 100 mcg/mL nasal solution): 10-40 mcg/day (0.1-0.4 mL) divided 1-3 times/day; adjust morning and evening doses separately for an adequate diurnal rhythm of water turnover. **Note:** The nasal spray pump can only deliver doses of 10 mcg (0.1 mL) or multiples of 10 mcg (0.1 mL); if doses other than this are needed, the rhinal tube delivery system is preferred.

Oral: Initial: 0.05 mg twice daily; total daily dose should be increased or decreased as needed to obtain adequate antidiuresis (range: 0.1-1.2 mg divided 2-3 times/day)

Hemophilia A and mild to moderate von Willebrand disease (type I):

I.V.: 0.3 mcg/kg by slow infusion, begin 30 minutes before procedure

Intranasal: Using high concentration spray (1.5 mg/mL): <50 kg: 150 mcg (1 spray); >50 kg: 300 mcg (1 spray each nostril); repeat use is determined by the patient's clinical condition and laboratory work; if using preoperatively, administer 2 hours before surgery

**Dosage Forms**

Injection, solution, as acetate (DDAVP®): 4 mcg/mL (1 mL, 10 mL)

Solution, intranasal, as acetate (DDAVP®): 100 mcg/mL (2.5 mL) [with rhinal tube]

Solution, intranasal spray, as acetate: 100 mcg/mL (5 mL) [delivers 10 mcg/spray]

DDAVP®: 100 mcg/mL (5 mL) [delivers 10 mcg/spray]

Stimate™: 1.5 mg/mL (2.5 mL) [delivers 150 mcg/spray]

Tablet, as acetate (DDAVP®): 0.1 mg, 0.2 mg

**Desocort® [Can]** see desonide on this page

**Desogen® [US]** see ethinyl estradiol and desogestrel on page 309

**desogestrel and ethinyl estradiol** see ethinyl estradiol and desogestrel on page 309

# desonide (DES oh nide)

**U.S./Canadian Brand Names** Desocort® [Can]; DesOwen® [US]; LoKara™ [US]; PMS-Desonide [Can]; Tridesilon® [US]

**Therapeutic Category** Corticosteroid, Topical

**Use** Adjunctive therapy for inflammation in acute and chronic corticosteroid responsive dermatosis (low potency corticosteroid)

**Usual Dosage** Corticosteroid responsive dermatoses: Topical: Apply 2-4 times/day sparingly. Therapy should be discontinued when control is achieved; if no improvement is seen, reassessment of diagnosis may be necessary.

**Dosage Forms**

Cream, topical: 0.05% (15 g, 60 g)

DesOwen®: 0.05% (15 g, 60 g, 90 g)

Tridesilon®: 0.05% (15 g)

Lotion, topical (DesOwen®, LoKara™): 0.05% (60 mL, 120 mL)

Ointment, topical: 0.05% (15 g, 60 g)

DesOwen®: 0.05% (15 g, 60 g)

Tridesilon®: 0.05% (15 g)

**DesOwen® [US]** see desonide on this page

## desoximetasone (des oks i MET a sone)

**Sound-Alike/Look-Alike Issues**
desoximetasone may be confused with dexamethasone
Topicort® may be confused with Topic®

**U.S./Canadian Brand Names** Taro-Desoximetasone [Can]; Topicort® [US/Can]; Topicort®-LP [US]

**Therapeutic Category** Corticosteroid, Topical

**Use** Relieves inflammation and pruritic symptoms of corticosteroid-responsive dermatosis (intermediate-to high-potency topical corticosteroid)

**Usual Dosage** Desoximetasone is a potent fluorinated topical corticosteroid. Therapy should be discontinued when control is achieved; if no improvement is seen, reassessment of diagnosis may be necessary.

Cream, gel: Children and Adults: Apply a thin film to affected area twice daily
Ointment: Children ≥10 years and Adults: Apply a thin film to affected area twice daily

**Dosage Forms**
Cream, topical: 0.25% (15 g, 60 g); 0.05% (15 g, 60 g)
Topicort®: 0.25% (15 g, 60 g)
Topicort®-LP: 0.05% (15 g, 60 g)
Gel, topical (Topicort®): 0.05% (15 g, 60 g) [contains alcohol 20%]
Ointment, topical (Topicort®): 0.25% (15 g, 60 g)

**desoxyephedrine hydrochloride** see methamphetamine on page 522

**Desoxyn®** **[US/Can]** see methamphetamine on page 522

**desoxyphenobarbital** see primidone on page 678

**Desquam-X®** **[US/Can]** see benzoyl peroxide on page 98

**Desquam-X® Wash** *(Discontinued)* see benzoyl peroxide on page 98

**Desquam-E™** **[US]** see benzoyl peroxide on page 98

**Desyrel®** **[US/Can]** see trazodone on page 817

**Detane®** **[US-OTC]** see benzocaine on page 95

**Detrol®** **[US/Can]** see tolterodine on page 810

**Detrol® LA** **[US]** see tolterodine on page 810

**Detuss** **[US]** see pseudoephedrine, hydrocodone, and chlorpheniramine on page 695

**Detussin® Expectorant** *(Discontinued)* see hydrocodone, pseudoephedrine, and guaifenesin on page 415

**Dex4 Glucose** **[US-OTC]** see glucose (instant) on page 377

**Dexacidin®** *(Discontinued)* see neomycin, polymyxin B, and dexamethasone on page 567

**Dexacine™** *(Discontinued)* see neomycin, polymyxin B, and dexamethasone on page 567

**Dexalone®** **[US-OTC]** see dextromethorphan on page 238

**dexamethasone and ciprofloxacin** see ciprofloxacin and dexamethasone on page 186

**dexamethasone and neomycin** see neomycin and dexamethasone on page 566

**dexamethasone and tobramycin** see tobramycin and dexamethasone on page 808

**Dexamethasone Intensol®** **[US]** see dexamethasone (systemic) on next page

**dexamethasone, neomycin, and polymyxin B** see neomycin, polymyxin B, and dexamethasone on page 567

## dexamethasone (ophthalmic) (deks a METH a sone op THAL mik)

**Sound-Alike/Look-Alike Issues**
dexamethasone may be confused with desoximetasone
Maxidex® may be confused with Maxzide®

**Synonyms** dexamethasone sodium phosphate

**U.S./Canadian Brand Names** Decadron® [US]; Maxidex® [US/Can]

**Therapeutic Category** Adrenal Corticosteroid

**Use** Inflammatory or allergic conjunctivitis

**Usual Dosage** Adults: Ophthalmic:
Ointment: Apply thin coating into conjunctival sac 3-4 times/day; gradually taper dose to discontinue

Suspension: Instill 2 drops into conjunctival sac every hour during the day and every other hour during the night; gradually reduce dose to every 3-4 hours, then to 3-4 times/day

**Dosage Forms**

Ointment, ophthalmic, as sodium phosphate: 0.05% (3.5 g)

Solution, ophthalmic, as sodium phosphate: 0.1% (5 mL)

Suspension, ophthalmic (Maxidex®): 0.1% (5 mL, 15 mL)

**dexamethasone sodium phosphate** *see* dexamethasone (ophthalmic) *on previous page*

# dexamethasone (systemic) (deks a METH a sone sis TEM ik)

**Sound-Alike/Look-Alike Issues**

dexamethasone may be confused with desoximetasone

Decadron® may be confused with Percodan®

**U.S./Canadian Brand Names** Apo-Dexamethasone® [Can]; Decadron® [US]; Dexamethasone Intensol® [US]; Dexasone® [Can]; DexPak® TaperPak® [US]; Diodex® [Can]; PMS-Dexamethasone [Can]

**Therapeutic Category** Adrenal Corticosteroid

**Use** Systemically and locally for chronic swelling; allergic, hematologic, neoplastic, and autoimmune diseases; may be used in management of cerebral edema, septic shock, as a diagnostic agent, antiemetic

**Usual Dosage**

Children:

Antiemetic (prior to chemotherapy): I.V. (should be given as sodium phosphate): 5-20 mg given 15-30 minutes before treatment

Antiinflammatory immunosuppressant: Oral, I.M., I.V. (injections should be given as sodium phosphate): 0.08-0.3 mg/kg/day **or** 2.5-10 mg/m²/day in divided doses every 6-12 hours

Extubation or airway edema: Oral, I.M., I.V. (injections should be given as sodium phosphate): 0.5-2 mg/kg/day in divided doses every 6 hours beginning 24 hours prior to extubation and continuing for 4-6 doses afterwards

Cerebral edema: I.V. (should be given as sodium phosphate): Loading dose: 1-2 mg/kg/dose as a single dose; maintenance: 1-1.5 mg/kg/day (maximum: 16 mg/day) in divided doses every 4-6 hours for 5 days then taper for 5 days, then discontinue

Bacterial meningitis in infants and children >2 months: I.V. (should be given as sodium phosphate): 0.6 mg/kg/day in 4 divided doses every 6 hours for the first 4 days of antibiotic treatment; start dexamethasone at the time of the first dose of antibiotic

Physiologic replacement: Oral, I.M., I.V.: 0.03-0.15 mg/kg/day **or** 0.6-0.75 mg/m²/day in divided doses every 6-12 hours

Adults:

Antiemetic:

Prophylaxis: Oral, I.V.: 10-20 mg 15-30 minutes before treatment on each treatment day

Continuous infusion regimen: Oral or I.V.: 10 mg every 12 hours on each treatment day

Mildly emetogenic therapy: Oral, I.M., I.V.: 4 mg every 4-6 hours

Delayed nausea/vomiting: Oral: 4-10 mg 1-2 times/day for 2-4 days **or**

8 mg every 12 hours for 2 days; then

4 mg every 12 hours for 2 days **or**

20 mg 1 hour before chemotherapy; then

10 mg 12 hours after chemotherapy; then

8 mg every 12 hours for 4 doses; then

4 mg every 12 hours for 4 doses

Anti-inflammatory:

Oral, I.M., I.V. (injections should be given as sodium phosphate): 0.75-9 mg/day in divided doses every 6-12 hours

Intra-articular, intralesional, or soft tissue (as sodium phosphate): 0.4-6 mg/day

Chemotherapy: Oral, I.V.: 40 mg every day for 4 days, repeated every 4 weeks (VAD regimen)

Cerebral edema: I.V. 10 mg stat, 4 mg I.M./I.V. (should be given as sodium phosphate) every 6 hours until response is maximized, then switch to oral regimen, then taper off if appropriate; dosage may be reduced after 24 days and gradually discontinued over 5-7 days

Cushing's syndrome, diagnostic: Oral: 1 mg at 11 PM, draw blood at 8 AM; greater accuracy for Cushing's syndrome may be achieved by the following:

Dexamethasone 0.5 mg by mouth every 6 hours for 48 hours (with 24-hour urine collection for 17-hydroxycorticosteroid excretion)

(Continued)

233

# dexamethasone (systemic) *(Continued)*

Differentiation of Cushing's syndrome due to ACTH excess from Cushing's due to other causes: Oral: Dexamethasone 2 mg every 6 hours for 48 hours (with 24-hour urine collection for 17-hydroxycortico-steroid excretion)

Multiple sclerosis (acute exacerbation): 30 mg/day for 1 week, followed by 4-12 mg/day for 1 month

Physiological replacement: Oral, I.M., I.V. (should be given as sodium phosphate): 0.03-0.15 mg/kg/day **or** 0.6-0.75 mg/m²/day in divided doses every 6-12 hours

Treatment of shock:

Addisonian crisis/shock (ie, adrenal insufficiency/responsive to steroid therapy): I.V. (given as sodium phosphate): 4-10 mg as a single dose, which may be repeated if necessary

Unresponsive shock (ie, unresponsive to steroid therapy): I.V. (given as sodium phosphate): 1-6 mg/kg as a single I.V. dose or up to 40 mg initially followed by repeat doses every 2-6 hours while shock persists

Hemodialysis: Supplemental dose is not necessary

Peritoneal dialysis: Supplemental dose is not necessary

**Dosage Forms** [DSC] = Discontinued product

Elixir, as base: 0.5 mg/5 mL (240 mL) [contains alcohol 5%; raspberry flavor]

Injection, solution, as sodium phosphate: 4 mg/mL (1 mL, 5 mL, 10 mL, 25 mL, 30 mL); 10 mg/mL (1 mL, 10 mL)

Decadron® Phosphate: 4 mg/mL (5 mL, 25 mL); 24 mg/mL (5 mL) [contains sodium bisulfite] [DSC]

Tablet: 0.25 mg, 0.5 mg, 0.75 mg, 1 mg, 1.5 mg, 2 mg, 4 mg, 6 mg [some 0.5 mg tablets may contain tartrazine]

Decadron®: 0.5 mg, 0.75 mg, 4 mg

DexPak® TaperPak®: 1.5 mg [51 tablets on taper dose card]

**Dexasone® [Can]** *see* dexamethasone (systemic) *on previous page*

**Dexasporin [US]** *see* neomycin, polymyxin B, and dexamethasone *on page 567*

**Dexatrim® Pre-Meal** *(Discontinued)*

# dexbrompheniramine and pseudoephedrine

(deks brom fen EER a meen & soo doe e FED rin)

**Synonyms** pseudoephedrine and dexbrompheniramine

**U.S./Canadian Brand Names** Drixoral® Cold & Allergy [US-OTC]; Drixoral® [Can]

**Therapeutic Category** Antihistamine/Decongestant Combination

**Use** Relief of symptoms of upper respiratory mucosal congestion in seasonal and perennial nasal allergies, acute rhinitis, rhinosinusitis and eustachian tube blockage

**Usual Dosage** Children >12 years and Adults: Oral: 1 timed release tablet every 12 hours, may require 1 tablet every 8 hours

**Dosage Forms** Tablet, sustained action: Dexbrompheniramine maleate 6 mg and pseudoephedrine sulfate 120 mg

**Dexchlor®** *(Discontinued)* *see* dexchlorpheniramine *on this page*

# dexchlorpheniramine (deks klor fen EER a meen)

**Synonyms** dexchlorpheniramine maleate

**Therapeutic Category** Antihistamine

**Use** Perennial and seasonal allergic rhinitis and other allergic symptoms including urticaria

**Usual Dosage** Oral:

Children:

2-5 years: 0.5 mg every 4-6 hours (do not use timed release)

6-11 years: 1 mg every 4-6 hours or 4 mg timed release at bedtime

Adults: 2 mg every 4-6 hours or 4-6 mg timed release at bedtime or every 8-10 hours

**Dosage Forms**

Syrup, as maleate: 2 mg/5 mL (480 mL, 3840 mL) [contains alcohol 6%; orange flavor]

Tablet, sustained action, as maleate: 4 mg, 6 mg

**dexchlorpheniramine maleate** *see* dexchlorpheniramine *on this page*

**dexchlorpheniramine tannate, pseudoephedrine tannate, and dextromethorphan tannate** *see* chlorpheniramine, pseudoephedrine, and dextromethorphan *on page 177*

**Dexedrine® [US/Can]** *see* dextroamphetamine *on page 237*

**Dexferrum®** **[US]** *see* iron dextran complex *on page 448*

**Dexiron™** **[Can]** *see* iron dextran complex *on page 448*

## dexmedetomidine (deks MED e toe mi deen)

**Sound-Alike/Look-Alike Issues**

Precedex™ may be confused with Peridex®

**Synonyms** dexmedetomidine hydrochloride

**U.S./Canadian Brand Names** Precedex™ [US/Can]

**Therapeutic Category** Alpha-Adrenergic Agonist - Central-Acting (Alpha$_2$-Agonists); Sedative

**Use** Sedation of initially intubated and mechanically ventilated patients during treatment in an intensive care setting; duration of infusion should not exceed 24 hours

**Usual Dosage** Individualized and titrated to desired clinical effect

Adults: I.V.: Solution must be diluted prior to administration. Initial: Loading infusion of 1 mcg/kg over 10 minutes, followed by a maintenance infusion of 0.2-0.7 mcg/kg/hour; not indicated for infusions lasting >24 hours

**Dosage Forms** Injection, solution [preservative free]: 100 mcg/mL (2 mL)

**dexmedetomidine hydrochloride** *see* dexmedetomidine *on this page*

## dexmethylphenidate (dex meth il FEN i date)

**Synonyms** dexmethylphenidate hydrochloride

**U.S./Canadian Brand Names** Focalin™ XR [US]; Focalin™ [US]

**Therapeutic Category** Central Nervous System Stimulant, Nonamphetamine

**Controlled Substance** C-II

**Use** Treatment of attention-deficit/hyperactivity disorder (ADHD)

**Usual Dosage** Treatment of ADHD: Oral:

Children ≥6 years: Patients not currently taking methylphenidate:

Tablet: Initial: 2.5 mg twice daily; dosage may be adjusted in increments of 2.5-5 mg  at weekly intervals (maximum dose: 20 mg/day); doses should be taken at least 4 hours apart

Capsule: Initial: 5 mg/day; dosage may be adjusted in increments of 5 mg/day at weekly intervals (maximum dose: 20 mg/day)

Adults: Patients not currently taking methylphenidate:

Tablet: Initial: 2.5 mg twice daily; dosage may be adjusted in increments of 2.5-5 mg  at weekly intervals (maximum dose: 20 mg/day); doses should be taken at least 4 hours apart

Capsule: Initial: 10 mg/day; dosage may be adjusted in increments of 10 mg/day at weekly intervals (maximum dose: 20 mg/day)

**Conversion to dexmethylphenidate from methylphenidate:**  Tablet, capsule: Initial: Half the total daily dose of racemic methylphenidate

**Conversion from dexmethylphenidate immediate release to dexmethylphenidate extended release:** When changing from Focalin™ tablets to Focalin™ XR capsules, patients may be switched to the same daily dose using Focalin™ XR (maximum dose: 20 mg/day)

Safety and efficacy for long-term use of dexmethylphenidate have not yet been established. Patients should be re-evaluated at appropriate intervals to assess continued need of the medication.

Dose reductions and discontinuation: Reduce dose or discontinue in patients with paradoxical aggravation. Discontinue if no improvement is seen after one month of treatment.

**Dosage Forms**

Capsule, extended release (Focalin™ XR): 5 mg, 10 mg, 20 mg [bimodal release]

Tablet, as hydrochloride (Focalin™): 2.5 mg, 5 mg, 10 mg

**dexmethylphenidate hydrochloride** *see* dexmethylphenidate *on this page*

**DexPak® TaperPak®** **[US]** *see* dexamethasone (systemic) *on page 233*

## dexpanthenol (deks PAN the nole)

**Synonyms** pantothenyl alcohol

**U.S./Canadian Brand Names** Panthoderm® [US-OTC]

**Therapeutic Category** Gastrointestinal Agent, Stimulant

**Use** Prophylactic use to minimize paralytic ileus; treatment of postoperative distention; topical to relieve itching and to aid healing of minor dermatoses

(Continued)

# dexpanthenol *(Continued)*

### Usual Dosage
Children and Adults: Relief of itching and aid in skin healing: Topical: Apply to affected area 1-2 times/day

Adults:
Prevention of postoperative ileus: I.M.: 250-500 mg stat, repeat in 2 hours, followed by doses every 6 hours until danger passes
Paralytic ileus: I.M.: 500 mg stat, repeat in 2 hours, followed by doses every 6 hours, if needed

### Dosage Forms
Cream, topical: 2% (30 g, 60 g)
Injection, solution: 250 mg/mL (2 mL)

**Dex PC [US]** *see* chlorpheniramine, phenylephrine, and dextromethorphan *on page 174*

# dexrazoxane (deks ray ZOKS ane)

### Sound-Alike/Look-Alike Issues
Zinecard® may be confused with Gemzar®

### Synonyms ICRF-187

### U.S./Canadian Brand Names Zinecard® [US/Can]

### Therapeutic Category Cardiovascular Agent, Other

**Use** Reduction of the incidence and severity of cardiomyopathy associated with doxorubicin administration in women with metastatic breast cancer who have received a cumulative doxorubicin dose of 300 mg/m$^2$ and who would benefit from continuing therapy with doxorubicin. It is not recommended for use with the initiation of doxorubicin therapy.

**Usual Dosage** Adults: I.V.: A 10:1 ratio of dexrazoxane:doxorubicin (500 mg/m$^2$ dexrazoxane: 50 mg/m$^2$ doxorubicin)

**Dosage Forms** Injection, powder for reconstitution: 250 mg, 500 mg [10 mg/mL when reconstituted]

# dextran (DEKS tran)

### Sound-Alike/Look-Alike Issues
dextran may be confused with Dexatrim®, Dexedrine®

### Synonyms dextran 40; dextran 70; dextran, high molecular weight; dextran, low molecular weight

### U.S./Canadian Brand Names Gentran® [US/Can]; LMD® [US]

### Therapeutic Category Plasma Volume Expander

**Use** Blood volume expander used in treatment of shock or impending shock when blood or blood products are not available; dextran 40 is also used as a priming fluid in cardiopulmonary bypass and for prophylaxis of venous thrombosis and pulmonary embolism in surgical procedures associated with a high risk of thromboembolic complications

**Usual Dosage** I.V. (requires an infusion pump): Dose and infusion rate are dependent upon the patient's fluid status and must be individualized:

**Volume expansion/shock:**
Children: Total dose should not exceed 20 mL/kg during first 24 hours
Adults: 500-1000 mL at a rate of 20-40 mL/minute; maximum daily dose: 20 mL/kg for first 24 hours; 10 mL/kg/day thereafter; therapy should not be continued beyond 5 days

**Pump prime (Dextran 40):** Varies with the volume of the pump oxygenator; generally, the 10% solution is added in a dose of 1-2 g/kg

**Prophylaxis of venous thrombosis/pulmonary embolism (Dextran 40):** Begin during surgical procedure and give 50-100 g on the day of surgery; an additional 50 g (500 mL) should be administered every 2-3 days during the period of risk (up to 2 weeks postoperatively); usual maximum infusion rate for nonemergency use: 4 mL/minute

### Dosage Forms
Infusion [premixed in D$_5$W; high molecular weight]: 6% Dextran 70 (500 mL)
Infusion [premixed in D$_5$W; low molecular weight] (Gentran®, LMD®): 10% Dextran 40 (500 mL)
Infusion [premixed in D$_{10}$W; high molecular weight]: 32% Dextran 70 (500 mL)
Infusion [premixed in NS; high molecular weight] (Gentran®): 6% Dextran 70 (500 mL)
Infusion [premixed in NS; low molecular weight] (Gentran®, LMD®): 10% Dextran (500 mL)

# dextran 1 (DEKS tran won)

### Sound-Alike/Look-Alike Issues
dextran may be confused with Dexatrim®, Dexedrine®

U.S./Canadian Brand Names Promit® [US]
Therapeutic Category Plasma Volume Expander
Use Prophylaxis of serious anaphylactic reactions to I.V. infusion of dextran
Usual Dosage I.V. (time between dextran 1 and dextran solution should not exceed 15 minutes):
  Children: 0.3 mL/kg 1-2 minutes before I.V. infusion of dextran
  Adults: 20 mL 1-2 minutes before I.V. infusion of dextran
Dosage Forms Injection, solution: 150 mg/mL (20 mL)

**dextran 40** *see dextran* *on previous page*

**dextran 70** *see dextran* *on previous page*

**dextran, high molecular weight** *see dextran* *on previous page*

**dextran, low molecular weight** *see dextran* *on previous page*

# dextroamphetamine (deks troe am FET a meen)
Sound-Alike/Look-Alike Issues
  Dexedrine® may be confused with dextran, Excedrin®
Synonyms dextroamphetamine sulfate
U.S./Canadian Brand Names Dexedrine® [US/Can]; Dextrostat® [US]
Therapeutic Category Amphetamine
Controlled Substance C-II
Use Narcolepsy; attention deficit/hyperactivity disorder (ADHD)
Usual Dosage Oral:
  Children:
  Narcolepsy: 6-12 years: Initial: 5 mg/day; may increase at 5 mg increments in weekly intervals until side effects appear (maximum dose: 60 mg/day)
  ADHD:
    3-5 years: Initial: 2.5 mg/day given every morning; increase by 2.5 mg/day in weekly intervals until optimal response is obtained; usual range: 0.1-0.5 mg/kg/dose every morning with maximum of 40 mg/day
    ≥6 years: 5 mg once or twice daily; increase in increments of 5 mg/day at weekly intervals until optimal response is obtained; usual range: 0.1-0.5 mg/kg/dose every morning (5-20 mg/day) with maximum of 40 mg/day
  Children >12 years and Adults: Narcolepsy: Initial: 10 mg/day, may increase at 10 mg increments in weekly intervals until side effects appear; maximum: 60 mg/day
Dosage Forms
  Capsule, sustained release, as sulfate: 5 mg, 10 mg, 15 mg
  Dexedrine® Spansule®: 5 mg, 10 mg, 15 mg
  Tablet, as sulfate: 5 mg, 10 mg
  Dexedrine®: 5 mg [contains tartrazine]
  Dextrostat®: 5 mg, 10 mg [contains tartrazine]

# dextroamphetamine and amphetamine (deks troe am FET a meen & am FET a meen)
Sound-Alike/Look-Alike Issues
  Adderall® may be confused with Inderal®
Synonyms amphetamine and dextroamphetamine
U.S./Canadian Brand Names Adderall XR® [US/Can]; Adderall® [US]
Therapeutic Category Amphetamine
Controlled Substance C-II
Use Attention deficit/hyperactivity disorder (ADHD); narcolepsy
Usual Dosage Oral: **Note:** Use lowest effective individualized dose; administer first dose as soon as awake
  ADHD:
  Children: <3 years: Not recommended
  Children: 3-5 years (Adderall®): Initial 2.5 mg/day given every morning; increase daily dose in 2.5 mg increments at weekly intervals until optimal response is obtained (maximum dose: 40 mg/day given in 1-3 divided doses); use intervals of 4-6 hours between additional doses
  Children: ≥6 years:
    Adderall®: Initial: 5 mg 1-2 times/day; increase daily dose in 5 mg increments at weekly intervals until optimal response is obtained (usual maximum dose: 40 mg/day given in 1-3 divided doses); use intervals of 4-6 hours between additional doses
(Continued)

# dextroamphetamine and amphetamine *(Continued)*

Adderall XR®: 5-10 mg once daily in the morning; if needed, may increase daily dose in 5-10 mg increments at weekly intervals (maximum dose: 30 mg/day)

Adolescents 13-17 years (Adderall XR®): 10 mg once daily in the morning; may be increased to 20 mg/day after 1 week if symptoms are not controlled; higher doses (up to 60 mg)/day have been evaluated; however, there is not adequate evidence that higher doses afforded additional benefit.

Adults: Adderall XR®: Initial: 20 mg once daily in the morning; higher doses (up to 60 mg once daily) have been evaluated; however, there is not adequate evidence that higher doses afforded additional benefit,

Narcolepsy (Adderall®):

Children: 6-12 years: Initial: 5 mg/day; increase daily dose in 5 mg at weekly intervals until optimal response is obtained (maximum dose: 60 mg/day given in 1-3 divided doses)

Children >12 years and Adults: Initial: 10 mg/day; increase daily dose in 10 mg increments at weekly intervals until optimal response is obtained (maximum dose: 60 mg/day given in 1-3 divided doses)

## Dosage Forms

Capsule, extended release (Adderall XR®):

5 mg [dextroamphetamine sulfate 1.25 mg, dextroamphetamine saccharate 1.25 mg, amphetamine aspartate monohydrate 1.25 mg, amphetamine sulfate 1.25 mg (equivalent to amphetamine base 3.1 mg)]

10 mg [dextroamphetamine sulfate 2.5 mg, dextroamphetamine saccharate 2.5 mg, amphetamine aspartate monohydrate 2.5 mg, amphetamine sulfate 2.5 mg (equivalent to amphetamine base 6.3 mg)]

15 mg [dextroamphetamine sulfate 3.75 mg, dextroamphetamine saccharate 3.75 mg, amphetamine aspartate monohydrate 3.75 mg, amphetamine sulfate 3.75 mg (equivalent to amphetamine base 9.4 mg)]

20 mg [dextroamphetamine sulfate 5 mg, dextroamphetamine saccharate 5 mg, amphetamine aspartate monohydrate 5 mg, amphetamine sulfate 5 mg (equivalent to amphetamine base 12.5 mg)]

25 mg [dextroamphetamine sulfate 6.25 mg, dextroamphetamine saccharate 6.25 mg, amphetamine aspartate monohydrate 6.25 mg, amphetamine sulfate 6.25 mg (equivalent to amphetamine base 15.6 mg)]

30 mg [dextroamphetamine sulfate 7.5 mg, dextroamphetamine saccharate 7.5 mg, amphetamine aspartate monohydrate 7.5 mg, amphetamine sulfate 7.5 mg (equivalent to amphetamine base 18.8 mg)]

Tablet (Adderall®):

5 mg [dextroamphetamine sulfate 1.25 mg, dextroamphetamine saccharate 1.25 mg, amphetamine aspartate 1.25 mg, amphetamine sulfate 1.25 mg (equivalent to amphetamine base 3.13 mg)]

7.5 mg [dextroamphetamine 1.875 mg, dextroamphetamine saccharate 1.875 mg, amphetamine aspartate 1.875 mg, amphetamine sulfate 1.875 mg (equivalent to amphetamine base 4.7 mg)]

10 mg [dextroamphetamine sulfate 2.5 mg, dextroamphetamine saccharate 2.5 mg, amphetamine aspartate 2.5 mg, amphetamine sulfate 2.5 mg (equivalent to amphetamine base 6.3 mg)]

12.5 mg [dextroamphetamine sulfate 3.125 mg, dextroamphetamine saccharate 3.125 mg, amphetamine aspartate 3.125 mg, amphetamine sulfate 3.125 mg (equivalent to amphetamine base 7.8 mg)]

15 mg [dextroamphetamine sulfate 3.75 mg, dextroamphetamine saccharate 3.75 mg, amphetamine aspartate 3.75 mg, amphetamine sulfate 3.75 mg (equivalent to amphetamine base 9.4 mg)]

20 mg [dextroamphetamine sulfate 5 mg, dextroamphetamine saccharate 5 mg, amphetamine aspartate 5 mg, amphetamine sulfate 5 mg (equivalent to amphetamine base 12.6 mg)]

30 mg [dextroamphetamine sulfate 7.5 mg, dextroamphetamine saccharate 7.5 mg, amphetamine aspartate 7.5 mg, amphetamine sulfate 7.5 mg (equivalent to amphetamine base 18.8 mg)]

**dextroamphetamine sulfate** *see* dextroamphetamine *on previous page*

# dextromethorphan (deks troe meth OR fan)

## Sound-Alike/Look-Alike Issues

Benylin® may be confused with Benadryl®, Ventolin®

Delsym® may be confused with Delfen®, Desyrel®

**U.S./Canadian Brand Names** Babee® Cof Syrup [US-OTC]; Benylin® Adult [US-OTC]; Benylin® Pediatric [US-OTC]; Creo-Terpin® [US-OTC]; Creomulsion® Cough [US-OTC]; Creomulsion® for Children [US-OTC]; Delsym® [US-OTC]; Dexalone® [US-OTC]; ElixSure™ Cough [US-OTC]; Hold® DM [US-OTC]; PediaCare® Children's Medicated Freezer Pops Long Acting Cough [US-OTC]; PediaCare® Infants' Long-Acting Cough [US-OTC]; Robitussin® CoughGels™ [US-OTC]; Robitussin® Honey Cough [US-OTC]; Robitussin® Maximum Strength Cough [US-OTC]; Robitussin® Pediatric Cough [US-OTC];

Scot-Tussin DM® Cough Chasers [US-OTC]; Silphen DM® [US-OTC]; Simply Cough® [US-OTC]; Triaminic® Thin Strips™ Long Acting Cough [US-OTC]; Vicks® 44® Cough Relief [US-OTC]

**Therapeutic Category** Antitussive

**Use** Symptomatic relief of coughs caused by minor viral upper respiratory tract infections or inhaled irritants; most effective for a chronic nonproductive cough

**Usual Dosage** Oral:

Children:

<2 years: Use only as directed by a physician

2-6 years (syrup): 2.5-7.5 mg every 4-8 hours; extended release is 15 mg twice daily (maximum: 30 mg/24 hours)

6-12 years: 5-10 mg every 4 hours or 15 mg every 6-8 hours; extended release is 30 mg twice daily (maximum: 60 mg/24 hours)

Children >12 years and Adults: 10-20 mg every 4 hours or 30 mg every 6-8 hours; extended release: 60 mg twice daily; maximum: 120 mg/day

**Dosage Forms**

Gelcap, as hydrobromide:

Dexalone®: 30 mg

Robitussin® CoughGels™: 15 mg [contains coconut oil]

Liquid, as hydrobromide:

Creo-Terpin®: 10 mg/15 mL (120 mL) [contains alcohol 25% and tartrazine]

Simply Cough®: 5 mg/5 mL (120 mL) [contains sodium benzoate; cherry berry flavor]

Vicks® 44® Cough Relief: 10 mg/5 mL (120 mL) [contains alcohol, sodium 10 mg/5 mL, sodium benzoate]

Liquid, oral, as hydrobromide [freezer pops] (PediaCare® Children's Medicated Freezer Pops Long Acting Cough): 7.5 mg/25 mL (8s) [alcohol free; contains sodium benzoate, berry flavor also contains benzyl alcohol; glacier grape™ and polar berry blue™ flavors]

Liquid, oral drops, as hydrobromide (PediaCare® Infants' Long-Acting Cough): 7.5 mg/0.8 mL (15 mL) [alcohol free, dye free; contains sodium benzoate; grape flavor]

Lozenge, as hydrobromide:

Hold® DM: 5 mg (10s) [cherry or original flavor]

Scot-Tussin DM® Cough Chasers: 5 mg (20s)

Strips, oral, as hydrobromide (Triaminic® Thin Strips™ Long Acting Cough): 7.5 mg [equivalent to dextromethorphan 5 mg; cherry flavor]

Suspension, extended release, as hydrobromide (Delsym®): 30 mg/5 mL (89 mL, 148 mL) [contains alcohol 0.26%, sodium 5 mg/5 mL; orange flavor]

Syrup, as hydrobromide:

Babee® Cof Syrup: 7.5 mg/5 mL (120 mL) [alcohol free, dye free; cherry flavor]

Benylin® Adult: 15 mg/5 mL (120 mL) [alcohol free, sugar free; contains sodium benzoate; raspberry flavor]

Benylin® Pediatric: 7.5 mg/mL (120 mL) [alcohol free, sugar free; contains sodium benzoate; grape flavor]

Creomulsion® Cough: 20 mg/15 mL (120 mL) [alcohol free; contains sodium benzoate]

Creomulsion® for Children: 5 mg/5 mL (120 mL) [alcohol free; contains sodium benzoate; cherry flavor]

ElixSure™ Cough: 7.5 mg/5 mL (120 mL) [cherry bubble gum flavor]

Robitussin® Honey Cough: 10 mg/5 mL (120 mL) [alcohol free; contains sodium benzoate]

Robitussin® Maximum Strength Cough: 15 mg/5 mL (120 mL, 240 mL) [contains alcohol, sodium benzoate]

Robitussin® Pediatric Cough: 7.5 mg/5mL (120 mL) [alcohol free; contains sodium benzoate; fruit punch flavor]

Silphen DM®: 10 mg/5 mL (120 mL) [strawberry flavor]

**dextromethorphan, acetaminophen, and pseudoephedrine** see acetaminophen, dextromethorphan, and pseudoephedrine on page 11

**dextromethorphan and guaifenesin** see guaifenesin and dextromethorphan on page 385

**dextromethorphan and promethazine** see promethazine and dextromethorphan on page 683

**dextromethorphan and pseudoephedrine** see pseudoephedrine and dextromethorphan on page 693

**dextromethorphan, brompheniramine, and pseudoephedrinc** see brompheniramine, pseudoephedrine, and dextromethorphan on page 116

**dextromethorphan, carbinoxamine, and pseudoephedrine** see carbinoxamine, pseudoephedrine, and dextromethorphan on page 145

**dextromethorphan, chlorpheniramine, and phenylephrine** *see* chlorpheniramine, phenylephrine, and dextromethorphan *on page 174*

**dextromethorphan, chlorpheniramine, and pseudoephedrine** *see* chlorpheniramine, pseudoephedrine, and dextromethorphan *on page 177*

**dextromethorphan, guaifenesin, and pseudoephedrine** *see* guaifenesin, pseudoephedrine, and dextromethorphan *on page 391*

**dextromethorphan, pseudoephedrine, and carbinoxamine** *see* carbinoxamine, pseudoephedrine, and dextromethorphan *on page 145*

**dextromethorphan tannate, pyrilamine tannate, and phenylephrine tannate** *see* phenylephrine, pyrilamine, and dextromethorphan *on page 644*

**dextropropoxyphene** *see* propoxyphene *on page 687*

**dextrose and tetracaine** *see* tetracaine and dextrose *on page 791*

**dextrose, levulose and phosphoric acid** *see* fructose, dextrose, and phosphoric acid *on page 362*

**Dextrostat**® **[US]** *see* dextroamphetamine *on page 237*

**Dey-Dose**® **Isoproterenol** *(Discontinued)* *see* isoproterenol *on page 450*

**Dey-Dose**® **Metaproterenol** *(Discontinued)*

**DFMO** *see* eflornithine *on page 281*

**DHAD** *see* mitoxantrone *on page 545*

**DHAQ** *see* mitoxantrone *on page 545*

**DHC**® *(Discontinued)* *see* hydrocodone and acetaminophen *on page 411*

**DHC Plus**® *(Discontinued)*

**DHE** *see* dihydroergotamine *on page 250*

**D.H.E. 45**® **[US]** *see* dihydroergotamine *on page 250*

**DHPG sodium** *see* ganciclovir *on page 366*

**DHS**™ **Sal [US-OTC]** *see* salicylic acid *on page 734*

**DHS**™ **Tar [US-OTC]** *see* coal tar *on page 201*

**DHS**™ **Targel [US-OTC]** *see* coal tar *on page 201*

**DHS**™ **Zinc [US-OTC]** *see* pyrithione zinc *on page 702*

**DHT**™ **[US]** *see* dihydrotachysterol *on page 250*

**DHT**™ **Intensol**™ **[US]** *see* dihydrotachysterol *on page 250*

**DiabetAid**™ **Antifungal Foot Bath [US-OTC]** *see* miconazole *on page 537*

**DiabetAid Gingivitis Mouth Rinse [US-OTC]** *see* cetylpyridinium *on page 164*

**Diabetic Tussin C**® **[US]** *see* guaifenesin and codeine *on page 384*

**Diabetic Tussin**® **Allergy Relief [US-OTC]** *see* chlorpheniramine *on page 171*

**Diabetic Tussin**® **DM [US-OTC]** *see* guaifenesin and dextromethorphan *on page 385*

**Diabetic Tussin**® **DM Maximum Strength [US-OTC]** *see* guaifenesin and dextromethorphan *on page 385*

**Diabetic Tussin**® **EX [US-OTC]** *see* guaifenesin *on page 383*

**Diabinese**® **[US]** *see* chlorpropamide *on page 179*

**Diaβeta**® **[US/Can]** *see* glyburide *on page 378*

**Dialose**® **Tablet** *(Discontinued)* *see* docusate *on page 263*

**Dialume**® *(Discontinued)* *see* aluminum hydroxide *on page 34*

**Diamicron**® **[Can]** *see* gliclazide *(Canada only)* *on page 375*

**Diamicron**® **MR [Can]** *see* gliclazide *(Canada only)* *on page 375*

**Diamine T.D.**® *(Discontinued)* *see* brompheniramine *on page 115*

**diaminocyclohexane oxalatoplatinum** *see* oxaliplatin *on page 605*

**diaminodiphenylsulfone** *see* dapsone *on page 224*

**Diamode [US-OTC]** *see* loperamide *on page 489*

Diamox® **[Can]** *see* acetazolamide *on page 13*

Diamox® **250 mg Tablet** *(Discontinued)* *see* acetazolamide *on page 13*

Diamox® **Sequels® [US]** *see* acetazolamide *on page 13*

Diane-35 **[Can]** *see* cyproterone and ethinyl estradiol *(Canada only) on page 217*

Diaparene® **[US-OTC]** *see* methylbenzethonium chloride *on page 528*

Diar-aid® *(Discontinued)* *see* loperamide *on page 489*

Diarr-Eze **[Can]** *see* loperamide *on page 489*

Diasorb® **[US-OTC]** *see* attapulgite *on page 81*

Diastat® **[US/Can]** *see* diazepam *on this page*

**diatrizoate meglumine** *see* radiological/contrast media (ionic) *on page 707*

**diatrizoate meglumine and diatrizoate sodium** *see* radiological/contrast media (ionic) *on page 707*

**diatrizoate meglumine and iodipamide meglumine** *see* radiological/contrast media (ionic) *on page 707*

**diatrizoate sodium** *see* radiological/contrast media (ionic) *on page 707*

Diatx™ **[US]** *see* vitamin B complex combinations *on page 849*

DiatxFe™ **[US]** *see* vitamin B complex combinations *on page 849*

Diazemuls® **[Can]** *see* diazepam *on this page*

Diazemuls® **Injection** *(Discontinued)* *see* diazepam *on this page*

## diazepam (dye AZ e pam)

**Sound-Alike/Look-Alike Issues**
diazepam may be confused with diazoxide, Ditropan®, lorazepam
Valium® may be confused with Valcyte™

**U.S./Canadian Brand Names** Apo-Diazepam® [Can]; Diastat® [US/Can]; Diazemuls® [Can]; Diazepam Intensol® [US]; Novo-Dipam [Can]; Valium® [US/Can]

**Therapeutic Category** Benzodiazepine

**Controlled Substance** C-IV

**Use** Management of anxiety disorders, ethanol withdrawal symptoms; skeletal muscle relaxant; treatment of convulsive disorders

**Orphan drug:** Viscous solution for rectal administration: Management of selected, refractory epilepsy patients on stable regimens of antiepileptic drugs (AEDs) requiring intermittent use of diazepam to control episodes of increased seizure activity

**Usual Dosage Oral absorption is more reliable than I.M.**
Children:
Conscious sedation for procedures: Oral: 0.2-0.3 mg/kg (maximum: 10 mg) 45-60 minutes prior to procedure
Sedation/muscle relaxant/anxiety:
Oral: 0.12-0.8 mg/kg/day in divided doses every 6-8 hours
I.M., I.V.: 0.04-0.3 mg/kg/dose every 2-4 hours to a maximum of 0.6 mg/kg within an 8-hour period if needed
Status epilepticus:
Infants 30 days to 5 years: I.V.: 0.05-0.3 mg/kg/dose given over 2-3 minutes, every 15-30 minutes to a maximum total dose of 5 mg; repeat in 2-4 hours as needed **or** 0.2-0.5 mg/dose every 2-5 minutes to a maximum total dose of 5 mg
>5 years: I.V.: 0.05-0.3 mg/kg/dose given over 2-3 minutes every 15-30 minutes to a maximum total dose of 10 mg; repeat in 2-4 hours as needed **or** 1 mg/dose given over 2-3 minutes, every 2-5 minutes to a maximum total dose of 10 mg
Rectal: 0.5 mg/kg, then 0.25 mg/kg in 10 minutes if needed
Anticonvulsant (acute treatment): Rectal gel formulation:
Infants <6 months: Not recommended
Children <2 years: Safety and efficacy have not been studied
Children 2-5 years: 0.5 mg/kg
Children 6-11 years: 0.3 mg/kg
Children ≥12 years and Adults: 0.2 mg/kg
(Continued)

# diazepam *(Continued)*

**Note:** Dosage should be rounded upward to the next available dose, 2.5, 5, 10, 15, and 20 mg/dose; dose may be repeated in 4-12 hours if needed; do not use more than 5 times per month or more than once every 5 days

Adolescents: Conscious sedation for procedures:

Oral: 10 mg

I.V.: 5 mg, may repeat with ½ dose if needed

Adults:

Anxiety/sedation/skeletal muscle relaxant:

Oral: 2-10 mg 2-4 times/day

I.M., I.V.: 2-10 mg, may repeat in 3-4 hours if needed

Sedation in the ICU patient: I.V.: 0.03-0.1 mg/kg every 30 minutes to 6 hours

Status epilepticus: I.V.: 5-10 mg every 10-20 minutes, up to 30 mg in an 8-hour period; may repeat in 2-4 hours if necessary

Rapid tranquilization of agitated patient (administer every 30-60 minutes): Oral: 5-10 mg; average total dose for tranquilization: 20-60 mg

### Dosage Forms

Gel, rectal:

Diastat®: Pediatric rectal tip [4.4 cm]: 5 mg/mL (2.5 mg, 5 mg) [contains ethyl alcohol 10%, sodium benzoate, benzyl alcohol 1.5%; twin pack]

Diastat® AcuDial™ delivery system:

10 mg: Pediatric/adult rectal tip [4.4 cm]: 5 mg/mL (delivers set doses of 5 mg, 7.5 mg, and 10 mg) [contains ethyl alcohol 10%, sodium benzoate, benzyl alcohol 1.5%; twin pack]

20 mg: Adult rectal tip [6 cm]: 5 mg/mL (delivers set doses of 10 mg, 12.5 mg, 15 mg, 17.5 mg, and 20 mg) [contains ethyl alcohol 10%, sodium benzoate, benzyl alcohol 1.5%; twin pack]

Injection, solution: 5 mg/mL (2 mL, 10 mL) [may contain benzyl alcohol, sodium benzoate, benzoic acid]

Solution, oral: 5 mg/5 mL (5 mL, 500 mL) [wintergreen-spice flavor]

Solution, oral concentrate (Diazepam Intensol®): 5 mg/mL (30 mL)

Tablet (Valium®): 2 mg, 5 mg, 10 mg

**Diazepam Intensol® [US]** *see* diazepam *on previous page*

# diazoxide *(dye az OKS ide)*

### Sound-Alike/Look-Alike Issues

diazoxide may be confused with diazepam, Dyazide®

Hyperstat® may be confused with Nitrostat®

**U.S./Canadian Brand Names** Hyperstat® [US]; Proglycem® [US/Can]

**Therapeutic Category** Antihypertensive Agent; Antihypoglycemic Agent

### Use

Oral: Hypoglycemia related to islet cell adenoma, carcinoma, hyperplasia, or adenomatosis, nesidioblastosis, leucine sensitivity, or extrapancreatic malignancy

I.V.: Severe hypertension

### Usual Dosage

Hypertension: Children and Adults: I.V.: 1-3 mg/kg up to a maximum of 150 mg in a single injection; repeat dose in 5-15 minutes until blood pressure adequately reduced; repeat administration at intervals of 4-24 hours; monitor the blood pressure closely; do not use longer than 10 days

Hyperinsulinemic hypoglycemia: Oral: **Note:** Use lower dose listed as initial dose

Newborns and Infants: 8-15 mg/kg/day in divided doses every 8-12 hours

Children and Adults: 3-8 mg/kg/day in divided doses every 8-12 hours

### Dosage Forms

Capsule (Proglycem®): 50 mg [not available in the U.S.]

Injection, solution (Hyperstat®): 15 mg/mL (20 mL)

Suspension, oral (Proglycem®): 50 mg/mL (30 mL) [contains alcohol 7.25%; chocolate-mint flavor]

**Dibent® Injection *(Discontinued)*** *see* dicyclomine *on page 245*

**Dibenzyline® [US/Can]** *see* phenoxybenzamine *on page 639*

# dibucaine *(DYE byoo kane)*

**U.S./Canadian Brand Names** Nupercainal® [US-OTC]

**Therapeutic Category** Local Anesthetic

**Use** Fast, temporary relief of pain and itching due to hemorrhoids, minor burns

**Usual Dosage** Children and Adults: Topical: Apply gently to the affected areas; no more than 30 g for adults or 7.5 g for children should be used in any 24-hour period

**Dosage Forms**
Ointment: 1% (30 g, 454 g)
Nupercainal®: 1% (30 g, 60g) [contains sodium bisulfite]

**DIC** *see* dacarbazine *on page 220*

**Dicarbosil®** *(Discontinued) see* calcium carbonate *on page 130*

**Dicetel® [Can]** *see* pinaverium *(Canada only) on page 648*

**dichloralphenazone, acetaminophen, and isometheptene** *see* acetaminophen, isometheptene, and dichloralphenazone *on page 12*

**dichloralphenazone, isometheptene, and acetaminophen** *see* acetaminophen, isometheptene, and dichloralphenazone *on page 12*

**6,7-dichloro-1,5-dihydroimidazo [2,1b] quinazolin-2(3H)-one monohydrochloride** *see* anagrelide *on page 52*

# dichlorodifluoromethane and trichloromonofluoromethane
(dye klor oh dye flor oh METH ane & tri klor oh mon oh flor oh METH ane)
**Synonyms** trichloromonofluoromethane and dichlorodifluoromethane
**U.S./Canadian Brand Names** Fluori-Methane® [US]
**Therapeutic Category** Analgesic, Topical
**Use** Management of pain associated with injections
**Usual Dosage** Invert bottle over treatment area approximately 12" away from site of application; open dispenseal spring valve completely, allowing liquid to flow in a stream from the bottle. The rate of spraying is approximately 10 cm/second and should be continued until entire muscle has been covered.
**Dosage Forms** Aerosol, topical: Dichlorodifluoromethane 15% and trichloromonofluoromethane 85% (103 mL) [contains chlorofluorocarbons]

**dichlorotetrafluoroethane and ethyl chloride** *see* ethyl chloride and dichlorotetrafluoroethane *on page 321*

# dichlorphenamide (dye klor FEN a mide)
**Sound-Alike/Look-Alike Issues**
Daranide® may be confused with Daraprim®
**Synonyms** diclofenamide
**U.S./Canadian Brand Names** Daranide® [US/Can]
**Therapeutic Category** Carbonic Anhydrase Inhibitor
**Use** Adjunct in treatment of open-angle glaucoma and perioperative treatment for angle-closure glaucoma
**Usual Dosage** Adults: Oral: 100-200 mg to start followed by 100 mg every 12 hours until desired response is obtained; maintenance dose: 25-50 mg 1-3 times/day
**Dosage Forms** Tablet: 50 mg

**dichysterol** *see* dihydrotachysterol *on page 250*

**Dickinson's® Witch Hazel [US-OTC]** *see* witch hazel *on page 855*

**Diclectin® [Can]** *see* doxylamine and pyridoxine *(Canada only) on page 273*

# diclofenac (dye KLOE fen ak)
**Sound-Alike/Look-Alike Issues**
diclofenac may be confused with Diflucan®, Duphalac®
Cataflam® may be confused with Catapres®
Voltaren® may be confused with tramadol, Ultram®, Verelan®
**Synonyms** diclofenac potassium; diclofenac sodium
**U.S./Canadian Brand Names** Apo-Diclo Rapide® [Can]; Apo-Diclo SR® [Can]; Apo-Diclo® [Can]; Cataflam® [US/Can]; Novo-Difenac K [Can]; Novo-Difenac [Can]; Novo-Difenac-SR [Can]; Nu-Diclo [Can]; Nu-Diclo-SR [Can]; Pennsaid® [Can]; PMS-Diclofenac SR [Can]; PMS-Diclofenac [Can]; Riva-Diclofenac [Can]; Riva-Diclofenac-K [Can]; Solaraze™ [US]; Voltaren Ophthalmic® [US]; Voltaren Ophtha® [Can]; Voltaren Rapide® [Can]; Voltaren® [US/Can]; Voltaren®-XR [US]
(Continued)

# diclofenac *(Continued)*

**Therapeutic Category** Analgesic, Nonnarcotic; Nonsteroidal Antiinflammatory Drug (NSAID)

**Use**

Immediate release: Ankylosing spondylitis; primary dysmenorrhea; acute and chronic treatment of rheumatoid arthritis, osteoarthritis

Delayed-release tablets: Acute and chronic treatment of rheumatoid arthritis, osteoarthritis, ankylosing spondylitis

Extended-release tablets: Chronic treatment of osteoarthritis, rheumatoid arthritis

Ophthalmic solution: Postoperative inflammation following cataract extraction; temporary relief of pain and photophobia in patients undergoing corneal refractive surgery

Topical gel: Actinic keratosis (AK) in conjunction with sun avoidance

**Usual Dosage** Adults:

Oral:

Analgesia/primary dysmenorrhea: Starting dose: 50 mg 3 times/day; maximum dose: 150 mg/day

Rheumatoid arthritis: 150-200 mg/day in 2-4 divided doses (100 mg/day of sustained release product)

Osteoarthritis: 100-150 mg/day in 2-3 divided doses (100-200 mg/day of sustained release product)

Ankylosing spondylitis: 100-125 mg/day in 4-5 divided doses

Ophthalmic:

Cataract surgery: Instill 1 drop into affected eye 4 times/day beginning 24 hours after cataract surgery and continuing for 2 weeks

Corneal refractive surgery: Instill 1-2 drops into affected eye within the hour prior to surgery, within 15 minutes following surgery, and then continue for 4 times/day, up to 3 days

Topical: Apply gel to lesion area twice daily for 60-90 days

**Dosage Forms**

Gel, as sodium (Solaraze®): 30 mg/g (50 g)

Solution, ophthalmic, as sodium (Voltaren Ophthalmic®): 0.1% (2.5 mL, 5 mL)

Tablet, as potassium (Cataflam®): 50 mg

Tablet, delayed release, enteric coated, as sodium (Voltaren®): 25 mg, 50 mg, 75 mg

Tablet, extended release, as sodium (Voltaren®-XR): 100 mg

# diclofenac and misoprostol *(dye KLOE fen ak & mye soe PROST ole)*

**Synonyms** misoprostol and diclofenac

**U.S./Canadian Brand Names** Arthrotec® [US/Can]

**Therapeutic Category** Analgesic, Nonnarcotic; Prostaglandin

**Use** The diclofenac component is indicated for the treatment of osteoarthritis and rheumatoid arthritis; the misoprostol component is indicated for the prophylaxis of NSAID-induced gastric and duodenal ulceration

**Usual Dosage** Oral: Adults:

Arthrotec® 50:

Osteoarthritis: 1 tablet 2-3 times/day

Rheumatoid arthritis: 1 tablet 3-4 times/day

For both regimens, if not tolerated by patient, the dose may be reduced to 1 tablet twice daily

Arthrotec® 75:

Patients who cannot tolerate full daily Arthrotec® 50 regimens: 1 tablet twice daily

**Note:** The use of these tablets may not be as effective at preventing GI ulceration

**Dosage Forms** Tablet: Diclofenac sodium 50 mg and misoprostol 200 mcg; diclofenac sodium 75 mg and misoprostol 200 mcg

# diclofenac potassium *see diclofenac on previous page*

# diclofenac sodium *see diclofenac on previous page*

# diclofenamide *see dichlorphenamide on previous page*

# dicloxacillin *(dye kloks a SIL in)*

**Synonyms** dicloxacillin sodium

**U.S./Canadian Brand Names** Dycill® [Can]; Pathocil® [Can]

**Therapeutic Category** Penicillin

**Use** Treatment of systemic infections such as pneumonia, skin and soft tissue infections, and osteomyelitis caused by penicillinase-producing staphylococci

**Usual Dosage** Oral:

Use in newborns not recommended

Children <40 kg: 12.5-25 mg/kg/day divided every 6 hours; doses of 50-100 mg/kg/day in divided doses every 6 hours have been used for therapy of osteomyelitis

Children >40 kg and Adults: 125-250 mg every 6 hours

**Dosage Forms** Capsule: 250 mg, 500 mg

**dicloxacillin sodium** *see* dicloxacillin *on previous page*

**dicumarol (all products) *(Discontinued)***

# dicyclomine (dye SYE kloe meen)

**Sound-Alike/Look-Alike Issues**

dicyclomine may be confused with diphenhydrAMINE, doxycycline, dyclonine

Bentyl® may be confused with Aventyl®, Benadryl®, Bontril®, Cantil®, Proventil®, Trental®

**Synonyms** dicyclomine hydrochloride; dicycloverine hydrochloride

**U.S./Canadian Brand Names** Bentylol® [Can]; Bentyl® [US]; Formulex® [Can]; Lomine [Can]; Riva-Dicyclomine [Can]

**Therapeutic Category** Anticholinergic Agent

**Use** Treatment of functional disturbances of GI motility such as irritable bowel syndrome

**Usual Dosage**

Oral:

Infants >6 months: 5 mg/dose 3-4 times/day

Children: 10 mg/dose 3-4 times/day

Adults: Begin with 80 mg/day in 4 equally divided doses, then increase up to 160 mg/day

I.M. **(should not be used I.V.)**: Adults: 80 mg/day in 4 divided doses (20 mg/dose)

**Dosage Forms**

Capsule, as hydrochloride: 10 mg

Injection, solution, as hydrochloride: 10 mg/mL (2 mL)

Syrup, as hydrochloride: 10 mg/5 mL (480 mL)

Tablet, as hydrochloride: 20 mg

**dicyclomine hydrochloride** *see* dicyclomine *on this page*

**dicycloverine hydrochloride** *see* dicyclomine *on this page*

**Di-Dak-Sol [US]** *see* sodium hypochlorite solution *on page 754*

# didanosine (dye DAN oh seen)

**Sound-Alike/Look-Alike Issues**

Videx® may be confused with Lidex®

**Synonyms** ddl; dideoxyinosine

**U.S./Canadian Brand Names** Videx® EC [US/Can]; Videx® [US/Can]

**Therapeutic Category** Antiviral Agent

**Use** Treatment of HIV infection; always to be used in combination with at least two other antiretroviral agents

**Usual Dosage** Treatment of HIV infection: Oral (administer on an empty stomach):

Children:

2 weeks to 8 months: 100 mg/m$^2$ twice daily is recommended by the manufacturer; 50 mg/m$^2$ may be considered in infants 2 weeks to 4 months

>8 months: 120 mg/m$^2$ twice daily; dosing range: 90-150 mg/m$^2$ twice daily; patients with CNS disease may require higher dose

**Note:** At least 2 tablets per dose should be administered for adequate buffering and absorption; tablets should be chewed or dispersed (in 1 ounce of water).

Adolescents and Adults: Dosing based on patient weight:

**Note:** Preferred dosing frequency is twice daily for didanosine tablets/oral solution

Chewable tablets, powder for oral solution:

<60 kg: 125 mg twice daily or 250 mg once daily

≥60 kg: 200 mg twice daily or 400 mg once daily

**Note:** Adults should receive 2-4 tablets per dose for adequate buffering and absorption; tablets should be chewed or dispersed (in 1 ounce of water).

Delayed release capsule (Videx® EC):

<60 kg: 250 mg once daily

≥60 kg: 400 mg once daily

(Continued)

# didanosine *(Continued)*

Dosing adjustment with tenofovir (didanosine tablets or delayed release capsules; based on tenofovir product labeling):
<60 kg: 200 mg once daily
≥60 kg: 250 mg once daily

**Dosage Forms**
Capsule, delayed release: 200 mg, 250 mg, 400 mg
Videx® EC: 125 mg, 200 mg, 250 mg, 400 mg
Powder for oral solution, pediatric (Videx®): 2 g, 4 g [makes 10 mg/mL solution after final mixing]
Tablet, buffered, chewable/dispersible (Videx®): 25 mg, 50 mg, 100 mg, 150 mg, 200 mg [all strengths contain phenylalanine 36.5 mg/tablet; orange flavor]

**dideoxycytidine** *see* zalcitabine *on page 857*

**dideoxyinosine** *see* didanosine *on previous page*

**Didrex® [US/Can]** *see* benzphetamine *on page 99*

**Didronel® [US/Can]** *see* etidronate disodium *on page 321*

**dietary supplements** *see* nutritional formula, enteral/oral *on page 591*

# diethylene triamine penta-acetic acid

(dye ETH i leen TRYE a meen PEN ta a SEE tik AS id)

**Synonyms** Ca-DTPA; diethylenetriamine pentaacetic acid; DTPA; pentetate calcium trisodium; pentetate zinc trisodium; trisodium calcium diethylenetriaminepentaacetate (Ca-DTPA); zinc diethylene-triaminepentaacetate (Zn-DTPA); Zn-DTPA

**Therapeutic Category** Antidote

**Use** Treatment of known or suspected internal contamination with plutonium, americium, or curium

**Usual Dosage** Internal contamination with plutonium, americium, or curium: Ca-DTPA is the preferred initial agent; sequential administration of Ca-DTPA then Zn-DTPA is recommended. I.V.:
Children <12 years:
Initial: Ca-DTPA: 14 mg/kg/day (maximum dose: 1 g/day)
Maintenance: Zn-DTPA: 14 mg/kg/day (maximum: 1 g/day); length of therapy depends on patient response and degree of contamination. **Note:** An equivalent dose of Ca-DTPA should be used for maintenance therapy only if Zn-DTPA is not available.
Children ≥12 years and Adults:
Initial: Ca-DTPA: 1 g/day
Pregnancy: Zn-DTPA 1 g/day should be used for the initial dose in pregnant women **except** in cases of high internal contamination,
Maintenance: Zn-DTPA: 1 g/day; length of therapy depends on patient response and degree of contamination. **Note:** An equivalent dose of Ca-DTPA should be used for maintenance therapy only if Zn-DTPA is not available.

**Dosage Forms** Injection, solution:
Ca-DTPA: 200 mg/mL (5 mL)
Zn-DTPA: 200 mg/mL (5 mL)

# diethylpropion (dye eth il PROE pee on)

**Synonyms** amfepramone; diethylpropion hydrochloride

**U.S./Canadian Brand Names** Tenuate® Dospan® [US/Can]; Tenuate® [US/Can]

**Therapeutic Category** Anorexiant

**Controlled Substance** C-IV

**Use** Short-term adjunct in a regimen of weight reduction based on exercise, behavioral modification, and caloric reduction in the management of exogenous obesity for patients with an initial body mass index ≥30 kg/m$^2$ or ≥27 kg/m$^2$ in the presence of other risk factors (diabetes, hypertension)

**Usual Dosage** Adults: Oral:
Tablet: 25 mg 3 times/day before meals or food
Tablet, controlled release: 75 mg at midmorning

**Dosage Forms**
Tablet, as hydrochloride (Tenuate®): 25 mg
Tablet, controlled release, as hydrochloride (Tenuate® Dospan®): 75 mg

**diethylpropion hydrochloride** *see* diethylpropion *on this page*

## difenoxin and atropine (dye fen OKS in & A troe peen)
**Synonyms** atropine and difenoxin
**U.S./Canadian Brand Names** Motofen® [US]
**Therapeutic Category** Antidiarrheal
**Controlled Substance** C-IV
**Use** Treatment of diarrhea
**Usual Dosage** Adults: Oral: Initial: 2 tablets, then 1 tablet after each loose stool; 1 tablet every 3-4 hours, up to 8 tablets in a 24-hour period; if no improvement after 48 hours, continued administration is not indicated
**Dosage Forms** Tablet: Difenoxin hydrochloride 1 mg and atropine sulfate 0.025 mg

**Differin® [US/Can]** *see* adapalene *on page 18*

## diflorasone (dye FLOR a sone)
**Sound-Alike/Look-Alike Issues**
Psorcon® may be confused with Proscar®, ProSom®, Psorion®
**Synonyms** diflorasone diacetate
**U.S./Canadian Brand Names** ApexiCon™ E [US]; ApexiCon™ [US]; Florone® [US/Can]; Psorcon® e™ [US]; Psorcon® [Can]
**Therapeutic Category** Corticosteroid, Topical
**Use** Relieves inflammation and pruritic symptoms of corticosteroid-responsive dermatosis (high to very high potency topical corticosteroid)

Maxiflor®: High potency topical corticosteroid
Psorcon®: Very high potency topical corticosteroid
**Usual Dosage** Topical: Apply ointment sparingly 1-3 times/day; apply cream sparingly 2-4 times/day. Therapy should be discontinued when control is achieved; if no improvement is seen, reassessment of diagnosis may be necessary.
**Dosage Forms** [DSC] = Discontinued product
Cream, as diacetate: 0.05% (15 g, 30 g, 60 g)
  ApexiCon™ E, Florone®: 0.05% (30 g, 60 g)
  Psorcon® e™: 0.05% (15 g, 30 g, 60 g)
Ointment, as diacetate: 0.05% (15 g, 30 g, 60 g)
  ApexiCon™: 0.05% (30 g, 60 g)
  Psorcon®: 0.05% (60 g) [DSC]
  Psorcon® e™: 0.05% (15 g, 30 g, 60 g)

**diflorasone diacetate** *see* diflorasone *on this page*

**Diflucan® [US/Can]** *see* fluconazole *on page 341*

## diflunisal (dye FLOO ni sal)
**Sound-Alike/Look-Alike Issues**
Dolobid® may be confused with Slo-Bid®
**U.S./Canadian Brand Names** Apo-Diflunisal® [Can]; Dolobid® [US]; Novo-Diflunisal [Can]; Nu-Diflunisal [Can]
**Therapeutic Category** Analgesic, Nonnarcotic; Nonsteroidal Antiinflammatory Drug (NSAID)
**Use** Management of inflammatory disorders usually including rheumatoid arthritis and osteoarthritis; can be used as an analgesic for treatment of mild to moderate pain
**Usual Dosage** Adults: Oral:
Osteoarthritis: 500-750 mg/day in divided doses
Pain: Initial: 500-1000 mg followed by 250-500 mg every 8-12 hours; maximum daily dose: 1.5 g
Inflammatory condition: 500-1000 mg/day in 2 divided doses; maximum daily dose: 1.5 g
**Dosage Forms** Tablet: 250 mg, 500 mg

**Digibind® [US/Can]** *see* digoxin immune Fab *on page 249*

**DigiFab™ [US]** *see* digoxin immune Fab *on page 249*

**Digitek® [US]** *see* digoxin *on this page*

## digoxin (di JOKS in)
**Sound-Alike/Look-Alike Issues**
digoxin may be confused with Desoxyn®, doxepin
(Continued)

# digoxin *(Continued)*

Lanoxin® may be confused with Lasix®, Levoxyl®, Levsinex®, Lomotil®, Lonox®, Mefoxin®, Xanax®

**U.S./Canadian Brand Names** Digitek® [US]; Digoxin CSD [Can]; Lanoxicaps® [US/Can]; Lanoxin® [US/Can]; Novo-Digoxin [Can]

**Therapeutic Category** Antiarrhythmic Agent, Miscellaneous; Cardiac Glycoside

**Use** Treatment of congestive heart failure and to slow the ventricular rate in tachyarrhythmias such as atrial fibrillation, atrial flutter, and supraventricular tachycardia (paroxysmal atrial tachycardia); cardiogenic shock

**Usual Dosage** When changing from oral (tablets or liquid) or I.M. to I.V. therapy, dosage should be reduced by 20% to 25%. Refer to the following:

Preterm infant[1]:
  Total digitalizing dose[2]:
    Oral: 20-30 mcg/kg[1]
    I.V. or I.M.: 15-25 mcg/kg[1]
  Daily maintenance dose[3]:
    Oral: 5-7.5 mcg/kg[1]
    I.V. or I.M.: 4-6 mcg/kg[1]
Full-term infant[1]:
  Total digitalizing dose[2]:
    Oral: 25-35 mcg/kg[1]
    I.V. or I.M.: 20-30 mcg/kg[1]
  Daily maintenance dose[3]:
    Oral: 6-10 mcg/kg[1]
    I.V. or I.M.: 5-8 mcg/kg[1]
1 month to 2 years[1]:
  Total digitalizing dose[2]:
    Oral: 35-60 mcg/kg[1]
    I.V. or I.M.: 30-50 mcg/kg[1]
  Daily maintenance dose[3]:
    Oral: 10-15 mcg/kg[1]
    I.V. or I.M.: 7.5-12 mcg/kg[1]
2-5 years[1]:
  Total digitalizing dose[2]:
    Oral: 30-40 mcg/kg[1]
    I.V. or I.M.: 25-35 mcg/kg[1]
  Daily maintenance dose[3]:
    Oral: 7.5-10 mcg/kg[1]
    I.V. or I.M.: 6-9 mcg/kg[1]
5-10 years[1]:
  Total digitalizing dose[2]:
    Oral: 20-35 mcg/kg[1]
    I.V. or I.M.: 15-30 mcg/kg[1]
  Daily maintenance dose[3]:
    Oral: 5-10 mcg/kg[1]
    I.V. or I.M.: 4-8 mcg/kg[1]
>10 years[1]:
  Total digitalizing dose[2]:
    Oral: 10-15 mcg/kg[1]
    I.V. or I.M.: 8-12 mcg/kg[1]
  Daily maintenance dose[3]:
    Oral: 2.5-5 mcg/kg[1]
    I.V. or I.M.: 2-3 mcg/kg[1]
Adults:
  Total digitalizing dose[2]:
    Oral: 0.75-1.5 mg
    I.V. or I.M.: 0.5-1 mg
  Daily maintenance dose[3]:
    Oral: 0.125-0.5 mg
    I.V. or I.M.: 0.1-0.4 mg

[1]Based on lean body weight and normal renal function for age. Decrease dose in patients with decreased renal function; digitalizing dose often not recommended in infants and children.

[2]Give one-half of the total digitalizing dose (TDD) in the initial dose, then give one-quarter of the TDD in each of two subsequent doses at 8- to 12-hour intervals. Obtain EKG 6 hours after each dose to assess potential toxicity.

[3]Divided every 12 hours in infants and children <10 years of age. Give once daily to children >10 years of age and adults.

**Dosage Forms** [DSC] = Discontinued product
Capsule (Lanoxicaps®): 50 mcg [DSC], 100 mcg, 200 mcg [contains ethyl alcohol]
Elixir: 50 mcg/mL (2.5 mL, 5 mL, 60 mL) [contains alcohol 10%; lime flavor]
  Lanoxin® (pediatric): 50 mcg/mL (60 mL) [contains alcohol 10%; lime flavor] [DSC]
Injection: 250 mcg/mL (1 mL, 2 mL) [contains alcohol 10% and propylene glycol 40%]
  Lanoxin®: 250 mcg/mL (2 mL) [contains alcohol 10% and propylene glycol 40%]
Injection, pediatric: 100 mcg/mL (1 mL) [contains alcohol 10% and propylene glycol 40%]
Tablet: 125 mcg, 250 mcg
  Digitek®, Lanoxin®: 125 mcg, 250 mcg

**Digoxin CSD [Can]** *see* digoxin *on page 247*

# digoxin immune Fab (di JOKS in i MYUN fab)

**Synonyms** antidigoxin fab fragments, ovlne
**U.S./Canadian Brand Names** Digibind® [US/Can]; DigiFab™ [US]
**Therapeutic Category** Antidote
**Use** Treatment of life-threatening or potentially life-threatening digoxin intoxication, including:
- acute digoxin ingestion (ie, >10 mg in adults or >4 mg in children)
- chronic ingestions leading to steady-state digoxin concentrations >6 ng/mL in adults or >4 ng/mL in children
- manifestations of digoxin toxicity due to overdose (life-threatening ventricular arrhythmias, progressive bradycardia, second- or third-degree heart block not responsive to atropine, serum potassium >5 mEq/L in adults or >6 mEq in children)

**Usual Dosage** Each vial of Digibind® 38 mg or DigiFab™ 40 mg will bind ~0.5 mg of digoxin or digitoxin.

Estimation of the dose is based on the body burden of digitalis. This may be calculated if the amount ingested is known or the postdistribution serum drug level is known (round dose to the nearest whole vial). Fab dose (in vials) based on number of tablets (0.25 mg) ingested.

5 tablets ingested: 2 vials
10 tablets ingested: 4 vials
25 tablets ingested: 10 vials
50 tablets ingested: 20 vials
75 tablets ingested: 30 vials
100 tablets ingested: 40 vials
150 tablets ingested: 60 vials
200 tablets ingested: 80 vials

**Fab dose based on serum drug level postdistribution:**
Digoxin: No. of vials = level (ng/mL) x body weight (kg) divided by 100
Digitoxin: No. of vials = digitoxin (ng/mL) x body weight (kg) divided by 1000
If neither amount ingested nor drug level are known, dose empirically as follows:
For acute toxicity: 20 vials, administered in 2 divided doses to decrease the possibility of a febrile reaction, and to avoid fluid overload in small children.
For chronic toxicity: 6 vials; for infants and small children (≤20kg), a single vial may be sufficient

**Dosage Forms** Injection, powder for reconstitution:
Digibind®: 38 mg
DigiFab™: 40 mg

**dihematoporphyrin ether** *see* porfimer *on page 661*

**Dihistine® DH [US]** *see* chlorpheniramine, pseudoephedrine, and codeine *on page 176*

# dihydrocodeine, aspirin, and caffeine (dye hye droe KOE deen, AS pir in, & KAF een)
**Sound-Alike/Look-Alike Issues**
Synalgos®-DC may be confused with Synagis®
(Continued)

## dihydrocodeine, aspirin, and caffeine (Continued)

**Synonyms** dihydrocodeine compound

**U.S./Canadian Brand Names** Synalgos®-DC [US]

**Therapeutic Category** Analgesic, Narcotic

**Controlled Substance** C-III

**Use** Management of mild to moderate pain that requires relaxation

**Usual Dosage** Adults: Oral: 1-2 capsules every 4-6 hours as needed for pain

**Dosage Forms** Capsule: Dihydrocodeine bitartrate 16 mg, aspirin 356.4 mg, and caffeine 30 mg

## dihydrocodeine bitartrate, phenylephrine hydrochloride, and chlorpheniramine maleate

*see* phenylephrine, hydrocodone, and chlorpheniramine *on page 643*

**dihydrocodeine compound** *see* dihydrocodeine, aspirin, and caffeine *on previous page*

## dihydroergotamine (dye hye droe er GOT a meen)

**Synonyms** DHE; dihydroergotamine mesylate

**U.S./Canadian Brand Names** D.H.E. 45® [US]; Migranal® [US/Can]

**Therapeutic Category** Ergot Alkaloid and Derivative

**Use** Treatment of migraine headache with or without aura; injection also indicated for treatment of cluster headaches

**Usual Dosage** Adults:

I.M., SubQ: 1 mg at first sign of headache; repeat hourly to a maximum dose of 3 mg total; maximum dose: 6 mg/week

I.V.: 1 mg at first sign of headache; repeat hourly up to a maximum dose of 2 mg total; maximum dose: 6 mg/week

Intranasal: 1 spray (0.5 mg) of nasal spray should be administered into each nostril; if needed, repeat after 15 minutes, up to a total of 4 sprays. **Note:** Do not exceed 3 mg (6 sprays) in a 24-hour period and no more than 8 sprays in a week.

**Dosage Forms**

Injection, solution, as mesylate (D.H.E. 45®): 1 mg/mL (1 mL) [contains ethanol 94%]

Solution, intranasal spray, as mesylate (Migranal®): 4 mg/mL [0.5 mg/spray] (1 mL) [contains caffeine 10 mg/mL]

**dihydroergotamine mesylate** *see* dihydroergotamine *on this page*

**dihydroergotoxine** *see* ergoloid mesylates *on page 293*

**dihydrogenated ergot alkaloids** *see* ergoloid mesylates *on page 293*

**dihydrohydroxycodeinone** *see* oxycodone *on page 608*

**dihydromorphinone** *see* hydromorphone *on page 418*

## dihydrotachysterol (dye hye droe tak ISS ter ole)

**Synonyms** dichysterol

**U.S./Canadian Brand Names** DHT™ Intensol™ [US]; DHT™ [US]; Hytakerol® [US/Can]

**Therapeutic Category** Vitamin D Analog

**Use** Treatment of hypocalcemia associated with hypoparathyroidism; prophylaxis of hypocalcemic tetany following thyroid surgery

**Usual Dosage** Oral:

Hypoparathyroidism:

Infants and young Children: Initial: 1-5 mg/day for 4 days, then 0.1-0.5 mg/day

Older Children and Adults: Initial: 0.8-2.4 mg/day for several days followed by maintenance doses of 0.2-1 mg/day

Nutritional rickets: 0.5 mg as a single dose or 13-50 mcg/day until healing occurs

Renal osteodystrophy: Maintenance: 0.25-0.6 mg/24 hours adjusted as necessary to achieve normal serum calcium levels and promote bone healing

**Dosage Forms** [DSC] = Discontinued product

Capsule (Hytakerol®): 0.125 mg [contains sesame oil] [DSC]

Solution, oral concentrate (DHT™ Intensol™): 0.2 mg/mL (30 mL) [contains alcohol 20%] [DSC]

Tablet (DHT™): 0.125 mg, 0.2 mg, 0.4 mg [DSC]

**dihydroxyanthracenedione dihydrochloride** *see* mitoxantrone *on page 545*

**1,25 dihydroxycholecalciferol** *see* calcitriol *on page 129*

**dihydroxydeoxynorvinkaleukoblastine** *see* vinorelbine *on page 847*

**dihydroxypropyl theophylline** *see* dyphylline *on page 277*

**Dihyrex® Injection** *(Discontinued)* *see* diphenhydramine *on page 254*

**diiodohydroxyquin** *see* iodoquinol *on page 445*

**Dilacor® XR [US]** *see* diltiazem *on this page*

**Dilantin® [US/Can]** *see* phenytoin *on page 645*

**Dilatrate®-SR [US]** *see* isosorbide dinitrate *on page 451*

**Dilaudid® [US/Can]** *see* hydromorphone *on page 418*

**Dilaudid® Cough Syrup** *(Discontinued)* *see* hydromorphone *on page 418*

**Dilaudid-HP® [US/Can]** *see* hydromorphone *on page 418*

**Dilaudid-HP-Plus® [Can]** *see* hydromorphone *on page 418*

**Dilaudid® Sterile Powder [Can]** *see* hydromorphone *on page 418*

**Dilaudid-XP® [Can]** *see* hydromorphone *on page 418*

**Dilocaine® Injection** *(Discontinued)* *see* lidocaine *on page 479*

**Dilomine® Injection** *(Discontinued)* *see* dicyclomine *on page 245*

**Dilor® [US/Can]** *see* dyphylline *on page 277*

**Diltia XT® [US]** *see* diltiazem *on this page*

## diltiazem (dil TYE a zem)

**Sound-Alike/Look-Alike Issues**
diltiazem may be confused with Dilantin®
Cardizem® may be confused with Cardene®, Cardene SR®, Cardizem CD®, Cardizem SR®, cardiem
Cartia XT™ may be confused with Procardia XL®
Tiazac® may be confused with Tigan®, Ziac®

**Synonyms** diltiazem hydrochloride

**U.S./Canadian Brand Names** Alti-Diltiazem CD [Can]; Apo-Diltiaz CD® [Can]; Apo-Diltiaz SR® [Can]; Apo-Diltiaz® [Can]; Cardizem® CD [US/Can]; Cardizem® LA [US]; Cardizem® SR [Can]; Cardizem® [US/Can]; Cartia XT™ [US]; Dilacor® XR [US]; Diltia XT® [US]; Gen-Diltiazem CD [Can]; Gen-Diltiazem [Can]; Med-Diltiazem [Can]; Novo-Diltazem [Can]; Novo-Diltazem-CD [Can]; Nu-Diltiaz [Can]; Nu-Diltiaz-CD [Can]; ratio-Diltiazem CD [Can]; Rhoxal-diltiazem CD [Can]; Rhoxal-diltiazem SR [Can]; Syn-Diltiazem® [Can]; Taztia XT™ [US]; Tiazac® XC [Can]; Tiazac® [US/Can]

**Therapeutic Category** Calcium Channel Blocker

**Use**
Oral: Essential hypertension; chronic stable angina or angina from coronary artery spasm
Injection: Atrial fibrillation or atrial flutter; paroxysmal supraventricular tachycardia (PSVT)

**Usual Dosage** Adults:
Oral:
Angina:
Capsule, extended release (Cardizem® CD, Cartia XT™, Dilacor® XR, Diltia XT®, Tiazac®): Initial: 120-180 mg once daily (maximum dose: 480 mg/day)
Tablet, extended release (Cardizem® LA): 180 mg once daily; may increase at 7- to 14-day intervals (maximum recommended dose: 360 mg/day)
Tablet, immediate release (Cardizem®): Usual starting dose: 30 mg 4 times/day; usual range: 180-360 mg/day
Hypertension:
Capsule, extended release (Cardizem® CD, Cartia XT™, Dilacor® XR, Diltia XT®, Tiazac®): Initial: 180-240 mg once daily; dose adjustment may be made after 14 days; usual dose range (JNC 7): 180-420 mg/day; Tiazac®: usual dose range: 120-540 mg/day
Capsule, sustained release (Cardizem® SR): Initial: 60-120 mg twice daily; dose adjustment may be made after 14 days; usual range: 240-360 mg/day
Tablet, extended release (Cardizem® LA): Initial: 180-240 mg once daily; dose adjustment may be made after 14 days; usual dose range (JNC 7): 120-540 mg/day
I.V.: Atrial fibrillation, atrial flutter, PSVT:
Initial bolus dose: 0.25 mg/kg actual body weight over 2 minutes (average adult dose: 20 mg)
Repeat bolus dose (may be administered after 15 minutes if the response is inadequate.): 0.35 mg/kg actual body weight over 2 minutes (average adult dose: 25 mg)
(Continued)

## diltiazem *(Continued)*

Continuous infusion (requires an infusion pump; infusions >24 hours or infusion rates >15 mg/hour are not recommended.): Initial infusion rate of 10 mg/hour; rate may be increased in 5 mg/hour increments up to 15 mg/hour as needed; some patients may respond to an initial rate of 5 mg/hour.

If diltiazem injection is administered by continuous infusion for >24 hours, the possibility of decreased diltiazem clearance, prolonged elimination half-life, and increased diltiazem and/or diltiazem metabolite plasma concentrations should be considered.

**Conversion from I.V. diltiazem to oral diltiazem:** Start oral approximately 3 hours after bolus dose. **Oral dose (mg/day) is approximately equal to [rate (mg/hour) x 3 + 3] x 10.**
3 mg/hour = 120 mg/day
5 mg/hour = 180 mg/day
7 mg/hour = 240 mg/day
11 mg/hour = 360 mg/day

**Dosage Forms** [DSC] = Discontinued product
Capsule, extended release, as hydrochloride [once-daily dosing]: 120 mg, 180 mg, 240 mg, 300 mg
Cardizem® CD: 120 mg, 180 mg, 240 mg, 300 mg, 360 mg
Cartia XT™: 120 mg, 180 mg, 240 mg, 300 mg
Dilacor® XR, Diltia XT®: 120 mg, 180 mg, 240 mg
Taztia XT™: 120 mg, 180 mg, 240 mg, 300 mg, 360 mg
Tiazac®: 120 mg, 180 mg, 240 mg, 300 mg, 360 mg, 420 mg
Capsule, sustained release, as hydrochloride [twice-daily dosing] (Cardizem® SR [DSC]): 60 mg, 90 mg, 120 mg
Injection, solution, as hydrochloride: 5 mg/mL (5 mL, 10 mL, 25 mL)
Injection, powder for reconstitution, as hydrochloride (Cardizem®): 25 mg
Tablet, as hydrochloride (Cardizem®): 30 mg, 60 mg, 90 mg, 120 mg
Tablet, extended release, as hydrochloride (Cardizem® LA): 120 mg, 180 mg, 240 mg, 300 mg, 360 mg, 420 mg

**diltiazem hydrochloride** *see* diltiazem *on previous page*

**Dimaphen DM [US-OTC]** *see* brompheniramine, pseudoephedrine, and dextromethorphan *on page 116*

## dimenhydrinate *(dye men HYE dri nate)*
**Sound-Alike/Look-Alike Issues**
dimenhyDRINATE may be confused with diphenhydrAMINE
**Tall-Man** dimenhyDRINATE
**U.S./Canadian Brand Names** Apo-Dimenhydrinate® [Can]; Dramamine® [US-OTC]; Gravol® [Can]; Novo-Dimenate [Can]; TripTone® [US-OTC]
**Therapeutic Category** Antihistamine
**Use** Treatment and prevention of nausea, vertigo, and vomiting associated with motion sickness
**Usual Dosage** Oral:
Children:
2-5 years: 12.5-25 mg every 6-8 hours, maximum: 75 mg/day
6-12 years: 25-50 mg every 6-8 hours, maximum: 150 mg/day
Adults: 50-100 mg every 4-6 hours, not to exceed 400 mg/day
**Dosage Forms**
Caplet (TripTone®): 50 mg
Tablet (Dramamine®): 50 mg
Tablet, chewable (Dramamine®): 50 mg [contains phenylalanine 1.5 mg/tablet and tartrazine; orange flavor]

## dimercaprol *(dye mer KAP role)*
**Synonyms** BAL; British anti-lewisite; dithioglycerol
**U.S./Canadian Brand Names** BAL in Oil® [US]
**Therapeutic Category** Chelating Agent
**Use** Antidote to gold, arsenic (except arsine), and mercury poisoning (except nonalkyl mercury); adjunct to edetate calcium disodium in lead poisoning; possibly effective for antimony, bismuth, chromium, copper, nickel, tungsten, or zinc

**Usual Dosage** Children and Adults: Deep I.M.:

Arsenic, mercury, and gold poisoning: 3 mg/kg every 4-6 hours for 2 days, then every 12 hours for 7-10 days or until recovery (initial dose may be up to 5 mg if severe poisoning)

Lead poisoning (in conjunction with calcium EDTA): For symptomatic acute encephalopathy or blood level >100 mcg/dL: 4-5 mg/kg every 4 hours for 3-5 days

**Dosage Forms** Injection, oil: 100 mg/mL (3 mL) [contains benzyl benzoate and peanut oil]

**Dimetabs®** Oral *(Discontinued)* see dimenhydrinate *on previous page*

**Dimetane®** Extentabs® [US-OTC] see brompheniramine *on page 115*

**Dimetapp®** 12-Hour Non-Drowsy Extentabs® [US-OTC] see pseudoephedrine *on page 692*

**Dimetapp®** Allergy [US-OTC] see brompheniramine *on page 115*

**Dimetapp®** Allergy Children's [US-OTC] see brompheniramine *on page 115*

**Dimetapp®** Children's ND [US-OTC] see loratadine *on page 491*

**Dimetapp®** Cold and Congestion [US-OTC] see guaifenesin, pseudoephedrine, and dextromethorphan *on page 391*

**Dimetapp®** Decongestant Infant [US-OTC] see pseudoephedrine *on page 692*

**Dimetapp®** DM Children's Cold and Cough [US-OTC] see brompheniramine, pseudoephedrine, and dextromethorphan *on page 116*

**Dimetapp®** Infant Decongestant Plus Cough [US-OTC] see pseudoephedrine and dextromethorphan *on page 693*

**Dimetapp®** Sinus Caplets *(Discontinued)* see pseudoephedrine and ibuprofen *on page 694*

$\beta,\beta$**-dimethylcysteine** see penicillamine *on page 627*

## dimethyl sulfoxide (dye meth il sul FOKS ide)

**Synonyms** DMSO

**U.S./Canadian Brand Names** Kemsol® [Can]; Rimso®-50 [US/Can]

**Therapeutic Category** Urinary Tract Product

**Use** Symptomatic relief of interstitial cystitis

**Usual Dosage** Instill 50 mL directly into bladder and allow to remain for 15 minutes; repeat every 2 weeks until maximum symptomatic relief is obtained

**Dosage Forms** Solution, intravesical: 50% [500 mg/mL] (50 mL)

**dimethyl triazeno imidazole carboxamide** see dacarbazine *on page 220*

**Dinate®** Injection *(Discontinued)* see dimenhydrinate *on previous page*

## dinoprostone (dye noe PROST one)

**Sound-Alike/Look-Alike Issues**

Prepidil® may be confused with Bepridil®

**Synonyms** PGE₂; prostaglandin E₂

**U.S./Canadian Brand Names** Cervidil® [US/Can]; Prepidil® [US/Can]; Prostin E₂® [US/Can]

**Therapeutic Category** Prostaglandin

**Use**

Gel: Promote cervical ripening prior to labor induction; usage for gel include any patient undergoing induction of labor with an unripe cervix, most commonly for pre-eclampsia, eclampsia, postdates, diabetes, intrauterine growth retardation, and chronic hypertension

Suppositories: Terminate pregnancy from 12th through 28th week of gestation; evacuate uterus in cases of missed abortion or intrauterine fetal death; manage benign hydatidiform mole

Vaginal insert: Initiation and/or cervical ripening in patients at or near term in whom there is a medical or obstetrical indication for the induction of labor

**Usual Dosage**

Abortifacient: Insert 1 suppository high in vagina, repeat at 3- to 5-hour intervals until abortion occurs up to 240 mg (maximum dose); continued administration for longer than 2 days is not advisable

Cervical ripening:

Gel:

Intracervical: 0.25-1 mg

Intravaginal: 2.5 mg

Suppositories: Intracervical: 2-3 mg

Vaginal Insert (Cervidil®): 10 mg (to be removed at the onset of active labor or after 12 hours)

(Continued)

## dinoprostone *(Continued)*

**Dosage Forms**
Gel, endocervical (Prepidil®): 0.5 mg/3 g syringe [each package contains a 10 mm and 20 mm shielded catheter]
Insert, vaginal (Cervidil®): 10 mg [releases 0.3 mg/hour]
Suppository, vaginal (Prostin E$_2$®): 20 mg

**Diocaine®** **[Can]** *see* proparacaine *on page 685*

**Diocarpine [Can]** *see* pilocarpine *on page 647*

**Diochloram®** **[Can]** *see* chloramphenicol *on page 167*

**Diocto®** **[US-OTC]** *see* docusate *on page 263*

**Diocto-K®** *(Discontinued)* *see* docusate *on page 263*

**Diocto-K Plus®** *(Discontinued)* *see* docusate *on page 263*

**dioctyl calcium sulfosuccinate** *see* docusate *on page 263*

**dioctyl sodium sulfosuccinate** *see* docusate *on page 263*

**Diodex®** **[Can]** *see* dexamethasone (systemic) *on page 233*

**Diodoquin®** **[Can]** *see* iodoquinol *on page 445*

**Diogent®** **[Can]** *see* gentamicin *on page 372*

**Diomycin®** **[Can]** *see* erythromycin *on page 295*

**Dionephrine®** **[Can]** *see* phenylephrine *on page 640*

**Dionosil Oily®** **[US]** *see* radiological/contrast media (ionic) *on page 707*

**Diopentolate®** **[Can]** *see* cyclopentolate *on page 214*

**Diopred®** **[Can]** *see* prednisolone (systemic) *on page 674*

**Dioptic's Atropine Solution [Can]** *see* atropine *on page 79*

**Dioptimyd®** **[Can]** *see* sulfacetamide and prednisolone *on page 771*

**Dioptrol®** **[Can]** *see* neomycin, polymyxin B, and dexamethasone *on page 567*

**Diosulf™** **[Can]** *see* sulfacetamide *on page 771*

**Diotame®** **[OTC]** *see* bismuth subsalicylate *on page 108*

**Diotrope®** **[Can]** *see* tropicamide *on page 829*

**Dioval® Injection** *(Discontinued)* *see* estradiol *on page 299*

**Diovan®** **[US/Can]** *see* valsartan *on page 838*

**Diovan HCT®** **[US/Can]** *see* valsartan and hydrochlorothiazide *on page 839*

**Diovol®** **[Can]** *see* aluminum hydroxide and magnesium hydroxide *on page 35*

**Diovol® Ex [Can]** *see* aluminum hydroxide and magnesium hydroxide *on page 35*

**Diovol Plus®** **[Can]** *see* aluminum hydroxide, magnesium hydroxide, and simethicone *on page 35*

**Dipentum®** **[US/Can]** *see* olsalazine *on page 597*

**Diphen®** **[US-OTC]** *see* diphenhydramine *on this page*

**Diphenacen 50® Injection** *(Discontinued)* *see* diphenhydramine *on this page*

**Diphen® AF [US-OTC]** *see* diphenhydramine *on this page*

**Diphenatol®** *(Discontinued)* *see* diphenoxylate and atropine *on page 257*

**Diphenhist [US-OTC]** *see* diphenhydramine *on this page*

## diphenhydramine *(dye fen HYE dra meen)*

**Sound-Alike/Look-Alike Issues**
diphenhydrAMINE may be confused with desipramine, dicyclomine, dimenhyDRINATE
Benadryl® may be confused with benazepril, Bentyl®, Benylin®, Caladryl®
**Synonyms** diphenhydramine citrate; diphenhydramine hydrochloride; diphenhydramine tannate
**Tall-Man** diphenhydr**AMINE**
**U.S./Canadian Brand Names** Aler-Cap [US-OTC]; Aler-Dryl [US-OTC]; Aler-Tab [US-OTC]; Allerdryl®
[Can]; AllerMax® [US-OTC]; Allernix [Can]; Altaryl [US-OTC]; Banophen® Anti-Itch [US-OTC];

Banophen® [US-OTC]; Benadryl® Allergy [US-OTC]; Benadryl® Children's Allergy Fastmelt® [US-OTC]; Benadryl® Children's Allergy [US-OTC]; Benadryl® Dye-Free Allergy [US-OTC]; Benadryl® Injection [US]; Benadryl® Itch Stopping Extra Strength [US-OTC]; Benadryl® Itch Stopping [US-OTC]; Benadryl® [Can]; Compoz® Nighttime Sleep Aid [US-OTC]; Dermamycin® [US-OTC]; Dermarest® Insect Bite [US-OTC]; Dermarest® Plus [US-OTC]; Diphenhist [US-OTC]; Diphen® AF [US-OTC]; Diphen® [US-OTC]; Dytan™ [US]; Genahist® [US-OTC]; Hydramine® [US-OTC]; Nytol® Extra Strength [Can]; Nytol® Quick Caps [US-OTC]; Nytol® Quick Gels [US-OTC]; Nytol® [Can]; PMS-Diphenhydramine [Can]; Q-Dryl [US-OTC]; Quenalin [US-OTC]; Siladryl® Allergy [US-OTC]; Siladryl® DAS [US-OTC]; Silphen® [US-OTC]; Simply Sleep® [US-OTC/Can]; Sleep-ettes D [US-OTC]; Sleepinal® [US-OTC]; Sominex® Maximum Strength [US-OTC]; Sominex® [US-OTC]; Triaminic® Thin Strips™ Cough and Runny Nose [US-OTC]; Twilite® [US-OTC]; Unisom® Maximum Strength SleepGels® [US-OTC]

**Therapeutic Category** Antihistamine

**Use** Symptomatic relief of allergic symptoms caused by histamine release which include nasal allergies and allergic dermatosis; can be used for mild nighttime sedation; prevention of motion sickness and as an antitussive; has antinauseant and topical anesthetic properties; treatment of antipsychotic-induced extrapyramidal symptoms

**Usual Dosage**

Children:

Oral, I.M., I.V.:

Treatment of moderate to severe allergic reactions: 5 mg/kg/day or 150 mg/m²/day in divided doses every 6-8 hours, not to exceed 300 mg/day

Minor allergic rhinitis or motion sickness:

2 to <6 years: 6.25 mg every 4-6 hours; maximum: 37.5 mg/day

6 to <12 years: 12.5-25 mg every 4-6 hours; maximum: 150 mg/day

≥12 years: 25-50 mg every 4-6 hours; maximum: 300 mg/day

Night-time sleep aid: 30 minutes before bedtime:

2 to <12 years: 1 mg/kg/dose; maximum: 50 mg/dose

≥12 years: 50 mg

Oral: Antitussive:

2 to <6 years: 6.25 mg every 4 hours; maximum 37.5 mg/day

6 to <12 years: 12.5 mg every 4 hours; maximum 75 mg/day

≥12 years: 25 mg every 4 hours; maximum 150 mg/day

I.M., I.V.: Treatment of dystonic reactions: 0.5-1 mg/kg/dose

Adults:

Oral: 25-50 mg every 6-8 hours

Minor allergic rhinitis or motion sickness: 25-50 mg every 4-6 hours; maximum: 300 mg/day

Moderate to severe allergic reactions: 25-50 mg every 4 hours, not to exceed 400 mg/day

Nighttime sleep aid: 50 mg at bedtime

I.M., I.V.: 10-50 mg in a single dose every 2-4 hours, not to exceed 400 mg/day

Dystonic reaction: 50 mg in a single dose; may repeat in 20-30 minutes if necessary

Topical: For external application, not longer than 7 days

**Dosage Forms**

Caplet, as hydrochloride: 25 mg, 50 mg

Aler-Dryl, AllerMax®, Compoz® Nighttime Sleep Aid, Sleep-ettes D, Sominex® Maximum Strength, Twilite®: 50 mg

Simply Sleep®, Nytol® Quick Caps: 25 mg

Capsule, as hydrochloride: 25 mg, 50 mg

Aler-Cap, Banophen®, Benadryl® Allergy, Diphen®, Diphenhist, Genahist®, Q-Dryl: 25 mg

Sleepinal®: 50 mg

Capsule, softgel, as hydrochloride: 50 mg

Benadryl® Dye-Free Allergy: 25 mg [dye-free]

Compoz® Nighttime Sleep Aid, Nytol® Quick Gels, Sleepinal®, Unisom® Maximum Strength Sleep-Gels®: 50 mg

Captab, as hydrochloride (Diphenhist®): 25 mg

Cream, as hydrochloride: 2% (30 g) [contains zinc acetate 0.1%]

Banophen® Anti-Itch: 2% (30 g) [contains zinc acetate 0.1%]

Benadryl® Itch Stopping: 1% (30 g) [contains zinc acetate 0.1%]

Benadryl® Itch Stopping Extra Strength: 2% (30 g) [contains zinc acetate 0.1%]

Diphenhist®: 2% (30 g) [contains zinc acetate 0.1%]

Elixir, as hydrochloride:

Altaryl: 12.5 mg/5 mL (120 mL, 480 mL, 3840 mL) [cherry flavor]

Banophen®: 12.5 mg/5 mL (120 mL)

(Continued)

## diphenhydramine *(Continued)*

Diphen AF: 12.5 mg/5 mL (120 mL, 240 mL, 480 mL) [alcohol free; cherry flavor]
Q-Dryl: 12.5 mg/5 mL (480 mL) [alcohol free]
Gel, topical, as hydrochloride:
Benadryl® Itch Stopping Extra Strength: 2% (120 mL)
Dermarest® Plus: 2% (28 g, 42 g) [contains menthol 1%]
Injection, solution, as hydrochloride: 50 mg/mL (1 mL)
Benadryl®: 50 mg/mL (1 mL, 10 mL)
Liquid, as hydrochloride:
AllerMax®: 12.5 mg/5 mL (120 mL)
Benadryl® Allergy: 12.5 mg/5 mL (120 mL, 240 mL) [alcohol free; contains sodium benzoate; cherry flavor]
Benadryl® Dye-Free Allergy: 12.5 mg/5 mL (120 mL) [alcohol free, dye free, sugar free; contains sodium benzoate; bubble gum flavor]
Genahist®: 12.5 mg/5 mL (120 mL) [alcohol free, sugar free; contains sodium benzoate; cherry flavor]
Hydramine®: 12.5 mg/5 mL (120 mL, 480 mL) [alcohol free]
Q-Dryl: 12.5 mg/5 mL (120 mL) [alcohol free; cherry flavor]
Quenalin: 12.5 mg/5 mL (120 mL) [fruit flavor]
Siladryl® Allergy: 12.5 mg/5 mL (120 mL, 240 mL, 480 mL) [alcohol free, sugar free; black cherry flavor]
Siladryl® DAS: 12.5 mg/5 mL (120 mL) [alcohol free, dye free, sugar free; black cherry flavor]
Liquid, topical, as hydrochloride [stick] (Benadryl® Itch Stopping Extra Strength): 2% (14 mL) [contains zinc acetate 0.1% and alcohol]
Solution, oral, as hydrochloride:
Banophen®: 12.5 mg/5mL (480 mL) [sugar free]
Diphenhist: 12.5 mg/5 mL (120 mL, 480 mL) [alcohol free; contains sodium benzoate]
Solution, topical, as hydrochloride [spray]:
Benadryl® Itch Stopping Extra Strength: 2% (60 mL) [contains zinc acetate 0.1% and alcohol]
Dermamycin®, Dermarest® Insect Bite: 2% (60 mL) [contains menthol 1%]
Strips, oral, as hydrochloride (Triaminic® Thin Strips™ Cough and Runny Nose): 12. 5 mg (16s) [grape flavor]
Suspension, as tannate (Dytan™): 25 mg/5 mL (120 mL) [strawberry flavor]
Syrup, as hydrochloride (Silphen® Cough): 12.5 mg/5 mL (120 mL, 240 mL, 480 mL) [contains alcohol; 5%; strawberry flavor]
Tablet, as hydrochloride: 25 mg, 50 mg
Aler-Tab, Benadryl® Allergy, Genahist®, Sleepinal®, Sominex®: 25 mg
Tablet, chewable, as hydrochloride (Benadryl® Children's Allergy): 12.5 mg [contains phenylalanine 4.2 mg/tablet; grape flavor]
Tablet, chewable, as tannate (Dytan™): 25 mg [contains phenylalanine; strawberry flavor]
Tablet, orally-disintegrating, as citrate (Benadryl® Children's Allergy Fastmelt®): 19 mg [equivalent to diphenhydramine hydrochloride 12.5 mg; contains phenylalanine 4.5 mg/tablet and soy protein isolate; cherry flavor]

**diphenhydramine and acetaminophen** *see* acetaminophen and diphenhydramine *on* page 7

## diphenhydramine and pseudoephedrine (dye fen HYE dra meen & soo doe e FED rin)

**Sound-Alike/Look-Alike Issues**
Benadryl® may be confused with benazepril, Bentyl®, Benylin®, Caladryl®
**Synonyms** pseudoephedrine and diphenhydramine
**U.S./Canadian Brand Names** Benadryl® Allergy and Sinus Fastmelt™ [US-OTC]; Benadryl® Allergy/Sinus [US-OTC]; Benadryl® Children's Allergy and Cold Fastmelt™ [US-OTC]; Benadryl® Children's Allergy and Sinus [US-OTC]
**Therapeutic Category** Antihistamine/Decongestant Combination
**Use** Relief of symptoms of upper respiratory mucosal congestion in seasonal and perennial nasal allergies, acute rhinitis, rhinosinusitis, and eustachian tube blockage
**Usual Dosage** Based on **pseudoephedrine** component: Adults: Oral: 60 mg every 4-6 hours, maximum: 240 mg/day
**Dosage Forms**
Liquid (Benadryl® Children's Allergy and Sinus): Diphenhydramine hydrochloride 12.5 mg and pseudoephedrine hydrochloride 30 mg per 5 mL [contains sodium benzoate; alcohol free, sugar free; grape flavor]

Tablet (Benadryl® Allergy/Sinus): Diphenhydramine hydrochloride 25 mg and pseudoephedrine hydrochloride 60 mg

Tablet, quick-dissolving (Benadryl® Children's Allergy and Cold Fastmelt™, Benadryl® Allergy and Sinus Fastmelt™): Diphenhydramine citrate 19 mg [equivalent to diphenhydramine hydrochloride 12.5 mg] and pseudoephedrine 30 mg [contains phenylalanine 4.6 mg/tablet; cherry flavor]

**diphenhydramine citrate** *see* diphenhydramine *on page 254*

**diphenhydramine hydrochloride** *see* diphenhydramine *on page 254*

**diphenhydramine, hydrocodone, and phenylephrine** *see* hydrocodone, phenylephrine, and diphenhydramine *on page 414*

**diphenhydramine tannate** *see* diphenhydramine *on page 254*

# diphenoxylate and atropine (dye fen OKS i late & A troe peen)
**Sound-Alike/Look-Alike Issues**
Lomotil® may be confused with Lamictal®, Lamisil®, lamotrigine, Lanoxin®, Lasix®, ludiomil
Lonox® may be confused with Lanoxin®, Loprox®
**Synonyms** atropine and diphenoxylate
**U.S./Canadian Brand Names** Lomotil® [US/Can]; Lonox® [US]
**Therapeutic Category** Antidiarrheal
**Controlled Substance** C-V
**Use** Treatment of diarrhea
**Usual Dosage** Oral:
Children (use with caution in young children due to variable responses): Liquid: 0.3-0.4 mg of diphenoxylate/kg/day in 2-4 divided doses **or**
<2 years: Not recommended
2-5 years: 2 mg of diphenoxylate 3 times/day
5-8 years: 2 mg of diphenoxylate 4 times/day
8-12 years: 2 mg of diphenoxylate 5 times/day
Adults: 15-20 mg/day of diphenoxylate in 3-4 divided doses; maintenance: 5-15 mg/day in 2-3 divided doses
**Dosage Forms**
Solution, oral: Diphenoxylate hydrochloride 2.5 mg and atropine sulfate 0.025 mg per 5 mL (5 mL, 10 mL, 60 mL)
Lomotil®: Diphenoxylate hydrochloride 2.5 mg and atropine sulfate 0.025 mg per 5 mL (60 mL) [contains alcohol 15%; cherry flavor]
Tablet (Lomotil®, Lonox®): Diphenoxylate hydrochloride 2.5 mg and atropine sulfate 0.025 mg

**Diphenylan Sodium®** *(Discontinued)* *see* phenytoin *on page 645*

**diphenylhydantoin** *see* phenytoin *on page 645*

# diphtheria and tetanus toxoid (dif THEER ee a & TET a nus TOKS oyd)
**Synonyms** DT; Td; tetanus and diphtheria toxoid
**U.S./Canadian Brand Names** Decavac™ [US]
**Therapeutic Category** Toxoid
**Use**
Diphtheria and tetanus toxoids adsorbed for pediatric use (DT): Infants and children through 6 years of age: Active immunity against diphtheria and tetanus when pertussis vaccine is contraindicated
Tetanus and diphtheria toxoids adsorbed for adult use (Td) (Decavac™): Children ≥7 years of age and Adults: Active immunity against diphtheria and tetanus; tetanus prophylaxis in wound management
**Usual Dosage** I.M.:
Infants and Children ≤6 years (DT): Primary immunization:
6 weeks to 1 year: Three 0.5 mL doses at least 4 weeks apart; administer a reinforcing dose 6-12 months after the third injection
1-6 years: Two 0.5 mL doses at least 4 weeks apart; reinforcing dose 6-12 months after second injection; if final dose is given after seventh birthday, use adult preparation
4-6 years (booster immunization): 0.5 mL; not necessary if the fourth dose was given after fourth birthday; routinely administer booster doses at 10-year intervals with the adult preparation
Children ≥7 years and Adults:
Primary immunization: Patients previously not immunized should receive 2 primary doses of 0.5 mL each, given at an interval of 4-6 weeks; third (reinforcing) dose of 0.5 mL 6-12 months later
(Continued)

## diphtheria and tetanus toxoid *(Continued)*

Booster immunization: 0.5 mL every 10 years; to be given to children 11-12 years of age if at least 5 years have elapsed since last dose of toxoid containing vaccine. Subsequent routine doses are not recommended more often than every 10 years.

Tetanus prophylaxis in wound management; use of tetanus toxoid (Td*) and/or tetanus immune globulin (TIG) depends upon the number of prior tetanus toxoid doses and type of wound:

Clean, minor wounds:
- Prior number of tetanus toxoid doses is unknown or <3: Td[1]
- Prior number of tetanus toxoid doses is ≥3: Td[1] only if >10 years since last dose
- If only three doses of fluid tetanus toxoid have been received, a fourth dose of toxoid, preferably an adsorbed toxoid, should be given

All other wounds:
- Prior number of tetanus toxoid doses is unknown or <3: Td[1] and TIG
- Prior number of tetanus toxoid doses is ≥3: Td[1] only if >5 years since last dose

[1]Adult tetanus and diphtheria toxoids; use pediatric preparations (DT or DTP) if the patient is <7 years old.

Adapted from Report of the Committee on Infectious Diseases, American Academy of Pediatrics, Elk Grove Village, IL: American Academy of Pediatrics, 1986.

### Dosage Forms

Injection, suspension, adult: Diphtheria 2 Lf units and tetanus 5 Lf units per 0.5 mL (5 mL)

Decavac™: Diphtheria 2 Lf units and tetanus 5 Lf units per 0.5 mL (0.5 mL) [latex free prefilled syringe; contains thimerosal]

Injection, suspension, pediatric [preservative free]: Diphtheria 6.7 Lf units and tetanus 5 Lf units per 0.5 mL (0.5 mL)

## diphtheria and tetanus toxoids and acellular pertussis adsorbed, hepatitis B (recombinant) and inactivated poliovirus vaccine combined *see* diphtheria, tetanus toxoids, acellular pertussis, hepatitis B (recombinant), and poliovirus (inactivated) vaccine *on this page*

## diphtheria antitoxin *(dif THEER ee a an tee TOKS in)*

**Therapeutic Category** Antitoxin

**Use** Treatment of diphtheria (neutralizes unbound toxin, available from CDC)

**Usual Dosage** I.M. or slow I.V. infusion: Dosage varies; range: 20,000-120,000 units

**Dosage Forms** Injection: ≥500 units/mL (40 mL) [20,000 units/vial]

## diphtheria CRM$_{197}$ protein *see* pneumococcal conjugate vaccine (7-valent) *on page 654*

## diphtheria CRM$_{197}$ protein conjugate *see Haemophilus* B conjugate vaccine *on page 394*

## diphtheria, tetanus toxoids, acellular pertussis, hepatitis B (recombinant), and poliovirus (inactivated) vaccine

(dif THEER ee a, TET a nus TOKS oyds, ay CEL yoo lar per TUS sis, hep a TYE tis bee ree KOM be nant, & POE lee oh VYE rus vak SEEN, in ak ti VAY ted vak SEEN)

**Synonyms** diphtheria and tetanus toxoids and acellular pertussis adsorbed, hepatitis B (recombinant) and inactivated poliovirus vaccine combined

**U.S./Canadian Brand Names** Pediarix™ [US]

**Therapeutic Category** Vaccine

**Use** Combination vaccine for the active immunization against diphtheria, tetanus, pertussis, hepatitis B virus (all known subtypes), and poliomyelitis (caused by poliovirus types 1, 2, and 3)

**Usual Dosage** I.M.: Children:

Immunization: 0.5 mL; repeat in 6-8 week intervals (preferably 8-week intervals) for a total of 3 doses. Vaccination usually begins at 2 months, but may be started as early as 6 weeks of age.

Use in children previously vaccinated with one or more component, and who are also scheduled to receive all vaccine components:

Hepatitis B vaccine: Infants born of HB$_s$Ag-negative mothers who received 1 dose of hepatitis B vaccine at birth may be given Pediarix™ (safety data limited); use in infants who received more than 1 dose of hepatitis B vaccine has not been studied. Infants who received 1 or more doses of hepatitis B vaccine (recombinant) may be given Pediarix™ to complete the hepatitis B series (safety and efficacy not established).

Diphtheria and tetanus toxoids, and acellular pertussis vaccine (DTaP): Infants previously vaccinated with 1 or 2 doses of Infanrix® may use Pediarix™ to complete the first 3 doses of the series (safety and efficacy not established); use of Pediarix™ to complete DTaP vaccination started with products other than Infanrix® is not recommended.

Inactivated polio vaccine (IPV): Infants previously vaccinated with 1 or 2 doses of IPV may use Pediarix™ to complete the first 3 doses of the series (safety and efficacy not established).

**Dosage Forms** Injection, suspension [single-dose]: Diphtheria toxoid 25 Lf, tetanus toxoid 10 Lf, inactivated PT 25 mcg, FHA 25 mcg, pertactin 8 mcg, $HB_sAg$ 10 mcg, poliovirus type 1 40 DU, poliovirus type 2 8 DU, and poliovirus type 3 32 DU per 0.5 mL [contains neomycin sulfate ≤0.05 ng/0.5 mL, polymyxin B ≤0.01 ng/0.5 mL, and yeast protein ≤5%; packaged in vials or prefilled syringes; the needleless prefilled syringes contain dry natural latex rubber in the tip cap and plunger]

# diphtheria, tetanus toxoids, and acellular pertussis vaccine

(dif THEER ee a, TET a nus TOKS oyds & ay CEL yoo lar per TUS sis vak SEEN)

**Synonyms** DTaP; dTpa; Tdap; tetanus toxoid, reduced diphtheria toxoid, and acellular pertussis, adsorbed

**U.S./Canadian Brand Names** Adacel™ [US/Can]; Boostrix® [US]; Daptacel® [US]; Infanrix® [US]; Tripedia® [US]

**Therapeutic Category** Toxoid

**Use**

Daptacel®, Infanrix®, Tripedia® (DTaP): Active immunization against diphtheria, tetanus, and pertussis from age 6 weeks through seventh birthday

Adacel™, Boostrix® (Tdap): Active booster immunization against diphtheria, tetanus, and pertussis

**Usual Dosage**

Primary immunization:

Children 6 weeks to <7 years: (Daptacel®, Infanrix®, Tripedia®): I.M.: 0.5 mL per dose, total of 5 doses administered as follows:

Three doses, usually given at 2-, 4-, and 6 months of age; may be given as early as 6 weeks of age and repeated every 4-8 weeks; use same product for all 3 doses

Fourth dose: Given at ~15-20 months of age, but at least 6 months after third dose

Fifth dose: Given at 5-6 years of age, prior to starting school or kindergarten; if the fourth dose is given at ≥4 years of age, the fifth dose may be omitted

Booster immunization:

Children 10-18 years (Boostrix®): I.M.: 0.5 mL as a single dose, administered 5 years after last dose of DTwP or DTaP vaccine.

Children ≥11 years and Adults ≤64 years (Adacel™): I.M.: 0.5 mL as a single dose, administered 5 years after last dose of DTwP or DTaP vaccine.

Adacel™ (in patients 11-64 years of age) or Boostrix® (in patients 10-18 years of age) may be used as an alternative to Td vaccine when a tetanus toxoid-containing vaccine is needed for wound management, and in whom the pertussis component is also indicated. Td vaccine is the preferred agent in children ≥7 years and adults.

**Dosage Forms** Injection, suspension:

Adacel™: Diphtheria 2 Lf units, tetanus 5 Lf units, and acellular pertussis 2.5 mcg per 0.5 mL (0.5 mL) [vial stopper is latex free]

Boostrix®: Diphtheria 2.5 Lf units, tetanus 5 Lf units, and acellular pertussis 8 mcg per 0.5 mL (0.5 mL) [available in vial and prefilled syringe; syringe cap and rubber plunger contain natural latex rubber]

Daptacel®: Diphtheria 15 Lf units, tetanus 5 Lf units, and acellular pertussis 10 mcg per 0.5 mL (0.5 mL) [vial stopper contains natural latex rubber]

Infanrix®: Diphtheria 25 Lf units, tetanus 10 Lf units, and acellular pertussis 25 mcg per 0.5 mL (0.5 mL) [available in vial and prefilled syringe; syringe cap and rubber plunger contain natural latex rubber]

Tripedia®: Diphtheria 6.7 Lf units, tetanus 5 Lf units, and acellular pertussis 46.8 mcg per 0.5 mL (7.5 mL) [contains trace amounts of thimerosal; vial stopper contains natural latex rubber]

**Note:** Tripedia® vaccine is also used to reconstitute ActHIB® to prepare TriHIBit® vaccine (diphtheria, tetanus toxoids, and acellular pertussis and *Haemophilus influenzae* b conjugate vaccine combination)

# diphtheria, tetanus toxoids, and acellular pertussis vaccine and *Haemophilus* b conjugate vaccine

(dif THEER ee a, TET a nus TOKS oyds & ay CEL yoo lar per TUS sis vak SEEN & hem OF fi lus in floo EN za bee KON joo gate vak SEEN)

**Synonyms** *Haemophilus influenzae* b conjugate vaccine and diphtheria, tetanus toxoids, and acellular pertussis vaccine

(Continued)

# diphtheria, tetanus toxoids, and acellular pertussis vaccine and *Haemophilus* b conjugate vaccine *(Continued)*

**U.S./Canadian Brand Names** TriHIBit® [US]

**Therapeutic Category** Toxoid; Vaccine, Inactivated Bacteria

**Use** Active immunization of children 15-18 months of age for prevention of diphtheria, tetanus, pertussis, and invasive disease caused by *H. influenzae* type b.

**Usual Dosage** Children >15 months of age: I.M.: 0.5 mL (as part of a general vaccination schedule; see individual vaccines). Vaccine should be used within 30 minutes of reconstitution.

**Dosage Forms** Injection, suspension: 5 Lf units tetanus toxoid, 6.7 Lf units diphtheria toxoid, 46.8 mcg pertussis antigens, and 10 mcg *H. influenzae* type b purified capsular polysaccharide per 0.5 mL (0.5 mL) [The combination of Tripedia® vaccine used to reconstitute ActHIB® forms TriHIBit®]

**diphtheria toxoid conjugate** *see Haemophilus* B conjugate vaccine *on page 394*

**dipivalyl epinephrine** *see* dipivefrin *on this page*

## dipivefrin (dye PI ve frin)

**Synonyms** dipivalyl epinephrine; dipivefrin hydrochloride; DPE

**U.S./Canadian Brand Names** Ophtho-Dipivefrin™ [Can]; PMS-Dipivefrin [Can]; Propine® [US/Can]

**Therapeutic Category** Adrenergic Agonist Agent

**Use** Reduces elevated intraocular pressure in chronic open-angle glaucoma; also used to treat ocular hypertension, low tension, and secondary glaucomas

**Usual Dosage** Adults: Ophthalmic: Instill 1 drop every 12 hours into the eyes

**Dosage Forms** Solution, ophthalmic, as hydrochloride: 0.1% (5 mL, 10 mL, 15 mL) [contains benzalkonium chloride]
Propine®: 0.1% (5 mL [DSC], 10 mL, 15 mL) [contains benzalkonium chloride]

**dipivefrin hydrochloride** *see* dipivefrin *on this page*

**Diprivan® [US/Can]** *see* propofol *on page 686*

**Diprolene® [US]** *see* betamethasone (topical) *on page 103*

**Diprolene® AF [US]** *see* betamethasone (topical) *on page 103*

**Diprolene® Glycol [Can]** *see* betamethasone (topical) *on page 103*

**dipropylacetic acid** *see* valproic acid and derivatives *on page 837*

**Diprosone® [Can]** *see* betamethasone (topical) *on page 103*

## dipyridamole (dye peer ID a mole)

**Sound-Alike/Look-Alike Issues**
dipyridamole may be confused with disopyramide
Persantine® may be confused with Periactin®, Permitil®

**U.S./Canadian Brand Names** Apo-Dipyridamole FC® [Can]; Persantine® [US/Can]

**Therapeutic Category** Antiplatelet Agent; Vasodilator

**Use**
Oral: Used with warfarin to decrease thrombosis in patients after artificial heart valve replacement
I.V.: Diagnostic agent in CAD

**Usual Dosage** Adults:
Oral: Adjunctive therapy for prophylaxis of thromboembolism with cardiac valve replacement: 75-100 mg 4 times/day
I.V.: Evaluation of coronary artery disease: 0.14 mg/kg/minute for 4 minutes; maximum dose: 60 mg

**Dosage Forms**
Injection, solution: 5 mg/mL (2 mL, 10 mL)
Tablet (Persantine®): 25 mg, 50 mg, 75 mg

**dipyridamole and aspirin** *see* aspirin and dipyridamole *on page 75*

## dirithromycin (dye RITH roe mye sin)

**Sound-Alike/Look-Alike Issues**
Dynabac® may be confused with Dynacin®, DynaCirc®, Dynapen®

U.S./Canadian Brand Names Dynabac® [US]

Therapeutic Category Macrolide (Antibiotic)

Use Treatment of mild to moderate upper and lower respiratory tract infections due to *Moraxella catarrhalis*, *Streptococcus pneumoniae*, *Legionella pneumophila*, *H. influenzae*, or *S. pyogenes*, ie, acute exacerbation of chronic bronchitis, secondary bacterial infection of acute bronchitis, community-acquired pneumonia, pharyngitis/tonsillitis, and uncomplicated infections of the skin and skin structure due to *Staphylococcus aureus*

Usual Dosage Adults: Oral: 500 mg once daily for 5-14 days (14 days required for treatment of community-acquired pneumonia due to *Legionella*, *Mycoplasma*, or *S. pneumoniae*; 10 days is recommended for treatment of *S. pyogenes* pharyngitis/tonsillitis)

Dosage Forms Tablet, enteric coated: 250 mg

**Disalcid®** *(Discontinued)* see salsalate *on page 738*

**disalicylic acid** see salsalate *on page 738*

**Disobrom®** *(Discontinued)* see dexbrompheniramine and pseudoephedrine *on page 234*

**disodium cromoglycate** see cromolyn sodium *on page 211*

**disodium thiosulfate pentahydrate** see sodium thiosulfate *on page 758*

***d*-isoephedrine hydrochloride** see pseudoephedrine *on page 692*

**Disonate®** *(Discontinued)* see docusate *on page 263*

## disopyramide (dye soe PEER a mide)

Sound-Alike/Look-Alike Issues

disopyramide may be confused with desipramine, dipyridamole

Norpace® may be confused with Norpramin®

Synonyms disopyramide phosphate

U.S./Canadian Brand Names Norpace® CR [US]; Norpace® [US/Can]; Rythmodan® [Can]; Rythmodan®-LA [Can]

Therapeutic Category Antiarrhythmic Agent, Class I-A

Use Suppression and prevention of unifocal and multifocal atrial and premature, ventricular premature complexes, coupled ventricular tachycardia; effective in the conversion of atrial fibrillation, atrial flutter, and paroxysmal atrial tachycardia to normal sinus rhythm and prevention of the recurrence of these arrhythmias after conversion by other methods

Usual Dosage Oral:

Children:

<1 year: 10-30 mg/kg/24 hours in 4 divided doses

1-4 years: 10-20 mg/kg/24 hours in 4 divided doses

4-12 years: 10-15 mg/kg/24 hours in 4 divided doses

12-18 years: 6-15 mg/kg/24 hours in 4 divided doses

Adults:

<50 kg: 100 mg every 6 hours or 200 mg every 12 hours (controlled release)

>50 kg: 150 mg every 6 hours or 300 mg every 12 hours (controlled release); if no response, increase to 200 mg every 6 hours. Maximum dose required for patients with severe refractory ventricular tachycardia is 400 mg every 6 hours.

Dosage Forms

Capsule (Norpace®): 100 mg, 150 mg

Capsule, controlled release (Norpace® CR): 100 mg, 150 mg

**disopyramide phosphate** see disopyramide *on this page*

**Disotate®** *(Discontinued)* see edetate disodium *on page 279*

**Di-Spaz® Injection** *(Discontinued)* see dicyclomine *on page 245*

**Di-Spaz® Oral** *(Discontinued)* see dicyclomine *on page 245*

**DisperMox™ [US]** see amoxicillin *on page 46*

## disulfiram (dye SUL fi ram)

Sound-Alike/Look-Alike Issues

disulfiram may be confused with Diflucan®

Antabuse® may be confused with Anturane®

(Continued)

## disulfiram *(Continued)*

**U.S./Canadian Brand Names** Antabuse® [US]
**Therapeutic Category** Aldehyde Dehydrogenase Inhibitor Agent
**Use** Management of chronic alcoholism
**Usual Dosage** Adults: Oral: Do not administer until the patient has abstained from ethanol for at least 12 hours

Initial: 500 mg/day as a single dose for 1-2 weeks; maximum daily dose is 500 mg
Average maintenance dose: 250 mg/day; range: 125-500 mg; duration of therapy is to continue until the patient is fully recovered socially and a basis for permanent self control has been established; maintenance therapy may be required for months or even years
**Dosage Forms** Tablet: 250 mg

**Dital® *(Discontinued)*** *see* phendimetrazine *on page 637*

**dithioglycerol** *see* dimercaprol *on page 252*

**dithranol** *see* anthralin *on page 54*

**Ditropan® [US/Can]** *see* oxybutynin *on page 607*

**Ditropan® XL [US/Can]** *see* oxybutynin *on page 607*

**Diurigen® *(Discontinued)*** *see* chlorothiazide *on page 170*

**Diuril® [US/Can]** *see* chlorothiazide *on page 170*

**divalproex sodium** *see* valproic acid and derivatives *on page 837*

**Dixarit® [Can]** *see* clonidine *on page 197*

**Dizac® Injectable Emulsion *(Discontinued)*** *see* diazepam *on page 241*

**Dizmiss® *(Discontinued)*** *see* meclizine *on page 506*

**5071-1DL(6)** *see* megestrol acetate *on page 508*

***dl*-alpha tocopherol** *see* vitamin E *on page 850*

**4-DMDR** *see* idarubicin *on page 429*

**D-Med® Injection *(Discontinued)*** *see* methylprednisolone *on page 531*

**DMSA** *see* succimer *on page 768*

**DMSO** *see* dimethyl sulfoxide *on page 253*

**DNA-derived humanized monoclonal antibody** *see* alemtuzumab *on page 26*

**DNase** *see* dornase alfa *on page 267*

**DNR** *see* daunorubicin hydrochloride *on page 225*

**Doak® Tar [US-OTC]** *see* coal tar *on page 201*

**Doan's® [US-OTC]** *see* magnesium salicylate *on page 499*

**Doan's® Extra Strength [US-OTC]** *see* magnesium salicylate *on page 499*

## dobutamine *(doe BYOO ta meen)*

**Sound-Alike/Look-Alike Issues**
DOBUTamine may be confused with DOPamine
**Synonyms** dobutamine hydrochloride
**Tall-Man** DOBUTamine
**U.S./Canadian Brand Names** Dobutrex® [Can]
**Therapeutic Category** Adrenergic Agonist Agent
**Use** Short-term management of patients with cardiac decompensation
**Usual Dosage** Administration requires the use of an infusion pump; I.V. infusion:
Neonates: 2-15 mcg/kg/minute, titrate to desired response
Children and Adults: 2.5-20 mcg/kg/minute; maximum: 40 mcg/kg/minute, titrate to desired response.
**Dosage Forms**
Infusion, as hydrochloride [premixed in dextrose]: 1 mg/mL (250 mL, 500 mL); 2 mg/mL (250 mL); 4 mg/mL (250 mL)
Injection, solution, as hydrochloride: 12.5 mg/mL (20 mL, 40 mL, 100 mL) [contains sodium bisulfite]

**dobutamine hydrochloride** *see* dobutamine *on this page*

**Dobutrex**® **[Can]** *see* dobutamine *on previous page*

# docetaxel (doe se TAKS el)

**Sound-Alike/Look-Alike Issues**

Taxotere® may be confused with Taxol®

**Synonyms** NSC-628503; RP-6976

**U.S./Canadian Brand Names** Taxotere® [US/Can]

**Therapeutic Category** Antineoplastic Agent

**Use** Treatment of locally-advanced or metastatic breast cancer; adjuvant treatment of operable node-positive breast cancer (in combination with doxorubicin and cyclophosphamide); treatment of locally-advanced or metastatic nonsmall cell lung cancer (NSCLC) in combination with cisplatin in treatment of patients who have not previously received chemotherapy for unresected NSCLC; treatment of prostate cancer (hormone refractory, metastatic)

**Usual Dosage** Children ≥16 years and Adults: I.V. infusion: Refer to individual protocols:

Breast cancer:

Locally-advanced or metastatic: 60-100 mg/m$^2$ every 3 weeks; patients initially started at 60 mg/m$^2$ who do not develop toxicity may tolerate higher doses

Operable, node-positive (adjuvant treatment): 75 mg/m$^2$ every 3 weeks for 6 courses

Nonsmall cell lung cancer: I.V.: 75 mg/m$^2$ every 3 weeks

Prostate cancer: 75 mg/m$^2$ every 3 weeks; prednisone (5 mg twice daily) is administered continuously

**Dosage Forms** Injection, solution [concentrate]: 20 mg/0.5 mL (0.5 mL, 2 mL) [contains Polysorbate 80®; diluent contains ethanol 13%]

# docosanol (doe KOE san ole)

**Synonyms** *n*-docosanol; behenyl alcohol

**U.S./Canadian Brand Names** Abreva® [US-OTC]

**Therapeutic Category** Antiviral Agent, Topical

**Use** Treatment of herpes simplex of the face or lips

**Usual Dosage** Children ≥12 years and Adults: Topical: Apply 5 times/day to affected area of face or lips. Start at first sign of cold sore or fever blister and continue until healed.

**Dosage Forms** Cream: 10% (2 g)

# docusate (DOK yoo sate)

**Sound-Alike/Look-Alike Issues**

docusate may be confused with Doxinate®

Colace® may be confused with Calan®

Surfak® may be confused with Surbex®

**Synonyms** dioctyl calcium sulfosuccinate; dioctyl sodium sulfosuccinate; docusate calcium; docusate potassium; docusate sodium; DOSS; DSS

**U.S./Canadian Brand Names** Apo-Docusate-Calcium® [Can]; Apo-Docusate-Sodium® [Can]; Colace® [US-OTC/Can]; Colax-C® [Can]; D-S-S® [US-OTC]; Diocto® [US-OTC]; Docusoft-S™ [US-OTC]; DOK™ [US-OTC]; DOS® [US-OTC]; Dulcolax® Stool Softener [US-OTC]; Enemeez® [US-OTC]; Fleet® Sof-Lax® [US-OTC]; Genasoft® [US-OTC]; Novo-Docusate Calcium [Can]; Novo-Docusate Sodium [Can]; Phillips'® Stool Softener Laxative [US-OTC]; PMS-Docusate Calcium [Can]; PMS-Docusate Sodium [Can]; Regulex® [Can]; Selax® [Can]; Silace [US-OTC]; Soflax™ [Can]; Surfak® [US-OTC]

**Therapeutic Category** Stool Softener

**Use** Stool softener in patients who should avoid straining during defecation and constipation associated with hard, dry stools; prophylaxis for straining (Valsalva) following myocardial infarction. A safe agent to be used in elderly; some evidence that doses <200 mg are ineffective; stool softeners are unnecessary if stool is well hydrated or "mushy" and soft; shown to be ineffective used long-term.

**Usual Dosage** Docusate salts are interchangeable; the amount of sodium or calcium per dosage unit is clinically insignificant

Infants and Children <3 years: Oral: 10-40 mg/day in 1-4 divided doses

Children: Oral:

3-6 years: 20-60 mg/day in 1-4 divided doses

6-12 years: 40-150 mg/day in 1-4 divided doses

Adolescents and Adults: Oral: 50-500 mg/day in 1-4 divided doses

Older Children and Adults: Rectal: Add 50-100 mg of docusate liquid to enema fluid (saline or water); administer as retention or flushing enema

(Continued)

## docusate *(Continued)*

### Dosage Forms

Capsule, as calcium (Surfak®): 240 mg

Capsule, as sodium: 100 mg, 250 mg

Colace®: 50 mg [contains sodium 3 mg], 100 mg [contains sodium 5 mg]

Docusoft-S™: 100 mg [contains sodium 5 mg]

DOK™, Genasoft®: 100 mg

DOS®, D-S-S®: 100 mg, 250 mg

Dulcolax® Stool Softener: 100 mg [contains sodium 5 mg]

Phillips'® Stool Softener Laxative: 100 mg [contains sodium 5.2 mg]

Enema, rectal, as sodium (Enemeez®): 283 mg/5 mL 5 mL

Gelcap, as sodium (Fleet® Sof-Lax®): 100 mg

Liquid, as sodium: 150 mg/15 mL (480 mL)

Colace®: 150 mg/15 mL (30 mL) [contains sodium 1 mg/mL]

Diocto®: 150 mg/15 mL (480 mL) [vanilla flavor]

Silace: 150 mg/15 mL (480 mL) [lemon-vanilla flavor]

Syrup, as sodium: 60 mg/15 mL (480 mL)

Colace®, Diocto®: 60 mg/15 mL (480 mL) [alcohol free, sugar free; contains sodium 36 mg/5 mL]

Silace: 20 mg/5 mL (480 mL) [peppermint flavor]

## docusate and senna (DOK yoo sate & SEN na)

### Sound-Alike/Look-Alike Issues

Senokot® may be confused with Depakote®

**Synonyms** senna and docusate; senna-S

**U.S./Canadian Brand Names** Peri-Colace® *(reformulation)* [US-OTC]; Senokot-S® [US-OTC]

**Therapeutic Category** Laxative, Stimulant;  Stool Softener

**Use** Short-term treatment of constipation

**Usual Dosage** Oral: Constipation: OTC ranges:

Children:

2-6 years: Initial: 4.3 mg sennosides plus 25 mg docusate (1/2 tablet) once daily (maximum: 1 tablet twice daily)

6-12 years: Initial: 8.6 sennosides plus 50 mg docusate (1 tablet) once daily (maximum: 2 tablets twice daily)

Children ≥12 years and Adults: Initial: 2 tablets (17.2 mg sennosides plus 100 mg docusate) once daily (maximum: 4 tablets twice daily)

### Dosage Forms

Tablet: Docusate sodium 50 mg and sennosides 8.6 mg

Peri-Colace® (reformulation): Docusate sodium 50 mg and sennosides 8.6 mg

Senokot-S®: Docusate sodium 50 mg and sennosides 8.6 mg [sugar free; contains sodium 3 mg/tablet]

## docusate calcium *see* docusate *on previous page*

## docusate potassium *see* docusate *on previous page*

## docusate sodium *see* docusate *on previous page*

## Docusoft-S™ [US-OTC] *see* docusate *on previous page*

## dofetilide (doe FET il ide)

**U.S./Canadian Brand Names** Tikosyn™ [US/Can]

**Therapeutic Category** Antiarrhythmic Agent, Class III

**Use** Maintenance of normal sinus rhythm in patients with chronic atrial fibrillation/atrial flutter of longer than 1-week duration who have been converted to normal sinus rhythm; conversion of atrial fibrillation and atrial flutter to normal sinus rhythm

**Usual Dosage** Adults: Oral:

**Note:** QT or $QT_c$ must be determined prior to first dose. If $QT_c$ >440 msec (>500 msec in patients with ventricular conduction abnormalities), dofetilide is contraindicated.

Initial: 500 mcg orally twice daily. Initial dosage must be adjusted in patients with estimated $Cl_{cr}$ <60 mL/minute. Dofetilide may be initiated at lower doses than recommended based on physician discretion.

Modification of dosage in response to initial dose: $QT_c$ interval should be measured 2-3 hours after the initial dose. If the $QT_c$ >15% of baseline, or if the $QT_c$ is >500 msec (550 msec in patients with ventricular conduction abnormalities) dofetilide should be adjusted. If the starting dose is 500 mcg twice

daily, then adjust to 250 mcg twice daily. If the starting dose was 250 mcg twice daily, then adjust to 125 mcg twice daily. If the starting dose was 125 mcg twice daily then adjust to 125 mcg every day. Continued monitoring for doses 2-5: $QT_c$ interval must be determined 2-3 hours after each subsequent dose of dofetilide for in-hospital doses 2-5. If the measured $QT_c$ is >500 msec (550 msec in patients with ventricular conduction abnormalities) at any time, dofetilide should be discontinued.
Chronic therapy (following the 5th dose):
QT or $QT_c$ and creatinine clearance should be evaluated every 3 months. If $QT_c$ >500 msec (>550 msec in patients with ventricular conduction abnormalities), dofetilide should be discontinued.
**Dosage Forms** Capsule: 125 mcg, 250 mcg, 500 mcg

**Dofus [US-OTC]** *see* Lactobacillus *on page 462*

**DOK™ [US-OTC]** *see* docusate *on page 263*

**Doktors® Nasal Solution *(Discontinued)*** *see* phenylephrine *on page 640*

**Dolacet® Forte *(Discontinued)*** *see* hydrocodone and acetaminophen *on page 411*

# dolasetron (dol A se tron)

**Sound-Alike/Look-Alike Issues**
dolasetron may be confused with granisetron, ondansetron, palonosetron
Anzemet® may be confused with Aldomet®

**Synonyms** dolasetron mesylate; MDL 73,147EF

**U.S./Canadian Brand Names** Anzemet® [US/Can]

**Therapeutic Category** Selective 5-HT$_3$ Receptor Antagonist

**Use** Prevention of nausea and vomiting associated with emetogenic cancer chemotherapy; prevention of postoperative nausea and vomiting; treatment of postoperative nausea and vomiting (injectable form only)

**Not recommended for treatment of existing chemotherapy-induced emesis (CIE).**

**Usual Dosage**
Nausea and vomiting prophylaxis, chemotherapy-induced (including initial and repeat courses):
Children 2-16 years:
Oral: 1.8 mg/kg within 1 hour before chemotherapy; maximum: 100 mg/dose
I.V.: 1.8 mg/kg ~30 minutes before chemotherapy; maximum: 100 mg/dose
Adults:
Oral:100 mg single dose 1 hour prior to chemotherapy
I.V.: 1.8 mg/kg or 100 mg 30 minutes prior to chemotherapy
Prevention of postoperative nausea and vomiting:
Children 2-16 years:
Oral: 1.2 mg/kg within 2 hours before surgery; maximum: 100 mg/dose
I.V.: 0.35 mg/kg (maximum: 12.5 mg) ~15 minutes before stopping anesthesia
Adults:
Oral: 100 mg within 2 hours before surgery
I.V.: 12.5 mg ~15 minutes before stopping anesthesia
Treatment of postoperative nausea and vomiting: I.V. (only):
Children: 0.35 mg/kg (maximum: 12.5 mg) as soon as needed
Adults: 12.5 mg as soon as needed

**Dosage Forms**
Injection, solution, as mesylate: 20 mg/mL (0.625 mL) [single-use ampul, Carpuject®, or vial]; 20 mg/mL (5 mL) [single-use vial]; 20 mg/mL (25 mL) [multidose vial]
Tablet, as mesylate: 50 mg, 100 mg

**dolasetron mesylate** *see* dolasetron *on this page*

**Dolene® *(Discontinued)*** *see* propoxyphene *on page 687*

**Dolgic® LQ [US]** *see* butalbital, acetaminophen, and caffeine *on page 124*

**Dolgic® Plus [US]** *see* butalbital, acetaminophen, and caffeine *on page 124*

**Dolobid® [US]** *see* diflunisal *on page 247*

**Dolophine® [US/Can]** *see* methadone *on page 521*

**Dolorac™ *(Discontinued)*** *see* capsaicin *on page 138*

**Dolorex® *(Discontinued)*** *see* capsaicin *on page 138*

**Dolsed® [US]** *see* methenamine, phenyl salicylate, atropine, hyoscyamine, benzoic acid, and methylene blue *on page 523*

**Dom-Benzydamine [Can]** *see* benzydamine *(Canada only) on page 100*

**Dom-Domperidone [Can]** *see* domperidone *(Canada only) on this page*

**Domeboro® [US-OTC]** *see* aluminum sulfate and calcium acetate *on page 36*

**dome paste bandage** *see* zinc gelatin *on page 861*

## domperidone *(Canada only)* (dom PE ri done)
**Synonyms** domperidone maleate
**U.S./Canadian Brand Names** Alti-Domperidone [Can]; Apo-Domperidone® [Can]; Dom-Domperidone [Can]; FTP-Domperidone Maleate [Can]; Motilium® [Can]; Novo-Domperidone [Can]; Nu-Domperidone [Can]; ratio-Domperidone [Can]
**Therapeutic Category** Dopamine Antagonist
**Use** Symptomatic management of upper GI motility disorders associated with chronic and subacute gastritis and diabetic gastroparesis; prevention of GI symptoms associated with use of dopamine-agonist anti-Parkinson agents
**Usual Dosage** Oral: Adults:
GI motility disorders: 10 mg 3-4 times/day, 15-30 minutes before meals; severe/resistant cases: 20 mg 3-4 times/day, 15-30 minutes before meals
Nausea/vomiting associated with dopamine-agonist anti-Parkinson agents: 20 mg 3-4 times/day
**Dosage Forms** Tablet: 10 mg [domperidone maleate 12.72 mg]

**domperidone maleate** *see* domperidone *(Canada only) on this page*

**Dom-Tiaprofenic® [Can]** *see* tiaprofenic acid *(Canada only) on page 801*

## donepezil (doh NEP e zil)
**Sound-Alike/Look-Alike Issues**
Aricept® may be confused with AcipHex®, Ascriptin®
**Synonyms** E2020
**U.S./Canadian Brand Names** Aricept® ODT [US]; Aricept® [US/Can]
**Therapeutic Category** Acetylcholinesterase Inhibitor; Cholinergic Agent
**Use** Treatment of mild to moderate dementia of the Alzheimer type
**Usual Dosage** Oral: Adults: Dementia of Alzheimer type: Initial: 5 mg/day at bedtime; may increase to 10 mg/day at bedtime after 4-6 weeks
**Dosage Forms**
Tablet, as hydrochloride (Aricept®): 5 mg, 10 mg
Tablet, orally-disintegrating, as hydrochloride (Aricept® ODT): 5 mg, 10 mg

**Donnamar® *(Discontinued)*** *see* hyoscyamine *on page 424*

**Donnapine® *(Discontinued)*** *see* hyoscyamine, atropine, scopolamine, and phenobarbital *on page 425*

**Donnatal® [US]** *see* hyoscyamine, atropine, scopolamine, and phenobarbital *on page 425*

**Donnatal Extentabs® [US]** *see* hyoscyamine, atropine, scopolamine, and phenobarbital *on page 425*

## dopamine (DOE pa meen)
**Sound-Alike/Look-Alike Issues**
DOPamine may be confused with DOBUTamine, Dopram®
**Synonyms** dopamine hydrochloride
**Tall-Man** DOPamine
**Therapeutic Category** Adrenergic Agonist Agent
**Use** Adjunct in the treatment of shock (eg, MI, open heart surgery, renal failure, cardiac decompensation) which persists after adequate fluid volume replacement
**Usual Dosage** I.V. infusion (administration requires the use of an infusion pump):
Neonates: 1-20 mcg/kg/minute continuous infusion, titrate to desired response.
Children: 1-20 mcg/kg/minute, maximum: 50 mcg/kg/minute continuous infusion, titrate to desired response.
Adults: 1-5 mcg/kg/minute up to 20 mcg/kg/minute, titrate to desired response. Infusion may be increased by 1-4 mcg/kg/minute at 10- to 30-minute intervals until optimal response is obtained.

If dosages >20-30 mcg/kg/minute are needed, a more direct-acting pressor may be more beneficial (ie, epinephrine, norepinephrine).

**Dosage Forms**
Infusion, as hydrochloride [premixed in $D_5W$]: 0.8 mg/mL (250 mL, 500 mL); 1.6 mg/mL (250 mL, 500 mL); 3.2 mg/mL (250 mL)
Injection, solution, as hydrochloride: 40 mg/mL (5 mL, 10 mL); 80 mg/mL (5 mL); 160 mg/mL (5 mL) [contains sodium metabisulfite]

**dopamine hydrochloride** *see dopamine on previous page*

**Dopram**® **[US]** *see doxapram on next page*

**Doral**® **[US/Can]** *see quazepam on page 703*

**Dormarex**® **2 Oral** *(Discontinued) see diphenhydramine on page 254*

## dornase alfa (DOOR nase AL fa)

**Synonyms** DNase; recombinant human deoxyribonuclease
**U.S./Canadian Brand Names** Pulmozyme® [US/Can]
**Therapeutic Category** Enzyme
**Use** Management of cystic fibrosis patients to reduce the frequency of respiratory infections that require parenteral antibiotics, and to improve pulmonary function
**Usual Dosage** Inhalation:
Children >3 months to Adults: 2.5 mg once daily through selected nebulizers; experience in children <5 years is limited
Patients unable to inhale or exhale orally throughout the entire treatment period may use Pari-Baby™ nebulizer. Some patients may benefit from twice daily administration.
**Dosage Forms** Solution for nebulization: 1 mg/mL (2.5 mL)

**Doryx**® **[US]** *see doxycycline on page 271*

## dorzolamide (dor ZOLE a mide)

**Synonyms** dorzolamide hydrochloride
**U.S./Canadian Brand Names** Trusopt® [US/Can]
**Therapeutic Category** Carbonic Anhydrase Inhibitor
**Use** Lowers intraocular pressure in patients with ocular hypertension or open-angle glaucoma
**Usual Dosage** Children and Adults: Reduction of intraocular pressure: Instill 1 drop in the affected eye(s) 3 times/day
**Dosage Forms** Solution, ophthalmic, as hydrochloride: 2% (5 mL, 10 mL) [contains benzalkonium chloride]

## dorzolamide and timolol (dor ZOLE a mide & TYE moe lole)

**Synonyms** timolol and dorzolamide
**U.S./Canadian Brand Names** Cosopt® [US/Can]
**Therapeutic Category** Beta-Adrenergic Blocker; Carbonic Anhydrase Inhibitor
**Use** Reduction of intraocular pressure in patients with ocular hypertension or open-angle glaucoma
**Usual Dosage** Ophthalmic: Children ≥2 years and Adults: Instill 1 drop in affected eye(s) twice daily
**Dosage Forms** Solution, ophthalmic: Dorzolamide hydrochloride 2% (as base) and timolol maleate 0.5% (as base) (5 mL, 10 mL) [contains benzalkonium chloride]

**dorzolamide hydrochloride** *see dorzolamide on this page*

**DOS**® **[US-OTC]** *see docusate on page 263*

**DOSS** *see docusate on page 263*

**Dostinex**® **[US/Can]** *see cabergoline on page 127*

**Dovobet**® **[Can]** *see betamethasone and calcipotriol (Canada only) on page 102*

**Dovonex**® **[US]** *see calcipotriene on page 128*

## doxacurium (doks a KYOO ri um)

**Sound-Alike/Look-Alike Issues**
doxacurium may be confused with doxapram, DOXOrubicin
(Continued)

# doxacurium *(Continued)*

**Synonyms** doxacurium chloride

**U.S./Canadian Brand Names** Nuromax® [US]

**Therapeutic Category** Skeletal Muscle Relaxant

**Use** Adjunct to general anesthesia to facilitate endotracheal intubation and to relax skeletal muscles during surgery; to facilitate mechanical ventilation in ICU patients; does not relieve pain or produce sedation; the characteristics of this agent make it especially useful in procedures requiring careful maintenance of hemodynamic stability for prolonged periods

**Usual Dosage** Administer I.V.; dose to effect; doses will vary due to interpatient variability; use ideal body weight for obese patients

Surgery:
 Children >2 years: Initial: 0.03-0.05 mg/kg followed by maintenance doses of 0.005-0.01 mg/kg after 30-45 minutes
 Adults: 0.05-0.08 mg/kg with thiopental/narcotic or 0.025 mg/kg after initial dose of succinylcholine for intubation; initial maintenance dose of 0.005-0.01 mg/kg after 100-160 minutes followed by repeat doses every 30-45 minutes
 Pretreatment/priming: 10% of intubating dose given 3-5 minutes before initial dose
 ICU: 0.05 mg/kg bolus followed by 0.025 mg/kg every 2-3 hours or 0.25-0.75 mcg/kg/minute once initial recovery from bolus dose observed

**Dosage Forms** Injection, solution, as chloride: 1 mg/mL (5 mL) [contains benzyl alcohol]

**doxacurium chloride** *see doxacurium on previous page*

# doxapram *(DOKS a pram)*

**Sound-Alike/Look-Alike Issues**
 doxapram may be confused with doxacurium, doxazosin, doxepin, Doxinate®, DOXOrubicin
 Dopram® may be confused with DOPamine

**Synonyms** doxapram hydrochloride

**U.S./Canadian Brand Names** Dopram® [US]

**Therapeutic Category** Respiratory Stimulant

**Use** Respiratory and CNS stimulant for respiratory depression secondary to anesthesia, drug-induced CNS depression; acute hypercapnia secondary to COPD

**Usual Dosage**

Respiratory depression following anesthesia:
 Intermittent injection: Initial: 0.5-1 mg/kg; may repeat at 5-minute intervals (only in patients who demonstrate initial response); maximum total dose: 2 mg/kg
 I.V. infusion: Initial: 5 mg/minute until adequate response or adverse effects seen; decrease to 1-3 mg/minute; maximum total dose: 4 mg/kg

Drug-induced CNS depression:
 Intermittent injection: Initial: Priming dose of 1-2 mg/kg, repeat after 5 minutes; may repeat at 1-2 hour intervals (until sustained consciousness); maximum: 3 g/day. May repeat in 24 hours if necessary.
 I.V. infusion: Initial: Priming dose of 1-2 mg/kg, repeat after 5 minutes. If no response, wait 1-2 hours and repeat. If some stimulation is noted, initiate infusion at 1-3 mg/minute (depending on size of patient/depth of CNS depression); suspend infusion if patient begins to awaken. Infusion should not be continued for >2 hours. May reinstitute infusion as described above, including bolus, after rest interval of 30 minutes to 2 hours; maximum: 3 g/day

Acute hypercapnia secondary to COPD: I.V. infusion: Initial: Initiate infusion at 1-2 mg/minute (depending on size of patient/depth of CNS depression); may increase to maximum rate of 3 mg/minute; infusion should not be continued for >2 hours. Monitor arterial blood gases prior to initiation of infusion and at 30-minute intervals during the infusion (to identify possible development of acidosis/$CO_2$ retention). Additional infusions are not recommended (per manufacturer).

**Dosage Forms** Injection, solution, as hydrochloride: 20 mg/mL (20 mL) [contains benzyl alcohol]

**doxapram hydrochloride** *see doxapram on this page*

# doxazosin *(doks AY zoe sin)*

**Sound-Alike/Look-Alike Issues**
 doxazosin may be confused with doxapram, doxepin, DOXOrubicin
 Cardura® may be confused with Cardene®, Cordarone®, Cordran®, Coumadin®, K-Dur®, Ridaura®

**Synonyms** doxazosin mesylate

**U.S./Canadian Brand Names** Alti-Doxazosin [Can]; Apo-Doxazosin® [Can]; Cardura-1™ [Can]; Cardura-2™ [Can]; Cardura-4™ [Can]; Cardura® [US]; Gen-Doxazosin [Can]; Novo-Doxazosin [Can]

**Therapeutic Category** Alpha-Adrenergic Blocking Agent

**Use** Treatment of hypertension alone or in conjunction with diuretics, cardiac glycosides, ACE inhibitors, or calcium antagonists (particularly appropriate for those with hypertension and other cardiovascular risk factors such as hypercholesterolemia and diabetes mellitus); treatment of urinary outflow obstruction and/or obstructive and irritative symptoms associated with benign prostatic hyperplasia (BPH), particularly useful in patients with troublesome symptoms who are unable or unwilling to undergo invasive procedures, but who require rapid symptomatic relief; can be used in combination with finasteride

**Usual Dosage** Oral:

Adults: 1 mg once daily in morning or evening; may be increased to 2 mg once daily. Thereafter titrate upwards, if needed, over several weeks, balancing therapeutic benefit with doxazosin-induced postural hypotension

Hypertension: Maximum dose: 16 mg/day

BPH: Goal: 4-8 mg/day; maximum dose: 8 mg/day

**Dosage Forms** Tablet: 1 mg, 2 mg, 4 mg, 8 mg

**doxazosin mesylate** *see doxazosin on previous page*

## doxepin (DOKS e pin)

**Sound-Alike/Look-Alike Issues**

doxepin may be confused with digoxin, doxapram, doxazosin, Doxidan®, doxycycline

Sinequan® may be confused with saquinavir, Serentil®, Seroquel®, Singulair®

Zonalon® may be confused with Zone-A Forte®

**Synonyms** doxepin hydrochloride

**U.S./Canadian Brand Names** Apo-Doxepin® [Can]; Novo-Doxepin [Can]; Prudoxin™ [US]; Sinequan® [US/Can]; Zonalon® [US/Can]

**Therapeutic Category** Antidepressant, Tricyclic (Tertiary Amine); Topical Skin Product

**Use**

Oral: Depression

Topical: Short-term (<8 days) management of moderate pruritus in adults with atopic dermatitis or lichen simplex chronicus

**Usual Dosage**

Oral: Topical: Burning mouth syndrome (dental use): Cream: Apply 3-4 times daily

Oral (entire daily dose may be given at bedtime):

Depression or anxiety:

Adolescents: Initial: 25-50 mg/day in single or divided doses; gradually increase to 100 mg/day

Adults: Initial: 25-150 mg/day at bedtime or in 2-3 divided doses; may gradually increase up to 300 mg/day; single dose should not exceed 150 mg; select patients may respond to 25-50 mg/day

Chronic urticaria, angioedema, nocturnal pruritus: Adults: 10-30 mg/day

Topical: Pruritus: Adults: Apply a thin film 4 times/day with at least 3- to 4-hour interval between applications; not recommended for use >8 days. **Note:** Low-dose (25-50 mg) oral administration has also been used to treat pruritus, but systemic effects are increased.

**Dosage Forms** [DSC] = Discontinued product

Capsule, as hydrochloride: 10 mg, 25 mg, 50 mg, 75 mg, 100 mg, 150 mg

Sinequan®: 10 mg, 25 mg, 50 mg, 75 mg, 100 mg [DSC], 150 mg [DSC]

Cream, as hydrochloride:

Prudoxin™: 5% (45 g) [contains benzyl alcohol]

Zonalon®: 5% (30 g, 45 g) [contains benzyl alcohol]

Solution, oral concentrate, as hydrochloride (Sinequan®): 10 mg/mL (120 mL)

**doxepin hydrochloride** *see doxepin on this page*

## doxercalciferol (doks er kal si fe FEER ole)

**Synonyms** 1α-hydroxyergocalciferol

**U.S./Canadian Brand Names** Hectorol® [US/Can]

**Therapeutic Category** Vitamin D Analog

**Use** Treatment of secondary hyperparathyroidism in patients with chronic kidney disease

*(Continued)*

## doxercalciferol *(Continued)*

### Usual Dosage

**Oral:**

Dialysis patients: Dose should be titrated to lower iPTH to 150-300 pg/mL; dose is adjusted at 8-week intervals (maximum dose: 20 mcg 3 times/week)

Initial dose: iPTH >400 pg/mL: 10 mcg 3 times/week at dialysis

Dose titration:

iPTH level decreased by 50% and >300 pg/mL: Dose can be increased to 12.5 mcg 3 times/week for 8 more weeks; this titration process can continue at 8-week intervals; each increase should be by 2.5 mcg/dose

iPTH level 150-300 pg/mL: Maintain current dose

iPTH level <100 pg/mL: Suspend doxercalciferol for 1 week; resume at a reduced dose; decrease each dose (not weekly dose) by at least 2.5 mcg

Predialysis patients: Dose should be titrated to lower iPTH to 35-70 pg/mL with stage 3 disease or to 70-110 pg/mL with stage 4 disease: Dose may be adjusted at 2-week intervals (maximum dose: 3.5 mcg/day)

Initial dose: 1 mcg/day

Dose titration:

iPTH level >70 pg/mL with stage 3 disease or >110 pg/mL with stage 4 disease: Increase dose by 0.5 mcg every 2 weeks as necessary

iPTH level 35-70 pg/mL with stage 3 disease or 70-110 pg/mL with stage 4 disease: Maintain current dose

iPTH level is <35 pg/mL with stage 3 disease or <70 pg/mL with stage 4 disease: Suspend doxercalciferol for 1 week, then resume at a reduced dose (at least 0.5 mcg lower)

**I.V.:**

Dialysis patients: Dose should be titrated to lower iPTH to 150-300 pg/mL; dose is adjusted at 8-week intervals (maximum dose: 18 mcg/week)

Initial dose: iPTH level >400 pg/mL: 4 mcg 3 times/week after dialysis, administered as a bolus dose

Dose titration:

iPTH level decreased by 50% and >300 pg/mL: Dose can be increased by 1-2 mcg at 8-week intervals, as necessary

iPTH level 150-300 pg/mL: Maintain the current dose

iPTH level <100 pg/mL: Suspend doxercalciferol for 1 week; resume at a reduced dose (at least 1 mcg lower)

### Dosage Forms

Capsule: 0.5 mcg, 2.5 mcg [contains coconut oil]

Injection, solution: 2 mcg/mL (2 mL) [contains disodium edetate]

**Doxidan® *(reformulation)* [US-OTC]** *see* bisacodyl *on page 107*

**Doxil® [US]** *see* doxorubicin (liposomal) *on next page*

## doxorubicin (doks oh ROO bi sin)

### Sound-Alike/Look-Alike Issues

DOXOrubicin may be confused with dactinomycin, DAUNOrubicin, doxacurium, doxapram, doxazosin, idarubicin

Adriamycin PFS® may be confused with achromycin, Aredia®, Idamycin®

Rubex® may be confused with Robaxin®

ADR is an error-prone abbreviation

conventional formulations (Adriamycin PFS®, Adriamycin RDF®, Rubex®) may be confused with liposomal formulations (DaunoXome®, Doxil®)

**Synonyms** adria; doxorubicin hydrochloride; hydroxydaunomycin hydrochloride; hydroxyldaunorubicin hydrochloride; NSC-123127

**Tall-Man** DOXOrubicin

**U.S./Canadian Brand Names** Adriamycin PFS® [US]; Adriamycin RDF® [US]; Adriamycin® [Can]; Rubex® [US]

**Therapeutic Category** Antineoplastic Agent

**Use** Treatment of leukemias, lymphomas, multiple myeloma, osseous and nonosseous sarcomas, mesotheliomas, germ cell tumors of the ovary or testis, and carcinomas of the head and neck, thyroid, lung, breast, stomach, pancreas, liver, ovary, bladder, prostate, uterus, and neuroblastoma

**Usual Dosage** Refer to individual protocols. I.V.:

Children:

35-75 mg/m$^2$ as a single dose, repeat every 21 days **or**

20-30 mg/m$^2$ once weekly **or**

60-90 mg/m$^2$ given as a continuous infusion over 96 hours every 3-4 weeks

Adults: Usual or typical dose: 60-75 mg/m$^2$ as a single dose, repeat every 21 days **or** other dosage regimens like 20-30 mg/m$^2$/day for 2-3 days, repeat in 4 weeks **or** 20 mg/m$^2$ once weekly

The lower dose regimen should be given to patients with decreased bone marrow reserve, prior therapy or marrow infiltration with malignant cells

**Dosage Forms**

Injection, powder for reconstitution, as hydrochloride: 10 mg, 20 mg, 50 mg [contains lactose]

Adriamycin RDF®: 10 mg, 20 mg, 50 mg, 150 mg [contains lactose; rapid dissolution formula]

Rubex®: 50 mg, 100 mg [contains lactose]

Injection, solution, as hydrochloride [preservative free]: 2 mg/mL (5 mL, 10 mL, 25 mL, 100 mL)

Adriamycin PFS® [preservative free]: 2 mg/mL (5 mL, 10 mL, 25 mL, 37.5 mL, 100 mL)

**doxorubicin hydrochloride** *see* doxorubicin *on previous page*

**doxorubicin hydrochloride (liposomal)** *see* doxorubicin (liposomal) *on this page*

# doxorubicin (liposomal) (doks oh ROO bi sin lip pah SOW mal)

**Sound-Alike/Look-Alike Issues**

DOXOrubicin may be confused with dactinomycin, DAUNOrubicin, doxacurium, doxapram, doxazosin, idarubicin

Doxil® may be confused with Doxy®, Paxil®

liposomal formulations (Doxil®) may be confused with conventional formulations (Adriamycin PFS®, Adriamycin RDF®, Cerubidine®, Rubex®).

**Synonyms** doxorubicin hydrochloride (liposomal)

**Tall-Man** DOXOrubicin (liposomal)

**U.S./Canadian Brand Names** Caelyx® [Can]; Doxil® [US]

**Therapeutic Category** Antineoplastic Agent

**Use** Treatment of AIDS-related Kaposi sarcoma, breast cancer, ovarian cancer, solid tumors

**Usual Dosage** Refer to individual protocols

AIDS-KS patients: I.V.: 20 mg/m$^2$/dose once every 3 weeks

Breast cancer: I.V.: 20-80 mg/m$^2$/dose every 8 weeks has been studied in a limited number of phase I/II trials

Ovarian cancer: I.V.: 50 mg/m$^2$/dose every 4 weeks

Solid tumors: I.V.: 50-60 mg/m$^2$/dose every 3-4 weeks

**Dosage Forms** Injection, solution, as hydrochloride: 2 mg/mL (10 mL, 25 mL)

**Doxy-100® [US]** *see* doxycycline *on this page*

**Doxycin [Can]** *see* doxycycline *on this page*

# doxycycline (doks i SYE kleen)

**Sound-Alike/Look-Alike Issues**

doxycycline may be confused with dicyclomine, doxepin, doxylamine

Doxy-100® may be confused with Doxil®

Monodox® may be confused with Maalox®

**Synonyms** doxycycline calcium; doxycycline hyclate; doxycycline monohydrate

**U.S./Canadian Brand Names** Adoxa™ [US]; Apo-Doxy Tabs® [Can]; Apo-Doxy® [Can]; Doryx® [US]; Doxy-100® [US]; Doxycin [Can]; Doxytec [Can]; Monodox® [US]; Novo-Doxylin [Can]; Nu-Doxycycline [Can]; Periostat® [US/Can]; Vibra-Tabs® [US/Can]; Vibramycin® [US]

**Therapeutic Category** Tetracycline Derivative

**Use** Principally in the treatment of infections caused by susceptible *Rickettsia*, *Chlamydia*, and *Mycoplasma*; alternative to mefloquine for malaria prophylaxis; treatment for syphilis, uncomplicated *Neisseria gonorrhoeae*, *Listeria*, *Actinomyces israelii*, and *Clostridium* infections in penicillin-allergic patients; used for community-acquired pneumonia and other common infections due to susceptible organisms; anthrax due to *Bacillus anthracis*, including inhalational anthrax (postexposure); treatment of infections caused by uncommon susceptible gram-negative and gram-positive organisms including *Borrelia recurrentis*, *Ureaplasma urealyticum*, *Haemophilus ducreyi*, *Yersinia pestis*, *Francisella tularensis*, *Vibrio cholerae*, *Campylobacter fetus*, *Brucella* spp, *Bartonella bacilliformis*, and *Calymmatobacterium granulomatis*

(Continued)

# doxycycline *(Continued)*

## Usual Dosage

Children:

Anthrax: Doxycycline should be used in children if antibiotic susceptibility testing, exhaustion of drug supplies, or allergic reaction preclude use of penicillin or ciprofloxacin. For treatment, the consensus recommendation does not include a loading dose for doxycycline.

Inhalational (postexposure prophylaxis) (*MMWR*, 2001, 50:889-893): Oral, I.V. (use oral route when possible):

≤8 years: 2.2 mg/kg every 12 hours for 60 days

>8 years and ≤45 kg: 2.2 mg/kg every 12 hours for 60 days

>8 years and >45 kg: 100 mg every 12 hours for 60 days

Cutaneous (treatment): Oral: See dosing for "Inhalational (postexposure prophylaxis)"

**Note:** In the presence of systemic involvement, extensive edema, and/or lesions on head/neck, doxycycline should initially be administered I.V.

Inhalational/gastrointestinal/oropharyngeal (treatment): I.V.: Refer to dosing for inhalational anthrax (postexposure prophylaxis); switch to oral therapy when clinically appropriate; refer to Adults dosing for "Note" on combined therapy and duration

Children ≥8 years (<45 kg): Susceptible infections: Oral, I.V.: 2-5 mg/kg/day in 1-2 divided doses, not to exceed 200 mg/day

Children >8 years (>45 kg) and Adults: Susceptible infections: Oral, I.V.: 100-200 mg/day in 1-2 divided doses

Acute gonococcal infection (PID) in combination with another antibiotic: 100 mg every 12 hours until improved, followed by 100 mg orally twice daily to complete 14 days

Community-acquired pneumonia: 100 mg twice daily

Lyme disease: Oral: 100 mg twice daily for 14-21 days

Early syphilis: 200 mg/day in divided doses for 14 days

Late syphilis: 200 mg/day in divided doses for 28 days

Uncomplicated chlamydial infections: 100 mg twice daily for ≥7 days

Endometritis, salpingitis, parametritis, or peritonitis: 100 mg I.V. twice daily with cefoxitin 2 g every 6 hours for 4 days and for ≥48 hours after patient improves; then continue with oral therapy 100 mg twice daily to complete a 10- to 14-day course of therapy

Periodontitis: Oral (Periostat®): 20 mg twice daily as an adjunct following scaling and root planing; may be administered for up to 9 months. Safety beyond 12 months of treatment and efficacy beyond 9 months of treatment have not been established.

Adults:

Anthrax:

Inhalational (postexposure prophylaxis): Oral, I.V. (use oral route when possible): 100 mg every 12 hours for 60 days (*MMWR*, 2001, 50:889-93); **Note:** Preliminary recommendation, FDA review and update is anticipated.

Cutaneous (treatment): Oral: 100 mg every 12 hours for 60 days. **Note:** In the presence of systemic involvement, extensive edema, lesions on head/neck, refer to I.V. dosing for treatment of inhalational/gastrointestinal/oropharyngeal anthrax

Inhalational/gastrointestinal/oropharyngeal (treatment): I.V.: Initial: 100 mg every 12 hours; switch to oral therapy when clinically appropriate; some recommend initial loading dose of 200 mg, followed by 100 mg every 8-12 hours (*JAMA*, 1997, 278:399-411). **Note:** Initial treatment should include two or more agents predicted to be effective (per CDC recommendations). Agents suggested for use in conjunction with doxycycline or ciprofloxacin include rifampin, vancomycin, imipenem, penicillin, ampicillin, chloramphenicol, clindamycin, and clarithromycin. May switch to oral antimicrobial therapy when clinically appropriate. Continue combined therapy for 60 days

## Dosage Forms [DSC] = Discontinued product

Capsule, as hyclate: 50 mg, 100 mg

Vibramycin®: 100 mg

Capsule, as monohydrate (Monodox®): 50 mg, 100 mg

Capsule, coated pellets, as hyclate (Doryx®): 75 mg, 100 mg [DSC]

Injection, powder for reconstitution, as hyclate (Doxy-100®): 100 mg

Powder for oral suspension, as monohydrate (Vibramycin®): 25 mg/5 mL (60 mL) [raspberry flavor]

Syrup, as calcium (Vibramycin®): 50 mg/5 mL (480 mL) [contains sodium metabisulfite; raspberry-apple flavor]

Tablet, as hyclate: 100 mg

Periostat®: 20 mg

Vibra-Tabs®: 100 mg

Tablet, as monohydrate (Adoxa™): 50 mg, 75 mg, 100 mg

Tablet, delayed-release coated pellets, as hyclate (Doryx®): 75 mg [contains sodium 4.5 mg (0.196 mEq)], 100 mg [contains sodium 6 mg (0.261 mEq)]

**doxycycline calcium** *see* doxycycline *on page 271*

**doxycycline hyclate** *see* doxycycline *on page 271*

**doxycycline monohydrate** *see* doxycycline *on page 271*

## doxylamine (dox IL a meen)
**Sound-Alike/Look-Alike Issues**
Sound-alike/look-alike issues:
doxylamine may be confused with doxycycline
**Synonyms** doxylamine succinate
**U.S./Canadian Brand Names** Medi-Sleep® [US-OTC]; Night-Time Sleep Aid [US-OTC]; Sleep-Aid® [US-OTC]; Unisom® [US-OTC]
**Therapeutic Category** Antihistamine
**Use** Sleep aid; antihistamine for hypersensitivity reactions and antiemetic
**Usual Dosage** Oral: Children >12 years and Adults: 25 mg at bedtime
**Dosage Forms** Tablet, as succinate: 25 mg

## doxylamine and pyridoxine *(Canada only)* (dox IL a meen & peer i DOX een)
**Sound-Alike/Look-Alike Issues**
doxylamine may be confused with doxycycline
**Synonyms** doxylamine succinate and pyridoxine hydrochloride; pyridoxine and doxylamine
**U.S./Canadian Brand Names** Diclectin® [Can]
**Therapeutic Category** Antihistamine; Vitamin
**Use** Treatment of pregnancy-associated nausea and vomiting
**Usual Dosage** Oral: Adults: Two delayed release tablets (a total of doxylamine 20 mg and pyridoxine 20 mg) at bedtime; in severe cases or in cases with nausea/vomiting during the day, dosage may be increased by 1 tablet in the morning and/or afternoon
**Dosage Forms** Tablet, delayed release: Doxylamine succinate 10 mg and pyridoxine hydrochloride 10 mg

**doxylamine succinate** *see* doxylamine *on this page*

**doxylamine succinate and pyridoxine hydrochloride** *see* doxylamine and pyridoxine *(Canada only)* *on this page*

**Doxytec [Can]** *see* doxycycline *on page 271*

**DPA** *see* valproic acid and derivatives *on page 837*

**D-Pan® *(Discontinued)*** *see* dexpanthenol *on page 235*

**DPE** *see* dipivefrin *on page 260*

**D-penicillamine** *see* penicillamine *on page 627*

**DPH** *see* phenytoin *on page 645*

**DPM™ [US-OTC]** *see* urea *on page 834*

**Dramamine® [US-OTC]** *see* dimenhydrinate *on page 252*

**Dramamine® Less Drowsy Formula [US-OTC]** *see* meclizine *on page 506*

**Dramilin® Injection *(Discontinued)*** *see* dimenhydrinate *on page 252*

**dried smallpox vaccine** *see* smallpox vaccine *on page 751*

**Drinex® *(Discontinued)*** *see* acetaminophen, chlorpheniramine, and pseudoephedrine *on page 10*

**Drisdol® [US/Can]** *see* ergocalciferol *on page 292*

**Dristan® Long Lasting Nasal [Can]** *see* oxymetazoline *on page 610*

**Dristan® Long Lasting Nasal Solution *(Discontinued)*** *see* oxymetazoline *on page 610*

**Dristan® N.D. [Can]** *see* acetaminophen and pseudoephedrine *on page 8*

**Dristan® N.D., Extra Strength [Can]** *see* acetaminophen and pseudoephedrine *on page 8*

**Dristan® Saline Spray *(Discontinued)*** *see* sodium chloride *on page 752*

**Dristan® Sinus [US-OTC]** *see* pseudoephedrine and ibuprofen *on page 694*

**Drithocreme® [US]** *see* anthralin *on page 54*

**Drithocreme® HP 1% (Discontinued)** *see* anthralin *on page 54*

**Dritho-Scalp® [US]** *see* anthralin *on page 54*

**Drituss DM [US]** *see* guaifenesin and dextromethorphan *on page 385*

**Drixoral® [Can]** *see* dexbrompheniramine and pseudoephedrine *on page 234*

**Drixoral® Cold & Allergy [US-OTC]** *see* dexbrompheniramine and pseudoephedrine *on page 234*

**Drixoral® Cough & Congestion Liquid Caps (Discontinued)** *see* pseudoephedrine and dextromethorphan *on page 693*

**Drixoral® Cough Liquid Caps (Discontinued)** *see* dextromethorphan *on page 238*

**Drixoral® Nasal [Can]** *see* oxymetazoline *on page 610*

**Drixoral® ND [Can]** *see* pseudoephedrine *on page 692*

**Drixoral® Non-Drowsy (Discontinued)** *see* pseudoephedrine *on page 692*

**Drize®-R [US]** *see* chlorpheniramine, phenylephrine, and methscopolamine *on page 175*

## dronabinol (droe NAB i nol)

**Sound-Alike/Look-Alike Issues**
dronabinol may be confused with droperidol
**Synonyms** delta-9 THC; delta-9-tetrahydro-cannabinol; tetrahydrocannabinol; THC
**U.S./Canadian Brand Names** Marinol® [US/Can]
**Therapeutic Category** Antiemetic
**Controlled Substance** C-III
**Use** Chemotherapy-associated nausea and vomiting refractory to other antiemetic; AIDS-related anorexia
**Usual Dosage** Refer to individual protocols. Oral:
Antiemetic: Children and Adults: 5 mg/m$^2$ 1-3 hours before chemotherapy, then 5 mg/m$^2$/dose every 2-4 hours after chemotherapy for a total of 4-6 doses/day; increase doses in increments of 2.5 mg/m$^2$ to a maximum of 15 mg/m$^2$/dose.
Appetite stimulant: Adults: Initial: 2.5 mg twice daily (before lunch and dinner); titrate up to a maximum of 20 mg/day.
**Dosage Forms** Capsule, gelatin: 2.5 mg, 5 mg, 10 mg [contains sesame oil]

## droperidol (droe PER i dole)

**Sound-Alike/Look-Alike Issues**
droperidol may be confused with dronabinol
Inapsine® may be confused with Nebcin®
**Synonyms** dehydrobenzperidol
**U.S./Canadian Brand Names** Inapsine® [US]
**Therapeutic Category** Antiemetic; Antipsychotic Agent, Butyrophenone
**Use** Antiemetic in surgical and diagnostic procedures; preoperative medication in patients when other treatments are ineffective or inappropriate
**Usual Dosage** Titrate carefully to desired effect
Children 2-12 years: Nausea and vomiting: I.M., I.V.: 0.05-0.06 mg/kg (maximum initial dose: 0.1 mg/kg); additional doses may be repeated to achieve effect; administer additional doses with caution
Adults: Nausea and vomiting: I.M., I.V.: Initial: 2.5 mg; additional doses of 1.25 mg may be administered to achieve desired effect; administer additional doses with caution
**Dosage Forms** Injection, solution: 2.5 mg/mL (1 mL, 2 mL)

**drospirenone and ethinyl estradiol** *see* ethinyl estradiol and drospirenone *on page 310*

## drotrecogin alfa (dro TRE coe jin AL fa)

**Synonyms** activated protein C, human, recombinant; drotrecogin alfa, activated; protein C (activated), human, recombinant
**U.S./Canadian Brand Names** Xigris® [US/Can]
**Therapeutic Category** Protein C (Activated)
**Use** Reduction of mortality from severe sepsis (associated with organ dysfunction) in adults at high risk of death (eg, APACHE II score ≥25)

Usual Dosage I.V.: Adults: Sepsis: 24 mcg/kg/hour for a total of 96 hours; stop infusion **immediately** if clinically-important bleeding is identified

Dosage Forms Injection, powder for reconstitution [preservative free]: 5 mg [contains sucrose 31.8 mg], 20 mg [contains sucrose 124.9 mg]

**drotrecogin alfa, activated** *see* drotrecogin alfa *on previous page*

**Droxia**™ **[US]** *see* hydroxyurea *on page 422*

**Dr. Scholl's® Callus Remover [US-OTC]** *see* salicylic acid *on page 734*

**Dr. Scholl's® Clear Away [US-OTC]** *see* salicylic acid *on page 734*

**Dry Eye® Therapy Solution *(Discontinued)*** *see* artificial tears *on page 71*

**Dryox® Gel *(Discontinued)*** *see* benzoyl peroxide *on page 98*

**Dryox® Wash *(Discontinued)*** *see* benzoyl peroxide *on page 98*

**Drysol**™ **[US]** *see* aluminum chloride hexahydrate *on page 34*

**Dryvax® [US]** *see* smallpox vaccine *on page 751*

**DSCG** *see* cromolyn sodium *on page 211*

**D-ser(bu$^t$)$^6$,Azgly$^{10}$-LHRH** *see* goserelin *on page 381*

**DSS** *see* docusate *on page 263*

**DT** *see* diphtheria and tetanus toxoid *on page 257*

**DTaP** *see* diphtheria, tetanus toxoids, and acellular pertussis vaccine *on page 259*

**DTIC** *see* dacarbazine *on page 220*

**DTIC-Dome® [US]** *see* dacarbazine *on page 220*

**DTPA** *see* diethylene triamine penta-acetic acid *on page 246*

**D-Trp(6)-LHRH** *see* triptorelin *on page 828*

**Duac**™ **[US]** *see* clindamycin and benzoyl peroxide *on page 193*

**Duet® [US]** *see* vitamins (multiple/prenatal) *on page 852*

**Duet**™ **DHA [US]** *see* vitamins (multiple/prenatal) *on page 852*

**Dulcolax® [US-OTC/Can]** *see* bisacodyl *on page 107*

**Dulcolax® Milk of Magnesia [US-OTC]** *see* magnesium hydroxide *on page 498*

**Dulcolax® Stool Softener [US-OTC]** *see* docusate *on page 263*

**Dull-C® [US-OTC]** *see* ascorbic acid *on page 71*

**duloxetine** (doo LOX e teen)

**Sound-Alike/Look-Alike Issues**
duloxetine may be confused with fluoxetine.

Synonyms (+)-(S)-N-methyl-γ-(1-naphthyloxy)-2-thiophenepropylamine hydrochloride; duloxetine hydrochloride; LY248686

U.S./Canadian Brand Names Cymbalta® [US]

Therapeutic Category Antidepressant, Serotonin/Norepinephrine Reuptake Inhibitor

Use Treatment of major depressive disorder; management of pain associated with diabetic neuropathy

Usual Dosage Oral: Adults:

Treatment of major depressive disorder: Initial: 40-60 mg/day; dose may be divided (ie, 20 or 30 mg twice daily) or given as a single daily dose of 60 mg; maximum dose: 60 mg/day

Management of diabetic neuropathy: 60 mg once daily; lower initial doses may be considered in patients where tolerability is a concern and/or renal impairment is present

Dosage Forms Capsule: 20 mg, 30 mg, 60 mg [contains enteric coated pellets]

**duloxetine hydrochloride** *see* duloxetine *on this page*

**DuoCet**™ ***(Discontinued)*** *see* hydrocodone and acetaminophen *on page 411*

**DuoFilm® [US-OTC/Can]** *see* salicylic acid *on page 734*

**Duoforte® 27 [Can]** *see* salicylic acid *on page 734*

**DuoNeb**™ **[US]** *see* ipratropium and albuterol *on page 446*

**DuoPlant® *(Discontinued)*** *see* salicylic acid *on page 734*

**Duo-Trach**® **Injection** *(Discontinued)* *see* lidocaine *on page 479*

**DuP 753** *see* losartan *on page 492*

**Duphalac**® *(Discontinued)* *see* lactulose *on page 464*

**Durabolin**® **[Can]** *see* nandrolone *on page 560*

**Duraclon**™ **[US]** *see* clonidine *on page 197*

**Duradrin**® **[US]** *see* acetaminophen, isometheptene, and dichloralphenazone *on page 12*

**Duradyne DHC**® *(Discontinued)* *see* hydrocodone and acetaminophen *on page 411*

**Duragesic**® **[US/Can]** *see* fentanyl *on page 332*

**Dura-Gest**® *(Discontinued)*

**Duralith**® **[Can]** *see* lithium *on page 486*

**Duralone**® **Injection** *(Discontinued)* *see* methylprednisolone *on page 531*

**Duramist**® **Plus [US-OTC]** *see* oxymetazoline *on page 610*

**Duramorph**® **[US]** *see* morphine sulfate *on page 549*

**Duratest**® **Injection** *(Discontinued)* *see* testosterone *on page 788*

**Durathate**® **Injection** *(Discontinued)* *see* testosterone *on page 788*

**Duration**® **[US-OTC]** *see* oxymetazoline *on page 610*

**Duratocin**™ **[Can]** *see* carbetocin *(Canada only) on page 143*

**Duratuss**® **DM [US]** *see* guaifenesin and dextromethorphan *on page 385*

**Dura-Vent**®**/DA** *(Discontinued)* *see* chlorpheniramine, phenylephrine, and methscopolamine *on page 175*

**Dura-Vent**® *(Discontinued)*

**Duricef**® **[US/Can]** *see* cefadroxil *on page 152*

**Duricef**® **Oral Suspension 125 mg/5 mL** *(Discontinued)* *see* cefadroxil *on page 152*

**Durolane**® **[Can]** *see* hyaluronate and derivatives *on page 406*

**Durrax**® **Oral** *(Discontinued)* *see* hydroxyzine *on page 423*

**dutasteride** (doo TAS teer ide)
U.S./Canadian Brand Names Avodart™ [US/Can]
Therapeutic Category Antineoplastic Agent, Anthracenedione
Use Treatment of symptomatic benign prostatic hyperplasia (BPH)
Usual Dosage Oral: Adults: Male: 0.5 mg once daily
Dosage Forms Capsule, softgel: 0.5 mg

**Duvoid**® **[Can]** *see* bethanechol *on page 104*

**Duvoid**® *(Discontinued)* *see* bethanechol *on page 104*

**D-Vi-Sol**® **[Can]** *see* cholecalciferol *on page 180*

**DW286** *see* gemifloxacin *on page 370*

**Dwelle**® **Ophthalmic Solution** *(Discontinued)* *see* artificial tears *on page 71*

**d-xylose** (dee-ZYE lose)
Synonyms wood sugar
Therapeutic Category Diagnostic Agent
Use Evaluating intestinal absorption and diagnosing malabsorptive states
Usual Dosage Oral:
Infants and young Children: 500 mg/kg as a 5% to 10% aqueous solution
Children: 5 g is dissolved in 250 mL water; additional fluids are permitted and are encouraged for children
Adults: 25 g dissolved in 200-300 mL water followed with an additional 200-400 mL water **or** 5 g dissolved in 200-300 mL water followed by an additional 200-400 mL water
Dosage Forms Powder for oral solution: 25 g

**Dyazide**® **[US]** *see* hydrochlorothiazide and triamterene *on page 410*

**Dycill**® **[Can]** *see* dicloxacillin *on page 244*

**Dycill**® *(Discontinued)* *see* dicloxacillin *on page 244*

**Dyclone**® *(Discontinued)* *see* dyclonine *on this page*

## dyclonine (DYE kloe neen)
**Sound-Alike/Look-Alike Issues**
dyclonine may be confused with dicyclomine
**Synonyms** dyclonine hydrochloride
**U.S./Canadian Brand Names** Cepacol® Dual Action Maximum Strength [US-OTC]; Sucrets® [US-OTC]
**Therapeutic Category** Local Anesthetic
**Use** Temporary relief of pain associated with oral mucosa
**Usual Dosage** Oral:
Lozenge: Children ≥2 years and Adults: One lozenge every 2 hours as needed (maximum: 10 lozenges/day)
Spray:
Children ≥3-12 years: 1-3 sprays, up to 4 times a day
Children ≥12 years and Adults: 1-4 sprays, up to 4 times a day
**Dosage Forms**
Lozenge, as hydrochloride (Sucrets®): 1.2 mg [children's cherry flavor]; 2 mg [wild cherry and assorted flavors]; 3 mg [vapor black cherry and wintergreen flavors]
Spray, oral, as hydrochloride (Cepacol® Dual Action Maximum Strength): 0.1% (120 mL) [contains glycerin 33%; cherry, honey lemon and cool menthol flavors]

**dyclonine hydrochloride** *see* dyclonine *on this page*

**Dygase [US]** *see* pancrelipase *on page 615*

**Dymelor**® *(Discontinued)* *see* acetohexamide *on page 14*

**Dymenate**® **Injection** *(Discontinued)* *see* dimenhydrinate *on page 252*

**Dynabac**® **[US]** *see* dirithromycin *on page 260*

**Dynacin**® **[US]** *see* minocycline *on page 542*

**DynaCirc**® **[US/Can]** *see* isradipine *on page 453*

**DynaCirc**® **CR [US]** *see* isradipine *on page 453*

**Dyna-Hex**® **[US-OTC]** *see* chlorhexidine gluconate *on page 168*

**Dynapen**® *(Discontinued)* *see* dicloxacillin *on page 244*

**Dynex [US]** *see* guaifenesin and pseudoephedrine *on page 388*

## dyphylline (DYE fi lin)
**Synonyms** dihydroxypropyl theophylline
**U.S./Canadian Brand Names** Dilor® [US/Can]; Lufyllin® [US/Can]
**Therapeutic Category** Theophylline Derivative
**Use** Bronchodilator in reversible airway obstruction due to asthma or COPD
**Usual Dosage**
Children: I.M.: 4.4-6.6 mg/kg/day in divided doses
Adults:
Oral: Up to 15 mg/kg 4 times/day, individualize dosage
I.M.: 250-500 mg, do not exceed total dosage of 15 mg/kg every 6 hours
**Dosage Forms** [DSC] = Discontinued product
Elixir (Lufyllin®): 100 mg/15 mL (473 mL) [contains alcohol 20%]
Injection, solution (Dilor®): 250 mg/mL (2 mL) [DSC]
Tablet (Dilor®, Lufyllin®): 200 mg, 400 mg

**Dyrenium**® **[US]** *see* triamterene *on page 821*

**Dyrexan-OD**® *(Discontinued)* *see* phendimetrazine *on page 637*

**Dytan**™ **[US]** *see* diphenhydramine *on page 254*

**E₂C and MPA** *see* estradiol cypionate and medroxyprogesterone acetate *on page 303*

**7E3** *see* abciximab *on page 3*

**E2020** *see* donepezil *on page 266*

**Easprin**® **[US]** *see* aspirin *on page 73*

**Ebixa**® **[Can]** *see* memantine *on page 510*

## echothiophate iodide (ek oh THYE oh fate EYE oh dide)
**Synonyms** ecostigmine iodide
**U.S./Canadian Brand Names** Phospholine Iodide® [US]
**Therapeutic Category** Cholinesterase Inhibitor
**Use** Used as miotic in treatment of open-angle glaucoma; may be useful in specific case of narrow-angle glaucoma; accommodative esotropia
**Usual Dosage** Adults:
Ophthalmic: Glaucoma: Instill 1 drop twice daily into eyes with 1 dose just prior to bedtime; some patients have been treated with 1 dose daily or every other day
Accommodative esotropia:
Diagnosis: Instill 1 drop of 0.125% once daily into both eyes at bedtime for 2-3 weeks
Treatment: Use lowest concentration and frequency which gives satisfactory response, with a maximum dose of 0.125% once daily, although more intensive therapy may be used for short periods of time
**Dosage Forms** Powder for reconstitution, ophthalmic: 6.25 mg [0.125%]

**EC-Naprosyn**® **[US]** *see* naproxen *on page 562*
*E. coli* **asparaginase** *see* asparaginase *on page 72*

## econazole (e KONE a zole)
**Synonyms** econazole nitrate
**U.S./Canadian Brand Names** Ecostatin® [Can]; Spectazole® [US/Can]
**Therapeutic Category** Antifungal Agent
**Use** Topical treatment of tinea pedis (athlete's foot), tinea cruris (jock itch), tinea corporis (ringworm), tinea versicolor, and cutaneous candidiasis
**Usual Dosage** Children and Adults: Topical:
Tinea pedis, tinea cruris, tinea corporis, tinea versicolor: Apply sufficient amount to cover affected areas once daily
Cutaneous candidiasis: Apply sufficient quantity twice daily (morning and evening)
Duration of treatment: Candidal infections and tinea cruris, versicolor, and corporis should be treated for 2 weeks and tinea pedis for 1 month; occasionally, longer treatment periods may be required
**Dosage Forms** Cream, topical, as nitrate: 1% (15 g, 30 g, 85 g)

**econazole nitrate** *see* econazole *on this page*
**Econopred**® **Plus [US]** *see* prednisolone (ophthalmic) *on page 673*
**Ecostatin**® **[Can]** *see* econazole *on this page*
**ecostigmine iodide** *see* echothiophate iodide *on this page*
**Ecotrin**® **[US-OTC]** *see* aspirin *on page 73*
**Ecotrin**® **Low Strength [US-OTC]** *see* aspirin *on page 73*
**Ecotrin**® **Maximum Strength [US-OTC]** *see* aspirin *on page 73*
**Ectosone [Can]** *see* betamethasone (topical) *on page 103*
**Ed A-Hist**® **[US]** *see* chlorpheniramine and phenylephrine *on page 171*
**edathamil disodium** *see* edetate disodium *on next page*
**Edecrin**® **[US/Can]** *see* ethacrynic acid *on page 307*

## edetate calcium disodium (ED e tate KAL see um dye SOW dee um)
**Synonyms** calcium disodium edetate; calcium EDTA
**U.S./Canadian Brand Names** Calcium Disodium Versenate® [US]
**Therapeutic Category** Chelating Agent
**Use** Treatment of symptomatic acute and chronic lead poisoning or for symptomatic patients with high blood lead levels; used as an aid in the diagnosis of lead poisoning; possibly useful in poisoning by zinc, manganese, and certain heavy radioisotopes
**Usual Dosage** Several regimens have been recommended:
Diagnosis of lead poisoning: Mobilization test (not recommended by AAP guidelines): I.M., I.V.:
Children: 500 mg/m$^2$/dose (maximum dose: 1 g) as a single dose or divided into 2 doses
Adults: 500 mg/m$^2$/dose

**Note:** Urine is collected for 24 hours after first EDTA dose and analyzed for lead content; if the ratio of mcg of lead in urine to mg calcium EDTA given is >1, then test is considered positive; for convenience, an 8-hour urine collection may be done after a single 50 mg/kg I.M. (maximum dose: 1 g) or 500 mg/m$^2$ I.V. dose; a positive test occurs if the ratio of lead excretion to mg calcium EDTA >0.5-0.6.

Treatment of lead poisoning: Children and Adults (each regimen is specific for route):

Symptoms of lead encephalopathy and/or blood lead level >70 mcg/dL: Treat 5 days; give in conjunction with dimercaprol; wait a minimum of 2 days with no treatment before considering a repeat course:

I.M.: 250 mg/m$^2$/dose every 4 hours

I.V.: 50 mg/kg/day as 24-hour continuous I.V. infusion **or** 1-1.5 g/m$^2$ I.V. as either an 8- to 24-hour infusion or divided into 2 doses every 12 hours

Symptomatic lead poisoning **without** encephalopathy **or** asymptomatic with blood lead level >70 mcg/dL: Treat 3-5 days; treatment with dimercaprol is recommended until the blood lead level concentration <50 mcg/dL:

I.M.: 167 mg/m$^2$ every 4 hours

I.V.: 1 g/m$^2$ as an 8- to 24-hour infusion or divided every 12 hours

Asymptomatic **children** with blood lead level 45-69 mcg/dL: I.V.: 25 mg/kg/day for 5 days as an 8- to 24-hour infusion or divided into 2 doses every 12 hours

Depending upon the blood lead level, additional courses may be necessary; repeat at least 2-4 days and preferably 2-4 weeks apart

Adults with lead nephropathy: An alternative dosing regimen reflecting the reduction in renal clearance is based upon the serum creatinine. Refer to the following:

Dose of Ca EDTA based on serum creatinine:

$S_{cr}$ ≤2 mg/dL: 1 g/m$^2$/day for 5 days*

$S_{cr}$ 2-3 mg/dL: 500 mg/m$^2$/day for 5 days*

$S_{cr}$ 3-4 mg/dL: 500 mg/m$^2$/dose every 48 hours for 3 doses*

$S_{cr}$ >4 mg/dL: 500 mg/m$^2$/week*

*Repeat these regimens monthly until lead excretion is reduced toward normal.

**Dosage Forms** Injection, solution: 200 mg/mL (5 mL)


# edetate disodium (ED e tate dye SOW dee um)

**Synonyms** edathamil disodium; EDTA; sodium edetate

**U.S./Canadian Brand Names** Endrate® [US]

**Therapeutic Category** Chelating Agent

**Use** Emergency treatment of hypercalcemia; control digitalis-induced cardiac dysrhythmias (ventricular arrhythmias)

**Usual Dosage** Hypercalcemia: I.V.:

Children: 40-70 mg/kg/day slow infusion over 3-4 hours or more to a maximum of 3 g/24 hours; administer for 5 days and allow 5 days between courses of therapy

Adults: 50 mg/kg/day over 3 or more hours to a maximum of 3 g/24 hours; a suggested regimen of 5 days followed by 2 days without drug and repeated courses up to 15 total doses

Digitalis-induced arrhythmias: Children and Adults: 15 mg/kg/hour (maximum dose: 60 mg/kg/day) as continuous infusion

**Dosage Forms** Injection, solution: 150 mg/mL (20 mL)


**Edex® [US]** *see* alprostadil *on page 31*


# edrophonium (ed roe FOE nee um)

**Synonyms** edrophonium chloride

**U.S./Canadian Brand Names** Enlon® [US/Can]; Reversol® [US]

**Therapeutic Category** Cholinergic Agent

**Use** Diagnosis of myasthenia gravis; differentiation of cholinergic crises from myasthenia crises; reversal of nondepolarizing neuromuscular blockers; adjunct treatment of respiratory depression caused by curare overdose

**Usual Dosage** Usually administered I.V., however, if not possible, I.M. or SubQ may be used:

Infants:

I.M.: 0.5-1 mg

I.V.: Initial: 0.1 mg, followed by 0.4 mg if no response; total dose = 0.5 mg

Children:

Diagnosis: Initial: 0.04 mg/kg over 1 minute followed by 0.16 mg/kg if no response, to a maximum total

(Continued)

# edrophonium (Continued)

dose of 5 mg for children <34 kg, or 10 mg for children >34 kg **or**

Alternative dosing (manufacturer's recommendation):

≤34 kg: 1 mg; if no response after 45 seconds, repeat dosage in 1 mg increments every 30-45 seconds, up to a total of 5 mg

>34 kg: 2 mg; if no response after 45 seconds, repeat dosage in 1 mg increments every 30-45 seconds, up to a total of 10 mg

I.M.:

<34 kg: 1 mg

>34 kg: 5 mg

Titration of oral anticholinesterase therapy: 0.04 mg/kg once given 1 hour after oral intake of the drug being used in treatment; if strength improves, an increase in neostigmine or pyridostigmine dose is indicated

Adults:

Diagnosis:

I.V.: 2 mg test dose administered over 15-30 seconds; 8 mg given 45 seconds later if no response is seen; test dose may be repeated after 30 minutes

I.M.: Initial: 10 mg; if no cholinergic reaction occurs, administer 2 mg 30 minutes later to rule out false-negative reaction

Titration of oral anticholinesterase therapy: 1-2 mg given 1 hour after oral dose of anticholinesterase; if strength improves, an increase in neostigmine or pyridostigmine dose is indicated

Reversal of nondepolarizing neuromuscular blocking agents (neostigmine with atropine usually preferred): I.V.: 10 mg over 30-45 seconds; may repeat every 5-10 minutes up to 40 mg

Termination of paroxysmal atrial tachycardia: I.V. rapid injection: 5-10 mg

Differentiation of cholinergic from myasthenic crisis: I.V.: 1 mg; may repeat after 1 minute. **Note:** Intubation and controlled ventilation may be required if patient has cholinergic crisis

**Dosage Forms** Injection, solution, as chloride:

Enlon®: 10 mg/mL (15 mL) [contains sodium sulfite]

Reversol®: 10 mg/mL (10 mL) [contains sodium sulfite]

**edrophonium chloride** see edrophonium on previous page

**ED-SPAZ® (Discontinued)** see hyoscyamine on page 424

**EDTA** see edetate disodium on previous page

**E.E.S.® [US/Can]** see erythromycin on page 295

# efalizumab (e fa li ZOO mab)

**Synonyms** anti-CD11a; hu1124

**U.S./Canadian Brand Names** Raptiva® [US]

**Therapeutic Category** Immunosuppressant Agent; Monoclonal Antibody

**Use** Treatment of chronic moderate-to-severe plaque psoriasis in patients who are candidates for systemic therapy or phototherapy

**Usual Dosage** SubQ: Adults: Psoriasis: Initial: 0.7 mg/kg, followed by weekly dose of 1 mg/kg (maximum: 200 mg/dose)

**Dosage Forms** Injection, powder for reconstitution: 150 mg [contains sucrose 123.2 mg/vial; delivers 125 mg/1.25 mL; packaged with prefilled syringe containing sterile water for injection]

# efavirenz (e FAV e renz)

**U.S./Canadian Brand Names** Sustiva® [US/Can]

**Therapeutic Category** Nonnucleoside Reverse Transcriptase Inhibitor (NNRTI)

**Use** Treatment of HIV-1 infections in combination with at least two other antiretroviral agents

**Usual Dosage** Oral: Dosing at bedtime is recommended to limit central nervous system effects; should not be used as single-agent therapy

Children: Dosage is based on body weight

10 kg to <15 kg: 200 mg once daily

15 kg to <20 kg: 250 mg once daily

20 kg to <25 kg: 300 mg once daily

25 kg to <32.5 kg: 350 mg once daily

32.5 kg to <40 kg: 400 mg once daily

≥40 kg: 600 mg once daily

Adults: 600 mg once daily

Dosage Forms
Capsule: 50 mg, 100 mg, 200 mg
Tablet: 600 mg

**Effer-K**™ **[US]** *see* potassium bicarbonate and potassium citrate, effervescent *on page 663*

**Effer-Syllium**® *(Discontinued)* *see* psyllium *on page 697*

**Effexor**® **[US]** *see* venlafaxine *on page 843*

**Effexor**® **XR [US/Can]** *see* venlafaxine *on page 843*

**Eflone**® *(Discontinued)* *see* fluorometholone *on page 348*

## eflornithine (ee FLOR ni theen)
Sound-Alike/Look-Alike Issues
Vaniqa™ may be confused with Viagra®
Synonyms DFMO; eflornithine hydrochloride
U.S./Canadian Brand Names Vaniqa™ [US]
Therapeutic Category Antiprotozoal; Topical Skin Product
Use Cream: Females ≥12 years: Reduce unwanted hair from face and adjacent areas under the chin
Orphan status: Injection: Treatment of meningoencephalitic stage of *Trypanosoma brucei gambiense* infection (sleeping sickness)
Usual Dosage
Children ≥12 years and Adults: Females: Topical: Apply thin layer of cream to affected areas of face and adjacent chin twice daily, at least 8 hours apart
Adults: I.V. infusion: 100 mg/kg/dose given every 6 hours (over at least 45 minutes) for 14 days
Dosage Forms
Cream, topical, as hydrochloride: 13.9% (30 g)
Injection, solution, as hydrochloride: 200 mg/mL (100 mL) [orphan drug status]

**eflornithine hydrochloride** *see* eflornithine *on this page*

**Efodine**® *(Discontinued)* *see* povidone-iodine *on page 668*

**eformoterol and budesonide** *see* budesonide and formoterol *(Canada only)* *on page 119*

**Efudex**® **[US/Can]** *see* fluorouracil *on page 349*

**E-Gems**® **[US-OTC]** *see* vitamin E *on page 850*

**EHDP** *see* etidronate disodium *on page 321*

**Elavil**® *(Discontinued)* *see* amitriptyline *on page 42*

**Eldepryl**® **[US]** *see* selegiline *on page 742*

**Eldopaque**® **[US-OTC/Can]** *see* hydroquinone *on page 420*

**Eldopaque Forte**® **[US]** *see* hydroquinone *on page 420*

**Eldoquin**® **[US-OTC/Can]** *see* hydroquinone *on page 420*

**Eldoquin Forte**® **[US]** *see* hydroquinone *on page 420*

**electrolyte lavage solution** *see* polyethylene glycol-electrolyte solution *on page 658*

**Elestat**™ **[US]** *see* epinastine *on page 287*

## eletriptan (el e TRIP tan)
Synonyms eletriptan hydrobromide
U.S./Canadian Brand Names Relpax® [US/Can]
Therapeutic Category Serotonin 5-HT$_{1B, 1D}$ Receptor Agonist
Use Acute treatment of migraine, with or without aura
Usual Dosage Oral: Adults: Acute migraine: 20-40 mg; if the headache improves but returns, dose may be repeated after 2 hours have elapsed since first dose; maximum 80 mg/day.
Note: If the first dose is ineffective, diagnosis needs to be re-evaluated. Safety of treating >3 headaches/month has not been established.
Dosage Forms Tablet, as hydrobromide [film coated]: 20 mg, 40 mg [as base]

**eletriptan hydrobromide** *see* eletriptan *on this page*

**Elidel**® **[US/Can]** *see* pimecrolimus *on page 648*

**Eligard**® **[US/Can]** *see* leuprolide acetate *on page 471*

**Elimite**® **[US]** *see* permethrin *on page 635*

**elipten** *see* aminoglutethimide *on page 40*

**Elitek**™ **[US]** *see* rasburicase *on page 712*

**Elixomin**® *(Discontinued) see* theophylline *on page 793*

**Elixophyllin**® **[US]** *see* theophylline *on page 793*

**Elixophyllin-GG**® **[US]** *see* theophylline and guaifenesin *on page 795*

**ElixSure**™ **Congestion [US-OTC]** *see* pseudoephedrine *on page 692*

**ElixSure**™ **Cough [US-OTC]** *see* dextromethorphan *on page 238*

**ElixSure**™ **Fever/Pain [US-OTC]** *see* acetaminophen *on page 4*

**ElixSure**™ **IB [US-OTC]** *see* ibuprofen *on page 427*

**Ellence**® **[US/Can]** *see* epirubicin *on page 289*

**Elmiron**® **[US/Can]** *see* pentosan polysulfate sodium *on page 632*

**Elocom**® **[Can]** *see* mometasone furoate *on page 547*

**Elocon**® **[US]** *see* mometasone furoate *on page 547*

**Eloxatin**™ **[US]** *see* oxaliplatin *on page 605*

**Elspar**® **[US/Can]** *see* asparaginase *on page 72*

**Eltor**® **[Can]** *see* pseudoephedrine *on page 692*

**Eltroxin**® **[Can]** *see* levothyroxine *on page 477*

**Emadine**® **[US]** *see* emedastine *on this page*

**Embeline**™ **[US]** *see* clobetasol *on page 194*

**Embeline**™ **E [US]** *see* clobetasol *on page 194*

**Emcyt**® **[US/Can]** *see* estramustine *on page 303*

**Emecheck**® *(Discontinued)*

**emedastine** (em e DAS teen)
  Synonyms emedastine difumarate
  U.S./Canadian Brand Names Emadine® [US]
  Therapeutic Category Antihistamine, H$_1$ Blocker, Ophthalmic
  Use Treatment of allergic conjunctivitis
  Usual Dosage Ophthalmic: Children ≥3 years and Adults: Instill 1 drop in affected eye up to 4 times/day
  Dosage Forms Solution, ophthalmic, as difumarate: 0.05% (5 mL) [contains benzalkonium chloride]

**emedastine difumarate** *see* emedastine *on this page*

**Emend**® **[US]** *see* aprepitant *on page 67*

**emetine hydrochloride** *(Discontinued)*

**Emetrol**® **[US-OTC]** *see* fructose, dextrose, and phosphoric acid *on page 362*

**Emitrip**® *(Discontinued) see* amitriptyline *on page 42*

**Emko**® *(Discontinued) see* nonoxynol 9 *on page 580*

**EMLA**® **[US/Can]** *see* lidocaine and prilocaine *on page 482*

**emtricitabine** (em trye SYE ta been)
  Synonyms BW524W91; coviracil; FTC
  U.S./Canadian Brand Names Emtriva™ [US]
  Therapeutic Category Antiretroviral Agent, Reverse Transcriptase Inhibitor (Nucleoside)
  Use Treatment of HIV infection in combination with at least two other antiretroviral agents
  Usual Dosage Oral: Adults: 200 mg once daily
  Dosage Forms
    Capsule: 200 mg
    Solution: 10 mg/mL (170 mL) [cotton candy flavor]

## emtricitabine and tenofovir (em trye SYE ta been & te NOE fo veer)

**Synonyms** tenofovir and emtricitabine

**U.S./Canadian Brand Names** Truvada™ [US]

**Therapeutic Category** Antiretroviral Agent, Reverse Transcriptase Inhibitor (Nucleoside); Antiretroviral Agent, Reverse Transcriptase Inhibitor (Nucleotide)

**Use** Treatment of HIV infection in combination with other antiretroviral agents

**Usual Dosage** Adults: Oral: One tablet (emtricitabine 200 mg and tenofovir 300 mg) once daily

**Dosage Forms** Tablet, film coated: Emtricitabine 200 mg and tenofovir disoproxil fumarate 300 mg

**Emtriva™ [US]** *see* emtricitabine *on previous page*

**Emulsoil®** *(Discontinued) see* castor oil *on page 151*

**E-Mycin®** *(Discontinued)*

**E-Mycin-E®** *(Discontinued)*

**ENA 713** *see* rivastigmine *on page 727*

**Enablex® [US]** *see* darifenacin *on page 225*

## enalapril (e NAL a pril)

**Sound-Alike/Look-Alike Issues**

enalapril may be confused with Anafranil®, Elavil®, Eldepryl®, nafarelin, ramipril

**Synonyms** enalapril maleate; enalaprilat

**U.S./Canadian Brand Names** Vasotec® [US/Can]

**Therapeutic Category** Angiotensin-Converting Enzyme (ACE) Inhibitor

**Use** Management of mild to severe hypertension; treatment of congestive heart failure, left ventricular dysfunction after myocardial infarction

**Usual Dosage** Use lower listed initial dose in patients with hyponatremia, hypovolemia, severe congestive heart failure, decreased renal function, or in those receiving diuretics.

Oral: **Enalapril:** Children 1 month to 16 years: Hypertension: Initial: 0.08 mg/kg (up to 5 mg) once daily; adjust dosage based on patient response; doses >0.58 mg/kg (40 mg) have not been evaluated in pediatric patients

Adults:

Oral: **Enalapril:**

Hypertension: 2.5-5 mg/day then increase as required, usually at 1- to 2-week intervals; usual dose range (JNC 7): 2.5-40 mg/day in 1-2 divided doses. **Note:** Initiate with 2.5 mg if patient is taking a diuretic which cannot be discontinued. May add a diuretic if blood pressure cannot be controlled with enalapril alone.

Heart failure: As standard therapy alone or with diuretics, beta-blockers, and digoxin, initiate with 2.5 mg once or twice daily (usual range: 5-20 mg/day in 2 divided doses; target: 40 mg). Titrate slowly at 1- to 2-week intervals.

Asymptomatic left ventricular dysfunction: 2.5 mg twice daily, titrated as tolerated to 20 mg/day

I.V.: **Enalaprilat:**

Hypertension: 1.25 mg/dose, given over 5 minutes every 6 hours; doses as high as 5 mg/dose every 6 hours have been tolerated for up to 36 hours. **Note:** If patients are concomitantly receiving diuretic therapy, begin with 0.625 mg I.V. over 5 minutes; if the effect is not adequate after 1 hour, repeat the dose and administer 1.25 mg at 6-hour intervals thereafter; if adequate, administer 0.625 mg I.V. every 6 hours.

Heart failure: Avoid I.V. administration in patients with unstable heart failure or those suffering acute myocardial infarction.

Conversion from I.V. to oral therapy if not concurrently on diuretics: 5 mg once daily; subsequent titration as needed; if concurrently receiving diuretics and responding to 0.625 mg I.V. every 6 hours, initiate with 2.5 mg/day.

**Dosage Forms**

Injection, solution, as enalaprilat: 1.25 mg/mL (1 mL, 2 mL) [contains benzyl alcohol]

Tablet, as maleate (Vasotec®): 2.5 mg, 5 mg, 10 mg, 20 mg

## enalapril and felodipine (e NAL a pril & fe LOE di peen)
**Synonyms** felodipine and enalapril
**U.S./Canadian Brand Names** Lexxel® [US/Can]
**Therapeutic Category** Antihypertensive Agent, Combination
**Use** Treatment of hypertension, however, not indicated for initial treatment of hypertension; replacement therapy in patients receiving separate dosage forms (for patient convenience); when monotherapy with one component fails to achieve desired antihypertensive effect, or when dose-limiting adverse effects limit upward titration of monotherapy
**Usual Dosage** Adults: Oral: 1 tablet daily
**Dosage Forms** Tablet, extended release:
Enalapril maleate 5 mg and felodipine 2.5 mg
Enalapril maleate 5 mg and felodipine 5 mg

## enalapril and hydrochlorothiazide (e NAL a pril & hye droe klor oh THYE a zide)
**Synonyms** hydrochlorothiazide and enalapril
**U.S./Canadian Brand Names** Vaseretic® [US/Can]
**Therapeutic Category** Antihypertensive Agent, Combination
**Use** Treatment of hypertension
**Usual Dosage** Oral: Dose is individualized
**Dosage Forms** Tablet:
5-12.5: Enalapril maleate 5 mg and hydrochlorothiazide 12.5 mg
10-25: Enalapril maleate 10 mg and hydrochlorothiazide 25 mg

**enalaprilat** *see* enalapril *on previous page*

**enalapril maleate** *see* enalapril *on previous page*

**Enbrel® [US/Can]** *see* etanercept *on page 307*

**Encare® [US-OTC]** *see* nonoxynol 9 *on page 580*

**EndaCof-DM [US]** *see* brompheniramine, pseudoephedrine, and dextromethorphan *on page 116*

**EndaCof-PD [US]** *see* brompheniramine, pseudoephedrine, and dextromethorphan *on page 116*

**Endagen™-HD [US]** *see* phenylephrine, hydrocodone, and chlorpheniramine *on page 643*

**Endal® [US]** *see* guaifenesin and phenylephrine *on page 387*

**Endal® HD [US]** *see* hydrocodone, phenylephrine, and diphenhydramine *on page 414*

**Endal® HD Plus [US]** *see* phenylephrine, hydrocodone, and chlorpheniramine *on page 643*

**Endantadine® [Can]** *see* amantadine *on page 37*

**EndoAvitene® [US]** *see* collagen hemostat *on page 206*

**Endocet® [US/Can]** *see* oxycodone and acetaminophen *on page 609*

**Endocodone® (Discontinued)** *see* oxycodone *on page 608*

**Endodan® [US/Can]** *see* oxycodone and aspirin *on page 610*

**Endo®-Levodopa/Carbidopa [Can]** *see* levodopa and carbidopa *on page 474*

**Endolor® (Discontinued)**

**Endrate® [US]** *see* edetate disodium *on page 279*

**Enduron® [Can]** *see* methyclothiazide *on page 528*

**Enduron® (Discontinued)** *see* methyclothiazide *on page 528*

**Enduronyl® [Can]** *see* methyclothiazide and deserpidine *on page 528*

**Enduronyl® Forte [US/Can]** *see* methyclothiazide and deserpidine *on page 528*

**Enecat® [US]** *see* radiological/contrast media (ionic) *on page 707*

**Enemeez® [US-OTC]** *see* docusate *on page 263*

**Ener-B® (Discontinued)** *see* cyanocobalamin *on page 212*

## enflurane (EN floo rane)
**Sound-Alike/Look-Alike Issues**
enflurane may be confused with isoflurane

**U.S./Canadian Brand Names** Ethrane® [US]

**Therapeutic Category** General Anesthetic

**Use** Maintenance of general anesthesia

**Usual Dosage** Minimum alveolar concentration (MAC), the concentration at which 50% of patients do not respond to surgical incision, is 1.6% for enflurane. The concentration at which amnesia and loss of awareness occur (MAC - awake) is 0.4%. Surgical levels of anesthesia are achieved with concentrations between 0.5% to 3%.

**Dosage Forms** Liquid, for inhalation: >99.9% (125 mL [DSC], 250 mL)

## enfuvirtide (en FYOO vir tide)

**Synonyms** T-20

**U.S./Canadian Brand Names** Fuzeon™ [US/Can]

**Therapeutic Category** Antiretroviral Agent, Fusion Protein Inhibitor

**Use** Treatment of HIV-1 infection in combination with other antiretroviral agents in treatment-experienced patients with evidence of HIV-1 replication despite ongoing antiretroviral therapy

**Usual Dosage** SubQ:

Children ≥6 years: 2 mg/kg twice daily (maximum dose: 90 mg twice daily)

Adults: 90 mg twice daily

**Dosage Forms** Injection, powder for reconstitution [single-use vial]: 108 mg [90 mg/mL following reconstitution; available in convenience kit of 60 vials, SWFI, syringes, alcohol wipes, patient instructions]

**Engerix-B® [US/Can]** see hepatitis B vaccine on page 401

**Engerix-B® and Havrix®** see hepatitis A inactivated and hepatitis B (recombinant) vaccine on page 400

**enhanced-potency inactivated poliovirus vaccine** see poliovirus vaccine (inactivated) on page 657

**Enisyl® (Discontinued)** see l-lysine on page 487

**Enlon® [US/Can]** see edrophonium on page 279

**Enomine® (Discontinued)**

**Enovil® (Discontinued)** see amitriptyline on page 42

## enoxaparin (ee noks a PA rin)

**Sound-Alike/Look-Alike Issues**

Lovenox® may be confused with Lotronex®, Protonix®

**Synonyms** enoxaparin sodium

**U.S./Canadian Brand Names** Lovenox® HP [Can]; Lovenox® [US/Can]

**Therapeutic Category** Anticoagulant (Other)

**Use**

DVT Treatment (acute): Inpatient treatment (patients with and without pulmonary embolism) and outpatient treatment (patients without pulmonary embolism)

DVT prophylaxis: Following hip or knee replacement surgery, abdominal surgery, or in medical patients with severely-restricted mobility during acute illness in patients at risk of thromboembolic complications

**Note:** High-risk patients include those with one or more of the following risk factors: >40 years of age, obesity, general anesthesia lasting >30 minutes, malignancy, history of deep vein thrombosis or pulmonary embolism

Unstable angina and non-Q-wave myocardial infarction (to prevent ischemic complications)

**Usual Dosage** Adults:

DVT prophylaxis:

Hip replacement surgery:

Twice-daily dosing: 30 mg twice daily, with initial dose within 12-24 hours after surgery, and every 12 hours until risk of DVT has diminished or the patient is adequately anticoagulated on warfarin.

Once-daily dosing: 40 mg once daily, with initial dose within 9-15 hours before surgery, and daily until risk of DVT has diminished or the patient is adequately anticoagulated on warfarin.

Knee replacement surgery: 30 mg twice daily, with initial dose within 12-24 hours after surgery, and every 12 hours until risk of DVT has diminished (usually 7-10 days).

Abdominal surgery: 40 mg once daily, with initial dose given 2 hours prior to surgery; continue until risk of DVT has diminished (usual 7-10 days).

Medical patients with severely-restricted mobility during acute illness: 40 mg once daily; continue until risk of DVT has diminished

(Continued)

# enoxaparin *(Continued)*

DVT treatment (acute): **Note:** Start warfarin within 72 hours and continue enoxaparin until INR is between 2.0 and 3.0 (usually 7 days).

Inpatient treatment (with or without pulmonary embolism): 1 mg/kg/dose every 12 hours or 1.5 mg/kg once daily.

Outpatient treatment (without pulmonary embolism): 1 mg/kg/dose every 12 hours.

Unstable angina or non-Q-wave MI: 1 mg/kg twice daily in conjunction with oral aspirin therapy (100-325 mg once daily); continue until clinical stabilization (a minimum of at least 2 days)

**Dosage Forms**

Injection, solution, as sodium [graduated prefilled syringe; preservative free]: 60 mg/0.6 mL (0.6 mL); 80 mg/0.8 mL (0.8 mL); 100 mg/mL (1 mL); 120 mg/0.8 mL (0.8 mL); 150 mg/mL (1 mL)

Injection, solution, as sodium [multidose vial]: 100 mg/mL (3 mL) [contains benzyl alcohol]

Injection, solution, as sodium [prefilled syringe; preservative free]: 30 mg/0.3 mL (0.3 mL); 40 mg/0.4 mL (0.4 mL)

**enoxaparin sodium** *see* enoxaparin *on previous page*

**Enpresse™ [US]** *see* ethinyl estradiol and levonorgestrel *on page 312*

**Ensure® [US-OTC]** *see* nutritional formula, enteral/oral *on page 591*

**Ensure Plus® [US-OTC]** *see* nutritional formula, enteral/oral *on page 591*

# entacapone *(en TA ka pone)*

**U.S./Canadian Brand Names** Comtan® [US/Can]

**Therapeutic Category** Anti-Parkinson Agent; Reverse COMT Inhibitor

**Use** Adjunct to levodopa/carbidopa therapy in patients with idiopathic Parkinson's disease who experience "wearing-off" symptoms at the end of a dosing interval

**Usual Dosage** Oral: Adults: 200 mg with each dose of levodopa/carbidopa, up to a maximum of 8 times/day (maximum daily dose: 1600 mg/day). To optimize therapy, the dosage of levodopa may need reduced or the dosing interval may need extended. Patients taking levodopa ≥800mg/day or who had moderate-to-severe dyskinesias prior to therapy required an average decrease of 25% in the daily levodopa dose.

**Dosage Forms** Tablet: 200 mg

**entacapone, carbidopa, and levodopa** *see* levodopa, carbidopa, and entacapone *on page 475*

# entecavir *(en TE ka veer)*

**U.S./Canadian Brand Names** Baraclude™ [US]

**Therapeutic Category** Antiretroviral Agent, Reverse Transcriptase Inhibitor (Nucleoside)

**Use** Treatment of chronic hepatitis B infection in adults with evidence of active viral replication and either evidence of persistent transaminase elevations or histologically-active disease

**Usual Dosage** Oral: Adolescents ≥16 years and Adults:

Nucleoside treatment naive: 0.5 mg daily

Lamivudine-resistant viremia (or known lamivudine-resistant mutations): 1 mg daily

**Dosage Forms**

Oral solution: 0.05 mg/mL (210 mL) [orange flavor]

Tablet: 0.5 mg, 1 mg

**Entertainer's Secret® [US-OTC]** *see* saliva substitute *on page 737*

**Entex® [US]** *see* guaifenesin and phenylephrine *on page 387*

**Entex® ER [US]** *see* guaifenesin and phenylephrine *on page 387*

**Entex® LA [US]** *see* guaifenesin and phenylephrine *on page 387*

**Entex® PSE [US]** *see* guaifenesin and pseudoephedrine *on page 388*

**Entocort® [Can]** *see* budesonide *on page 118*

**Entocort™ EC [US]** *see* budesonide *on page 118*

**Entrobar® [US]** *see* radiological/contrast media (ionic) *on page 707*

**Entrophen® [Can]** *see* aspirin *on page 73*

**Entsol® [US-OTC]** *see* sodium chloride *on page 752*

**Entuss-D® Liquid *(Discontinued)*** *see* hydrocodone and pseudoephedrine *on page 413*

**Enulose® [US]** *see* lactulose *on page 464*

**Enzone® [US]** *see* pramoxine and hydrocortisone *on page 671*

## ephedrine (e FED rin)
**Sound-Alike/Look-Alike Issues**
ephedrine may be confused with Epifrin®, epinephrine
**Synonyms** ephedrine sulfate
**U.S./Canadian Brand Names** Pretz-D® [US-OTC]
**Therapeutic Category** Adrenergic Agonist Agent
**Use** Treatment of bronchial asthma, nasal congestion, acute bronchospasm, idiopathic orthostatic hypotension
**Usual Dosage**
Children:
Oral, SubQ: 3 mg/kg/day or 25-100 mg/m$^2$/day in 4-6 divided doses every 4-6 hours
I.M., slow I.V. push: 0.2-0.3 mg/kg/dose every 4-6 hours
Adults:
Oral: 25-50 mg every 3-4 hours as needed
I.M., SubQ: 25-50 mg, parenteral adult dose should not exceed 150 mg in 24 hours
I.V.: 5-25 mg/dose slow I.V. push repeated after 5-10 minutes as needed, then every 3-4 hours not to exceed 150 mg/24 hours

Nasal spray:
Children 6-12 years: 1-2 sprays into each nostril, not more frequently than every 4 hours
Children ≥12 years and Adults: 2-3 sprays into each nostril, not more frequently than every 4 hours
**Dosage Forms**
Capsule, as sulfate: 25 mg
Injection, solution, as sulfate: 50 mg/mL (1 mL, 10 mL)
Solution, intranasal spray, as sulfate (Pretz-D®): 0.25% (50 mL)

**ephedrine, chlorpheniramine, phenylephrine, and carbetapentane** *see* chlorpheniramine, ephedrine, phenylephrine, and carbetapentane *on page 173*

**ephedrine sulfate** *see* ephedrine *on this page*

**Epi-C® [US]** *see* radiological/contrast media (ionic) *on page 707*

**epidermal thymocyte activating factor** *see* aldesleukin *on page 25*

**Epifoam® [US]** *see* pramoxine and hydrocortisone *on page 671*

**Epifrin® *(Discontinued)*** *see* epinephrine *on this page*

## epinastine (ep i NAS teen)
**Synonyms** epinastine hydrochloride
**U.S./Canadian Brand Names** Elestat™ [US]
**Therapeutic Category** Antihistamine, H$_1$ Blocker, Ophthalmic
**Use** Treatment of allergic conjunctivitis
**Usual Dosage** Ophthalmic: Allergic conjunctivitis: Children ≥3 years and Adults: Instill 1 drop into each eye twice daily; continue throughout period of exposure, even in the absence of symptoms
**Dosage Forms** Solution, ophthalmic, as hydrochloride: 0.05% (5 mL) [contains benzalkonium chloride]

**epinastine hydrochloride** *see* epinastine *on this page*

## epinephrine (ep i NEF rin)
**Sound-Alike/Look-Alike Issues**
epinephrine may be confused with ephedrine
Epifrin® may be confused with ephedrine, EpiPen®
EpiPen® may be confused with Epifrin®
**Synonyms** adrenaline; epinephrine bitartrate; epinephrine hydrochloride
**U.S./Canadian Brand Names** Adrenalin® [US/Can]; EpiPen® Jr [US/Can]; EpiPen® [US/Can]; Primatene® Mist [US-OTC]; Twinject™ [US]; Vaponefrin® [Can]
(Continued)

# epinephrine *(Continued)*

**Therapeutic Category** Adrenergic Agonist Agent

**Use** Treatment of bronchospasms, anaphylactic reactions, cardiac arrest; added to local anesthetics to decrease systemic absorption, increase duration of action, and decrease toxicity of the local anesthetic

**Usual Dosage**

Neonates: Cardiac arrest: I.V.: Intratracheal: 0.01-0.03 mg/kg (0.1-0.3 mL/kg of **1:10,000** solution) every 3-5 minutes as needed; dilute intratracheal doses to 1-2 mL with normal saline

Infants and Children:

Bronchodilator: SubQ: 10 mcg/kg (0.01 mL/kg of **1:1000**) (single doses not to exceed 0.5 mg) **or** suspension (1:200): 0.005 mL/kg/dose (0.025 mg/kg/dose) to a maximum of 0.15 mL (0.75 mg for single dose) every 8-12 hours

Bradycardia:

I.V.: 0.01 mg/kg (0.1 mL/kg of **1:10,000** solution) every 3-5 minutes as needed (maximum: 1 mg/10 mL)

Intratracheal: 0.1 mg/kg (0.1 mL/kg of **1:1000** solution every 3-5 minutes); doses as high as 0.2 mg/kg may be effective

Asystole or pulseless arrest:

I.V. or intraosseous: **First dose:** 0.01 mg/kg (0.1 mL/kg of a **1:10,000** solution); **subsequent doses:** 0.1 mg/kg (0.1 mL/kg of a **1:1000** solution); doses as high as 0.2 mg/kg may be effective; repeat every 3-5 minutes

Intratracheal: 0.1 mg/kg (0.1 mL/kg of a **1:1000** solution); doses as high as 0.2 mg/kg may be effective

Hypersensitivity reaction: SubQ: 0.01 mg/kg every 15 minutes for 2 doses then every 4 hours as needed (single doses not to exceed 0.5 mg)

Refractory hypotension (refractory to dopamine/dobutamine): Continuous I.V. infusions of 0.1-1 mcg/kg/minute; titrate dosage to desired effect

Nebulization: 0.25-0.5 mL of 2.25% **racemic epinephrine** solution diluted in 3 mL normal saline, or L-epinephrine at an equivalent dose; racemic epinephrine 10 mg = 5 mg L-epinephrine; use lower end of dosing range for younger infants

Intranasal: Children ≥6 years and Adults: Apply locally as drops or spray or with sterile swab

Adults:

Asystole:

I.V.: 1 mg every 3-5 minutes; if this approach fails, higher doses of epinephrine (up to 0.2 mg/kg) may be used, but are not recommended (Class Indeterminate; 2000 ACLS guidelines)

Intratracheal: Administer 2-2.5 times the recommended I.V. dose; dilute in 10 mL NS or distilled water. **Note:** Absorption is greater with distilled water, but causes more adverse effects on $PaO_2$.

Bronchodilator: I.M., SubQ (**1:1000**): 0.1-0.5 mg every 10-15 minutes to 4 hours

Hypersensitivity reaction: I.M., SubQ: 0.3-0.5 mg every 15-20 minutes if condition requires; if hypotension is present: 0.1 mg I.V. slowly over 5-10 minutes followed by continuous infusion 1-10 mcg/minute

Symptomatic bradycardia or heart block (not responsive to atropine or pacing): I.V. infusion: 1-10 mcg/minute; titrate to desired effect

Refractory hypotension (refractory to dopamine/dobutamine): Continuous I.V. infusion 1 mcg/minute (range: 1-10 mcg/minute); titrate dosage to desired effect; severe cardiac dysfunction may require doses >10 mcg/minute (up to 0.1 mcg/kg/minute)

Nebulization: Instill 8-15 drops into nebulizer reservoirs; administer 1-3 inhalations 4-6 times/day

**Dosage Forms**

Aerosol for oral inhalation (Primatene® Mist): 0.22 mg/inhalation (15 mL, 22.5 mL) [contains CFCs]

Injection, solution [prefilled auto injector]:

EpiPen®: 0.3 mg/0.3 mL [1:1000] (2 mL) [contains sodium metabisulfite; available as single unit or in double-unit pack with training unit]

EpiPen® Jr: 0.15 mg/0.3 mL [1:2000] (2 mL) [contains sodium metabisulfite; available as single unit or in double-unit pack with training unit]

Twinject™: 0.15 mg/0.15 mL [1:1000] (1.1 mL) [contains sodium bisulfite; two 0.15 mg doses per injector]; 0.3 mg/0.3 mL [1:1000] (1.1 mL) [contains sodium bisulfite; two 0.3 mg doses per injector]

Injection, solution, as hydrochloride: 0.1 mg/mL [1:10,000] (10 mL); 1 mg/mL [1:1000] (1 mL) [products may contain sodium metabisulfite]

Adrenalin®: 1 mg/mL [1:1000] (1 mL, 30 mL) [contains sodium bisulfite]

Solution for oral inhalation, as hydrochloride (Adrenalin®): 1% [10 mg/mL, 1:100] (7.5 mL) [contains sodium bisulfite]

## epinephrine and chlorpheniramine (ep i NEF rin & klor fen IR a meen)
**Synonyms** insect sting kit
**U.S./Canadian Brand Names** Ana-Kit® [US]
**Therapeutic Category** Antidote
**Use** Anaphylaxis emergency treatment of insect bites or stings by the sensitive patient that may occur within minutes of insect sting or exposure to an allergic substance
**Usual Dosage** Children and Adults: I.M. or SubQ:
Epinephrine:
&lt;2 years: 0.05-0.1 mL
2-6 years: 0.15 mL
6-12 years: 0.2 mL
&gt;12 years : 0.3 mL
Chlorpheniramine:
&lt;6 years: 1 tablet
6-12 years: 2 tablets
&gt;12 years: 4 tablets
**Dosage Forms** Kit: Epinephrine hydrochloride 1:1000 [prefilled syringe, delivers two 0.3 mL doses; contains sodium bisulfite] (1 mL), chlorpheniramine maleate chewable tablet 2 mg (4), sterile alcohol pads [isopropyl alcohol 70%] (2), tourniquet (1)

**epinephrine and lidocaine** *see* lidocaine and epinephrine *on page 480*

**epinephrine bitartrate** *see* epinephrine *on page 287*

**epinephrine hydrochloride** *see* epinephrine *on page 287*

**EpiPen® [US/Can]** *see* epinephrine *on page 287*

**EpiPen® Jr [US/Can]** *see* epinephrine *on page 287*

**epipodophyllotoxin** *see* etoposide *on page 322*

**EpiQuin™ Micro [US]** *see* hydroquinone *on page 420*

## epirubicin (ep i ROO bi sin)
**Sound-Alike/Look-Alike Issues**
epirubicin may be confused with DAUNOrubicin
Ellence® may be confused with Elase®
**Synonyms** pidorubicin hydrochloride; pidorubicin
**U.S./Canadian Brand Names** Ellence® [US/Can]; Pharmorubicin® [Can]
**Therapeutic Category** Antineoplastic Agent, Anthracycline; Antineoplastic Agent, Antibiotic
**Use** Adjuvant therapy for primary breast cancer
**Usual Dosage** Adults: I.V.: 100-120 mg/m$^2$ once every 3-4 weeks **or** 50-60 mg/m$^2$ days 1 and 8 every 3-4 weeks
Breast cancer:
CEF-120: 60 mg/m$^2$ on days 1 and 8 every 28 days for 6 cycles
FEC-100: 100 mg/m$^2$ on day 1 every 21 days for 6 cycles
**Note:** Patients receiving 120 mg/m$^2$/cycle as part of combination therapy should also receive prophylactic therapy with sulfamethoxazole/trimethoprim or a fluoroquinolone.
Dosage modifications:
Delay day 1 dose until platelets are ≥100,000/mm$^3$, ANC ≥1500/mm$^3$, and nonhematologic toxicities have recovered to ≤grade 1
Reduce day 1 dose in subsequent cycles to 75% of previous day 1 dose if patient experiences nadir platelet counts &lt;50,000/mm$^3$, ANC &lt;250/mm$^3$, neutropenic fever, or grade 3/4 nonhematologic toxicity during the previous cycle
For divided doses (day 1 and day 8), reduce day 8 dose to 75% of day 1 dose if platelet counts are 75,000-100,000/mm$^3$ and ANC is 1000-1499/mm$^3$; omit day 8 dose if platelets are &lt;75,000/mm$^3$, ANC &lt;1000/mm$^3$, or grade 3/4 nonhematologic toxicity
Dosage adjustment in bone marrow dysfunction: Heavily-treated patients, patients with pre-existing bone marrow depression or neoplastic bone marrow infiltration: Lower starting doses (75-90 mg/mm$^2$) should be considered.
**Dosage Forms** Injection, solution [preservative free]: 2 mg/mL (25 mL, 100 mL)

**Epitol® [US]** *see* carbamazepine *on page 140*

**Epival® I.V. [Can]** *see* valproic acid and derivatives *on page 837*

**Epivir**® **[US]** *see* lamivudine *on page 464*

**Epivir-HBV**® **[US]** *see* lamivudine *on page 464*

## eplerenone (e PLER en one)

**Sound-Alike/Look-Alike Issues**
Inspra™ may be confused with Spiriva®

**U.S./Canadian Brand Names** Inspra™ [US]

**Therapeutic Category** Antihypertensive Agent; Selective Aldosterone Blocker

**Use** Treatment of hypertension (may be used alone or in combination with other antihypertensive agents); treatment of CHF following acute MI

**Usual Dosage** Oral: Adults:

Hypertension: Initial: 50 mg once daily; may increase to 50 mg twice daily if response is not adequate; may take up to 4 weeks for full therapeutic response. Doses >100 mg/day are associated with increased risk of hyperkalemia and no greater therapeutic effect.

Concurrent use with moderate CYP3A4 inhibitors: Initial: 25 mg once daily

Congestive heart failure (post-MI): Initial: 25 mg once daily; dosage goal: titrate to 50 mg once daily within 4 weeks, as tolerated

**Dosage adjustment per serum potassium concentrations for CHF:**

<5.0 mEq/L:
Increase dose from 25 mg every other day to 25 mg daily **or**
Increase dose from 25 mg daily to 50 mg daily

5.0-5.4 mEq/L: No adjustment needed

5.5-5.9 mEq/L:
Decrease dose from 50 mg daily to 25 mg daily **or**
Decrease dose from 25 mg daily to 25 mg every other day **or**
Decrease does from 25 mg every other day to withhold medication

≥6.0 mEq/L: Withhold medication until potassium <5.5 mEq/L, then restart at 25 mg every other day

**Dosage Forms** Tablet [film coated]: 25 mg, 50 mg

**EPO** *see* epoetin alfa *on this page*

## epoetin alfa (e POE e tin AL fa)

**Sound-Alike/Look-Alike Issues**
epoetin alfa may be confused with darbepoetin alfa
Epogen® may be confused with Neupogen®

**Synonyms** rHuEPO-α; EPO; erythropoietin

**U.S./Canadian Brand Names** Epogen® [US]; Eprex® [Can]; Procrit® [US]

**Therapeutic Category** Colony-Stimulating Factor

**Use** Treatment of anemia related to HIV therapy, chronic renal failure, antineoplastic therapy; reduction of allogeneic blood transfusion for elective, noncardiac, nonvascular surgery

**Usual Dosage**

**Chronic renal failure patients:** I.V., SubQ:

Children: Initial dose: 50 units/kg 3 times/week

Adults: Initial dose: 50-100 units/kg 3 times/week

*Dose adjustment:* Children and Adults: Reduce dose by 25% when hemoglobin approaches 12 g/dL **or** hemoglobin increases 1 g/dL in any 2-week period. Increase dose by 25% if hemoglobin does not increase by 2 g/dL after 8 weeks of therapy and hemoglobin is below suggested target range. Suggested target hemoglobin range: 10-12 g/dL.

*Maintenance dose:* Individualize to target range; limit additional dosage increases to every 4 weeks (or longer)

Dialysis patients: Median dose:
Children: 167 units/kg/week **or** 76 units/kg 2-3 times/week
Adults: 75 units/kg 3 times/week

Nondialysis patients:
Children: Dosing range: 50-250 units/kg 1-3 times/week
Adults: Median dose: 75-150 units/kg

**Zidovudine-treated, HIV-infected patients** (patients with erythropoietin levels >500 mU/mL are **unlikely** to respond): I.V., SubQ:

Children: Initial dose: Reported dosing range: 50-400 units/kg 2-3 times/week

Adults: 100 units/kg 3 times/week for 8 weeks. **Dose adjustment:** Increase dose by 50-100 units/kg 3 times/week if response is not satisfactory in terms of reducing transfusion requirements or increasing hemoglobin after 8 weeks of therapy. Evaluate response every 4-8 weeks thereafter and adjust the dose accordingly by 50-100 units/kg increments 3 times/week. If patient has not responded satisfactorily to a 300 unit/kg dose 3 times/week, a response to higher doses is unlikely. Stop dose if hemoglobin exceeds 13 g/dL and resume treatment at a 25% dose reduction when hemoglobin drops to 12 g/dL.

**Cancer patient on chemotherapy:** Treatment of patients with erythropoietin levels >200 mU/mL is **not recommended**

Children: I.V., SubQ: Dosing range: 25-300 units/kg 3-7 times/week; commonly reported initial dose: 150 units/kg

Adults: SubQ: Initial dose: 150 units/kg 3 times/week or 40,000 units once weekly; commonly used doses range from 10,000 units 3 times/week to 40,000-60,000 units once weekly.

*Dose adjustment:* Children and Adults: If response is not satisfactory after a sufficient period of evaluation (8 weeks of 3 times/week and 4 weeks of once-weekly therapy), the dose may be increased every 4 weeks (or longer) up to 300 units/kg 3 times/week, **or** when dosed weekly, increased all at once to 60,000 units weekly. If patient does not respond, a response to higher doses is unlikely. Stop dose if hemoglobin exceeds 13 g/dL and resume treatment at a 25% dose reduction when hemoglobin drops to 12 g/dL; reduce dose by 25% if hemoglobin increases by 1 g/dL in any 2-week period, or if hemoglobin approaches 12 g/dL.

**Surgery patients:** Prior to initiating treatment, obtain a hemoglobin to establish that is >10 mg/dL or ≤13 mg/dL: Adults: SubQ: Initial dose: 300 units/kg/day for 10 days before surgery, on the day of surgery, and for 4 days after surgery

Alternative dose: 600 units/kg in once weekly doses (21, 14, and 7 days before surgery) plus a fourth dose on the day of surgery

### Dosage Forms

Injection, solution [preservative free]: 2000 units/mL (1 mL); 3000 units/mL (1 mL); 4000 units/mL (1 mL); 10,000 units/mL (1 mL); 40,000 units/mL (1 mL) [contains human albumin]

Injection, solution [with preservative]: 10,000 units/mL (2 mL); 20,000 units/mL (1 mL) [contains human albumin and benzyl alcohol]

**Epogen® [US]** *see* epoetin alfa *on previous page*

## epoprostenol (e poe PROST en ole)

**Synonyms** epoprostenol sodium; PGI$_2$; PGX; prostacyclin

**U.S./Canadian Brand Names** Flolan® [US/Can]

**Therapeutic Category** Platelet Inhibitor

**Use Orphan drug:** Treatment of primary pulmonary hypertension; treatment of secondary pulmonary hypertension due to intrinsic precapillary pulmonary vascular disease

**Usual Dosage** I.V.: The drug is administered by continuous intravenous infusion via a central venous catheter using an ambulatory infusion pump; during dose ranging it may be administered peripherally

**Acute dose ranging:** The initial infusion rate should be 2 ng/kg/minute by continuous I.V. and increased in increments of 2 ng/kg/minute every 15 minutes or longer until dose-limiting effects are elicited (such as chest pain, anxiety, dizziness, changes in heart rate, dyspnea, nausea, vomiting, headache, hypotension and/or flushing)

**Continuous chronic infusion:** Initial: 4 ng/kg/minute **less** than the maximum-tolerated infusion rate determined during acute dose ranging

If maximum-tolerated infusion rate is <5 ng/kg/minute, the chronic infusion rate should be 1/2 the maximum-tolerated acute infusion rate

**Dosage Forms** Injection, powder for reconstitution, as sodium: 0.5 mg, 1.5 mg [provided with 50 mL sterile diluent]

**epoprostenol sodium** *see* epoprostenol *on this page*

**Eprex® [Can]** *see* epoetin alfa *on previous page*

## eprosartan (ep roe SAR tan)

**U.S./Canadian Brand Names** Teveten® [US/Can]

**Therapeutic Category** Angiotensin II Receptor Antagonist

**Use** Treatment of hypertension; may be used alone or in combination with other antihypertensives

**Usual Dosage** Adults: Oral: Dosage must be individualized; can administer once or twice daily with total daily doses of 400-800 mg. Usual starting dose is 600 mg once daily as monotherapy in patients who are euvolemic. Limited clinical experience with doses >800 mg.

**Dosage Forms** Tablet: 400 mg, 600 mg

## eprosartan and hydrochlorothiazide (ep roe SAR tan & hye droe klor oh THYE a zide)

**Synonyms** eprosartan mesylate and hydrochlorothiazide; hydrochlorothiazide and eprosartan

**U.S./Canadian Brand Names** Teveten® HCT [US/Can]; Teveten® Plus [Can]

**Therapeutic Category** Angiotensin II Antagonist Combination; Antihypertensive Agent, Combination; Diuretic, Thiazide

**Use** Treatment of hypertension (not indicated for initial treatment)

**Usual Dosage** Oral: Adults: Dose is individualized (combination substituted for individual components)
Usual recommended dose: Eprosartan 600 mg/hydrochlorothiazide 12.5 mg once daily (maximum dose: Eprosartan 600 mg/hydrochlorothiazide 25 mg once daily)

**Dosage Forms** Tablet:
600 mg/12.5 mg: Eprosartan 600 mg and hydrochlorothiazide 12.5 mg
600 mg/25 mg: Eprosartan 600 mg and hydrochlorothiazide 25 mg

**eprosartan mesylate and hydrochlorothiazide** *see* eprosartan and hydrochlorothiazide *on this page*

**epsilon aminocaproic acid** *see* aminocaproic acid *on page 40*

**epsom salts** *see* magnesium sulfate *on page 500*

**EPT** *see* teniposide *on page 785*

**eptacog alfa (activated)** *see* factor VIIa (recombinant) *on page 325*

## eptifibatide (ep TIF i ba tide)

**Synonyms** intrifiban

**U.S./Canadian Brand Names** Integrilin® [US/Can]

**Therapeutic Category** Antiplatelet Agent

**Use** Treatment of patients with acute coronary syndrome (UA/NQMI), including patients who are to be managed medically and those undergoing percutaneous coronary intervention (PCI including PTCA; intracoronary stenting)

**Usual Dosage** I.V.: Adults:
Acute coronary syndrome: Bolus of 180 mcg/kg (maximum: 22.6 mg) over 1-2 minutes, begun as soon as possible following diagnosis, followed by a continuous infusion of 2 mcg/kg/minute (maximum: 15 mg/hour) until hospital discharge or initiation of CABG surgery, up to 72 hours. Concurrent aspirin (160-325 mg initially and daily thereafter) and heparin therapy (target aPTT 50-70 seconds) are recommended.

Percutaneous coronary intervention (PCI) with or without stenting: Bolus of 180 mcg/kg (maximum: 22.6 mg) administered immediately before the initiation of PCI, followed by a continuous infusion of 2 mcg/kg/minute (maximum: 15 mg/hour). A second 180 mcg/kg bolus (maximum: 22.6 mg) should be administered 10 minutes after the first bolus. Infusion should be continued until hospital discharge or for up to 18-24 hours, whichever comes first. Concurrent aspirin (160-325 mg 1-24 hours before PCI and daily thereafter) and heparin therapy (ACT 200-300 seconds during PCI) are recommended. Heparin infusion after PCI is discouraged. In patients who undergo coronary artery bypass graft surgery, discontinue infusion prior to surgery.

**Dosage Forms** Injection, solution: 0.75 mg/mL (100 mL); 2 mg/mL (10 mL, 100 mL)

**Epzicom™ [US]** *see* abacavir and lamivudine *on page 2*

**Equagesic® [US]** *see* aspirin and meprobamate *on page 75*

**Equalactin® [US-OTC]** *see* polycarbophil *on page 657*

**Equalizer Gas Relief [US-OTC]** *see* simethicone *on page 748*

**Equanil® *(Discontinued)*** *see* meprobamate *on page 514*

**Equetro™ [US]** *see* carbamazepine *on page 140*

**Equilet® *(Discontinued)*** *see* calcium carbonate *on page 130*

**Erbitux™ [US]** *see* cetuximab *on page 163*

**Ercaf® *(Discontinued)*** *see* ergotamine *on page 294*

## ergocalciferol (er goe kal SIF e role)

**Sound-Alike/Look-Alike Issues**
Calciferol™ may be confused with calcitriol
Drisdol® may be confused with Drysol™

**Synonyms** activated ergosterol; viosterol; vitamin $D_2$

**U.S./Canadian Brand Names** Calciferol™ [US]; Drisdol® [US/Can]; Ostoforte® [Can]

**Therapeutic Category** Vitamin D Analog

**Use** Treatment of refractory rickets, hypophosphatemia, hypoparathyroidism; dietary supplement

**Usual Dosage** Oral dosing is preferred; I.M. therapy required with GI, liver, or biliary disease associated with malabsorption

Dietary supplementation (each 1 mcg = 40 int. units):
Infants and Children: 5 mcg/day (200 int. units/day)
Adults:
18-50 years: 5 mcg/day (200 int. units/day)
51-70 years: 10 mcg/day (400 int. units/day)
Renal failure:
Children: 100-1000 mcg/day (4000-40,000 int. units)
Adults: 500 mcg/day (20,000 int. units)
Hypoparathyroidism:
Children: 1.25-5 mg/day (50,000-200,000 int. units) and calcium supplements
Adults: 625 mcg to 5 mg/day (25,000-200,000 int. units) and calcium supplements
Vitamin D-dependent rickets:
Children: 75-125 mcg/day (3000-5000 int. units); maximum: 1500 mcg/day
Adults: 250 mcg to 1.5 mg/day (10,000-60,000 int. units)
Nutritional rickets and osteomalacia:
Children and Adults (with normal absorption): 25-125 mcg/day (1000-5000 int. units)
Children with malabsorption: 250-625 mcg/day (10,000-25,000 int. units)
Adults with malabsorption: 250-7500 mcg (10,000-300,000 int. units)
Vitamin D-resistant rickets:
Children: Initial: 1000-2000 mcg/day (40,000-80,000 int. units) with phosphate supplements; daily dosage is increased at 3- to 4-month intervals in 250-500 mcg (10,000-20,000 int. units) increments
Adults: 250-1500 mcg/day (10,000-60,000 int. units) with phosphate supplements
Familial hypophosphatemia: 10,000-80,000 int. units daily plus 1-2 g/day elemental phosphorus
Osteoporosis prophylaxis: Adults:
51-70 years: 400 int. units/day
>70 years: 600 int. units/day
Maximum daily dose: 2000 int. units/day

**Dosage Forms** [DSC] = Discontinued product
Capsule (Drisdol®): 50,000 int. units [1.25 mg; contains tartrazine and soybean oil]
Injection, solution (Calciferol™): 500,000 int. units/mL [12.5 mg/mL] (1 mL) [contains sesame oil] [DSC]
Liquid, drops (Calciferol™, Drisdol®): 8000 int. units/mL [200 mcg/mL] (60 mL) [OTC]

## ergoloid mesylates (ER goe loid MES i lates)

**Synonyms** dihydroergotoxine; dihydrogenated ergot alkaloids

**U.S./Canadian Brand Names** Hydergine® [Can]

**Therapeutic Category** Ergot Alkaloid and Derivative

**Use** Treatment of cerebrovascular insufficiency in primary progressive dementia, Alzheimer dementia, and senile onset

**Usual Dosage** Adults: Oral: 1 mg 3 times/day up to 4.5-12 mg/day; up to 6 months of therapy may be necessary

**Dosage Forms**
Tablet: 1 mg
Tablet, sublingual: 1 mg

## Ergomar® [US] see ergotamine on next page

## ergometrine maleate see ergonovine on this page

## ergonovine (er goe NOE veen)

**Synonyms** ergometrine maleate; ergonovine maleate

**Therapeutic Category** Ergot Alkaloid and Derivative

**Use** Prevention and treatment of postpartum and postabortion hemorrhage caused by uterine atony or subinvolution

**Usual Dosage** Adults: I.M., I.V. (I.V. should be reserved for emergency use only): 0.2 mg, repeat dose in 2-4 hours as needed

**Dosage Forms** Injection, as maleate: 0.2 mg/mL (1 mL)

**ergonovine maleate** *see* ergonovine *on previous page*

# ergotamine (er GOT a meen)
**Synonyms** ergotamine tartrate
**U.S./Canadian Brand Names** Ergomar® [US]
**Therapeutic Category** Ergot Alkaloid and Derivative
**Use** Abort or prevent vascular headaches, such as migraine, migraine variants, or so-called "histaminic cephalalgia"
**Usual Dosage** Sublingual: One tablet under tongue at first sign, then 1 tablet every 30 minutes if needed; maximum dose: 3 tablets/24 hours, 5 tablets/week
**Dosage Forms** Tablet, sublingual: Ergotamine tartrate 2 mg

**ergotamine tartrate** *see* ergotamine *on this page*

**Ergotamine Tartrate and Caffeine Cafatine®** *(Discontinued) see* ergotamine *on this page*

**ergotamine tartrate, belladonna, and phenobarbital** *see* belladonna, phenobarbital, and ergotamine tartrate *on page 92*

# erlotinib (er LOE tye nib)
**Sound-Alike/Look-Alike Issues**
erlotinib may be confused with gefitinib
**Synonyms** CP358774; erlotinib hydrochloride; NSC-718781; OSI-774; R 14-15
**U.S./Canadian Brand Names** Tarceva™ [US]
**Therapeutic Category** Antineoplastic, Tyrosine Kinase Inhibitor
**Use** Salvage therapy of advanced or metastatic nonsmall cell lung cancer
**Usual Dosage** Oral: Adults: 150 mg/day until disease progression or unacceptable toxicity occurs; dose reduction (if required) should be done in increments of 50 mg
**Note:** Dose reductions are more likely to be needed when erlotinib is administered concomitantly with strong CYP3A4 inhibitors. Likewise, the CYP3A4 inducers may require increased doses; doses of >150 mg/day should be considered with rifampin.
**Dosage Forms** Tablet: 25 mg, 100 mg, 150 mg

**erlotinib hydrochloride** *see* erlotinib *on this page*

**Errin™ [US]** *see* norethindrone *on page 582*

**Ertaczo™ [US]** *see* sertaconazole *on page 744*

# ertapenem (er ta PEN em)
**Sound-Alike/Look-Alike Issues**
Invanz® may be confused with Avinza™
**Synonyms** ertapenem sodium; L-749,345; MK0826
**U.S./Canadian Brand Names** Invanz® [US/Can]
**Therapeutic Category** Antibiotic, Carbapenem
**Use** Treatment of the following moderate-severe infections: Complicated intraabdominal infections, complicated skin and skin structure infections (including diabetic foot infections without osteomyelitis), complicated UTI (including pyelonephritis), acute pelvic infections, and community-acquired pneumonia. Antibacterial coverage includes aerobic gram-positive organisms, aerobic gram-negative organisms, anaerobic organisms.

**Note:** Methicillin-resistant *Staphylococcus*, *Enterococcus* spp, penicillin-resistant strains of *Streptococcus pneumoniae*, beta-lactamase-positive strains of *Haemophilus influenzae* are **resistant** to ertapenem, as are most *Pseudomonas aeruginosa*.

**Usual Dosage Note:** I.V. therapy may be administered for up to 14 days; I.M. therapy for up to 7 days
Children 3 months to 12 years: I.M., I.V.:
Intraabdominal infection: 15 mg/kg twice daily (maximum: 1 g/day) for 5-14 days
Skin and skin structure infections: 15 mg/kg twice daily (maximum: 1 g/day) for 7-14 days
Community-acquired pneumonia: 15 mg/kg twice daily (maximum: 1 g/day); duration of total antibiotic treatment: 10-14 days*
Urinary tract infections/pyelonephritis: 15 mg/kg twice daily (maximum: 1 g/day); duration of total antibiotic treatment: 10-14 days*
Acute pelvic infections: 15 mg/kg twice daily (maximum: 1 g/day) for 3-10 days

Children ≥13 years and Adults: I.M., I.V.:
Intraabdominal infection: 1 g/day for 5-14 days
Skin and skin structure infections: 1 g/day for 7-14 days
Community-acquired pneumonia: 1 g/day; duration of total antibiotic treatment: 10-14 days*
Urinary tract infections/pyelonephritis: 1 g/day; duration of total antibiotic treatment: 10-14 days*
Acute pelvic infections: 1 g/day for 3-10 days
*Duration includes possible switch to appropriate oral therapy after at least 3 days of parenteral treatment, once clinical improvement demonstrated.

**Dosage Forms** Injection, powder for reconstitution: 1 g [contains sodium 137 mg/g (~6 mEq/g)]

**ertapenem sodium** see ertapenem on previous page

**Erwinia asparaginase** see asparaginase on page 72

**Erybid™ [Can]** see erythromycin on this page

**Eryc® [US/Can]** see erythromycin on this page

**Eryderm® [US]** see erythromycin on this page

**Erygel® [US]** see erythromycin on this page

**EryPed® [US]** see erythromycin on this page

**Ery-Tab® [US]** see erythromycin on this page

**Erythrocin® [US]** see erythromycin on this page

# erythromycin (er ith roe MYE sin)

## Sound-Alike/Look-Alike Issues
erythromycin may be confused with azithromycin, clarithromycin, Ethmozine®
Akne-Mycin® may be confused with AK-Mycin®
E.E.S.® may be confused with DES®
Eryc® may be confused with Emcyt®, Ery-Tab®
Ery-Tab® may be confused with Eryc®
Erythrocin® may be confused with Ethmozine®

**Synonyms** erythromycin base; erythromycin estolate; erythromycin ethylsuccinate; erythromycin glucep-tate; erythromycin lactobionate; erythromycin stearate

**U.S./Canadian Brand Names** A/T/S® [US]; Akne-Mycin® [US]; Apo-Erythro Base® [Can]; Apo-Erythro E-C® [Can]; Apo-Erythro-ES® [Can]; Apo-Erythro-S® [Can]; Diomycin® [Can]; E.E.S.® [US/Can]; Ery-Tab® [US]; Erybid™ [Can]; Eryc® [US/Can]; Eryderm® [US]; Erygel® [US]; EryPed® [US]; Erythrocin® [US]; Novo-Rythro Estolate [Can]; Novo-Rythro Ethylsuccinate [Can]; Nu-Erythromycin-S [Can]; PCE® [US/Can]; PMS-Erythromycin [Can]; Romycin® [US]; Sans Acne® [Can]; Theramycin Z® [US]

**Therapeutic Category** Acne Products; Antibiotic, Ophthalmic; Antibiotic, Topical; Macrolide (Antibiotic)

## Use
Systemic: Treatment of susceptible bacterial infections including *S. pyogenes*, some *S. pneumoniae*, some *S. aureus*, *M. pneumoniae*, *Legionella pneumophila*, diphtheria, pertussis, chancroid, *Chlamydia*, erythrasma, *N. gonorrhoeae*, *E. histolytica*, syphilis and nongonococcal urethritis, and *Campylobacter* gastroenteritis; used in conjunction with neomycin for decontaminating the bowel
Ophthalmic: Treatment of superficial eye infections involving the conjunctiva or cornea; neonatal ophthalmia
Topical: Treatment of acne vulgaris

## Usual Dosage
Neonates: Ophthalmic: Prophylaxis of neonatal gonococcal or chlamydial conjunctivitis: 0.5-1 cm ribbon of ointment should be instilled into each conjunctival sac
Infants and Children:
Treatment of susceptible infections:
Oral: (**Note:** Due to differences in absorption, 400 mg erythromycin ethylsuccinate produces the same serum levels as 250 mg erythromycin base, sterate or estolate)
Base: 30-50 mg/kg/day in 2-4 divided doses; do not exceed 2 g/day
Estolate: 30-50 mg/kg/day in 2-4 divided doses; do not exceed 2 g/day
Ethylsuccinate: 30-50 mg/kg/day in 2-4 divided doses; do not exceed 3.2 g/day
Stearate: 30-50 mg/kg/day in 2-4 divided doses; do not exceed 2 g/day
I.V.: Lactobionate: 15-50 mg/kg/day divided every 6 hours, not to exceed 4 g/day
Preop bowel preparation: 20 mg/kg erythromycin base at 1, 2, and 11 PM on the day before surgery combined with mechanical cleansing of the large intestine and oral neomycin
(Continued)

# erythromycin *(Continued)*

Children and Adults:
Ophthalmic: Instill 1/2" (1.25 cm) 2-6 times/day depending on the severity of the infection
Topical: Apply over the affected area twice daily after the skin has been thoroughly washed and patted dry

Adults:
Treatment of susceptible infections:
Oral:
Base: 250-500 mg every 6-12 hours
Ethylsuccinate: 400-800 mg every 6-12 hours
I.V. (lactobionate): 15-20 mg/kg/day divided every 6 hours or 500 mg to 1 g every 6 hours, or given as a continuous infusion over 24 hours (maximum: 4 g/24 hours)
Preop bowel preparation: Oral: 1 g erythromycin base at 1, 2, and 11 PM on the day before surgery combined with mechanical cleansing of the large intestine and oral neomycin

**Dosage Forms** [DSC] = Discontinued product; [CAN] = Canadian brand name
Capsule, delayed release, enteric-coated pellets, as base (Eryc®): 250 mg
Gel, topical: 2% (30 g, 60 g)
A/T/S®: 2% (30 g) [contains alcohol 92%]
Erygel®: 2% (30 g, 60 g) [contains alcohol 92%]
Granules for oral suspension, as ethylsuccinate (E.E.S.®): 200 mg/5 mL (100 mL, 200 mL) [cherry flavor]
Injection, powder for reconstitution, as lactobionate (Erythrocin®): 500 mg, 1 g
Ointment, ophthalmic: 0.5% [5 mg/g] (1 g, 3.5 g)
Romycin®: 0.5% [5 mg/g] (3.5 g)
Ointment, topical (Akne-Mycin®): 2% (25 g)
Powder for oral suspension, as ethylsuccinate (EryPed®): 200 mg/5 mL (100 mL, 200 mL) [fruit flavor]; 400 mg/5 mL (100 mL, 200 mL) [banana flavor]
Powder for oral suspension, as ethylsuccinate [drops] (EryPed®): 100 mg/2.5 mL (50 mL) [fruit flavor]
Solution, topical: 2% (60 mL)
A/T/S®: 2% (60 mL) [contains alcohol 66%]
Eryderm®, T-Stat® [DSC], Theramycin Z®: 2% (60 mL) [contain alcohol]
Sans Acne® [CAN]: 2% (60 mL) [contains ethyl alcohol 44%; not available in U.S.]
Staticin®: 1.5% (60 mL) [DSC]
Suspension, oral, as estolate: 125 mg/5 mL (480 mL); 250 mg/5 mL (480 mL)
Suspension, oral, as ethylsuccinate: 200 mg/5 mL (480 mL); 400 mg/5 mL (480 mL)
E.E.S.®: 200 mg/5 mL (100 mL, 480 mL) [fruit flavor]; 400 mg/5 mL (100 mL, 480 mL) [orange flavor]
Swab (T-Stat® [DSC]): 2% (60s)
Tablet, chewable, as ethylsuccinate (EryPed®): 200 mg [fruit flavor] [DSC]
Tablet, delayed release, enteric coated, as base (Ery-Tab®): 250 mg, 333 mg, 500 mg
Tablet [film coated], as base: 250 mg, 500 mg
Tablet [film coated], as ethylsuccinate (E.E.S.®): 400 mg
Tablet [film coated], as stearate: 250 mg
Erythrocin®: 250 mg, 500 mg
Tablet [polymer-coated particles], as base (PCE®): 333 mg, 500 mg

# erythromycin and benzoyl peroxide *(er ith roe MYE sin & BEN zoe il per OKS ide)*

**Synonyms** benzoyl peroxide and erythromycin
**U.S./Canadian Brand Names** Benzamycin® Pak [US]; Benzamycin® [US]
**Therapeutic Category** Acne Products
**Use** Topical control of acne vulgaris
**Usual Dosage** Apply twice daily, morning and evening
**Dosage Forms** Gel, topical:
Benzamycin®: Erythromycin 30 mg and benzoyl peroxide 50 mg per g (47 g)
Benzamycin® Pak: Erythromycin 30 mg and benzoyl peroxide 50 mg per 0.8 g packet (60s) [supplied with diluent containing alcohol]

# erythromycin and sulfisoxazole *(er ith roe MYE sin & sul fi SOKS a zole)*

**Sound-Alike/Look-Alike Issues**
Pediazole® may be confused with Pediapred®

**Synonyms** sulfisoxazole and erythromycin

**U.S./Canadian Brand Names** Pediazole® [US/Can]

**Therapeutic Category** Macrolide (Antibiotic); Sulfonamide

**Use** Treatment of susceptible bacterial infections of the upper and lower respiratory tract, otitis media in children caused by susceptible strains of *Haemophilus influenzae*, and many other infections in patients allergic to penicillin

**Usual Dosage** Oral (dosage recommendation is based on the product's erythromycin content):
Children ≥2 months: 50 mg/kg/day erythromycin and 150 mg/kg/day sulfisoxazole in divided doses every 6 hours; not to exceed 2 g erythromycin/day or 6 g sulfisoxazole/day for 10 days
Adults >45 kg: 400 mg erythromycin and 1200 mg sulfisoxazole every 6 hours

**Dosage Forms** Powder for oral suspension: Erythromycin ethylsuccinate 200 mg and sulfisoxazole acetyl 600 mg per 5 mL (100 mL, 150 mL, 200 mL) [strawberry-banana flavor]

**erythromycin base** *see* erythromycin *on page 295*

**erythromycin estolate** *see* erythromycin *on page 295*

**erythromycin ethylsuccinate** *see* erythromycin *on page 295*

**erythromycin gluceptate** *see* erythromycin *on page 295*

**erythromycin lactobionate** *see* erythromycin *on page 295*

**erythromycin stearate** *see* erythromycin *on page 295*

**erythropoiesis stimulating protein** *see* darbepoetin alfa *on page 224*

**erythropoietin** *see* epoetin alfa *on page 290*

## escitalopram (es sye TAL oh pram)

**Synonyms** escitalopram oxalate; Lu-26-054; S-citalopram

**U.S./Canadian Brand Names** Cipralex® [Can]; Lexapro™ [US]

**Therapeutic Category** Antidepressant, Selective Serotonin Reuptake Inhibitor

**Use** Treatment of major depressive disorder; generalized anxiety disorders (GAD)

**Usual Dosage** Oral: Adults: Depression, GAD: Initial: 10 mg/day; dose may be increased to 20 mg/day after at least 1 week

**Dosage Forms**
Solution, oral: 1 mg/mL (240 mL) [peppermint flavor]
Tablet: 5 mg, 10 mg, 20 mg
**Note:** Cipralex® [CAN] is available only in 10 mg and 20 mg strengths.

**escitalopram oxalate** *see* escitalopram *on this page*

**Esclim® [US]** *see* estradiol *on page 299*

**Eserine® [Can]** *see* physostigmine *on page 646*

**eserine salicylate** *see* physostigmine *on page 646*

**Esgic® [US]** *see* butalbital, acetaminophen, and caffeine *on page 124*

**Esgic-Plus™ [US]** *see* butalbital, acetaminophen, and caffeine *on page 124*

**Eskalith® [US]** *see* lithium *on page 486*

**Eskalith CR® [US]** *see* lithium *on page 486*

## esmolol (ES moe lol)

**Sound-Alike/Look-Alike Issues**
esmolol may be confused with Osmitrol®
Brevibloc® may be confused with bretylium, Brevital®, Bumex®, Buprenex®

**Synonyms** esmolol hydrochloride

**U.S./Canadian Brand Names** Brevibloc® [US/Can]

**Therapeutic Category** Antiarrhythmic Agent, Class II; Beta-Adrenergic Blocker

**Use** Treatment of supraventricular tachycardia and atrial fibrillation/flutter (primarily to control ventricular rate); treatment of tachycardia and/or hypertension (especially intraoperative or postoperative)

**Usual Dosage I.V. infusion requires an infusion pump** (must be adjusted to individual response and tolerance):

Children: A limited amount of information regarding esmolol use in pediatric patients is currently available. Some centers have utilized doses of 100-500 mcg/kg given over 1 minute for control of supraventricular tachycardias.
(Continued)

## esmolol *(Continued)*

Loading doses of 500 mcg/kg/minute over 1 minute with maximal doses of 50-250 mcg/kg/minute (mean = 173) have been used in addition to nitroprusside to treat postoperative hypertension after coarctation of aorta repair.

Adults:

Intraoperative tachycardia and/or hypertension (immediate control): Initial bolus: 80 mg (~1 mg/kg) over 30 seconds, followed by a 150 mcg/kg/minute infusion, if necessary. Adjust infusion rate as needed to maintain desired heart rate and/or blood pressure, up to 300 mcg/kg/minute.

Supraventricular tachycardia or gradual control of postoperative tachycardia/hypertension: Loading dose: 500 mcg/kg over 1 minute; follow with a 50 mcg/kg/minute infusion for 4 minutes; response to this initial infusion rate may be a rough indication of the responsiveness of the ventricular rate.

Infusion may be continued at 50 mcg/kg/minute or, if the response is inadequate, titrated upward in 50 mcg/kg/minute increments (increased no more frequently than every 4 minutes) to a maximum of 200 mcg/kg/minute.

To achieve more rapid response, following the initial loading dose and 50 mcg/kg/minute infusion, rebolus with a second 500 mcg/kg loading dose over 1 minute, and increase the maintenance infusion to 100 mcg/kg/minute for 4 minutes. If necessary, a third (and final) 500 mcg/kg loading dose may be administered, prior to increasing to an infusion rate of 150 mcg/minute. After 4 minutes of the 150 mcg/kg/minute infusion, the infusion rate may be increased to a maximum rate of 200 mcg/kg/minute (without a bolus dose).

Usual dosage range (SVT): 50-200 mcg/kg/minute with average dose of 100 mcg/kg/minute. For control of postoperative hypertension, as many as one-third of patients may require higher doses (250-300 mcg/kg/minute) to control blood pressure; the safety of doses >300 mcg/kg/minute has not been studied.

Esmolol: Hemodynamic effects of beta-blockade return to baseline within 20-30 minutes after discontinuing esmolol infusions.

Guidelines for withdrawal of therapy:

Transfer to alternative antiarrhythmic drug (propranolol, digoxin, verapamil).

Infusion should be reduced by 50% 30 minutes following the first dose of the alternative agent.

Following the second dose of the alternative drug, patient's response should be monitored and if control is adequate for the first hours, esmolol may be discontinued.

**Dosage Forms**

Infusion [premixed in sodium chloride; preservative free] (Brevibloc®): 2000 mg (100 mL) [20 mg/mL; double strength]; 2500 mg (250 mL) [10 mg/mL]

Injection, solution, as hydrochloride: 10 mg/mL (10 mL) [premixed in sodium chloride]

Brevibloc®: 10 mg/mL (10 mL) [alcohol free; premixed in sodium chloride]; 20 mg/mL (5 mL) [alcohol free; double strength; premixed in sodium chloride]; 250 mg/mL (10 mL) [contains alcohol 25%; concentrate]

**esmolol hydrochloride** *see* esmolol *on previous page*

**E-Solve-2® Topical** *(Discontinued)*

## esomeprazole *(es oh ME pray zol)*

**Synonyms** esomeprazole magnesium

**U.S./Canadian Brand Names** Nexium® [US/Can]

**Therapeutic Category** Proton Pump Inhibitor

**Use** Oral: Short-term (4-8 weeks) treatment of erosive esophagitis; maintaining symptom resolution and healing of erosive esophagitis; treatment of symptomatic gastroesophageal reflux disease (GERD); as part of a multidrug regimen for *Helicobacter pylori* eradication in patients with duodenal ulcer disease (active or history of within the past 5 years); prevention of gastric ulcers associated with continuous NSAID therapy

I.V.: Short-term (≤10 weeks) treatment of gastroesophageal reflux disease (GERD) when oral therapy is not possible or appropriate

**Usual Dosage Note:** Delayed-release capsules should be swallowed whole and taken at least 1 hour before eating

Children: Safety and efficacy have not been established in pediatric patients

Adults:

Oral:

Erosive esophagitis (healing): 20-40 mg once daily for 4-8 weeks; maintenance: 20 mg once daily

Symptomatic GERD: 20 mg once daily for 4 weeks

*Helicobacter pylori* eradication: 40 mg once daily; requires combination therapy

Prevention of NSAID-induced gastric ulcers: 20-40 mg once daily for up to 6 months

I.V.: GERD: 20 mg or 40 mg once daily for ≤10 days; change to oral therapy as soon as appropriate

**Dosage Forms**

Capsule, delayed release: 20 mg, 40 mg

Injection, powder for reconstitution: 20 mg, 40 mg [contains edetate sodium]

**esomeprazole magnesium** *see* esomeprazole *on previous page*

**Esoterica® Regular [US-OTC]** *see* hydroquinone *on page 420*

**Especol® [US-OTC]** *see* fructose, dextrose, and phosphoric acid *on page 362*

**Estalis® [Can]** *see* estradiol and norethindrone *on page 302*

**Estalis-Sequi® [Can]** *see* estradiol and norethindrone *on page 302*

**Estar® [US-OTC/Can]** *see* coal tar *on page 201*

**estazolam** (es TA zoe lam)

**Sound-Alike/Look-Alike Issues**

ProSom® may be confused with PhosLo®, Proscar®, Pro-Sof® Plus, Prozac®, Psorcon®

**U.S./Canadian Brand Names** ProSom® [US]

**Therapeutic Category** Benzodiazepine

**Controlled Substance** C-IV

**Use** Short-term management of insomnia

**Usual Dosage** Adults: Oral: 1 mg at bedtime, some patients may require 2 mg; start at doses of 0.5 mg in debilitated patients

**Dosage Forms** Tablet: 1 mg, 2 mg

**esterified estrogen and methyltestosterone** *see* estrogens (esterified) and methyltestosterone *on page 306*

**esterified estrogens** *see* estrogens (esterified) *on page 305*

**Estivin® II Ophthalmic *(Discontinued)*** *see* naphazoline *on page 561*

**Estra-L® Injection *(Discontinued)*** *see* estradiol *on this page*

**Estrace® [US/Can]** *see* estradiol *on this page*

**Estraderm® [US/Can]** *see* estradiol *on this page*

**estradiol** (es tra DYE ole)

**Sound-Alike/Look-Alike Issues**

Alora® may be confused with Aldara™

Estraderm® may be confused with Testoderm®

**Synonyms** estradiol acetate; estradiol cypionate; estradiol hemihydrate; estradiol transdermal; estradiol valerate

**U.S./Canadian Brand Names** Alora® [US]; Climara® [US/Can]; Delestrogen® [US]; Depo®-Estradiol [US/Can]; Esclim® [US]; Estrace® [US/Can]; Estraderm® [US/Can]; Estradot® [Can]; Estrasorb™ [US]; Estring® [US/Can]; EstroGel® [US/Can]; Femring™ [US]; Femtrace® [US]; Gynodiol® [US]; Menostar™ [US]; Oesclim® [Can]; Vagifem® [US/Can]; Vivelle-Dot® [US]; Vivelle® [US]

**Therapeutic Category** Estrogen Derivative

**Use** Treatment of moderate-to-severe vasomotor symptoms associated with menopause; treatment of vulvar and vaginal atrophy; hypoestrogenism (due to hypogonadism, castration, or primary ovarian failure); prostatic cancer (palliation), breast cancer (palliation), osteoporosis (prophylaxis); abnormal uterine bleeding due to hormonal imbalance; postmenopausal urogenital symptoms of the lower urinary tract (urinary urgency, dysuria)

**Usual Dosage** All dosage needs to be adjusted based upon the patient's response

Oral:

Prostate cancer (androgen-dependent, inoperable, progressing): 10 mg 3 times/day for at least 3 months

Breast cancer (inoperable, progressing in appropriately selected patients): 10 mg 3 times/day for at least 3 months

Osteoporosis prophylaxis in postmenopausal females: 0.5 mg/day in a cyclic regimen (3 weeks on and 1 week off)

Female hypoestrogenism (due to hypogonadism, castration, or primary ovarian failure): 1-2 mg/day; titrate as necessary to control symptoms using minimal effective dose for maintenance therapy

(Continued)

# estradiol (Continued)

Moderate to severe vasomotor symptoms associated with menopause: 1-2 mg/day, adjusted as necessary to limit symptoms; administration should be cyclic (3 weeks on, 1 week off). Patients should be re-evaluated at 3- to 6-month intervals to determine if treatment is still necessary.

I.M.

Prostate cancer: Valerate: ≥30 mg or more every 1-2 weeks

Moderate to severe vasomotor symptoms associated with menopause:

Cypionate: 1-5 mg every 3-4 weeks

Valerate: 10-20 mg every 4 weeks

Female hypoestrogenism (due to hypogonadism):

Cypionate: 1.5-2 mg monthly

Valerate: 10-20 mg every 4 weeks

Topical:

Emulsion: Moderate-to-severe vasomotor symptoms associated with menopause: 3.84 g applied once daily in the morning

Gel: Moderate-to-severe vasomotor symptoms associated with menopause, vulvar and vaginal atrophy: 1.25 g/day applied at the same time each day

Transdermal: Indicated dose may be used continuously in patients without an intact uterus. May be given continuously or cyclically (3 weeks on, 1 week off) in patients with an intact uterus **(exception - Menostar™, see specific dosing instructions).** When changing patients from oral to transdermal therapy, start transdermal patch 1 week after discontinuing oral hormone (may begin sooner if symptoms reappear within 1 week):

**Once-weekly patch:**

Moderate to severe vasomotor symptoms associated with menopause (Climara®): Apply 0.025 mg/day patch once weekly. Adjust dose as necessary to control symptoms. Patients should be re-evaluated at 3- to 6-month intervals to determine if treatment is still necessary.

Osteoporosis prophylaxis in postmenopausal women:

Climara®: Apply patch once weekly; minimum effective dose 0.025 mg/day; adjust response to therapy by biochemical markers and bone mineral density

Menostar™: Apply patch once weekly. In women with a uterus, also administer a progestin for 14 days every 6-12 months

**Twice-weekly patch:**

Moderate to severe vasomotor symptoms associated with menopause, vulvar/vaginal atrophy, female hypogonadism: Titrate to lowest dose possible to control symptoms, adjusting initial dose after the first month of therapy; re-evaluate therapy at 3- to 6-month intervals to taper or discontinue medication:

Alora®, Esclim®, Estraderm®, Vivelle-Dot®: Apply 0.05 mg patch twice weekly

Vivelle®: Apply 0.0375 mg patch twice weekly

Prevention of osteoporosis in postmenopausal women:

Alora®, Vivelle®, Vivelle-Dot®: Apply 0.025 mg patch twice weekly, increase dose as necessary

Estraderm®: Apply 0.05 mg patch twice weekly

**Vaginal cream:** Vulvar and vaginal atrophy: Insert 2-4 g/day intravaginally for 2 weeks, then gradually reduce to 1/2 the initial dose for 2 weeks, followed by a maintenance dose of 1 g 1-3 times/week

**Vaginal ring:**

Postmenopausal vaginal atrophy, urogenital symptoms: Estring®: 2 mg intravaginally; following insertion, ring should remain in place for 90 days

Moderate to severe vasomotor symptoms associated with menopause; vulvar/vaginal atrophy: Femring™: 0.05 mg intravaginally; following insertion, ring should remain in place for 3 months; dose may be increased to 0.1 mg if needed

**Vaginal tablets:** Atrophic vaginitis: Vagifem®: Initial: Insert 1 tablet once daily for 2 weeks; maintenance: Insert 1 tablet twice weekly; attempts to discontinue or taper medication should be made at 3- to 6-month intervals

## Dosage Forms

Cream, vaginal (Estrace®): 0.1 mg/g (12 g) [refill tube]: 0.1 mg/g (42.5 g) [tube with applicator]

Emulsion, topical, as hemihydrate (Estrasorb™): 2.5 mg/g (56s) [each pouch contains 4.35 mg estradiol hemihydrate; contents of two pouches delivers estradiol 0.05 mg/day]

Gel, topical (EstroGel®): 0.06% (93 g) [pump; delivers estradiol 0.75 mg/1.25 g; 64 doses]

Injection, oil, as cypionate (Depo®-Estradiol): 5 mg/mL (5 mL) [contains chlorobutanol; in cottonseed oil]

Injection, oil, as valerate (Delestrogen®):

10 mg/mL (5 mL) [contains chlorobutanol; in sesame oil]

20 mg/mL (5 mL) [contains benzyl alcohol; in castor oil]

40 mg/mL (5 mL) [contains benzyl alcohol; in castor oil]

Ring, vaginal, as base (Estring®): 2 mg [total estradiol 2 mg; releases 7.5 mcg/day over 90 days] (1s)

Ring, vaginal, as acetate (Femring™): 0.05 mg [total estradiol 12.4 mg; releases 0.05 mg/day over 3 months] (1s); 0.1 mg [total estradiol 24.8 mg; releases 0.1 mg/day over 3 months] (1s)

Tablet, oral, as acetate (Femtrace®): 0.45 mg, 0.9 mg, 1.8 mg

Tablet, oral, micronized: 0.5 mg, 1 mg, 2 mg

 Estrace®: 0.5 mg, 1 mg, 2 mg [2 mg tablets contain tartrazine]

 Gynodiol®: 0.5 mg, 1 mg, 1.5 mg, 2 mg

Tablet, vaginal, as base (Vagifem®): 25 mcg [contains lactose]

Transdermal system: 0.025 mg/24 hours [once-weekly patch]; 0.05 mg/24 hours (4s) [once-weekly patch]; 0.075 mg/24 hours [once-weekly patch]; 0.1 mg/24 hours (4s) [once-weekly patch]

Alora® [twice-weekly patch]:
 0.025 mg/24 hours [9 cm$^2$, total estradiol 0.77 mg] (8s)
 0.05 mg/24 hours [18 cm$^2$, total estradiol 1.5 mg] (8s, 24s)
 0.075 mg/24 hours [27 cm$^2$, total estradiol 2.3 mg] (8s)
 0.1 mg/24 hours [36 cm$^2$, total estradiol 3.1 mg] (8s)

Climara® [once-weekly patch]:
 0.025 mg/24 hours [6.5 cm$^2$, total estradiol 2.04 mg] (4s)
 0.0375 mg/24 hours [9.375 cm$^2$, total estradiol 2.85 mg] (4s)
 0.05 mg/24 hours [12.5 cm$^2$, total estradiol 3.8 mg] (4s)
 0.06 mg/24 hours [15 cm$^2$, total estradiol 4.55 mg] (4s)
 0.075 mg/24 hours [18.75 cm$^2$, total estradiol 5.7 mg] (4s)
 0.1 mg/24 hours [25 cm$^2$, total estradiol 7.6 mg] (4s)

Esclim® [twice-weekly patch]:
 0.025 mg/day [11 cm$^2$, total estradiol 5 mg] (8s)
 0.0375 mg/day [16.5 cm$^2$, total estradiol 7.5 mg] (8s)
 0.05 mg/day [22 cm$^2$, total estradiol 10 mg] (8s)
 0.075 mg/day [33 cm$^2$, total estradiol 15 mg] (8s)
 0.1 mg/day [44 cm$^2$, total estradiol 20 mg] (8s)

Estraderm® [twice-weekly patch]:
 0.05 mg/24 hours [10 cm$^2$, total estradiol 4 mg] (8s)
 0.1 mg/24 hours [20 cm$^2$, total estradiol 8 mg] (8s)

Menostar™ [once-weekly patch]: 0.014 mg/24 hours [3.25 cm$^2$, total estradiol 1 mg] (4s)

Vivelle® [twice-weekly patch]:
 0.05 mg/24 hours [14.5 cm$^2$, total estradiol 4.33 mg] (8s)
 0.1 mg/24 hours [29 cm$^2$, total estradiol 8.66 mg] (8s)

Vivelle-Dot® [twice-weekly patch]:
 0.025 mg/day [2.5 cm$^2$, total estradiol 0.39 mg] (8s)
 0.0375 mg/day [3.75 cm$^2$, total estradiol 0.585 mg] (8s)
 0.05 mg/day [5 cm$^2$, total estradiol 0.78 mg] (8s)
 0.075 mg/day [7.5 cm$^2$, total estradiol 1.17 mg] (8s)
 0.1 mg/day [10 cm$^2$, total estradiol 1.56 mg] (8s)

**estradiol acetate** *see* estradiol *on page 299*

# estradiol and levonorgestrel (es tra DYE ole & LEE voe nor jes trel)

**Synonyms** levonorgestrel and estradiol

**U.S./Canadian Brand Names** ClimaraPro™ [US]

**Therapeutic Category** Estrogen and Progestin Combination

**Use** Treatment of moderate-to-severe vasomotor symptoms associated with menopause in women with an intact uterus

**Usual Dosage** Topical: Adults: Treatment of moderate to severe vasomotor symptoms associated with menopause in females with an intact uterus:

Estradiol 0.045 mg/levonorgestrel 0.015 mg: Apply one patch weekly; patients should be re-evaluated at 3- to 6-month Intervals to determine if treatment is still necessary

**Dosage Forms** Transdermal system: Estradiol 0.045 mg/24 hours and levonorgestrel 0.015 mg/24 hours (4s) [once-weekly patch; 22 cm$^2$; contains estradiol 4.4 mg and levonorgestrel 1.39 mg]

**estradiol and NGM** *see* estradiol and norgestimate *on next page*

# estradiol and norethindrone (es tra DYE ole & nor eth IN drone)

**Synonyms** norethindrone and estradiol

**U.S./Canadian Brand Names** Activella® [US]; CombiPatch® [US]; Estalis-Sequi® [Can]; Estalis® [Can]

**Therapeutic Category** Estrogen and Progestin Combination

**Use** Women with an intact uterus:

Tablet: Treatment of moderate-to-severe vasomotor symptoms associated with menopause; treatment of vulvar and vaginal atrophy; prophylaxis for postmenopausal osteoporosis

Transdermal patch: Treatment of moderate-to-severe vasomotor symptoms associated with menopause; treatment of vulvar and vaginal atrophy; treatment of hypoestrogenism due to hypogonadism, castration, or primary ovarian failure

**Usual Dosage** Adults:

Oral (Activella®): 1 tablet daily

Transdermal patch (CombiPatch®):

Continuous combined regimen: Apply one patch twice weekly

Continuous sequential regimen: Apply estradiol-only patch for first 14 days of cycle, followed by one CombiPatch® applied twice weekly for the remaining 14 days of a 28-day cycle

Transdermal patch, combination pack (product-specific dosing for Canadian formulation):

Estalis®: Continuous combined regimen: Apply a new patch twice weekly during a 28-day cycle

Estalis-Sequi®: Continuous sequential regimen: Apply estradiol-only patch (Vivelle®) for first 14 days, followed by one Estalis® patch applied twice weekly during the last 14 days of a 28-day cycle

**Note:** In women previously receiving oral estrogens, initiate upon reappearance of menopausal symptoms following discontinuation of oral therapy.

**Dosage Forms** [CAN] = Canadian brand name

Combination pack (Estalis-Sequi® [CAN; not available in U.S.]):

140/50:

Transdermal system (Vivelle®): Estradiol 50 mcg per day (4s) [14.5 sq cm; total estradiol 4.33 mg]

Transdermal system (Estalis®): Norethindrone acetate 140 mcg and estradiol 50 mcg per day (4s) [9 sq cm; total norethindrone acetate 2.7 mg, total estradiol 0.62 mg; not available in U.S.]

250/50:

Transdermal system (Vivelle®): Estradiol 50 mcg per day (4s) [14.5 sq cm; total estradiol 4.33 mg]

Transdermal system (Estalis®): Norethindrone acetate 250 mcg and estradiol 50 mcg per day (4s) [16 sq cm; total norethindrone acetate 4.8 mg, total estradiol 0.51 mg; not available in U.S.]

Tablet (Activella®): Estradiol 1 mg and norethindrone acetate 0.5 mg (28s)

Transdermal system:

CombiPatch®:

0.05/0.14: Estradiol 0.05 mg and norethindrone acetate 0.14 mg per day (8s) [9 sq cm]

0.05/0.25: Estradiol 0.05 mg and norethindrone acetate 0.25 mg per day (8s) [16 sq cm]

Estalis® [CAN]:

140/50: Norethindrone acetate 140 mcg and estradiol 50 mcg per day (8s) [9 sq cm; total norethindrone acetate 2.7 mg, total estradiol 0.62 mg; not available in U.S.]

250/50 Norethindrone acetate 250 mcg and estradiol 50 mcg per day (8s) [16 sq cm; total norethindrone acetate 4.8 mg, total estradiol 0.51 mg; not available in U.S.]

# estradiol and norgestimate (es tra DYE ole & nor JES ti mate)

**Synonyms** estradiol and NGM; norgestimate and estradiol; ortho prefest

**U.S./Canadian Brand Names** Prefest™ [US]

**Therapeutic Category** Estrogen and Progestin Combination

**Use** Women with an intact uterus: Treatment of moderate to severe vasomotor symptoms associated with menopause; treatment of atrophic vaginitis; prevention of osteoporosis

**Usual Dosage** Oral: Adults: Females with an intact uterus:

Treatment of menopausal symptoms, atrophic vaginitis, prevention of osteoporosis: Treatment is cyclical and consists of the following: One tablet of estradiol 1 mg (pink tablet) once daily for 3 days, followed by 1 tablet of estradiol 1 mg and norgestimate 0.09 mg (white tablet) once daily for 3 days; repeat sequence continuously. **Note:** This dose may not be the lowest effective combination for these indications. In case of a missed tablet, restart therapy with next available tablet in sequence (taking only 1 tablet each day).

**Dosage Forms** Tablet: Estradiol 1 mg [15 pink tablets] and estradiol 1 mg and norgestimate 0.09 mg [15 white tablets] (supplied in blister card of 30)

**estradiol cypionate** *see* estradiol *on page 299*

## estradiol cypionate and medroxyprogesterone acetate
(es tra DYE ole sip pe OH nate & me DROKS ee proe JES te rone AS e tate)

**Synonyms** $E_2C$ and MPA; medroxyprogesterone acetate and estradiol cypionate

**U.S./Canadian Brand Names** Lunelle™ [US]

**Therapeutic Category** Contraceptive

**Use** Prevention of pregnancy

**Usual Dosage** Adults: Female: I.M.: 0.5 mL

First dose: Within first 5 days of menstrual period or within 5 days of a complete 1st trimester abortion; do not administer <4 weeks postpartum **if not breast-feeding** or <6 weeks postpartum **if breast-feeding**

Maintenance dose: Monthly, every 28-30 days following previous injection; do not exceed 33 days; pregnancy must be ruled out if >33 days have past between injections; bleeding episodes cannot be used to guide injection schedule; shortening schedule may lead to menstrual pattern changes

Switching from other forms of contraception: First injection should be given within 7 days of last active oral contraceptive pill; when switching from other methods, timing of injection should ensure continuous contraceptive coverage

**Dosage Forms** Injection, suspension: Estradiol cypionate 5 mg and medroxyprogesterone acetate 25 mg per 0.5 mL (0.5 mL)

**estradiol hemihydrate** *see* estradiol *on page 299*

**estradiol transdermal** *see* estradiol *on page 299*

**estradiol valerate** *see* estradiol *on page 299*

**Estradot**® **[Can]** *see* estradiol *on page 299*

## estramustine (es tra MUS teen)
**Sound-Alike/Look-Alike Issues**

Emcyt® may be confused with Eryc®

**Synonyms** estramustine phosphate sodium; NSC-89199

**U.S./Canadian Brand Names** Emcyt® [US/Can]

**Therapeutic Category** Antineoplastic Agent

**Use** Palliative treatment of prostatic carcinoma (progressive or metastatic)

**Usual Dosage** Refer to individual protocols.

Oral: 10-16 mg/kg/day (14 mg/kg/day is most common) or 140 mg 4 times/day (some patients have been maintained for >3 years on therapy)

**Dosage Forms** Capsule, as phosphate sodium: 140 mg

**estramustine phosphate sodium** *see* estramustine *on this page*

**Estrasorb**™ **[US]** *see* estradiol *on page 299*

**Estratab**® **[Can]** *see* estrogens (esterified) *on page 305*

**Estratab**® ***(Discontinued)*** *see* estrogens (esterified) *on page 305*

**Estratest**® **[US/Can]** *see* estrogens (esterified) and methyltestosterone *on page 306*

**Estratest**® **H.S. [US]** *see* estrogens (esterified) and methyltestosterone *on page 306*

**Estring**® **[US/Can]** *see* estradiol *on page 299*

**Estro-Cyp**® **Injection** ***(Discontinued)*** *see* estradiol *on page 299*

**EstroGel**® **[US/Can]** *see* estradiol *on page 299*

**estrogenic substances, conjugated** *see* estrogens (conjugated/equine) *on next page*

## estrogens (conjugated A/synthetic) (ES troe jenz, KON joo gate ed, aye, sin THET ik)
**Sound-Alike/Look-Alike Issues**

Cenestin® may be confused with Senexon®

**U.S./Canadian Brand Names** Cenestin® [US]

**Therapeutic Category** Estrogen Derivative

**Use** Treatment of moderate to severe vasomotor symptoms of menopause; treatment of vulvar and vaginal atrophy

**Usual Dosage** The lowest dose that will control symptoms should be used; medication should be discontinued as soon as possible.

(Continued)

303

## estrogens (conjugated A/synthetic) *(Continued)*

Oral: Adults:

Moderate to severe vasomotor symptoms: 0.45 mg/day; may be titrated up to 1.25 mg/day. Attempts to discontinue medication should be made at 3- to 6-month intervals.

Vulvar and vaginal atrophy: 0.3 mg/day

**Dosage Forms** Tablet: 0.3 mg, 0.45 mg, 0.625 mg, 0.9 mg, 1.25 mg

## estrogens (conjugated/equine) (ES troe jenz KON joo gate ed, EE kwine)

**Sound-Alike/Look-Alike Issues**

Premarin® may be confused with Primaxin®, Provera®, Remeron®

**Synonyms** C.E.S.; CEE; estrogenic substances, conjugated

**U.S./Canadian Brand Names** C.E.S.® [Can]; Cenestin [Can]; Premarin® [US/Can]

**Therapeutic Category** Estrogen Derivative

**Use** Treatment of moderate to severe vasomotor symptoms associated with menopause; treatment of vulvar and vaginal atrophy; hypoestrogenism (due to hypogonadism, castration, or primary ovarian failure); prostatic cancer (palliation); breast cancer (palliation); osteoporosis (prophylaxis, postmenopausal women at significant risk only); abnormal uterine bleeding

**Usual Dosage** Adults:

**Male:** Androgen-dependent prostate cancer: Oral: 1.25-2.5 mg 3 times/day

**Female:**

Prevention of osteoporosis in postmenopausal women: Oral: Initial: 0.3 mg/day cyclically* or daily, depending on medical assessment of patient. Dose may be adjusted based on bone mineral density and clinical response. The lowest effective dose should be used.

Moderate to severe vasomotor symptoms associated with menopause: Oral: Initial: 0.3 mg/day, cyclically* or daily, depending on medical assessment of patient. The lowest dose that will control symptoms should be used. Medication should be discontinued as soon as possible.

Vulvar and vaginal atrophy:

Oral: Initial: 0.3 mg/day; the lowest dose that will control symptoms should be used. May be given cyclically* or daily, depending on medical assessment of patient. Medication should be discontinued as soon as possible.

Vaginal cream: Intravaginal: 1/2 to 2 g/day given cyclically*

Abnormal uterine bleeding:

Acute/heavy bleeding:

I.M., I.V.: 25 mg, may repeat in 6-12 hours if needed

**Note:** Treatment should be followed by a low-dose oral contraceptive; medroxyprogesterone acetate along with or following estrogen therapy can also be given

Female hypogonadism: Oral: 0.3-0.625 mg/day given cyclically*; dose may be titrated in 6- to 12-month intervals; progestin treatment should be added to maintain bone mineral density once skeletal maturity is achieved.

Female castration, primary ovarian failure: Oral: 1.25 mg/day given cyclically*; adjust according to severity of symptoms and patient response. For maintenance, adjust to the lowest effective dose.

***Cyclic administration:** Either 3 weeks on, 1 week off **or** 25 days on, 5 days off

**Male and Female:** Breast cancer palliation, metastatic disease in selected patients: Oral: 10 mg 3 times/day for at least 3 months

**Dosage Forms**

Cream, vaginal: 0.625 mg/g (42.5 g)

Injection, powder for reconstitution: 25 mg [contains lactose 200 mg; diluent contains benzyl alcohol]

Tablet: 0.3 mg, 0.45 mg, 0.625 mg, 0.9 mg, 1.25 mg

## estrogens (conjugated/equine) and medroxyprogesterone

(ES troe jenz KON joo gate ed/EE kwine & me DROKS ee proe JES te rone)

**Sound-Alike/Look-Alike Issues**

Premphase® may be confused with Prempro™

Prempro™ may be confused with Premphase®

**Synonyms** medroxyprogesterone and estrogens (conjugated); MPA and estrogens (conjugated)

**U.S./Canadian Brand Names** Premphase® [US/Can]; Premplus® [Can]; Prempro™ [US/Can]

**Therapeutic Category** Estrogen and Progestin Combination

**Use** Women with an intact uterus: Treatment of moderate to severe vasomotor symptoms associated with menopause; treatment of atrophic vaginitis; osteoporosis (prophylaxis)

**Usual Dosage** Oral: Adults:

Treatment of moderate to severe vasomotor symptoms associated with menopause or treatment of atrophic vaginitis in females with an intact uterus. (The lowest dose that will control symptoms should be used; medication should be discontinued as soon as possible):

Premphase®: One maroon conjugated estrogen 0.625 mg tablet daily on days 1 through 14 and one light blue conjugated estrogen 0.625 mg/MPA 5 mg tablet daily on days 15 through 28; re-evaluate patients at 3- and 6-month intervals to determine if treatment is still necessary; monitor patients for signs of endometrial cancer; rule out malignancy if unexplained vaginal bleeding occurs

Prempro™: One conjugated estrogen 0.3 mg/MPA 1.5 mg tablet daily; re-evaluate at 3-and 6-month intervals to determine if therapy is still needed; dose may be increased to a maximum of one conjugated estrogen 0.625 mg/MPA 5 mg tablet daily in patients with bleeding or spotting, once malignancy has been ruled out

Osteoporosis prophylaxis in females with an intact uterus:

Premphase®: One maroon conjugated estrogen 0.625 tablet daily on days 1 through 14 and one light blue conjugated estrogen 0.625 mg/MPA 5 mg tablet daily on days 15 through 28; monitor patients for signs of endometrial cancer; rule out malignancy if unexplained vaginal bleeding occurs

Prempro™: One conjugated estrogen 0.3 mg/MPA 1.5 mg tablet daily; dose may be increased to one conjugated estrogen 0.625 mg/MPA 5 mg tablet daily; in patients with bleeding or spotting, once malignancy has been ruled out

**Dosage Forms** Tablet:

Premphase® [therapy pack contains 2 separate tablet formulations]: Conjugated estrogens 0.625 mg [14 maroon tablets] and conjugated estrogen 0.625 mg/medroxyprogesterone acetate 5 mg [14 light blue tablets] (28s)

Prempro™:

0.3/1.5: Conjugated estrogens 0.3 mg and medroxyprogesterone acetate 1.5 mg (28s)
0.45/1.5: Conjugated estrogens 0.45 mg and medroxyprogesterone acetate 1.5 mg (28s)
0.625/2.5: Conjugated estrogens 0.625 mg and medroxyprogesterone acetate 2.5 mg (28s)
0.625/5: Conjugated estrogens 0.625 mg and medroxyprogesterone acetate 5 mg (28s)

# estrogens (esterified) (ES troe jenz, es TER i fied)

**Sound-Alike/Look-Alike Issues**

Estratab® may be confused with Estratest®, Estratest® H.S.

**Synonyms** esterified estrogens

**U.S./Canadian Brand Names** Estratab® [Can]; Menest® [US/Can]

**Therapeutic Category** Estrogen Derivative

**Use** Treatment of moderate to severe vasomotor symptoms associated with menopause; treatment of vulvar and vaginal atrophy; hypoestrogenism (due to hypogonadism, castration, or primary ovarian failure); prostatic cancer (palliation); breast cancer (palliation); osteoporosis (prophylaxis, in women at significant risk only)

**Usual Dosage** Oral: Adults:

Prostate cancer (palliation): 1.25-2.5 mg 3 times/day

Female hypogonadism: 2.5-7.5 mg of estrogen daily for 20 days followed by a 10-day rest period. Administer cyclically (3 weeks on and 1 week off). If bleeding does not occur by the end of the 10-day period, repeat the same dosing schedule; the number of courses is dependent upon the responsiveness of the endometrium. If bleeding occurs before the end of the 10-day period, begin an estrogen-progestin cyclic regimen of 2.5-7.5 mg esterified estrogens daily for 20 days. During the last 5 days of estrogen therapy, give an oral progestin. If bleeding occurs before regimen is concluded, discontinue therapy and resume on the fifth day of bleeding.

Moderate to severe vasomotor symptoms associated with menopause: 1.25 mg/day administered cyclically (3 weeks on and 1 week off). If patient has not menstruated within the last 2 months or more, cyclic administration is started arbitrary. If the patient is menstruating, cyclical administration is started on day 5 of the bleeding. For short-term use only and should be discontinued as soon as possible. Re-evaluate at 3- to 6-month intervals for tapering or discontinuation of therapy.

Atopic vaginitis and kraurosis vulvae: 0.3 to ≥1.25 mg/day, depending on the tissue response of the individual patient. Administer cyclically. For short-term use only and should be discontinued as soon as possible. Re-evaluate at 3- to 6-month intervals for tapering or discontinuation of therapy.

Breast cancer (palliation): 10 mg 3 times/day for at least 3 months

Osteoporosis in postmenopausal women: Initial: 0.3 mg/day and increase to a maximum daily dose of 1.25 mg/day; initiate therapy as soon as possible after menopause; cyclically or daily, depending on medical assessment of patient. Monitor patients with an intact uterus for signs of endometrial cancer; rule out malignancy if unexplained vaginal bleeding occurs

(Continued)

## estrogens (esterified) *(Continued)*

Female castration and primary ovarian failure: 1.25 mg/day, cyclically. Adjust dosage upward or downward, according to the severity of symptoms and patient response. For maintenance, adjust dosage to lowest level that will provide effective control.

**Dosage Forms** Tablet: 0.3 mg, 0.625 mg, 1.25 mg, 2.5 mg

## estrogens (esterified) and methyltestosterone

(ES troe jenz es TER i fied & meth il tes TOS te rone)

**Sound-Alike/Look-Alike Issues**

Estratest® may be confused with Eskalith®, Estratab®, Estratest® H.S.

Estratest® H.S. may be confused with Eskalith®, Estratab®, Estratest®

**Synonyms** conjugated estrogen and methyltestosterone; esterified estrogen and methyltestosterone

**U.S./Canadian Brand Names** Estratest® H.S. [US]; Estratest® [US/Can]; Syntest D.S. [US]; Syntest H.S. [US]

**Therapeutic Category** Estrogen and Androgen Combination

**Use** Vasomotor symptoms of menopause

**Usual Dosage** Adults: Female: Oral: Lowest dose that will control symptoms should be chosen, normally given 3 weeks on and 1 week off

**Dosage Forms** Tablet:

Estratest®: Esterified estrogen 1.25 mg and methyltestosterone 2.5 mg [contains sodium benzoate]

Estratest® H.S.: Esterified estrogen 0.625 mg and methyltestosterone 1.25 mg [contains sodium benzoate]

Syntest D.S.: Esterified estrogen 1.25 mg and methyltestosterone 2.5 mg

Syntest H.S.: Esterified estrogen 0.625 mg and methyltestosterone 1.25 mg

## estropipate (ES troe pih pate)

**Synonyms** ortho est; piperazine estrone sulfate

**U.S./Canadian Brand Names** Ogen® [US/Can]; Ortho-Est® [US]

**Therapeutic Category** Estrogen Derivative

**Use** Treatment of moderate to severe vasomotor symptoms associated with menopause; treatment of vulvar and vaginal atrophy; hypoestrogenism (due to hypogonadism, castration, or primary ovarian failure); osteoporosis (prophylaxis, in women at significant risk only)

**Usual Dosage** Adults: Oral:

Moderate to severe vasomotor symptoms associated with menopause: Usual dosage range: 0.75-6 mg estropipate daily; use the lowest dose and regimen that will control symptoms, and discontinue as soon as possible. Attempt to discontinue or taper medication at 3- to 6-month intervals. If a patient with vasomotor symptoms has not menstruated within the last ≥2 months, start the cyclic administration arbitrarily. If the patient has menstruated, start cyclic administration on day 5 of bleeding.

Female hypogonadism: 1.5-9 mg estropipate daily for the first 3 weeks, followed by a rest period of 8-10 days; use the lowest dose and regimen that will control symptoms. Repeat if bleeding does not occur by the end of the rest period. The duration of therapy necessary to product the withdrawal bleeding will vary according to the responsiveness of the endometrium. If satisfactory withdrawal bleeding does not occur, give an oral progestin in addition to estrogen during the third week of the cycle.

Female castration or primary ovarian failure: 1.5-9 mg estropipate daily for the first 3 weeks of a theoretical cycle, followed by a rest period of 8-10 days; use the lowest dose and regimen that will control symptoms

Osteoporosis prophylaxis: 0.75 mg estropipate daily for 25 days of a 31-day cycle

Atrophic vaginitis or kraurosis vulvae: 0.75-6 mg estropipate daily; administer cyclically. Use the lowest dose and regimen that will control symptoms; discontinue as soon as possible.

**Dosage Forms**

Tablet: 0.625 mg [estropipate 0.75 mg]; 1.25 mg [estropipate 1.5 mg]; 2.5 mg [estropipate 3 mg]

Ogen®: 0.625 mg [estropipate 0.75 mg]; 1.25 mg [estropipate 1.5 mg]; 2.5 mg [estropipate 3 mg]

Ortho-Est®: 0.625 mg [estropipate 0.75 mg]; 1.25 mg [estropipate 1.5 mg]

**Estrostep® 21 *(Discontinued)*** see ethinyl estradiol and norethindrone on page 314

**Estrostep® Fe [US]** see ethinyl estradiol and norethindrone on page 314

## eszopiclone (es zoe PIK lone)
**U.S./Canadian Brand Names** Lunesta™ [US]
**Therapeutic Category** Hypnotic, Nonbenzodiazepine
**Controlled Substance** C-IV
**Use** Treatment of insomnia
**Usual Dosage** Oral: Adults: Insomnia: Initial: 2 mg before bedtime (maximum dose: 3 mg)
Concurrent use with strong CYP3A4 inhibitor: 1 mg before bedtime; if needed, dose may be increased to 2 mg
**Dosage Forms** Tablet [film coated]: 1 mg, 2 mg, 3 mg

**ETAF** *see* aldesleukin *on page 25*

## etanercept (et a NER sept)
**U.S./Canadian Brand Names** Enbrel® [US/Can]
**Therapeutic Category** Antirheumatic, Disease Modifying
**Use** Treatment of moderately- to severely-active rheumatoid arthritis, moderately- to severely-active polyarticular juvenile arthritis (in patients with inadequate response to at least one disease-modifying antirheumatic drug), psoriatic arthritis, active ankylosing spondylitis (AS); moderate-to-severe chronic plaque psoriasis
**Usual Dosage** SubQ:
Children 4-17 years: Juvenile rheumatoid arthritis:
 Once-weekly dosing: 0.8 mg/kg (maximum: 50 mg/dose) once weekly
 Twice-weekly dosing: 0.4 mg/kg (maximum: 25 mg/dose) twice weekly (individual doses should be separated by 72-96 hours)
Adults:
 Rheumatoid arthritis, psoriatic arthritis, ankylosing spondylitis:
 Once-weekly dosing: 50 mg once weekly
 Twice weekly dosing: 25 mg given twice weekly (individual doses should be separated by 72-96 hours)
 **Note:** If the physician determines that it is appropriate, patients may self-inject after proper training in injection technique.
 Plaque psoriasis:
 Initial: 50 mg twice weekly, 3-4 days apart (starting doses of 25 or 50 mg once weekly have also been used successfully); maintain initial dose for 3 months
 Maintenance dose: 50 mg weekly
**Dosage Forms**
Injection, powder for reconstitution: 25 mg [diluent contains benzyl alcohol; packaging may contain dry natural rubber (latex)]
Injection, solution: 50 mg/mL (0.98 mL) [prefilled syringe with 27-gauge ½ inch needle]

**ethacrynate sodium** *see* ethacrynic acid *on this page*

## ethacrynic acid (eth a KRIN ik AS id)
**Sound-Alike/Look-Alike Issues**
Edecrin® may be confused with Eulexin®, Ecotrin®
**Synonyms** ethacrynate sodium
**U.S./Canadian Brand Names** Edecrin® [US/Can]
**Therapeutic Category** Diuretic, Loop
**Use** Management of edema associated with congestive heart failure; hepatic cirrhosis or renal disease; short-term management of ascites due to malignancy, idiopathic edema, and lymphedema
**Usual Dosage** I.V. formulation should be diluted in $D_5W$ or NS (1 mg/mL) and infused over several minutes.

Children: Oral: 1 mg/kg/dose once daily; increase at intervals of 2-3 days as needed, to a maximum of 3 mg/kg/day.
Adults:
 Oral: 50-200 mg/day in 1-2 divided doses; may increase in increments of 25-50 mg at intervals of several days; doses up to 200 mg twice daily may be required with severe, refractory edema.
 I.V.: 0.5-1 mg/kg/dose (maximum: 100 mg/dose); repeat doses not routinely recommended; however, if indicated, repeat doses every 8-12 hours.
**Dosage Forms**
Injection, powder for reconstitution, as ethacrynate sodium: 50 mg
Tablet: 25 mg

## ethambutol (e THAM byoo tole)
**Sound-Alike/Look-Alike Issues**
Myambutol® may be confused with Nembutal®
**Synonyms** ethambutol hydrochloride
**U.S./Canadian Brand Names** Etibi® [Can]; Myambutol® [US]
**Therapeutic Category** Antimycobacterial Agent
**Use** Treatment of tuberculosis and other mycobacterial diseases in conjunction with other anti-tuberculosis agents
**Usual Dosage** Oral:
Treatment of tuberculosis: **Note:** Used as part of a multidrug regimen. Treatment regimens consist of an initial 2 month phase, followed by a continuation phase of 4 or 7 additional months; frequency of dosing may differ depending on phase of therapy.
Children:
Daily therapy: 15-20 mg/kg/day (maximum: 1 g/day)
Twice weekly directly observed therapy (DOT): 50 mg/kg (maximum: 4 g/dose)
Adults (suggested doses by lean body weight):
Daily therapy: 15-25 mg/kg
40-55 kg: 800 mg
56-75 kg: 1200 mg
76-90 kg: 1600 mg (maximum dose regardless of weight)
Twice weekly directly observed therapy (DOT): 50 mg/kg
40-55 kg: 2000 mg
56-75 kg: 2800 mg
76-90 kg: 4000 mg (maximum dose regardless of weight)
Three times/week DOT: 25-30 mg/kg (maximum: 2.5 g)
40-55 kg: 1200 mg
56-75 kg: 2000 mg
76-90 kg: 2400 mg (maximum dose regardless of weight)
**Disseminated *Mycobacterium avium* complex (MAC) in patients with advanced HIV infection:** 15 mg/kg ethambutol in combination with azithromycin 600 mg daily
**Dosage Forms** Tablet, as hydrochloride: 100 mg, 400 mg

**ethambutol hydrochloride** *see* ethambutol *on this page*

**Ethamolin® [US]** *see* ethanolamine oleate *on this page*

**ethanoic acid** *see* acetic acid *on page 13*

**ethanol** *see* alcohol (ethyl) *on page 24*

## ethanolamine oleate (ETH a nol a meen OH lee ate)
**Sound-Alike/Look-Alike Issues**
Ethamolin® may be confused with ethanol
**Synonyms** monoethanolamine
**U.S./Canadian Brand Names** Ethamolin® [US]
**Therapeutic Category** Sclerosing Agent
**Use Orphan drug:** Sclerosing agent used for bleeding esophageal varices
**Usual Dosage** Adults: 1.5-5 mL per varix, up to 20 mL total or 0.4 mL/kg for a 50 kg patient; doses should be decreased in patients with severe hepatic dysfunction and should receive less than recommended maximum dose
**Dosage Forms** Injection, solution: 5% [50 mg/mL] (2 mL) [contains benzyl alcohol]

## ethaverine (eth AV er een)
**Synonyms** ethaverine hydrochloride
**Therapeutic Category** Vasodilator
**Use** Peripheral and cerebral vascular insufficiency associated with arterial spasm
**Usual Dosage** Adults: Oral: 100 mg 3 times/day
**Dosage Forms** Tablet, as hydrochloride: 100 mg

**ethaverine hydrochloride** *see* ethaverine *on this page*

**ethinyl estradiol and cyproterone acetate** *see* cyproterone and ethinyl estradiol *(Canada only)*
*on page 217*

# ethinyl estradiol and desogestrel (ETH in il es tra DYE ole & des oh JES trel)

**Sound-Alike/Look-Alike Issues**
Ortho-Cept® may be confused with Ortho-Cyclen®

**Synonyms** desogestrel and ethinyl estradiol; ortho cept

**U.S./Canadian Brand Names** Apri® [US]; Cyclessa® [US]; Desogen® [US]; Kariva™ [US]; Marvelon® [Can]; Mircette® [US]; Ortho-Cept® [US/Can]; Solia™ [US]; Velivet™ [US]

**Therapeutic Category** Contraceptive, Oral

**Use** Prevention of pregnancy

**Usual Dosage** Oral: Adults: Female: Contraception:

Schedule 1 (Sunday starter): Dose begins on first Sunday after onset of menstruation; if the menstrual period starts on Sunday, take first tablet that very same day. **With a Sunday start, an additional method of contraception should be used until after the first 7 days of consecutive administration.**

For 21-tablet package: Dosage is 1 tablet daily for 21 consecutive days, followed by 7 days off of the medication; a new course begins on the 8th day after the last tablet is taken.

For 28-tablet package: Dosage is 1 tablet daily without interruption.

Schedule 2 (Day 1 starter): Dose starts on first day of menstrual cycle taking 1 tablet daily.

For 21-tablet package: Dosage is 1 tablet daily for 21 consecutive days, followed by 7 days off of the medication; a new course begins on the 8th day after the last tablet is taken.

For 28-tablet package: Dosage is 1 tablet daily without interruption.

If all doses have been taken on schedule and one menstrual period is missed, continue dosing cycle. If two consecutive menstrual periods are missed, pregnancy test is required before new dosing cycle is started.

Missed doses **monophasic formulations** (refer to package insert for complete information):

One dose missed: Take as soon as remembered or take 2 tablets next day

Two consecutive doses missed in the first 2 weeks: Take 2 tablets as soon as remembered or 2 tablets next 2 days. **An additional method of contraception should be used for 7 days after missed dose.**

Two consecutive doses missed in week 3 or three consecutive doses missed at any time:

Schedule 1 (Sunday starter): Continue to take 1 tablet daily until Sunday, then discard the rest of the pack, and a new pack is started that same day.

Schedule 2 (Day 1 starter): Current pack should be discarded, and a new pack started that same day. **An additional method of contraception should be used for 7 days after missed dose.**

Missed doses **biphasic/triphasic formulations** (refer to package insert for complete information):

One dose missed: Take as soon as remembered or take 2 tablets next day.

Two consecutive doses missed in week 1 or week 2 of the pack: Take 2 tablets as soon as remembered and 2 tablets the next day. Resume taking 1 tablet daily until the pack is empty. **An additional method of contraception should be used for 7 days after a missed dose.**

Two consecutive doses missed in week 3 of the pack; **an additional method of contraception must be used for 7 days after a missed dose**:

Schedule 1 (Sunday starter): Take 1 tablet every day until Sunday. Discard the remaining pack and start a new pack of pills on the same day.

Schedule 2 (Day 1 starter): Discard the remaining pack and start a new pack the same day.

Three or more consecutive doses missed; **an additional method of contraception must be used for 7 days after a missed dose**:

Schedule 1 (Sunday starter): Take 1 tablet every day until Sunday; on Sunday, discard the pack and start a new pack.

Schedule 2 (Day 1 starter): Discard the remaining pack and begin new pack of tablets starting on the same day.

**Dosage Forms**

Tablet, low-dose formulations:

Kariva™:

Day 1-21: Ethinyl estradiol 0.02 mg and desogestrel 0.15 mg [21 white tablets]

Day 22-23: 2 inactive light green tablets

Day 24-28: Ethinyl estradiol 0.01 mg [5 light blue tablets] (28s)

Mircette®:

Day 1-21: Ethinyl estradiol 0.02 mg and desogestrel 0.15 mg [21 white tablets]

Day 22-23: 2 inactive green tablets

Day 24-28: Ethinyl estradiol 0.01 mg [5 yellow tablets] (28s)

(Continued)

## ethinyl estradiol and desogestrel *(Continued)*

Tablet, monophasic formulations:

Apri® 28: Ethinyl estradiol 0.03 mg and desogestrel 0.15 mg [21 rose tablets and 7 white inactive tablets] (28s)

Desogen®, Reclipsen™, Solia™: Ethinyl estradiol 0.03 mg and desogestrel 0.15 mg [21 white tablets and 7 green inactive tablets] (28s)

Ortho-Cept® 28: Ethinyl estradiol 0.03 mg and desogestrel 0.15 mg [21 orange tablets and 7 green inactive tablets] (28s)

Tablet, triphasic formulations:

Cyclessa®:
Day 1-7:Ethinyl estradiol 0.025 mg and desogestrel 0.1 mg [7 light yellow tablets]
Day 8-14: Ethinyl estradiol 0.025 mg and desogestrel 0.125 mg [7 orange tablets]
Day 14-21: Ethinyl estradiol 0.025 mg and desogestrel 0.15 mg [7 red tablets]
Day 21-28: 7 green inactive tablets (28s)

Velivet™:
Day 1-7: Ethinyl estradiol 0.025 mg and desogestrel 0.1 mg [7 beige tablets]
Day 8-14: Ethinyl estradiol 0.025 mg and desogestrel 0.125 mg [7 orange tablets]
Day 14-21: Ethinyl estradiol 0.025 mg and desogestrel 0.15 mg [7 pink tablets]
Day 21-28: 7 white inactive tablets (28s)

## ethinyl estradiol and drospirenone (ETH in il es tra DYE ole & droh SPYE re none)

**Synonyms** drospirenone and ethinyl estradiol

**U.S./Canadian Brand Names** Yasmin® [US/Can]

**Therapeutic Category** Contraceptive

**Use** Prevention of pregnancy

**Usual Dosage** Oral: Adults: Female: Contraception: Dosage is 1 tablet daily for 28 consecutive days. Dose should be taken at the same time each day, either after the evening meal or at bedtime. Dosing may be started on the first day of menstrual period (Day 1 starter) or on the first Sunday after the onset of the menstrual period (Sunday starter).

Day 1 starter: Dose starts on first day of menstrual cycle taking 1 tablet daily.

Sunday starter: Dose begins on first Sunday after onset of menstruation; if the menstrual period starts on Sunday, take first tablet that very same day. **With a Sunday start, an additional method of contraception should be used until after the first 7 days of consecutive administration.**

If all doses have been taken on schedule and one menstrual period is missed, continue dosing cycle. If two consecutive menstrual periods are missed, pregnancy test is required before new dosing cycle is started.

If doses have been missed during the first 3 weeks and the menstrual period is missed, pregnancy should be ruled out prior to continuing treatment.

**Missed doses (monophasic formulations)** (refer to package insert for complete information):

One dose missed: Take as soon as remembered or take 2 tablets next day

Two consecutive doses missed in the first 2 weeks: Take 2 tablets as soon as remembered or 2 tablets next 2 days. **An additional method of contraception should be used for 7 days after missed dose.**

Two consecutive doses missed in week 3 or three consecutive doses missed at any time: **An additional method of contraception must be used for 7 days after a missed dose.**

Day 1 starter: Current pack should be discarded, and a new pack should be started that same day.

Sunday starter: Continue dose of 1 tablet daily until Sunday, then discard the rest of the pack, and a new pack should be started that same day.

Any number of doses missed in week 4: Continue taking one pill each day until pack is empty; no back-up method of contraception is needed

**Dosage Forms** Tablet: Ethinyl estradiol 0.03 mg and drospirenone 3 mg [21 yellow active tablets and 7 white inactive tablets] (28s)

## ethinyl estradiol and ethynodiol diacetate

(ETH in il es tra DYE ole & e thye noe DYE ole dye AS e tate)

**Sound-Alike/Look-Alike Issues**

Demulen® may be confused with Dalmane®, Demerol®

**Synonyms** ethynodiol diacetate and ethinyl estradiol

**U.S./Canadian Brand Names** Demulen® 30 [Can]; Demulen® [US]; Zovia™ [US]

**Therapeutic Category** Contraceptive, Oral

**Use** Prevention of pregnancy

**Usual Dosage** Oral: Adults: Female: Contraception:

Schedule 1 (Sunday starter): Dose begins on first Sunday after onset of menstruation; if the menstrual period starts on Sunday, take first tablet that very same day. **With a Sunday start, an additional method of contraception should be used until after the first 7 days of consecutive administration.**

For 21-tablet package: 1 tablet/day for 21 consecutive days, followed by 7 days off of the medication; a new course begins on the 8th day after the last tablet is taken.

For 28-tablet package: 1 tablet/day without interruption.

Schedule 2 (Day 1 starter): Dose starts on first day of menstrual cycle taking 1 tablet daily.

For 21-tablet package: 1 tablet/day for 21 consecutive days, followed by 7 days off of the medication; a new course begins on the 8th day after the last tablet is taken.

For 28-tablet package: 1 tablet/day without interruption.

If all doses have been taken on schedule and one menstrual period is missed, continue dosing cycle. If two consecutive menstrual periods are missed, pregnancy test is required before new dosing cycle is started.

Missed doses **monophasic formulations** (refer to package insert for complete information):

One dose missed: Take as soon as remembered or take 2 tablets next day

Two consecutive doses missed in the first 2 weeks: Take 2 tablets as soon as remembered or 2 tablets next 2 days. **An additional method of contraception should be used for 7 days after missed dose.**

Two consecutive doses missed in week 3 or three consecutive doses missed at any time: **An additional method of contraception should be used for 7 days after missed dose:**

Schedule 1 (Sunday starter): Continue dose of 1 tablet daily until Sunday, then discard the rest of the pack, and a new pack should be started that same day.

Schedule 2 (Day 1 starter): Current package should be discarded, and a new pack should be started that same day.

**Dosage Forms**

Tablet, monophasic formulations:

Demulen® 1/35-28: Ethinyl estradiol 0.035 mg and ethynodiol diacetate 1 mg [21 white tablets and 7 blue inactive tablets] (28s)

Kelnor™ 1/35: Ethinyl estradiol 0.035 mg and ethynodiol diacetate 1 mg [21 light yellow tablets and 7 white inactive tablets] (28s)

Zovia™ 1/35-28: Ethinyl estradiol 0.035 mg and ethynodiol diacetate 1 mg [21 light pink tablets and 7 white inactive tablets] (28s)

Zovia™ 1/50-28: Ethinyl estradiol 0.05 mg and ethynodiol diacetate 1 mg [21 pink tablets and 7 white inactive tablets] (28s)

# ethinyl estradiol and etonogestrel (ETH in il es tra DYE ole & et oh noe JES trel)

**Synonyms** etonogestrel and ethinyl estradiol

**U.S./Canadian Brand Names** NuvaRing® [US/Can]

**Therapeutic Category** Contraceptive; Estrogen and Progestin Combination

**Use** Prevention of pregnancy

**Usual Dosage** Vaginal: Adults: Female: Contraception: One ring, inserted vaginally and left in place for 3 consecutive weeks, then removed for 1 week. A new ring is inserted 7 days after the last was removed (even if bleeding is not complete) and should be inserted at approximately the same time of day the ring was removed the previous week.

**Initial treatment should begin as follows (pregnancy should always be ruled out first):**

No hormonal contraceptive use in the past month: Using the first day of menstruation as "Day 1," insert the ring on or prior to "Day 5," even if bleeding is not complete. **An additional form of contraception should be used for the following 7 days.**\*

Switching from combination oral contraceptive: Ring should be inserted within 7 days after the last active tablet was taken and no later than the first day a new cycle of tablets would begin. Additional forms of contraception are not needed.

Switching from progestin-only contraceptive: **An additional form of contraception should be used for the following 7 days with any of the following.**\*

If previously using a progestin-only mini-pill, insert the ring on any day of the month; do not skip days between the last pill and insertion of the ring.

If previously using an implant, insert the ring on the same day of implant removal.

(Continued)

# ethinyl estradiol and etonogestrel *(Continued)*

If previously using a progestin-containing IUD, insert the ring on day of IUD removal.

If previously using a progestin injection, insert the ring on the day the next injection would be given.

Following complete 1st trimester abortion: Insert ring within the first five days of abortion. If not inserted within five days, follow instructions for "No hormonal contraceptive use within the past month" and instruct patient to use a nonhormonal contraceptive in the interim.

Following delivery or 2nd trimester abortion: Insert ring 4 weeks postpartum (in women who are not breast-feeding) or following 2nd trimester abortion. **An additional form of contraception should be used for the following 7 days.***

If the ring is accidentally removed from the vagina at anytime during the 3-week period of use, it may be rinsed with cool or lukewarm water (not hot) and reinserted as soon as possible. If the ring is not reinserted within three hours, contraceptive effectiveness will be decreased. **An additional form of contraception should be used until the ring has been inserted for 7 continuous days.***

If the ring has been removed for longer than 1 week, pregnancy must be ruled out prior to restarting therapy. **An additional form of contraception should be used for the following 7 days.***

If the ring has been left in place for >3 weeks, a new ring should be inserted following a 1-week (ring-free) interval. Pregnancy must be ruled out prior to insertion and **an additional form of contraception should be used for the following 7 days.***

***Note:** Diaphragms may interfere with proper ring placement, and therefore, are not recommended for use as an additional form of contraception.

**Dosage Forms** Ring, vaginal: Ethinyl estradiol 0.015 mg/day and etonogestrel 0.12 mg/day (1s) [3-week duration]

# ethinyl estradiol and levonorgestrel (ETH in il es tra DYE ole & LEE voe nor jes trel)

**Sound-Alike/Look-Alike Issues**

Alesse® may be confused with Aleve®

Nordette® may be confused with Nicorette®

PREVEN® may be confused with Prevnar®

Tri-Levlen® may be confused with Trilafon®

Triphasil® may be confused with Tri-Norinyl®

**Synonyms** levonorgestrel and ethinyl estradiol

**U.S./Canadian Brand Names** Alesse® [US/Can]; Aviane™ [US]; Enpresse™ [US]; Lessina™ [US]; Levlen® [US]; Levlite™ [US]; Levora® [US]; Lutera™ [US]; Min-Ovral® [Can]; Nordette® [US]; Portia™ [US]; PREVEN® [US]; Seasonale® [US]; Tri-Levlen® [US]; Triphasil® [US/Can]; Triquilar® [Can]; Trivora® [US]

**Therapeutic Category** Contraceptive, Oral

**Use** Prevention of pregnancy; postcoital contraception

**Usual Dosage** Oral: Adults: Female:

Contraception, 28-day cycle:

Schedule 1 (Sunday starter): Dose begins on first Sunday after onset of menstruation; if the menstrual period starts on Sunday, take first tablet that very same day. With a Sunday start, an additional method of contraception should be used until after the first 7 days of consecutive administration:

For 21-tablet package: 1 tablet/day for 21 consecutive days, followed by 7 days off of the medication; a new course begins on the 8th day after the last tablet is taken

For 28-tablet package: 1 tablet/day without interruption

Schedule 2 (Day 1 starter): Dose starts on first day of menstrual cycle taking 1 tablet/day:

For 21-tablet package: 1 tablet/day for 21 consecutive days, followed by 7 days off of the medication; a new course begins on the 8th day after the last tablet is taken

For 28-tablet package: 1 tablet/day without interruption

If all doses have been taken on schedule and one menstrual period is missed, continue dosing cycle. If two consecutive menstrual periods are missed, pregnancy test is required before new dosing cycle is started.

Missed doses **monophasic formulations** (refer to package insert for complete information):

One dose missed: Take as soon as remembered or take 2 tablets next day

Two consecutive doses missed in the first 2 weeks: Take 2 tablets as soon as remembered or 2 tablets next 2 days. An additional method of contraception should be used for 7 days after missed dose.

Two consecutive doses missed in week 3 or three consecutive doses missed at any time: An additional method of contraception must be used for 7 days after a missed dose:

Schedule 1 (Sunday starter): Continue dose of 1 tablet daily until Sunday, then discard the rest of the pack, and a new pack should be started that same day.

Schedule 2 (Day 1 starter): Current pack should be discarded, and a new pack should be started that same day.

Missed doses **biphasic/triphasic formulations** (refer to package insert for complete information):

One dose missed: Take as soon as remembered or take 2 tablets next day.

Two consecutive doses missed in week 1 or week 2 of the pack: Take 2 tablets as soon as remembered and 2 tablets the next day. Resume taking 1 tablet daily until the pack is empty. An additional method of contraception should be used for 7 days after a missed dose.

Two consecutive doses missed in week 3 of the pack: An additional method of contraception must be used for 7 days after a missed dose.

Schedule 1 (Sunday starter): Take 1 tablet every day until Sunday. Discard the remaining pack and start a new pack of pills on the same day.

Schedule 2 (Day 1 starter): Discard the remaining pack and start a new pack the same day.

Three or more consecutive doses missed: An additional method of contraception must be used for 7 days after a missed dose.

Schedule 1 (Sunday starter): Take 1 tablet every day until Sunday; on Sunday, discard the pack and start a new pack.

Schedule 2 (Day 1 starter): Discard the remaining pack and begin new pack of tablets starting on the same day.

Contraception, 91-day cycle (Seasonale®): One active tablet/day for 84 consecutive days, followed by 1 inactive tablet/day for 7 days; if all doses have been taken on schedule and one menstrual period is missed, pregnancy should be ruled out prior to continuing therapy.

Missed doses:

One dose missed: Take as soon as remembered or take 2 tablets the next day

Two consecutive doses missed: Take 2 tablets as soon as remembered or 2 tablets the next 2 days. An additional nonhormonal method of contraception should be used for 7 consecutive days after the missed dose.

Three or more consecutive doses missed: Do not take the missed doses; continue taking 1 tablet/day until pack is complete. Bleeding may occur during the following week. An additional nonhormonal method of contraception should be used for 7 consecutive days after the missed dose.

Emergency contraception (PREVEN®): Initial: 2 tablets as soon as possible (but within 72 hours of unprotected intercourse), followed by a second dose of 2 tablets 12 hours later. Repeat dose or use antiemetic if vomiting occurs within 1 hour of dose.

## Dosage Forms

Tablet (PREVEN®): Ethinyl estradiol 0.05 mg and levonorgestrel 0.25 mg (4s) [also available as a kit containing 4 tablets and a pregnancy test]

Tablet, low-dose formulations:

Alesse® 28: Ethinyl estradiol 0.02 mg and levonorgestrel 0.1 mg [21 pink tablets and 7 light green inactive tablets] (28s)

Aviane™ 28: Ethinyl estradiol 0.02 mg and levonorgestrel 0.1 mg [21 orange tablets and 7 light green inactive tablets] (28s)

Lessina™ 28, Levlite™ 28: Ethinyl estradiol 0.02 mg and levonorgestrel 0.1 mg [21 pink tablets and 7 white inactive tablets] (28s)

Lutera™: Ethinyl estradiol 0.02 mg and levonorgestrel 0.1 mg [21 white tablets and 7 peach inactive tablets] (28s)

Tablet, monophasic formulations:

Levlen® 28: Ethinyl estradiol 0.03 mg and levonorgestrel 0.15 mg [21 light orange tablets and 7 pink inactive tablets] (28s)

Levora® 28: Ethinyl estradiol 0.03 mg and levonorgestrel 0.15 mg [21 white tablets and 7 peach inactive tablets] (28s)

Nordette® 21: Ethinyl estradiol 0.03 mg and levonorgestrel 0.15 mg [light orange tablets] (21s)

Nordette® 28: Ethinyl estradiol 0.03 mg and levonorgestrel 0.15 mg [21 light orange tablets and 7 pink inactive tablets] (28s)

Portia™ 28: Ethinyl estradiol 0.03 mg and levonorgestrel 0.15 mg [21 pink tablets and 7 white inactive tablets] (28s)

Seasonale®: Ethinyl estradiol 0.03 mg and levonorgestrel 0.15 mg [84 pink tablets and 7 white inactive tablets; extended cycle regimen]

Tablet, triphasic formulations:

Enpresse™:

Day 1-6: Ethinyl estradiol 0.03 mg and levonorgestrel 0.05 mg [6 pink tablets]

Day 7-11: Ethinyl estradiol 0.04 mg and levonorgestrel 0.075 mg [5 white tablets]

Day 12-21: Ethinyl estradiol 0.03 mg and levonorgestrel 0.125 mg [10 orange tablets]

(Continued)

## ethinyl estradiol and levonorgestrel *(Continued)*

Day 22-28: 7 light green inactive tablets (28s)

Tri-Levlen® 28, Triphasil® 28:

Day 1-6: Ethinyl estradiol 0.03 mg and levonorgestrel 0.05 mg [6 brown tablets]

Day 7-11: Ethinyl estradiol 0.04 mg and levonorgestrel 0.075 mg [5 white tablets]

Day 12-21: Ethinyl estradiol 0.03 mg and levonorgestrel 0.125 mg [10 light yellow tablets]

Day 22-28: 7 light green inactive tablets (28s)

Trivora® 28:

Day 1-6: Ethinyl estradiol 0.03 mg and levonorgestrel 0.05 mg [6 blue tablets]

Day 7-11: Ethinyl estradiol 0.04 mg and levonorgestrel 0.075 mg [5 white tablets]

Day 12-21: Ethinyl estradiol 0.03 mg and levonorgestrel 0.125 mg [10 pink tablets]

Day 22-28: 7 peach inactive tablets (28s)

**ethinyl estradiol and NGM** *see* ethinyl estradiol and norgestimate *on page 317*

## ethinyl estradiol and norelgestromin (ETH in il es tra DYE ole & nor el JES troe min)

**Synonyms** norelgestromin and ethinyl estradiol

**U.S./Canadian Brand Names** Evra™ [Can]; Ortho Evra™ [US]

**Therapeutic Category** Contraceptive; Estrogen and Progestin Combination

**Use** Prevention of pregnancy

**Usual Dosage** Topical: Adults: Female:

Contraception: Apply one patch each week for 3 weeks (21 total days); followed by one week that is patch-free. Each patch should be applied on the same day each week ("patch change day") and only one patch should be worn at a time. No more than 7 days should pass during the patch-free interval.

Schedule 1 (Sunday starter): Dose begins on first Sunday after onset of menstruation; if the menstrual period starts on Sunday, apply one patch that very same day. **With a Sunday start, an additional method of contraception (nonhormonal) should be used until after the first 7 days of consecutive administration.** Each patch change will then occur on Sunday.

Schedule 2 (Day 1 starter): Dose starts on first day of menstrual cycle, applying one patch during the first 24 hours of menstrual cycle. No back-up method of contraception is needed as long as the patch is applied on the first day of cycle. Each patch change will then occur on that same day of the week.

Additional dosing considerations:

No bleeding during patch-free week/missed menstrual period: If patch has been applied as directed, continue treatment on usual "patch change day". If used correctly, no bleeding during patch-free week does not necessarily indicate pregnancy. However, if no withdrawal bleeding occurs for 2 consecutive cycles, pregnancy should be ruled out. If patch has not been applied as directed, and one menstrual period is missed, pregnancy should be ruled out prior to continuing treatment.

If a patch becomes partially or completely detached for <24 hours: Try to reapply to same place, or replace with a new patch immediately. Do not reapply if patch is no longer sticky, if it is sticking to itself or another surface, or if it has material sticking to it.

If a patch becomes partially or completely detached for >24 hours (or time period is unknown): Apply a new patch and use this day of the week as the new "patch change day" from this point on. **An additional method of contraception (nonhormonal) should be used until after the first 7 days of consecutive administration.**

Switching from oral contraceptives: Apply first patch on the first day of withdrawal bleeding. If there is no bleeding within 5 days of taking the last active tablet, pregnancy must first be ruled out. If patch is applied later than the first day of bleeding, **an additional method of contraception (nonhormonal) should be used until after the first 7 days of consecutive administration**

Use after childbirth: Therapy should not be started <4 weeks after childbirth. Pregnancy should be ruled out prior to treatment if menstrual periods have not restarted. **An additional method of contraception (nonhormonal) should be used until after the first 7 days of consecutive administration.**

Use after abortion or miscarriage: Therapy may be started immediately if abortion/miscarriage occur within the first trimester. If therapy is not started within 5 days, follow instructions for first time use. If abortion/miscarriage occur during the second trimester, therapy should not be started for at least 4 weeks. Follow directions for use after childbirth.

**Dosage Forms** Patch, transdermal: Ethinyl estradiol 0.75 mg and norelgestromin 6 mg [releases ethinyl estradiol 20 mcg and norelgestromin 150 mcg per day] (1s, 3s)

## ethinyl estradiol and norethindrone (ETH in il es tra DYE ole & nor eth IN drone)

**Sound-Alike/Look-Alike Issues**

femhrt® may be confused with Femara®

Modicon® may be confused with Mylicon®

Norinyl® may be confused with Nardil®

Tri-Norinyl® may be confused with Triphasil®

**Synonyms** norethindrone acetate and ethinyl estradiol

**U.S./Canadian Brand Names** Aranelle™ [US]; Brevicon® 0.5/35 [Can]; Brevicon® 1/35 [Can]; Brevicon® [US]; Estrostep® Fe [US]; femhrt® [US/Can]; Junel™ Fe [US]; Junel™ [US]; Loestrin® Fe [US]; Loestrin® [US]; Loestrin™ 1.5.30 [Can]; Microgestin™ Fe [US]; Microgestin™ [US]; Minestrin™ 1/20 [Can]; Modicon® [US]; Necon® 0.5/35 [US]; Necon® 1/35 [US]; Necon® 10/11 [US]; Necon® 7/7/7 [US]; Norinyl® 1+35 [US]; Nortrel™ 7/7/7 [US]; Nortrel™ [US]; Ortho-Novum® [US]; Ortho® 0.5/35 [Can]; Ortho® 1/35 [Can]; Ortho® 7/7/7 [Can]; Ovcon® [US]; Select™ 1/35 [Can]; Synphasic® [Can]; Tri-Norinyl® [US]

**Therapeutic Category** Contraceptive, Oral

**Use** Prevention of pregnancy; treatment of acne; moderate to severe vasomotor symptoms associated with menopause; prevention of osteoporosis (in women at significant risk only)

**Usual Dosage** Oral:

Adolescents ≥15 years and Adults: Female: Acne: Estrostep®: Refer to dosing for contraception

Adults: Female:

Moderate-to-severe vasomotor symptoms associated with menopause: Initial: femhrt® 0.5/2.5: 1 tablet daily; patient should be re-evaluated at 3- to 6-month intervals to determine if treatment is still necessary; patient should be maintained at the lowest effective dose

Prevention of osteoporosis: Initial: femhrt® 0.5/2.5: 1 tablet daily; patient should be maintained on the lowest effective dose

Contraception:

Schedule 1 (Sunday starter): Dose begins on first Sunday after onset of menstruation; if the menstrual period starts on Sunday, take first tablet that very same day. With a Sunday start, an additional method of contraception should be used until after the first 7 days of consecutive administration.

For 21-tablet package: Dosage is 1 tablet daily for 21 consecutive days, followed by 7 days off of the medication; a new course begins on the 8th day after the last tablet is taken.

For 28-tablet package: Dosage is 1 tablet daily without interruption.

Schedule 2 (Day 1 starter): Dose starts on first day of menstrual cycle taking 1 tablet daily.

For 21-tablet package: Dosage is 1 tablet daily for 21 consecutive days, followed by 7 days off of the medication; a new course begins on the 8th day after the last tablet is taken.

For 28-tablet package: Dosage is 1 tablet daily without interruption.

If all doses have been taken on schedule and one menstrual period is missed, continue dosing cycle. If two consecutive menstrual periods are missed, pregnancy test is required before new dosing cycle is started.

Missed doses **monophasic formulations** (refer to package insert for complete information):

One dose missed: Take as soon as remembered or take 2 tablets next day Two consecutive doses missed in the first 2 weeks: Take 2 tablets as soon as remembered or 2 tablets next 2 days. An additional method of contraception should be used for 7 days after missed dose.

Two consecutive doses missed in week 3 or three consecutive doses missed at any time: An additional method of contraception must be used for 7 days after a missed dose.

Schedule 1 (Sunday starter): Continue dose of 1 tablet daily until Sunday, then discard the rest of the pack, and a new pack should be started that same day.

Schedule 2 (Day 1 starter): Current pack should be discarded, and a new pack should be started that same day.

Missed doses **biphasic/triphasic formulations** (refer to package insert for complete information):

One dose missed: Take as soon as remembered or take 2 tablets next day.

Two consecutive doses missed in week 1 or week 2 of the pack: Take 2 tablets as soon as remembered and 2 tablets the next day. Resume taking 1 tablet daily until the pack is empty. An additional method of contraception should be used for 7 days after a missed dose.

Two consecutive doses missed in week 3 of the pack: An additional method of contraception must be used for 7 days after a missed dose.

Schedule 1 (Sunday Starter): Take 1 tablet every day until Sunday. Discard the remaining pack and start a new pack of pills on the same day.

Schedule 2 (Day 1 starter): Discard the remaining pack and start a new pack the same day.

Three or more consecutive doses missed: An additional method of contraception must be used for 7 days after a missed dose.

Schedule 1 (Sunday Starter): Take 1 tablet every day until Sunday; on Sunday, discard the pack and start a new pack.

Schedule 2 (Day 1 Starter): Discard the remaining pack and begin new pack of tablets starting on the same day.

(Continued)

# ethinyl estradiol and norethindrone *(Continued)*

## Dosage Forms

Tablet (femhrt®):
1/5: Ethinyl estradiol 5 mcg and norethindrone acetate 1 mg [white tablets]
0.5/2.5: Ethinyl estradiol 2.5 mcg and norethindrone acetate 0.5 mg [white tablets]

Tablet, monophasic formulations:
Brevicon®: Ethinyl estradiol 0.035 mg and norethindrone 0.5 mg [21 blue tablets and 7 orange inactive tablets] (28s)
Junel™ 21 1/20: Ethinyl estradiol 0.02 mg and norethindrone acetate 1 mg [yellow tablets] (21s)
Junel™ 21 1.5/30: Ethinyl estradiol 0.03 mg and norethindrone acetate 1.5 mg [pink tablets] (21s)
Junel™ Fe 1/20: Ethinyl estradiol 0.02 mg and norethindrone acetate 1 mg [21 yellow tablets] and ferrous fumarate 75 mg [7 brown tablets] (28s)
Junel™ Fe 1.5/30: Ethinyl estradiol 0.03 mg and norethindrone acetate 1.5 mg [21 pink tablets] and ferrous fumarate 75 mg [7 brown tablets] (28s)
Loestrin® 21 1/20, Microgestin™ 1/20: Ethinyl estradiol 0.02 mg and norethindrone acetate 1 mg [white tablets] (21s)
Loestrin® 21 1.5/30, Microgestin™ 1.5/30: Ethinyl estradiol 0.03 mg and norethindrone acetate 1.5 mg [green tablets] (21s)
Loestrin® Fe 1/20, Microgestin™ Fe 1/20: Ethinyl estradiol 0.02 mg and norethindrone acetate 1 mg [21 white tablets] and ferrous fumarate 75 mg [7 brown tablets] (28s)
Loestrin® Fe 1.5/30, Microgestin™ Fe 1.5/30: Ethinyl estradiol 0.03 mg and norethindrone acetate 1.5 mg [21 green tablets] and ferrous fumarate 75 mg [7 brown tablets] (28s)
Modicon® 28: Ethinyl estradiol 0.035 mg and norethindrone 0.5 mg [21 white tablets and 7 green inactive tablets] (28s)
Necon® 0.5/35-28: Ethinyl estradiol 0.035 mg and norethindrone 0.5 mg [21 light yellow tablets and 7 white inactive tablets] (28s)
Necon® 1/35-28: Ethinyl estradiol 0.035 mg and norethindrone 1 mg [21 dark yellow tablets and 7 white inactive tablets] (28s)
Norinyl® 1+35: Ethinyl estradiol 0.035 mg and norethindrone 1 mg [21 yellow-green tablets and 7 orange inactive tablets] (28s)
Nortrel™ 0.5/35 mg:
Ethinyl estradiol 0.035 mg and norethindrone 0.5 mg [light yellow tablets] (21s)
Ethinyl estradiol 0.035 mg and norethindrone 0.5 mg [21 light yellow tablets and 7 white inactive tablets] (28s)
Nortrel™ 1/35 mg:
Ethinyl estradiol 0.035 mg and norethindrone 1 mg [yellow tablets] (21s)
Ethinyl estradiol 0.035 mg and norethindrone 1 mg [21 yellow tablets and 7 white inactive tablets] (28s)
Ortho-Novum® 1/35 28: Ethinyl estradiol 0.035 mg and norethindrone 1 mg [21 peach tablets and 7 green inactive tablets] (28s)
Ovcon® 35 21-day: Ethinyl estradiol 0.035 mg and norethindrone 0.4 mg [peach tablets] (21s)
Ovcon® 35 28-day: Ethinyl estradiol 0.035 mg and norethindrone 0.4 mg [21 peach tablets and 7 green inactive tablets] (28s)
Ovcon® 50: Ethinyl estradiol 0.05 mg and norethindrone 1 mg [21 yellow tablets and 7 green inactive tablets] (28s)

Tablet, biphasic formulations:
Necon® 10/11-28:
Day 1-10: Ethinyl estradiol 0.035 mg and norethindrone 0.5 mg [10 light yellow tablets]
Day 11-21: Ethinyl estradiol 0.035 mg and norethindrone 1 mg [11 dark yellow tablets]
Day 22-28: 7 white inactive tablets (28s)
Ortho-Novum® 10/11-28:
Day 1-10: Ethinyl estradiol 0.035 mg and norethindrone 0.5 mg [10 white tablets]
Day 11-21: Ethinyl estradiol 0.035 mg and norethindrone 1 mg [11 peach tablets]
Day 22-28: 7 green inactive tablets (28s)

Tablet, triphasic formulations:
Aranelle™:
Day 1-7: Ethinyl estradiol 0.035 mg and norethindrone 0.5 mg [7 light yellow tablets]
Day 8-16: Ethinyl estradiol 0.035 mg and norethindrone 1 mg [9 white tablets]
Day 17-21: Ethinyl estradiol 0.035 mg and norethindrone 0.5 mg [5 light yellow tablets]
Day 22-28: 7 peach inactive tablets (28s)

Estrostep® Fe:
   Day 1-5: Ethinyl estradiol 0.02 mg and norethindrone acetate 1 mg [5 white triangular tablets]
   Day 6-12: Ethinyl estradiol 0.03 mg and norethindrone acetate 1 mg [7 white square tablets]
   Day 13-21: Ethinyl estradiol 0.035 mg and norethindrone acetate 1 mg [9 white round tablets]
   Day 22-28: Ferrous fumarate 75 mg [7 brown tablets] (28s)
Leena™:
   Day 1-7: Ethinyl estradiol 0.035 mg and norethindrone 0.5 mg [7 light blue tablets]
   Day 8-16: Ethinyl estradiol 0.035 mg and norethindrone 1 mg [9 light yellow-green tablets]
   Day 17-21: Ethinyl estradiol 0.035 mg and norethindrone 0.5 mg [5 light blue tablets]
   Day 22-28: 7 orange inactive tablets (28s)
Necon® 7/7/7, Ortho-Novum® 7/7/7 28:
   Day 1-7: Ethinyl estradiol 0.035 mg and norethindrone 0.5 mg [7 white tablets]
   Day 8-14: Ethinyl estradiol 0.035 mg and norethindrone 0.75 mg [7 light peach tablets]
   Day 15-21: Ethinyl estradiol 0.035 mg and norethindrone 1 mg [7 peach tablets]
   Day 22-28: 7 green inactive tablets (28s)
Nortrel™ 7/7/7 28:
   Day 1-7: Ethinyl estradiol 0.035 mg and norethindrone 0.5 mg [7 light yellow tablets]
   Day 8-14: Ethinyl estradiol 0.035 mg and norethindrone 0.75 mg [7 blue tablets]
   Day 15-21: Ethinyl estradiol 0.035 mg and norethindrone 1 mg [7 peach tablets]
   Day 22-28: 7 white inactive tablets (28s)
Ortho-Novum® 7/7/7 28:
   Day 1-7: Ethinyl estradiol 0.035 mg and norethindrone 0.5 mg [7 white tablets]
   Day 8-14: Ethinyl estradiol 0.035 mg and norethindrone 0.75 mg [7 light peach tablets]
   Day 15-21: Ethinyl estradiol 0.035 mg and norethindrone 1 mg [7 peach tablets]
   Day 22-28: 7 green inactive tablets (28s)
Tri-Norinyl® 28:
   Day 1-7: Ethinyl estradiol 0.035 mg and norethindrone 0.5 mg [7 blue tablets]
   Day 8-16: Ethinyl estradiol 0.035 mg and norethindrone 1 mg [9 yellow-green tablets]
   Day 17-21: Ethinyl estradiol 0.035 mg and norethindrone 0.5 mg [5 blue tablets]
   Day 22-28: 7 orange inactive tablets (28s)

## ethinyl estradiol and norgestimate (ETH in il es tra DYE ole & nor JES ti mate)

**Sound-Alike/Look-Alike Issues**
   Ortho-Cyclen® may be confused with Ortho-Cept®
**Synonyms** ethinyl estradiol and NGM; norgestimate and ethinyl estradiol
**U.S./Canadian Brand Names** Cyclen® [Can]; MonoNessa™ [US]; Ortho Tri-Cyclen® Lo [US]; Ortho Tri-Cyclen® [US]; Ortho-Cyclen® [US]; Previfem™ [US]; Sprintec™ [US]; Tri-Cyclen® Lo [Can]; Tri-Cyclen® [Can]; Tri-Previfem™ [US]; Tri-Sprintec™ [US]; TriNessa™ [US]
**Therapeutic Category** Contraceptive, Oral
**Use** Prevention of pregnancy; treatment of acne
**Usual Dosage** Oral:
   Children ≥15 years and Adults: Female: Acne (Ortho Tri-Cyclen®): Refer to dosing for contraception

   Adults: Female:
   Contraception:
   Schedule 1 (Sunday starter): Dose begins on first Sunday after onset of menstruation; if the menstrual period starts on Sunday, take first tablet that very same day. **With a Sunday start, an additional method of contraception should be used until after the first 7 days of consecutive administration.**
      For 21-tablet package: Dosage is 1 tablet daily for 21 consecutive days, followed by 7 days off of the medication; a new course begins on the 8th day after the last tablet is taken.
      For 28-tablet package: Dosage is 1 tablet daily without interruption.
   Schedule 2 (Day 1 starter): Dose starts on first day of menstrual cycle taking 1 tablet daily.
      For 21-tablet package: Dosage is 1 tablet daily for 21 consecutive days, followed by 7 days off of the medication; a new course begins on the 8th day after the last tablet is taken.
      For 28-tablet package: Dosage is 1 tablet daily without interruption.
   If all doses have been taken on schedule and one menstrual period is missed, continue dosing cycle. If two consecutive menstrual periods are missed, pregnancy test is required before new dosing cycle is started.
   Missed doses **monophasic formulations** (refer to package insert for complete information):
   One dose missed: Take as soon as remembered or take 2 tablets next day
(Continued)

## ethinyl estradiol and norgestimate *(Continued)*

Two consecutive doses missed in the first 2 weeks: Take 2 tablets as soon as remembered or 2 tablets next 2 days. **An additional method of contraception should be used for 7 days after missed dose.**

Two consecutive doses missed in week 3 or three consecutive doses missed at any time: **An additional method of contraception must be used for 7 days after a missed dose:**

Schedule 1 (Sunday starter): Continue dose of 1 tablet daily until Sunday, then discard the rest of the pack, and a new pack should be started that same day.

Schedule 2 (Day 1 starter): Current pack should be discarded, and a new pack should be started that same day.

Missed doses **biphasic/triphasic formulations** (refer to package insert for complete information):

One dose missed: Take as soon as remembered or take 2 tablets next day.

Two consecutive doses missed in week 1 or week 2 of the pack: Take 2 tablets as soon as remembered and 2 tablets the next day. Resume taking 1 tablet daily until the pack is empty. **An additional method of contraception must be used for 7 days after a missed dose.**

Two consecutive doses missed in week 3 of the pack. **An additional method of contraception must be used for 7 days after a missed dose.**

Schedule 1 (Sunday starter): Take 1 tablet every day until Sunday. Discard the remaining pack and start a new pack of pills on the same day.

Schedule 2 (Day 1 starter): Discard the remaining pack and start a new pack the same day.

Three or more consecutive doses missed. **An additional method of contraception must be used for 7 days after a missed dose.**

Schedule 1 (Sunday starter): Take 1 tablet every day until Sunday; on Sunday, discard the pack and start a new pack.

Schedule 2 (Day 1 starter): Discard the remaining pack and begin new pack of tablets starting on the same day.

### Dosage Forms

Tablet, monophasic formulations:

MonoNessa™, Ortho-Cyclen®: Ethinyl estradiol 0.035 mg and norgestimate 0.25 mg [21 blue tablets and 7 green inactive tablets] (28s)

Previfem™: Ethinyl estradiol 0.035 mg and norgestimate 0.25 mg [21 blue tablets and 7 teal inactive tablets] (28s)

Sprintec™: Ethinyl estradiol 0.035 mg and norgestimate 0.25 mg [21 blue tablets and 7 white inactive tablets] (28s)

Tablet, triphasic formulations:

Ortho Tri-Cyclen®, TriNessa™:
Day 1-7: Ethinyl estradiol 0.035 mg and norgestimate 0.18 mg [7 white tablets]
Day 8-14: Ethinyl estradiol 0.035 mg and norgestimate 0.215 mg [7 light blue tablets]
Day 15-21: Ethinyl estradiol 0.035 mg and norgestimate 0.25 mg [7 blue tablets]
Day 22-28: 7 green inactive tablets (28s)

Tri-Previfem™:
Day 1-7: Ethinyl estradiol 0.035 mg and norgestimate 0.18 mg [7 white tablets]
Day 8-14: Ethinyl estradiol 0.035 mg and norgestimate 0.215 mg [7 light blue tablets]
Day 15-21: Ethinyl estradiol 0.035 mg and norgestimate 0.25 mg [7 blue tablets]
Day 22-28: 7 teal inactive tablets (28s)

Tri-Sprintec™:
Day 1-7: Ethinyl estradiol 0.035 mg and norgestimate 0.18 mg [7 gray tablets]
Day 8-14: Ethinyl estradiol 0.035 mg and norgestimate 0.215 mg [7 light blue tablets]
Day 15-21: Ethinyl estradiol 0.035 mg and norgestimate 0.25 mg [7 blue tablets]
Day 22-28: 7 white inactive tablets (28s)

Ortho Tri-Cyclen® Lo:
Day 1-7: Ethinyl estradiol 0.025 mg and norgestimate 0.18 mg [7 white tablets]
Day 8-14: Ethinyl estradiol 0.025 mg and norgestimate 0.215 mg [7 light blue tablets]
Day 15-21: Ethinyl estradiol 0.025 mg and norgestimate 0.25 mg [7 dark blue tablets]
Day 22-28: 7 green inactive tablets (28s)

## ethinyl estradiol and norgestrel (ETH in il es tra DYE ole & nor JES trel)

**Synonyms** morning after pill; norgestrel and ethinyl estradiol

**U.S./Canadian Brand Names** Cryselle™ [US]; Lo/Ovral® [US]; Low-Ogestrel® [US]; Ogestrel® [US]; Ovral® [Can]

**Therapeutic Category** Contraceptive, Oral

**Use** Prevention of pregnancy; postcoital contraceptive or "morning after" pill

**Usual Dosage** Oral: Adults: Female:

Contraception:

Schedule 1 (Sunday starter): Dose begins on first Sunday after onset of menstruation; if the menstrual period starts on Sunday, take first tablet that very same day. **With a Sunday start, an additional method of contraception should be used until after the first 7 days of consecutive administration.**

For 21-tablet package: Dosage is 1 tablet daily for 21 consecutive days, followed by 7 days off of the medication; a new course begins on the 8th day after the last tablet is taken.

For 28-tablet package: Dosage is 1 tablet daily without interruption.

Schedule 2 (Day 1 starter): Dose starts on first day of menstrual cycle taking 1 tablet daily.

For 21-tablet package: Dosage is 1 tablet daily for 21 consecutive days, followed by 7 days off of the medication; a new course begins on the 8th day after the last tablet is taken.

For 28-tablet package: Dosage is 1 tablet daily without interruption.

If all doses have been taken on schedule and one menstrual period is missed, continue dosing cycle. If two consecutive menstrual periods are missed, pregnancy test is required before new dosing cycle is started.

Missed doses **monophasic formulations** (refer to package insert for complete information):

One dose missed: Take as soon as remembered or take 2 tablets next day

Two consecutive doses missed in the first 2 weeks: Take 2 tablets as soon as remembered or 2 tablets next 2 days. **An additional method of contraception should be used for 7 days after missed dose.**

Two consecutive doses missed in week 3 or three consecutive doses missed at any time:

Schedule 1 (Sunday starter): Continue to take 1 tablet daily until Sunday, then discard the rest of the pack, and a new pack is started that same day.

Schedule 2 (Day 1 starter): Current pack should be discarded, and a new pack started that same day. **An additional method of contraception should be used for 7 days after missed dose.**

Postcoital contraception:

Ethinyl estradiol 0.03 mg and norgestrel 0.3 mg formulation: 4 tablets within 72 hours of unprotected intercourse and 4 tablets 12 hours after first dose

Ethinyl estradiol 0.05 mg and norgestrel 0.5 mg formulation: 2 tablets within 72 hours of unprotected intercourse and 2 tablets 12 hours after first dose

**Dosage Forms**

Tablet, monophasic formulations:

Cryselle™: Ethinyl estradiol 0.03 mg and norgestrel 0.3 mg [21 white tablets and 7 light green inactive tablets] (28s)

Low-Ogestrel® 28: Ethinyl estradiol 0.03 mg and norgestrel 0.3 mg [21 white tablets and 7 peach inactive tablets] (28s)

Lo/Ovral® 28: Ethinyl estradiol 0.03 mg and norgestrel 0.3 mg [21 white tablets and 7 pink inactive tablets] (28s)

Ogestrel® 28: Ethinyl estradiol 0.05 mg and norgestrel 0.5 mg [21 white tablets and 7 peach inactive tablets] (28s)

**ethiodized oil** *see* radiological/contrast media (ionic) *on page 707*

**Ethiodol® [US]** *see* radiological/contrast media (ionic) *on page 707*

**ethiofos** *see* amifostine *on page 38*

# ethionamide (e thye on AM ide)

**U.S./Canadian Brand Names** Trecator® [US/Can]

**Therapeutic Category** Antimycobacterial Agent

**Use** Treatment of tuberculosis and other mycobacterial diseases, in conjunction with other antituberculosis agents, when first-line agents have failed or resistance has been demonstrated

**Usual Dosage** Oral:

Children: 15-20 mg/kg/day in 2-3 divided doses, not to exceed 1 g/day

Adults: 15-20 mg/kg/day; initiate dose at 250 mg/day for 1-2 days, then increase to 250 mg twice daily for 1-2 days, with gradual increases to highest tolerated dose; average adult dose: 750 mg/day (maximum: 1 g/day in 3-4 divided doses)

**Dosage Forms** Tablet: 250 mg

**Ethmozine® [US/Can]** *see* moricizine *on page 549*

## ethopropazine *(Canada only)* (eth oh PROE pa zeen)

**Therapeutic Category** Anti-Parkinson Agent

**Use** Symptomatic treatment of drug induced extrapyramidal manifestations and of Parkinson disease of postencephalitic, arteriosclerotic or idiopathic etiology.

**Usual Dosage** Must be adapted to each individual. In drug induced extrapyramidal reactions 100 mg twice daily usually brings about good control of symptoms. In post encephalitic, arteriosclerotic or idiopathic parkinsonism, initiate treatment at a low dose of 50 mg 3 times a day and increase from 50 to 100 mg daily every 2 to 3 days until the optimum effect is obtained or the limit of tolerance is attained. Drowsiness and anticholinergic effects which may appear at the beginning of treatment generally subside after a few days. The normal daily dose usually ranges between 100 and 500 mg but it may reach 1 g or more per day in certain patients.

**Dosage Forms** Tablet, as hydrochloride: 50 mg

## ethosuximide (eth oh SUKS i mide)

**Sound-Alike/Look-Alike Issues**

ethosuximide may be confused with methsuximide

Zarontin® may be confused with Xalatan®, Zantac®, Zaroxolyn®

**U.S./Canadian Brand Names** Zarontin® [US/Can]

**Therapeutic Category** Anticonvulsant

**Use** Management of absence (petit mal) seizures

**Usual Dosage** Oral:

Children 3-6 years: Initial: 250 mg/day (or 15 mg/kg/day) in 2 divided doses; increase every 4-7 days; usual maintenance dose: 15-40 mg/kg/day in 2 divided doses

Children >6 years and Adults: Initial: 250 mg twice daily; increase by 250 mg as needed every 4-7 days, up to 1.5 g/day in 2 divided doses; usual maintenance dose: 20-40 mg/kg/day in 2 divided doses

**Dosage Forms**

Capsule: 250 mg

Syrup: 250 mg/5 mL (473 mL) [contains sodium benzoate; raspberry flavor]

## ethotoin (ETH oh toyn)

**Synonyms** ethylphenylhydantoin

**U.S./Canadian Brand Names** Peganone® [US/Can]

**Therapeutic Category** Hydantoin

**Use** Generalized tonic-clonic or complex-partial seizures

**Usual Dosage** Oral:

Children: 30-60 mg/kg/day or 250 mg twice daily, may be increased up to 2-3 g/day

Adults: 250 mg 4 times/day after meals, may be increased up to 3 g/day in divided doses 4 times/day

**Dosage Forms** Tablet: 250 mg

**ethoxynaphthamido penicillin sodium** *see* nafcillin *on page 557*

**Ethrane® [US]** *see* enflurane *on page 284*

**ethyl alcohol** *see* alcohol (ethyl) *on page 24*

**ethyl aminobenzoate** *see* benzocaine *on page 95*

## ethyl chloride (ETH il KLOR ide)

**Synonyms** chloroethane

**U.S./Canadian Brand Names** Gebauer's Ethyl Chloride® [US]

**Therapeutic Category** Local Anesthetic

**Use** Local anesthetic in minor operative procedures and to relieve pain caused by insect stings and burns, and irritation caused by myofascial and visceral pain syndromes

**Usual Dosage** Dosage varies with use

**Dosage Forms** Aerosol: 100% (103 mL) [available as a fine-point or medium spray]

# ethyl chloride and dichlorotetrafluoroethane
(ETH il KLOR ide & dye klor oh te tra floo or oh ETH ane)
**Synonyms** dichlorotetrafluoroethane and ethyl chloride
**U.S./Canadian Brand Names** Fluro-Ethyl® [US]
**Therapeutic Category** Local Anesthetic
**Use** Topical refrigerant anesthetic to control pain associated with minor surgical procedures, dermabrasion, injections, contusions, and minor strains
**Usual Dosage** Press gently on side of spray valve allowing the liquid to emerge as a fine mist approximately 2" to 4" from site of application
**Dosage Forms** Aerosol: Ethyl chloride 25% and dichlorotetrafluoroethane 75% (148 mL)

**ethyl esters of omega-3 fatty acids** *see* omega-3-acid ethyl esters *on page 598*

**ethylphenylhydantoin** *see* ethotoin *on previous page*

**ethynodiol diacetate and ethinyl estradiol** *see* ethinyl estradiol and ethynodiol diacetate *on page 310*

**Ethyol® [US/Can]** *see* amifostine *on page 38*

**Etibi® [Can]** *see* ethambutol *on page 308*

# etidronate disodium (e ti DROE nate dye SOW dee um)
**Sound-Alike/Look-Alike Issues**
etidronate may be confused with etidocaine, etomidate, etretinate
**Synonyms** EHDP; sodium etidronate
**U.S./Canadian Brand Names** Didronel® [US/Can]; Gen-Etidronate [Can]
**Therapeutic Category** Bisphosphonate Derivative
**Use** Symptomatic treatment of Paget disease and heterotopic ossification due to spinal cord injury or after total hip replacement, hypercalcemia associated with malignancy
**Usual Dosage** Adults: Oral formulation should be taken on an empty stomach 2 hours before any meal.
Paget's disease: Oral:
Initial: 5-10 mg/kg/day (not to exceed 6 months) or 11-20 mg/kg/day (not to exceed 3 months). Doses >10 mg/kg/day are **not** recommended.
Retreatment: Initiate only after etidronate-free period ≥90 days. Monitor patients every 3-6 months. Retreatment regimens are the same as for initial treatment.
Heterotopic ossification: Oral:
Caused by spinal cord injury: 20 mg/kg/day for 2 weeks, then 10 mg/kg/day for 10 weeks; total treatment period: 12 weeks
Complicating total hip replacement: 20 mg/kg/day for 1 month preoperatively then 20 mg/kg/day for 3 months postoperatively; total treatment period is 4 months
Hypercalcemia associated with malignancy:
I.V. (dilute dose in at least 250 mL NS): 7.5 mg/kg/day for 3 days; there should be at least 7 days between courses of treatment
Oral: Start 20 mg/kg/day on the last day of infusion and continue for 30-90 days
**Dosage Forms**
Injection, solution: 50 mg/mL (6 mL)
Tablet: 200 mg, 400 mg

# etodolac (ee toe DOE lak)
**Sound-Alike/Look-Alike Issues**
Lodine® may be confused with codeine, iodine, Iopidine®, Lopid®
**Synonyms** etodolic acid
**U.S./Canadian Brand Names** Apo-Etodolac® [Can]; Lodine® [US/Can]; Utradol™ [Can]
**Therapeutic Category** Analgesic, Nonnarcotic; Nonsteroidal Antiinflammatory Drug (NSAID)
**Use** Acute and long-term use in the management of signs and symptoms of osteoarthritis; rheumatoid arthritis and juvenile rheumatoid arthritis; management of acute pain
**Usual Dosage Note:** For chronic conditions, response is usually observed within 2 weeks.
Children 6-16 years: Oral: Juvenile rheumatoid arthritis (Lodine® XL):
20-30 kg: 400 mg once daily
31-45 kg: 600 mg once daily
46-60 kg: 800 mg once daily
>60 kg: 1000 mg once daily
(Continued)

# etodolac *(Continued)*

Adults: Oral:
Acute pain: 200-400 mg every 6-8 hours, as needed, not to exceed total daily doses of 1000 mg
Rheumatoid arthritis, osteoarthritis: 400 mg 2 times/day **or** 300 mg 2-3 times/day **or** 500 mg 2 times/day (doses >1000 mg/day have not been evaluated)
Lodine® XL: 400-1000 mg once daily
**Dosage Forms** [DSC] = Discontinued product
Capsule: 200 mg, 300 mg
Lodine®: 200 mg [DSC], 300 mg
Tablet: 400 mg, 500 mg
Tablet, extended release (Lodine® XL): 400 mg, 500 mg [DSC]

**etodolic acid** *see* etodolac *on previous page*

**EtOH** *see* alcohol (ethyl) *on page 24*

# etomidate (e TOM i date)

**Sound-Alike/Look-Alike Issues**
etomidate may be confused with etidronate
**U.S./Canadian Brand Names** Amidate® [US/Can]
**Therapeutic Category** General Anesthetic
**Use** Induction and maintenance of general anesthesia
**Usual Dosage** Children >10 years and Adults: I.V.: Initial: 0.2-0.6 mg/kg over 30-60 seconds for induction of anesthesia; maintenance: 5-20 mcg/kg/minute
**Dosage Forms** Injection, solution: 2 mg/mL (10 mL, 20 mL) [contains propylene glycol 35% v/v]

**etonogestrel and ethinyl estradiol** *see* ethinyl estradiol and etonogestrel *on page 311*

**Etopophos® [US]** *see* etoposide phosphate *on next page*

# etoposide (e toe POE side)

**Sound-Alike/Look-Alike Issues**
etoposide may be confused with teniposide
VePesid® may be confused with Versed
**Synonyms** epipodophyllotoxin; VP-16-213; VP-16
**U.S./Canadian Brand Names** Toposar® [US]; VePesid® [US/Can]
**Therapeutic Category** Antineoplastic Agent
**Use** Treatment of lymphomas, ANLL, lung, testicular, bladder, and prostate carcinoma, hepatoma, rhabdomyosarcoma, uterine carcinoma, neuroblastoma, mycosis fungoides, Kaposi sarcoma, histiocytosis, gestational trophoblastic disease, Ewing sarcoma, Wilms tumor, and brain tumors
**Usual Dosage** Refer to individual protocols.
Children: I.V.: 60-120 mg/m$^2$/day for 3-5 days every 3-6 weeks
AML:
Remission induction: 150 mg/m$^2$/day for 2-3 days for 2-3 cycles
Intensification or consolidation: 250 mg/m$^2$/day for 3 days, courses 2-5
Brain tumor: 150 mg/m$^2$/day on days 2 and 3 of treatment course
Neuroblastoma: 100 mg/m$^2$/day over 1 hour on days 1-5 of cycle; repeat cycle every 4 weeks
BMT conditioning regimen used in patients with rhabdomyosarcoma or neuroblastoma: I.V. continuous infusion: 160 mg/m$^2$/day for 4 days
Conditioning regimen for allogenic BMT: 60 mg/kg/dose as a single dose
Adults:
Small cell lung cancer:
Oral: Twice the I.V. dose rounded to the nearest 50 mg given once daily if total dose ≤400 mg or in divided doses if >400 mg
I.V.: 35 mg/m$^2$/day for 4 days or 50 mg/m$^2$/day for 5 days every 3-4 weeks total dose ≤400 mg/day or in divided doses if >400 mg/day
IVPB: 60-100 mg/m$^2$/day for 3 days (with cisplatin)
CIV: 500 mg/m$^2$ over 24 hours every 3 weeks
Testicular cancer:
IVPB: 50-100 mg/m$^2$/day for 5 days repeated every 3-4 weeks
I.V.: 100 mg/m$^2$ every other day for 3 doses repeated every 3-4 weeks
BMT/relapsed leukemia: I.V.: 2.4-3.5 g/m$^2$ or 25-70 mg/kg administered over 4-36 hours

Dosage Forms [DSC] = Discontinued product
Capsule, softgel (VePesid®): 50 mg
Injection, solution: 20 mg/mL (5 mL, 25 mL, 50 mL) [may contain benzyl alcohol or alcohol]
Toposar®: 20 mg/mL (5 mL, 10 mL, 25 mL) [contains benzyl alcohol]
VePesid®: 20 mg/mL (5 mL, 7.5 mL, 25 mL, 50 mL) [contains benzyl alcohol and alcohol 30%] [DSC]

## etoposide phosphate (e toe POE side FOS fate)
Sound-Alike/Look-Alike Issues
etoposide may be confused with teniposide
U.S./Canadian Brand Names Etopophos® [US]
Therapeutic Category Antineoplastic Agent
Use Treatment of refractory testicular tumors and small cell lung cancer
Usual Dosage Refer to individual protocols. Adults:
Small cell lung cancer: I.V. (in combination with other approved chemotherapeutic drugs): **Equivalent doses of etoposide phosphate to an etoposide dosage** range of 35 mg/m$^2$/day for 4 days to 50 mg/m$^2$/day for 5 days. Courses are repeated at 3- to 4-week intervals after adequate recovery from any toxicity.
Testicular cancer: I.V. (in combination with other approved chemotherapeutic agents): **Equivalent dose of etoposide phosphate to etoposide dosage** range of 50-100 mg/m$^2$/day on days 1-5 to 100 mg/m$^2$/day on days 1, 3, and 5. Courses are repeated at 3- to 4-week intervals after adequate recovery from any toxicity.
Dosage Forms Injection, powder for reconstitution, as base: 100 mg

**Etrafon® [Can]** see amitriptyline and perphenazine on page 43

**ETS-2% Topical (Discontinued)**

**Eudal®-SR [US]** see guaifenesin and pseudoephedrine on page 388

**Euflex® [Can]** see flutamide on page 353

**Euglucon® [Can]** see glyburide on page 378

**Eulexin® [US/Can]** see flutamide on page 353

**Eurax® [US]** see crotamiton on page 212

**Eutron® (Discontinued)**

**Evac-Q-Mag® (Discontinued)** see magnesium citrate on page 498

**Evac-U-Gen [US-OTC]** see senna on page 743

**Evalose® (Discontinued)** see lactulose on page 464

**Everone® 200 [Can]** see testosterone on page 788

**Everone® Injection (Discontinued)** see testosterone on page 788

**Evista® [US/Can]** see raloxifene on page 710

**Evoclin™ [US]** see clindamycin on page 192

**Evoxac® [US/Can]** see cevimeline on page 164

**Evra™ [Can]** see ethinyl estradiol and norelgestromin on page 314

**Exact® Acne Medication [US-OTC]** see benzoyl peroxide on page 98

**Excedrin® Extra Strength [US-OTC]** see acetaminophen, aspirin, and caffeine on page 9

**Excedrin® IB (Discontinued)** see ibuprofen on page 427

**Excedrin® Migraine [US-OTC]** see acetaminophen, aspirin, and caffeine on page 9

**Excedrin® P.M. [US-OTC]** see acetaminophen and diphenhydramine on page 7

**Exelderm® [US/Can]** see sulconazole on page 770

**Exelon® [US/Can]** see rivastigmine on page 727

## exemestane (ex e MES tane)
U.S./Canadian Brand Names Aromasin® [US/Can]
Therapeutic Category Antineoplastic Agent, Miscellaneous
Use Treatment of advanced breast cancer in postmenopausal women whose disease has progressed following tamoxifen therapy
Usual Dosage Adults: Oral: 25 mg once daily after a meal
Dosage Forms Tablet: 25 mg

## exenatide (ex EN a tide)
Synonyms AC 2993; AC002993; exendin-4 ; LY2148568
U.S./Canadian Brand Names Byetta™ [US]
Therapeutic Category Antidiabetic Agent, Incretin Mimetic
Use
   Management (adjunctive) of type 2 diabetes mellitus (noninsulin dependent, NIDDM)
Usual Dosage SubQ: Adults: Initial: 5 mcg twice daily within 60 minutes prior to a meal (morning and evening); after 1 month, may be increased to 10 mcg twice daily (based on response)
Dosage Forms Injection, solution [prefilled pen]: 250 mcg/mL (1.2 mL [provides 5 mcg/dose]; 2.4 mL [provides 10 mcg/dose])

exendin-4 *see* exenatide *on this page*

Exidine® Scrub *(Discontinued)* *see* chlorhexidine gluconate *on page 168*

Ex-lax® [US-OTC] *see* senna *on page 743*

Ex-lax® Maximum Strength [US-OTC] *see* senna *on page 743*

Exorex® [US] *see* coal tar *on page 201*

Exsel® *(Discontinued)* *see* selenium sulfide *on page 742*

Extendryl [US] *see* chlorpheniramine, phenylephrine, and methscopolamine *on page 175*

Extendryl JR [US] *see* chlorpheniramine, phenylephrine, and methscopolamine *on page 175*

Extendryl SR [US] *see* chlorpheniramine, phenylephrine, and methscopolamine *on page 175*

Extra Action Cough Syrup *(Discontinued)* *see* guaifenesin and dextromethorphan *on page 385*

EYE001 *see* pegaptanib *on page 623*

Eye-Lube-A® Solution *(Discontinued)* *see* artificial tears *on page 71*

Eye-Sed® Ophthalmic *(Discontinued)* *see* zinc sulfate *on page 861*

Eye-Sine™ [US-OTC] *see* tetrahydrozoline *on page 792*

Eyestil [Can] *see* hyaluronate and derivatives *on page 406*

Eye-Stream® [Can] *see* balanced salt solution *on page 88*

EZ-Char™ [US-OTC] *see* charcoal *on page 165*

## ezetimibe (ez ET i mibe)
Sound-Alike/Look-Alike Issues
   Zetia™ may be confused with Zestril®
U.S./Canadian Brand Names Ezetrol® [Can]; Zetia™ [US]
Therapeutic Category Antilipemic Agent, 2-Azetidinone
Use Use in combination with dietary therapy for the treatment of primary hypercholesterolemia (as monotherapy or in combination with HMG-CoA reductase inhibitors); homozygous sitosterolemia; homozygous familial hypercholesterolemia (in combination with atorvastatin or simvastatin)
Usual Dosage Oral:
   Hyperlipidemias: Children ≥10 years and Adults: 10 mg/day
   Sitosterolemia: Adults: 10 mg/day
Dosage Forms Tablet: 10 mg [capsule shaped]

## ezetimibe and simvastatin (ez ET i mibe & SIM va stat in)
U.S./Canadian Brand Names Vytorin™ [US]
Therapeutic Category Antilipemic Agent, 2-Azetidinone
Use Used in combination with dietary modification for the treatment of primary hypercholesterolemia and homozygous familial hypercholesterolemia
Usual Dosage Oral: Adults:
   Homozygous familial hypercholesterolemia: Ezetimibe 10 mg and simvastatin 40 mg once daily or ezetimibe 10 mg and simvastatin 80 mg once daily in the evening
   Hyperlipidemias: Initial: Ezetimibe 10 mg and simvastatin 20 mg once daily in the evening

Patients who require >55% reduction in LDL-C: Initial: Ezetimibe 10 mg and simvastatin 40 mg once daily

**Dosage Forms** Tablet:

10/10: Ezetimibe 10 mg and simvastatin 10 mg
10/20: Ezetimibe 10 mg and simvastatin 20 mg
10/40: Ezetimibe 10 mg and simvastatin 40 mg
10/80: Ezetimibe 10 mg and simvastatin 80 mg

**Ezetrol**® **[Can]** *see* ezetimibe *on previous page*

**Ezide**® *(Discontinued) see* hydrochlorothiazide *on page 409*

**E•R•O [US-OTC]** *see* carbamide peroxide *on page 141*

**F₃T** *see* trifluridine *on page 823*

**Fabrazyme**® **[US/Can]** *see* agalsidase beta *on page 20*

**Factive**® **[US]** *see* gemifloxacin *on page 370*

**factor VIII (human)** *see* antihemophilic factor (human) *on page 55*

**factor VIII (porcine)** *see* antihemophilic factor (porcine) *on page 56*

**factor VIII (recombinant)** *see* antihemophilic factor (recombinant) *on page 57*

# factor VIIa (recombinant) (FAK ter SEV en ree KOM be nant)

**Sound-Alike/Look-Alike Issues**

NovoSeven® may be confused with Novacet®

**Synonyms** coagulation factor VIIa; eptacog alfa (activated); rFVIIa

**U.S./Canadian Brand Names** Niastase® [Can]; NovoSeven® [US]

**Therapeutic Category** Antihemophilic Agent; Blood Product Derivative

**Use** Treatment of bleeding episodes in patients with hemophilia A or B when inhibitors to factor VIII or factor IX are present

**Usual Dosage** Children and Adults: I.V. administration only: 90 mcg/kg every 2 hours until hemostasis is achieved or until the treatment is judged ineffective. The dose and interval may be adjusted based upon the severity of bleeding and the degree of hemostasis achieved. The duration of therapy following hemostasis has not been fully established; for patients experiencing severe bleeds, dosing should be continued at 3-6 hour intervals after hemostasis has been achieved and the duration of dosing should be minimized.

In clinical trials, dosages have ranged from 35-120 mcg/kg and a decision on the final therapeutic dosages was reached within 8 hours in the majority of patients

**Dosage Forms** Injection, powder for reconstitution [preservative free]: 1.2 mg, 2.4 mg, 4.8 mg [latex free; contains sodium 0.44 mEq/mg rFVIIa, polysorbate 80]

# factor IX (FAK ter nyne)

**U.S./Canadian Brand Names** AlphaNine® SD [US]; BeneFix® [US/Can]; Immunine® VH [Can]; Mononine® [US/Can]

**Therapeutic Category** Antihemophilic Agent

**Use** Control bleeding in patients with factor IX deficiency (hemophilia B or Christmas disease)

**Usual Dosage** Dosage is expressed in units of factor IX activity and must be individualized. I.V. only:

**Formula for units required to raise blood level %:**

AlphaNine® SD, Mononine®: Children and Adults:

Number of Factor IX Units Required = body weight (in kg) x desired Factor IX level increase (% normal) x 1 unit/kg

For example, for a 100% level a patient who has an actual level of 20%: Number of Factor IX Units needed = 70 kg x 80% x 1 Unit/kg = 5600 Units

BeneFix®:

Children <15 years:

Number of Factor IX Units Required = body weight (in kg) x desired Factor IX level increase (% normal) x 1.4 units/kg

Adults:

Number of Factor IX Units Required = body weight (in kg) x desired Factor IX level increase (% normal) x 1.2 units/kg

(Continued)

# factor IX *(Continued)*

**Guidelines:** As a general rule, the level of factor IX required for treatment of different conditions is listed below:

Minor spontaneous hemorrhage, prophylaxis:
Desired levels of factor IX for hemostasis: 15% to 25%
Initial loading dose to achieve desired level: 20-30 units/kg
Frequency of dosing: Every 12-24 hours if necessary
Duration of treatment: 1-2 days

Moderate hemorrhage:
Desired levels of factor IX for hemostasis: 25% to 50%
Initial loading dose to achieve desired level: 25-50 units/kg
Frequency of dosing: Every 12-24 hours
Duration of treatment: 2-7 days

Major hemorrhage:
Desired levels of factor IX for hemostasis: >50%
Initial loading dose to achieve desired level: 30-50 units/kg
Frequency of dosing: Every 12-24 hours, depending on half-life and measured factor IX levels (after 3-5 days, maintain at least 20% activity)
Duration of treatment: 7-10 days, depending upon nature of insult

Surgery:
Desired levels of factor IX for hemostasis: 50% to 100%
Initial loading dose to achieve desired level: 50-100 units/kg
Frequency of dosing: Every 12-24 hours, depending on half-life and measured factor IX levels
Duration of treatment: 7-10 days, depending upon nature of insult

**Dosage Forms** Injection, powder for reconstitution (**Note:** Exact potency labeled on each vial):
AlphaNine® SD [human derived; solvent detergent treated; virus filtered; contains nondetectable levels of factors II, VII, X; supplied with diluent]
BeneFix® [recombinant formulation; supplied with diluent]
Mononine® [human derived; monoclonal antibody purified; contains nondetectable levels of factors II, VII, X; supplied with diluent]

# factor IX complex (human) (FAK ter nyne KOM pleks HYU man)

**Synonyms** prothrombin complex concentrate

**U.S./Canadian Brand Names** Bebulin® VH [US]; Profilnine® SD [US]; Proplex® T [US]

**Therapeutic Category** Antihemophilic Agent

**Use**
Control bleeding in patients with factor IX deficiency (hemophilia B or Christmas disease) **Note:** Factor IX concentrate containing **only** factor IX is also available and preferable for this indication.
Prevention/control of bleeding in hemophilia A patients with inhibitors to factor VIII
Prevention/control of bleeding in patients with factor VII deficiency
Emergency correction of the coagulopathy of warfarin excess in critical situations.

**Usual Dosage** Children and Adults: Dosage is expressed in units of factor IX activity and must be individualized. I.V. only:

**Formula for units required to raise blood level %:**
Total blood volume (mL blood/kg) = 70 mL/kg (adults), 80 mL/kg (children)
Plasma volume = total blood volume (mL) x [1 - Hct (in decimals)]
For example, for a 70 kg adult with a Hct = 40%: Plasma volume = [70 kg x 70 mL/kg] x [1 - 0.4] = 2940 mL
To calculate number of units needed to increase level to desired range (highly individualized and dependent on patient's condition): Number of units = desired level increase [desired level - actual level] x plasma volume (in mL)
For example, for a 100% level in the above patient who has an actual level of 20%: Number of units needed = [1 (for a 100% level) - 0.2] x 2940 mL = 2352 units

As a general rule, the level of factor IX required for treatment of different conditions is listed below:

Minor Spontaneous Hemorrhage, Prophylaxis:
Desired levels of factor IX for hemostasis: 15% to 25%
Initial loading dose to achieve desired level: <20-30 units/kg
Frequency of dosing: Once; repeated in 24 hours if necessary
Duration of treatment: Once; repeated if necessary

Major Trauma or Surgery:
Desired levels of factor IX for hemostasis: 25% to 50%

Initial loading dose to achieve desired level: <75 units/kg
Frequency of dosing: Every 18-30 hours, depending on half-life and measured factor IX levels
Duration of treatment: Up to 10 days, depending upon nature of insult

**Factor VIII inhibitor patients:** 75 units/kg/dose; may be given every 6-12 hours
**Anticoagulant overdosage:** I.V.: 15 units/kg

**Dosage Forms** Injection, powder for reconstitution (**Note:** Exact potency labeled on each vial):
Bebulin® VH [single-dose vial; vapor heated; supplied with sterile water for injection]
Profilnine® SD [single-dose vial; solvent detergent treated]
Proplex® T [single-dose vial; heat treated; supplied with sterile water for injection]

**Factrel® [US]** *see* gonadorelin *on page 381*

# famciclovir (fam SYE kloe veer)

**U.S./Canadian Brand Names** Famvir® [US/Can]
**Therapeutic Category** Antiviral Agent
**Use** Management of acute herpes zoster (shingles) and recurrent episodes of genital herpes; treatment of recurrent herpes simplex in immunocompetent patients
**Usual Dosage Initiate therapy as soon as herpes zoster is diagnosed:** Adults: Oral:
Acute herpes zoster: 500 mg every 8 hours for 7 days
Recurrent herpes simplex in immunocompetent patients: 125 mg twice daily for 5 days
Genital herpes:
First episode: 250 mg 3 times/day for 7-10 days
Recurrent episodes: 125 mg twice daily for 5 days
Prophylaxis: 250 mg twice daily
Severe (hospitalized patients): 250 mg twice daily
**Dosage Forms** Tablet: 125 mg, 250 mg, 500 mg

# famotidine (fa MOE ti deen)

**U.S./Canadian Brand Names** Apo-Famotidine® [Can]; Famotidine Omega [Can]; Fluxid™ [US]; Gen-Famotidine [Can]; Novo-Famotidine [Can]; Nu-Famotidine [Can]; Pepcid® AC [US-OTC/Can]; Pepcid® I.V. [Can]; Pepcid® [US/Can]; ratio-Famotidine [Can]; Riva-Famotidine [Can]
**Therapeutic Category** Histamine $H_2$ Antagonist
**Use** Therapy and treatment of duodenal ulcer, gastric ulcer, control gastric pH in critically-ill patients, symptomatic relief in gastritis, gastroesophageal reflux, active benign ulcer, and pathological hypersecretory conditions
OTC labeling: Relief of heartburn, acid indigestion, and sour stomach
**Usual Dosage**
Children: Treatment duration and dose should be individualized
Peptic ulcer: 1-16 years:
Oral: 0.5 mg/kg/day at bedtime or divided twice daily (maximum dose: 40 mg/day); doses of up to 1 mg/kg/day have been used in clinical studies
I.V.: 0.25 mg/kg every 12 hours (maximum dose: 40 mg/day); doses of up to 0.5 mg/kg have been used in clinical studies
GERD: Oral:
<3 months: 0.5 mg/kg once daily
3-12 months: 0.5 mg/kg twice daily
1-16 years: 1 mg/kg/day divided twice daily (maximum dose: 40 mg twice daily); doses of up to 2 mg/kg/day have been used in clinical studies

Children ≥12 years and Adults: Heartburn, indigestion, sour stomach: OTC labeling: Oral: 10-20 mg every 12 hours; dose may be taken 15-60 minutes before eating foods known to cause heartburn

Adults:
Duodenal ulcer: Oral: Acute therapy: 40 mg/day at bedtime for 4-8 weeks; maintenance therapy: 20 mg/day at bedtime
Gastric ulcer: Oral: Acute therapy: 40 mg/day at bedtime
Hypersecretory conditions: Oral: Initial: 20 mg every 6 hours, may increase in increments up to 160 mg every 6 hours
GERD: Oral: 20 mg twice daily for 6 weeks
Esophagitis and accompanying symptoms due to GERD: Oral: 20 mg or 40 mg twice daily for up to 12 weeks
Patients unable to take oral medication: I.V.: 20 mg every 12 hours
**Dosage Forms** [DSC] = Discontinued product
(Continued)

## famotidine *(Continued)*

Gelcap (Pepcid® AC): 10 mg

Infusion [premixed in NS] (Pepcid®): 20 mg (50 mL)

Injection, solution: 10 mg/mL (4 mL, 20 mL, 50 mL) [contains benzyl alcohol]

Pepcid®: 10 mg/mL (4 mL [DSC], 20 mL)

Injection, solution [preservative free] (Pepcid®): 10 mg/mL (2 mL)

Powder for oral suspension (Pepcid®): 40 mg/5 mL (50 mL) [contains sodium benzoate; cherry-banana-mint flavor]

Tablet: 10 mg [OTC], 20 mg, 40 mg

Pepcid®: 20 mg, 40 mg [film coated]

Pepcid® AC: 10 mg, 20 mg

Tablet, chewable (Pepcid® AC): 10 mg [contains phenylalanine 1.4 mg/tablet; mint flavor]

Tablet, orally-disintegrating (Fluxid™): 20 mg, 40 mg [cherry flavor]

## famotidine, calcium carbonate, and magnesium hydroxide

(fa MOE ti deen, KAL see um KAR bun ate, & mag NEE zhum hye DROKS ide)

**Synonyms** calcium carbonate, magnesium hydroxide, and famotidine; magnesium hydroxide, famotidine, and calcium carbonate

**U.S./Canadian Brand Names** Pepcid® Complete [US-OTC/Can]

**Therapeutic Category** Antacid; Histamine $H_2$ Antagonist

**Use** Relief of heartburn due to acid indigestion

**Usual Dosage** Children ≥12 years and Adults: Relief of heartburn due to acid indigestion: Oral: Pepcid® Complete: 1 tablet as needed; no more than 2 tablets in 24 hours; do **not** swallow whole, chew tablet completely before swallowing; do not use for longer than 14 days

**Dosage Forms** Tablet, chewable: Famotidine 10 mg, calcium carbonate 800 mg, and magnesium hydroxide 165 mg [berry blend and mint flavors]

**Famotidine Omega [Can]** *see* famotidine *on previous page*

**Famvir® [US/Can]** *see* famciclovir *on previous page*

**Fansidar® [US]** *see* sulfadoxine and pyrimethamine *on page 773*

**Fareston® [US/Can]** *see* toremifene *on page 812*

**Faslodex® [US]** *see* fulvestrant *on page 363*

**Fasturtec® [Can]** *see* rasburicase *on page 712*

## fat emulsion *(fat e MUL shun)*

**Synonyms** intravenous fat emulsion

**U.S./Canadian Brand Names** Intralipid® [US/Can]; Liposyn® III [US]

**Therapeutic Category** Intravenous Nutritional Therapy

**Use** Source of calories and essential fatty acids for patients requiring parenteral nutrition of extended duration

**Usual Dosage** Fat emulsion should not exceed 60% of the total daily calories

Premature Infants: Initial dose: 0.25-0.5 g/kg/day, increase by 0.25-0.5 g/kg/day to a maximum of 3 g/kg/day depending on needs/nutritional goals; limit to 1 g/kg/day if on phototherapy; maximum rate of infusion: 0.15 g/kg/hour (0.75 mL/kg/hour of 20% solution)

Infants and Children: Initial dose: 0.5-1 g/kg/day, increase by 0.5 g/kg/day to a maximum of 3 g/kg/day depending on needs/nutritional goals; maximum rate of infusion: 0.25 g/kg/hour (1.25 mL/kg/hour of 20% solution)

Adolescents and Adults: Initial dose: 1 g/kg/day, increase by 0.5-1 g/kg/day to a maximum of 2.5 g/kg/day of 10% and 3 g/kg/day of 20% depending on needs/nutritional goals; maximum rate of infusion: 0.25 g/kg/hour (1.25 mL/kg/hour of 20% solution); do not exceed 50 mL/hour (20%) or 100 mL/hour (10%)

Prevention of essential fatty acid deficiency (8% to 10% of total caloric intake): 0.5-1 g/kg/24 hours

Children: 5-10 mL/kg/day at 0.1 mL/minute then up to 100 mL/hour

Adults: 500 mL (10%) twice weekly at rate of 1 mL/minute for 30 minutes, then increase to 42 mL/hour (500 mL over 12 hours)

**Note:** At the onset of therapy, the patient should be observed for any immediate allergic reactions such as dyspnea, cyanosis, and fever; slower initial rates of infusion may be used for the first 10-15 minutes of the infusion (eg, 0.1 mL/minute of 10% or 0.05 mL/minute of 20% solution)

Dosage Forms Injection, emulsion [soybean oil]:

Intralipid®: 10% [100 mg/mL] (100 mL, 250 mL, 500 mL); 20% [200 mg/mL] (50 mL, 100 mL, 250 mL, 500 mL, 1000 mL); 30% [300 mg/mL] (500 mL)

Liposyn® III: 10% [100 mg/mL] (200 mL, 500 mL); 20% [200 mg/mL] (200 mL, 500 mL); 30% [300 mg/mL] (500 mL)

**FazaClo® [US]** *see* clozapine *on page 200*

**5-FC** *see* flucytosine *on page 342*

**FC1157a** *see* toremifene *on page 812*

**Fedahist® Expectorant *(Discontinued)*** *see* guaifenesin and pseudoephedrine *on page 388*

**Fedahist® Expectorant Pediatric *(Discontinued)*** *see* guaifenesin and pseudoephedrine *on page 388*

**Fedahist® Tablet *(Discontinued)*** *see* chlorpheniramine and pseudoephedrine *on page 172*

**Feen-A-Mint® *(Discontinued)*** *see* bisacodyl *on page 107*

**Feiba VH® [US]** *see* anti-inhibitor coagulant complex *on page 58*

**Feiba® VH Immuno [Can]** *see* anti-inhibitor coagulant complex *on page 58*

## felbamate (FEL ba mate)

**U.S./Canadian Brand Names** Felbatol® [US]

**Therapeutic Category** Anticonvulsant

**Use** Not as a first-line antiepileptic treatment; only in those patients who respond inadequately to alternative treatments and whose epilepsy is so severe that a substantial risk of aplastic anemia and/or liver failure is deemed acceptable in light of the benefits conferred by its use. Patient must be fully advised of risk and provide signed written informed consent. Felbamate can be used as either monotherapy or adjunctive therapy in the treatment of partial seizures (with and without generalization) and in adults with epilepsy.

**Orphan drug:** Adjunctive therapy in the treatment of partial and generalized seizures associated with Lennox-Gastaut syndrome in children

**Usual Dosage** Anticonvulsant:

Monotherapy: Children >14 years and Adults:

Initial: 1200 mg/day in divided doses 3 or 4 times/day; titrate previously untreated patients under close clinical supervision, increasing the dosage in 600 mg increments every 2 weeks to 2400 mg/day based on clinical response and thereafter to 3600 mg/day as clinically indicated

Conversion to monotherapy: Initiate at 1200 mg/day in divided doses 3 or 4 times/day, reduce the dosage of the concomitant anticonvulsant(s) by 20% to 33% at the initiation of felbamate therapy; at week 2, increase the felbamate dosage to 2400 mg/day while reducing the dosage of the other anticonvulsant(s) up to an additional 33% of their original dosage; at week 3, increase the felbamate dosage up to 3600 mg/day and continue to reduce the dosage of the other anticonvulsant(s) as clinically indicated

Adjunctive therapy: Children with Lennox-Gastaut and ages 2-14 years:

Week 1:

Felbamate: 15 mg/kg/day divided 3-4 times/day

Concomitant anticonvulsant(s): Reduce original dosage by 20% to 30%

Week 2:

Felbamate: 30 mg/kg/day divided 3-4 times/day

Concomitant anticonvulsant(s): Reduce original dosage up to an additional 33%

Week 3:

Felbamate: 45 mg/kg/day divided 3-4 times/day

Concomitant anticonvulsant(s): Reduce dosage as clinically indicated

Adjunctive therapy: Children >14 years and Adults:

Week 1:

Felbamate: 1200 mg/day initial dose

Concomitant anticonvulsant(s): Reduce original dosage by 20% to 33%

Week 2:

Felbamate: 2400 mg/day (therapeutic range)

Concomitant anticonvulsant(s): Reduce original dosage by up to an additional 33%

Week 3:

Felbamate: 3600 mg/day (therapeutic range)

Concomitant anticonvulsant(s): Reduce original dosage as clinically indicated

(Continued)

# felbamate *(Continued)*

### Dosage Forms
Suspension, oral: 600 mg/5 mL (240 mL, 960 mL)
Tablet: 400 mg, 600 mg

**Felbatol®** **[US]** *see* felbamate *on previous page*

**Feldene®** **[US]** *see* piroxicam *on page 650*

## felodipine *(fe LOE di peen)*
### Sound-Alike/Look-Alike Issues
Plendil® may be confused with Isordil®, pindolol, Pletal®, Prilosec®, Prinivil®
**U.S./Canadian Brand Names** Plendil® [US/Can]; Renedil® [Can]
**Therapeutic Category** Calcium Channel Blocker
**Use** Treatment of hypertension
### Usual Dosage
Adults: Oral: 2.5-10 mg once daily; usual initial dose: 5 mg; increase by 5 mg at 2-week intervals, as needed; maximum: 10 mg
Usual dose range (JNC 7) for hypertension: 2.5-20 mg once daily
**Dosage Forms** Tablet, extended release: 2.5 mg, 5 mg, 10 mg

**felodipine and enalapril** *see* enalapril and felodipine *on page 284*

**Femara®** **[US/Can]** *see* letrozole *on page 470*

**Femcet®** *(Discontinued)*

**Femguard®** *(Discontinued) see* sulfabenzamide, sulfacetamide, and sulfathiazole *on page 771*

**femhrt®** **[US/Can]** *see* ethinyl estradiol and norethindrone *on page 314*

**Femilax™** **[US-OTC]** *see* bisacodyl *on page 107*

**Femiron®** **[US-OTC]** *see* ferrous fumarate *on page 334*

**Fem-Prin®** **[US-OTC]** *see* acetaminophen, aspirin, and caffeine *on page 9*

**Femring™** **[US]** *see* estradiol *on page 299*

**Femstat® One [Can]** *see* butoconazole *on page 126*

**Femtrace®** **[US]** *see* estradiol *on page 299*

## fenofibrate *(fen oh FYE brate)*
### Synonyms procetofene; proctofene
**U.S./Canadian Brand Names** Antara™ [US]; Apo-Feno-Micro® [Can]; Apo-Fenofibrate® [Can]; Gen-Fenofibrate Micro [Can]; Lipidil EZ® [Can]; Lipidil Micro® [Can]; Lipidil Supra® [Can]; Lofibra™ [US]; Novo-Fenofibrate [Can]; Nu-Fenofibrate [Can]; PMS-Fenofibrate Micro [Can]; ratio-Fenofibrate MC [Can]; TriCor® [US/Can]; Triglide™ [US]
**Therapeutic Category** Antihyperlipidemic Agent, Miscellaneous
**Use** Adjunct to dietary therapy for the treatment of adults with elevations of serum triglyceride levels (types IV and V hyperlipidemia); adjunct to dietary therapy for the reduction of low density lipoprotein cholesterol (LDL-C), total cholesterol (total-C), triglycerides, and apolipoprotein B (apo B) in adult patients with primary hypercholesterolemia or mixed dyslipidemia (Fredrickson types IIa and IIb)
**Usual Dosage** Oral: Adults:
Hypertriglyceridemia: Initial:
Antara™: 43-130 mg/day
Lofibra™: 67 mg/day with meals, up to 200 mg/day
TriCor®: 48 mg/day, up to 145 mg/day
Previously dosed as 54 mg/day with meals (up to 160 mg/day) using the old tablet formulation
Triglide™: 50-160 mg/day
Hypercholesterolemia or mixed hyperlipidemia:
Antara™: 130 mg/day
Lofibra™: 200 mg/day with meals
TriCor®: 145 mg/day
Previously dosed as 160 mg/day with meals using the old tablet formulation
Triglide™: 160 mg/day
**Dosage Forms** [DSC] = Discontinued product

Capsule [micronized]:
Antara™: 43 mg, 87 mg, 130 mg
Lofibra™: 67 mg, 134 mg, 200 mg
Tablet :
TriCor®: 54 mg [DSC], 160 mg [DSC]
TriCor® [new formulation]: 48 mg, 145 mg
Triglide™: 50 mg, 160 mg

## fenoldopam (fe NOL doe pam)

**Synonyms** fenoldopam mesylate

**U.S./Canadian Brand Names** Corlopam® [US/Can]

**Therapeutic Category** Antihypertensive Agent

**Use** Treatment of severe hypertension (up to 48 hours in adults), including in patients with renal compromise; short-term (up to 4 hours) blood pressure reduction in pediatric patients

**Usual Dosage** I.V.: Hypertension, severe:

Children: Initial: 0.2 mcg/kg/minute; may be increased to dosages of 0.3-0.5 mcg/kg/minute every 20-30 minutes (maximum dose: 0.8 mcg/kg/minute); limited to short-term (4 hours) use

Adults: Initial: 0.1-0.3 mcg/kg/minute (lower initial doses may be associated with less reflex tachycardia); may be increased in increments of 0.05-0.1 mcg/kg/minute every 15 minutes until target blood pressure is reached; the maximal infusion rate reported in clinical studies was 1.6 mcg/kg/minute

**Dosage Forms** Injection, solution: 10 mg/mL (1 mL, 2 mL) [contains sodium metabisulfite and propylene glycol]

**fenoldopam mesylate** *see* fenoldopam *on this page*

## fenoprofen (fen oh PROE fen)

**Sound-Alike/Look-Alike Issues**

fenoprofen may be confused with flurbiprofen

Nalfon® may be confused with Naldecon®

**Synonyms** fenoprofen calcium

**U.S./Canadian Brand Names** Nalfon® [US/Can]

**Therapeutic Category** Analgesic, Nonnarcotic; Nonsteroidal Antiinflammatory Drug (NSAID)

**Use** Symptomatic treatment of acute and chronic rheumatoid arthritis and osteoarthritis; relief of mild to moderate pain

**Usual Dosage** Adults: Oral:

Rheumatoid arthritis: 300-600 mg 3-4 times/day up to 3.2 g/day

Mild to moderate pain: 200 mg every 4-6 hours as needed

**Dosage Forms**

Capsule, as calcium (Nalfon®): 200 mg, 300 mg

Tablet, as calcium: 600 mg

**fenoprofen calcium** *see* fenoprofen *on this page*

## fenoterol *(Canada only)* (fen oh TER ole)

**Synonyms** fenoterol hydrobromide

**U.S./Canadian Brand Names** Berotec® [Can]

**Therapeutic Category** Beta$_2$-Adrenergic Agonist Agent

**Use** Treatment and prevention of symptoms of reversible obstructive pulmonary disease (including asthma and acute bronchospasm), chronic bronchitis, emphysema

**Usual Dosage** Inhalation: Children ≥12 years of age and Adults:

MDI:

Acute treatment: 1 puff initially; may repeat in 5 minutes; if relief is not evident, additional doses and/or other therapy may be necessary

Intermittent/long-term treatment: 1-2 puffs 3-4 times/day (maximum of 8 puffs/24 hours)

Solution: 0.5-1 mg (up to maximum of 2.5 mg)

**Dosage Forms**

Aerosol for inhalation, as hydrobromide: MDI: 100 mcg/dose [200 doses]

Solution for inhalation, as hydrobromide: 0.625 mg/mL (2 mL); 0.25 mg/mL (2 mL)

**fenoterol hydrobromide** *see* fenoterol *(Canada only) on this page*

# fentanyl (FEN ta nil)

**Sound-Alike/Look-Alike Issues**
fentanyl may be confused with alfentanil, sufentanil

**Synonyms** fentanyl citrate

**U.S./Canadian Brand Names** Actiq® [US/Can]; Duragesic® [US/Can]; Sublimaze® [US]

**Therapeutic Category** Analgesic, Narcotic; General Anesthetic

**Controlled Substance** C-II

**Use**
Injection: Sedation, relief of pain, preoperative medication, adjunct to general or regional anesthesia

Transdermal: Management of moderate-to-severe chronic pain

Transmucosal (Actiq®): Management of breakthrough cancer pain

**Usual Dosage Note:** These are guidelines and do not represent the maximum doses that may be required in all patients. Doses should be titrated to pain relief/prevention. Monitor vital signs routinely. Single I.M. doses have a duration of 1-2 hours, single I.V. doses last 0.5-1 hour.

**Sedation for minor procedures/analgesia:**
Children 1-12 years:
Sedation for minor procedures/analgesia: I.M., I.V.: 1-2 mcg/kg/dose; may repeat at 30- to 60-minute intervals. **Note:** Children 18-36 months of age may require 2-3 mcg/kg/dose

Continuous sedation/analgesia: Initial I.V. bolus: 1-2 mcg/kg; then 1-3 mcg/kg/hour to a maximum dose of 5 mcg/kg/hour

Children >12 years and Adults: I.V.: 25-50 mcg; may repeat every 3-5 minutes to desired effect or adverse event; maximum dose of 500 mcg/4 hours; higher doses are used for major procedures

**Surgery:** Adults:
Premedication: I.M., slow I.V.: 25-100 mcg/dose 30-60 minutes prior to surgery

Adjunct to regional anesthesia: Slow I.V.: 25-100 mcg/dose over 1-2 minutes. **Note:** An I.V. should be in place with regional anesthesia so the I.M. route is rarely used but still maintained as an option in the package labeling.

Adjunct to general anesthesia: Slow I.V.:
Low dose: 0.5-2 mcg/kg/dose depending on the indication. For example, 0. 5 mcg/kg will provide analgesia or reduce the amount of propofol needed for laryngeal mask airway insertion with minimal respiratory depression. However, to blunt the hemodynamic response to intubation 2 mcg/kg is often necessary.

Moderate dose: Initial: 2-15 mcg/kg/dose; maintenance (bolus or infusion): 1-2 mcg/kg/hour. Discontinuing fentanyl infusion 30-60 minutes prior to the end of surgery will usually allow adequate ventilation upon emergence from anesthesia. For "fast-tracking" and early extubation following major surgery, total fentanyl doses are limited to 10-15 mcg/kg.

High dose: **Note:** High-dose (20-50 mcg/kg/dose) fentanyl is rarely used, but is still maintained in the package labeling.

**Acute pain management:** Adults:
Severe: I.M, I.V.: 50-100 mcg/dose every 1-2 hours as needed; patients with prior opiate exposure may tolerate higher initial doses

Patient-controlled analgesia (PCA): I.V.: Usual concentration: 10 mcg/mL
Demand dose: Usual: 10 mcg; range: 10-50 mcg
Lockout interval: 5-8 minutes

**Breakthrough cancer pain:**
Adults: Transmucosal: Actiq® dosing should be individually titrated to provide adequate analgesia with minimal side effects. For patients who are tolerant to and currently receiving opioid therapy for persistent cancer pain. Initial starting dose: 200 mcg; the second dose may be started 15 minutes after completion of the first dose. Consumption should be limited to 4 units/day or less. Patients needing more than 4 units/day should have the dose of their long-term opioid re-evaluated.

**Chronic pain management:** Children ≥2 years and Adults (opioid-tolerant patients): Transdermal:
Initial: To convert patients from oral or parenteral opioids to transdermal formulation, a 24-hour analgesic requirement should be calculated (based on prior opiate use). Using the tables, the appropriate initial dose can be determined. The initial fentanyl dosage may be approximated from the 24-hour morphine dosage and titrated to minimize adverse effects and provide analgesia. Change patch every 72 hours.

Titration: Short-acting agents may be required until analgesic efficacy is established and/or as supplements for "breakthrough" pain. The amount of supplemental doses should be closely monitored. Appropriate dosage increases may be based on daily supplemental dosage using the ratio of 45 mg/24 hours of oral morphine to a 12.5 mcg/hour increase in fentanyl dosage.

*Frequency of adjustment:* The dosage should not be titrated more frequently than every 3 days after the initial dose or every 6 days thereafter. Patients should wear a consistent fentanyl dosage through two applications (6 days) before dosage increase based on supplemental opiate dosages can be estimated.

*Frequency of application:* The majority of patients may be controlled on every 72-hour administration; however, a small number of patients require every 48-hour administration.

### Dosage Forms

Infusion [premixed in NS]: 0.05 mg (10 mL); 1 mg (100 mL); 1.25 mg (250 mL); 2 mg (100 mL); 2.5 mg (250 mL)

Injection, solution, as citrate [preservative free]: 0.05 mg/mL (2 mL, 5 mL, 10 mL, 20 mL, 30 mL, 50 mL)
Sublimaze®: 0.05 mg/mL (2 mL, 5 mL, 10 mL, 20 mL)

Lozenge, oral transmucosal, as citrate (Actiq®): 200 mcg, 400 mcg, 600 mcg, 800 mcg, 1200 mcg, 1600 mcg [mounted on a plastic radiopaque handle; raspberry flavor]

Transdermal system: 25 mcg/hour [6.25 cm$^2$] (5s); 50 mcg/hour [12.5 cm$^2$] (5s); 75 mcg/hour [18.75 cm$^2$]; 100 mcg/hour [25 cm$^2$] (5s)
Duragesic®: 12 [delivers 12.5 mcg/hour; 5 cm$^2$] (5s); 25 [delivers 25 mcg/hour; 10 cm$^2$] (5s); 50 [delivers 50 mcg/hour; 20 cm$^2$] (5s); 75 [delivers 75 mcg/hour; 30 cm$^2$]; 100 [delivers 100 mcg/hour; 40 cm$^2$] (5s)

**fentanyl citrate** *see* fentanyl *on previous page*

**Fentanyl Oralet® *(Discontinued)*** *see* fentanyl *on previous page*

**Feosol® [US-OTC]** *see* ferrous sulfate *on page 335*

**Feosol® Elixir *(Discontinued)*** *see* ferrous sulfate *on page 335*

**Feostat® [US-OTC]** *see* ferrous fumarate *on next page*

**Ferancee® *(Discontinued)*** *see* ferrous sulfate and ascorbic acid *on page 335*

**Feratab® [US-OTC]** *see* ferrous sulfate *on page 335*

**Fer-Gen-Sol [US-OTC]** *see* ferrous sulfate *on page 335*

**Fergon® [US-OTC]** *see* ferrous gluconate *on page 335*

**Feridex I.V.® [US]** *see* ferumoxides *on page 336*

**Fer-In-Sol® [US-OTC/Can]** *see* ferrous sulfate *on page 335*

**Fer-In-Sol® Syrup *(Discontinued)*** *see* ferrous sulfate *on page 335*

**Fer-Iron® [US-OTC]** *see* ferrous sulfate *on page 335*

**Fermalac [Can]** *see* Lactobacillus *on page 462*

**Ferodan™ [Can]** *see* ferrous sulfate *on page 335*

**Fero-Grad 500® [US-OTC]** *see* ferrous sulfate and ascorbic acid *on page 335*

**Fero-Gradumet® *(Discontinued)*** *see* ferrous sulfate *on page 335*

**Ferospace® *(Discontinued)*** *see* ferrous sulfate *on page 335*

**Ferralet® *(Discontinued)*** *see* ferrous gluconate *on page 335*

**Ferralyn® Lanacaps® *(Discontinued)*** *see* ferrous sulfate *on page 335*

**Ferra-TD® *(Discontinued)*** *see* ferrous sulfate *on page 335*

**Ferretts [US-OTC]** *see* ferrous fumarate *on next page*

**Ferrex 150 [US-OTC]** *see* polysaccharide-iron complex *on page 660*

**ferric (III) hexacyanoferrate (II)** *see* ferric hexacyanoferrate *on next page*

## ferric gluconate (FER ik GLOO koe nate)

### Sound-Alike/Look-Alike Issues
Ferrlecit® may be confused with Ferralet®

**Synonyms** sodium ferric gluconate

**U.S./Canadian Brand Names** Ferrlecit® [US/Can]

**Therapeutic Category** Iron Salt

**Use** Repletion of total body iron content in patients with iron-deficiency anemia who are undergoing hemodialysis in conjunction with erythropoietin therapy

(Continued)

## ferric gluconate *(Continued)*

**Usual Dosage** I.V.: Repletion of iron in hemodialysis patients:

Children ≥6 years: 1.5 mg/kg (maximum: 125 mg/dose) diluted in NS 25 mL, administered over 60 minutes at 8 sequential dialysis sessions

Adults: **Note:** A test dose of 2 mL diluted in NS 50 mL administered over 60 minutes was previously recommended (not in current manufacturer labeling).

125 mg elemental iron per 10 mL (either by I.V. infusion or slow I.V. injection). Most patients will require a cumulative dose of 1 g elemental iron over approximately 8 sequential dialysis treatments to achieve a favorable response.

**Dosage Forms** Injection, solution: Elemental iron 12.5 mg/mL (5 mL) [contains benzyl alcohol and sucrose 20%]

## ferric hexacyanoferrate (FER ik hex a SYE an oh fer ate)

**Synonyms** ferric (III) hexacyanoferrate (II); insoluble prussian blue; prussian blue

**U.S./Canadian Brand Names** Radiogardase™ [US]

**Therapeutic Category** Antidote

**Use** Treatment of known or suspected internal contamination with radioactive cesium and/or radioactive or nonradioactive thallium

**Usual Dosage** Oral: Internal contamination with radioactive cesium and/or radioactive or nonradioactive thallium:

Children 2-12 years: 1 g 3 times/day; treatment should begin as soon as possible following exposure, but is also effective if therapy is delayed

Children >12 years and Adults: 3 g 3 times/day; treatment should begin as soon as possible following exposure, but is also effective if therapy is delayed

**Note:** Cesium exposure: Once internal radioactivity is substantially decreased, dosage may be reduced to 1-2 g 3 times/day to improve gastrointestinal tolerance

**Dosage Forms** Capsule: 0.5 g

**Ferrlecit®** **[US/Can]** *see* ferric gluconate *on previous page*

**Ferro-Sequels®** **[US-OTC]** *see* ferrous fumarate *on this page*

## ferrous fumarate (FER us FYOO ma rate)

**Sound-Alike/Look-Alike Issues**

Feostat® may be confused with Feosol®

**Synonyms** iron fumarate

**U.S./Canadian Brand Names** Femiron® [US-OTC]; Feostat® [US-OTC]; Ferretts [US-OTC]; Ferro-Sequels® [US-OTC]; Hemocyte® [US-OTC]; Ircon® [US-OTC]; Nephro-Fer® [US-OTC]; Palafer® [Can]

**Therapeutic Category** Electrolyte Supplement, Oral

**Use** Prevention and treatment of iron-deficiency anemias

**Usual Dosage** Oral **(dose expressed in terms of elemental iron):**

Children:

Severe iron-deficiency anemia: 4-6 mg Fe/kg/day in 3 divided doses

Mild to moderate iron deficiency anemia: 3 mg Fe/kg/day in 1-2 divided doses

Prophylaxis: 1-2 mg Fe/kg/day

Adults:

Iron deficiency: 60-100 mg twice daily up to 60 mg 2 times/day

Prophylaxis: 60-100 mg/day

To avoid GI upset, start with a single daily dose and increase by 1 tablet/day each week or as tolerated until desired daily dose is achieved

**Dosage Forms**

Tablet: 324 mg [elemental iron 106 mg]

Femiron®: 63 mg [elemental iron 20 mg]

Ferretts: 325 mg [elemental iron 106 mg]

Hemocyte®: 324 mg [elemental iron 106 mg]

Ircon®: 200 mg [elemental iron 66 mg]

Nephro-Fer®: 350 mg [elemental iron 115 mg; contains tartrazine]

Tablet, chewable (Feostat®): 100 mg [elemental iron 33 mg; chocolate flavor]

Tablet, timed release (Ferro-Sequels®): 150 mg [elemental iron 50 mg; contains docusate sodium and sodium benzoate]

## ferrous gluconate (FER us GLOO koe nate)

**Synonyms** iron gluconate

**U.S./Canadian Brand Names** Apo-Ferrous Gluconate® [Can]; Fergon® [US-OTC]; Novo-Ferrogluc [Can]

**Therapeutic Category** Electrolyte Supplement, Oral

**Use** Prevention and treatment of iron-deficiency anemias

**Usual Dosage** Oral **(dose expressed in terms of elemental iron):**
Children:
Severe iron-deficiency anemia: 4-6 mg Fe/kg/day in 3 divided doses
Mild to moderate iron deficiency anemia: 3 mg Fe/kg/day in 1-2 divided doses
Prophylaxis: 1-2 mg Fe/kg/day
Adults:
Iron deficiency: 60 mg twice daily up to 60 mg 4 times/day
Prophylaxis: 60 mg/day

**Dosage Forms**
Tablet: 246 mg [elemental iron 28 mg]; 300 mg [elemental iron 34 mg]; 325 mg [elemental iron 36 mg]
Fergon®: 240 mg [elemental iron 27 mg]

## ferrous sulfate (FER us SUL fate)

**Sound-Alike/Look-Alike Issues**
Feosol® may be confused with Feostat®, Fer-In-Sol®
Fer-In-Sol® may be confused with Feosol®
Slow FE® may be confused with Slow-K®

**Synonyms** $FeSO_4$; iron sulfate

**U.S./Canadian Brand Names** Apo-Ferrous Sulfate® [Can]; Feosol® [US-OTC]; Fer-Gen-Sol [US-OTC]; Fer-In-Sol® [US-OTC/Can]; Fer-Iron® [US-OTC]; Feratab® [US-OTC]; Ferodan™ [Can]; Slow FE® [US-OTC]

**Therapeutic Category** Electrolyte Supplement, Oral

**Use** Prevention and treatment of iron-deficiency anemias

**Usual Dosage** Oral:
Children **(dose expressed in terms of elemental iron)**:
Severe iron-deficiency anemia: 4-6 mg Fe/kg/day in 3 divided doses
Mild to moderate iron deficiency anemia: 3 mg Fe/kg/day in 1-2 divided doses
Prophylaxis: 1-2 mg Fe/kg/day up to a maximum of 15 mg/day
Adults **(dose expressed in terms of ferrous sulfate)**:
Iron deficiency: 300 mg twice daily up to 300 mg 4 times/day or 250 mg (extended release) 1-2 times/day
Prophylaxis: 300 mg/day

**Dosage Forms**
Elixir: 220 mg/5 mL (480 mL) [elemental iron 44 mg/5 mL; contains alcohol]
Liquid, oral drops: 75 mg/0.6 mL (50 mL) [elemental iron 15 mg/0.6 mL]
Fer-Gen-Sol: 75 mg/0.6 mL (50 mL) [elemental iron 15 mg/0.6 mL]
Fer-In-Sol®: 75 mg/0.6 mL (50 mL) [elemental iron 15 mg/0.6 mL; contains alcohol 0.2% and sodium bisulfite]
Fer-Iron®: 75 mg/0.6 mL (50 mL) [elemental iron 15 mg/0.6 mL]
Tablet: 324 mg [elemental iron 65 mg]; 325 mg [elemental iron 65 mg]
Feratab®: 300 mg [elemental iron 60 mg]
Tablet, exsiccated (Feosol®): 200 mg [elemental iron 65 mg]
Tablet, exsiccated, timed release (Slow FE®): 160 mg [elemental iron 50 mg]

## ferrous sulfate and ascorbic acid (FER us SUL fate & a SKOR bik AS id)

**Synonyms** ascorbic acid and ferrous sulfate; iron sulfate and vitamin C

**U.S./Canadian Brand Names** Fero-Grad 500® [US-OTC]

**Therapeutic Category** Vitamin

**Use** Treatment of iron deficiency in nonpregnant adults; treatment and prevention of iron deficiency in pregnant adults

**Usual Dosage** Adults: Oral: 1 tablet daily

**Dosage Forms** [DSC] = Discontinued product
Capsule, extended release (Vitelle™ Irospan®): Ferrous sulfate [elemental iron 65 mg] and ascorbic acid 150 mg [DSC]
(Continued)

## ferrous sulfate and ascorbic acid *(Continued)*

Tablet, controlled release (Fero-Grad 500®): Ferrous sulfate 525 mg [elemental iron 105 mg] and ascorbic acid 500 mg

Tablet, extended release (Vitelle™ Irospan®): Ferrous sulfate [elemental iron 65 mg] and ascorbic acid 150 mg [DSC]

## ferrous sulfate, ascorbic acid, and vitamin B-complex

(FER us SUL fate, a SKOR bik AS id, & VYE ta min bee KOM pleks)

**Therapeutic Category** Vitamin

**Use** Conditions of iron deficiency with an increased needed for B-complex vitamins and vitamin C

**Usual Dosage** Oral:

Children 1-3 years: 5 mL twice daily after meals

Children >4 years and Adults: 10 mL 3 times/day after meals

**Dosage Forms**

Liquid (components all per 15 mL):

Iberet®-Liquid:

Ascorbic acid: 112.5 mg

$B_1$: 4.5 mg

$B_2$: 4.5 mg

$B_3$: 22.5 mg

$B_5$: 7.5 mg

$B_6$: 3.75 mg

$B_{12}$: 18.75 mg

Ferrous sulfate: 78.75 mg

Iberet®-Liquid 500:

Ascorbic acid: 375 mg

$B_1$: 4.5 mg

$B_2$: 4.5 mg

$B_3$: 22.5 mg

$B_5$: 7.5 mg

$B_6$: 3.75 mg

$B_{12}$: 18.75 mg

Ferrous sulfate: 78.75 mg

## ferrous sulfate, ascorbic acid, vitamin B-complex, and folic acid

(FER us SUL fate, a SKOR bik AS id, VYE ta min bee-KOM pleks, & FOE lik AS id)

**Therapeutic Category** Vitamin

**Use** Treatment of iron deficiency and prevention of concomitant folic acid deficiency where there is an associated deficient intake or increased need for B complex vitamins

**Usual Dosage** Adults: Oral: 1 tablet daily

**Dosage Forms**

Tablet, controlled release:

Ascorbic acid: 500 mg

$B_1$: 6 mg

$B_2$: 6 mg

$B_3$: 30 mg

$B_5$: 10 mg

$B_6$: 5 mg

$B_{12}$: 25 mcg

Ferrous sulfate: 105 mg

Folic acid: 800 mcg

**Fertinorm® H.P. [Can]** *see* urofollitropin *on page 835*

## ferumoxides (fer yoo MOX ides)

**Sound-Alike/Look-Alike Issues**

Feridex I.V.® may be confused with Fertinex®

**U.S./Canadian Brand Names** Feridex I.V.® [US]

**Therapeutic Category** Radiopaque Agents

**Use** For I.V. administration as an adjunct to MRI (in adult patients) to enhance the T2 weighted images used in the detection and evaluation of lesions of the liver

Usual Dosage Adults: 0.56 mg of iron (0.05 mL Feridex I.V.®)/kg body weight diluted in 100 mL of 5% dextrose and infused over 30 minutes; a 5-micron filter is recommended; do not administer undiluted
Dosage Forms Injection, solution: Iron 11.2 mg/mL (5 mL) [contains mannitol 61.3 mg/mL]

**FeSO₄** *see* ferrous sulfate *on page 335*

**Fe-Tinic™ 150 (Discontinued)** *see* polysaccharide-iron complex *on page 660*

**FeverALL® [US-OTC]** *see* acetaminophen *on page 4*

## fexofenadine (feks oh FEN a deen)

**Sound-Alike/Look-Alike Issues**
Allegra® may be confused with Viagra®
**Synonyms** fexofenadine hydrochloride
**U.S./Canadian Brand Names** Allegra® [US/Can]
**Therapeutic Category** Antihistamine
**Use** Relief of symptoms associated with seasonal allergic rhinitis; treatment of chronic idiopathic urticaria
**Usual Dosage** Oral:
Children 6-11 years: 30 mg twice daily
Children ≥12 years and Adults:
Seasonal allergic rhinitis: 60 mg twice daily **or** 180 mg once daily
Chronic idiopathic urticaria: 60 mg twice daily
**Dosage Forms** Tablet, as hydrochloride: 30 mg, 60 mg, 180 mg

## fexofenadine and pseudoephedrine (feks oh FEN a deen & soo doe e FED rin)

**Sound-Alike/Look-Alike Issues**
Allegra-D® may be confused with Viagra®
**Synonyms** pseudoephedrine and fexofenadine
**U.S./Canadian Brand Names** Allegra-D® 12 Hour [US]; Allegra-D® 24 Hour [US]; Allegra-D® [Can]
**Therapeutic Category** Antihistamine/Decongestant Combination
**Use** Relief of symptoms associated with seasonal allergic rhinitis in adults and children ≥12 years of age
**Usual Dosage** Oral: Children ≥12 years and Adults:
Allegra-D® 12 Hour: One tablet twice daily
Allegra-D® 24 Hour: One tablet once daily
**Dosage Forms** Tablet, extended release:
Allegra-D® 12 Hour: Fexofenadine hydrochloride 60 mg [immediate release] and pseudoephedrine hydrochloride 120 mg [extended release]
Allegra-D® 24 Hour: Fexofenadine hydrochloride 180 mg [immediate release] and pseudoephedrine hydrochloride 240 mg [extended release]

**fexofenadine hydrochloride** *see* fexofenadine *on this page*

**Fiberall® [US]** *see* psyllium *on page 697*

**FiberCon® [US-OTC]** *see* polycarbophil *on page 657*

**FiberEase™ [US-OTC]** *see* methylcellulose *on page 529*

**Fiber-Lax® [US-OTC]** *see* polycarbophil *on page 657*

## fibrin sealant kit (FI brin SEEL ent kit)

**Synonyms** FS
**U.S./Canadian Brand Names** Crosseal™ [US]; Tisseel® VH [US/Can]
**Therapeutic Category** Hemostatic Agent
**Use**
Crosseal™: Adjunct to hemostasis in liver surgery
Tisseel® VH: Adjunct to hemostasis in cardiopulmonary bypass surgery and splenic injury (due to blunt or penetrating trauma to the abdomen) when the control of bleeding by conventional surgical techniques is ineffective or impractical; adjunctive sealant for closure of colostomies; hemostatic agent in heparinized patients undergoing cardiopulmonary bypass
**Usual Dosage** Adjunct to hemostasis: Apply topically; actual dose is based on size of surface to be covered:
Crosseal™: Children and Adults. To cover a layer of 1 mm thickness:
Maximum area to be sealed: 20 cm²
Required size of Crosseal™ kit: 1 mL
(Continued)

# fibrin sealant kit (Continued)

Maximum area to be sealed: 40 cm$^2$
Required size of Crosseal™ kit: 2 mL
Maximum area to be sealed: 100 cm$^2$
Required size of Crosseal™ kit: 5 mL
**Note:** If hemostatic effect is not complete, apply a second layer.

Tisseel® VH: Adults:
Maximum area to be sealed: 4 cm$^2$
Required size of Tisseel® VH kit: 0.5 mL
Maximum area to be sealed: 8 cm$^2$
Required size of Tisseel® VH kit: 1 mL
Maximum area to be sealed: 16 cm$^2$
Required size of Tisseel® VH kit: 2 mL
Maximum area to be sealed: 40 cm$^2$
Required size of Tisseel® VH kit: 5 mL
Apply in thin layers to avoid excess formation of granulation tissue and slow absorption of the sealant. Following application, hold the sealed parts in the desired position for 3-5 minutes. To prevent sealant from adhering to gloves or surgical instruments, wet them with saline prior to contact.

**Dosage Forms** Topical: Kit [each kit contains]:
Crosseal™: Fibrinogen 40-60 mg/mL [human; also contains tranexamic acid]; thrombin 800-1200 int. units/mL [human; also contains human albumin and mannitol]; spray application device (1 mL, 2 mL, 5 mL)
Tisseel® VH: Fibrinogen 75-115 mg/mL [sealer protein concentrate, human]; aprotinin 3000 KIU/mL [fibrinolysis inhibitor solution, bovine]; thrombin 500 int. units/mL [human]; calcium chloride solution 40 micromoles/mL (0.5 mL, 1 mL, 2 mL, 5 mL)

**Fibro-XL [US-OTC]** see psyllium on page 697
**Fibro-Lax [US-OTC]** see psyllium on page 697

# filgrastim (fil GRA stim)

**Sound-Alike/Look-Alike Issues**
Neupogen® may be confused with Epogen®, Neumega®, Nutramigen®
**Synonyms** G-CSF; granulocyte colony stimulating factor
**U.S./Canadian Brand Names** Neupogen® [US/Can]
**Therapeutic Category** Colony-Stimulating Factor
**Use** Stimulation of granulocyte production in patients with malignancies, including myeloid malignancies; receiving myelosuppressive therapy associated with a significant risk of neutropenia; severe chronic neutropenia (SCN); receiving bone marrow transplantation (BMT); undergoing peripheral blood progenitor cell (PBPC) collection
**Usual Dosage** Refer to individual protocols.
**Dosing, even in morbidly obese patients, should be based on actual body weight. Rounding doses to the nearest vial size often enhances patient convenience and reduces costs without compromising clinical response.**
Myelosuppressive therapy: 5 mcg/kg/day - doses may be increased by 5 mcg/kg according to the duration and severity of the neutropenia.
Bone marrow transplantation: 5-10 mcg/kg/day - doses may be increased by 5 mcg/kg according to the duration and severity of neutropenia; recommended steps based on neutrophil response:
When ANC >1000/mm$^3$ for 3 consecutive days: Reduce filgrastim dose to 5 mcg/kg/day
If ANC remains >1000/mm$^3$ for 3 more consecutive days: Discontinue filgrastim
If ANC decreases to <1000/mm$^3$: Resume at 5 mcg/kg/day
If ANC decreases <1000/mm$^3$ during the 5 mcg/kg/day dose, increase filgrastim to 10 mcg/kg/day and follow the above steps
Peripheral blood progenitor cell (PBPC) collection: 10 mcg/kg/day **or** 5-8 mcg/kg twice daily in donors. The optimal timing and duration of growth factor stimulation has not been determined.
Severe chronic neutropenia:
Congenital: 6 mcg/kg twice daily
Idiopathic/cyclic: 5 mcg/kg/day

**Dosage Forms**
Injection, solution [preservative free]: 300 mcg/mL (1 mL, 1.6 mL) [vial; contains sodium 0.035 mg/mL and sorbitol]

Injection, solution [preservative free]: 600 mcg/mL (0.5 mL, 0.8 mL) [prefilled Singleject® syringe; contains sodium 0.035 mg/mL and sorbitol]

**Finacea**™ **[US]** *see* azelaic acid *on page 83*

## finasteride (fi NAS teer ide)
**Sound-Alike/Look-Alike Issues**
Proscar® may be confused with ProSom®, Prozac®, Psorcon®
**U.S./Canadian Brand Names** Propecia® [US/Can]; Proscar® [US/Can]
**Therapeutic Category** Antiandrogen
**Use**
Propecia®: Treatment of male pattern hair loss in **men only**. Safety and efficacy were demonstrated in men between 18-41 years of age.
Proscar®: Treatment of symptomatic benign prostatic hyperplasia (BPH); can be used in combination with an alpha blocker, doxazosin
**Usual Dosage** Oral: Adults: Male:
Benign prostatic hyperplasia (Proscar®): 5 mg/day as a single dose; clinical responses occur within 12 weeks to 6 months of initiation of therapy; long-term administration is recommended for maximal response
Male pattern baldness (Propecia®): 1 mg daily
**Dosage Forms** Tablet [film coated]:
Propecia®: 1 mg
Proscar®: 5 mg

**Fiorgen PF**® *(Discontinued)*

**Fioricet**® **[US]** *see* butalbital, acetaminophen, and caffeine *on page 124*

**Fiorinal**® **[US/Can]** *see* butalbital, aspirin, and caffeine *on page 125*

**Fiorinal**®**-C 1/2 [Can]** *see* butalbital, aspirin, caffeine, and codeine *on page 125*

**Fiorinal**®**-C 1/4 [Can]** *see* butalbital, aspirin, caffeine, and codeine *on page 125*

**Fiorinal**® **With Codeine [US]** *see* butalbital, aspirin, caffeine, and codeine *on page 125*

**Fiorital**® *(Discontinued)*

**First**® **Testosterone [US]** *see* testosterone *on page 788*

**First**® **Testosterone MC [US]** *see* testosterone *on page 788*

**fisalamine** *see* mesalamine *on page 516*

**fish oil** *see* omega-3-acid ethyl esters *on page 598*

**FK506** *see* tacrolimus *on page 778*

**Flagyl**® **[US/Can]** *see* metronidazole *on page 535*

**Flagyl ER**® **[US]** *see* metronidazole *on page 535*

**Flagyl**® **I.V. RTU**™ **[US]** *see* metronidazole *on page 535*

**Flamazine**® **[Can]** *see* silver sulfadiazine *on page 747*

**Flarex**® **[US/Can]** *see* fluorometholone *on page 348*

**Flavorcee**® *(Discontinued)* *see* ascorbic acid *on page 71*

## flavoxate (fla VOKS ate)
**Sound-Alike/Look-Alike Issues**
flavoxate may be confused with fluvoxamine
Urispas® may be confused with Urised®
**Synonyms** flavoxate hydrochloride
**U.S./Canadian Brand Names** Apo-Flavoxate® [Can]; Urispas® [US/Can]
**Therapeutic Category** Antispasmodic Agent, Urinary
**Use** Antispasmodic to provide symptomatic relief of dysuria, nocturia, suprapubic pain, urgency, and incontinence due to detrusor instability and hyper-reflexia in elderly with cystitis, urethritis, urethrocystitis, urethrotrigonitis, and prostatitis
**Usual Dosage** Children >12 years and Adults: Oral: 100-200 mg 3-4 times/day; reduce the dose when symptoms improve
**Dosage Forms** Tablet [film coated], as hydrochloride: 100 mg

**flavoxate hydrochloride** *see* flavoxate *on previous page*

**flecainide** (fle KAY nide)
### Sound-Alike/Look-Alike Issues
flecainide may be confused with fluconazole
Tambocor™ may be confused with tamoxifen
### Synonyms flecainide acetate
### U.S./Canadian Brand Names Tambocor™ [US/Can]
### Therapeutic Category Antiarrhythmic Agent, Class I-C
### Use Prevention and suppression of documented life-threatening ventricular arrhythmias (eg, sustained ventricular tachycardia); controlling symptomatic, disabling supraventricular tachycardias in patients without structural heart disease in whom other agents fail
### Usual Dosage Oral:
Children:
Initial: 3 mg/kg/day or 50-100 mg/m$^2$/day in 3 divided doses
Usual: 3-6 mg/kg/day or 100-150 mg/m$^2$/day in 3 divided doses; up to 11 mg/kg/day or 200 mg/m$^2$/day for uncontrolled patients with subtherapeutic levels
Adults:
Life-threatening ventricular arrhythmias:
Initial: 100 mg every 12 hours
Increase by 50-100 mg/day (given in 2 doses/day) every 4 days; maximum: 400 mg/day.
Use of higher initial doses and more rapid dosage adjustments have resulted in an increased incidence of proarrhythmic events and congestive heart failure, particularly during the first few days. Do not use a loading dose. Use very cautiously in patients with history of congestive heart failure or myocardial infarction.
Prevention of paroxysmal supraventricular arrhythmias in patients with disabling symptoms but no structural heart disease:
Initial: 50 mg every 12 hours
Increase by 50 mg twice daily at 4-day intervals; maximum: 300 mg/day.
### Dosage Forms Tablet, as acetate: 50 mg, 100 mg, 150 mg

**flecainide acetate** *see* flecainide *on this page*

**Fleet® Accu-Prep® [US-OTC]** *see* sodium phosphates *on page 756*

**Fleet® Babylax® [US-OTC]** *see* glycerin *on page 379*

**Fleet® Bisacodyl Enema [US-OTC]** *see* bisacodyl *on page 107*

**Fleet Enema® [Can]** *see* sodium phosphates *on page 756*

**Fleet® Flavored Castor Oil *(Discontinued)*** *see* castor oil *on page 151*

**Fleet® Glycerin Suppositories [US-OTC]** *see* glycerin *on page 379*

**Fleet® Glycerin Suppositories Maximum Strength [US-OTC]** *see* glycerin *on page 379*

**Fleet® Laxative *(Discontinued)*** *see* bisacodyl *on page 107*

**Fleet® Liquid Glycerin Suppositories [US-OTC]** *see* glycerin *on page 379*

**Fleet® Phospho-Soda® [US-OTC]** *see* sodium phosphates *on page 756*

**Fleet® Phospho-Soda® Oral Laxative [Can]** *see* sodium phosphates *on page 756*

**Fleet® Sof-Lax® [US-OTC]** *see* docusate *on page 263*

**Fleet® Stimulant Laxative [US-OTC]** *see* bisacodyl *on page 107*

**Fletcher's® Castoria® [US-OTC]** *see* senna *on page 743*

**Flexaphen® *(Discontinued)*** *see* chlorzoxazone *on page 179*

**Flexeril® [US/Can]** *see* cyclobenzaprine *on page 213*

**Flexitec [Can]** *see* cyclobenzaprine *on page 213*

**Flex-Power [US-OTC]** *see* triethanolamine salicylate *on page 823*

**Flintstones® Complete [US-OTC]** *see* vitamins (multiple/pediatric) *on page 852*

**Flintstones® Plus Calcium [US-OTC]** *see* vitamins (multiple/pediatric) *on page 852*

**Flintstones® Plus Extra C [US-OTC]** *see* vitamins (multiple/pediatric) *on page 852*

**Flintstones® Plus Iron [US-OTC]** *see* vitamins (multiple/pediatric) *on page 852*

**Flo-Coat**® **[US]** *see* radiological/contrast media (ionic) *on page 707*

## floctafenine *(Canada only)* (flok ta FEN een)
**U.S./Canadian Brand Names** Idarac® [Can]
**Therapeutic Category** Nonsteroidal Antiinflammatory Drug (NSAID), Oral
**Use** Short-term use in acute pain of mild and moderate severity
**Usual Dosage** Adults: Oral: 200-400 mg every 6-8 hours as required; maximum recommended daily dose: 1200 mg
**Dosage Forms** Tablet: 200 mg, 400 mg

**Flolan**® **[US/Can]** *see* epoprostenol *on page 291*

**Flomax**® **[US/Can]** *see* tamsulosin *on page 780*

**Flonase**® **[US/Can]** *see* fluticasone (nasal) *on page 354*

**Flora-Q**™ **[US-OTC]** *see* Lactobacillus *on page 462*

**Florazole**® **ER [Can]** *see* metronidazole *on page 535*

**Florical**® **[US-OTC]** *see* calcium carbonate *on page 130*

**Florinef**® **[US/Can]** *see* fludrocortisone *on page 343*

**Florone**® **[US/Can]** *see* diflorasone *on page 247*

**Florone E**® *(Discontinued)* *see* diflorasone *on page 247*

**Flovent**® **Diskus**® **[Can]** *see* fluticasone (oral inhalation) *on page 354*

**Flovent**® **HFA [US/Can]** *see* fluticasone (oral inhalation) *on page 354*

**Floxin**® **[US/Can]** *see* ofloxacin *on page 594*

## floxuridine (floks YOOR i deen)
**Sound-Alike/Look-Alike Issues**
floxuridine may be confused with fludarabine
FUDR® may be confused with Fludara®
**Synonyms** 5-FUDR; fluorodeoxyuridine; NSC-27640
**U.S./Canadian Brand Names** FUDR® [US/Can]
**Therapeutic Category** Antineoplastic Agent
**Use** Management of hepatic metastases of colorectal and gastric cancers
**Usual Dosage** Refer to individual protocols.
Intra-arterial:
0.1-0.6 mg/kg/day
4-20 mg/day
I.V.:
0.15 mg/kg/day for 7-14 days
0.5-1 mg/kg/day for 6-15 days
30 mg/kg/day for 5 days, then 15 mg/kg/day every other day, up to 11 days
**Dosage Forms** Injection, powder for reconstitution: 500 mg

**Fluanxol**® **[Can]** *see* flupenthixol *(Canada only)* *on page 350*

**Fluarix**™ **[US]** *see* influenza virus vaccine *on page 437*

**flubenisolone** *see* betamethasone (topical) *on page 103*

**Flucaine**® **[US]** *see* proparacaine and fluorescein *on page 686*

## fluconazole (floo KOE na zole)
**Sound-Alike/Look-Alike Issues**
fluconazole may be confused with flecainide
Diflucan® may be confused with diclofenac, Diprivan®, disulfiram
**U.S./Canadian Brand Names** Apo-Fluconazole® [Can]; Diflucan® [US/Can]; Fluconazole Omega [Can]; Gen-Fluconazole [Can]; Novo-Fluconazole [Can]
**Therapeutic Category** Antifungal Agent
**Use** Treatment of candidiasis (vaginal, oropharyngeal, esophageal, urinary tract infections, peritonitis, pneumonia, and systemic infections); cryptococcal meningitis; antifungal prophylaxis in allogeneic bone marrow transplant recipients
**Usual Dosage** The daily dose of fluconazole is the same for oral and I.V. administration
(Continued)

## fluconazole *(Continued)*

Neonates: First 2 weeks of life, especially premature neonates: Same dose as older children every 72 hours

Children: Once-daily dosing by indication:

Oropharyngeal candidiasis: Day 1: 6 mg/kg, then 3 mg/kg/day for at least 14 days

Esophageal candidiasis: Day 1: 6 mg/kg, then 3-12 mg/kg/day for a minimum of 21 days and for at least 2 weeks following resolution of symptoms

Systemic candidiasis: 6 mg/kg every 12 hours for at least 28 days

Cryptococcal meningitis, acute: Day 1: 12 mg/kg, then 6-12 mg/kg/day for at least 10-12 weeks after CSF culture becomes negative

Cryptococcal meningitis, relapse suppression: Day 1: 6 mg/kg, then 6 mg/kg/day

Adults: Oral, I.V.: **Note:** Susceptibility for *Candida* is divided into susceptible, susceptible-dose dependent (SDD), and resistant. Increased dose (up to 400 mg/day) may be used to treat SDD strains, especially when there has been treatment failure at lower doses. Once-daily dosing by indication:

Oropharyngeal candidiasis (OPC) (long-term suppression): Day 1: 200 mg, then 200 mg/day; chronic therapy in AIDS patients with history of OPC

Esophageal candidiasis: Day 1: 200 mg, then 100-200 mg/day; continue 14-21 days after clinical improvement

Prevention of candidiasis in bone marrow transplant: Day 1: 400 mg, then 400 mg/day for a minimum of 3 days before neutropenia, 7 days after neutrophils >1000 cells/mm$^3$

Urinary candidiasis: 200 mg/day for 14 days

Candididemia, primary therapy, non-neutropenic: 400-800 mg/day for 14 days after last positive blood-culture and resolution of signs/symptoms

Candididemia, alternative therapy, non-neutropenic: 800 mg/day (with conventional amphotericin B) for 4-7 days, then 800 mg/day for 14 days after last positive blood culture and resolution of signs/symptoms

Candididemia, secondary, neutropenic: 6-12 mg/kg/day for 14 days after last positive bloodculture and resolution of signs/symptoms

Cryptococcal meningitis, consolidation (after induction with amphotericin plus flucytosine): 400 mg for at least 10 weeks

Cryptococcal meningitis, relapse suppression (maintenance): 200-400 mg/day

Vaginal candidiasis: Day 1: 150 mg single dose

### Dosage Forms

Infusion [premixed in sodium chloride]: 2 mg/mL (100 mL, 200 mL)

Diflucan® [premixed in sodium chloride or dextrose] 2 mg/mL (100 mL, 200 mL)

Powder for oral suspension (Diflucan®): 10 mg/mL (35 mL); 40 mg/mL (35 mL) [contains sodium benzoate; orange flavor]

Tablet (Diflucan®): 50 mg, 100 mg, 150 mg, 200 mg

## Fluconazole Omega [Can] *see* fluconazole *on previous page*

## flucytosine *(floo SYE toe seen)*

### Sound-Alike/Look-Alike Issues

flucytosine may be confused with fluorouracil

Ancobon® may be confused with Oncovin®

### Synonyms 5-FC; 5-fluorocytosine; 5-flurocytosine

### U.S./Canadian Brand Names Ancobon® [US/Can]

### Therapeutic Category Antifungal Agent

### Use Adjunctive treatment of susceptible fungal infections (usually *Candida* or *Cryptococcus*); synergy with amphotericin B for certain fungal infections (*Cryptococcus* spp., *Candida* spp.)

### Usual Dosage Children and Adults: Oral: 50-150 mg/kg/day in divided doses every 6 hours

### Dosage Forms Capsule: 250 mg, 500 mg

## Fludara® [US/Can] *see* fludarabine *on this page*

## fludarabine *(floo DARE a been)*

### Sound-Alike/Look-Alike Issues

fludarabine may be confused with floxuridine, Flumadine®

Fludara® may be confused with FUDR®

**Synonyms** fludarabine phosphate
**U.S./Canadian Brand Names** Fludara® [US/Can]
**Therapeutic Category** Antineoplastic Agent
**Use** Treatment of chronic lymphocytic leukemia (CLL) (including refractory CLL); non-Hodgkin's lymphoma in adults
**Usual Dosage** Adults:
Chronic lymphocytic leukemia: 25 mg/m²/day for 5 days every 28 days
Non-Hodgkin's lymphoma: Loading dose: 20 mg/m² followed by 30 mg/m²/day for 48 hours
**Dosage Forms** Injection, powder for reconstitution, as phosphate: 50 mg

**fludarabine phosphate** *see* fludarabine *on previous page*

# fludrocortisone (floo droe KOR ti sone)
**Sound-Alike/Look-Alike Issues**
Florinef® may be confused with Fiorinal®
**Synonyms** 9α-fluorohydrocortisone acetate; fludrocortisone acetate; fluohydrisone acetate; fluohydrocortisone acetate
**U.S./Canadian Brand Names** Florinef® [US/Can]
**Therapeutic Category** Adrenal Corticosteroid (Mineralocorticoid)
**Use** Partial replacement therapy for primary and secondary adrenocortical insufficiency in Addison's disease; treatment of salt-losing adrenogenital syndrome
**Usual Dosage** Oral:
Infants and Children: 0.05-0.1 mg/day
Adults: 0.1-0.2 mg/day with ranges of 0.1 mg 3 times/week to 0.2 mg/day
Addison's disease: Initial: 0.1 mg/day; if transient hypertension develops, reduce the dose to 0.05 mg/day. Preferred administration with cortisone (10-37.5 mg/day) or hydrocortisone (10-30 mg/day).
Salt-losing adrenogenital syndrome: 0.1-0.2 mg/day
**Dosage Forms** Tablet, as acetate: 0.1 mg

**fludrocortisone acetate** *see* fludrocortisone *on this page*
**Flumadine® [US/Can]** *see* rimantadine *on page 724*

# flumazenil (FLOO may ze nil)
**U.S./Canadian Brand Names** Anexate® [Can]; Romazicon® [US/Can]
**Therapeutic Category** Antidote
**Use** Benzodiazepine antagonist; reverses sedative effects of benzodiazepines used in conscious sedation and general anesthesia; treatment of benzodiazepine overdose
**Usual Dosage** I.V.:
Children: Reversal of conscious sedation and general anesthesia:
Initial: 0.01 mg/kg over 15 seconds (maximum: 0.2 mg)
Repeat doses (maximum: 4 doses): 0.005-0.01 mg/kg (maximum: 0.2 mg) repeated at 1-minute intervals
Maximum total cumulative dose: 1 mg or 0.05 mg/kg (whichever is lower)
Adults:
Reversal of conscious sedation and general anesthesia:
Initial: 0.2 mg over 15 seconds
Repeat doses: If desired level of consciousness is not obtained, 0.2 mg may be repeated at 1-minute intervals.
Maximum total cumulative dose: 1 mg (usual dose: 0.6-1 mg). In the event of resedation: Repeat doses may be given at 20-minute intervals with maximum of 1 mg/dose and 3 mg/hour
Suspected benzodiazepine overdose:
Initial: 0.2 mg over 30 seconds; if the desired level of consciousness is not obtained, 0.3 mg can be given over 30 seconds
Repeat doses: 0.5 mg over 30 seconds repeated at 1-minute intervals
Maximum total cumulative dose: 3 mg (usual dose: 1-3 mg). Patients with a partial response at 3 mg may require additional titration up to a total dose of 5 mg. If a patient has not responded 5 minutes after cumulative dose of 5 mg, the major cause of sedation is not likely due to benzodiazepines. In the event of resedation: May repeat doses at 20-minute intervals with maximum of 1 mg/dose and 3 mg/hour.
Resedation: Repeated doses may be given at 20-minute intervals as needed; repeat treatment doses of 1 mg (at a rate of 0.5 mg/minute) should be given at any time and no more than 3 mg should be given in
(Continued)

## flumazenil *(Continued)*

any hour. After intoxication with high doses of benzodiazepines, the duration of a single dose of flumazenil is not expected to exceed 1 hour; if desired, the period of wakefulness may be prolonged with repeated low intravenous doses of flumazenil, or by an infusion of 0.1-0.4 mg/hour. Most patients with benzodiazepine overdose will respond to a cumulative dose of 1-3 mg and doses >3 mg do not reliably produce additional effects. Rarely, patients with a partial response at 3 mg may require additional titration up to a total dose of 5 mg. **If a patient has not responded 5 minutes after receiving a cumulative dose of 5 mg, the major cause of sedation is not likely to be due to benzodiazepines.**

**Dosage Forms** Injection, solution: 0.1 mg/mL (5 mL, 10 mL) [contains edetate sodium]

**flumethasone and clioquinol** *see* clioquinol and flumethasone *(Canada only) on page 193*

**fluMist® [US]** *see* influenza virus vaccine *on page 437*

## flunarizine *(Canada only)* (floo NAR i zeen)

**U.S./Canadian Brand Names** Sibelium® [Can]

**Therapeutic Category** Calcium-Entry Blocker (Selective)

**Use** Prophylaxis of migraine with and without aura; the safety of flunarizine in long-term use (ie, >4 months) has not been systematically evaluated in controlled clinical trials. Flunarizine is not indicated in the treatment of acute migraine attacks.

**Usual Dosage** The usual adult dosage is 10 mg/day administered in the evening. Patients who experience side effects may be maintained on 5 mg at bedtime.

Duration of therapy: Clinical experience indicates that the onset of effect of flunarizine is gradual and maximum benefits may not be seen before the patient has completed several weeks of continuous treatment. Therapy, therefore, should not be discontinued for lack of response before an adequate time period has elapsed (ie, 6-8 weeks).

**Dosage Forms** Capsule, as hydrochloride: 5 mg

## flunisolide (floo NISS oh lide)

**Sound-Alike/Look-Alike Issues**

flunisolide may be confused with Flumadine®, fluocinonide

Nasarel® may be confused with Nizoral®

**U.S./Canadian Brand Names** AeroBid® [US]; AeroBid®-M [US]; Alti-Flunisolide [Can]; Apo-Flunisolide® [Can]; Nasalide® [Can]; Nasarel® [US]; Rhinalar® [Can]

**Therapeutic Category** Adrenal Corticosteroid

**Use** Steroid-dependent asthma; nasal solution is used for seasonal or perennial rhinitis

**Usual Dosage**

Children >6 years:

Oral inhalation: 2 inhalations twice daily (morning and evening) up to 4 inhalations/day

Nasal: 1 spray each nostril twice daily (morning and evening), not to exceed 4 sprays/day each nostril

Adults:

Oral inhalation: 2 inhalations twice daily (morning and evening) up to 8 inhalations/day maximum

Nasal: 2 sprays each nostril twice daily (morning and evening); maximum dose: 8 sprays/day in each nostril

**Dosage Forms**

Aerosol for oral inhalation:

AeroBid®: 250 mcg/actuation (7 g) [100 metered doses; contains CFCs]

AeroBid®-M: 250 mcg/actuation (7 g) [100 metered doses; contains CFCs; menthol flavor]

Solution, intranasal spray (Nasarel®): 29 mcg/actuation (25 mL) [200 sprays; contains benzalkonium chloride]

## fluocinolone (floo oh SIN oh lone)

**Sound-Alike/Look-Alike Issues**

fluocinolone may be confused with fluocinonide

**Synonyms** fluocinolone acetonide

**U.S./Canadian Brand Names** Capex™ [US/Can]; Derma-Smoothe/FS® [US/Can]; Retisert™ [US]; Synalar® [US/Can]

**Therapeutic Category** Corticosteroid, Topical

**Use** Relief of susceptible inflammatory dermatosis [low, medium, high potency topical corticosteroid]; psoriasis of the scalp; atopic dermatitis in children ≥2 years of age

Ocular implant (Retisert™): Treatment of chronic, noninfectious uveitis affecting the posterior segment of the eye.

**Usual Dosage**

Children ≥2 years: Topical: Atopic dermatitis (Derma-Smoothe/FS®): Moisten skin; apply to affected area twice daily; do not use for longer than 4 weeks

Children and Adults: Topical: Corticosteroid-responsive dermatoses: Cream, ointment, solution: Apply a thin layer to affected area 2-4 times/day; may use occlusive dressings to manage psoriasis or recalcitrant conditions

Adults:

Topical:

Atopic dermatitis (Derma-Smoothe/FS®): Apply thin film to affected area 3 times/day

Inflammatory and pruritic manifestations (dental use): Apply to oral lesion 4 times/day , after meals and at bedtime

Scalp psoriasis (Derma-Smoothe/FS®): Massage thoroughly into wet or dampened hair/scalp; cover with shower cap. Leave on overnight (or for at least 4 hours). Remove by washing hair with shampoo and rinsing thoroughly.

Seborrheic dermatitis of the scalp (Capex™): Apply no more than 1 ounce to scalp once daily; work into lather and allow to remain on scalp for ~5 minutes. Remove from hair and scalp by rinsing thoroughly with water.

Ocular implant: Chronic uveitis: One silicone-encased tablet (0.59 mg) surgically implanted into the posterior segment of the eye is designed to release 0.6 mcg/day, decreasing over 30 days to a steady-state release rate of 0.3-0.4 mcg/day for 30 months. Recurrence of uveitis denotes depletion of tablet, requiring reimplantation.

**Dosage Forms**

Cream, as acetonide: 0.01% (15 g, 60 g); 0.025% (15 g, 60 g)

Synalar®: 0.025% (15 g, 60 g)

Oil, as acetonide:

Derma-Smoothe/FS® [eczema oil]: 0.01% (120 mL) [contains peanut oil]

Derma-Smoothe/FS® [scalp oil]: 0.01% (120 mL) [contains peanut oil; packaged with shower caps]

Ointment, as acetonide (Synalar®): 0.025% (15 g, 60 g)

Shampoo, as acetonide (Capex™): 0.01% (120 mL)

Solution, as acetonide: 0.01% (60 mL)

Synalar®: 0.01% (20 mL, 60 mL)

Tablet, ocular implant, as acetonide (Retisert™): 0.59 mg [enclosed in silicone elastomer]

**fluocinolone acetonide** *see* fluocinolone *on previous page*

# fluocinolone, hydroquinone, and tretinoin

(floo oh SIN oh lone, HYE droe kwin one, & TRET i noyn)

**Synonyms** hydroquinone, fluocinolone acetonide, and tretinoin; tretinoin, fluocinolone acetonide, and hydroquinone

**U.S./Canadian Brand Names** Tri-Luma™ [US]

**Therapeutic Category** Corticosteroid, Topical; Depigmenting Agent; Retinoic Acid Derivative

**Use** Short-term treatment of moderate to severe melasma of the face

**Usual Dosage** Topical: Adults: Melasma: Apply a thin film once daily to hyperpigmented areas of melasma (including ½ inch of normal-appearing surrounding skin). Apply 30 minutes prior to bedtime; not indicated for use beyond 8 weeks. Do not use occlusive dressings.

**Dosage Forms** Cream, topical: Hydroquinone 4%, tretinoin 0.05%, fluocinolone acetonide 0.01% (30 g) [contains sodium metabisulfite]

# fluocinonide (floo oh SIN oh nide)

**Sound-Alike/Look-Alike Issues**

fluocinonide may be confused with flunisolide, fluocinolone

Lidex® may be confused with Lasix®, Videx®, Wydase®

**U.S./Canadian Brand Names** Lidemol® [Can]; Lidex-E® [US]; Lidex® [US/Can]; Lyderm® [Can]; Tiamol® [Can]; Topsyn® [Can]; Vanos™ [US]

**Therapeutic Category** Corticosteroid, Topical

**Use** Anti-inflammatory, antipruritic; treatment of plaque-type psoriasis (up to 10% of body surface area) [high-potency topical corticosteroid]

(Continued)

345

## fluocinonide *(Continued)*

### Usual Dosage

Children and Adults: Pruritus and inflammation: Topical (0.5% cream): Apply thin layer to affected area 2-4 times/day depending on the severity of the condition. Therapy should be discontinued when control is achieved; if no improvement is seen, reassessment of diagnosis may be necessary.

Adults: Plaque-type psoriasis (Vanos™): Topical (0.1% cream): Apply a thin layer once or twice daily to affected areas (limited to <10% of body surface area). **Note:** Not recommended for use >2 consecutive weeks or >60 g/week total exposure. Discontinue when control is achieved.

### Dosage Forms

Cream, anhydrous, emollient (Lidex®): 0.05% (15 g, 30 g, 60 g)
Cream, aqueous, emollient (Lidex-E®): 0.05% (15 g, 30 g, 60 g)
Cream (Vanos™): 0.1% (30 g, 60 g)
Gel (Lidex®): 0.05% (15 g, 30 g, 60 g)
Ointment (Lidex®): 0.05% (15 g, 30 g, 60 g)
Solution (Lidex®): 0.05% (60 mL) [contains alcohol 35%]

**fluohydrisone acetate** *see* fludrocortisone *on page 343*

**fluohydrocortisone acetate** *see* fludrocortisone *on page 343*

**Fluonid® Topical *(Discontinued)*** *see* fluocinolone *on page 344*

**Fluor-I-Strip® [US]** *see* fluorescein sodium *on this page*

**Fluor-I-Strip-AT® [US]** *see* fluorescein sodium *on this page*

**Fluoracaine® [US]** *see* proparacaine and fluorescein *on page 686*

**Fluor-A-Day [US-OTC/Can]** *see* fluoride *on next page*

**FluorCare® Neutral *(Discontinued)*** *see* fluoride *on next page*

**fluorescein and proparacaine** *see* proparacaine and fluorescein *on page 686*

## fluorescein sodium *(FLURE e seen SOW dee um)*

**Synonyms** soluble fluorescein

**U.S./Canadian Brand Names** AK-Fluor [US]; Angiscein® [US]; Fluor-I-Strip-AT® [US]; Fluor-I-Strip® [US]; Fluorescite® [US/Can]; Fluorets® [US]; Ful-Glo® [US]

**Therapeutic Category** Diagnostic Agent

**Use** Demonstrates defects of corneal epithelium; diagnostic aid in ophthalmic angiography

### Usual Dosage

Ophthalmic:

Solution: Instill 1-2 drops of 2% solution and allow a few seconds for staining; wash out excess with sterile water or irrigating solution

Strips: Moisten strip with sterile water. Place moistened strip at the fornix into the lower cul-de-sac close to the punctum. For best results, patient should close lid tightly over strip until desired amount of staining is obtained. Patient should blink several times after application.

Removal of foreign bodies, sutures or tonometry (Fluress®): Instill 1 or 2 drops (single instillations) into each eye before operating

Deep ophthalmic anesthesia (Fluress®): Instill 2 drops into each eye every 90 seconds up to 3 doses

Injection: Prior to use, perform intradermal skin test; have epinephrine 1:1000, an antihistamine, and oxygen available

Children: 3.5 mg/lb (7.5 mg/kg) injected rapidly into antecubital vein

Adults: 500-750 mg injected rapidly into antecubital vein

### Dosage Forms

Injection, solution:
AK-Fluor, Fluorescite®: 10% (5 mL); 25% (2 mL)
Angiscein®: 10% (5 mL)
Strip, ophthalmic:
Fluorets®, Fluor-I-Strip-AT®: 1 mg
Fluor-I-Strip®: 9 mg
Ful-Glo®: 0.6 mg

**Fluorescite® [US/Can]** *see* fluorescein sodium *on this page*

**Fluorets® [US]** *see* fluorescein sodium *on this page*

# fluoride (FLOR ide)

## Sound-Alike/Look-Alike Issues
Luride® may be confused with Lortab®

Phos-Flur® may be confused with PhosLo®

Thera-Flur-N® may be confused with Thera-Flu®

**Synonyms** acidulated phosphate fluoride; sodium fluoride; stannous fluoride

**U.S./Canadian Brand Names** ACT® [US-OTC]; Fluor-A-Day [US-OTC/Can]; Fluorigard® [US-OTC]; Fluorinse® [US]; Fluotic® [Can]; Flura-Drops® [US]; Flura-Loz® [US]; Gel-Kam® Rinse [US]; Gel-Kam® [US-OTC]; Lozi-Flur™ [US]; Luride® Lozi-Tab® [US]; Luride® [US]; NeutraCare® [US]; NeutraGard® [US-OTC]; Pediaflor® [US]; Pharmaflur® 1.1 [US]; Pharmaflur® [US]; Phos-Flur® Rinse [US-OTC]; Phos-Flur® [US]; PreviDent® 5000 Plus™ [US]; PreviDent® [US]; Stan-gard® [US]; Stop® [US]; Thera-Flur-N® [US]

**Therapeutic Category** Mineral, Oral

**Use** Prevention of dental caries

## Usual Dosage Oral:
The recommended daily dose of oral fluoride supplement (mg), based on fluoride ion content (ppm) in drinking water (2.2 mg of sodium fluoride is equivalent to 1 mg of fluoride ion): Adapted from Recommeded Dosage Schedule of The American Dental Association, The American Academy of Pediatric Dentistry, and The American Academy of Pediatrics:

Less than 0.3 ppm:

Birth to 6 months: 0 mg

6 months to 3 years: 0.25 mg

3-6 years: 0.5 mg

6-16 years: 1 mg

0.3-0.6 ppm:

Birth to 3 years: 0 mg

3-6 years: 0.25 mg

6-16 years: 0.5 mg

Cream: Children ≥6 years and Adults: Brush teeth with cream once daily regardless of fluoride content of drinking water

Dental rinse or gel:

Children 6-12 years: 5-10 mL rinse or apply to teeth and spit daily after brushing

Adults: 10 mL rinse or apply to teeth and spit daily after brushing

PreviDent® rinse: Children >6 years and Adults: Once weekly, rinse 10 mL vigorously around and between teeth for 1 minute, then spit; this should be done preferably at bedtime, after thoroughly brushing teeth; for maximum benefit, do not eat, drink, or rinse mouth for at least 30 minutes after treatment; do not swallow

Fluorinse®: Children >6 years and Adults: Once weekly, vigorously swish 5-10 mL in mouth for 1 minute, then spit

Lozenge (Lozi-Flur™): Adults: One lozenge daily regardless of fluoride content of drinking water

## Dosage Forms [DSC] = Discontinued product
Cream, oral, as sodium [toothpaste]: 1.1% (51 g) [fluoride 2.5 mg/dose]

Denta 5000 Plus: 1.1% (51g) [fluoride 2.5 mg/dose; spearmint flavor]

EtheDent™: 1.1% (51g) [fluoride 2.5 mg/dose]

Gel-drops, as sodium fluoride (Thera-Flur-N®): 1.1% (24 mL) [fluoride 0.5%; neutral pH; no artificial color or flavor]

Gel, topical, as acidulated phosphate fluoride (Phos-Flur®): 1.1% (60 g) [fluoride 0.5%; cherry and mint flavors]

Gel, topical, as sodium fluoride: 1.1% (56 g) [fluoride 2 mg/dose]

DentaGel, EtheDent™: 1.1% (56 g) [fluoride 2 mg/dose; fresh mint flavor]

NeutraCare®: 1.1% (60 g) [neutral pH; grape and mint flavors]

NeutraGard® Advanced: 1.1% (60 g) [cinnamon and mint flavors]

PreviDent®: 1.1% (60 g) [fluoride 2 mg/dose; berry, cherry, and mint flavors]

Gel, topical, as stannous fluoride:

Gel-Kam®: 0.4% (129 g) [bubble gum, cinnamon, fruit/berry, and mint flavors]

Just for Kids™: 0.4% (122 g) [bubble gum, fruit punch, and grapey grape flavors]

Omnii Gel™: 0.4% (122 g) [cinnamon, grape, natural, mint, and raspberry flavors]

StanGard®: 0.4% (122 g) [bubble gum, cherry, mint, and raspberry flavors]

Stop®: 0.4% (120 g) [bubble gum, cinnamon, grape, and mint flavors]

Lozenge, as sodium (Lozi-Flur™): 2.21 mg [fluoride 1 mg; cherry flavor]

Paste, oral, as sodium [toothpaste] (ControlRx®): 1.1% (56 g) [vanilla mint flavor]

Solution, oral drops, as sodium: 1.1 mg/mL (50 mL) [fluoride 0.5 mg/mL]

(Continued)

## fluoride *(Continued)*

Flura-Drops®: 0.55 mg/drop (24 mL) [fluoride 0.25 mg/drop; dye free, sugar free]

Luride®: 1.1 mg/mL (50 mL) [fluoride 0.5 mg/mL; sugar free]

Pediaflor®: 1.1 mg/mL (50 mL) [fluoride 0.5 mg/mL; contains alcohol <0.5%; sugar free; cherry flavor] [DSC]

Solution, oral rinse, as sodium:

ACT®: 0.05% (530 mL) [fluoride 0.02%; bubble gum, cinnamon (contains tartrazine), and mint flavors]

ACT® Plus: 0.05% (530 mL) [fluoride 0.02%; alcohol free; icy cool mint flavor]

ACT® x2™: 0.5% (530 mL) [fluoride 0.02%; contains alcohol 11%; icy cool mint and spearmint flavors]

CaviRinse™: 0.2% (240 mL) [mint flavor]

Fluorigard®: 0.05% (480 mL) [alcohol free, sugar free; contains sodium benzoate and tartrazine; mint flavor]

Fluorinse®: 0.2% (480 mL) [alcohol free; cinnamon and mint flavors]

NeutraGard®: 0.05% (480 mL) [neutral pH; mint and tropical blast flavors]

NeutraGard® Plus: 0.2% (480 mL) [neutral pH; mint and tropical blast flavors]

Phos-Flur®: 0.44% (500 mL) [bubble gum, cherry, grape, and mint flavors]

PreviDent®: 0.2% (250 mL) [contains alcohol; mint flavor]

Solution, oral rinse concentrate, as stannous fluoride:

Gel-Kam®: 0.63% (300 mL) [fluoride 0.1%/dose; cinnamon and mint flavors]

PerioMed™: 0.63% (284 mL) [fluoride 7 mg/30 mL; alcohol free; cinnamon, mint and tropical fruit flavors]

StanGard® Perio: 0.63% (284 mL) [mint flavor]

Tablet, chewable, as sodium: 0.5 mg [fluoride 0.25 mg]; 1.1 mg [fluoride 0.5 mg]; 2.2 mg [fluoride 1 mg]

EtheDent™:

0.55 mg [fluoride 0.25 mg; sugar free; contains aspartame; vanilla flavor]

1.1 mg [fluoride 0.5 mg; sugar free; contains aspartame; grape flavor]

2.2 mg [fluoride 1 mg; sugar free; contains aspartame; cherry flavor]

Fluor-A-Day:

0.56 mg [fluoride 0.25 mg; raspberry flavor]

1.1 mg [fluoride 0.5 mg; raspberry flavor]

2.21 mg [fluoride 1 mg; raspberry flavor]

Luride® Lozi-Tab®:

0.55 mg [fluoride 0.25 mg; sugar free; vanilla flavor]

1.1 mg [fluoride 0.5 mg; sugar free; grape flavor]

2.2 mg [fluoride 1 mg; sugar free; cherry flavor]

Pharmaflur®: 2.2 mg [fluoride 1 mg; dye free, sugar free; cherry flavor]

Pharmaflur® 1.1: 1.1 mg [fluoride 0.5 mg; dye free, sugar free; grape flavor]

**Fluorigard® [US-OTC]** *see* fluoride *on previous page*

**Fluori-Methane® [US]** *see* dichlorodifluoromethane and trichloromonofluoromethane *on page 243*

**Fluorinse® [US]** *see* fluoride *on previous page*

**Fluoritab® *(Discontinued)*** *see* fluoride *on previous page*

**5-fluorocytosine** *see* flucytosine *on page 342*

**fluorodeoxyuridine** *see* floxuridine *on page 341*

**9α-fluorohydrocortisone acetate** *see* fludrocortisone *on page 343*

## fluorometholone (flure oh METH oh lone)

**U.S./Canadian Brand Names** Flarex® [US/Can]; FML® Forte [US/Can]; FML® [US/Can]; PMS-Fluorometholone [Can]

**Therapeutic Category** Adrenal Corticosteroid

**Use** Treatment of steroid-responsive inflammatory conditions of the eye

**Usual Dosage** Children >2 years and Adults: Ophthalmic: Re-evaluate therapy if improvement is not seen within 2 days; use care not to discontinue prematurely; in chronic conditions, gradually decrease dosing frequency prior to discontinuing treatment

Ointment: Apply small amount (~½ inch ribbon) to conjunctival sac every 4 hours in severe cases; 1-3 times/day in mild to moderate cases

Solution: Instill 1-2 drops into conjunctival sac every hour during day, every 2 hours at night until favorable response is obtained, then use 1 drop every 4 hours; for mild to moderate inflammation, instill 1-2 drops into conjunctival sac 2-4 times/day

**Dosage Forms** [DSC] = Discontinued product
Ointment, ophthalmic, as base (FML®): 0.1% (3.5 g)
Suspension, ophthalmic, as base: (5 mL, 10 mL, 15 mL)
Fluor-Op®: 0.1% (5 mL, 10 mL, 15 mL) [contains benzalkonium chloride and polyvinyl alcohol] [DSC]
FML®: 0.1% (5 mL, 10 mL, 15 mL) [contains benzalkonium chloride]
FML® Forte: 0.25% (2 mL, 5 mL, 10 mL, 15 mL) [contains benzalkonium chloride]
Suspension, ophthalmic, as acetate:
Eflone®: 0.1% (5 mL, 10 mL) [DSC]
Flarex®: 0.1% (5 mL, 10 mL) [contains benzalkonium chloride]

**fluorometholone and sulfacetamide** *see* sulfacetamide sodium and fluorometholone *on page 772*

**Fluor-Op®** *(Discontinued)* *see* fluorometholone *on previous page*

**Fluoroplex® [US]** *see* fluorouracil *on this page*

## fluorouracil (flure oh YOOR a sil)
**Sound-Alike/Look-Alike Issues**
fluorouracil may be confused with flucytosine
Efudex® may be confused with Efidac (Efidac 24®), Eurax®
**Synonyms** 5-fluorouracil; 5-FU; FU
**U.S./Canadian Brand Names** Adrucil® [US]; Carac™ [US]; Efudex® [US/Can]; Fluoroplex® [US]
**Therapeutic Category** Antineoplastic Agent
**Use** Treatment of carcinomas of the breast, colon, head and neck, pancreas, rectum, or stomach; topically for the management of actinic or solar keratoses and superficial basal cell carcinomas
**Usual Dosage** Adults:
Refer to individual protocols:
I.V. bolus: 500-600 mg/m$^2$ every 3-4 weeks **or** 425 mg/m$^2$ on days 1-5 every 4 weeks
Continuous I.V. infusion: 1000 mg/m$^2$/day for 4-5 days every 3-4 weeks **or**
2300-2600 mg/m$^2$ on day 1 every week **or**
300-400 mg/m$^2$/day **or**
225 mg/m$^2$/day for 5-8 weeks (with radiation therapy)
Actinic keratoses: Topical:
Carac™: Apply thin film to lesions once daily for up to 4 weeks, as tolerated
Efudex®: Apply to lesions twice daily for 2-4 weeks; complete healing may not be evident for 1-2 months following treatment
Fluoroplex®: Apply to lesions twice daily for 2-6 weeks
Basal cell carcinoma: Topical: Efudex®: Apply to affected lesions twice daily for 3-6 weeks; treatment may be continued for up to 10-12 weeks
**Dosage Forms**
Cream, topical:
Carac™: 0.5% (30 g)
Efudex®: 5% (25 g, 40 g)
Fluoroplex®: 1% (30 g) [contains benzyl alcohol]
Injection, solution: 50 mg/mL (10 mL, 20 mL, 50 mL, 100 mL)
Adrucil®: 50 mg/mL (10 mL, 50 mL, 100 mL)
Solution, topical (Efudex®): 2% (10 mL); 5% (10 mL)

**5-fluorouracil** *see* fluorouracil *on this page*

**Fluothane®** *(Discontinued)* *see* halothane *on page 397*

**Fluotic® [Can]** *see* fluoride *on page 347*

## fluoxetine (floo OKS e teen)
**Sound-Alike/Look-Alike Issues**
fluoxetine may be confused with duloxetine, fluvastatin
Prozac® may be confused with Prilosec®, Proscar®, ProSom®, ProStep®
Sarafem™ may be confused with Serophene®
**Synonyms** fluoxetine hydrochloride
**U.S./Canadian Brand Names** Alti-Fluoxetine [Can]; Apo-Fluoxetine® [Can]; CO Fluoxetine [Can]; FXT [Can]; Gen-Fluoxetine [Can]; Novo-Fluoxetine [Can]; Nu-Fluoxetine [Can]; PMS-Fluoxetine [Can]; Prozac® Weekly™ [US]; Prozac® [US/Can]; Rhoxal-fluoxetine [Can]; Sarafem™ [US]
(Continued)

## fluoxetine *(Continued)*

**Therapeutic Category** Antidepressant, Selective Serotonin Reuptake Inhibitor

**Use** Treatment of major depressive disorder; treatment of binge-eating and vomiting in patients with moderate-to-severe bulimia nervosa; obsessive-compulsive disorder (OCD); premenstrual dysphoric disorder (PMDD); panic disorder with or without agoraphobia

**Usual Dosage** Oral:

Children:

Depression: 8-18 years: 10-20 mg/day; lower-weight children can be started at 10 mg/day, may increase to 20 mg/day after 1 week if needed

OCD: 7-18 years: Initial: 10 mg/day; in adolescents and higher-weight children, dose may be increased to 20 mg/day after 2 weeks. Range: 10-60 mg/day

Adults: 20 mg/day in the morning; may increase after several weeks by 20 mg/day increments; maximum: 80 mg/day; doses >20 mg may be given once daily or divided twice daily. **Note:** Lower doses of 5-10 mg/day have been used for initial treatment.

Usual dosage range:

Bulimia nervosa: 60-80 mg/day

Depression: 20-40 mg/day; patients maintained on Prozac® 20 mg/day may be changed to Prozac® Weekly™ 90 mg/week, starting dose 7 days after the last 20 mg/day dose

OCD: 40-80 mg/day

Panic disorder: Initial: 10 mg/day; after 1 week, increase to 20 mg/day; may increase after several weeks; doses >60 mg/day have not been evaluated

PMDD (Sarafem™): 20 mg/day continuously, **or** 20 mg/day starting 14 days prior to menstruation and through first full day of menses (repeat with each cycle)

**Dosage Forms** [DSC] = Discontinued product

Capsule, as hydrochloride: 10 mg, 20 mg, 40 mg

Prozac®: 10 mg, 20 mg, 40 mg

Sarafem®: 10 mg, 20 mg

Capsule, delayed release, as hydrochloride (Prozac® Weekly™): 90 mg

Solution, oral, as hydrochloride (Prozac®): 20 mg/5 mL (120 mL) [contains alcohol 0.23% and benzoic acid; mint flavor]

Tablet, as hydrochloride: 10 mg, 20 mg

Prozac® [scored]: 10 mg [DSC]

**fluoxetine and olanzapine** *see* olanzapine and fluoxetine *on page 596*

**fluoxetine hydrochloride** *see* fluoxetine *on previous page*

## fluoxymesterone (floo oks i MES te rone)

**Sound-Alike/Look-Alike Issues**

Halotestin® may be confused with Haldol®, haloperidol, halothane, Halotussin®

**U.S./Canadian Brand Names** Halotestin® [US]

**Therapeutic Category** Androgen

**Controlled Substance** C-III

**Use** Replacement of endogenous testicular hormone; in females, used as palliative treatment of breast cancer

**Usual Dosage** Adults: Oral:

Male:

Hypogonadism: 5-20 mg/day

Delayed puberty: 2.5-20 mg/day for 4-6 months

Female: Inoperable breast carcinoma: 10-40 mg/day in divided doses for 1-3 months

**Dosage Forms** [DSC] = Discontinued product

Tablet: 10 mg

Halotestin®: 2 mg, 5 mg, 10 mg [contains tartrazine; 10 mg tablet DSC]

## flupenthixol *(Canada only)* (floo pen THIKS ol)

**Synonyms** flupenthixol decanoate; flupenthixol dihydrochloride

**U.S./Canadian Brand Names** Fluanxol® [Can]

**Therapeutic Category** Antipsychotic Agent; Thioxanthene Derivative

**Use** Maintenance therapy of chronic schizophrenic patients whose main manifestations do **not** include excitement, agitation, or hyperactivity

### Usual Dosage

I.M. (depot): Flupenthixol is administered by deep I.M. injection, preferably in the gluteus maximus, **NOT for I.V. use**; maintenance dosages are given at 2- to 3-week intervals

Patients not previously treated with long-acting depot neuroleptics should be given an initial test dose of 5-20 mg. An initial dose of 20 mg is usually well tolerated; however, a 5 mg test dose is recommended in elderly, frail, and cachectic patients, and in patients whose individual or family history suggests a predisposition to extrapyramidal reactions. In the subsequent 5-10 days, the therapeutic response and the appearance of extrapyramidal symptoms should be carefully monitored. Oral neuroleptic drugs may be continued, but dosage should be reduced during this overlapping period and eventually discontinued.

Oral: Initial: 1 mg 3 times/day; dose must be individualized. May be increased by 1 mg every 2-3 days based on tolerance and control of symptoms. Usual maintenance dosage: 3-6 mg/day in divided doses (doses ≥12 mg/day used in some patients).

### Dosage Forms

Injection, solution, as decanoate [depot]: 20 mg/mL (10 mL); 100 mg/mL (2 mL)
Tablet, as dihydrochloride: 0.5 mg, 3 mg

**flupenthixol decanoate** see flupenthixol *(Canada only)* on previous page

**flupenthixol dihydrochloride** see flupenthixol *(Canada only)* on previous page

## fluphenazine (floo FEN a zeen)

### Sound-Alike/Look-Alike Issues

Prolixin® may be confused with Proloprim®

**Synonyms** fluphenazine decanoate

**U.S./Canadian Brand Names** Apo-Fluphenazine Decanoate® [Can]; Apo-Fluphenazine® [Can]; Modecate® [Can]; PMS-Fluphenazine Decanoate [Can]; Prolixin Decanoate® [US]

**Therapeutic Category** Phenothiazine Derivative

**Use** Management of manifestations of psychotic disorders and schizophrenia; depot formulation may offer improved outcome in individuals with psychosis who are nonadherent with oral antipsychotics

**Usual Dosage** Adults: Psychoses:

Oral: 0.5-10 mg/day in divided doses at 6- to 8-hour intervals; some patients may require up to 40 mg/day

I.M.: 2.5-10 mg/day in divided doses at 6- to 8-hour intervals (parenteral dose is $^1/_3$ to $^1/_2$ the oral dose for the hydrochloride salts)

I.M. (decanoate): 12.5 mg every 2 weeks

Conversion from hydrochloride to decanoate I.M. 0.5 mL (12.5 mg) decanoate every 3 weeks is approximately equivalent to 10 mg hydrochloride/day

**Dosage Forms** [DSC] = Discontinued product

Elixir, as hydrochloride (Prolixin®): 2.5 mg/5 mL (60 mL) [contains alcohol 14% and sodium benzoate] [DSC]

Injection, oil, as decanoate: 25 mg/mL (5 mL) [may contain benzyl alcohol, sesame oil]

Prolixin Decanoate®: 25 mg/mL (5 mL) [contains benzyl alcohol, sesame oil]

Injection, solution, as hydrochloride (Prolixin® [DSC]): 2.5 mg/mL (10 mL)

Solution, oral concentrate, as hydrochloride (Prolixin®): 5 mg/mL (120 mL) [contains alcohol 14%] [DSC]

Tablet, as hydrochloride: 1 mg, 2.5 mg, 5 mg, 10 mg

Prolixin®: 1 mg, 2.5 mg, 5 mg [contains tartrazine], 10 mg [DSC]

**fluphenazine decanoate** see fluphenazine on this page

**Flura®** *(Discontinued)* see fluoride on page 347

**Flura-Drops®** [US] see fluoride on page 347

**Flura-Loz®** [US] see fluoride on page 347

## flurandrenolide (flure an DREN oh lide)

### Sound-Alike/Look-Alike Issues

Cordran® may be confused with Cardura®, codeine, Cordarone®

**Synonyms** flurandrenolone

**U.S./Canadian Brand Names** Cordran® SP [US]; Cordran® [US/Can]

**Therapeutic Category** Corticosteroid, Topical

**Use** Inflammation of corticosteroid-responsive dermatoses [medium potency topical corticosteroid]

(Continued)

## flurandrenolide *(Continued)*

**Usual Dosage** Topical: Therapy should be discontinued when control is achieved; if no improvement is seen, reassessment of diagnosis may be necessary.
Children:
  Ointment, cream: Apply sparingly 1-2 times/day
  Tape: Apply once daily
Adults: Cream, lotion, ointment: Apply sparingly 2-3 times/day

**Dosage Forms**
  Cream, emulsified, as base (Cordran® SP): 0.025% (30 g, 60 g); 0.05% (15 g, 30 g, 60 g)
  Lotion (Cordran®): 0.05% (15 mL, 60 mL)
  Ointment (Cordran®): 0.025% (30 g, 60 g); 0.05% (15 g, 30 g, 60 g)
  Tape, topical [roll] (Cordran®): 4 mcg/cm$^2$ (7.5 cm x 60 cm, 7.5 cm x 200 cm)

**flurandrenolone** *see* flurandrenolide *on previous page*

**Flurate® Ophthalmic Solution *(Discontinued)*** *see* fluorescein sodium *on page 346*

## flurazepam *(flure AZ e pam)*

**Sound-Alike/Look-Alike Issues**
  flurazepam may be confused with temazepam
  Dalmane® may be confused with Demulen®, Dialume®
**Synonyms** flurazepam hydrochloride
**U.S./Canadian Brand Names** Apo-Flurazepam® [Can]; Dalmane® [US]
**Therapeutic Category** Benzodiazepine
**Controlled Substance** C-IV
**Use** Short-term treatment of insomnia
**Usual Dosage** Oral:
  Children: Insomnia:
    ≤15 years: Dose not established
    >15 years: 15 mg at bedtime
  Adults: Insomnia: 15-30 mg at bedtime
**Dosage Forms** Capsule, as hydrochloride: 15 mg, 30 mg

**flurazepam hydrochloride** *see* flurazepam *on this page*

## flurbiprofen *(flure BI proe fen)*

**Sound-Alike/Look-Alike Issues**
  flurbiprofen may be confused with fenoprofen
  Ansaid® may be confused with Asacol®, Axid®
  Ocufen® may be confused with Ocuflox®, Ocupress®
**Synonyms** flurbiprofen sodium
**U.S./Canadian Brand Names** Alti-Flurbiprofen [Can]; Ansaid® [Can]; Apo-Flurbiprofen® [Can]; Froben-SR® [Can]; Froben® [Can]; Novo-Flurprofen [Can]; Nu-Flurprofen [Can]; Ocufen® [US/Can]
**Therapeutic Category** Analgesic, Nonnarcotic; Nonsteroidal Antiinflammatory Drug (NSAID)
**Use**
  Oral: Treatment of rheumatoid arthritis and osteoarthritis
  Ophthalmic: Inhibition of intraoperative miosis
**Usual Dosage**
  Oral:
    Rheumatoid arthritis and osteoarthritis: 200-300 mg/day in 2-, 3-, or 4 divided doses; do not administer more than 100 mg for any single dose; maximum: 300 mg/day
    Dental: Management of postoperative pain: 100 mg every 12 hours
  Ophthalmic: Instill 1 drop every 30 minutes, beginning 2 hours prior to surgery (total of 4 drops in each affected eye)
**Dosage Forms** [DSC] = Discontinued product
  Solution, ophthalmic, as sodium (Ocufen®): 0.03% (2.5 mL) [contains thimerosal]
  Tablet: 50 mg, 100 mg
  Ansaid®: 50 mg, 100 mg [DSC]

**flurbiprofen sodium** *see* flurbiprofen *on this page*

**5-flurocytosine** *see* flucytosine *on page 342*

**Fluro-Ethyl**® **[US]** *see* ethyl chloride and dichlorotetrafluoroethane *on page 321*

**Flurosyn**® **Topical** *(Discontinued)* *see* fluocinolone *on page 344*

**FluShield**® *(Discontinued)* *see* influenza virus vaccine *on page 437*

## flutamide (FLOO ta mide)

**Sound-Alike/Look-Alike Issues**
flutamide may be confused with Flumadine®, thalidomide
Eulexin® may be confused with Edecrin®, Eurax®

**Synonyms** 4'-nitro-3'-trifluoromethylisobutyrantide; niftolid; NSC-147834; SCH 13521

**U.S./Canadian Brand Names** Apo-Flutamide® [Can]; Euflex® [Can]; Eulexin® [US/Can]; Novo-Flutamide [Can]

**Therapeutic Category** Antiandrogen

**Use** Treatment of metastatic prostatic carcinoma in combination therapy with LHRH agonist analogues

**Usual Dosage** Oral: Adults: Prostatic carcinoma: 250 mg 3 times/day

**Dosage Forms** Capsule: 125 mg

## Flutex® Topical *(Discontinued)*

## fluticasone and salmeterol (floo TIK a sone & sal ME te role)

**Sound-Alike/Look-Alike Issues**
Advair may be confused with Advicor®

**Synonyms** salmeterol and fluticasone

**U.S./Canadian Brand Names** Advair Diskus® [US/Can]

**Therapeutic Category** Beta$_2$-Adrenergic Agonist Agent; Corticosteroid, Inhalant

**Use** Maintenance treatment of asthma in adults and children ≥4 years; **not** for use for relief of acute bronchospasm; maintenance treatment of COPD associated with chronic bronchitis

**Usual Dosage** Oral inhalation: **Note:** Do not use to transfer patients from systemic corticosteroid therapy.

COPD: Adults: Fluticasone 250 mcg/salmeterol 50 mcg twice daily, 12 hours apart

Asthma:
Children 4-11 years: Fluticasone 100 mcg/salmeterol 50 mcg twice daily, 12 hours apart
Children ≥12 and Adults: One inhalation twice daily, morning and evening, 12 hours apart
**Note:** Advair Diskus® is available in 3 strengths, initial dose prescribed should be based upon previous asthma therapy. Dose should be increased after 2 weeks if adequate response is not achieved. Patients should be titrated to lowest effective dose once stable. (Because each strength contains salmeterol 50 mcg/inhalation, dose adjustments should be made by changing inhaler strength. No more than 1 inhalation of any strength should be taken more than twice a day). Maximum dose: Fluticasone 500 mcg/salmeterol 50 mcg, one inhalation twice daily.
Patients not currently on inhaled corticosteroids: Fluticasone 100 mcg/salmeterol 50 mcg
Patients currently using inhaled beclomethasone dipropionate:
≤420 mcg/day: Fluticasone 100 mcg/salmeterol 50 mcg
462-840 mcg/day: Fluticasone 250 mcg/salmeterol 50 mcg
Patients currently using inhaled budesonide:
≤400 mcg/day: Fluticasone 100 mcg/salmeterol 50 mcg
800-1200 mcg/day: Fluticasone 250 mcg/salmeterol 50 mcg
1600 mcg/day: Fluticasone 500 mcg/salmeterol 50 mcg
Patients currently using inhaled flunisolide:
≤1000 mcg/day: Fluticasone 100 mcg/salmeterol 50 mcg
1250-2000 mcg/day: Fluticasone 250 mcg/salmeterol 50 mcg
Patients currently using inhaled fluticasone propionate aerosol:
≤176 mcg/day: Fluticasone 100 mcg/salmeterol 50 mcg
440 mcg/day: Fluticasone 250 mcg/salmeterol 50 mcg
660-880 mcg/day: Fluticasone 500 mcg/salmeterol 50 mcg
Patients currently using inhaled fluticasone propionate powder:
≤200 mcg/day: Fluticasone 100 mcg/salmeterol 50 mcg
500 mcg/day: Fluticasone 250 mcg/salmeterol 50 mcg
1000 mcg/day: Fluticasone 500 mcg/salmeterol 50 mcg
Patients currently using inhaled triamcinolone acetonide:
≤1000 mcg/day: Fluticasone 100 mcg/salmeterol 50 mcg
1100-1600 mcg/day: Fluticasone 250 mcg/salmeterol 50 mcg
(Continued)

## fluticasone and salmeterol *(Continued)*

**Dosage Forms** Powder for oral inhalation:
100/50: Fluticasone propionate 100 mcg and salmeterol xinafoate 50 mcg (28s, 60s) [contains lactose]
250/50: Fluticasone propionate 250 mcg and salmeterol xinafoate 50 mcg (28s, 60s) [contains lactose]
500/50: Fluticasone propionate 500 mcg and salmeterol xinafoate 50 mcg (28s, 60s) [contains lactose]

## fluticasone (nasal) (floo TIK a sone NAY sal)

**U.S./Canadian Brand Names** Flonase® [US/Can]
**Therapeutic Category** Adrenal Corticosteroid
**Use** Intranasal: Management of seasonal and perennial allergic rhinitis and nonallergic rhinitis in patients ≥4 years of age
**Usual Dosage** Rhinitis: Intranasal:
Children ≥4 years and Adolescents: Initial: 1 spray (50 mcg/spray) per nostril once daily; patients not adequately responding or patients with more severe symptoms may use 2 sprays (100 mcg) per nostril. Depending on response, dosage may be reduced to 100 mcg daily. Total daily dosage should not exceed 2 sprays in each nostril (200 mcg)/day. Dosing should be at regular intervals.
Adults: Initial: 2 sprays (50 mcg/spray) per nostril once daily; may also be divided into 100 mcg twice a day. After the first few days, dosage may be reduced to 1 spray per nostril once daily for maintenance therapy. Dosing should be at regular intervals.
**Dosage Forms** Spray, intranasal: 50 mcg/actuation (16 g = 120 actuations)

## fluticasone (oral inhalation) (floo TIK a sone or al in ha LAY shun)

**U.S./Canadian Brand Names** Flovent® Diskus® [Can]; Flovent® HFA [US/Can]
**Therapeutic Category** Adrenal Corticosteroid
**Use** Inhalation: Maintenance treatment of asthma as prophylactic therapy. It is also indicated for patients requiring oral corticosteroid therapy for asthma to assist in total discontinuation or reduction of total oral dose. NOT indicated for the relief of acute bronchospasm.
**Usual Dosage** Inhalation, oral: Asthma:
Flovent®, Flovent® HFA: Children ≥12 years: Refer to Adults dosing.
Flovent® Diskus® [Can]:
Children 4-16 years: Usual starting dose: 50-100 mcg twice daily; may increase to 200 mcg twice daily in patients not adequately controlled; titrate to the lowest effective dose once asthma stability is achieved
Children ≥16 years: Refer to Adults dosing.
Adults: **Note:** Titrate to the lowest effective dose once asthma stability is achieved
Flovent®, Flovent® HFA: Manufacturers labeling: Dosing based on previous therapy
Bronchodilator alone: Recommended starting dose: 88 mcg twice daily; highest recommended dose: 440 mcg twice daily
Inhaled corticosteroids: Recommended starting dose: 88-220 mcg twice daily; highest recommended dose: 440 mcg twice daily; a higher starting dose may be considered in patients previously requiring higher doses of inhaled corticosteroids
Oral corticosteroids: Recommended starting dose:
Flovent®: 880 mcg twice daily
Flovent® HFA: 440 mcg twice daily
Highest recommended dose: 880 mcg twice daily; starting dose is patient dependent. In patients on chronic oral corticosteroids therapy, reduce prednisone dose no faster than 2.5-5 mg/day on a weekly basis; begin taper after 1 week of fluticasone therapy
NIH Asthma Guidelines (administer in divided doses twice daily).
"Low" dose: 88-264 mcg/day
"Medium" dose: 264-660 mcg/day
"High" dose: >660 mcg/day
Flovent® Diskus® [CAN]:
Mild asthma: 100-250 mcg twice daily
Moderate asthma: 250-500 mcg twice da
Severe asthma: 500 mcg twice daily; may increase to 1000 mcg twice daily in very severe patients requiring high doses of corticosteroids
**Dosage Forms** [DSC] = Discontinued product; [CAN] = Canadian brand name
Aerosol for oral inhalation, as propionate [contains CFCs] (Flovent®):
44 mcg/inhalation (7.9 g) [60 metered doses], (13 g) [120 metered doses] [DSC]
110 mcg/inhalation (7.9 g) [60 metered doses], (13 g) [120 metered doses] [DSC]
220 mcg/inhalation (7.9 g) [60 metered doses], (13 g) [120 metered doses] [DSC]

Aerosol for oral inhalation, as propionate [CFC free] (Flovent® HFA):
44 mcg/inhalation (10.6 g) [120 metered doses]
110 mcg/inhalation (12 g) [120 metered doses]
220 mcg/inhalation (12 g) [120 metered doses]
Powder for oral inhalation, as propionate [prefilled blister pack] (Flovent® Diskus®) [CAN; not available in the United States]:
50 mcg (28s, 60s) [contains lactose]
100 mcg (28s, 60s) [contains lactose]
250 mcg (28s, 60s) [contains lactose]
500 mcg (28s, 60s) [contains lactose]

## fluticasone (topical) (floo TIK a sone TOP i kal)

**Sound-Alike/Look-Alike Issues**
Cutivate® may be confused with Ultravate®
**U.S./Canadian Brand Names** Cutivate® [US]
**Therapeutic Category** Adrenal Corticosteroid; Corticosteroid, Topical
**Use** Relief of inflammation and pruritus associated with corticosteroid-responsive dermatoses; atopic dermatitis
**Usual Dosage** Topical:
Corticosteroid-responsive dermatoses:
Children ≥3 months: Cream: Apply sparingly to affected area twice daily. If no improvement is seen within 2 weeks, reassessment of diagnosis may be necessary
Adults: Cream, lotion, ointment: Apply sparingly to affected area twice daily. If no improvement is seen within 2 weeks, reassessment of diagnosis may be necessary.
Atopic dermatitis:
Children ≥3 months: Cream: Apply sparingly to affected area twice daily. If no improvement is seen within 2 weeks, reassessment of diagnosis may be necessary.
Children ≥1 year: Lotion: Apply sparingly to affected area twice daily
Adults: Cream, lotion: Apply sparingly to affected area once or twice daily. If no improvement is seen within 2 weeks, reassessment of diagnosis may be necessary
**Dosage Forms**
Cream, as propionate (Cutivate®): 0.05% (15 g, 30 g, 60 g)
Lotion, as propionate (Cutivate®): 0.05% (60 mL)
Ointment, as propionate (Cutivate®): 0.005% (15 g, 30 g, 60 g)

## fluvastatin (FLOO va sta tin)

**Sound-Alike/Look-Alike Issues**
fluvastatin may be confused with fluoxetine
**U.S./Canadian Brand Names** Lescol® XL [US]; Lescol® [US/Can]
**Therapeutic Category** HMG-CoA Reductase Inhibitor
**Use** To be used as a component of multiple risk factor intervention in patients at risk for atherosclerosis vascular disease due to hypercholesterolemia

Adjunct to dietary therapy to reduce elevated total cholesterol (total-C), LDL-C, triglyceride, and apolipoprotein B (apo-B) levels and to increase HDL-C in primary hypercholesterolemia and mixed dyslipidemia (Fredrickson types IIa and IIb); to slow the progression of coronary atherosclerosis in patients with coronary heart disease; reduce risk of coronary revascularization procedures in patients with coronary heart disease
**Usual Dosage** Adults: Oral:
Patients requiring ≥25% decrease in LDL-C: 40 mg capsule or 80 mg extended release tablet once daily in the evening; may also use 40 mg capsule twice daily
Patients requiring <25% decrease in LDL-C: 20 mg capsule once daily in the evening
**Note:** Dosing range: 20-80 mg/day; adjust dose based on response to therapy; maximum response occurs within 4-6 weeks
**Dosage Forms**
Capsule (Lescol®): 20 mg, 40 mg
Tablet, extended release (Lescol® XL): 80 mg

**Fluviral S/F® [Can]** see influenza virus vaccine on page 437
**Fluvirin® [US]** see influenza virus vaccine on page 437

## fluvoxamine (floo VOKS a meen)
**Sound-Alike/Look-Alike Issues**
fluvoxamine may be confused with flavoxate
Luvox® may be confused with Lasix®, Levoxyl®
**U.S./Canadian Brand Names** Alti-Fluvoxamine [Can]; Apo-Fluvoxamine® [Can]; Luvox® [Can]; Novo-Fluvoxamine [Can]; Nu-Fluvoxamine [Can]; PMS-Fluvoxamine [Can]; Rhoxal-fluvoxamine [Can]
**Therapeutic Category** Antidepressant, Selective Serotonin Reuptake Inhibitor
**Use** Treatment of obsessive-compulsive disorder (OCD) in children ≥8 years of age and adults
**Usual Dosage** Oral: **Note:** When total daily dose exceeds 50 mg, the dose should be given in 2 divided doses:
Children 8-17 years: Initial: 25 mg at bedtime; adjust in 25 mg increments at 4- to 7-day intervals, as tolerated, to maximum therapeutic benefit: Range: 50-200 mg/day
Maximum: Children: 8-11 years: 200 mg/day, adolescents: 300 mg/day; lower doses may be effective in female versus male patients
Adults: Initial: 50 mg at bedtime; adjust in 50 mg increments at 4- to 7-day intervals; usual dose range: 100-300 mg/day; divide total daily dose into 2 doses; administer larger portion at bedtime
**Dosage Forms** Tablet: 25 mg, 50 mg, 100 mg

**Fluxid**™ **[US]** *see* famotidine *on page 327*

**Fluzone**® **[US]** *see* influenza virus vaccine *on page 437*

**FML**® **[US/Can]** *see* fluorometholone *on page 348*

**FML**® **Forte [US/Can]** *see* fluorometholone *on page 348*

**FML-S**® **[US]** *see* sulfacetamide sodium and fluorometholone *on page 772*

**Focalin**™ **[US]** *see* dexmethylphenidate *on page 235*

**Focalin**™ **XR [US]** *see* dexmethylphenidate *on page 235*

**Foille**® **[US-OTC]** *see* benzocaine *on page 95*

**folacin** *see* folic acid *on this page*

**folacin, vitamin B₁₂, and vitamin B₆** *see* folic acid, cyanocobalamin, and pyridoxine *on next page*

**folate** *see* folic acid *on this page*

**Folbee [US]** *see* folic acid, cyanocobalamin, and pyridoxine *on next page*

**Folex**® **PFS**™ *(Discontinued) see* methotrexate *on page 524*

**Folgard**® **[US-OTC]** *see* folic acid, cyanocobalamin, and pyridoxine *on next page*

**Folgard RX 2.2**® **[US]** *see* folic acid, cyanocobalamin, and pyridoxine *on next page*

## folic acid (FOE lik AS id)
**Sound-Alike/Look-Alike Issues**
folic acid may be confused with folinic acid
**Synonyms** folacin; folate; pteroylglutamic acid
**U.S./Canadian Brand Names** Apo-Folic® [Can]
**Therapeutic Category** Vitamin, Water Soluble
**Use** Treatment of megaloblastic and macrocytic anemias due to folate deficiency; dietary supplement to prevent neural tube defects
**Usual Dosage**
Oral, I.M., I.V., SubQ: Anemia:
Infants: 0.1 mg/day
Children <4 years: Up to 0.3 mg/day
Children >4 years and Adults: 0.4 mg/day
Pregnant and lactating women: 0.8 mg/day
Oral:
RDA: Expressed as dietary folate equivalents:
Children:
1-3 years: 150 mcg/day
4-8 years: 200 mcg/day
9-13 years: 300 mcg/day
Children ≥14 years and Adults: 400 mcg/day

Prevention of neural tube defects:
Females of childbearing potential: 400 mcg/day
Females at high risk or with family history of neural tube defects: 4 mg/day

**Dosage Forms**
Injection, solution, as sodium folate: 5 mg/mL (10 mL) [contains benzyl alcohol]
Tablet: 0.4 mg, 0.8 mg, 1 mg

# folic acid, cyanocobalamin, and pyridoxine
(FOE lik AS id, sye an oh koe BAL a min, & peer i DOKS een)

**Synonyms** cyanocobalamin, folic acid, and pyridoxine; folacin, vitamin $B_{12}$, and vitamin $B_6$; pyridoxine, folic acid, and cyanocobalamin

**U.S./Canadian Brand Names** Folbee [US]; Folgard RX 2.2® [US]; Folgard® [US-OTC]; Foltx® [US]; Tricardio B [US]

**Therapeutic Category** Vitamin

**Use** Nutritional supplement in end-stage renal failure, dialysis, hyperhomocysteinemia, homocystinuria, malabsorption syndromes, dietary deficiencies

**Usual Dosage** Oral: Adults: 1 tablet daily

**Dosage Forms** [DSC] = Discontinued product
Tablet: Folic acid 0.8 mg, cyanocobalamin 1000 mcg, and pyridoxine hydrochloride 50 mg
Folbee: Folic acid 2.5 mg, cyanocobalamin 1000 mcg, and pyridoxine hydrochloride 25 mg [dye free, lactose free, and sugar free]
Folgard®: Folic acid 0.8 mg, cyanocobalamin 115 mcg, and pyridoxine hydrochloride 10 mg
Folgard RX 2.2®: Folic acid 2.2 mg, cyanocobalamin 500 mcg, and pyridoxine hydrochloride 25 mg
Foltx®: Folic acid 2.5 mg, cyanocobalamin 1000 mcg, and pyridoxine hydrochloride 25 mg [DSC]; folic acid 2.5 mg, cyanocobalamin 2000 mcg, and pyridoxine hydrochloride 25 mg [new strength]
Tricardio B: Folic acid 0.4 mg, cyanocobalamin 250 mcg, and pyridoxine hydrochloride 25 mg

**folinic acid** *see* leucovorin *on page 470*

**Follistim® [US]** *see* follitropin beta *on this page*

# follitropin alfa (foe li TRO pin AL fa)
**Therapeutic Category** Ovulation Stimulator

**Use** Induction of ovulation in the anovulatory infertile patient in whom the cause of infertility is functional and not caused by primary ovarian failure

**Usual Dosage** Adults (women): SubQ.: Initial: 75 units/day for the first cycle; an incremental dose adjustment of up to 37.5 units may be considered after 14 days; treatment duration should not exceed 35 days unless an E2 rise indicates follicular development

**Dosage Forms** Injection: 37.5 FSH units, 75 FSH units, 150 FSH units

# follitropin beta (foe li TRO pin BAY ta)
**U.S./Canadian Brand Names** Follistim® [US]

**Therapeutic Category** Ovulation Stimulator

**Use** The development of multiple follicles in infertility patients treated in Assisted Reproductive Technology (ART) program and for the induction of ovulation

**Usual Dosage** Adults (female): I.M./SubQ:
Ovulation: In general, a sequential treatment scheme is recommended. This usually starts with daily administration of 75 int. units (International Units) FSH activity. The starting dose is maintained for at least seven days. If there is no ovarian response, the daily dose is then gradually increased until follicle growth and/or plasma estradiol levels indicate an adequate pharmacodynamic response. A daily increase in estradiol levels of 40% to 100% is considered to be optimal. The daily dose is then maintained until preovulatory conditions are reached. Preovulatory conditions are reached when there ultrasonographic evidence of a dominant follicle of at least 18 mm in diameter and/or when plasma estradiol levels of 300-900 picograms/mL (1000-3000 pmol/L) are attained; usually, 7-14 days of treatment are sufficient to reach this state. The administration is then discontinued and ovulation can be induced by administering human chorionic gonadotropin (hCG). If the number of responding follicles is too high or estradiol levels increase too rapidly (ie, more than a daily doubling of estradiol for 2-3 consecutive days), the daily dose should be decreased. Since follicles of >14 mm may lead to pregnancies, multiple preovulatory follicles exceeding 14 mm carry the risk of multiple gestations. In that case, hCG should be withheld and pregnancy should be avoided in order to prevent multiple gestations.
(Continued)

## follitropin beta *(Continued)*

ART: Various stimulation protocols are applied; starting dose of 150-225 units is recommended for at least the first four days; thereafter, the dose may be adjusted individually, based upon ovarian response. In clinical studies, it was shown that maintenance dosages ranging from 75-375 units for 6-12 days are sufficient, although longer treatment may be necessary. May be given either alone, or in combination with a GnRH agonist to prevent premature luteinization; in the latter case, a higher total treatment dose of Follistim® may be required. Ovarian response is monitored by ultrasonography and measurement of plasma estradiol levels; when ultrasonographic evaluation indicates the presence of at least three follicles of 16-20 mm, and there is evidence of a good estradiol (plasma levels of about 300-400 picogram/mL (1000-1300 pmol/L) for each follicle with a diameter >18 mm), the final phase of maturation of the follicles is induced by administration of hCG. Oocyte retrieval is performed 34-35 hours later.

**Dosage Forms** Injection: 75 FSH units

**Foltx® [US]** *see* folic acid, cyanocobalamin, and pyridoxine *on previous page*

**Folvite® *(Discontinued)*** *see* folic acid *on page 356*

## fomepizole *(foe ME pi zole)*

**Synonyms** 4-methylpyrazole; 4-MP

**U.S./Canadian Brand Names** Antizol® [US]

**Therapeutic Category** Antidote

**Use Orphan drug:** Treatment of methanol or ethylene glycol poisoning alone or in combination with hemodialysis

**Usual Dosage** Adults: Ethylene glycol and methanol toxicity: I.V.: A loading dose of 15 mg/kg should be administered, followed by doses of 10 mg/kg every 12 hours for 4 doses, then 15 mg/kg every 12 hours thereafter until ethylene glycol levels have been reduced <20 mg/dL and patient is asymptomatic with normal pH

**Dosage Forms** Injection, solution [preservative free]: 1 g/mL (1.5 mL)

## fomivirsen *(Canada only)* *(foe MI vir sen)*

**Synonyms** fomivirsen sodium

**U.S./Canadian Brand Names** Vitravene™ [Can]

**Therapeutic Category** Antiviral Agent, Ophthalmic

**Use** Local treatment of cytomegalovirus (CMV) retinitis in patients with acquired immunodeficiency syndrome who are intolerant or insufficiently responsive to other treatments for CMV retinitis or when other treatments for CMV retinitis are contraindicated

**Usual Dosage** Adults: Intravitreal injection: Induction: 330 mcg (0.05 mL) every other week for 2 doses, followed by maintenance dose of 330 mcg (0.05 mL) every 4 weeks

If progression occurs during maintenance, a repeat of the induction regimen may be attempted to establish resumed control. Unacceptable inflammation during therapy may be managed by temporary interruption, provided response has been established. Topical corticosteroids have been used to reduce inflammation.

**Dosage Forms** [DSC] = Discontinued product

Injection, solution, intravitreal, as sodium: 6.6 mg/mL (0.25 mL) [DSC]

**fomivirsen sodium** *see* fomivirsen *(Canada only)* *on this page*

## fondaparinux *(fon da PARE i nuks)*

**Synonyms** fondaparinux sodium

**U.S./Canadian Brand Names** Arixtra® [US/Can]

**Therapeutic Category** Factor Xa Inhibitor

**Use** Prophylaxis of deep vein thrombosis (DVT) in patients undergoing surgery for hip replacement, knee replacement, hip fracture (including extended prophylaxis following hip fracture surgery), or abdominal surgery (in patients at risk for thromboembolic complications); treatment of acute pulmonary embolism (PE); treatment of acute DVT without PE

**Usual Dosage** SubQ:

DVT prophylaxis: Adults ≥50 kg: 2.5 mg once daily. **Note:** Initiate dose after hemostasis has been established, 6-8 hours postoperatively.

Usual duration: 5-9 days (up to 10 days following abdominal surgery or up to 11 days following hip replacement or knee replacement)

Extended prophylaxis is recommended following hip fracture surgery (has been tolerated for up to 32 days).

Acute DVT/PE treatment: SubQ: Adults: **Note:** Concomitant treatment with warfarin sodium should be initiated as soon as possible, usually within 72 hours:

<50 kg: 5 mg once daily

50-100 kg: 7.5 mg once daily

>100 kg: 10 mg once daily

Usual duration: 5-9 days  (has been administered up to 26 days)

Dosage Forms Injection, solution, as sodium [preservative free]: 2.5 mg/0.5 mL (0.5 mL); 5 mg/0.4mL (0.4 mL); 7.5 mg/0.6 mL (0.6 mL); 10 mg/0.8 mL (0.8 mL) [prefilled syringe]

**fondaparinux sodium** see fondaparinux on previous page

**Foradil® [Can]** see formoterol on this page

**Foradil® Aerolizer™ [US]** see formoterol on this page

**Forane® [US/Can]** see isoflurane on page 449

## formoterol (for MOH te rol)

Sound-Alike/Look-Alike Issues

Foradil® may be confused with Toradol®

Synonyms formoterol fumarate

U.S./Canadian Brand Names Foradil® Aerolizer™ [US]; Foradil® [Can]; Oxeze® Turbuhaler® [Can]

Therapeutic Category Beta₂-Adrenergic Agonist Agent

Use Maintenance treatment of asthma and prevention of bronchospasm in patients ≥5 years of age with reversible obstructive airway disease, including patients with symptoms of nocturnal asthma, who require regular treatment with inhaled, short-acting beta₂ agonists; maintenance treatment of broncho-constriction in patients with COPD; prevention of exercise-induced bronchospasm in patients ≥5 years of age

**Note:** Oxeze® is also approved in Canada for acute relief of symptoms ("on demand" treatment) in patients ≥6 years of age.

Usual Dosage

Asthma maintenance treatment: Children ≥5 years and Adults: Inhalation: 12 mcg capsule every 12 hours

Oxeze® (CAN): **Note:** Not labeled for use in the U.S.: Children ≥6 years and Adults: Inhalation: 6 mcg or 12 mcg every 12 hours. Maximum dose: Children: 24 mcg/day; Adults: 48 mcg/day

Prevention of exercise-induced bronchospasm: Children ≥5 years and Adults: Inhalation: 12 mcg capsule at least 15 minutes before exercise on an "as needed" basis; additional doses should not be used for another 12 hours. **Note:** If already using for asthma maintenance then should not use additional doses for exercise-induced bronchospasm.

Oxeze® (CAN): **Note:** Not labeled for use in the U.S.: Children ≥6 years and Adults: Inhalation: 6 mcg or 12 mcg at least 15 minutes before exercise.

COPD maintenance treatment: Adults: Inhalation: 12 mcg capsule every 12 hours

**Additional indication for Oxeze® (approved in Canada):** Acute ("on demand") relief of bronchocon-striction: Children ≥12 years and Adults: 6 mcg or 12 mcg as a single dose (maximum dose: 72 mcg in any 24-hour period). The prolonged use of high dosages (48 mcg/day for ≥3 consecutive days) may be a sign of suboptimal control, and should prompt the re-evaluation of therapy.

Dosage Forms [CAN] = Canadian brand name

Aerosol, oral (Oxeze® [CAN]): 6 mcg/dose (60 doses), 12 mcg/dose (60 doses) [contains lactose 600 mcg/dose]

Powder for oral inhalation, as fumarate [capsule]: 12 mcg (12s, 60s) [contains lactose 25 mg]

**formoterol fumarate** see formoterol on this page

**formoterol fumarate dehydrate and budesonide** see budesonide and formoterol (Canada only) on page 119

**Formula EM [US-OTC]** see fructose, dextrose, and phosphoric acid on page 362

**Formula Q® (Discontinued)** see quinine on page 705

**Formulation R™ [US-OTC]** see phenylephrine on page 640

**Formulex® [Can]** see dicyclomine on page 245

**5-formyl tetrahydrofolate** see leucovorin on page 470

**Fortamet**™ **[US]** *see* metformin *on page 519*

**Fortaz**® **[US/Can]** *see* ceftazidime *on page 157*

**Forteo**™ **[US/Can]** *see* teriparatide *on page 787*

**Fortovase**® **[Can]** *see* saquinavir *on page 738*

**Fortovase**® *(Discontinued)* *see* saquinavir *on page 738*

**Fosamax**® **[US/Can]** *see* alendronate *on page 26*

**Fosamax Plus D**™ **[US]** *see* alendronate and cholecalciferol *on page 26*

## fosamprenavir (FOS am pren a veer)

**Sound-Alike/Look-Alike Issues**
Lexiva™ may be confused with Levitra®
**Synonyms** fosamprenavir calcium; GW433908G
**U.S./Canadian Brand Names** Lexiva™ [US]; Telzir® [Can]
**Therapeutic Category** Antiretroviral Agent, Protease Inhibitor
**Use** Treatment of HIV infections in combination with at least two other antiretroviral agents
**Usual Dosage** Oral: Adults: HIV infection:
**Antiretroviral therapy-naive patients:**
Unboosted regimen: 1400 mg twice daily (without ritonavir)
Ritonavir-boosted regimens:
Once-daily regimen: Fosamprenavir 1400 mg plus ritonavir 200 mg once daily
Twice-daily regimen: Fosamprenavir 700 mg plus ritonavir 100 mg twice daily. **Note:** Also used in protease inhibitor-experienced patients
**Protease inhibitor-experienced patients:** Fosamprenavir 700 mg plus ritonavir 100 mg twice daily.
**Note:** Once-daily administration is not recommended in protease inhibitor-experienced patients.
**Combination therapy with efavirenz (ritonavir-boosted regimen):**
Once-daily regimen: Fosamprenavir 1400 mg daily plus ritonavir 300 mg once daily
Twice-daily regimen: No dosage adjustment recommended for twice-daily regimen
**Combination therapy with nevirapine (ritonavir-boosted regimen):** Fosampranavir 700 mg plus ritonavir 100 mg twice daily
**Dosage Forms** Tablet, as calcium: 700 mg
Dosage formulation available in Canada (not in U.S.):
Suspension, oral, as calcium (Telzir®): 50 mg/mL (225 mL)

**fosamprenavir calcium** *see* fosamprenavir *on this page*

## foscarnet (fos KAR net)

**Synonyms** PFA; phosphonoformate; phosphonoformic acid
**U.S./Canadian Brand Names** Foscavir® [US/Can]
**Therapeutic Category** Antiviral Agent
**Use**
Treatment of herpes virus infections suspected to be caused by acyclovir-resistant (HSV, VZV) or ganciclovir-resistant (CMV) strains; this occurs almost exclusively in immunocompromised persons (eg, with advanced AIDS) who have received prolonged treatment for a herpes virus infection
Treatment of CMV retinitis in persons with AIDS
**Usual Dosage**
CMV retinitis: I.V.:
Induction treatment: 60 mg/kg/dose every 8 hours **or** 100 mg/kg every 12 hours for 14-21 days
Maintenance therapy: 90-120 mg/kg/day as a single infusion
Herpes simplex infections (acyclovir-resistant): Induction: I.V.: 40 mg/kg/dose every 8-12 hours for 14-21 days
**Dosage Forms** Injection, solution: 24 mg/mL (250 mL, 500 mL)

**Foscavir**® **[US/Can]** *see* foscarnet *on this page*

## fosfomycin (fos foe MYE sin)

**Sound-Alike/Look-Alike Issues**
Monurol™ may be confused with Monopril®

**Synonyms** fosfomycin tromethamine

**U.S./Canadian Brand Names** Monurol™ [US/Can]

**Therapeutic Category** Antibiotic, Miscellaneous

**Use** Single oral dose in the treatment of uncomplicated urinary tract infections in women due to suscep-tible strains of *E. coli* and *Enterococcus*; may have an advantage over other agents since it maintains high concentration in the urine for up to 48 hours

**Usual Dosage** Adults: Oral: Female: Uncomplicated UTI: Single dose of 3 g in 4 oz of water

**Dosage Forms** Powder, as tromethamine: 3 g

**fosfomycin tromethamine** *see* fosfomycin *on previous page*

## fosinopril (foe SIN oh pril)

**Sound-Alike/Look-Alike Issues**

fosinopril may be confused with lisinopril

Monopril® may be confused with Accupril®, minoxidil, moexipril, Monoket®, Monurol™, ramipril

**Synonyms** fosinopril sodium

**U.S./Canadian Brand Names** Monopril® [US/Can]; Novo-Fosinopril [Can]

**Therapeutic Category** Angiotensin-Converting Enzyme (ACE) Inhibitor

**Use** Treatment of hypertension, either alone or in combination with other antihypertensive agents; treatment of congestive heart failure, left ventricular dysfunction after myocardial infarction

**Usual Dosage** Oral:

Children >50 kg: Hypertension: Initial: 5-10 mg once daily

Adults:

Hypertension: Initial: 10 mg/day; most patients are maintained on 20-40 mg/day. May need to divide the dose into two if trough effect is inadequate; discontinue the diuretic, if possible 2-3 days before initiation of therapy; resume diuretic therapy carefully, if needed.

Heart failure: Initial: 10 mg/day (5 mg if renal dysfunction present) and increase, as needed, to a maximum of 40 mg once daily over several weeks; usual dose: 20-40 mg/day. If hypotension, orthostasis, or azotemia occur during titration, consider decreasing concomitant diuretic dose, if any.

**Dosage Forms** Tablet, as sodium: 10 mg, 20 mg, 40 mg

## fosinopril and hydrochlorothiazide (foe SIN oh pril & hye droe klor oh THYE a zide)

**Sound-Alike/Look-Alike Issues**

Monopril® may be confused with Accupril®, minoxidil, moexipril, Monoket®, Monurol™, ramipril

**Synonyms** hydrochlorothiazide and fosinopril

**U.S./Canadian Brand Names** Monopril-HCT® [US/Can]

**Therapeutic Category** Angiotensin-Converting Enzyme (ACE) Inhibitor

**Use** Treatment of hypertension; not indicated for first-line treatment

**Usual Dosage Note:** A patient whose blood pressure is not adequately controlled with fosinopril or hydrochlorothiazide monotherapy may be switched to combination therapy; **not** for initial treatment.

Adults: Oral: Hypertension: Fosinopril 10-80 mg per day, hydrochlorothiazide 12.5-50 mg per day

**Dosage Forms** Tablet:

10/12.5: Fosinopril 10 mg and hydrochlorothiazide 12.5 mg

20/12.5: Fosinopril 20 mg and hydrochlorothiazide 12.5 mg

**fosinopril sodium** *see* fosinopril *on this page*

## fosphenytoin (FOS fen i toyn)

**Sound-Alike/Look-Alike Issues**

Cerebyx® may be confused with Celebrex®, Celexa™, Cerezyme®

**Synonyms** fosphenytoin sodium

**U.S./Canadian Brand Names** Cerebyx® [US/Can]

**Therapeutic Category** Hydantoin

**Use** Used for the control of generalized convulsive status epilepticus and prevention and treatment of seizures occurring during neurosurgery; indicated for short-term parenteral administration when other means of phenytoin administration are unavailable, inappropriate or deemed less advantageous (the safety and effectiveness of fosphenytoin in this use has not been systematically evaluated for more than 5 days)

**Usual Dosage The dose, concentration in solutions, and infusion rates for fosphenytoin are expressed as phenytoin sodium equivalents (PE); fosphenytoin should always be prescribed and dispensed in phenytoin sodium equivalents (PE)**

(Continued)

## fosphenytoin *(Continued)*

Adults:

Status epilepticus: I.V.: Loading dose: 15-20 mg PE/kg I.V. administered at 100-150 mg PE/minute

Nonemergent loading and maintenance dosing: I.V. or I.M.:

Loading dose: 10-20 mg PE/kg I.V. or I.M. (maximum I.V. rate: 150 mg PE/minute)

Initial daily maintenance dose: 4-6 mg PE/kg/day I.V. or I.M.

I.M. or I.V. substitution for oral phenytoin therapy: May be substituted for oral phenytoin sodium at the same total daily dose; however, Dilantin® capsules are ~90% bioavailable by the oral route; phenytoin, supplied as fosphenytoin, is 100% bioavailable by both the I.M. and I.V. routes; for this reason, plasma phenytoin concentrations may increase when I.M. or I.V. fosphenytoin is substituted for oral phenytoin sodium therapy; in clinical trials I.M. fosphenytoin was administered as a single daily dose utilizing either 1 or 2 injection sites; some patients may require more frequent dosing

**Dosage Forms** Injection, solution, as sodium: 75 mg/mL [equivalent to phenytoin sodium 50 mg/mL] (2 mL, 10 mL)

**fosphenytoin sodium** *see* fosphenytoin *on previous page*

**Fosrenol™ [US]** *see* lanthanum *on page 468*

**Fostex® 10% BPO [US-OTC]** *see* benzoyl peroxide *on page 98*

**Fragmin® [US/Can]** *see* dalteparin *on page 221*

## framycetin *(Canada only)* (fra mye CEE tin)

**U.S./Canadian Brand Names** Sofra-Tulle® [Can]

**Therapeutic Category** Antibiotic, Topical

**Use** Treatment of infected or potentially infected burns, wounds, ulcers, and graft sites

**Usual Dosage** A single layer to be applied directly to the wound and covered with an appropriate dressing. If exudative, dressings should be changed at least daily. In case of leg ulcers, cut dressing accurately to size of ulcer to decrease the risk of sensitization and to avoid contact with surrounding healthy skin.

**Dosage Forms** Dressing, gauze: 1% (10 cm x 10 cm, 10 cm x 30 cm)

**Fraxiparine™ [Can]** *see* nadroparin *(Canada only) on page 557*

**Fraxiparine™ Forte [Can]** *see* nadroparin *(Canada only) on page 557*

**Freezone® [US-OTC]** *see* salicylic acid *on page 734*

**Frisium® [Can]** *see* clobazam *(Canada only) on page 194*

**Froben® [Can]** *see* flurbiprofen *on page 352*

**Froben-SR® [Can]** *see* flurbiprofen *on page 352*

**Frova® [US]** *see* frovatriptan *on this page*

## frovatriptan (froe va TRIP tan)

**Synonyms** frovatriptan succinate

**U.S./Canadian Brand Names** Frova® [US]

**Therapeutic Category** Antimigraine Agent; Serotonin 5-HT$_{1B, 1D}$ Receptor Agonist

**Use** Acute treatment of migraine with or without aura in adults

**Usual Dosage** Oral: Adults: Migraine: 2.5 mg; if headache recurs, a second dose may be given if first dose provided some relief and at least 2 hours have elapsed since the first dose (maximum daily dose: 7.5 mg)

**Dosage Forms** Tablet, as base: 2.5 mg

**frovatriptan succinate** *see* frovatriptan *on this page*

## fructose, dextrose, and phosphoric acid (FRUK tose, DEKS trose, & foss FOR ik AS id)

**Sound-Alike/Look-Alike Issues**

Emetrol® may be confused with emetine

**Synonyms** dextrose, levulose and phosphoric acid; levulose, dextrose and phosphoric acid; phosphorated carbohydrate solution; phosphoric acid, levulose and dextrose

**U.S./Canadian Brand Names** Emetrol® [US-OTC]; Especol® [US-OTC]; Formula EM [US-OTC]; Kalmz [US-OTC]; Nausea Relief [US-OTC]; Nausetrol® [US-OTC]

**Therapeutic Category** Antiemetic

**Use** Relief of nausea associated with upset stomach that occurs with intestinal flu, food indiscretions, and emotional upsets

**Usual Dosage** Oral:

Motion sickness and vomiting due to drug therapy: 5 mL doses for young children; 15 mL doses for older children and adults

Regurgitation in infants: 5 or 10 mL, 10-15 minutes before each feeding; in refractory cases: 10-15 mL, 30 minutes before each feeding

Vomiting due to psychogenic factors:

Children: 5-10 mL; repeat dose every 15 minutes until distress subsides; do not take for more than 1 hour

Adults: 15-30 mL; repeat dose every 15 minutes until distress subsides; do not take for more than 1 hour

**Dosage Forms**

Liquid, oral: Fructose 1.87 g, dextrose 1.87 g, and phosphoric acid 21.5 mg per 5 mL (120 mL)

Emetrol®: Fructose 1.87 g, dextrose 1.87 g, and phosphoric acid 21.5 mg per 5 mL (120 mL, 240 mL) [cherry and lemon mint flavors]

Especol®: Fructose 1.87 g, dextrose 1.87 g, and phosphoric acid 21.5 mg per 5 mL (120 mL) [cherry and lemon-lime flavors]

Formula EM, Nausea Relief: Fructose 1.87 g, dextrose 1.87 g, and phosphoric acid 21.5 mg per 5 mL (120 mL)

Kalmz, Nausetrol®: Fructose 1.87 g, dextrose 1.87 g, and phosphoric acid 21.5 mg per 5 mL (120 mL) [cherry flavor]

**frusemide** *see* furosemide *on next page*

**FS** *see* fibrin sealant kit *on page 337*

**FS Shampoo® Topical *(Discontinued)*** *see* fluocinolone *on page 344*

**FTC** *see* emtricitabine *on page 282*

**FTP-Domperidone Maleate [Can]** *see* domperidone *(Canada only) on page 266*

**FU** *see* fluorouracil *on page 349*

**5-FU** *see* fluorouracil *on page 349*

**Fucidin® [Can]** *see* fusidic acid *(Canada only) on next page*

**Fucithalmic® [Can]** *see* fusidic acid *(Canada only) on next page*

**FUDR® [US/Can]** *see* floxuridine *on page 341*

**5-FUDR** *see* floxuridine *on page 341*

**Ful-Glo® [US]** *see* fluorescein sodium *on page 346*

**fulvestrant** (fool VES trant)

**Synonyms** ICI-182,780; zeneca 182,780; ZM-182,780

**U.S./Canadian Brand Names** Faslodex® [US]

**Therapeutic Category** Antineoplastic Agent, Estrogen Receptor Antagonist

**Use** Treatment of hormone receptor positive metastatic breast cancer in postmenopausal women with disease progression following antiestrogen therapy.

**Usual Dosage** I.M.: Adults (postmenopausal women): 250 mg at 1-month intervals

**Dosage Forms** Injection, solution: 50 mg/mL (2.5 mL, 5 mL) [prefilled syringe; contains alcohol, benzyl alcohol, benzyl stearate, castor oil]

**Fumasorb® *(Discontinued)*** *see* ferrous fumarate *on page 334*

**Fumerin® *(Discontinued)*** *see* ferrous fumarate *on page 334*

**Funduscein® Injection *(Discontinued)*** *see* fluorescein sodium *on page 346*

**Fungi-Guard [US-OTC]** *see* tolnaftate *on page 809*

**Fungi-Nail® [US-OTC]** *see* undecylenic acid and derivatives *on page 833*

**Fungizone® [Can]** *see* amphotericin B (conventional) *on page 49*

**Fung-O® [US-OTC]** *see* salicylic acid *on page 734*

**Fungoid® Tincture [US-OTC]** *see* miconazole *on page 537*

**Furacin® Topical *(Discontinued)*** *see* nitrofurazone *on page 578*

**Furadantin**® **[US]** *see* nitrofurantoin *on page 577*

**Furalan**® *(Discontinued) see* nitrofurantoin *on page 577*

**Furan**® *(Discontinued) see* nitrofurantoin *on page 577*

**Furanite**® *(Discontinued) see* nitrofurantoin *on page 577*

**furazosin** *see* prazosin *on page 672*

## furosemide (fyoor OH se mide)

**Sound-Alike/Look-Alike Issues**
furosemide may be confused with torsemide
Lasix® may be confused with Esidrix®, Lanoxin®, Lidex®, Lomotil®, Luvox®, Luxiq®

**Synonyms** frusemide

**U.S./Canadian Brand Names** Apo-Furosemide® [Can]; Lasix® Special [Can]; Lasix® [US/Can]; Novo-Semide [Can]

**Therapeutic Category** Diuretic, Loop

**Use** Management of edema associated with congestive heart failure and hepatic or renal disease; alone or in combination with antihypertensives in treatment of hypertension

**Usual Dosage**
Infants and Children:
Oral: 1-2 mg/kg/dose increased in increments of 1 mg/kg/dose with each succeeding dose until a satisfactory effect is achieved to a maximum of 6 mg/kg/dose no more frequently than 6 hours.
I.M., I.V.: 1 mg/kg/dose, increasing by each succeeding dose at 1 mg/kg/dose at intervals of 6-12 hours until a satisfactory response up to 6 mg/kg/dose.
Adults:
Oral: 20-80 mg/dose initially increased in increments of 20-40 mg/dose at intervals of 6-8 hours; usual maintenance dose interval is twice daily or every day; may be titrated up to 600 mg/day with severe edematous states.
Hypertension (JNC 7): 20-80 mg/day in 2 divided doses
I.M., I.V.: 20-40 mg/dose, may be repeated in 1-2 hours as needed and increased by 20 mg/dose until the desired effect has been obtained. Usual dosing interval: 6-12 hours; for acute pulmonary edema, the usual dose is 40 mg I.V. over 1-2 minutes. If not adequate, may increase dose to 80 mg.
Continuous I.V. infusion: Initial I.V. bolus dose of 0.1 mg/kg followed by continuous I.V. infusion doses of 0.1 mg/kg/hour doubled every 2 hours to a maximum of 0.4 mg/kg/hour if urine output is <1 mL/kg/hour have been found to be effective and result in a lower daily requirement of furosemide than with intermittent dosing. Other studies have used a rate of ≤4 mg/minute as a continuous I.V. infusion.
Refractory heart failure: Oral, I.V.: Doses up to 8 g/day have been used.

**Dosage Forms**
Injection, solution: 10 mg/mL (2 mL, 4 mL, 8 mL, 10 mL)
Solution, oral: 10 mg/mL (60 mL, 120 mL) [orange flavor]; 40 mg/5 mL (5 mL, 500 mL) [pineapple-peach flavor]
Tablet (Lasix®): 20 mg, 40 mg, 80 mg

## fusidic acid *(Canada only)* (fyoo SI dik AS id)

**Synonyms** sodium fusidate

**U.S./Canadian Brand Names** Fucidin® [Can]; Fucithalmic® [Can]

**Therapeutic Category** Antifungal Agent, Systemic

**Use**
Systemic: Treatment of skin and soft tissue infections, or osteomyelitis, caused by susceptible organisms, including *Staphylococcus aureus* (penicillinase-producing or nonpenicillinase strains); may be used in the treatment of pneumonia, septicemia, endocarditis, burns, and cystic fibrosis caused by susceptible organisms when other antibiotics have failed
Topical: Treatment of primary and secondary skin infections caused by susceptible organisms
Ophthalmic: Treatment of superficial infections of the eye and conjunctiva caused by susceptible organisms

**Usual Dosage**
I.V.:
Children ≤12 years: 20 mg/kg/day in 3 divided doses
Children >12 years and Adults: 500 mg sodium fusidate 3 times/day
Ophthalmic: Children ≥2 years and Adults: Instill 1 drop in each eye every 12 hours for 7 days
Topical: Children and Adults: Apply to affected area 3-4 times/day until favorable results are achieved. If a gauze dressing is used, frequency of application may be reduced to 1-2 times/day.

Oral: Adults: 500 mg sodium fusidate 3 times/day. (**Note:** Oral dosage may be increased to 1000 mg 3 times/day in fulminating infections.)

**Dosage Forms**
Cream, as fusidic acid (Fucidin®): 2% (15 g, 30 g)
Injection, powder for reconstitution, as sodium fusidate (Fucidin®): 500 mg [packaged with 10 mL diluent/buffer solution]
Ointment, topical, as sodium fusidate (Fucidin®): 2% (15 g, 30 g) [contains lanolin]
Suspension, ophthalmic, as fusidic acid (Fucithalmic®): 10 mg/g [1%] (0.2 g) [unit-dose, without preservative]; (3 g, 5 g) [multidose, contains benzalkonium chloride]
Tablet [film coated], as sodium fusidate (Fucidin®): 250 mg

**Fuzeon™ [US/Can]** *see* enfuvirtide *on page 285*

**FXT [Can]** *see* fluoxetine *on page 349*

**G-1® *(Discontinued)***

# gabapentin (GA ba pen tin)
**Sound-Alike/Look-Alike Issues**
Neurontin® may be confused with Neoral®, Noroxin®
**U.S./Canadian Brand Names** Apo-Gabapentin® [Can]; Gen-Gabapentin [Can]; Neurontin® [US/Can]; Novo-Gabapentin [Can]; Nu-Gabapentin [Can]; PMS-Gabapentin [Can]
**Therapeutic Category** Anticonvulsant
**Use** Adjunct for treatment of partial seizures with and without secondary generalized seizures in patients >12 years of age with epilepsy; adjunct for treatment of partial seizures in pediatric patients 3-12 years of age; management of postherpetic neuralgia (PHN) in adults
**Usual Dosage** Oral:
Children: Anticonvulsant:
3-12 years: Initial: 10-15 mg/kg/day in 3 divided doses; titrate to effective dose over ~3 days; dosages of up to 50 mg/kg/day have been tolerated in clinical studies
3-4 years: Effective dose: 40 mg/kg/day in 3 divided doses
≥5-12 years: Effective dose: 25-35 mg/kg/day in 3 divided doses
See "Note" in Adults dosing.
Children >12 years and Adults:
Anticonvulsant: Initial: 300 mg 3 times/day; if necessary the dose may be increased up to 1800 mg/day. Doses of up to 2400 mg/day have been tolerated in long-term clinical studies; up to 3600 mg/day has been tolerated in short-term studies.
**Note:** If gabapentin is discontinued or if another anticonvulsant is added to therapy, it should be done slowly over a minimum of 1 week
Adults: Postherpetic neuralgia or neuropathic pain: Day 1: 300 mg, Day 2: 300 mg twice daily, Day 3: 300 mg 3 times/day; dose may be titrated as needed for pain relief (range: 1800-3600 mg/day, daily doses >1800 mg do not generally show greater benefit)
**Dosage Forms**
Capsule (Neurontin®): 100 mg, 300 mg, 400 mg
Solution, oral (Neurontin®): 250 mg/5 mL (480 mL) [cool strawberry anise flavor]
Tablet: 100 mg, 300 mg, 400 mg
Neurontin®: 600 mg, 800 mg

**Gabitril® [US/Can]** *see* tiagabine *on page 801*

**gadopentetate dimeglumine** *see* radiological/contrast media (ionic) *on page 707*

**gadoteridol** *see* radiological/contrast media (nonionic) *on page 709*

# galantamine (ga LAN ta meen)
**Sound-Alike/Look-Alike Issues**
Reminyl® may be confused with Amaryl®
**Synonyms** galantamine hydrobromide
**U.S./Canadian Brand Names** Razadyne™ ER [US]; Razadyne™ [US]; Reminyl® [US/Can]
**Therapeutic Category** Acetylcholinesterase Inhibitor (Central)
**Use** Treatment of mild-to-moderate dementia of Alzheimer disease
**Usual Dosage** Oral: Adults:
**Note:** Oral solution and tablet should be taken with breakfast and dinner; capsule should be taken with breakfast. If therapy is interrupted for ≥3 days, restart at the lowest dose and increase to current dose.
(Continued)

## galantamine *(Continued)*

Immediate release tablet or solution: Mild-to-moderate dementia of Alzheimer: Initial: 4 mg twice a day for 4 weeks; if tolerated, increase to 8 mg twice daily for ≥4 weeks; if tolerated, increase to 12 mg twice daily

Range: 16-24 mg/day in 2 divided doses

Extended-release capsule: Initial: 8 mg once daily for 4 weeks; if tolerated, increase to 16 mg once daily for ≥4 weeks; if tolerated, increase to 24 mg once daily

Range: 16-24 mg once daily

**Conversion to galantamine from other cholinesterase inhibitors:** Patients experiencing poor tolerability with donepezil or rivastigmine should wait until side effects subside or allow a 7-day washout period prior to beginning galantamine. Patients not experiencing side effects with donepezil or rivastigmine may begin galantamine therapy the day immediately following discontinuation of previous therapy.

**Dosage Forms**

Capsule, extended release, as hydrobromide: 8 mg, 16 mg, 24 mg [contains gelatin]

Solution, oral, as hydrobromide: 4 mg/mL (100 mL) [with calibrated pipette]

Tablet, as hydrobromide: 4 mg, 8 mg, 12 mg

**galantamine hydrobromide** *see* galantamine *on previous page*

## galsulfase *(gal SUL fase)*

**Synonyms** recombinant N-acetylgalactosamine 4-sulfatase; rhASB

**U.S./Canadian Brand Names** Naglazyme™ [US]

**Therapeutic Category** Enzyme

**Use** Replacement therapy in mucopolysaccharidosis VI (MPS VI; Maroteaux-Lamy Syndrome) for improvement of walking and stair-climbing capacity

**Usual Dosage** MPS VI: Children >5 years: I.V.: 1 mg/kg once weekly

**Dosage Forms** Injection, solution [preservative free]: 5 mg/5 mL (5 mL)

**Gamimune® N [US/Can]** *see* immune globulin (intravenous) *on page 433*

**gamma benzene hexachloride** *see* lindane *on page 483*

**Gammagard® Liquid [US]** *see* immune globulin (intravenous) *on page 433*

**Gammagard® S/D [US/Can]** *see* immune globulin (intravenous) *on page 433*

**gamma globulin** *see* immune globulin (intramuscular) *on page 432*

**gamma hydroxybutyric acid** *see* sodium oxybate *on page 755*

**gammaphos** *see* amifostine *on page 38*

**Gammar®-P I.V. [US]** *see* immune globulin (intravenous) *on page 433*

**Gamulin® Rh *(Discontinued)***

**Gamunex® [US/Can]** *see* immune globulin (intravenous) *on page 433*

## ganciclovir *(gan SYE kloe veer)*

**Sound-Alike/Look-Alike Issues**

Cytovene® may be confused with Cytosar®, Cytosar-U®

**Synonyms** DHPG sodium; GCV sodium; nordeoxyguanosine

**U.S./Canadian Brand Names** Cytovene® [US/Can]; Vitrasert® [US/Can]

**Therapeutic Category** Antiviral Agent

**Use**

Parenteral: Treatment of CMV retinitis in immunocompromised individuals, including patients with acquired immunodeficiency syndrome; prophylaxis of CMV infection in transplant patients

Oral: Alternative to the I.V. formulation for maintenance treatment of CMV retinitis in immunocompromised patients, including patients with AIDS, in whom retinitis is stable following appropriate induction therapy and for whom the risk of more rapid progression is balanced by the benefit associated with avoiding daily I.V. infusions.

Implant: Treatment of CMV retinitis

**Usual Dosage**

CMV retinitis: Slow I.V. infusion (dosing is based on total body weight):

Children >3 months and Adults:

Induction therapy: 5 mg/kg/dose every 12 hours for 14-21 days followed by maintenance therapy

Maintenance therapy: 5 mg/kg/day as a single daily dose for 7 days/week or 6 mg/kg/day for 5 days/week

CMV retinitis: Oral: 1000 mg 3 times/day with food **or** 500 mg 6 times/day with food

Prevention of CMV disease in patients with advanced HIV infection and normal renal function: Oral: 1000 mg 3 times/day with food

Prevention of CMV disease in transplant patients: Same initial and maintenance dose as CMV retinitis except duration of initial course is 7-14 days, duration of maintenance therapy is dependent on clinical condition and degree of immunosuppression

Intravitreal implant: One implant for 5- to 8-month period; following depletion of ganciclovir, as evidenced by progression of retinitis, implant may be removed and replaced

**Dosage Forms**

Capsule: 250 mg, 500 mg

Cytovene®: 250 mg, 500 mg [DSC]

Implant, intravitreal (Vitrasert®): 4.5 mg [released gradually over 5-8 months]

Injection, powder for reconstitution, as sodium (Cytovene®): 500 mg

**Ganidin NR [US]** *see* guaifenesin *on page 383*

## ganirelix (ga ni REL ix)

**Synonyms** ganirelix acetate

**U.S./Canadian Brand Names** Antagon® [US/Can]; Orgalutran® [Can]

**Therapeutic Category** Antigonadotropic Agent

**Use** Inhibits premature luteinizing hormone (LH) surges in women undergoing controlled ovarian hyperstimulation in fertility clinics.

**Usual Dosage** Adult: SubQ: 250 mcg/day during the mid-to-late phase after initiating follicle-stimulating hormone on day 2 or 3 of cycle. Treatment should be continued daily until the day of chorionic gonadotropin administration.

**Dosage Forms** Injection, solution, as acetate: 250 mcg/0.5 mL [prefilled glass syringe with 27-gauge x 1/2 inch needle]

**ganirelix acetate** *see* ganirelix *on this page*

**Gani-Tuss® DM NR [US]** *see* guaifenesin and dextromethorphan *on page 385*

**Gani-Tuss® NR [US]** *see* guaifenesin and codeine *on page 384*

**Gantrisin® [US]** *see* sulfisoxazole *on page 775*

**GAR-936** *see* tigecycline *on page 803*

**Garamycin® *(Discontinued)*** *see* gentamicin *on page 372*

**Gas-X® [US-OTC]** *see* simethicone *on page 748*

**Gas-X® Extra Strength [US-OTC]** *see* simethicone *on page 748*

**Gas-X® Maximum Strength [US-OTC]** *see* simethicone *on page 748*

**Gas Ban™ [US-OTC]** *see* calcium carbonate and simethicone *on page 132*

**Gas-Ban DS® *(Discontinued)*** *see* aluminum hydroxide, magnesium hydroxide, and simethicone *on page 35*

**Gastrocrom® [US]** *see* cromolyn sodium *on page 211*

**Gastrografin® [US]** *see* radiological/contrast media (ionic) *on page 707*

**Gastrosed™ *(Discontinued)*** *see* hyoscyamine *on page 424*

## gatifloxacin (gat i FLOKS a sin)

**U.S./Canadian Brand Names** Tequin® [US/Can]; Zymar™ [US/Can]

**Therapeutic Category** Antibiotic, Quinolone

**Use**

Oral, I.V.: Treatment of the following infections when caused by susceptible bacteria: Acute bacterial exacerbation of chronic bronchitis; acute sinusitis; community-acquired pneumonia including pneumonia caused by multidrug-resistant *S. pneumoniae* (MDRSP); uncomplicated skin and skin structure infection; uncomplicated urinary tract infections (cystitis); complicated urinary tract infections; pyelonephritis; uncomplicated urethral and cervical gonorrhea; acute, uncomplicated rectal infections in women

Ophthalmic: Bacterial conjunctivitis

(Continued)

## gatifloxacin *(Continued)*

**Usual Dosage**
Children ≥1 year and Adults: Ophthalmic: Bacterial conjunctivitis:
Days 1 and 2: Instill 1 drop into affected eye(s) every 2 hours while awake (maximum: 8 times/day)
Days 3-7: Instill 1 drop into affected eye(s) up to 4 times/day while awake
Adults: Oral, I.V.:
Acute bacterial exacerbation of chronic bronchitis: 400 mg every 24 hours for 5 days
Acute sinusitis: 400 mg every 24 hours for 10 days
Community-acquired pneumonia: 400 mg every 24 hours for 7-14 days
Uncomplicated skin/skin structure infections: 400 mg every 24 hours for 7-10 days
Uncomplicated urinary tract infections (cystitis): 400 mg single dose or 200 mg every 24 hours for 3 days
Complicated urinary tract infections: 400 mg every 24 hours for 7-10 days
Acute pyelonephritis: 400 mg every 24 hours for 7-10 days
Uncomplicated urethral gonorrhea in men, cervical or rectal gonorrhea in women: 400 mg single dose
**Dosage Forms**
Injection, infusion [premixed in $D_5W$] (Tequin®): 200 mg (100 mL); 400 mg (200 mL)
Injection, solution [preservative free] (Tequin®): 10 mg/mL (40 mL)
Solution, ophthalmic (Zymar™): 0.3% (2.5 mL, 5 mL) [contains benzalkonium chloride]
Tablet (Tequin®): 200 mg, 400 mg
Tequin® Teq-paq™ [unit-dose pack]: 400 mg (5s)

**Gaviscon® Extra Strength [US-OTC]** *see* aluminum hydroxide and magnesium carbonate *on page 35*

**Gaviscon® Liquid [US-OTC]** *see* aluminum hydroxide and magnesium carbonate *on page 35*

**G-CSF** *see* filgrastim *on page 338*

**G-CSF (PEG conjugate)** *see* pegfilgrastim *on page 623*

**GCV sodium** *see* ganciclovir *on page 366*

**Gebauer's Ethyl Chloride® [US]** *see* ethyl chloride *on page 320*

**Gee Gee®** *(Discontinued)* *see* guaifenesin *on page 383*

## gefitinib *(ge FI tye nib)*

**Sound-Alike/Look-Alike Issues**
gefitinib may be confused with erlotinib
**Synonyms** NSC-715055; ZD1839
**U.S./Canadian Brand Names** IRESSA® [US]
**Therapeutic Category** Antineoplastic, Tyrosine Kinase Inhibitor
**Use U.S. Labeling:** Monotherapy for continued treatment of locally advanced or metastatic nonsmall cell lung cancer after failure of platinum-based and docetaxel therapies. Treatment is limited to patients who are benefiting or have benefited from treatment with gefitinib.
**Note:** Due to the lack of improved survival data from clinical trials of gefitinib, and in response to positive survival data with another EGFR inhibitor, physicians are advised to use other treatment options in advanced nonsmall cell lung cancer patients following one or two prior chemotherapy regimens when they are refractory/intolerant to their most recent regimen.

**Canada labeling:** Approved indication is limited to NSCLC patients with epidermal growth factor receptor (EGFR) expression status positive or unknown.
**Usual Dosage Note:** In response to the lack of improved survival data from the ISEL trial, AstraZeneca has temporarily suspended promotion of this drug.
Oral: Adults: 250 mg/day; consider 500 mg/day in patients receiving effective CYP3A4 inducers (eg, rifampin, phenytoin)
**Dosage Forms** Tablet: 250 mg

## gelatin (absorbable) *(JEL a tin, ab SORB a ble)*

**Synonyms** absorbable gelatin sponge
**U.S./Canadian Brand Names** Gelfilm® [US]; Gelfoam® [US]
**Therapeutic Category** Hemostatic Agent
**Use** Adjunct to provide hemostasis in surgery; open prostatic surgery
**Usual Dosage** Hemostasis: Apply packs or sponges dry or saturated with sodium chloride. When applied dry, hold in place with moderate pressure. When applied wet, squeeze to remove air bubbles. The

powder is applied as a paste prepared by adding approximately 4 mL of sterile saline solution to the powder.

**Dosage Forms**
Film, ophthalmic (Gelfilm®): 25 mm x 50 mm (6s)
Film, topical (Gelfilm®): 100 mm x 125 mm (1s)
Powder, topical (Gelfoam®): 1 g
Sponge, dental (Gelfoam®): Size 4 (12s)
Sponge, topical (Gelfoam®):
  Size 50 (4s)
  Size 100 (6s)
  Size 200 (6s)
  Size 2 cm (1s)
  Size 6 cm (6s)
  Size 12-7 mm (12s)

## gelatin, pectin, and methylcellulose (JEL a tin, PEK tin, & meth il SEL yoo lose)
**Synonyms** methylcellulose, gelatin, and pectin; pectin, gelatin, and methylcellulose
**Therapeutic Category** Protectant, Topical
**Use** Temporary relief from minor oral irritations
**Usual Dosage** Press small dabs into place until the involved area is coated with a thin film; do not try to spread onto area; may be used as often as needed

**Gelclair® [US]** see maltodextrin on page 501

**Gelfilm® [US]** see gelatin (absorbable) on previous page

**Gelfoam® [US]** see gelatin (absorbable) on previous page

**Gel-Kam® [US-OTC]** see fluoride on page 347

**Gel-Kam® Rinse [US]** see fluoride on page 347

**Gel-Tin® (Discontinued)** see fluoride on page 347

**Gelucast® [US]** see zinc gelatin on page 861

**Gelusil® [US-OTC/Can]** see aluminum hydroxide, magnesium hydroxide, and simethicone on page 35

**Gelusil® Extra Strength [Can]** see aluminum hydroxide and magnesium hydroxide on page 35

## gemcitabine (jem SITE a been)
**Sound-Alike/Look-Alike Issues**
  Gemzar® may be confused with Zinecard®
**Synonyms** gemcitabine hydrochloride
**U.S./Canadian Brand Names** Gemzar® [US/Can]
**Therapeutic Category** Antineoplastic Agent
**Use**
  Adenocarcinoma of the pancreas: First-line therapy in locally-advanced (nonresectable stage II or stage III) or metastatic (stage IV) adenocarcinoma of the pancreas
  Breast cancer: First-line therapy in metastatic breast cancer
  Nonsmall-cell lung cancer: First-line therapy in locally-advanced (stage IIIA or IIIB) or metastatic (stage IV) nonsmall-cell lung cancer
**Usual Dosage** Refer to individual protocols. **Note**: Prolongation of the infusion time >60 minutes and administration more frequently than once weekly have been shown to increase toxicity. I.V.:
  Pancreatic cancer: Initial: 1000 mg/m$^2$ over 30 minutes once weekly for up to 7 weeks followed by 1 week rest; subsequent cycles once weekly for 3 consecutive weeks out of every 4 weeks.
    Dose adjustment: Patients who complete an entire cycle of therapy may have the dose in subsequent cycles increased by 25% as long as the absolute granulocyte count (AGC) nadir is >1500 x 10$^6$/L, platelet nadir is >100,000 x 10$^6$/L, and nonhematologic toxicity is less than WHO Grade 1. If the increased dose is tolerated (with the same parameters) the dose in subsequent cycles may again be increased by 20%.
  Nonsmall cell lung cancer:
    28-day cycle: 1000 mg/m$^2$ over 30 minutes on days 1, 8, 15; repeat every 28 days
    **or**
    21-day cycle: 1250 mg/m$^2$ over 30 minutes on days 1, 8; repeat every 21 days
  (Continued)

## gemcitabine *(Continued)*

Breast cancer: 1250 mg/m$^2$ over 30 minutes on days 1 and 8 of each 21-day cycle

**Dosage Forms** Injection, powder for reconstitution, as hydrochloride: 200 mg, 1 g

**gemcitabine hydrochloride** *see gemcitabine on previous page*

## gemfibrozil (jem Fl broe zil)

**Sound-Alike/Look-Alike Issues**

Lopid® may be confused with Levbid®, Lodine®, Lorabid®, Slo-bid™

**Synonyms** CI-719

**U.S./Canadian Brand Names** Apo-Gemfibrozil® [Can]; Gen-Gemfibrozil [Can]; Lopid® [US/Can]; Novo-Gemfibrozil [Can]; Nu-Gemfibrozil [Can]; PMS-Gemfibrozil [Can]

**Therapeutic Category** Antihyperlipidemic Agent, Miscellaneous

**Use** Treatment of hypertriglyceridemia in types IV and V hyperlipidemia for patients who are at greater risk for pancreatitis and who have not responded to dietary intervention

**Usual Dosage** Adults: Oral: 1200 mg/day in 2 divided doses, 30 minutes before breakfast and dinner

**Dosage Forms** Tablet [film coated]: 600 mg

## gemifloxacin (je mi FLOKS a sin)

**Synonyms** DW286; gemifloxacin mesylate; LA 20304a; SB-265805

**U.S./Canadian Brand Names** Factive® [US]

**Therapeutic Category** Antibiotic, Quinolone

**Use** Treatment of acute exacerbation of chronic bronchitis; treatment of community-acquired pneumonia, including pneumonia caused by multidrug-resistant strains of *S. pneumoniae* (MDRSP)

**Usual Dosage** Oral: Adults: 320 mg once daily

Duration of therapy:

Acute exacerbations of chronic bronchitis: 5 days

Community-acquired pneumonia (mild to moderate severity): 7 days

**Dosage Forms** Tablet, as mesylate: 320 mg

**gemifloxacin mesylate** *see gemifloxacin on this page*

## gemtuzumab ozogamicin (gem TOO zoo mab oh zog a MY sin)

**U.S./Canadian Brand Names** Mylotarg® [US/Can]

**Therapeutic Category** Antineoplastic Agent, Natural Source (Plant) Derivative

**Use** Treatment of relapsed acute myeloid leukemia (CD33 positive)

**Usual Dosage** I.V.: Adults ≥60 years: 9 mg/m$^2$, infused over 2 hours. A full treatment course is a total of two doses administered with 14 days between doses. Full hematologic recovery is not necessary for administration of the second dose. There has been only limited experience with repeat courses of gemtuzumab ozogamicin.

**Note:** The patient should receive diphenhydramine 50 mg orally and acetaminophen 650-1000 mg orally 1 hour prior to administration of each dose. Acetaminophen dosage should be repeated as needed every 4 hours for two additional doses. Pretreatment with methylprednisolone may ameliorate infusion-related symptoms.

**Dosage Forms** Injection, powder for reconstitution: 5 mg

**Gemzar® [US/Can]** *see gemcitabine on previous page*

**Genabid® *(Discontinued)***

**Genac® [US-OTC]** *see triprolidine and pseudoephedrine on page 827*

**Gen-Acebutolol [Can]** *see acebutolol on page 4*

**Genaced™ [US-OTC]** *see acetaminophen, aspirin, and caffeine on page 9*

**Gen-Acyclovir [Can]** *see acyclovir on page 17*

**Genagesic® *(Discontinued)***

**Genahist® [US-OTC]** *see diphenhydramine on page 254*

**Gen-Alprazolam [Can]** *see alprazolam on page 30*

**Genamin® Expectorant *(Discontinued)***

**Gen-Amiodarone [Can]** *see amiodarone on page 41*

**Gen-Amoxicillin [Can]** *see* amoxicillin *on page 46*

**Genapap® [US-OTC]** *see* acetaminophen *on page 4*

**Genapap® Children [US-OTC]** *see* acetaminophen *on page 4*

**Genapap® Extra Strength [US-OTC]** *see* acetaminophen *on page 4*

**Genapap® Infant [US-OTC]** *see* acetaminophen *on page 4*

**Genapap® Sinus Maximum Strength [US-OTC]** *see* acetaminophen and pseudoephedrine *on page 8*

**Genaphed® [US-OTC]** *see* pseudoephedrine *on page 692*

**Genasal [US-OTC]** *see* oxymetazoline *on page 610*

**Genasoft® [US-OTC]** *see* docusate *on page 263*

**Genasyme® [US-OTC]** *see* simethicone *on page 748*

**Gen-Atenolol [Can]** *see* atenolol *on page 76*

**Genatuss® *(Discontinued)*** *see* guaifenesin *on page 383*

**Genatuss DM® [US-OTC]** *see* guaifenesin and dextromethorphan *on page 385*

**Gen-Azathioprine [Can]** *see* azathioprine *on page 83*

**Gen-Baclofen [Can]** *see* baclofen *on page 88*

**Gen-Beclo [Can]** *see* beclomethasone *on page 91*

**Gen-Bromazepam [Can]** *see* bromazepam *(Canada only) on page 114*

**Gen-Budesonide AQ [Can]** *see* budesonide *on page 118*

**Gen-Buspirone [Can]** *see* buspirone *on page 123*

**Gencalc® 600 *(Discontinued)*** *see* calcium carbonate *on page 130*

**Gen-Captopril [Can]** *see* captopril *on page 139*

**Gen-Carbamazepine CR [Can]** *see* carbamazepine *on page 140*

**Gen-Cimetidine [Can]** *see* cimetidine *on page 183*

**Gen-Ciprofloxacin [Can]** *see* ciprofloxacin *on page 184*

**Gen-Citalopram [Can]** *see* citalopram *on page 188*

**Gen-Clobetasol [Can]** *see* clobetasol *on page 194*

**Gen-Clomipramine [Can]** *see* clomipramine *on page 196*

**Gen-Clonazepam [Can]** *see* clonazepam *on page 197*

**Gen-Clozapine [Can]** *see* clozapine *on page 200*

**Gen-Cyclobenzaprine [Can]** *see* cyclobenzaprine *on page 213*

**Gen-Cyproterone [Can]** *see* cyproterone *(Canada only) on page 218*

**Gen-Diltiazem [Can]** *see* diltiazem *on page 251*

**Gen-Diltiazem CD [Can]** *see* diltiazem *on page 251*

**Gen-Divalproex [Can]** *see* valproic acid and derivatives *on page 837*

**Gen-Doxazosin [Can]** *see* doxazosin *on page 268*

**Genebs® [US-OTC]** *see* acetaminophen *on page 4*

**Genebs® Extra Strength [US-OTC]** *see* acetaminophen *on page 4*

**Generlac [US]** *see* lactulose *on page 464*

**Genesec® [US-OTC]** *see* acetaminophen and phenyltoloxamine *on page 8*

**Gen-Etidronate [Can]** *see* etidronate disodium *on page 321*

**Geneye® [US-OTC]** *see* tetrahydrozoline *on page 792*

**Gen-Famotidine [Can]** *see* famotidine *on page 327*

**Gen-Fenofibrate Micro [Can]** *see* fenofibrate *on page 330*

**Genfiber® [US-OTC]** *see* psyllium *on page 697*

**Gen-Fluconazole [Can]** *see* fluconazole *on page 341*

**Gen-Fluoxetine [Can]** *see* fluoxetine *on page 349*

**Gen-Gabapentin [Can]** *see* gabapentin *on page 365*

**Gen-Gemfibrozil [Can]** *see* gemfibrozil *on page 370*

**Gen-Glybe [Can]** *see* glyburide *on page 378*

**Gengraf**® **[US]** *see* cyclosporine *on page 215*

**Gen-Hydroxychloroquine [Can]** *see* hydroxychloroquine *on page 421*

**Gen-Hydroxyurea [Can]** *see* hydroxyurea *on page 422*

**Gen-Indapamide [Can]** *see* indapamide *on page 434*

**Gen-Ipratropium [Can]** *see* ipratropium *on page 446*

**Gen-K**® ***(Discontinued)*** *see* potassium chloride *on page 663*

**Gen-Lovastatin [Can]** *see* lovastatin *on page 494*

**Gen-Medroxy [Can]** *see* medroxyprogesterone acetate *on page 507*

**Gen-Meloxicam [Can]** *see* meloxicam *on page 509*

**Gen-Metformin [Can]** *see* metformin *on page 519*

**Gen-Minocycline [Can]** *see* minocycline *on page 542*

**Gen-Mirtazapine [Can]** *see* mirtazapine *on page 543*

**Gen-Nabumetone [Can]** *see* nabumetone *on page 556*

**Gen-Naproxen EC [Can]** *see* naproxen *on page 562*

**Gen-Nitro [Can]** *see* nitroglycerin *on page 578*

**Gen-Nizatidine [Can]** *see* nizatidine *on page 580*

**Gen-Nortriptyline [Can]** *see* nortriptyline *on page 583*

**Genoptic**® **[US]** *see* gentamicin *on this page*

**Genora**® **0.5/35** ***(Discontinued)*** *see* ethinyl estradiol and norethindrone *on page 314*

**Genora**® **1/35** ***(Discontinued)*** *see* ethinyl estradiol and norethindrone *on page 314*

**Genora**® **1/50** ***(Discontinued)*** *see* mestranol and norethindrone *on page 517*

**Genotropin**® **[US]** *see* somatropin *on page 760*

**Genotropin Miniquick**® **[US]** *see* somatropin *on page 760*

**Gen-Oxybutynin [Can]** *see* oxybutynin *on page 607*

**Gen-Paroxetine [Can]** *see* paroxetine *on page 620*

**Gen-Pindolol [Can]** *see* pindolol *on page 648*

**Gen-Piroxicam [Can]** *see* piroxicam *on page 650*

**Genpril**® **[US-OTC]** *see* ibuprofen *on page 427*

**Gen-Ranidine [Can]** *see* ranitidine hydrochloride *on page 710*

**Gen-Salbutamol [Can]** *see* albuterol *on page 22*

**Gen-Selegiline [Can]** *see* selegiline *on page 742*

**Gen-Sertraline [Can]** *see* sertraline *on page 744*

**Gen-Simvastatin [Can]** *see* simvastatin *on page 748*

**Gen-Sotalol [Can]** *see* sotalol *on page 762*

**Gentacidin**® ***(Discontinued)*** *see* gentamicin *on this page*

**Gentak**® **[US]** *see* gentamicin *on this page*

## gentamicin (jen ta MYE sin)

### Sound-Alike/Look-Alike Issues
gentamicin may be confused with kanamycin
Garamycin® may be confused with kanamycin, Terramycin®

**Synonyms** gentamicin sulfate

**U.S./Canadian Brand Names** Alcomicin® [Can]; Diogent® [Can]; Genoptic® [US]; Gentak® [US]; SAB-Gentamicin [Can]

**Therapeutic Category** Aminoglycoside (Antibiotic); Antibiotic, Ophthalmic; Antibiotic, Topical

**Use** Treatment of susceptible bacterial infections, normally gram-negative organisms including *Pseudomonas*, *Proteus*, *Serratia*, and gram-positive *Staphylococcus*; treatment of bone infections, respiratory tract infections, skin and soft tissue infections, as well as abdominal and urinary tract infections, endocarditis, and septicemia; used topically to treat superficial infections of the skin or ophthalmic infections caused by susceptible bacteria; prevention of bacterial endocarditis prior to dental or surgical procedures®

**Usual Dosage** Individualization is **critical** because of the low therapeutic index.

**Use of ideal body weight (IBW) for determining the mg/kg/dose appears to be more accurate than dosing on the basis of total body weight (TBW).** In morbid obesity, dosage requirement may best be estimated using a dosing weight of IBW + 0.4 (TBW - IBW).

Initial and periodic plasma drug levels (eg, peak and trough with conventional dosing) should be determined, particularly in critically-ill patients with serious infections or in disease states known to significantly alter aminoglycoside pharmacokinetics (eg, cystic fibrosis, burns, or major surgery).

Infants and Children <5 years: I.M., I.V.: 2.5 mg/kg/dose every 8 hours*

Children ≥5 years: I.M., I.V.: 2-2.5 mg/kg/dose every 8 hours*

Prevention of bacterial endocarditis: Dental, oral, upper respiratory procedures, GI/GU procedures: 1.5 mg/kg with ampicillin (50 mg/kg) 30 minutes prior to procedure

*Note: Higher individual doses and/or more frequent intervals (eg, every 6 hours) may be required in selected clinical situations (cystic fibrosis) or serum levels document the need

Children and Adults:
Intrathecal: 4-8 mg/day
Ophthalmic:
Ointment: Instill 1/2" (1.25 cm) 2-3 times/day to every 3-4 hours
Solution: Instill 1-2 drops every 2-4 hours, up to 2 drops every hour for severe infections
Topical: Apply 3-4 times/day to affected area

Adults: I.M., I.V.: Systemic infections:
Severe, life-threatening infections:
Conventional dosing: 2-2.5 mg/kg/dose every 8-12 hours; to ensure adequate peak concentrations early in therapy, higher initial dosages may be considered in selected patients when extracellular water is increased (edema, septic shock, postsurgical, or trauma)
Once-daily dosing: Some clinicians suggest a daily dose of 4-7 mg/kg once daily for all patients with normal renal function; this dose is at least as efficacious with similar, if not less, toxicity than conventional dosing.
Urinary tract infections: 1.5 mg/kg/dose every 8 hours
Synergy (for gram-positive infections): 1 mg/kg/dose
Prevention of bacterial endocarditis:
Dental, oral, or upper respiratory procedures: 1.5 mg/kg (not to exceed 80 mg) with ampicillin (1-2 g) 30 minutes prior to procedure
GI/GU surgery: 1.5 mg/kg (not to exceed 80 mg) with ampicillin (2 g) 30 minutes prior to procedure

**Dosage Forms** [DSC] = Discontinued product
Cream, topical, as sulfate: 0.1% (15 g, 30 g)
Infusion, as sulfate [premixed in NS]: 40 mg (50 mL); 60 mg (50 mL, 100 mL); 70 mg (50 mL); 80 mg (50 mL, 100 mL); 90 mg (100 mL); 100 mg (50 mL, 100 mL); 120 mg (100 mL)
Injection, solution, as sulfate [ADD-Vantage® vial]: 10 mg/mL (6 mL, 8 mL, 10 mL)
Injection, solution, as sulfate: 40 mg/mL (2 mL, 20 mL) [may contain sodium metabisulfite]
Injection, solution, pediatric, as sulfate: 10 mg/mL (2 mL) [may contain sodium metabisulfite]
Injection, solution, pediatric, as sulfate [preservative free]: 10 mg/mL (2 mL)
Ointment, ophthalmic, as sulfate (Gentak®): 0.3% [3 mg/g] (3.5 g)
Ointment, topical, as sulfate: 0.1% (15 g, 30 g)
Solution, ophthalmic, as sulfate: 0.3% (5 mL, 15 mL) [contains benzalkonium chloride]
Genoptic®: 0.3% (1 mL) [contains benzalkonium chloride]
Gentacidin®: 0.3% (5 mL) [contains benzalkonium chloride] [DSC]
Gentak®: 0.3% (5 mL, 15 mL) [contains benzalkonium chloride]

**gentamicin and prednisolone** *see* prednisolone and gentamicin *on page 673*

**gentamicin sulfate** *see* gentamicin *on previous page*

**Gen-Tamoxifen [Can]** *see* tamoxifen *on page 780*

**Genteal® [Can]** *see* hydroxypropyl methylcellulose *on page 422*

**GenTeal® Mild [US-OTC]** *see* hydroxypropyl methylcellulose *on page 422*

**Gen-Temazepam [Can]** *see* temazepam *on page 784*

**Gen-Ticlopidine [Can]** *see* ticlopidine *on page 802*

**Gen-Timolol [Can]** *see* timolol *on page 803*

**Gentlax**® **[Can]** *see* bisacodyl *on page 107*

**Gentran**® **[US/Can]** *see* dextran *on page 236*

**Gentrasul**® *(Discontinued)* *see* gentamicin *on page 372*

**Gen-Trazodone [Can]** *see* trazodone *on page 817*

**Gen-Triazolam [Can]** *see* triazolam *on page 821*

**Gen-Verapamil [Can]** *see* verapamil *on page 843*

**Gen-Verapamil SR [Can]** *see* verapamil *on page 843*

**Gen-Warfarin [Can]** *see* warfarin *on page 854*

**Gen-Zopiclone [Can]** *see* zopiclone *(Canada only)* *on page 864*

**Geocillin**® **[US]** *see* carbenicillin *on page 141*

**Geodon**® **[US]** *see* ziprasidone *on page 862*

**Geref**® **Diagnostic [US]** *see* sermorelin acetate *on page 744*

**Geref**® *(Discontinued)* *see* sermorelin acetate *on page 744*

**Geriation [US-OTC]** *see* vitamins (multiple/oral) *on page 852*

**Geridium**® *(Discontinued)* *see* phenazopyridine *on page 636*

**Geri-Hydrolac**™ **[US-OTC]** *see* lactic acid and ammonium hydroxide *on page 462*

**Geri-Hydrolac**™**-12 [US-OTC]** *see* lactic acid and ammonium hydroxide *on page 462*

**Geritol Complete**® **[US-OTC]** *see* vitamins (multiple/oral) *on page 852*

**Geritol Extend**® **[US-OTC]** *see* vitamins (multiple/oral) *on page 852*

**Geritol**® **Tonic [US-OTC]** *see* vitamins (multiple/oral) *on page 852*

**German measles vaccine** *see* rubella virus vaccine (live) *on page 733*

**Gevrabon**® **[US-OTC]** *see* vitamin B complex combinations *on page 849*

**GF196960** *see* tadalafil *on page 779*

**GG** *see* guaifenesin *on page 383*

**GG-Cen**® *(Discontinued)* *see* guaifenesin *on page 383*

**GHB** *see* sodium oxybate *on page 755*

**GI87084B** *see* remifentanil *on page 714*

**glargine, insulin** *see* insulin preparations *on page 438*

## glatiramer acetate (gla TIR a mer AS e tate)

**Sound-Alike/Look-Alike Issues**
Copaxone® may be confused with Compazine®

**Synonyms** copolymer-1

**U.S./Canadian Brand Names** Copaxone® [US/Can]

**Therapeutic Category** Biological, Miscellaneous

**Use** Treatment of relapsing-remitting type multiple sclerosis; studies indicate that it reduces the frequency of attacks and the severity of disability; appears to be most effective for patients with minimal disability

**Usual Dosage** Adults: SubQ: 20 mg daily

**Dosage Forms** Injection, solution [preservative free]: 20 mg/mL (1 mL) [prefilled syringe; contains mannitol; packaged with alcohol pads]

**Glaucon**® *(Discontinued)* *see* epinephrine *on page 287*

**Gleevec**® **[US/Can]** *see* imatinib *on page 430*

**Gliadel**® **[US]** *see* carmustine *on page 149*

**glibenclamide** *see* glyburide *on page 378*

## gliclazide *(Canada only)* (GLYE kla zide)

**U.S./Canadian Brand Names** Apo-Gliclazide® [Can]; Diamicron® MR [Can]; Diamicron® [Can]; Novo-Gliclazide [Can]; Rhoxal-gliclazide [Can]

**Therapeutic Category** Antidiabetic Agent; Hypoglycemic Agent, Oral; Sulfonylurea Agent

**Use** Management of type 2 diabetes mellitus (noninsulin-dependent, NIDDM)

**Usual Dosage** Oral: Adults:

Immediate release tablet: Initial: 80-160 mg/day; typical dose range 80-320 mg/day; dosage of ≥160 mg should be divided into 2 equal parts for twice-daily administration; maximum dose: 320 mg/day; should be taken with meals

Sustained release tablet: 30-120 mg once daily

**Note:** There is no fixed dosage regimen for the management of diabetes mellitus with gliclazide or any other hypoglycemic agent. Dose must be individualized based on frequent determinations of blood glucose during dose titration and throughout maintenance.

**Dosage Forms**

Tablet (Diamicron®): 80 mg

Tablet, sustained release (Diamicron® MR): 30 mg

## glimepiride (GLYE me pye ride)

**Sound-Alike/Look-Alike Issues**

glimepiride may be confused with glipiZIDE

Amaryl® may be confused with Altace®, Amerge®, Reminyl®

**U.S./Canadian Brand Names** Amaryl® [US/Can]

**Therapeutic Category** Antidiabetic Agent, Oral

**Use** Management of type 2 diabetes mellitus (noninsulin-dependent, NIDDM) as an adjunct to diet and exercise to lower blood glucose; may be used in combination with metformin or insulin in patients whose hyperglycemia cannot be controlled by diet and exercise in conjunction with a single oral hypoglycemic agent

**Usual Dosage** Oral (allow several days between dose titrations):

Adults: Initial: 1-2 mg once daily, administered with breakfast or the first main meal; usual maintenance dose: 1-4 mg once daily; after a dose of 2 mg once daily, increase in increments of 2 mg at 1- to 2-week intervals based upon the patient's blood glucose response to a maximum of 8 mg once daily

Combination with insulin therapy (fasting glucose level for instituting combination therapy is in the range of >150 mg/dL in plasma or serum depending on the patient): initial recommended dose: 8 mg once daily with the first main meal

After starting with low-dose insulin, upward adjustments of insulin can be done approximately weekly as guided by frequent measurements of fasting blood glucose. Once stable, combination-therapy patients should monitor their capillary blood glucose on an ongoing basis, preferably daily.

**Dosage Forms** Tablet: 1 mg, 2 mg, 4 mg

## glipizide (GLIP i zide)

**Sound-Alike/Look-Alike Issues**

glipiZIDE may be confused with glimepiride, glyBURIDE

Glucotrol® may be confused with Glucophage®, Glucotrol® XL, glyBURIDE

Glucotrol® XL may be confused with Glucotrol®

**Synonyms** glydiazinamide

**Tall-Man** glipiZIDE

**U.S./Canadian Brand Names** Glucotrol® XL [US]; Glucotrol® [US]

**Therapeutic Category** Antidiabetic Agent, Oral

**Use** Management of type 2 diabetes mellitus (noninsulin-dependent, NIDDM)

**Usual Dosage** Oral (allow several days between dose titrations): Adults: Initial: 5 mg/day; adjust dosage at 2.5-5 mg daily increments as determined by blood glucose response at intervals of several days.

Immediate release tablet: Maximum recommended once-daily dose: 15 mg; maximum recommended total daily dose: 40 mg

Extended release tablet (Glucotrol® XL): Maximum recommended dose: 20 mg

When transferring from insulin to glipizide:

Current insulin requirement ≤20 units: Discontinue insulin and initiate glipizide at usual dose

Current insulin requirement >20 units: Decrease insulin by 50% and initiate glipizide at usual dose; gradually decrease insulin dose based on patient response. Several days should elapse between dosage changes.

**Dosage Forms**

Tablet (Glucotrol®): 5 mg, 10 mg

(Continued)

## glipizide *(Continued)*

Tablet, extended release: 5 mg, 10 mg
(Glucotrol® XL): 2.5 mg, 5 mg, 10 mg

## glipizide and metformin (GLIP i zide & met FOR min)

**Synonyms** glipizide and metformin hydrochloride; metformin and glipizide
**U.S./Canadian Brand Names** Metaglip™ [US]
**Therapeutic Category** Antidiabetic Agent (Biguanide); Antidiabetic Agent (Sulfonylurea)
**Use** Initial therapy for management of type 2 diabetes mellitus (noninsulin-dependent, NIDDM) when hyperglycemia cannot be managed with diet and exercise alone. Second-line therapy for management of type 2 diabetes (NIDDM) when hyperglycemia cannot be managed with a sulfonylurea or metformin along with diet and exercise.
**Usual Dosage** Oral: Adults:

Type 2 diabetes, first-line therapy: Initial: Glipizide 2.5 mg/metformin 250 mg once daily with a meal. Dose adjustment: Increase dose by 1 tablet/day every 2 weeks, up to a maximum of glipizide 10 mg/metformin 1000 mg daily

Patients with fasting plasma glucose (FPG) 280-320 mg/dL: Consider glipizide 2.5 mg/metformin 500 mg twice daily. Dose adjustment: Increase dose by 1 tablet/day every 2 weeks, up to a maximum of glipizide 10 mg/metformin 2000 mg daily in divided doses

Type 2 diabetes, second-line therapy: Glipizide 2.5 mg/metformin 500 mg **or** glipizide 5 mg/metformin 500 mg twice daily with morning and evening meals; starting dose should not exceed current daily dose of glipizide (or sulfonylurea equivalent) or metformin. Dose adjustment: Titrate dose in increments of no more than glipizide 5 mg/metformin 500 mg, up to a maximum dose of glipizide 20 mg/metformin 2000 mg daily.

**Dosage Forms** Tablet [film coated]:
2.5/250: Glipizide 2.5 mg and metformin 250 mg
2.5/500: Glipizide 2.5 mg and metformin 500 mg
5/500: Glipizide 5 mg and metformin 500 mg

**glipizide and metformin hydrochloride** *see* glipizide and metformin *on this page*

**glivec** *see* imatinib *on page 430*

**GlucaGen® [US]** *see* glucagon *on this page*

**GlucaGen® Diagnostic Kit [US]** *see* glucagon *on this page*

**GlucaGen® HypoKit™ [US]** *see* glucagon *on this page*

## glucagon (GLOO ka gon)

**Sound-Alike/Look-Alike Issues**
glucagon may be confused with Glaucon®
**Synonyms** glucagon hydrochloride
**U.S./Canadian Brand Names** GlucaGen® Diagnostic Kit [US]; GlucaGen® HypoKit™ [US]; GlucaGen® [US]; Glucagon Emergency Kit [US]
**Therapeutic Category** Antihypoglycemic Agent
**Use** Management of hypoglycemia; diagnostic aid in radiologic examinations to temporarily inhibit GI tract movement
**Usual Dosage**

Hypoglycemia or insulin shock therapy: I.M., I.V., SubQ:
Children <20 kg: 0.5 mg or 20-30 mcg/kg/dose; repeated in 20 minutes as needed
Children ≥20 kg and Adults: 1 mg; may repeat in 20 minutes as needed
**Note:** If patient fails to respond to glucagon, I.V. dextrose must be given.
Diagnostic aid: Adults: I.M., I.V.: 0.25-2 mg 10 minutes prior to procedure

**Dosage Forms** Injection, powder for reconstitution, as hydrochloride:
GlucaGen®: 1 mg [equivalent to 1 unit; contains lactose 107 mg]
GlucaGen® Diagnostic Kit: 1 mg [equivalent to 1 unit; contains lactose 107 mg; packaged with sterile water]
GlucaGen® HypoKit™: 1 mg [equivalent to 1 unit; contains lactose 107 mg; packaged with prefilled syringe containing sterile water]
Glucagon®: 1 mg [equivalent to 1 unit; contains lactose 49 mg]
Glucagon Diagnostic Kit, Glucagon Emergency Kit: 1 mg [equivalent to 1 unit; contains lactose 49 mg; packaged with diluent syringe containing glycerin 12 mg/mL and water for injection]

**Glucagon Diagnostic Kit** *(Discontinued)* *see* glucagon *on previous page*

**Glucagon Emergency Kit [US]** *see* glucagon *on previous page*

**glucagon hydrochloride** *see* glucagon *on previous page*

**glucocerebrosidase** *see* alglucerase *on page 27*

**GlucoNorm® [Can]** *see* repaglinide *on page 715*

**Glucophage® [US/Can]** *see* metformin *on page 519*

**Glucophage® XR [US]** *see* metformin *on page 519*

## glucose (instant) (GLOO kose IN stant)

**Sound-Alike/Look-Alike Issues**
Glutose™ may be confused with Glutofac®
**U.S./Canadian Brand Names** B-D™ Glucose [US-OTC]; Dex4 Glucose [US-OTC]; Glutol™ [US-OTC]; Glutose™ [US-OTC]; Insta-Glucose® [US-OTC]
**Therapeutic Category** Antihypoglycemic Agent
**Use** Management of hypoglycemia
**Usual Dosage** Adults: Oral: 10-20 g
**Dosage Forms**
Gel, oral:
Glutose™: 40% (15 g, 45 g)
Insta-Glucose®: 40% (30 g)
Solution, oral (Glutol™): 55% [100 g dextrose/180 mL] (180 mL)
Tablet, chewable:
B-D™ Glucose: 5 g
Dex4 Glucose: 4 g

## glucose polymers (GLOO kose POL i merz)

**U.S./Canadian Brand Names** Moducal® [US-OTC]; Polycose® [US-OTC]
**Therapeutic Category** Nutritional Supplement
**Use** Supplies calories for those persons not able to meet the caloric requirement with usual food intake
**Usual Dosage** Adults: Oral: Add to foods or beverages or mix in water
**Dosage Forms**
Liquid (Polycose®): 43% (126 mL)
Powder:
Moducal®: 368 g
Polycose®: 350 g

**Glucotrol® [US]** *see* glipizide *on page 375*

**Glucotrol® XL [US]** *see* glipizide *on page 375*

**Glucovance® [US]** *see* glyburide and metformin *on next page*

**Glu-K® [US-OTC]** *see* potassium gluconate *on page 665*

**glulisine, insulin** *see* insulin preparations *on page 438*

## glutamic acid (gloo TAM ik AS id)

**Synonyms** glutamic acid hydrochloride
**Therapeutic Category** Gastrointestinal Agent, Miscellaneous
**Use** Treatment of hypochlorhydria and achlorhydria
**Usual Dosage** Adults: Oral:
Tablet/powder: 500-1000 mg/day before meals or food
Capsule: 1-3 capsules 3 times/day before meals
**Dosage Forms**
Capsule, as hydrochloride: 340 mg
Tablet: 500 mg

**glutamic acid hydrochloride** *see* glutamic acid *on this page*

**Glutofac®-MX [US]** *see* vitamins (multiple/oral) *on page 852*

**Glutofac®-ZX [US]** *see* vitamins (multiple/oral) *on page 852*

**Glutol™ [US-OTC]** *see* glucose (instant) *on this page*

**Glutose™ [US-OTC]** *see* glucose (instant) *on previous page*

**Glyate® *(Discontinued)*** *see* guaifenesin *on page 383*

**glybenclamide** *see* glyburide *on this page*

**glybenzcyclamide** *see* glyburide *on this page*

## glyburide (GLYE byoor ide)

**Sound-Alike/Look-Alike Issues**
glyBURIDE may be confused with glipiZIDE, Glucotrol®
Diaβeta® may be confused with Diabinese®, Zebeta®
Micronase® may be confused with microK®, miconazole, Micronor®

**Synonyms** glibenclamide; glybenclamide; glybenzcyclamide

**Tall-Man** glyBURIDE

**U.S./Canadian Brand Names** Albert® Glyburide [Can]; Apo-Glyburide® [Can]; Diaβeta® [US/Can]; Euglucon® [Can]; Gen-Glybe [Can]; Glynase® PresTab® [US]; Micronase® [US]; Novo-Glyburide [Can]; Nu-Glyburide [Can]; PMS-Glyburide [Can]; ratio-Glyburide [Can]

**Therapeutic Category** Antidiabetic Agent, Oral

**Use** Management of type 2 diabetes mellitus (noninsulin-dependent, NIDDM)

**Usual Dosage** Oral:
Adults:
Initial: 2.5-5 mg/day, administered with breakfast or the first main meal of the day. In patients who are more sensitive to hypoglycemic drugs, start at 1.25 mg/day.
Increase in increments of no more than 2.5 mg/day at weekly intervals based on the patient's blood glucose response
Maintenance: 1.25-20 mg/day given as single or divided doses; maximum: 20 mg/day
Micronized tablets (Glynase® PresTab®): Adults:
Initial: 1.5-3 mg/day, administered with breakfast or the first main meal of the day in patients who are more sensitive to hypoglycemic drugs, start at 0.75 mg/day. Increase in increments of no more than 1.5 mg/day in weekly intervals based on the patient's blood glucose response.
Maintenance: 0.75-12 mg/day given as a single dose or in divided doses. Some patients (especially those receiving >6 mg/day) may have a more satisfactory response with twice-daily dosing.

**Dosage Forms** [DSC] = Discontinued product
Tablet (Diaβeta®, Micronase®): 1.25 mg, 2.5 mg, 5 mg
Tablet, micronized: 1.5 mg, 3 mg, 6 mg
Glynase® PresTab®: 1.5 mg [DSC], 3 mg, 6 mg

## glyburide and metformin (GLYE byoor ide & met FOR min)

**Synonyms** glyburide and metformin hydrochloride; metformin and glyburide

**U.S./Canadian Brand Names** Glucovance® [US]

**Therapeutic Category** Antidiabetic Agent (Sulfonylurea); Antidiabetic Agent, Oral

**Use** Initial therapy for management of type 2 diabetes mellitus (noninsulin-dependent, NIDDM). Second-line therapy for management of type 2 diabetes (NIDDM) when hyperglycemia cannot be managed with a sulfonylurea or metformin; combination therapy with a thiazolidinedione may be required to achieve additional control.

**Usual Dosage Note:** Dose must be individualized. Dosages expressed as glyburide/metformin components.
Adults: Oral:
Initial therapy (no prior treatment with sulfonylurea or metformin): 1.25 mg/250 mg once daily with a meal; patients with Hb $A_{1c}$ >9% or fasting plasma glucose (FPG) >200 mg/dL may start with 1.25 mg/250 mg twice daily
Dosage may be increased in increments of 1.25 mg/250 mg, at intervals of not less than 2 weeks; maximum daily dose: 10 mg/2000 mg (limited experience with higher doses)
Previously treated with a sulfonylurea or metformin alone: Initial: 2.5 mg/500 mg or 5 mg/500 mg twice daily; increase in increments no greater than 5 mg/500 mg; maximum daily dose: 20 mg/2000 mg
When switching patients previously on a sulfonylurea and metformin together, do not exceed the daily dose of glyburide (or glyburide equivalent) or metformin.
**Note:** May combine with a thiazolidinedione in patients with an inadequate response to glyburide/metformin therapy (risk of hypoglycemia may be increased).

**Dosage Forms** Tablet [film coated]:
1.25 mg/250 mg: Glyburide 1.25 mg and metformin hydrochloride 250 mg
2.5 mg/500 mg: Glyburide 2.5 mg and metformin hydrochloride 500 mg
5 mg/500 mg: Glyburide 5 mg and metformin hydrochloride 500 mg

**glyburide and metformin hydrochloride** *see* glyburide and metformin *on previous page*

## glycerin (GLIS er in)

**Synonyms** glycerol

**U.S./Canadian Brand Names** Bausch & Lomb® Computer Eye Drops [US-OTC]; Colace® Adult/Children Suppositories [US-OTC]; Colace® Infant/Children Suppositories [US-OTC]; Fleet® Babylax® [US-OTC]; Fleet® Glycerin Suppositories Maximum Strength [US-OTC]; Fleet® Glycerin Suppositories [US-OTC]; Fleet® Liquid Glycerin Suppositories [US-OTC]; Sani-Supp® [US-OTC]

**Therapeutic Category** Laxative; Ophthalmic Agent, Miscellaneous

**Use** Constipation; reduction of intraocular pressure; reduction of corneal edema; glycerin has been administered orally to reduce intracranial pressure

**Usual Dosage**

Constipation: Rectal:

Children <6 years: 1 infant suppository 1-2 times/day as needed or 2-5 mL as an enema

Children >6 years and Adults: 1 adult suppository 1-2 times/day as needed or 5-15 mL as an enema

Children and Adults:

Reduction of intraocular pressure: Oral: 1-1.8 g/kg 1-1$^1$/$_2$ hours preoperatively; additional doses may be administered at 5-hour intervals

Reduction of intracranial pressure: Oral: 1.5 g/kg/day divided every 4 hours; 1 g/kg/dose every 6 hours has also been used

Reduction of corneal edema: Ophthalmic solution: Instill 1-2 drops in eye(s) prior to examination OR for lubricant effect, instill 1-2 drops in eye(s) every 3-4 hours

**Dosage Forms** [DSC] = Discontinued product

Solution, ophthalmic, sterile (Bausch & Lomb® Computer Eye Drops): 1% (15 mL) [contains benzalkonium chloride]

Solution, oral (Osmoglyn®): 50% (220 mL) [lime flavor] [DSC]

Solution, rectal:

Fleet® Babylax®: 2.3 g/2.3 mL (4 mL) [6 units per box]

Fleet® Liquid Glycerin Suppositories: 5.6 g/5.5 mL (7.5 mL) [4 units per box]

Suppository, rectal: 82.5% (12s, 25s) [pediatric size]; 82.5% (12s, 24s, 25s, 50s, 100s) [adult size]

Colace® Adult/Children: 2.1 g (12s, 24s, 48s, 100s)

Colace® Infant/Children: 1.2 g (12s, 24s)

Fleet® Glycerin Suppositories: 1 g (12s) [pediatric size]; 2g (12s, 24s, 50s) [adult size]

Fleet® Glycerin Suppositories Maximum Strength: 3g (18s) [adult size]

Sani-Supp®: 82.5% (10s, 25s) [pediatric size]; 82.5% (10s, 25s, 50s) [adult size]

## glycerin, lanolin, and peanut oil (GLIS er in, LAN oh lin, & PEE nut oyl)

**Therapeutic Category** Topical Skin Product

**Use** Nipple care of pregnant and nursing women

**Usual Dosage** Topical: Apply as often as needed

**Dosage Forms** Cream: 2 oz

**glycerol** *see* glycerin *on this page*

**glycerol guaiacolate** *see* guaifenesin *on page 383*

**Glycerol-T® *(Discontinued)*** *see* theophylline and guaifenesin *on page 795*

**glycerol triacetate** *see* triacetin *on page 818*

**glyceryl trinitrate** *see* nitroglycerin *on page 578*

**Glycofed® *(Discontinued)*** *see* guaifenesin and pseudoephedrine *on page 388*

**GlycoLax™ [US]** *see* polyethylene glycol-electrolyte solution *on page 658*

**Glycon [Can]** *see* metformin *on page 519*

## glycopyrrolate (glye koe PYE roe late)

**Synonyms** glycopyrronium bromide

**U.S./Canadian Brand Names** Robinul® Forte [US]; Robinul® [US]

**Therapeutic Category** Anticholinergic Agent

**Use** Inhibit salivation and excessive secretions of the respiratory tract preoperatively; reversal of neuromuscular blockade; control of upper airway secretions; adjunct in treatment of peptic ulcer

(Continued)

## glycopyrrolate *(Continued)*

### Usual Dosage
Children:
Reduction of secretions (preanesthetic):
Oral: 40-100 mcg/kg/dose 3-4 times/day
I.M., I.V.: 4-10 mcg/kg/dose every 3-4 hours; maximum: 0.2 mg/dose or 0.8 mg/24 hours
Intraoperative: I.V.: 4 mcg/kg not to exceed 0.1 mg; repeat at 2- to 3-minute intervals as needed
Preoperative: I.M.:
<2 years: 4-9 mcg/kg 30-60 minutes before procedure
>2 years: 4 mcg/kg 30-60 minutes before procedure
Children and Adults: Reverse neuromuscular blockade: I.V.: 0.2 mg for each 1 mg of neostigmine or 5 mg of pyridostigmine administered or 5-15 mcg/kg glycopyrrolate with 25-70 mcg/kg of neostigmine or 0.1-0.3 mg/kg of pyridostigmine (agents usually administered simultaneously, but glycopyrrolate may be administered first if bradycardia is present)
Adults:
Reduction of secretions:
Intraoperative: I.V.: 0.1 mg repeated as needed at 2- to 3-minute intervals
Preoperative: I.M.: 4 mcg/kg 30-60 minutes before procedure
Peptic ulcer:
Oral: 1-2 mg 2-3 times/day
I.M., I.V.: 0.1-0.2 mg 3-4 times/day

### Dosage Forms
Injection, solution (Robinul®): 0.2 mg/mL (1 mL, 2 mL, 5 mL, 20 mL) [contains benzyl alcohol]
Tablet:
Robinul®: 1 mg
Robinul® Forte: 2 mg

**glycopyrronium bromide** *see* glycopyrrolate *on previous page*

**Glycotuss®** *(Discontinued) see* guaifenesin *on page 383*

**Glycotuss-dM®** *(Discontinued) see* guaifenesin and dextromethorphan *on page 385*

**glydiazinamide** *see* glipizide *on page 375*

**Glynase® PresTab® [US]** *see* glyburide *on page 378*

**Gly-Oxide® [US-OTC]** *see* carbamide peroxide *on page 141*

**Glyquin® [US]** *see* hydroquinone *on page 420*

**Glyquin-XM™ [US]** *see* hydroquinone *on page 420*

**Glyset® [US/Can]** *see* miglitol *on page 541*

**GM-CSF** *see* sargramostim *on page 739*

**G-myticin®** *(Discontinued) see* gentamicin *on page 372*

**GnRH** *see* gonadorelin *on next page*

**Gold Bond® Antifungal [US-OTC]** *see* tolnaftate *on page 809*

## gold sodium thiomalate *(gold SOW dee um thye oh MAL ate)*
**U.S./Canadian Brand Names** Aurolate® [US]; Myochrysine® [Can]
**Therapeutic Category** Gold Compound
**Use** Treatment of progressive rheumatoid arthritis
**Usual Dosage** I.M.:
Children: Initial: Test dose of 10 mg is recommended, followed by 1 mg/kg/week for 20 weeks; maintenance: 1 mg/kg/dose at 2- to 4-week intervals thereafter for as long as therapy is clinically beneficial and toxicity does not develop. Administration for 2-4 months is usually required before clinical improvement is observed.
Adults: 10 mg first week; 25 mg second week; then 25-50 mg/week until 1 g cumulative dose has been given; if improvement occurs without adverse reactions, administer 25-50 mg every 2-3 weeks for 2-20 weeks, then every 3-4 weeks indefinitely
**Dosage Forms** Injection, solution: 50 mg/mL (1 mL, 10 mL) [contains benzyl alcohol]

**GoLYTELY® [US]** *see* polyethylene glycol-electrolyte solution *on page 658*

# gonadorelin (goe nad oh RELL in)
**Sound-Alike/Look-Alike Issues**
gonadorelin may be confused with gonadotropin, guanadrel
Factrel® may be confused with Sectral®
Gonadotropin may be confused with gonadorelin
**Synonyms** GnRH; gonadorelin acetate; gonadorelin hydrochloride; gonadotropin releasing hormone; LHRH; LRH; luteinizing hormone releasing hormone
**U.S./Canadian Brand Names** Factrel® [US]; Lutrepulse™ [Can]
**Therapeutic Category** Diagnostic Agent; Gonadotropin
**Use** Evaluation of functional capacity and response of gonadotrophic hormones; evaluate abnormal gonadotropin regulation as in precocious puberty and delayed puberty.
**Orphan drug:** Lutrepulse®: Induction of ovulation in females with hypothalamic amenorrhea
**Usual Dosage**
Diagnostic test: Children >12 years and Female Adults: I.V., SubQ hydrochloride salt: 100 mcg administered in women during early phase of menstrual cycle (day 1-7)
Primary hypothalamic amenorrhea: Female Adults: Acetate: I.V.: 5 mcg every 90 minutes via Lutrepulse® pump kit at treatment intervals of 21 days (pump will pulsate every 90 minutes for 7 days)
**Dosage Forms** Injection, powder for reconstitution, as hydrochloride: 100 mcg [diluent contains benzyl alcohol]

**gonadorelin acetate** *see* gonadorelin *on this page*

**gonadorelin hydrochloride** *see* gonadorelin *on this page*

**gonadotropin releasing hormone** *see* gonadorelin *on this page*

**Gonak™ [US-OTC]** *see* hydroxypropyl methylcellulose *on page 422*

**gonioscopic ophthalmic solution** *see* hydroxypropyl methylcellulose *on page 422*

**Goniosoft™ [US]** *see* hydroxypropyl methylcellulose *on page 422*

**Goniosol® (Discontinued)** *see* hydroxypropyl methylcellulose *on page 422*

**Goody's® Extra Strength Headache Powder [US-OTC]** *see* acetaminophen, aspirin, and caffeine *on page 9*

**Goody's® Extra Strength Pain Relief [US-OTC]** *see* acetaminophen, aspirin, and caffeine *on page 9*

**Goody's PM® Powder [US-OTC]** *see* acetaminophen and diphenhydramine *on page 7*

**Gordofilm® [US-OTC]** *see* salicylic acid *on page 734*

**Gormel® [US-OTC]** *see* urea *on page 834*

# goserelin (GOE se rel in)
**Synonyms** D-ser(bu^t)^6,Azgly^10-LHRH; goserelin acetate; ICI-118630; NSC-606864
**U.S./Canadian Brand Names** Zoladex® LA [Can]; Zoladex® [US/Can]
**Therapeutic Category** Gonadotropin-Releasing Hormone Analog
**Use** Palliative treatment of advanced breast cancer and carcinoma of the prostate; treatment of endometriosis, including pain relief and reduction of endometriotic lesions; endometrial thinning agent as part of treatment for dysfunctional uterine bleeding
**Usual Dosage** SubQ: Adults:
Prostate cancer:
Monthly implant: 3.6 mg injected into upper abdomen every 28 days
3-month implant: 10.8 mg injected into the upper abdominal wall every 12 weeks
Breast cancer, endometriosis, endometrial thinning: Monthly implant: 3.6 mg injected into upper abdomen every 28 days
**Note:** For breast cancer, treatment may continue indefinitely; for endometriosis, it is recommended that duration of treatment not exceed 6 months. Only 1-2 doses are recommended for endometrial thinning.
**Dosage Forms**
Injection, solution, 1-month implant [disposable syringe; single-dose]: 3.6 mg [with 16-gauge hypodermic needle]
Injection, solution, 3-month implant [disposable syringe; single-dose]: 10.8 mg [with 14-gauge hypodermic needle]

**goserelin acetate** *see* goserelin *on this page*

**GP 47680** *see* oxcarbazepine *on page 606*

**G-Phed [US]** *see* guaifenesin and pseudoephedrine *on page 388*

**GR38032R** *see* ondansetron *on page 599*

**gramicidin, neomycin, and polymyxin B** *see* neomycin, polymyxin B, and gramicidin *on page 568*

## granisetron (gra NI se tron)

**Sound-Alike/Look-Alike Issues**
granisetron may be confused with dolasetron, ondansetron, palonosetron

**Synonyms** BRL 43694

**U.S./Canadian Brand Names** Kytril® [US/Can]

**Therapeutic Category** Selective 5-HT$_3$ Receptor Antagonist

**Use** Prophylaxis of chemotherapy-related emesis; prophylaxis of nausea and vomiting associated with radiation therapy, including total body irradiation and fractionated abdominal radiation; prophylaxis of postoperative nausea and vomiting (PONV)

Generally **not** recommended for treatment of existing chemotherapy-induced emesis (CIE) or for prophylaxis of nausea from agents with a low emetogenic potential.

**Usual Dosage**
Oral: Adults:
Prophylaxis of chemotherapy-related emesis: 2 mg once daily up to 1 hour before chemotherapy or 1 mg twice daily; the first 1 mg dose should be given up to 1 hour before chemotherapy.
Prophylaxis of radiation therapy-associated emesis: 2 mg once daily given 1 hour before radiation therapy.
I.V.:
Children ≥2 years and Adults: Prophylaxis of chemotherapy-related emesis:
Within U.S.: 10 mcg/kg/dose (or 1 mg/dose) administered IVPB over 5 minutes given within 30 minutes of chemotherapy: for some drugs (eg, carboplatin, cyclophosphamide) with a later onset of emetic action, 10 mcg/kg every 12 hours may be necessary.
Outside U.S.: 40 mcg/kg/dose (or 3 mg/dose); maximum: 9 mg/24 hours
Breakthrough: Repeat the dose 2-3 times within the first 24 hours as necessary **(not based on controlled trials, or generally recommended)**
Adults: PONV:
Prevention: 1 mg given undiluted over 30 seconds; administer before induction of anesthesia or before reversal of anesthesia
Treatment: 1 mg given undiluted over 30 seconds

**Dosage Forms**
Injection, solution: 1 mg/mL (4 mL) [contains benzyl alcohol]
Injection, solution [preservative free]: 0.1 mg/mL (1 mL); 1 mg/mL (1 mL)
Solution, oral: 2 mg/10 mL (30 mL) [contains sodium benzoate; orange flavor]
Tablet: 1 mg

**Granulex® [US]** *see* trypsin, balsam peru, and castor oil *on page 830*

**granulocyte colony stimulating factor** *see* filgrastim *on page 338*

**granulocyte colony stimulating factor (PEG conjugate)** *see* pegfilgrastim *on page 623*

**granulocyte-macrophage colony stimulating factor** *see* sargramostim *on page 739*

**Gravol® [Can]** *see* dimenhydrinate *on page 252*

**Grifulvin® V [US]** *see* griseofulvin *on this page*

**Grifulvin® V Tablet 250 mg and 500 mg (Discontinued)** *see* griseofulvin *on this page*

**Grisactin® Ultra (Discontinued)** *see* griseofulvin *on this page*

## griseofulvin (gri see oh FUL vin)

**Sound-Alike/Look-Alike Issues**
Fulvicin® may be confused with Furacin®

**Synonyms** griseofulvin microsize; griseofulvin ultramicrosize

**U.S./Canadian Brand Names** Grifulvin® V [US]; Gris-PEG® [US]

**Therapeutic Category** Antifungal Agent

**Use** Treatment of susceptible tinea infections of the skin, hair, and nails

**Usual Dosage** Oral:
Children >2 years:
Microsize: 10-20 mg/kg/day in single or 2 divided doses.
Ultramicrosize: >2 years: 5-10 mg/kg/day in single or 2 divided doses.
Adults:
Microsize: 500-1000 mg/day in single or divided doses
Ultramicrosize: 330-375 mg/day in single or divided doses; doses up to 750 mg/day have been used for infections more difficult to eradicate such as tinea unguium
Duration of therapy depends on the site of infection:
Tinea corporis: 2-4 weeks
Tinea capitis: 4-6 weeks or longer (up to 8-12 weeks)
Tinea pedis: 4-8 weeks
Tinea unguium: 3-6 months or longer
**Dosage Forms**
Suspension, oral, microsize (Grifulvin® V): 125 mg/5 mL (120 mL) [contains alcohol 0.2%]
Tablet, microsize (Grifulvin® V): 500 mg
Tablet, ultramicrosize: 125 mg, 250 mg, 330 mg
Gris-PEG®: 125 mg, 250 mg

**griseofulvin microsize** *see* griseofulvin *on previous page*

**griseofulvin ultramicrosize** *see* griseofulvin *on previous page*

**Gris-PEG® [US]** *see* griseofulvin *on previous page*

**Guaicon DM® [US-OTC]** *see* guaifenesin and dextromethorphan *on page 385*

**Guaifed® [US]** *see* guaifenesin and phenylephrine *on page 387*

**Guaifed-PD® [US]** *see* guaifenesin and phenylephrine *on page 387*

**Guaifen-C [US]** *see* guaifenesin and codeine *on next page*

# guaifenesin (gwye FEN e sin)
**Sound-Alike/Look-Alike Issues**
guaifenesin may be confused with guanfacine
Mucinex® may be confused with Mucomyst®
Naldecon® may be confused with Nalfon®
**Synonyms** GG; glycerol guaiacolate
**U.S./Canadian Brand Names** Allfen Jr [US]; Balminil Expectorant [Can]; Benylin® E Extra Strength [Can]; Diabetic Tussin® EX [US-OTC]; Ganidin NR [US]; Guiatuss™ [US-OTC]; Humibid® e [US-OTC]; Iophen NR [US]; Koffex Expectorant [Can]; Mucinex® [US-OTC]; Naldecon Senior EX® [US-OTC]; Organ-1 NR [US]; Organidin® NR [US]; Phanasin [US-OTC]; Phanasin® Diabetic Choice [US-OTC]; Q-Tussin [US-OTC]; Robitussin® [US-OTC/Can]; Scot-Tussin® Expectorant [US-OTC]; Siltussin DAS [US-OTC]; Siltussin SA [US-OTC]; Tussin [US-OTC]
**Therapeutic Category** Expectorant
**Use** Help loosen phlegm and thin bronchial secretions to make coughs more productive
**Usual Dosage** Oral:
Children:
6 months to 2 years: 25-50 mg every 4 hours, not to exceed 300 mg/day
2-5 years: 50-100 mg every 4 hours, not to exceed 600 mg/day
6-11 years: 100-200 mg every 4 hours, not to exceed 1.2 g/day
Children >12 years and Adults: 200-400 mg every 4 hours to a maximum of 2.4 g/day
Extended release tablet: 600-1200 mg every 12 hours, not to exceed 2.4 g/day
**Dosage Forms** [DSC] = Discontinued product
Liquid: 100 mg/5 mL (120 mL, 480 mL)
Diabetic Tussin EX®: 100 mg/5 mL (120 mL) [alcohol free, sugar free, dye free; contains phenylalanine 8.4 mg/5 mL]
Ganidin NR: 100 mg/5 mL (480 mL) [raspberry flavor]
Iophen NR: 100 mg/5 mL (480 mL)
Naldecon Senior EX®: 200 mg/5 mL (120 mL) [alcohol free, sugar free; contains sodium benzoate] [DSC]
Organidin® NR: 100 mg/5 mL (480 mL) [contains sodium benzoate; raspberry flavor]
Q-Tussin: 100 mg/5 mL (120 mL, 240 mL, 480 mL, 3840 mL) [alcohol free; cherry flavor]
Siltussin DAS: 100 mg/5 mL (120 mL) [alcohol free, dye free, sugar free; strawberry flavor]
Syrup: 100 mg/5 mL (120 mL, 480 mL)
(Continued)

## guaifenesin (Continued)

Guiatuss™: 100 mg/5 mL (120 mL, 480 mL) [alcohol free; fruit-mint flavor]

Phanasin: 100 mg/5 mL (120 mL, 240 mL) [alcohol free, sugar free; mint flavor]

Phanasin® Diabetic Choice: 100 mg/5 mL (120 mL) [alcohol free, sugar free; mint flavor]

Robitussin®: 100 mg/5 mL (5 mL, 10 mL, 15 mL, 30 mL, 120 mL, 240 mL, 480 mL) [alcohol free; contains sodium benzoate]

Scot-Tussin® Expectorant: 100 mg/5 mL (120 mL) [alcohol free, dye free, sugar free; contains benzoic acid; grape flavor]

Siltussin SA: 100 mg/5 mL (120 mL, 240 mL, 480 mL) [alcohol free, sugar free; strawberry flavor]

Tussin: 100 mg/5 mL (120 mL, 240 mL)

Syrup, oral drops (Phanasin®): 50 mg/mL (50 mL) [alcohol free, sugar free; fruit flavor]

Tablet: 200 mg

Allfen Jr: 400 mg [dye free]

Humibid® e: 400 mg

Organ-1 NR, Organidin® NR: 200 mg

Tablet, extended release (Mucinex®): 600 mg

**Guaifenesin AC [US]** *see* guaifenesin and codeine *on this page*

## guaifenesin and codeine (gwye FEN e sin & KOE deen)

**Sound-Alike/Look-Alike Issues**

Halotussin® may be confused with Halotestin®

**Synonyms** codeine and guaifenesin

**U.S./Canadian Brand Names** Brontex® [US]; Cheracol® [US]; Cheratussin AC [US]; Diabetic Tussin C® [US]; Gani-Tuss® NR [US]; Guaifen-C [US]; Guaifenesin AC [US]; Guaituss AC® [US]; Iophen-C NR [US]; Kolephrin® #1 [US]; Mytussin® AC [US]; Robafen® AC [US]; Romilar® AC [US]; Tussi-Organidin® NR [US]; Tussi-Organidin® S-NR [US]

**Therapeutic Category** Antitussive/Expectorant

**Controlled Substance** C-V

**Use** Temporary control of cough due to minor throat and bronchial irritation

**Usual Dosage** Oral:

Children:

2-6 years: 1-1.5 mg/kg codeine/day divided into 4 doses administered every 4-6 hours (maximum: 30 mg/24 hours)

6-12 years: 5 mL every 4 hours, not to exceed 30 mL/24 hours

Children >12 years and Adults: 5-10 mL every 6 hours not to exceed 60 mL/24 hours

**Dosage Forms**

Liquid:

Brontex®: Guaifenesin 75 mg and codeine phosphate 2.5 mg per 5 mL (480 mL) [alcohol free; strawberry mint flavor]

Diabetic Tussin C®: Guaifenesin 200 mg and codeine phosphate 10 mg per 5 mL (480 mL) [contains phenylalanine 0.03 mcg/5 mL; cherry vanilla flavor]

Gani-Tuss® NR: Guaifenesin 100 mg and codeine phosphate 10 mg per 5 mL (480 mL) [raspberry flavor]

Guaifen-C: Guaifenesin 75 mg and codeine phosphate 2.5 mg per 5 mL (480 mL) [cherry flavor]

Guaifenesin AC: Guaifenesin 100 mg and codeine phosphate 10 mg per 5 mL (120 mL, 480 mL) [alcohol free, sugar free; raspberry flavor]

Iophen-C NR: Guaifenesin 100 mg and codeine phosphate 10 mg per 5 mL (480 mL) [raspberry flavor]

Kolephrin® #1: Guaifenesin 100 mg and codeine phosphate 10 mg per 5 mL (120 mL) [contains sodium 1.1 mg/5 mL and sodium benzoate]

Tussi-Organidin® NR: Guaifenesin 100 mg and codeine phosphate 10 mg per 5 mL (480 mL) [contains sodium benzoate; raspberry flavor]

Tussi-Organidin® S-NR: Guaifenesin 100 mg and codeine phosphate 10 mg per 5 mL (120 mL) [contains sodium benzoate; raspberry flavor]

Syrup:

Cheracol®: Guaifenesin 100 mg and codeine phosphate 10 mg per 5 mL (120 mL) [contains alcohol 4.75% and benzoic acid]

Cheratussin AC: Guaifenesin 100 mg and codeine phosphate 10 mg per 5 mL (120 mL, 240 mL, 480 mL)

Guaituss AC®: Guaifenesin 100 mg and codeine phosphate 10 mg per 5 mL (120 mL, 480 mL) [contains alcohol; sugar free; fruit-mint flavor]

Mytussin® AC: Guaifenesin 100 mg and codeine phosphate 10 mg per 5 mL (120 mL, 480 mL) [contains alcohol; sugar free; fruit flavor]

Robafen® AC: Guaifenesin 100 mg and codeine phosphate 10 mg per 5 mL (120 mL, 480 mL)

Romilar® AC: Guaifenesin 100 mg and codeine phosphate 10 mg per 5 mL (480 mL) [contains benzoic acid and phenylalanine; alcohol free, sugar free, dye free; grape flavor]

Tablet (Brontex®): Guaifenesin 300 mg and codeine phosphate 10 mg

# guaifenesin and dextromethorphan (gwye FEN e sin & deks troe meth OR fan)

## Sound-Alike/Look-Alike Issues
Benylin® may be confused with Benadryl®, Ventolin®

**Synonyms** dextromethorphan and guaifenesin

**U.S./Canadian Brand Names** Allfen-DM [US]; Altarussin DM [US-OTC]; Amibid DM [US]; Balminil DM E [Can]; Benylin® DM-E [Can]; Benylin® Expectorant [US-OTC]; Cheracol® D [US-OTC]; Cheracol® Plus [US-OTC]; Coricidin HBP® Chest Congestion and Cough [US-OTC]; Diabetic Tussin® DM Maximum Strength [US-OTC]; Diabetic Tussin® DM [US-OTC]; Drituss DM [US]; Duratuss® DM [US]; Gani-Tuss® DM NR [US]; Genatuss DM® [US-OTC]; Guaicon DM® [US-OTC]; Guaifenex® DM [US]; Guia-D [US]; Guiacon DMS® [US-OTC]; Guiatuss-DM® [US-OTC]; Hydro-Tussin™ DM [US]; Iophen DM NR [US]; Koffex DM-Expectorant [Can]; Kolephrin® GG/DM [US-OTC]; Mindal DM [US]; Mintab DM [US]; Mucinex® DM [US-OTC]; Phanatuss® DM [US-OTC]; Q-Bid DM [US]; Q-Tussin DM [US-OTC]; Respa-DM® [US], Robafen DM [US-OTC]; Robitussin® Cough and Congestion [US-OTC]; Robitussin® DM Infant [US-OTC]; Robitussin® DM [US-OTC/Can]; Robitussin® Sugar Free Cough [US-OTC]; Safe Tussin® 30 [US-OTC]; Scot-Tussin® Senior [US-OTC]; Silexin® [US-OTC]; Siltussin DM DAS [US-OTC]; Siltussin DM [US-OTC]; Su-Tuss DM [US]; Touro® DM [US]; Vicks® 44E [US-OTC]; Vicks® Pediatric Formula 44E [US-OTC]; Z-Cof LA™ [US]

**Therapeutic Category** Antitussive/Expectorant

**Use** Temporary control of cough due to minor throat and bronchial irritation

**Usual Dosage** Oral:

Children 2-6 years:
General dosing guidelines: Guaifenesin 50-100 mg and dextromethorphan 2.5-5 mg every 4 hours (maximum dose: Guaifenesin 600 mg and dextromethorphan 30 mg per day)
Product-specific labeling:
Benylin®: 5 mL every 4 hour (maximum: 6 doses/24 hours)
Guaifenex® DM, Touro® DM: 1/2 tablet every 12 hours (maximum: 1 tablet/24 hour)
Robitussin® DM, Robitussin® DM Infant, Robitussin® Sugar Free Cough: 2.5 mL every 4 hours (maximum: 6 doses/24 hours)
Vicks® Pediatric Formula 44E: 7.5 mL every 4 hours (maximum: 6 doses/24 hours)

Children: 6-12 years:
General dosing guidelines: Guaifenesin 100-200 mg and dextromethorphan 5-10 mg every 4 hours (maximum dose: Guaifenesin 1200 mg and dextromethorphan 60 mg per day)
Product-specific labeling:
Benylin®: 10 mL every 4 hours (maximum: 6 doses/24 hours)
Guaifenex® DM, Touro® DM: 1 tablet every 12 hours (maximum: 2 tablets/24 hours)
Humibid® CS: 1/2 tablet every 4 hours (maximum: 6 doses/24 hours)
Robitussin® DM, Robitussin® Sugar Free Cough: 5 mL every 4 hours (maximum: 6 doses/24 hours)
Vicks® 44E: 7.5 mL every 4 hours (maximum: 6 doses/24 hours)
Vicks® Pediatric Formula 44E: 15 mL every 4 hours (maximum: 6 doses/24 hours)
Z-Cof LA™: 1/2 tablet very 12 hours

Children ≥12 years and Adults:
General dosing guidelines: Guaifenesin 200-400 mg and dextromethorphan 10-20 mg every 4 hours (maximum dose: Guaifenesin 2400 mg and dextromethorphan 120 mg per day)
Product-specific labeling:
Benylin®: 20 mL every 4 hours (maximum: 6 doses/24 hours)
Guaifenex® DM, Mucinex® DM, Touro® DM: 1-2 tablets every 12 hours (maximum: 4 tablets/24 hours)
Humibid® CD: 1 tablet every 4 hours (maximum: 6 tablets/24 hours)
Robitussin® DM, Robitussin® Sugar Free Cough: 10 mL every 4 hours (maximum: 6 doses/24 hours)
Vicks® 44E: 15 mL every 4 hours (maximum: 6 doses/24 hours)
Vicks® Pediatric Formula 44E: 30 mL every 4 hours (maximum: 6 doses/24 hours)
Z-Cof LA™: 1 tablet every 12 hours

**Dosage Forms** [DSC] = Discontinued product
Caplet, sustained release (Mindal DM): Guaifenesin 500 mg and dextromethorphan hydrobromide 30 mg
(Continued)

## guaifenesin and dextromethorphan *(Continued)*

Capsule, softgel (Coricidin HBP® Chest Congestion and Cough): Guaifenesin 200 mg and dextromethorphan hydrobromide 10 mg

Elixir:

Duratuss DM®: Guaifenesin 225 mg and dextromethorphan hydrobromide 25 mg per 5 mL (480 mL) [contains sodium benzoate; grape flavor]

Drituss DM: Guaifenesin 200 mg and dextromethorphan hydrobromide 20 mg per 5 mL (480 mL) [grape flavor]

Su-Tuss DM: Guaifenesin 200 mg and dextromethorphan hydrobromide 20 mg per 5 mL (480 mL) [fruit flavor]

Liquid: Guaifenesin 100 mg and dextromethorphan hydrobromide 10 mg per 5 mL (480 mL)

Diabetic Tussin® DM: Guaifenesin 100 mg and dextromethorphan hydrobromide 10 mg per 5 mL (120 mL) [alcohol free, sugar free, dye free; contains phenylalanine 8.4 mg/5 mL]

Diabetic Tussin® DM Maximum Strength: Guaifenesin 200 mg and dextromethorphan hydrobromide 10 mg per 5 mL (120 mL) [alcohol free, sugar free, dye free; contains phenylalanine 8.4 mg/5 mL]

Gani-Tuss® DM NR: Guaifenesin 100 mg and dextromethorphan hydrobromide 10 mg per 5 mL (480 mL) [raspberry flavor]

Hydro-Tussin™ DM: Guaifenesin 200 mg and dextromethorphan hydrobromide 20 mg per 5 mL (480 mL) [alcohol free, sugar free; contains sodium benzoate]

Iophen DM NR: Guaifenesin 100 mg and dextromethorphan hydrobromide 10 mg per 5 mL (480 mL) [raspberry flavor]

Kolephrin® GG/DM: Guaifenesin 150 mg and dextromethorphan hydrobromide 10 mg per 5 mL (120 mL) [alcohol free; cherry flavor]

Q-Tussin DM: Guaifenesin 100 mg and dextromethorphan hydrobromide 10 mg per 5 mL (120 mL, 240 mL, 480 mL, 3840 mL) [cherry flavor]

Safe Tussin®: Guaifenesin 100 mg and dextromethorphan hydrobromide 15 mg per 5 mL (120 mL) [alcohol free, sodium free, sugar free, dye free; mint flavor]

Scot-Tussin® Senior: Guaifenesin 200 mg and dextromethorphan hydrobromide 15 mg per 5 mL (120 mL) [alcohol free, sodium free, sugar free]

Tussi-Organidin® DM NR: Guaifenesin 100 mg and dextromethorphan hydrobromide 10 mg per 5 mL (120 mL, 480 mL) [contains sodium benzoate; raspberry flavor] [DSC]

Vicks® 44E: Guaifenesin 200 mg and dextromethorphan hydrobromide 20 mg per 15 mL (120 mL, 235 mL) [contains sodium 31 mg/15 mL, alcohol, sodium benzoate]

Vicks® Pediatric Formula 44E: Guaifenesin 100 mg and dextromethorphan hydrobromide 10 mg per 15 mL (120 mL) [alcohol free; contains sodium 30 mg/15 mL, sodium benzoate; cherry flavor]

Liquid, oral drops (Robitussin® DM Infant): Guaifenesin 100 mg and dextromethorphan hydrobromide 5 mg per 2.5 mL (30 mL) [alcohol free; contains sodium benzoate; fruit punch flavor]

Syrup: Guaifenesin 100 mg and dextromethorphan hydrobromide 10 mg per 5 mL (120 mL, 480 mL)

Altarussin DM: Guaifenesin 100 mg and dextromethorphan hydrobromide 10 mg per 5 mL (120 mL, 240 mL, 480 mL, 3840 mL)

Benylin® Expectorant: Guaifenesin 100 mg and dextromethorphan hydrobromide 5 mg per 5 mL (120 mL) [alcohol free, sugar free; contains sodium benzoate; raspberry flavor]

Cheracol® D: Guaifenesin 100 mg and dextromethorphan hydrobromide 10 mg per 5 mL (120 mL, 180 mL) [contains alcohol 4.75%, benzoic acid]

Cheracol® Plus: Guaifenesin 100 mg and dextromethorphan hydrobromide 10 mg per 5 mL (120 mL) [contains alcohol 4.75%, benzoic acid]

Genatuss DM®: Guaifenesin 100 mg and dextromethorphan hydrobromide 10 mg per 5 mL (120 mL)

Guiatuss® DM: Guaifenesin 100 mg and dextromethorphan hydrobromide 10 mg per 5 mL (120 mL, 480 mL, 3840 mL) [alcohol free; contains sodium benzoate]

Guaicon DM®: Guaifenesin 100 mg and dextromethorphan hydrobromide 10 mg per 5 mL (10 mL) [alcohol free]

Guaicon DMS®: Guaifenesin 100 mg and dextromethorphan hydrobromide 10 mg per 5 mL (10 mL) [alcohol free, sugar free]

Mintab DM: Guaifenesin 200 mg and dextromethorphan hydrobromide 10 mg per 5 mL (480 mL) [alcohol free, dye free; cherry vanilla flavor]

Phanatuss® DM: Guaifenesin 100 mg and dextromethorphan hydrobromide 10 mg per 5 mL (120 mL) [alcohol free, sugar free]

Robafen® DM: Guaifenesin 100 mg and dextromethorphan hydrobromide 10 mg per 5 mL (120 mL, 240 mL, 480 mL) [cherry flavor]

Robitussin® Cough and Congestion: Guaifenesin 100 mg and dextromethorphan hydrobromide 10 mg per 5 mL (120 mL) [alcohol free; contains sodium benzoate]

Robitussin®-DM: Guaifenesin 100 mg and dextromethorphan hydrobromide 10 mg per 5 mL (5 mL, 120 mL, 340 mL, 360 mL) [alcohol free; contains sodium benzoate]

Robitussin® Sugar Free Cough: Guaifenesin 100 mg and dextromethorphan hydrobromide 10 mg per 5 mL (120 mL) [alcohol free, sugar free; contains sodium benzoate]

Silexin®: Guaifenesin 100 mg and dextromethorphan hydrobromide 10 mg per 5 mL (45 mL) [alcohol free, sugar free)]

Siltussin DM: Guaifenesin 100 mg and dextromethorphan hydrobromide 10 mg per 5 mL (120 mL, 240 mL, 480 mL) [strawberry flavor]

Siltussin DM DAS: Guaifenesin 100 mg and dextromethorphan hydrobromide 10 mg per 5 mL (120 mL) [alcohol free, dye free, sugar free; strawberry flavor]

Tablet:

Humibid® CS: Guaifenesin 400 mg and dextromethorphan hydrobromide 20 mg [DSC]

Silexin®: Guaifenesin 100 mg and dextromethorphan hydrobromide 10 mg

Tablet, extended release: Guaifenesin 500 mg and dextromethorphan hydrobromide 30 mg

Amibid DM, Guaifenex® DM, Humibid® DM [DSC], Mucinex® DM, Q-Bid DM, Respa-DM®: Guaifenesin 600 mg and dextromethorphan hydrobromide 30 mg

Aquatab® DM: Guaifenesin 1200 mg and dextromethorphan hydrobromide 60 mg [DSC]

Mucophen® DM: Guaifenesin 1000 mg and dextromethorphan hydrobromide 60 mg

Touro® DM: Guaifenesin 575 mg and dextromethorphan hydrobromide 30 mg

Tablet, long-acting: Guaifenesin 500 mg and dextromethorphan hydrobromide 30 mg; guaifenesin 1000 mg and dextromethorphan hydrobromide 50 mg; guaifenesin 1000 mg and dextromethorphan hydrobromide 60 mg

Z-Cof LA: Guaifenesin 650 mg and dextromethorphan hydrobromide 30 mg [scored]

Tablet, sustained release: Guaifenesin 800 mg and dextromethorphan hydrobromide 30 mg; guaifenesin 1000 mg and dextromethorphan hydrobromide 60 mg; guaifenesin 1200 mg and dextromethorphan hydrobromide 60 mg

Allfen-DM: Guaifenesin 1000 mg and dextromethorphan hydrobromide 55  mg

Tussi-Bid®: Guaifenesin 1200 mg and dextromethorphan hydrobromide 60 mg

Tablet, timed release [scored] (Guia-D): Guaifenesin 1000 mg and dextromethorphan hydrobromide 60mg [dye free]

**guaifenesin and hydrocodone** *see* hydrocodone and guaifenesin *on page 412*

# guaifenesin and phenylephrine (gwye FEN e sin & fen il EF rin)

## Sound-Alike/Look-Alike Issues
Endal® may be confused with Depen®, Intal®

Entex® may be confused with Tenex®

**Synonyms** guaifenesin and phenylephrine tannate; phenylephrine hydrochloride and guaifenesin

**U.S./Canadian Brand Names** Aldex™ [US]; Ami-Tex LA [US]; Amidal [US]; Crantex ER [US]; Crantex LA [US]; Deconsal® II [US]; Endal® [US]; Entex® ER [US]; Entex® LA [US]; Entex® [US]; Guaifed-PD® [US]; Guaifed® [US]; Liquibid-D [US]; Liquibid-PD [US]; PhenaVent™ D [US]; PhenaVent™ Ped [US]; PhenaVent™ [US]; Prolex™-D [US]; Rescon GG [US]; Sil-Tex [US]; Sina-12X [US]; SINUvent® PE [US]

**Therapeutic Category** Cold Preparation

**Use** Temporary relief of nasal congestion, sinusitis, rhinitis and hay fever; temporary relief of cough associated with upper respiratory tract conditions, especially when associated with dry, nonproductive cough

**Usual Dosage** Oral:

Children 2-6 years:

Entex®, Rescon GG, Sil-Tex: 2.5 mL every 4-6 hours; maximum 10 mL/24 hours

Sina-12X suspension: 2.5-5 mL every 12 hours

Children 6-12 years:

Aldex™, Crantex LA, Liquibid-D, PhenaVent™ D, Sina-12X tablet: One-half tablet every 12 hours (maximum: 1 tablet/24 hours)

Deconsal® II: One capsule daily

Entex®, Rescon GG: 5 mL every 4-6 hours (maximum: 20 mL/24 hours)

Guaifed-PD®, PhenaVent™ Ped: One capsule every 12 hours

Liquibid-PD, SINUvent® PE: One tablet every 12 hours (maximum: 2 tablets/24 hours)

Prolex™-D: One-half to 1 tablet every 12 hours

Sina-12X suspension: Refer to Adults dosing.

(Continued)

# guaifenesin and phenylephrine *(Continued)*

Children ≥12 years:

Aldex™, Crantex LA, Deconsal® II, Entex®, Entex® LA, Guaifed®, Guaifed-PD®, Liquibid-D, Liquibid-PD, PhenaVent™, PhenaVent™ D, PhenaVent™ Ped, Prolex™-D, Rescon GG, Sil-Tex, Sina-12X, SINUvent® PE: Refer to Adults dosing

Crantex ER, Entex® ER: One capsule every 12 hours

Adults:

Aldex™, Crantex LA, Liquibid-D, PhenaVent™ D: One tablet every 12 hours

Crantex ER, Entex® ER, Guaifed-PD®, PhenaVent™ Ped: 1-2 capsules every 12 hours

Deconsal® II: 1-2 capsules every 12 hours (maximum: 3 capsules/24 hours)

Endal®, Prolex™-D: 1-2 tablets every 12 hours

Entex®, Sil-Tex: 5-10 mL every 4-6 hours (maximum: 40 mL/24 hours)

Entex® LA, Guaifed®, PhenaVent™: One capsule every 12 hours (maximum: 2 capsules/24 hours)

Liquibid-PD, Sina-12X tablet: 1-2 tablets every 12 hours (maximum: 4 tablets/24 hours)

Rescon GG: 10 mL every 4-6 hours (maximum: 40 mL/24 hours)

Sina-12X suspension: 5-10 mL every 12 hours

SINUvent® PE: Two tablets every 12 hours

## Dosage Forms

Capsule, variable release:

Crantex ER, Entex® ER: Guaifenesin 300 mg [immediate release] and phenylephrine hydrochloride 10 mg [extended release]

Deconsal® II: Guaifenesin 375 mg [immediate release] and phenylephrine hydrochloride 20 mg [extended release] [contains tartrazine]

Entex® LA: Guaifenesin 400 mg [immediate release] and phenylephrine hydrochloride 30 mg [extended release]

Guaifed®, PhenaVent™: Guaifenesin 400 mg [immediate release] and phenylephrine hydrochloride 15 mg [extended release]

Guaifed-PD®, PhenaVent™ Ped: Guaifenesin 200 mg [immediate release] and phenylephrine hydrochloride 7.5 mg [extended release]

Liquid: Guaifenesin 100 mg and phenylephrine hydrochloride 7.5 mg per 5 mL (480 mL)

Entex®, Sil-Tex: Guaifenesin 100 mg and phenylephrine hydrochloride 7.5 mg per 5 mL (480 mL) [alcohol free, dye-free, sugar free; punch flavor]

Rescon GG: Guaifenesin 100 mg and phenylephrine hydrochloride 5 mg per 5 mL (120 mL, 480 mL) [cherry orange-pineapple flavor]

Suspension (Sina-12X): Guaifenesin 100 mg and phenylephrine tannate 5 mg per 5 mL (120 mL) [contains benzoic acid; grape flavor]

Tablet:

Amidal: Guaifenesin 300 mg and phenylephrine hydrochloride 20 mg

Sina-12X: Guaifenesin 200 mg and phenylephrine tannate 25 mg

Tablet, extended release: Guaifenesin 600 mg and phenylephrine hydrochloride 20 mg; Guaifenesin 600 mg and phenylephrine hydrochloride 40 mg; Guaifenesin 1200 mg and phenylephrine hydrochloride 40 mg

Aldex™: Guaifenesin 650 mg and phenylephrine hydrochloride 25 mg

Ami-Tex LA: Guaifenesin 600 mg and phenylephrine hydrochloride 30 mg

Liquibid-D: Guaifenesin 600 mg and phenylephrine hydrochloride 40 mg

Liquibid-PD: Guaifenesin 275 mg and phenylephrine hydrochloride 25 mg

PhenaVent™ D: Guaifenesin 1200 mg and phenylephrine hydrochloride 40 mg

SINUvent® PE: Guaifenesin 600 mg and phenylephrine hydrochloride 15 mg

Tablet, sustained release: Guaifenesin 600 mg and phenylephrine hydrochloride 30 mg

Crantex LA: Guaifenesin 600 mg and phenylephrine hydrochloride 30 mg [dye-free]

Prolex™-D: Guaifenesin 600 mg and phenylephrine hydrochloride 20 mg [dye-free]

Tablet, timed release (Endal®): Guaifenesin 300 mg and phenylephrine hydrochloride 20 mg

**guaifenesin and phenylephrine tannate** *see* guaifenesin and phenylephrine *on previous page*

# guaifenesin and pseudoephedrine (gwye FEN e sin & soo doe e FED rin)

## Sound-Alike/Look-Alike Issues

Entex® may be confused with Tenex®

Profen II® may be confused with Profen II DM®, Profen Forte®, Profen Forte™ DM

Profen Forte® may be confused with Profen II®, Profen II DM®, Profen Forte™ DM

**Synonyms** pseudoephedrine and guaifenesin

**U.S./Canadian Brand Names** Ambifed-G [US]; Ami-Tex PSE [US]; Congestac® [US-OTC]; Contac® Cold-Chest Congestion, Non Drowsy, Regular Strength [Can]; Dynex [US]; Entex® LA [Can]; Entex® PSE [US]; Eudal®-SR [US]; G-Phed [US]; Guaifenex® GP [US]; Guaifenex® PSE [US]; Guaimax-D® [US]; Levall G [US]; Maxifed-G® [US]; Maxifed® [US]; Miraphen PSE [US]; Mucinex®-D [US-OTC]; Nasatab® LA [US]; Novahistex® Expectorant with Decongestant [Can]; PanMist®-JR [US]; PanMist®-LA [US]; PanMist®-S [US]; Profen Forte® [US]; Profen II® [US]; Pseudo GG TR [US]; Pseudovent™ 400 [US]; Pseudovent™ [US]; Pseudovent™-Ped [US]; Refenesen Plus [US-OTC]; Respaire®-120 SR [US]; Respaire®-60 SR [US]; Robitussin-PE® [US-OTC]; Robitussin® Severe Congestion [US-OTC]; Sudafed® Non-Drying Sinus [US-OTC]; Touro LA® [US]; Zephrex LA® [US]; Zephrex® [US]

**Therapeutic Category** Expectorant/Decongestant

**Use** Temporary relief of nasal congestion and to help loosen phlegm and thin bronchial secretions in the treatment of cough

**Usual Dosage** Oral:

Children 2-6 years:
Guaifenex® PSE 60: One-half tablet every 12 hours (maximum: 1 tablet/12 hours)
Maxifed-G®: One-third to 1/2 tablet every 12 hours (maximum: 1 tablet/12 hours)
PanMist®-S: 2.5 mL 4 times/day (maximum: Pseudoephedrine 4 mg/kg/day)
Robitussin® PE: 2.5 mL every 4-6 hours (maximum: 4 doses/24 hours)

Children 6-12 years:
Ambifed-G, Dynex, Eudal®-SR, Guaimax-D®, Guaifenex® PSE 80, Guaifenex® PSE 120, Maxifed®, Miraphen PSE, Nasatab® LA, PanMist®-LA, Profen II®, Profen Forte®, Zephrex® LA: One-half caplet or tablet every 12 hours (maximum: 1 tablet/24 hours)
Congestac®: One-half caplet every 4-6 hours (maximum: 2 caplets/24 hours)
Guaifenex® PSE 60, PanMist®-JR, Pseudovent™-Ped, Respaire®-60 SR: One tablet or capsule every 12 hours (maximum: 2 tablets or capsules every 24 hours)
Levall G: One capsule every 24 hours
Maxifed-G®: One-half to 1 tablet every 12 hours (maximum: 2 tablets/24 hours)
PanMist®-S: 5 mL 4 times/day (maximum: Pseudoephedrine 4 mg/kg/day)
Robitussin® PE: 5 mL every 4-6 hours (maximum: 4 doses/24 hours)
Robitussin® Severe Congestion: One capsule every 4 hours (maximum: 4 doses/24 hours)
Zephrex®: One-half tablet every 6 hours

Children >12 years and Adults:
Ambifed-G, Aquatab® D, Dynex, Entex® PSE, Eudal®- SR, G-Phed, Guaifenex® GP, Guaifenex® PSE 120, Guaimax-D®, Levall G, Miraphen PSE, Mucinex®-D 1200/120, Nasatab® LA, PanMist®-LA, Profen Forte®, Pseudovent™, Respaire®-120 SR, Touro LA, Zephrex® LA: One tablet or capsule every 12 hours (maximum: 2 tablets or capsules in 24 hours)
Congestac®: One caplet every 4-6 hours (maximum: 4 caplets in 24 hours)
Guaifenex® PSE 60, Maxifed-G®, Mucinex®-D 600/60, PanMist®-JR, Pseudovent™-Ped, Respaire®-60 SR: 1-2 tablets or capsules every 12 hours (maximum: 4 tablets or capsules/24 hours)
Guaifenex® PSE 80, PanMist®-LA: One tablet every twelve hours (maximum: 3 tablets/24 hours)
Guaifenex™ RX: 1-2 of the AM tablets every morning and 1-2 of the PM tablets 12 hours following morning dose
Maxifed®, Profen II®: One to 1 1/2 tablets every 12 hours (maximum: 3 tablets/24 hours)
PanMist®-S: Up to 10 mL 4 times/day
Robitussin® PE: 10 mL every 4-6 hours (maximum: 4 doses/24 hours)
Robitussin® Severe Congestion, Sudafed® Non-Drying Sinus: Two capsules every 4 hours (maximum: 4 doses/24 hours)
Zephrex®: One tablet every 6 hours

**Dosage Forms** [DSC] = Discontinued product
Caplet (Congestac®, Refenesen Plus): Guaifenesin 400 mg and pseudoephedrine hydrochloride 60 mg
Caplet, long-acting (Touro LA®): Guaifenesin 500 mg and pseudoephedrine hydrochloride 120 mg
Caplet, prolonged release (Ambifed-G): Guaifenesin 1000 mg and pseudoephedrine hydrochloride 60 mg
Capsule, extended release:
Respaire®-60 SR: Guaifenesin 200 mg and pseudoephedrine hydrochloride 60 mg
Respaire®-120 SR: Guaifenesin 250 mg and pseudoephedrine hydrochloride 120 mg
Capsule, liquicap (Sudafed® Non-Drying Sinus): Guaifenesin 200 mg and pseudoephedrine hydrochloride 30 mg
Capsule, softgel (Robitussin® Severe Congestion): Guaifenesin 200 mg and pseudoephedrine hydrochloride 30 mg
(Continued)

## guaifenesin and pseudoephedrine *(Continued)*

Capsule, variable release:

Entex® PSE: Guaifenesin 400 mg [immediate release] and pseudoephedrine hydrochloride 120 mg [extended release]

G-Phed: Guaifenesin 250 mg [immediate release] and pseudoephedrine hydrochloride 120 mg [prolonged release]

Levall G: Guaifenesin 400 mg [immediate release] and pseudoephedrine hydrochloride 90 mg [extended release]

Pseudovent™: Guaifenesin 250 mg [immediate release] and pseudoephedrine hydrochloride 120 mg [prolonged release]

Pseudovent™-Ped: Guaifenesin 300 mg [immediate release] and pseudoephedrine hydrochloride 60 mg [prolonged release]

Pseudovent™ 400: Guaifenesin 400 mg [immediate release] and pseudoephedrine hydrochloride 1200 mg [extended release]

Combination package (Guaifenex™-Rx) [14-day treatment package; each package contains] [DSC]:

Tablet, extended release: Guaifenesin 600 mg and pseudoephedrine hydrochloride 60 mg (28s) [for AM dose]

Tablet, extended release: Guaifenesin 600 mg (28s) [for PM dose]

Syrup: Guaifenesin 200 mg and pseudoephedrine hydrochloride 40 mg per 5 mL (480 mL)

PanMist®-S: Guaifenesin 200 mg and pseudoephedrine hydrochloride 40 mg per 5 mL (480 mL) [alcohol free; grape flavor]

Robitussin-PE®: Guaifenesin 100 mg and pseudoephedrine hydrochloride 30 mg per 5 mL (120 mL, 240 mL) [alcohol free; contains sodium benzoate]

Tablet (Zephrex®): Guaifenesin 400 mg and pseudoephedrine hydrochloride 60 mg

Tablet, extended release: Guaifenesin 550 mg and pseudoephedrine hydrochloride 60 mg; guaifenesin 595 mg and pseudoephedrine hydrochloride 48 mg; guaifenesin 600 mg and pseudoephedrine hydrochloride 60 mg; guaifenesin 600 mg and pseudoephedrine hydrochloride 120 mg; guaifenesin 795 mg and pseudoephedrine hydrochloride 85 mg; guaifenesin 800 mg and pseudoephedrine hydrochloride 45 mg; guaifenesin 800 mg and pseudoephedrine hydrochloride 60 mg; guaifenesin 800 mg and pseudoephedrine hydrochloride 90 mg; guaifenesin 1200 mg and pseudoephedrine hydrochloride 50 mg; guaifenesin 1200 mg and pseudoephedrine hydrochloride 60 mg; guaifenesin 1200 mg and pseudoephedrine hydrochloride 75 mg; guaifenesin 1200 mg and pseudoephedrine hydrochloride 90 mg; guaifenesin 1200 mg and pseudoephedrine hydrochloride 120 mg

Ami-Tex PSE, Guaimax-D®, Zephrex LA®: Guaifenesin 600 mg and pseudoephedrine hydrochloride 120 mg

Aquatab® D: Guaifenesin 1200 mg and pseudoephedrine hydrochloride 75 mg [DSC]

Guaifenex® GP: Guaifenesin 1200 mg and pseudoephedrine hydrochloride 120 mg [dye free]

Guaifenex® PSE 60: Guaifenesin 600 mg and pseudoephedrine hydrochloride 60 mg

Guaifenex® PSE 80: Guaifenesin 800 mg and pseudoephedrine hydrochloride 80 mg

Maxifed®: Guaifenesin 700 mg and pseudoephedrine hydrochloride 80 mg

Maxifed-G®: Guaifenesin 550 mg and pseudoephedrine hydrochloride 60 mg

Mucinex®-D 600/60: Guaifenesin 600 mg and pseudoephedrine hydrochloride 60 mg

Mucinex®-D 1200/120: Guaifenesin 1200 mg and pseudoephedrine hydrochloride 120 mg

PanMist®-JR, Pseudo GG TR: Guaifenesin 595 mg and pseudoephedrine hydrochloride 48 mg

PanMist®-LA: Guaifenesin 795 mg and pseudoephedrine hydrochloride 85 mg

Profen II®: Guaifenesin 800 mg and pseudoephedrine hydrochloride 45 mg

Profen Forte®: Guaifenesin 800 mg and pseudoephedrine hydrochloride 90 mg

Tablet, long acting:

Dynex: Guaifenesin 1200 mg and pseudoephedrine hydrochloride 90 mg

Guaifenex® PSE 120: Guaifenesin 600 mg and pseudoephedrine hydrochloride 120 mg [dye free]

Miraphen PSE: Guaifenesin 600 mg and pseudoephedrine hydrochloride 120 mg

Tablet, sustained release (Nasatab® LA): Guaifenesin 500 mg and pseudoephedrine hydrochloride 120 mg

**guaifenesin and theophylline** *see* theophylline and guaifenesin *on page 795*

**guaifenesin, hydrocodone, and pseudoephedrine** *see* hydrocodone, pseudoephedrine, and guaifenesin *on page 415*

## guaifenesin, pseudoephedrine, and codeine

(gwye FEN e sin, soo doe e FED rin, & KOE deen)

**Sound-Alike/Look-Alike Issues**

Halotussin® may be confused with Halotestin®

**Synonyms** codeine, guaifenesin, and pseudoephedrine; pseudoephedrine, guaifenesin, and codeine

**U.S./Canadian Brand Names** Benylin® 3.3 mg-D-E [Can]; Calmylin with Codeine [Can]; Guiatuss™ DAC® [US]; Mytussin® DAC [US]; Nucofed® Expectorant [US]; Nucofed® Pediatric Expectorant [US]

**Therapeutic Category** Antitussive/Decongestant/Expectorant

**Controlled Substance** C-III; C-V

**Use** Temporarily relieves nasal congestion and controls cough due to minor throat and bronchial irritation; helps loosen phlegm and thin bronchial secretions to make coughs more productive

**Usual Dosage** Oral:

Children 6-12 years: 5 mL every 4 hours, not to exceed 40 mL/24 hours

Children >12 years and Adults: 10 mL every 4 hours, not to exceed 40 mL/24 hours

**Dosage Forms** [DSC] = Discontinued product

Syrup:

Guiatuss™ DAC: Guaifenesin 100 mg, pseudoephedrine hydrochloride 30 mg, and codeine phosphate 10 mg per 5 mL (480 mL)

Mytussin® DAC: Guaifenesin 100 mg, pseudoephedrine hydrochloride 30 mg, and codeine phosphate 10 mg per 5 mL (120 mL, 480 mL) [sugar free; contains alcohol 1.7%; strawberry-raspberry flavor]

Nucofed® Expectorant: Guaifenesin 200 mg, pseudoephedrine hydrochloride 60 mg, and codeine phosphate 20 mg per 5 mL (480 mL) [contains alcohol 12.5%; cherry flavor]

Nucofed® Pediatric Expectorant: Guaifenesin 100 mg, pseudoephedrine hydrochloride 30 mg, and codeine phosphate 10 mg per 5 mL (480 mL) [contains alcohol 6%; strawberry flavor]

## guaifenesin, pseudoephedrine, and dextromethorphan

(gwye FEN e sin, soo doe e FED rin, & deks troe meth OR fan)

**Sound-Alike/Look-Alike Issues**

Profen II DM® may be confused with Profen II®, Profen Forte®, Profen Forte™ DM

Profen Forte™ DM may be confused with Profen II®, Profen II DM®, Profen Forte®

**Synonyms** dextromethorphan, guaifenesin, and pseudoephedrine; pseudoephedrine, dextromethorphan, and guaifenesin

**U.S./Canadian Brand Names** Ambifed-G DM [US]; Balminil DM + Decongestant + Expectorant [Can]; Benylin® DM-D-E [Can]; Dimetapp® Cold and Congestion [US-OTC]; Koffex DM + Decongestant + Expectorant [Can]; Maxifed® DM [US]; Novahistex® DM Decongestant Expectorant [Can]; Novahistine® DM Decongestant Expectorant [Can]; PanMist®-DM [US]; Profen Forte™ DM [US]; Profen II DM® [US]; Pseudovent™ DM [US]; Relacon-DM [US]; Robitussin® CF [US-OTC]; Robitussin® Cold and Congestion [US-OTC]; Robitussin® Cough & Cold® [Can]; Robitussin® Cough and Cold Infant [US-OTC]; Touro™ CC [US]; Tri-Vent™ DM [US]; Z-Cof DM [US]

**Therapeutic Category** Cold Preparation

**Use** Temporarily relieves nasal congestion and controls cough due to minor throat and bronchial irritation; helps loosen phlegm and thin bronchial secretions to make coughs more productive

**Usual Dosage Note:** Also refer to specific product labeling.

Children 2-6 years:

Maxifed® DM: 1/3 to 1/2 tablet every 12 hours, not to exceed 1 tablet/24 hours

PanMist®-DM (syrup), Tri-Vent™ DM: 2.5 mL up to 3-4 times/day, not to exceed pseudoephedrine 4 mg/kg/day

Profen II DM (syrup): 1.25-2.5 mL every 4 hours, not to exceed 15 mL/24 hours

Robitussin® Pediatric Cough and Cold Infant: 2.5 mL every 4-6 hours, not to exceed 4 doses/24 hours

Touro™ CC: 1/2 tablet every 12 hour, not to exceed 1 tablet/24 hours

Z-Cof DM: 2.5 mL 2-3 times/day, not to exceed 7.5 mL/24 hours

Children 6-12 years:

Ambifed-G DM, Profen Forte™ DM, Profen II DM®: 1/2 tablet every 12 hours not to exceed 1 tablet/24 hours

Dimetapp® Cold and Congestion, Robitussin® Cold and Congestion: 1 caplet every 4-6 hours, not to exceed 4 doses/24 hours

Maxifed® DM: 1/2 to 1 tablet every 12 hours, not to exceed 2 tablets/24 hours

PanMist®-DM (syrup), Tri-Vent™ DM: 5 mL up to 3-4 times/day, not to exceed pseudoephedrine 4 mg/kg/day

PanMist®-DM (tablet), Touro™ CC, Pseudovent™ DM: 1 tablet every 12 hours, not to exceed 2 tablets/24 hours

(Continued)

# guaifenesin, pseudoephedrine, and dextromethorphan *(Continued)*

Profen II DM (syrup): 2.5-5 mL every 4 hours, not to exceed 30 mL/24 hours

Z-Cof DM: 5 mL 2-3 times/day, not to exceed 15 mL/24 hours

Children ≥12 years and Adults:

Ambifed-G DM, Aquatab® C, Profen Forte™ DM: 1 tablet every 12 hours not to exceed 2 tablets/24 hours

Dimetapp® Cold and Congestion, Robitussin® Cold and Congestion: 2 caplets every 4-6 hours not to exceed 4 doses in 24 hours

Guaifenex™-Rx DM: 1-2 of the "AM" tablets in the morning and 1-2 of the "PM" tablets 12 hours later

Maxifed® DM, PanMist®-DM (tablet), Touro™ CC, Pseudovent™ DM: 1-2 tablets every 12 hours, not to exceed 4 tablets/24 hours

PanMist®-DM (syrup), Tri-Vent™ DM: Up to 10 mL 3-4 times/day, not to exceed pseudoephedrine 240 mg/24 hours

Profen II DM (tablet): 1 to 1¹/₂ tablets every 12 hours, not to exceed 3 tablets/24 hours

Profen II DM (syrup): 5-10 mL every 4 hours, not to exceed 60 mL/24 hours

Z-Cof DM: 10 mL 2-3 times/day, not to exceed 30 mL/24 hours

**Dosage Forms** [DSC] = Discontinued product

Caplet (Dimetapp® Cold and Congestion, Robitussin® Cold and Congestion): Guaifenesin 200 mg, pseudoephedrine hydrochloride 30 mg, and dextromethorphan hydrobromide 10 mg

Caplet, prolonged release (Ambifed-G DM): Guaifenesin 1000 mg, pseudoephedrine hydrochloride 60 mg, and dextromethorphan hydrobromide 30 mg

Caplet, sustained release (Touro™ CC): Guaifenesin 575 mg, pseudoephedrine hydrochloride 60 mg, and dextromethorphan hydrobromide 30 mg [dye free]

Capsule, softgel (Robitussin® Cold and Congestion): Guaifenesin 200 mg, pseudoephedrine hydrochloride 30 mg, and dextromethorphan hydrobromide 10 mg

Combination package (Guaifenex™-Rx DM) [14 day treatment package] [DSC]:

Tablet, extended release: Guaifenesin 600 mg, and pseudoephedrine hydrochloride 60 mg (28s) [for AM dose]

Tablet, extended release: Guaifenesin 600 mg, and dextromethorphan hydrobromide 30 mg (28s) [for PM dose]

Liquid: Guaifenesin 100 mg, pseudoephedrine hydrochloride 30 mg, and dextromethorphan hydrobromide 10 mg per 5 mL (120 mL)

Profen II DM®: Guaifenesin 200 mg, pseudoephedrine hydrochloride 15 mg, and dextromethorphan hydrobromide 10 mg per 5 mL (480 mL) [alcohol free, dye free, sugar free; cherry flavor]

Relacon-DM: Guaifenesin 200 mg, pseudoephedrine hydrochloride 40 mg, and dextromethorphan hydrobromide 15 mg (480 mL) [grape flavor]

Liquid, oral drops (Robitussin® Cough and Cold Infant): Guaifenesin 100 mg, pseudoephedrine hydrochloride 15 mg, and dextromethorphan hydrobromide 5 mg per 2.5 mL (30 mL) [alcohol free; contains sodium benzoate]

Syrup: Guaifenesin 100 mg, pseudoephedrine hydrochloride 45 mg, and dextromethorphan hydrobromide 15 mg per 5 mL (480 mL)

PanMist®-DM: Guaifenesin 100 mg, pseudoephedrine hydrochloride 40 mg, and dextromethorphan hydrobromide 15 mg per 5 mL (480 mL) [alcohol free, dye free, sugar free; strawberry flavor]

Robitussin® CF: Guaifenesin 100 mg, pseudoephedrine hydrochloride 30 mg, and dextromethorphan hydrobromide 10 mg per 5 mL (120 mL, 240 mL, 360 mL) [alcohol free; contains sodium benzoate]

Tri-Vent™ DM: Guaifenesin 100 mg, pseudoephedrine hydrochloride 40 mg, and dextromethorphan hydrobromide 15 mg per 5 mL (480 mL) [alcohol free, dye free, sugar free; strawberry flavor]

Tablet, extended release: Guaifenesin 800 mg, pseudoephedrine hydrochloride 60 mg, and dextromethorphan hydrobromide 30 mg; guaifenesin 1200 mg, pseudoephedrine hydrochloride 60 mg, and dextromethorphan hydrobromide 60 mg; guaifenesin 1200 mg, pseudoephedrine hydrochloride 120 mg, and dextromethorphan hydrobromide 60 mg; guaifenesin 800 mg, pseudoephedrine hydrochloride 90 mg, and dextromethorphan hydrobromide 60 mg; guaifenesin 550 mg, pseudoephedrine hydrochloride 60 mg, and dextromethorphan hydrobromide 30 mg; guaifenesin 595 mg, pseudoephedrine hydrochloride 48 mg, and dextromethorphan hydrobromide 32 mg; guaifenesin 600 mg, pseudoephedrine hydrochloride 60 mg, and dextromethorphan hydrobromide 30 mg

Aquatab® C: Guaifenesin 1200 mg, pseudoephedrine hydrochloride 60 mg, and dextromethorphan hydrobromide 60 mg [DSC]

PanMist®-DM, Pseudovent™ DM: Guaifenesin 595 mg, pseudoephedrine hydrochloride 48 mg, and dextromethorphan hydrobromide 32 mg

Profen Forte™ DM: Guaifenesin 800 mg, pseudoephedrine hydrochloride 90 mg, and dextromethorphan hydrobromide 60 mg

Profen II DM®: Guaifenesin 800 mg, pseudoephedrine hydrochloride 45 mg, and dextromethorphan hydrobromide 30 mg

Tablet, sustained release (Maxifed® DM): Guaifenesin 550 mg, pseudoephedrine hydrochloride 60 mg, and dextromethorphan hydrobromide 30 mg [dye free]

**Guaifenex®** *(Discontinued)*

**Guaifenex® DM [US]** *see* guaifenesin and dextromethorphan *on page 385*

**Guaifenex® GP [US]** *see* guaifenesin and pseudoephedrine *on page 388*

**Guaifenex® PPA 75** *(Discontinued)*

**Guaifenex® PSE [US]** *see* guaifenesin and pseudoephedrine *on page 388*

**Guaifenex™-Rx** *(Discontinued)* *see* guaifenesin and pseudoephedrine *on page 388*

**Guaifenex™-Rx DM** *(Discontinued)* *see* guaifenesin, pseudoephedrine, and dextromethorphan *on page 391*

**Guaimax-D® [US]** *see* guaifenesin and pseudoephedrine *on page 388*

**Guaipax®** *(Discontinued)*

**Guaitab®** *(Discontinued)* *see* guaifenesin and pseudoephedrine *on page 388*

**Guaituss AC® [US]** *see* guaifenesin and codeine *on page 384*

**Guaituss CF®** *(Discontinued)*

**Guaivent®** *(Discontinued)* *see* guaifenesin and pseudoephedrine *on page 388*

## guanabenz (GWAHN a benz)
**Sound-Alike/Look-Alike Issues**
guanabenz may be confused with guanadrel, guanfacine
**Synonyms** guanabenz acetate
**U.S./Canadian Brand Names** Wytensin® [Can]
**Therapeutic Category** Alpha-Adrenergic Agonist
**Use** Management of hypertension
**Usual Dosage** Adults: Oral: Initial: 4 mg twice daily; increase in increments of 4-8 mg/day every 1-2 weeks to a maximum of 32 mg twice daily.
**Dosage Forms** Tablet: 4 mg, 8 mg

**guanabenz acetate** *see* guanabenz *on this page*

## guanfacine (GWAHN fa seen)
**Sound-Alike/Look-Alike Issues**
guanfacine may be confused with guaifenesin, guanabenz, guanidine
Tenex® may be confused with Entex®, Ten-K®, Xanax®
**Synonyms** guanfacine hydrochloride
**U.S./Canadian Brand Names** Tenex® [US/Can]
**Therapeutic Category** Alpha-Adrenergic Agonist
**Use** Management of hypertension
**Usual Dosage** Oral: Adults: Hypertension: 1 mg usually at bedtime, may increase if needed at 3- to 4-week intervals; usual dose range (JNC 7): 0.5-2 mg once daily
**Dosage Forms** Tablet: 1 mg, 2 mg

**guanfacine hydrochloride** *see* guanfacine *on this page*

## guanidine (GWAHN i deen)
**Sound-Alike/Look-Alike Issues**
guanidine may be confused with guanfacine, guanethidine
**Synonyms** guanidine hydrochloride
**Therapeutic Category** Cholinergic Agent
**Use** Reduction of the symptoms of muscle weakness associated with the myasthenic syndrome of Eaton-Lambert, not for myasthenia gravis
**Usual Dosage** Adults: Oral: Eaton-Lambert syndrome: Initial: 10-15 mg/kg/day in 3-4 divided doses, gradually increase to 35 mg/kg/day or up to development of side effects
**Dosage Forms** Tablet, as hydrochloride: 125 mg

**guanidine hydrochloride** *see* guanidine *on previous page*

**Guia-D [US]** *see* guaifenesin and dextromethorphan *on page 385*

**Guiacon DMS**® **[US-OTC]** *see* guaifenesin and dextromethorphan *on page 385*

**GuiaCough**® *(Discontinued)* *see* guaifenesin and dextromethorphan *on page 385*

**GuiaCough**® **Expectorant** *(Discontinued)* *see* guaifenesin *on page 383*

**Guiatex**® *(Discontinued)*

**Guiatuss**™ **[US-OTC]** *see* guaifenesin *on page 383*

**Guiatuss**™ **DAC**® **[US]** *see* guaifenesin, pseudoephedrine, and codeine *on page 391*

**Guiatuss-DM**® **[US-OTC]** *see* guaifenesin and dextromethorphan *on page 385*

**gum benjamin** *see* benzoin *on page 98*

**GW433908G** *see* fosamprenavir *on page 360*

**G-well**® *(Discontinued)* *see* lindane *on page 483*

**Gynazole-1**® **[US/Can]** *see* butoconazole *on page 126*

**Gyne-Lotrimin**® **3 [US-OTC]** *see* clotrimazole *on page 199*

**Gyne-Sulf**® *(Discontinued)* *see* sulfabenzamide, sulfacetamide, and sulfathiazole *on page 771*

**Gynodiol**® **[US]** *see* estradiol *on page 299*

**Gynogen L.A.**® **Injection** *(Discontinued)* *see* estradiol *on page 299*

**Gynol II**® **[US-OTC]** *see* nonoxynol 9 *on page 580*

**Gynovite**® **Plus [US-OTC]** *see* vitamins (multiple/oral) *on page 852*

**H-C Tussive [US]** *see* phenylephrine, hydrocodone, and chlorpheniramine *on page 643*

# *Haemophilus* B conjugate and hepatitis B vaccine
(he MOF i lus bee KON joo gate & hep a TYE tis bee vak SEEN)
**Sound-Alike/Look-Alike Issues**
Comvax® may be confused with Recombivax [Recombivax HB®]
**Synonyms** *Haemophilus* b (meningococcal protein conjugate) conjugate vaccine; hepatitis b vaccine (recombinant); Hib
**U.S./Canadian Brand Names** Comvax® [US]
**Therapeutic Category** Vaccine, Inactivated Virus
**Use**
Immunization against invasive disease caused by *H. influenzae* type b and against infection caused by all known subtypes of hepatitis B virus in infants 6 weeks to 15 months of age born of hepatitis B surface antigen (HB$_s$Ag) negative mothers

Infants born of HB$_s$Ag-positive mothers or mothers of unknown HB$_s$Ag status should receive hepatitis B immune globulin and hepatitis B vaccine (recombinant) at birth and should complete the hepatitis B vaccination series given according to a particular schedule
**Usual Dosage** Infants: I.M.: 0.5 mL at 2, 4, and 12-15 months of age (total of 3 doses)
If the recommended schedule cannot be followed, the interval between the first two doses should be at least 6 weeks and the interval between the second and third dose should be as close as possible to 8-11 months. Minimum age for first dose is 6 weeks.
*Modified Schedule:* Children who receive one dose of hepatitis B vaccine at or shortly after birth may receive Comvax® on a schedule of 2, 4, and 12-15 months of age
**Dosage Forms** Injection, suspension [preservative free]: *Haemophilus* b PRP 7.5 mcg and HB$_s$Ag 5 mcg per 0.5 mL (0.5 mL) [vial stopper contains latex]

## *Haemophilus* B conjugate vaccine (he MOF fi lus bee KON joo gate vak SEEN)
**Synonyms** *Haemophilus* b oligosaccharide conjugate vaccine; *Haemophilus* b polysaccharide vaccine; diphtheria CRM$_{197}$ protein conjugate; diphtheria toxoid conjugate; HbCV; HbOC; Hib polysaccharide conjugate; PRP-OMP; PRP-T
**U.S./Canadian Brand Names** ActHIB® [US/Can]; HibTITER® [US]; PedvaxHIB® [US/Can]
**Therapeutic Category** Vaccine, Inactivated Bacteria
**Use** Routine immunization of children 2 months to 5 years of age against invasive disease caused by *H. influenzae*

Unimmunized children ≥5 years of age with a chronic illness known to be associated with increased risk of *Haemophilus influenzae* type b disease, specifically, persons with anatomic or functional asplenia or sickle cell anemia or those who have undergone splenectomy, should receive *Haemophilus influenzae* type b (Hib) vaccine.

*Haemophilus* b conjugate vaccines are not indicated for prevention of bronchitis or other infections due to *H. influenzae* in adults; adults with specific dysfunction or certain complement deficiencies who are at especially high risk of *H. influenzae* type b infection (HIV-infected adults); patients with Hodgkin's disease (vaccinated at least 2 weeks before the initiation of chemotherapy or 3 months after the end of chemotherapy)

**Usual Dosage** Children: I.M.: 0.5 mL as a single dose should be administered; do not inject I.V.

**Dosage Forms**
Injection, powder for reconstitution (ActHIB®) [preservative free]: *Haemophilus* b capsular polysaccharide 10 mcg and tetanus toxoid 24 mcg per dose [may be reconstituted with provided diluent (forms solution; vial stopper contains latex) or TriHIBit® (forms suspension)]
Injection, solution [preservative free] (HibTITER®): *Haemophilus* b saccharide 10 mcg and diphtheria CRM 197 protein 25 mcg per 0.5 mL (0.5 mL) [vial stopper contains latex]
Injection, suspension (PedvaxHIB®): *Haemophilus* b capsular polysaccharide 7.5 mcg and *Neisseria meningitidis* OMPC 125 mcg per 0.5 mL (0.5 mL) [contains aluminum 225 mcg/0.5 mL]

**Haemophilus b (meningococcal protein conjugate) conjugate vaccine** *see Haemophilus* B conjugate and hepatitis B vaccine *on previous page*

**Haemophilus b oligosaccharide conjugate vaccine** *see Haemophilus* B conjugate vaccine *on previous page*

**Haemophilus b polysaccharide vaccine** *see Haemophilus* B conjugate vaccine *on previous page*

**Haemophilus influenzae b conjugate vaccine and diphtheria, tetanus toxoids, and acellular pertussis vaccine** *see* diphtheria, tetanus toxoids, and acellular pertussis vaccine and *Haemophilus* b conjugate vaccine *on page 259*

**halazone tablet** *(Discontinued)*

# halcinonide (hal SIN oh nide)
**Sound-Alike/Look-Alike Issues**
halcinonide may be confused with Halcion®
Halog® may be confused with Haldol®, Mycolog®
**U.S./Canadian Brand Names** Halog® [US/Can]
**Therapeutic Category** Corticosteroid, Topical
**Use** Inflammation of corticosteroid-responsive dermatoses [high potency topical corticosteroid]
**Usual Dosage** Children and Adults: Topical: Steroid-responsive dermatoses: Apply sparingly 1-3 times/day, occlusive dressing may be used for severe or resistant dermatoses; a thin film is effective; do not overuse. Therapy should be discontinued when control is achieved; if no improvement is seen, reassessment of diagnosis may be necessary.
**Dosage Forms** [DSC] = Discontinued product
Cream (Halog®): 0.1% (15 g, 30 g, 60 g, 240 g)
Ointment (Halog®): 0.1% (15 g, 30 g, 60 g, 240 g) [DSC]
Solution, topical (Halog®): 0.1% (20 mL, 60 mL)

**Halcion® [US/Can]** *see* triazolam *on page 821*

**Haldol® [US]** *see* haloperidol *on next page*

**Haldol® Decanoate [US]** *see* haloperidol *on next page*

**Haley's M-O** *see* magnesium hydroxide and mineral oil emulsion *on page 499*

**HalfLytely® and Bisacodyl [US]** *see* polyethylene glycol-electrolyte solution and bisacodyl *on page 659*

**Halfprin® [US-OTC]** *see* aspirin *on page 73*

# halobetasol (hal oh BAY ta sol)
**Sound-Alike/Look-Alike Issues**
Ultravate® may be confused with Cutivate®
**Synonyms** halobetasol propionate
**U.S./Canadian Brand Names** Ultravate® [US/Can]
**Therapeutic Category** Corticosteroid, Topical
**Use** Relief of inflammatory and pruritic manifestations of corticosteroid-response dermatoses [super high potency topical corticosteroid]
(Continued)

# halobetasol *(Continued)*

Usual Dosage Children ≥12 years and Adults: Topical:

Inflammatory and pruritic manifestations (dental use): Cream: Apply sparingly to lesion twice daily. Treatment should not exceed 2 consecutive weeks and total dosage should not exceed 50 g/week. Therapy should be discontinued when control is achieved; if no improvement is seen, reassessment of diagnosis may be necessary.

Steroid-responsive dermatoses: Apply sparingly to skin twice daily, rub in gently and completely; treatment should not exceed 2 consecutive weeks and total dosage should not exceed 50 g/week. Therapy should be discontinued when control is achieved; if no improvement is seen, reassessment of diagnosis may be necessary.

Dosage Forms

Cream, as propionate: 0.05% (15 g, 50 g)
Ointment, as propionate: 0.05% (15 g, 50 g)

**halobetasol propionate** *see* halobetasol *on previous page*

**Halog® [US/Can]** *see* halcinonide *on previous page*

**Halog®-E *(Discontinued)*** *see* halcinonide *on previous page*

# haloperidol (ha loe PER i dole)

Sound-Alike/Look-Alike Issues

haloperidol may be confused Halotestin®
Haldol® may be confused with Halcion®, Halenol®, Halog®, Halotestin®, Stadol®

Synonyms haloperidol decanoate; haloperidol lactate

U.S./Canadian Brand Names Apo-Haloperidol LA® [Can]; Apo-Haloperidol® [Can]; Haldol® Decanoate [US]; Haldol® [US]; Haloperidol Long Acting [Can]; Haloperidol-LA Omega [Can]; Novo-Peridol [Can]; Peridol [Can]; PMS-Haloperidol LA [Can]

Therapeutic Category Antipsychotic Agent, Butyrophenone

Use Management of schizophrenia; control of tics and vocal utterances of Tourette disorder in children and adults; severe behavioral problems in children

Usual Dosage

Children: 3-12 years (15-40 kg): Oral:

Initial: 0.05 mg/kg/day or 0.25-0.5 mg/day given in 2-3 divided doses; increase by 0.25-0.5 mg every 5-7 days; maximum: 0.15 mg/kg/day

Usual maintenance:

Agitation or hyperkinesia: 0.01-0.03 mg/kg/day once daily
Nonpsychotic disorders: 0.05-0.075 mg/kg/day in 2-3 divided doses
Psychotic disorders: 0.05-0.15 mg/kg/day in 2-3 divided doses

Children 6-12 years: Sedation/psychotic disorders: I.M. (as lactate): 1-3 mg/dose every 4-8 hours to a maximum of 0.15 mg/kg/day; change over to oral therapy as soon as able

Adults: Psychosis:

Oral: 0.5-5 mg 2-3 times/day; usual maximum: 30 mg/day
I.M. (as lactate): 2-5 mg every 4-8 hours as needed
I.M. (as decanoate): Initial: 10-20 times the daily oral dose administered at 4-week intervals
Maintenance dose: 10-15 times initial oral dose; used to stabilize psychiatric symptoms

Dosage Forms [DSC] = Discontinued product. **Note:** Strength expressed as base.

Injection, oil, as decanoate (Haldol® Decanoate): 50 mg/mL (1 mL, 5 mL); 100 mg/mL (1 mL, 5 mL) [contains benzyl alcohol, sesame oil]
Injection, solution, as lactate: 5 mg/mL (1 mL, 10 mL)
Haldol®: 5 mg/mL (1 mL; 10 mL [DSC])
Solution, oral concentrate, as lactate: 2 mg/mL (15 mL, 120 mL)
Tablet: 0.5 mg, 1 mg, 2 mg, 5 mg, 10 mg, 20 mg

**haloperidol decanoate** *see* haloperidol *on this page*

**haloperidol lactate** *see* haloperidol *on this page*

**Haloperidol-LA Omega [Can]** *see* haloperidol *on this page*

**Haloperidol Long Acting [Can]** *see* haloperidol *on this page*

**Halotestin® [US]** *see* fluoxymesterone *on page 350*

# halothane (HA loe thane)

**Sound-Alike/Look-Alike Issues**
halothane may be confused with Halotestin®

**Therapeutic Category** General Anesthetic

**Use** Induction and maintenance of general anesthesia

**Usual Dosage** Minimum alveolar concentration (MAC), the concentration at which 50% of patients do not respond to surgical incision, is 0.74% for halothane. The concentration at which amnesia and loss of awareness occur (MAC - awake) is 0.41%. Surgical levels of anesthesia are maintained with concentrations between 0.5% to 2%; inspired concentrations of up to 3% required for induction of anesthesia.

**Dosage Forms** Liquid: 125 mL, 250 mL

**Halotussin®** *(Discontinued)* *see* guaifenesin *on page 383*

**Halotussin® DM** *(Discontinued)* *see* guaifenesin and dextromethorphan *on page 385*

**Halotussin® PE** *(Discontinued)* *see* guaifenesin and pseudoephedrine *on page 388*

**Haltran®** *(Discontinued)* *see* ibuprofen *on page 427*

**hamamelis water** *see* witch hazel *on page 855*

**HandClens® [US-OTC]** *see* benzalkonium chloride *on page 95*

**Havrix® [US/Can]** *see* hepatitis A vaccine *on page 400*

**Havrix® and Engerix-B®** *see* hepatitis A inactivated and hepatitis B (recombinant) vaccine *on page 400*

**HbCV** *see* Haemophilus B conjugate vaccine *on page 394*

**HBIG** *see* hepatitis B immune globulin *on page 401*

**H-BIG®** *(Discontinued)* *see* hepatitis B immune globulin *on page 401*

**hBNP** *see* nesiritide *on page 570*

**HbOC** *see* Haemophilus B conjugate vaccine *on page 394*

**hCG** *see* chorionic gonadotropin (human) *on page 181*

**HD 85® [US]** *see* radiological/contrast media (ionic) *on page 707*

**HD 200 Plus® [US]** *see* radiological/contrast media (ionic) *on page 707*

**HDA® Toothache [US-OTC]** *see* benzocaine *on page 95*

**HDCV** *see* rabies virus vaccine *on page 707*

**Head & Shoulders® Classic Clean [US-OTC]** *see* pyrithione zinc *on page 702*

**Head & Shoulders® Classic Clean 2-In-1 [US-OTC]** *see* pyrithione zinc *on page 702*

**Head & Shoulders® Dry Scalp Care [US-OTC]** *see* pyrithione zinc *on page 702*

**Head & Shoulders® Extra Fullness [US-OTC]** *see* pyrithione zinc *on page 702*

**Head & Shoulders® Intensive Treatment [US-OTC]** *see* selenium sulfide *on page 742*

**Head & Shoulders® Refresh [US-OTC]** *see* pyrithione zinc *on page 702*

**Head & Shoulders® Smooth & Silky 2-In-1 [US-OTC]** *see* pyrithione zinc *on page 702*

**Healon® [US/Can]** *see* hyaluronate and derivatives *on page 406*

**Healon®5 [US]** *see* hyaluronate and derivatives *on page 406*

**Healon GV® [US/Can]** *see* hyaluronate and derivatives *on page 406*

**Hectorol® [US/Can]** *see* doxercalciferol *on page 269*

**Helidac® [US]** *see* bismuth subsalicylate, metronidazole, and tetracycline *on page 108*

**Helistat® [US]** *see* collagen hemostat *on page 206*

**Helitene® [US]** *see* collagen hemostat *on page 206*

**Helixate® FS [US/Can]** *see* antihemophilic factor (recombinant) *on page 57*

**Hemabate® [US/Can]** *see* carboprost tromethamine *on page 147*

**hemiacidrin** *see* citric acid, magnesium carbonate, and glucono-delta-lactone *on page 188*

# hemin (HEE min)

**U.S./Canadian Brand Names** Panhematin® [US]

**Therapeutic Category** Blood Modifiers

**Use Orphan drug:** Treatment of recurrent attacks of acute intermittent porphyria (AIP) only after an appropriate period of alternate therapy has been tried

**Usual Dosage** I.V.: 1-4 mg/kg/day administered over 10-15 minutes for 3-14 days; may be repeated no earlier than every 12 hours; not to exceed 6 mg/kg in any 24-hour period

**Dosage Forms** Injection, powder for reconstitution [preservative free]: 313 mg [provides 7 mg/mL when reconstituted]

**Hemocyte®** [US-OTC] *see* ferrous fumarate *on page 334*

**Hemocyte Plus®** [US] *see* vitamins (multiple/oral) *on page 852*

**Hemofil® M [US/Can]** *see* antihemophilic factor (human) *on page 55*

**Hemorrhoidal HC** *see* hydrocortisone (topical) *on page 417*

**Hemril®-30 [US]** *see* hydrocortisone (topical) *on page 417*

**Hepalean® [Can]** *see* heparin *on this page*

**Hepalean® Leo [Can]** *see* heparin *on this page*

**Hepalean®-LOK [Can]** *see* heparin *on this page*

# heparin (HEP a rin)

**Sound-Alike/Look-Alike Issues**

heparin may be confused with Hespan®

**Synonyms** heparin calcium; heparin lock flush; heparin sodium

**U.S./Canadian Brand Names** Hep-Lock® [US]; Hepalean® Leo [Can]; Hepalean® [Can]; Hepalean®-LOK [Can]; HepFlush®-10 [US]

**Therapeutic Category** Anticoagulant (Other)

**Use** Prophylaxis and treatment of thromboembolic disorders

**Note:** Heparin lock flush solution is intended only to maintain patency of I.V. devices and is **not** to be used for anticoagulant therapy.

**Usual Dosage**

Children:

Intermittent I.V.: Initial: 50-100 units/kg, then 50-100 units/kg every 4 hours

I.V. infusion: Initial: 50 units/kg, then 15-25 units/kg/hour; increase dose by 2-4 units/kg/hour every 6-8 hours as required

Adults:

Prophylaxis (low-dose heparin): SubQ: 5000 units every 8-12 hours

Intermittent I.V.: Initial: 10,000 units, then 50-70 units/kg (5000-10,000 units) every 4-6 hours

I.V. infusion (weight-based dosing per institutional nomogram recommended):

Acute coronary syndromes: MI: Fibrinolytic therapy:

Alteplase, reteplase, or tenecteplase with dosing as follows: Concurrent bolus of 60 units/kg (maximum: 4000 units), then 12 units/kg/hour (maximum: 1000 units/hour) as continuous infusion. Check aPTT every 4-6 hours; adjust to target of 1.5-2 times the upper limit of control (50-70 seconds in clinical trials); usual range 10-30 units/kg/hour. Duration of heparin therapy depends on concurrent therapy and the specific patient risks for systemic or venous thromboembolism.

Streptokinase: Heparin use optional depending on concurrent therapy and specific patient risks for systemic or venous thromboembolism (anterior MI, CHF, previous embolus, atrial fibrillation, LV thrombus): If heparin is administered, start when aPTT <2 times the upper limit of control; do not use a bolus, but initiate infusion adjusted to a target aPTT of 1.5-2 times the upper limit of control (50-70 seconds in clinical trials). If heparin is not administered by infusion, 7500-12,500 units SubQ every 12 hours (when aPTT <2 times the upper limit of control) is recommended.

Percutaneous coronary intervention: Heparin bolus and infusion may be administered to an activated clotting time (ACT) of 300-350 seconds if no concurrent GPIIb/IIIa receptor antagonist is administered or 200-250 seconds if a GPIIb/IIIa receptor antagonist is administered.

Treatment of unstable angina (high-risk and some intermediate-risk patients): Initial bolus of 60-70 units/kg (maximum: 5000 units), followed by an initial infusion of 12-15 units/kg/hour (maximum: 1000 units/hour). The American College of Chest Physicians consensus conference has recommended dosage adjustments to correspond to a therapeutic range equivalent to heparin levels of 0.3-0.7 units/mL by antifactor Xa determinations.

Treatment of venous thromboembolism:

DVT/PE: I.V. push: 80 units/kg followed by continuous infusion of 18 units/kg/hour

DVT: SubQ: 17,500 units every 12 hours

Line flushing: When using daily flushes of heparin to maintain patency of single and double lumen central catheters, 10 units/mL is commonly used for younger infants (eg, <10 kg) while 100 units/mL is used for older infants, children, and adults. Capped PVC catheters and peripheral heparin locks require flushing more frequently (eg, every 6-8 hours). Volume of heparin flush is usually similar to volume of catheter (or slightly greater). Additional flushes should be given when stagnant blood is observed in catheter, after catheter is used for drug or blood administration, and after blood withdrawal from catheter.

Addition of heparin (0.5-3 unit/mL) to peripheral and central parenteral nutrition has not been shown to decrease catheter-related thrombosis. The final concentration of heparin used for TPN solutions may need to be decreased to 0.5 units/mL in small infants receiving larger amounts of volume in order to avoid approaching therapeutic amounts. Arterial lines are heparinized with a final concentration of 1 unit/mL.

Using a standard heparin solution (25,000 units/500 mL $D_5W$), the following infusion rates can be used to achieve the listed doses.

For a dose of:

400 units/hour: Infuse at 8 mL/hour

500 units/hour: Infuse at 10 mL/hour

600 units/hour: Infuse at 12 mL/hour

700 units/hour: Infuse at 14 mL/hour

800 units/hour: Infuse at 16 mL/hour

900 units/hour: Infuse at 18 mL/hour

1000 units/hour: Infuse at 20 mL/hour

1100 units/hour: Infuse at 22 mL/hour

1200 units/hour: Infuse at 24 mL/hour

1300 units/hour: Infuse at 26 mL/hour

1400 units/hour: Infuse at 28 mL/hour

1500 units/hour: Infuse at 30 mL/hour

1600 units/hour: Infuse at 32 mL/hour

1700 units/hour: Infuse at 34 mL/hour

1800 units/hour: Infuse at 36 mL/hour

1900 units/hour: Infuse at 38 mL/hour

2000 units/hour: Infuse at 40 mL/hour

**Dosage Forms** [DSC] = Discontinued product

Infusion, as sodium [premixed in NaCl 0.45%; porcine intestinal mucosa source]: 12,500 units (250 mL); 25,000 units (250 mL, 500 mL)

Infusion, as sodium [preservative free; premixed in $D_5W$; porcine intestinal mucosa source]: 10,000 units (100 mL) [contains sodium metabisulfite]; 12,500 units (250 mL) [contains sodium metabisulfite]; 20,000 units (500 mL) [contains sodium metabisulfite]; 25,000 units (250 mL, 500 mL) [contains sodium metabisulfite]

Infusion, as sodium [preservative free; premixed in NaCl 0.9%; porcine intestinal mucosa source]: 1000 units (500 mL); 2000 units (1000 mL)

Injection, solution, as sodium [beef lung source; multidose vial]: 1000 units/mL (10 mL, 30 mL); 5000 units/mL (10 mL), 10,000 units/mL (1 mL, 4 mL) [contains benzyl alcohol] [DSC]

Injection, solution, as sodium [lock flush preparation; porcine intestinal mucosa source; multidose vial]: 10 units/mL (1 mL, 10 mL, 30 mL) [contains parabens]; 100 units/mL (1 mL, 5 mL) [contains parabens]

Injection, solution, as sodium [lock flush preparation; porcine intestinal mucosa source; multidose vial]: 10 units/mL (10 mL, 30 mL); 100 units/mL (10 mL, 30 mL) [contains benzyl alcohol]

Hep-Lock®: 10 units/mL (1 mL, 2 mL, 10 mL, 30 mL); 100 units/mL (1 mL, 2 mL, 10 mL, 30 mL) [contains benzyl alcohol]

Injection, solution, as sodium [lock flush preparation; porcine intestinal mucosa source; prefilled syringe]: 10 units/mL (1 mL, 2 mL, 3 mL, 5 mL); 100 units/mL (1 mL, 2 mL, 3 mL, 5 mL) [contains benzyl alcohol]

Injection, solution, as sodium [preservative free; lock flush preparation; porcine intestinal mucosa source; prefilled syringe]: 100 units/mL (5 mL)

Injection, solution, as sodium [preservative free; lock flush preparation; porcine intestinal mucosa source; vial] (HepFlush®-10): 10 units/mL (10 mL)

Injection, solution, as sodium [porcine intestinal mucosa source; multidose vial]: 1000 units/mL (1 mL, 10 mL, 30 mL) [contains benzyl alcohol]; 1000 units/mL (1 mL, 10 mL, 30 mL) [contains (Continued)

# heparin *(Continued)*

methylparabens]; 5000 units/mL (1 mL, 10 mL) [contains benzyl alcohol]; 5000 units/mL (1 mL) [contains methylparabens]; 10,000 units/mL (1 mL, 4 mL) [contains benzyl alcohol]; 10,000 units/mL (1 mL, 5 mL) [contains methylparabens]; 20,000 units/mL (1 mL) [contains methylparabens]

Injection, solution, as sodium [porcine intestinal mucosa source; prefilled syringe]: 5000 units/mL (1 mL) [contains benzyl alcohol]

Injection, solution, as sodium [preservative free; porcine intestinal mucosa source; prefilled syringe]: 10,000 units/mL (0.5 mL)

Injection, solution, as sodium [preservative free; porcine intestinal mucosa source; vial]: 1000 units/mL (2 mL); 2000 units/mL (5 mL); 2500 units/mL (10 mL)

**heparin calcium** *see* heparin *on page 398*

**heparin cofactor I** *see* antithrombin III *on page 58*

**heparin lock flush** *see* heparin *on page 398*

**heparin sodium** *see* heparin *on page 398*

# hepatitis A inactivated and hepatitis B (recombinant) vaccine

(hep a TYE tis aye in ak ti VAY ted & hep a TYE tis bee ree KOM be nant vak SEEN)

**Synonyms** Engerix-B® and Havrix®; Havrix® and Engerix-B®; hepatitis B (recombinant) and hepatitis A inactivated vaccine

**U.S./Canadian Brand Names** Twinrix® [US/Can]

**Therapeutic Category** Vaccine

**Use** Active immunization against disease caused by hepatitis A virus and hepatitis B virus (all known subtypes) in populations desiring protection against or at high risk of exposure to these viruses.

Populations include travelers to areas of intermediate/high endemicity for **both** HAV and HBV; those at increased risk of HBV infection due to behavioral or occupational factors; patients with chronic liver disease; laboratory workers who handle live HAV and HBV; healthcare workers, police, and other personnel who render first-aid or medical assistance; workers who come in contact with sewage; employees of day care centers and correctional facilities; patients/staff of hemodialysis units; male homosexuals; patients frequently receiving blood products; military personnel; users of injectable illicit drugs; close household contacts of patients with hepatitis A and hepatitis B infection.

**Usual Dosage** I.M.: Adults: Primary immunization: Three doses (1 mL each) given on a 0-, 1-, and 6-month schedule

**Dosage Forms** Injection, suspension: Inactivated hepatitis A virus 720 ELISA units and hepatitis B surface antigen 20 mcg per mL (1 mL) [prefilled syringe; single-dose vial]

# hepatitis A vaccine (hep a TYE tis aye vak SEEN)

**U.S./Canadian Brand Names** Avaxim® [Can]; Avaxim®-Pediatric [Can]; Havrix® [US/Can]; VAQTA® [US/Can]

**Therapeutic Category** Vaccine, Inactivated Virus

**Use**

Active immunization against disease caused by hepatitis A virus in populations desiring protection against or at high risk of exposure

Populations at high risk of exposure to hepatitis A virus may include children and adolescents in selected states and regions, travelers to developing countries, household and sexual contacts of persons infected with hepatitis A, child day care employees, patients with chronic liver disease, illicit drug users, male homosexuals, institutional workers (eg, institutions for the mentally and physically handicapped persons, prisons), and healthcare workers who may be exposed to hepatitis A virus (eg, laboratory employees)

**Usual Dosage** I.M.:

Havrix®:

Children 2-18 years: 720 ELISA units (0.5 mL) with a booster dose of 720 ELISA units 6-12 months following primary immunization

Adults: 1440 ELISA units (1 mL) with a booster 6-12 months following primary immunization

VAQTA®:

Children 12 months to 18 years: 25 units (0.5 mL) with 25 units (0.5 mL) booster to be given 6-18 months after primary immunization (6-12 months if initial dose was with Havrix®)

Adults: 50 units (1 mL) with 50 units (1 mL) booster to be given 6-18 months after primary immunization (6-12 months if initial dose was with Havrix®)

Dosage Forms

Injection, suspension, adult:

Havrix®: Viral antigen 1440 ELISA units/mL (1 mL) [contains trace amounts of neomycin; syringe plunger contains latex rubber; available in prefilled syringe or single-dose vial]

VAQTA®: HAV antigen 50 units/mL (1 mL) [vial stopper and syringe plunger contain latex rubber; available in prefilled syringe or single-dose vial]

Injection, suspension, pediatric (Havrix®): Viral antigen 720 ELISA units/0.5 mL (0.5 mL) [contains trace amounts of neomycin; syringe plunger contains latex rubber; available in prefilled syringe or single-dose vial]

Injection, suspension, pediatric/adolescent (VAQTA®): HAV antigen 25 units/0.5 mL (0.5 mL) [vial stopper and syringe plunger contain latex rubber; available in prefilled syringe or single-dose vial]

## hepatitis B immune globulin (hep a TYE tis bee i MYUN GLOB yoo lin)

Synonyms HBIG

U.S./Canadian Brand Names BayHep B® [US/Can]; Nabi-HB® [US]

Therapeutic Category Immune Globulin

Use Provide prophylactic passive immunity to hepatitis B infection to those individuals exposed; newborns of mothers known to be hepatitis B surface antigen positive; hepatitis B immune globulin is not indicated for treatment of active hepatitis B infections and is ineffective in the treatment of chronic active hepatitis B infection

Usual Dosage I.M.:

Newborns: Hepatitis B: 0.5 mL as soon after birth as possible (within 12 hours); may repeat at 3 months in order for a higher rate of prevention of the carrier state to be achieved; at this time an active vaccination program with the vaccine may begin

Adults: Postexposure prophylaxis: 0.06 mL/kg as soon as possible after exposure (ie, within 24 hours of needlestick, ocular, or mucosal exposure or within 14 days of sexual exposure); usual dose: 3-5 mL; repeat at 28-30 days after exposure

Note: HBIG may be administered at the same time (but at a different site) or up to 1 month preceding hepatitis B vaccination without impairing the active immune response

Dosage Forms Note: Potency expressed in international units as compared to the WHO standard

Injection, solution [preservative free]:

BayHepB®: 217 int. units/mL (0.5 mL) [neonatal single-dose syringe]; (1 mL) [single-dose syringe or single-dose vial]; (5 mL) [single-dose vial]

Nabi-HB®: 208 int. units/mL (1 mL, 5 mL) [single-dose vial]

## hepatitis B inactivated virus vaccine (plasma derived) see hepatitis B vaccine on this page

## hepatitis B inactivated virus vaccine (recombinant DNA) see hepatitis B vaccine on this page

## hepatitis B (recombinant) and hepatitis A inactivated vaccine see hepatitis A inactivated and hepatitis B (recombinant) vaccine on previous page

## hepatitis B vaccine (hep a TYE tis bee vak SEEN)

Sound-Alike/Look-Alike Issues

Recombivax HB® may be confused with Comvax®

Synonyms hepatitis B inactivated virus vaccine (plasma derived); hepatitis B inactivated virus vaccine (recombinant DNA)

U.S./Canadian Brand Names Engerix-B® [US/Can]; Recombivax HB® [US/Can]

Therapeutic Category Vaccine, Inactivated Virus

Use Immunization against infection caused by all known subtypes of hepatitis B virus, in individuals considered at high risk of potential exposure to hepatitis B virus or HB$_s$Ag-positive materials:

Healthcare workers[1]

Special patient groups (eg, adolescents, infants born to HB$_s$ Ag-positive mothers, children born after 11/21/91, military personnel)

Hemodialysis patients[2] (see dosing recommendations), recipients of certain blood products[3]

Lifestyle factors: Homosexual and bisexual men, intravenous drug abusers, heterosexually-active persons with multiple sexual partners or recently acquired sexually-transmitted diseases

Environmental factors: Household and sexual contacts of HBV carriers; prison inmates; clients and staff of institutions for the mentally handicapped; residents, immigrants, and refugees from areas with endemic HBV infection; international travelers at increased risk of acquiring HBV infection

(Continued)

## hepatitis B vaccine *(Continued)*

[1]The risk of hepatitis B virus (HBV) infection for healthcare workers varies both between hospitals and within hospitals. Hepatitis B vaccination is recommended for all healthcare workers with blood exposure.

[2]Hemodialysis patients often respond poorly to hepatitis B vaccination; higher vaccine doses or increased number of doses are required. A special formulation of one vaccine is now available for such persons (Recombivax HB®, 40 mcg/mL). The anti-HB$_s$(antibody to hepatitis B surface antigen) response of such persons should be tested after they are vaccinated, and those who have not responded should be revaccinated with 1-3 additional doses. Patients with chronic renal disease should be vaccinated as early as possible, ideally before they require hemodialysis. In addition, their anti-HB$_s$ levels should be monitored at 6- to 12-month intervals to assess the need for revaccination.

[3]Patients with hemophilia should be immunized subcutaneously, not intramuscularly.

**Usual Dosage** I.M.:

Immunization regimen: Regimen consists of 3 doses (0, 1, and 6 months): First dose given on the elected date, second dose given 1 month later, third dose given 6 months after the first dose.

**Initial dose:**

Birth (infants born of HB$_s$ Ag-negative mothers) to 19 years:

Recombivax HB®: 0.5 mL (5 mcg/0.5 mL pediatric/adolescent formulation) **or**

Engerix-B®: 0.5 mL (10 mcg/0.5 mL formulation)

20 years and older:

Recombivax HB®: 1 mL (10 mcg/mL adult formulation) **or**

Engerix-B®: 1 mL (20 mcg/mL formulation)

Dialysis or immunocompromised patients (revaccinate if anti-HB$_s$ <10 mIU/mL ≥1-2 months after third dose):

Recombivax HB®: 1 mL (40 mcg/mL dialysis formulation) **or**

Engerix-B®: 2 mL (two 1 mL doses given at different sites using the 40 mcg/2 mL dialysis formulation)

**1-month dose:**

Birth (infants born of HB$_s$Ag-negative mothers) to 19 years:

Recombivax HB®: 0.5 mL (5 mcg/0.5 mL pediatric/adolescent formulation) **or**

Engerix-B®: 0.5 mL (10 mcg/0.5 mL formulation)

20 years and older:

Recombivax HB®: 1 mL (10 mcg/mL adult formulation) **or**

Engerix-B®: 1 mL (20 mcg/mL formulation)

Dialysis or immunocompromised patients (revaccinate if anti-HB$_s$ <10 mIU/mL ≥1-2 months after third dose):

Recombivax HB®: 1 mL (40 mcg/mL dialysis formulation) **or**

Engerix-B®: 2 mL (two 1 mL doses given at different sites using the 40 mcg/2 mL dialysis formulation)

**6-month dose:**

Birth (infants born of HB$_s$Ag-negative mothers) to 19 years: 0.5 mL (5 mcg/0.5 mL pediatric/adolescent formulation) Recombivax HB® **or**  0.5 mL (10 mcg/0.5 mL formulation) Engerix-B®

20 years and older:

Recombivax HB®: 1 mL (10 mcg/mL adult formulation) **or**

Engerix-B®: 1 mL (20 mcg/mL formulation)

Dialysis or immunocompromised patients (revaccinate if anti-HB$_s$ <10 mIU/mL ≥1-2 months after third dose):

Recombivax HB®: 1 mL (40 mcg/mL dialysis formulation) **or**

Engerix-B®: 2 mL (two 1 mL doses given at different sites using the 40 mcg/2 mL dialysis formulation)

Alternative dosing schedule for **Recombivax HB®**: Children 11-15 years (10 mcg/mL adult formulation): First dose of 1 mL given on the elected date, second dose given 4-6 months later

Alternative dosing schedules for **Engerix-B®**:

Children ≤10 years (10 mcg/0.5 mL formulation): High-risk children: 0.5 mL at 0, 1, 2, and 12 months; lower-risk children ages 5-10 who are candidates for an extended administration schedule may receive an alternative regimen of 0.5 mL at 0, 12, and 24 months. If booster dose is needed, revaccinate with 0.5 mL.

Adolescents 11-19 years (20 mcg/mL formulation): 1 mL at 0, 1, and 6 months. High-risk adolescents: 1 mL at 0, 1, 2, and 12 months; lower-risk adolescents 11-16 years who are candidates for an extended administration schedule may receive an alternative regimen of 0.5 mL (using the 10 mcg/ 0.5 mL) formulation at 0, 12, and 24 months. If booster dose is needed, revaccinate with 20 mcg.

Adults ≥20 years: High-risk adults (20 mcg/mL formulation): 1 mL at 0, 1, 2, and 12 months. If booster dose is needed, revaccinate with 1 mL.

Postexposure prophylaxis recommended dosage for infants born to $HB_s$ Ag-positive mothers (by product /age):

**Engerix-B**® (pediatric formulation 10 mcg/0.5 mL):

Give 0.5 mL within 7 days; repeat 0.5 mL at 1 month and 6 months.

Alternately, the first dose may be given at birth at the same time as HBIG, but give in the opposite anterolateral thigh. This may better ensure vaccine absorption.

An alternate regimen is administration of the vaccine at birth, within 7 days of birth, and at 1, 2, and 12 months later.

**Recombivax HB**® (pediatric/adolescent formulation 5 mcg/0.5 mL):

Give 0.5 mL within 7 days; repeat 0.5 mL at 1 month and 6 months

Alternately, the first dose may be given at birth at the same time as HBIG, but give in the opposite anterolateral thigh. This may better ensure vaccine absorption.

**Hepatitis B immune globulin:** Give 0.5 mL at birth.

**Dosage Forms** Injection, suspension [recombinant DNA]:

Engerix-B®:

Adult: Hepatitis B surface antigen 20 mcg/mL (1 mL) [contains trace amounts of thimerosal]

Pediatric/adolescent: Hepatitis B surface antigen 10 mcg/0.5 mL (0.5 mL) [contains trace amounts of thimerosal]

Recombivax HB®:

Adult [preservative free]: Hepatitis B surface antigen 10 mcg/mL (1 mL, 3 mL)

Dialysis [preservative free]: Hepatitis B surface antigen 40 mcg/mL (1 mL)

Pediatric/adolescent [preservative free]: Hepatitis B surface antigen 5 mcg/0.5 mL (0.5 mL)

**hepatitis b vaccine (recombinant)** *see Haemophilus* B conjugate and hepatitis B vaccine *on page 394*

**HepFlush**®**-10 [US]** *see* heparin *on page 398*

**Hep-Lock**® **[US]** *see* heparin *on page 398*

**Hepsera**™ **[US]** *see* adefovir *on page 18*

**Heptalac**® ***(Discontinued)*** *see* lactulose *on page 464*

**Heptovir**® **[Can]** *see* lamivudine *on page 464*

**Herceptin**® **[US/Can]** *see* trastuzumab *on page 816*

**HES** *see* hetastarch *on this page*

**Hespan**® **[US]** *see* hetastarch *on this page*

**hetastarch** (HET a starch)

**Sound-Alike/Look-Alike Issues**

Hespan® may be confused with heparin

**Synonyms** HES; hydroxyethyl starch

**U.S./Canadian Brand Names** Hespan® [US]; Hextend® [US/Can]

**Therapeutic Category** Plasma Volume Expander

**Use** Blood volume expander used in treatment of hypovolemia

Hespan®: Adjunct in leukapheresis to improve harvesting and increasing the yield of granulocytes by centrifugal means

**Usual Dosage** I.V. infusion (requires an infusion pump):

Children: Safety and efficacy have not been established

Plasma volume expansion:

Adults: 500-1000 mL (up to 1500 mL/day) or 20 mL/kg/day (up to 1500 mL/day); larger volumes (15,000 mL/24 hours) have been used safely in small numbers of patients

Leukapheresis: 250-700 mL; **Note:** Citrate anticoagulant is added before use.

**Dosage Forms**

Infusion [premixed in lactated electrolyte injection] (Hextend®): 6% (500 mL)

Infusion, solution [premixed in NaCl 0.9%] (Hespan®): 6% (500 mL)

**Hexabrix**™ **[US]** *see* radiological/contrast media (ionic) *on page 707*

**hexachlorocyclohexane** *see* lindane *on page 483*

**hexachlorophene** (heks a KLOR oh feen)

**Sound-Alike/Look-Alike Issues**

pHisoHex® may be confused with Fostex®, pHisoDerm®

(Continued)

## hexachlorophene *(Continued)*

**U.S./Canadian Brand Names** pHisoHex® [US/Can]
**Therapeutic Category** Antibacterial, Topical
**Use** Surgical scrub and as a bacteriostatic skin cleanser; control an outbreak of gram-positive infection when other procedures have been unsuccessful
**Usual Dosage** Children and Adults: Topical: Apply 5 mL cleanser and water to area to be cleansed; lather and rinse thoroughly under running water
**Dosage Forms** Liquid, topical: 3% (150 mL, 500 mL, 3840 mL)

**Hexalen®** [US/Can] *see* altretamine *on page 34*

**hexamethylenetetramine** *see* methenamine *on page 522*

**hexamethylmelamine** *see* altretamine *on page 34*

**Hexit™** [Can] *see* lindane *on page 483*

**HEXM** *see* altretamine *on page 34*

**Hextend®** [US/Can] *see* hetastarch *on previous page*

## hexylresorcinol *(heks il re ZOR si nole)*

**U.S./Canadian Brand Names** S.T. 37® [US-OTC]; Sucrets® Original [US-OTC]
**Therapeutic Category** Local Anesthetic
**Use** Minor antiseptic and local anesthetic for sore throat; topical antiseptic for minor cuts or abrasions
**Usual Dosage** Children ≥2 years and Adults:
  Antiseptic: Topical: Solution: Apply to affected area 1-3 times/day
  Sore throat: Oral:
    Lozenge: May be used as needed, allow to dissolve slowly in mouth (maximum: 10 lozenges/day)
    Solution: Gargle or swish in mouth up to 4 times/day
**Dosage Forms**
  Lozenge (Sucrets® Original): 2.4 mg [mint flavor]
  Solution (S.T. 37®): 0.1% (480 mL) [contains sodium bisulfite]

**Hib** *see* *Haemophilus* B conjugate and hepatitis B vaccine *on page 394*

**Hibiclens®** [US-OTC] *see* chlorhexidine gluconate *on page 168*

**Hibidil®** 1:2000 [Can] *see* chlorhexidine gluconate *on page 168*

**Hibistat®** [US-OTC] *see* chlorhexidine gluconate *on page 168*

**Hib polysaccharide conjugate** *see* *Haemophilus* B conjugate vaccine *on page 394*

**HibTITER®** [US] *see* *Haemophilus* B conjugate vaccine *on page 394*

**Hi-Kovite** [US-OTC] *see* vitamins (multiple/oral) *on page 852*

**Hiprex®** [US/Can] *see* methenamine *on page 522*

**hirulog** *see* bivalirudin *on page 109*

**Histade™** [US] *see* chlorpheniramine and pseudoephedrine *on page 172*

**Histalet®** X *(Discontinued)* *see* guaifenesin and pseudoephedrine *on page 388*

## histamine *(HIS ta meen)*

**Therapeutic Category** Diagnostic Agent
**Use** To test the ability of the gastric mucosa to produce hydrochloric acid
**Usual Dosage** Adults: SubQ: Gastric acid test:
  The patient fasts for 12 hours. A plastic duodenal tube is passed into the stomach, the gastric content withdrawn, and its acidity determined. Care should be taken to prevent the patient from swallowing salivary secretions during administration of the test results. The alkalinity of the saliva may interfere with the test results. Histamine phosphate 500 to 750 mcg is then injected.
  Gastric content is again removed after 5 minutes and at 15 minute intervals thereafter on 3 occasions The volume and acidity of each specimen is determined. If no acidity is detected, a maximum histamine stimulation test can be performed using 40 mcg/kg histamine phosphate. Pulse rate and blood pressure should be determined immediately after histamine injection.
**Dosage Forms** Injection, as phosphate: 0.275 mg/mL (5 mL)

**Histatab®** **Plus** *(Discontinued)* *see* chlorpheniramine and phenylephrine *on page 171*

**Hista-Vent**® **DA [US]** *see* chlorpheniramine, phenylephrine, and methscopolamine *on page 175*

**Histerone**® **Injection** *(Discontinued)* *see* testosterone *on page 788*

**Histex**™ **[US]** *see* chlorpheniramine and pseudoephedrine *on page 172*

**Histex**™ **I/E [US]** *see* carbinoxamine *on page 144*

**Histex**™ **CT [US]** *see* carbinoxamine *on page 144*

**Histex**™ **HC [US]** *see* hydrocodone, carbinoxamine, and pseudoephedrine *on page 414*

**Histex**™ **PD [US]** *see* carbinoxamine *on page 144*

**Histex**™ **PD-12 [US]** *see* carbinoxamine *on page 144*

**Histex**™ **SR [US]** *see* brompheniramine and pseudoephedrine *on page 115*

**Histinex**® **D Liquid** *(Discontinued)* *see* hydrocodone and pseudoephedrine *on page 413*

**Histinex**® **HC [US]** *see* phenylephrine, hydrocodone, and chlorpheniramine *on page 643*

**Histinex**® **PV [US]** *see* pseudoephedrine, hydrocodone, and chlorpheniramine *on page 695*

**Histor-D**® **Syrup** *(Discontinued)* *see* chlorpheniramine and phenylephrine *on page 171*

**Histor-D**® **Timecelles**® *(Discontinued)* *see* chlorpheniramine, phenylephrine, and methscopola-mine *on page 175*

**Histrodrix**® *(Discontinued)* *see* dexbrompheniramine and pseudoephedrine *on page 234*

**Histussin D**® **[US]** *see* hydrocodone and pseudoephedrine *on page 413*

**Histussin**® **HC [US]** *see* phenylephrine, hydrocodone, and chlorpheniramine *on page 643*

**Hi-Vegi-Lip [US]** *see* pancrelipase *on page 615*

**Hivid**® **[US/Can]** *see* zalcitabine *on page 857*

**HMM** *see* altretamine *on page 34*

**HMR 3647** *see* telithromycin *on page 783*

**HMS Liquifilm**® *(Discontinued)* *see* medrysone *on page 508*

**HN₂** *see* mechlorethamine *on page 505*

**Hold**® **DM [US-OTC]** *see* dextromethorphan *on page 238*

## homatropine (hoe MA troe peen)

**Synonyms** homatropine hydrobromide
**U.S./Canadian Brand Names** Isopto® Homatropine [US]
**Therapeutic Category** Anticholinergic Agent
**Use** Producing cycloplegia and mydriasis for refraction; treatment of acute inflammatory conditions of the uveal tract
**Usual Dosage** Ophthalmic:
Children:
Mydriasis and cycloplegia for refraction: Instill 1 drop of 2% solution immediately before the procedure; repeat at 10-minute intervals as needed
Uveitis: Instill 1 drop of 2% solution 2-3 times/day
Adults:
Mydriasis and cycloplegia for refraction: Instill 1-2 drops of 2% solution or 1 drop of 5% solution before the procedure; repeat at 5- to 10-minute intervals as needed; maximum of 3 doses for refraction
Uveitis: Instill 1-2 drops of 2% or 5% 2-3 times/day up to every 3-4 hours as needed
**Dosage Forms** Solution, ophthalmic, as hydrobromide: 2% (5 mL); 5% (5 mL, 15 mL) [contains benzal-konium chloride]

**homatropine and hydrocodone** *see* hydrocodone and homatropine *on page 413*

**homatropine hydrobromide** *see* homatropine *on this page*

**horse antihuman thymocyte gamma globulin** *see* antithymocyte globulin (equine) *on page 59*

**H.P. Acthar**® **Gel [US]** *see* corticotropin *on page 208*

**Hp-PAC**® **[Can]** *see* lansoprazole, amoxicillin, and clarithromycin *on page 468*

**HTF919** *see* tegaserod *on page 782*

**hu1124** *see* efalizumab *on page 280*

**Humalog**® **[US/Can]** *see* insulin preparations *on page 438*

**Humalog**® **Mix 25**™ **[Can]** *see* insulin preparations *on page 438*

**Humalog**® **Mix 50/50 Insulin** *(Discontinued)*

**Humalog**® **Mix 75/25**™ **[US]** *see* insulin preparations *on page 438*

**human antitumor necrosis factor-alpha** *see* adalimumab *on page 18*

**human diploid cell cultures rabies vaccine** *see* rabies virus vaccine *on page 707*

**human growth hormone** *see* somatropin *on page 760*

**humanized IgG1 anti-CD52 monoclonal antibody** *see* alemtuzumab *on page 26*

**human LFA-3/IgG(1) fusion protein** *see* alefacept *on page 25*

**human thyroid stimulating hormone** *see* thyrotropin alpha *on page 800*

**Humate-P**® **[US/Can]** *see* antihemophilic factor (human) *on page 55*

**Humatin**® **[US/Can]** *see* paromomycin *on page 620*

**Humatrope**® **[US/Can]** *see* somatropin *on page 760*

**Humegon**® **[Can]** *see* chorionic gonadotropin (human) *on page 181*

**Humegon**™ *(Discontinued)* *see* menotropins *on page 511*

**Humibid**® **CS** *(Discontinued)* *see* guaifenesin and dextromethorphan *on page 385*

**Humibid**® **DM** *(Discontinued)* *see* guaifenesin and dextromethorphan *on page 385*

**Humibid**® ***e* [US-OTC]** *see* guaifenesin *on page 383*

**Humibid**® **LA** *(Discontinued)* *see* guaifenesin *on page 383*

**Humibid**® **Pediatric** *(Discontinued)* *see* guaifenesin *on page 383*

**Humibid**® **Sprinkle** *(Discontinued)* *see* guaifenesin *on page 383*

**Humira**® **[US/Can]** *see* adalimumab *on page 18*

**Humulin**® **[Can]** *see* insulin preparations *on page 438*

**Humulin**® **50/50 [US]** *see* insulin preparations *on page 438*

**Humulin**® **L** *(Discontinued)* *see* insulin preparations *on page 438*

**Humulin**® **70/30 [US]** *see* insulin preparations *on page 438*

**Humulin**® **N [US]** *see* insulin preparations *on page 438*

**Humulin**® **R [US]** *see* insulin preparations *on page 438*

**Humulin**® **R (Concentrated) U-500 [US]** *see* insulin preparations *on page 438*

**Humulin**® **U** *(Discontinued)* *see* insulin preparations *on page 438*

**Hurricaine**® **[US]** *see* benzocaine *on page 95*

**HXM** *see* altretamine *on page 34*

**Hyalgan**® **[US]** *see* hyaluronate and derivatives *on this page*

**hyaluronan** *see* hyaluronate and derivatives *on this page*

## hyaluronate and derivatives (hye al yoor ON ate & dah RIV ah tives)

**Sound-Alike/Look-Alike Issues**
Synvisc® may be confused with Synagis®

**Synonyms** hyaluronan; hyaluronic acid; hylan polymers; sodium hyaluronate

**U.S./Canadian Brand Names** Biolon™ [US]; Cystistat® [Can]; Durolane® [Can]; Eyestil [Can]; Healon GV® [US/Can]; Healon® [US/Can]; Healon®5 [US]; Hyalgan® [US]; Hylaform® Plus [US]; Hylaform® [US]; IPM Wound Gel™ [US-OTC]; OrthoVisc® [US/Can]; Provisc® [US]; Restylane® [US]; Supartz™ [US]; Suplasyn® [Can]; Synvisc® [US]; Vitrax® [US]

**Therapeutic Category** Antirheumatic Miscellaneous; Ophthalmic Agent, Viscoelastic; Skin and Mucous Membrane Agent

**Use**
Intraarticular injection: Treatment of pain in osteoarthritis in knee in patients who have failed nonpharmacologic treatment and simple analgesics
Intradermal: Correction of moderate-to-severe facial wrinkles or folds
Ophthalmic: Surgical aid in cataract extraction, intraocular implantation, corneal transplant, glaucoma filtration, and retinal attachment surgery

Topical: Management of skin ulcers and wounds

**Usual Dosage** Adults:

Osteoarthritis of the knee: Intra-articular:

Hyalgan®: Inject 20 mg (2 mL) once weekly for 5 weeks; some patients may benefit with a total of 3 injections

Orthovisc®: Inject 30 mg (2 mL) once weekly for 3-4 weeks

Supartz™: Inject 25 mg (2.5 mL) once weekly for 5 weeks

Synvisc®: Inject 2 mL once weekly for 3 weeks (total of 3 injections)

Facial wrinkles: Intradermal (Hylaform®, Hylaform® Plus, Restylane®): Inject as required for cosmetic result; typical treatment regimen requires <2 mL; limit injection to ≤1.5 mL per injection site. Hylaform®, Hylaform® Plus: Maximum: 20 mL/60 kg/year

Ophthalmic (Biolon™, Healon®, Provisc®, Vitrax®): Depends upon procedure (slowly introduce a sufficient quantity into eye)

Topical (IPM Wound Gel™): Apply to clean dry ulcer or wound, and cover with nonstick dressing; repeat daily. Discontinue if wound size increase after 3-4 applications.

**Dosage Forms**

Hylan B: Injection, gel:

Hylaform® [500 micron particle]: 5.5 mg/mL (0.75 mL) [prefilled syringe; derived from avian source]

Hylaform® Plus [700 micron particle]: 5.5 mg/mL (0.75 mL) [prefilled syringe; derived from avian source]

Hylan polymers A and B (Hylan G-F 20): Injection, solution, intra-articular (Synvisc®): 8 mg/mL (2 mL) [prefilled syringe; contains trace amounts of *Streptococcus*]

**Sodium Hyaluronate:**

Gel, topical (IPM Wound Gel™): 2.5% (10 g)

Injection, gel, intradermal (Restylane®): 20 mg/mL [prefilled syringe]

Injection, solution, intra-articular:

Hyalgan®: 10 mg/mL (2 mL)

Orthovisc®: 15 mg/mL (2 mL) [prefilled syringe; derived from avian source]

Supartz™: 10 mg/mL (2.5 mL) [derived from avian source]

Injection, solution, intraocular:

Biolon™: 10 mg/mL (0.5 mL, 1 mL)

Healon®: 10 mg/mL (0.4 mL, 0.55 mL, 0.85 mL, 2 mL)

Healon®5: 23 mg/mL

Healon GV®: 14 mg/mL (0.55 mL, 0.85 mL)

Provisc®: 10 mg/mL (0.4 mL, 0.55 mL, 0.8 mL) [prefilled syringe; contains lactose]

Vitrax®: 30 mg/mL (0.65 mL)

**hyaluronic acid** *see* hyaluronate and derivatives *on previous page*

# hyaluronidase (hye al yoor ON i dase)

**Sound-Alike/Look-Alike Issues**

Wydase® may be confused with Lidex®, Wyamine®

**U.S./Canadian Brand Names** Amphadase™ [US]; Vitrase® [US]

**Therapeutic Category** Enzyme

**Use** Increase the dispersion and absorption of other drugs; increase rate of absorption of parenteral fluids given by hypodermoclysis; adjunct in subcutaneous urography for improving resorption of radiopaque agents

**Usual Dosage Note:** A preliminary skin test for hypersensitivity can be performed. ACTH, antihistamines, corticosteroids, estrogens, and salicylates, when used in large doses, may cause tissues to be partly resistant to hyaluronidase. May require larger doses of hyaluronidase for the same effect.

Skin test: Intradermal: 0.02 mL (3 units) of a 150 units/mL solution. Positive reaction consists of a wheal with pseudopods appearing within 5 minutes and persisting for 20-30 minutes with localized itching.

Hypodermoclysis: SubQ: 15 units is added to each 100 mL of I.V. fluid to be administered

Premature Infants and Neonates: Volume of a single clysis should not exceed 25 mL/kg and the rate of administration should not exceed 2 mL/minute

Children <3 years: Volume of a single clysis should not exceed 200 mL

Children ≥3 years and Adults: Rate and volume of a single clysis should not exceed those used for infusion of I.V. fluids

**Dosage Forms**

Injection, powder for reconstitution (Vitrase®): 6200 units [ovine derived; contains lactose]

Injection, solution (Amphadase™): 150 units/mL (2 mL) [bovine derived; contains edetate disodium 1 mg, thimerosal ≤0.1 mg]

Injection, solution [preservative free] (Vitrase®): 200 units/mL (2 mL) [ovine derived; contains lactulose]

**Hyate:C**® **[US]** *see* antihemophilic factor (porcine) *on page 56*

**hycamptamine** *see* topotecan *on page 811*

**Hycamtin**® **[US/Can]** *see* topotecan *on page 811*

**hycet**™ **[US]** *see* hydrocodone and acetaminophen *on page 411*

**HycoClear Tuss**® *(Discontinued) see* hydrocodone and guaifenesin *on page 412*

**Hycodan**® **[US]** *see* hydrocodone and homatropine *on page 413*

**Hycomine**® **Compound [US]** *see* hydrocodone, chlorpheniramine, phenylephrine, acetaminophen, and caffeine *on page 414*

**Hycomine**® *(Discontinued)*

**Hycomine**® **Pediatric** *(Discontinued)*

**Hycort**™ **[Can]** *see* hydrocortisone (topical) *on page 417*

**Hycotuss**® **[US]** *see* hydrocodone and guaifenesin *on page 412*

**Hydeltra T.B.A.**® **[Can]** *see* prednisolone (systemic) *on page 674*

**Hydergine**® **[Can]** *see* ergoloid mesylates *on page 293*

**Hydergine**® *(Discontinued) see* ergoloid mesylates *on page 293*

**Hyderm [Can]** *see* hydrocortisone (topical) *on page 417*

## hydralazine (hye DRAL a zeen)

### Sound-Alike/Look-Alike Issues
hydrALAZINE may be confused with hydrOXYzine

**Synonyms** hydralazine hydrochloride

**Tall-Man** hydr**ALAZINE**

**U.S./Canadian Brand Names** Apo-Hydralazine® [Can]; Apresoline® [Can]; Novo-Hylazin [Can]; Nu-Hydral [Can]

**Therapeutic Category** Vasodilator

**Use** Management of moderate to severe hypertension, congestive heart failure, hypertension secondary to pre-eclampsia/eclampsia; treatment of primary pulmonary hypertension

### Usual Dosage
Children:
Oral: Initial: 0.75-1 mg/kg/day in 2-4 divided doses; increase over 3-4 weeks to maximum of 7.5 mg/kg/day in 2-4 divided doses; maximum daily dose: 200 mg/day
I.M., I.V.: 0.1-0.2 mg/kg/dose (not to exceed 20 mg) every 4-6 hours as needed, up to 1.7-3.5 mg/kg/day in 4-6 divided doses
Adults:
Oral: Hypertension:
Initial dose: 10 mg 4 times/day for first 2-4 days; increase to 25 mg 4 times/day for the balance of the first week
Increase by 10-25 mg/dose gradually to 50 mg 4 times/day (maximum: 300 mg/day); usual dose range (JNC 7): 25-100 mg/day in 2 divided doses
Oral: Congestive heart failure:
Initial dose: 10-25 mg 3-4 times/day
Adjustment: Dosage must be adjusted based on individual response
Target dose: 75 mg 4 times/day in combination with isosorbide dinitrate (40 mg 4 times/day)
Range: Typically 200-600 mg daily in 2-4 divided doses; dosages as high as 3 g/day have been used in some patients for symptomatic and hemodynamic improvement. Hydralazine 75 mg 4 times/day combined with isosorbide dinitrate 40 mg 4 times/day were shown in clinical trials to provide a mortality benefit in the treatment of CHF. Higher doses may be used for symptomatic and hemodynamic improvement following optimization of standard therapy.
I.M., I.V.:
Hypertension: Initial: 10-20 mg/dose every 4-6 hours as needed, may increase to 40 mg/dose; change to oral therapy as soon as possible.
Pre-eclampsia/eclampsia: 5 mg/dose then 5-10 mg every 20-30 minutes as needed.

### Dosage Forms
Injection, solution, as hydrochloride: 20 mg/mL (1 mL)
Tablet, as hydrochloride: 10 mg, 25 mg, 50 mg, 100 mg

## hydralazine and hydrochlorothiazide (hye DRAL a zeen & hye droe klor oh THYE a zide)
**Synonyms** hydrochlorothiazide and hydralazine
**Therapeutic Category** Antihypertensive Agent, Combination
**Use** Management of moderate to severe hypertension and treatment of congestive heart failure
**Usual Dosage** Adults: Oral: Take as directed; not to exceed 50 mg hydrochlorothiazide per day
**Dosage Forms** Capsule:
25/25: Hydralazine hydrochloride 25 mg and hydrochlorothiazide 25 mg
50/50: Hydralazine hydrochloride 50 mg and hydrochlorothiazide 50 mg
100/50: Hydralazine hydrochloride 100 mg and hydrochlorothiazide 50 mg

**hydralazine and isosorbide dinitrate** *see* isosorbide dinitrate and hydralazine *on page 451*

**hydralazine hydrochloride** *see* hydralazine *on previous page*

## hydralazine, hydrochlorothiazide, and reserpine
(hye DRAL a zeen, hye droe klor oh THYE a zide, & re SER peen)
**Synonyms** hydrochlorothiazide, hydralazine, and reserpine; reserpine, hydralazine, and hydrochlorothiazide
**Therapeutic Category** Antihypertensive Agent, Combination
**Use** Hypertensive disorders
**Usual Dosage** Adults: Oral: 1-2 tablets 3 times/day
**Dosage Forms** Tablet: Hydralazine 25 mg, hydrochlorothiazide 15 mg, and reserpine 0.1 mg

**Hydramine® [US-OTC]** *see* diphenhydramine *on page 254*

**hydrated chloral** *see* chloral hydrate *on page 166*

**Hydrate® *(Discontinued)*** *see* dimenhydrinate *on page 252*

**Hydrea® [US/Can]** *see* hydroxyurea *on page 422*

**Hydrisalic™ [US-OTC]** *see* salicylic acid *on page 734*

**Hydrocet® *(Discontinued)*** *see* hydrocodone and acetaminophen *on page 411*

## hydrochlorothiazide (hye droe klor oh THYE a zide)
**Sound-Alike/Look-Alike Issues**
hydrochlorothiazide may be confused with hydrocortisone, hydroflumethiazide
Esidrix may be confused with Lasix®
HCTZ is an error-prone abbreviation
**U.S./Canadian Brand Names** Apo-Hydro® [Can]; Microzide™ [US]; Novo-Hydrazide [Can]; PMS-Hydrochlorothiazide [Can]
**Therapeutic Category** Diuretic, Thiazide
**Use** Management of mild to moderate hypertension; treatment of edema in congestive heart failure and nephrotic syndrome
**Usual Dosage** Oral (effect of drug may be decreased when used every day):
Children (in pediatric patients, chlorothiazide may be preferred over hydrochlorothiazide as there are more dosage formulations [eg, suspension] available):
<6 months: 2-3 mg/kg/day in 2 divided doses
>6 months: 2 mg/kg/day in 2 divided doses
Adults:
Edema: 25-100 mg/day in 1-2 doses; maximum: 200 mg/day
Hypertension: 12.5-50 mg/day; minimal increase in response and more electrolyte disturbances are seen with doses >50 mg/day
**Dosage Forms**
Capsule (Microzide™): 12.5 mg
Tablet: 25 mg, 50 mg

**hydrochlorothiazide and amiloride** *see* amiloride and hydrochlorothiazide *on page 40*

**hydrochlorothiazide and benazepril** *see* benazepril and hydrochlorothiazide *on page 93*

**hydrochlorothiazide and bisoprolol** *see* bisoprolol and hydrochlorothiazide *on page 109*

**hydrochlorothiazide and captopril** *see* captopril and hydrochlorothiazide *on page 139*

**hydrochlorothiazide and enalapril** *see* enalapril and hydrochlorothiazide *on page 284*

**hydrochlorothiazide and eprosartan** *see* eprosartan and hydrochlorothiazide *on page 292*

**hydrochlorothiazide and fosinopril** *see* fosinopril and hydrochlorothiazide *on page 361*

**hydrochlorothiazide and hydralazine** *see* hydralazine and hydrochlorothiazide *on previous page*

**hydrochlorothiazide and irbesartan** *see* irbesartan and hydrochlorothiazide *on page 447*

**hydrochlorothiazide and lisinopril** *see* lisinopril and hydrochlorothiazide *on page 486*

**hydrochlorothiazide and losartan** *see* losartan and hydrochlorothiazide *on page 493*

**hydrochlorothiazide and methyldopa** *see* methyldopa and hydrochlorothiazide *on page 529*

**hydrochlorothiazide and moexipril** *see* moexipril and hydrochlorothiazide *on page 547*

**hydrochlorothiazide and olmesartan medoxomil** *see* olmesartan and hydrochlorothiazide *on page 596*

**hydrochlorothiazide and propranolol** *see* propranolol and hydrochlorothiazide *on page 689*

**hydrochlorothiazide and quinapril** *see* quinapril and hydrochlorothiazide *on page 704*

## hydrochlorothiazide and spironolactone

(hye droe klor oh THYE a zide & speer on oh LAK tone)

**Sound-Alike/Look-Alike Issues**
Aldactazide® may be confused with Aldactone®

**Synonyms** spironolactone and hydrochlorothiazide

**U.S./Canadian Brand Names** Aldactazide 25® [Can]; Aldactazide 50® [Can]; Aldactazide® [US]; Novo-Spirozine [Can]

**Therapeutic Category** Antihypertensive Agent, Combination

**Use** Management of mild to moderate hypertension; treatment of edema in congestive heart failure and nephrotic syndrome, and cirrhosis of the liver accompanied by edema and/or ascites

**Usual Dosage** Oral:
Children: 1.66-3.3 mg/kg/day (of spironolactone) in 2-4 divided doses
Adults:
Hydrochlorothiazide 25 mg and spironolactone 25 mg: $^1/_2$-8 tablets daily
Hydrochlorothiazide 50 mg and spironolactone 50 mg: $^1/_2$-4 tablets daily in 1-2 doses

**Dosage Forms**
Tablet: Hydrochlorothiazide 25 mg and spironolactone 25 mg
Aldactazide®:
25/25: Hydrochlorothiazide 25 mg and spironolactone 25 mg
50/50: Hydrochlorothiazide 50 mg and spironolactone 50 mg

**hydrochlorothiazide and telmisartan** *see* telmisartan and hydrochlorothiazide *on page 783*

## hydrochlorothiazide and triamterene (hye droe klor oh THYE a zide & trye AM ter een)

**Sound-Alike/Look-Alike Issues**
Dyazide® may be confused with diazoxide, Dynacin®
Maxzide® may be confused with Maxidex®

**Synonyms** triamterene and hydrochlorothiazide

**U.S./Canadian Brand Names** Apo-Triazide® [Can]; Dyazide® [US]; Maxzide® [US]; Maxzide®-25 [US]; Novo-Triamzide [Can]; Nu-Triazide [Can]; Penta-Triamterene HCTZ [Can]; Riva-Zide [Can]

**Therapeutic Category** Antihypertensive Agent, Combination

**Use** Management of mild to moderate hypertension; treatment of edema in congestive heart failure and nephrotic syndrome

**Usual Dosage** Adults: Oral:
Hydrochlorothiazide 25 mg and triamterene 37.5 mg: 1-2 tablets/capsules once daily
Hydrochlorothiazide 50 mg and triamterene 75 mg: $^1/_2$-1 tablet daily

**Dosage Forms**
Capsule (Dyazide®): Hydrochlorothiazide 25 mg and triamterene 37.5 mg
Tablet:
Maxzide®: Hydrochlorothiazide 50 mg and triamterene 75 mg
Maxzide®-25: Hydrochlorothiazide 25 mg and triamterene 37.5 mg

**hydrochlorothiazide and valsartan** *see* valsartan and hydrochlorothiazide *on page 839*

**hydrochlorothiazide, hydralazine, and reserpine** *see* hydralazine, hydrochlorothiazide, and reserpine *on previous page*

**Hydrocil® Instant [US-OTC]** *see* psyllium *on page 697*

# hydrocodone and acetaminophen (hye droe KOE done & a seet a MIN oh fen)

**Sound-Alike/Look-Alike Issues**
Lorcet® may be confused with Fioricet®
Lortab® may be confused with Cortef®, Lorabid®, Luride®
Vicodin® may be confused with Hycodan®, Hycomine®, Indocin®, Uridon®
Zydone® may be confused with Vytone®

**Synonyms** acetaminophen and hydrocodone

**U.S./Canadian Brand Names** Anexsia® [US]; Bancap HC® [US]; Ceta-Plus® [US]; Co-Gesic® [US]; hycet™ [US]; Lorcet® 10/650 [US]; Lorcet® Plus [US]; Lortab® [US]; Margesic® H [US]; Maxidone™ [US]; Norco® [US]; Stagesic® [US]; Vicodin® ES [US]; Vicodin® HP [US]; Vicodin® [US]; Zydone® [US]

**Therapeutic Category** Analgesic, Narcotic

**Controlled Substance** C-III

**Use** Relief of moderate to severe pain

**Usual Dosage** Oral (doses should be titrated to appropriate analgesic effect): Analgesic:
Children 2-13 years or <50 kg: Hydrocodone 0.135 mg/kg/dose every 4-6 hours; do not exceed 6 doses/day or the maximum recommended dose of acetaminophen
Children and Adults ≥50 kg: Average starting dose in opioid naive patients: Hydrocodone 5-10 mg 4 times/day; the dosage of acetaminophen should be limited to ≤4 g/day (and possibly less in patients with hepatic impairment or ethanol use).
Dosage ranges (based on specific product labeling): Hydrocodone 2.5-10 mg every 4-6 hours; maximum: 60 mg hydrocodone/day (maximum dose of hydrocodone may be limited by the acetaminophen content of specific product)

**Dosage Forms**
Capsule (Bancap HC®, Ceta-Plus®, Margesic® H, Stagesic®): Hydrocodone bitartrate 5 mg and acetaminophen 500 mg
Elixir: Hydrocodone bitartrate 7.5 mg and acetaminophen 500 mg per 15 mL (480 mL)
Lortab®: Hydrocodone bitartrate 7.5 mg and acetaminophen 500 mg per 15 mL (480 mL) [contains alcohol 7%; tropical fruit punch flavor]
Solution, oral (hycet™): Hydrocodone bitartrate 7.5 mg and acetaminophen 325 mg per 15 mL (480 mL) [contains alcohol 7%; tropical fruit punch flavor]
Tablet:
Hydrocodone bitartrate 2.5 mg and acetaminophen 500 mg
Hydrocodone bitartrate 5 mg and acetaminophen 325 mg
Hydrocodone bitartrate 5 mg and acetaminophen 500 mg
Hydrocodone bitartrate 7.5 mg and acetaminophen 325 mg
Hydrocodone bitartrate 7.5 mg and acetaminophen 500 mg
Hydrocodone bitartrate 7.5 mg and acetaminophen 650 mg
Hydrocodone bitartrate 7.5 mg and acetaminophen 750 mg
Hydrocodone bitartrate 10 mg and acetaminophen 325 mg
Hydrocodone bitartrate 10 mg and acetaminophen 500 mg
Hydrocodone bitartrate 10 mg and acetaminophen 650 mg
Hydrocodone bitartrate 10 mg and acetaminophen 660 mg
Anexsia®:
5/500: Hydrocodone bitartrate 5 mg and acetaminophen 500 mg
7.5/650: Hydrocodone bitartrate 7.5 mg and acetaminophen 650 mg
Co-Gesic® 5/500: Hydrocodone bitartrate 5 mg and acetaminophen 500 mg
Lorcet® 10/650: Hydrocodone bitartrate 10 mg and acetaminophen 650 mg
Lorcet® Plus: Hydrocodone bitartrate 7.5 mg and acetaminophen 650 mg
Lortab®:
2.5/500: Hydrocodone bitartrate 2.5 mg and acetaminophen 500 mg
5/500: Hydrocodone bitartrate 5 mg and acetaminophen 500 mg
7.5/500: Hydrocodone bitartrate 7.5 mg and acetaminophen 500 mg
10/500: Hydrocodone bitartrate 10 mg and acetaminophen 500 mg
Maxidone™: Hydrocodone bitartrate 10 mg and acetaminophen 750 mg
Norco®:
Hydrocodone bitartrate 5 mg and acetaminophen 325 mg
Hydrocodone bitartrate 7.5 mg and acetaminophen 325 mg
Hydrocodone bitartrate 10 mg and acetaminophen 325 mg
Vicodin®: Hydrocodone bitartrate 5 mg and acetaminophen 500 mg
Vicodin® ES: Hydrocodone bitartrate 7.5 mg and acetaminophen 750 mg
Vicodin® HP: Hydrocodone bitartrate 10 mg and acetaminophen 660 mg
(Continued)

## hydrocodone and acetaminophen *(Continued)*

Zydone®:
Hydrocodone bitartrate 5 mg and acetaminophen 400 mg
Hydrocodone bitartrate 7.5 mg and acetaminophen 400 mg
Hydrocodone bitartrate 10 mg and acetaminophen 400 mg

## hydrocodone and aspirin (hye droe KOE done & AS pir in)

**Synonyms** aspirin and hydrocodone
**U.S./Canadian Brand Names** Damason-P® [US]
**Therapeutic Category**  Analgesic, Narcotic
**Controlled Substance** C-III
**Use** Relief of moderate to moderately severe pain
**Usual Dosage** Adults: Oral: 1-2 tablets every 4-6 hours as needed for pain
**Dosage Forms** Tablet: Hydrocodone bitartrate 5 mg and aspirin 500 mg

## hydrocodone and chlorpheniramine (hye droe KOE done & klor fen IR a meen)

**Synonyms** chlorpheniramine and hydrocodone
**U.S./Canadian Brand Names** Tussionex® [US]
**Therapeutic Category**  Antihistamine/Antitussive
**Controlled Substance** C-III
**Use** Symptomatic relief of cough and allergy
**Usual Dosage** Oral:
Children 6-12 years: 2.5 mL every 12 hours; do not exceed 5 mL/24 hours
Adults: 5 mL every 12 hours; do not exceed 10 mL/24 hours
**Dosage Forms** Suspension, extended release: Hydrocodone polistirex (as bitartrate) 10 mg and chlorpheniramine polistirex (as maleate) 8 mg per 5 mL (480 mL)

## hydrocodone and guaifenesin (hye droe KOE done & gwye FEN e sin)

**Sound-Alike/Look-Alike Issues**
Vicodin® may be confused with Hycodan®, Hycomine®, Indocin®, Uridon®
**Synonyms** guaifenesin and hydrocodone
**U.S./Canadian Brand Names** Codiclear® DH [US]; Hycotuss® [US]; Kwelcof® [US]; Maxi-Tuss HCG [US]; Pneumotussin® [US]; Vitussin [US]
**Therapeutic Category**  Antitussive/Expectorant
**Controlled Substance** C-III
**Use** Symptomatic relief of nonproductive coughs associated with upper and lower respiratory tract congestion
**Usual Dosage**
Children:
6-12 years:
Codiclear® DH, Hycotuss®, Kwelcof®, Maxi-Tuss HCG: 2.5-5 mL every 4 hours, after meals and at bedtime
Pneumotussin®: One tablet or 5 mL every 4-6 hours (maximum: 4 doses/24 hours)
>12 years:
Codiclear® DH, Hycotuss®, Kwelcof®, Maxi-Tuss HCG: 5-10 mL every 4 hours, after meals and at bedtime
Pneumotussin®: 1-2 tablets or 10 mL every 4-6 hours (maximum: 4 doses/24 hours)
Adults:
Codiclear® DH, Kwelcof®, Hycotuss®: 5-15 mL every 4 hours, after meals and at bedtime (maximum: 30 mL/24 hours)
Maxi-Tuss HCG: 5-10 mL every 4 hours, after meals and at bedtime
Pneumotussin®: 1-2 tablets or 10 mL every 4-6 hours (maximum: 4 doses/24 hours)
**Dosage Forms**
Liquid: Hydrocodone bitartrate 5 mg and guaifenesin 100 mg per 5 mL (480 mL, 960 mL) [may contain benzoic acid]
Hycotuss®: Hydrocodone bitartrate 5 mg and guaifenesin 100 mg per 5 mL (480 mL) [contains alcohol 10%; butterscotch flavor]
Kwelcof®: Hydrocodone bitartrate 5 mg and guaifenesin 100 mg per 5 mL (480 mL) [alcohol free, dye free, sugar free; contains benzoic acid; fruit flavor]

Vitussin: Hydrocodone bitartrate 5 mg and guaifenesin 100 mg per 5 mL (480 mL) [alcohol free, sugar free, dye free; cherry flavor]

Tablet (Pneumotussin®): Hydrocodone bitartrate 2.5 mg and guaifenesin 300 mg [dye free]

Syrup:

Codiclear® DH: Hydrocodone bitartrate 5 mg and guaifenesin 100 mg per 5 mL (120 mL, 480 mL) [alcohol free, dye free, sugar free; contains benzoic acid; cherry flavor]

Maxi-Tuss HCG: Hydrocodone bitartrate 6 mg and guaifenesin 200 mg per 5 mL (480 mL) [alcohol free, sugar free; contains aspartame; butterscotch flavor]

Pneumotussin®: Hydrocodone bitartrate 2.5 mg and guaifenesin 200 mg per 5 mL (480 mL) [alcohol free, dye free, sugar free; cherry punch flavor]

## hydrocodone and homatropine (hye droe KOE done & hoe MA troe peen)

**Sound-Alike/Look-Alike Issues**

Hycodan® may be confused with Hycomine®, Vicodin®

**Synonyms** homatropine and hydrocodone

**U.S./Canadian Brand Names** Hycodan® [US]; Hydromet® [US]; Hydropane® [US]; Tussigon® [US]

**Therapeutic Category** Antitussive

**Controlled Substance** C-III

**Use** Symptomatic relief of cough

**Usual Dosage** Oral (based on hydrocodone component):

Children: 0.6 mg/kg/day in 3-4 divided doses; do not administer more frequently than every 4 hours

A single dose should not exceed 1.25 mg in children <2 years of age, 5 mg in children 2-12 years, and 10 mg in children >12 years

Adults: 10 mg every 4-6 hours, a single dose should not exceed 15 mg; do not administer more frequently than every 4 hours

**Dosage Forms**

Syrup (Hycodan®, Hydromet®, Hydropane®): Hydrocodone bitartrate 5 mg and homatropine methylbromide 1.5 mg per 5 mL (480 mL) [cherry flavor]

Tablet (Hycodan®, Tussigon®): Hydrocodone bitartrate 5 mg and homatropine methylbromide 1.5 mg

## hydrocodone and ibuprofen (hye droe KOE done & eye byoo PROE fen)

**Synonyms** ibuprofen and hydrocodone

**U.S./Canadian Brand Names** Reprexain™ [US]; Vicoprofen® [US/Can]

**Therapeutic Category** Analgesic, Narcotic

**Controlled Substance** C-III

**Use** Short-term (generally <10 days) management of moderate to severe acute pain; is not indicated for treatment of such conditions as osteoarthritis or rheumatoid arthritis

**Usual Dosage** Adults: Oral: 1-2 tablets every 4-6 hours as needed for pain; maximum: 5 tablets/day

**Dosage Forms**

Tablet: Hydrocodone bitartrate 5 mg and ibuprofen 200 mg; hydrocodone bitartrate 7.5 mg and ibuprofen 200 mg

Reprexain™: Hydrocodone bitartrate 5 mg and ibuprofen 200 mg

Vicoprofen®: Hydrocodone bitartrate 7.5 mg and ibuprofen 200 mg

## hydrocodone and pseudoephedrine (hye droe KOE done & soo doe e FED rin)

**Synonyms** pseudoephedrine and hydrocodone

**U.S./Canadian Brand Names** Histussin D® [US]; P-V Tussin Tablet [US]

**Therapeutic Category** Cough and Cold Combination

**Controlled Substance** C-III

**Use** Symptomatic relief of cough due to colds, nasal congestion, and cough

**Usual Dosage** Oral: Adults: 5 mL 4 times/day

**Dosage Forms**

Syrup (Histussin D®): Hydrocodone bitartrate 5 mg and pseudoephedrine hydrochloride 60 mg per 5 mL (480 mL)

Tablet (P-V Tussin): Hydrocodone bitartrate 5 mg and pseudoephedrine hydrochloride 60 mg

## hydrocodone bitartrate, carbinoxamine maleate, and pseudoephedrine hydrochloride

see hydrocodone, carbinoxamine, and pseudoephedrine on next page

## hydrocodone bitartrate, phenylephrine hydrochloride, and diphenhydramine hydrochloride

see hydrocodone, phenylephrine, and diphenhydramine on next page

## hydrocodone, carbinoxamine, and pseudoephedrine
(hye droe KOE done, kar bi NOKS a meen, & soo doe e FED rin)

**Synonyms** carbinoxamine, pseudoephedrine, and hydrocodone; hydrocodone bitartrate, carbinoxamine maleate, and pseudoephedrine hydrochloride; pseudoephedrine, hydrocodone, and carbinoxamine

**U.S./Canadian Brand Names** Histex™ HC [US]; Tri-Vent™ HC [US]

**Therapeutic Category** Antihistamine/Decongestant/Antitussive

**Controlled Substance** C-III

**Use** Symptomatic relief of cough, congestion, and rhinorrhea associated with the common cold, influenza, bronchitis, or sinusitis

**Usual Dosage** Oral: Relief of cough, congestion, and runny nose:
Children:
2-10 years: Dosing based on hydrocodone content: 0.6 mg/kg/day given in 4 divided doses. Alternately, the following dosing may be used based on age:
2-4 years: 1.25 mL every 4-6 hours; maximum dose: 7.5 mL/24 hours
4-10 years: 2.5 mL every 4-6 hours; maximum dose: 15 mL/24 hours
>10 years: Refer to Adults dosing
Adults: 5-10 mL every 4-6 hours; maximum dose: 30 mL/24 hours

**Dosage Forms**
Liquid: Hydrocodone bitartrate 5 mg, carbinoxamine maleate 2 mg, and pseudoephedrine hydrochloride 30 mg per 5 mL (480 mL)
Histex™ HC, Tri-Vent™ HC: Hydrocodone bitartrate 5 mg, carbinoxamine maleate 2 mg, and pseudoephedrine hydrochloride 30 mg per 5 mL (480 mL) [alcohol free, sugar free; peach flavor]

**hydrocodone, chlorpheniramine, and pseudoephedrine** *see* pseudoco-done, and chlorpheniramine *on page 695*

## hydrocodone, chlorpheniramine, phenylephrine, acetaminophen, and caffeine (hye droe KOE done, klor fen IR a meen, fen il EF rin, a seet a MIN oh fen, & KAF een)

**Sound-Alike/Look-Alike Issues**
Hycomine® may be confused with Byclomine®, Hycamtin®, Hycodan®, Vicodin®

**Synonyms** acetaminophen, caffeine, hydrocodone, chlorpheniramine, and phenylephrine; caffeine, hydrocodone, chlorpheniramine, phenylephrine, and acetaminophen; chlorpheniramine, hydrocodone, phenylephrine, acetaminophen, and caffeine; phenylephrine, hydrocodone, chlorpheniramine, acetaminophen, and caffeine

**U.S./Canadian Brand Names** Hycomine® Compound [US]

**Therapeutic Category** Antitussive

**Controlled Substance** C-III

**Use** Symptomatic relief of cough and symptoms of upper respiratory infection

**Usual Dosage** Adults: Oral: 1 tablet every 4 hours, up to 4 times/day

**Dosage Forms** Tablet: Hydrocodone bitartrate 5 mg, chlorpheniramine maleate 2 mg, phenylephrine hydrochloride 10 mg, acetaminophen 250 mg, and caffeine 30 mg [cherry flavor]

### Hydrocodone PA® Syrup (Discontinued)

**hydrocodone, phenylephrine, and chlorpheniramine** *see* phenylephrine, hydrocodone, and chlorpheniramine *on page 643*

## hydrocodone, phenylephrine, and diphenhydramine
(hye droe KOE done, fen il EF rin, & dye fen HYE dra meen)

**Sound-Alike/Look-Alike Issues**
Endal® may be confused with Depen®, Intal®

**Synonyms** diphenhydramine, hydrocodone, and phenylephrine; hydrocodone bitartrate, phenylephrine hydrochloride, and diphenhydramine hydrochloride; phenylephrine, diphenhydramine, and hydrocodone

**U.S./Canadian Brand Names** Endal® HD [US]; Hydro DP [US]; TussiNate™ [US]

**Therapeutic Category** Antihistamine/Decongestant/Antitussive; Antitussive; Decongestant

**Controlled Substance** C-III

**Use** Symptomatic relief of cough and congestion associated with the common cold, sinusitis, or acute upper respiratory tract infections

**Usual Dosage** Oral: Relief of cough, congestion:
Children 6-12 years: 5 mL every 4 hours (maximum: 20 mL/24 hours)
Children >12 years and Adults: 10 mL every 4 hours (maximum: 40 mL/24 hours)

**Dosage Forms** Syrup:

Endal® HD: Hydrocodone bitartrate 2 mg, phenylephrine hydrochloride 7.5 mg, and diphenhydramine hydrochloride 12.5 mg per 5 mL (480 mL) [alcohol free, sugar free; contains sodium benzoate; cherry flavor]

Hydro DP: Hydrocodone bitartrate 2 mg, phenylephrine hydrochloride 7.5 mg, and diphenhydramine hydrochloride 12.5 mg per 5 mL (480 mL) [cherry flavor]

TussiNate™: Hydrocodone bitartrate 3.5 mg, phenylephrine hydrochloride 5 mg, and diphenhydramine hydrochloride 12.5 mg per 5 mL (480 mL) [alcohol free; contains sodium benzoate; black raspberry flavor]

# hydrocodone, pseudoephedrine, and guaifenesin

(hye droe KOE done, soo doe e FED rin & gwye FEN e sin)

**Synonyms** guaifenesin, hydrocodone, and pseudoephedrine; pseudoephedrine, hydrocodone, and guaifenesin

**U.S./Canadian Brand Names** Hydro-Tussin™ HD [US]; Hydro-Tussin™ XP [US]; Su-Tuss®-HD [US]; Tussend® Expectorant [US]; Ztuss™ Tablet [US]

**Therapeutic Category** Antitussive/Decongestant/Expectorant

**Controlled Substance** C-III

**Use** Symptomatic relief of irritating, nonproductive cough associated with upper respiratory conditions and allergies

**Usual Dosage** Oral: Cough/congestion:

Children:

2-6 years: Hydro-Tussin™ XP: 1.25-2.5 mL 4 times/day as needed

6-12 years:

Hydro-Tussin™ XP: 2.5-5 mL 4 times/day as needed

Tussend®, Hydro-Tussin™ HD: 5 mL every 4-6 hours as needed

Ztuss™: One-half to 1 tablet every 4-6 hours (maximum: 6 tablets/24 hours)

Children ≥12 years and Adults:

Hydro-Tussin™ XP: 5-10 mL 4 times/day as needed

Tussend®, Hydro-Tussin™ HD: 10 mL every 4-6 hours as needed

Ztuss™: 1-1½ tablets every 4-6 hours (maximum: 8 tablets/24 hours)

**Dosage Forms**

Elixir (Su-Tuss®-HD): Hydrocodone bitartrate 2.5 mg, pseudoephedrine hydrochloride 30 mg, and guaifenesin 100 mg per 5 mL (480 mL) [contains alcohol; fruit punch flavor]

Liquid:

Hydro-Tussin™ HD: Hydrocodone bitartrate 2.5 mg, pseudoephedrine hydrochloride 30 mg, and guaifenesin 100 mg per 5 mL (480 mL) [alcohol free; contains sodium benzoate]

Hydro-Tussin® XP: Hydrocodone bitartrate 3 mg, pseudoephedrine hydrochloride 15 mg, and guaifenesin 100 mg per 5 mL (480 mL) [alcohol free, dye free]

Tussend® Expectorant: Hydrocodone bitartrate 2.5 mg, pseudoephedrine hydrochloride 30 mg, and guaifenesin 100 mg per 5 mL (480 mL) [contains alcohol; fruit punch flavor]

Tablet (Ztuss™): Hydrocodone bitartrate 5 mg, pseudoephedrine hydrochloride 30 mg, and guaifenesin 300 mg [sugar free]

**hydrocortisone acetate** *see* hydrocortisone (systemic) *on next page*

**hydrocortisone, acetic acid, and propylene glycol diacetate** *see* acetic acid, propylene glycol diacetate, and hydrocortisone *on page 14*

**hydrocortisone and benzoyl peroxide** *see* benzoyl peroxide and hydrocortisone *on page 99*

**hydrocortisone and ciprofloxacin** *see* ciprofloxacin and hydrocortisone *on page 186*

**hydrocortisone and iodoquinol** *see* iodoquinol and hydrocortisone *on page 445*

**hydrocortisone and lidocaine** *see* lidocaine and hydrocortisone *on page 482*

**hydrocortisone and pramoxine** *see* pramoxine and hydrocortisone *on page 671*

**hydrocortisone and urea** *see* urea and hydrocortisone *on page 835*

**hydrocortisone, bacitracin, neomycin, and polymyxin B** *see* bacitracin, neomycin, polymyxin B, and hydrocortisone *on page 87*

**hydrocortisone butyrate** *see* hydrocortisone (topical) *on page 417*

**hydrocortisone, neomycin, and polymyxin B** *see* neomycin, polymyxin B, and hydrocortisone *on page 568*

**hydrocortisone, neomycin, colistin, and thonzonium** *see* neomycin, colistin, hydrocortisone, and thonzonium *on page 567*

**hydrocortisone, propylene glycol diacetate, and acetic acid** *see* acetic acid, propylene glycol diacetate, and hydrocortisone *on page 14*

## hydrocortisone (rectal) (hye droe KOR ti sone REK tal)

**Sound-Alike/Look-Alike Issues**

hydrocortisone may be confused with hydrocodone, hydroxychloroquine, hydrochlorothiazide

**U.S./Canadian Brand Names** Anucort-HC® [US]; Anusol®-HC [US]; Anusol® HC-1 [US-OTC]; Cortenema® [Can]; Corticool® [US-OTC]; Cortifoam® [US/Can]; Hemril®-30 [US]; Preparation H® Hydrocortisone [US-OTC]; Procto-Kit™ [US]; Procto-Pak™ [US]; Proctocort® [US]; ProctoCream® HC [US]; Proctosert [US]; Proctosol-HC® [US]; Proctozone-HC™ [US]; Tucks® Anti-Itch [US-OTC]

**Therapeutic Category** Adrenal Corticosteroid

**Use** Adjunctive treatment of ulcerative colitis

**Usual Dosage** Adults: Rectal: Ulcerative colitis: 10-100 mg 1-2 times/day for 2-3 weeks

**Dosage Forms** [DSC] = Discontinued product

Aerosol, rectal, as acetate (Cortifoam®): 10% (15 g) [90 mg/applicator]

Cream, rectal, as acetate (Nupercainal® Hydrocortisone Cream): 1% (30 g) [strength expressed as base]

Cream, rectal, as base:

Cortizone®-10: 1% (30 g) [contains aloe]

Preparation H® Hydrocortisone: 1% (27 g)

Suppository, rectal, as acetate:  25 mg (12s, 24s, 100s)

Anucort-HC®, Tucks® Anti-Itch: 25 mg (12s, 24s, 100s) [strength expressed as base; Anucort-HC® *renamed* Tucks® Anti-Itch]

Anusol-HC®, Proctosol-HC®: 25 mg (12s, 24s)

Encort™: 30 mg (12s)

Hemril®-30, Proctocort®, Proctosert: 30 mg (12s, 24s)

Suspension, rectal, as base: 100 mg/60 mL (7s)

Colocort®: 100 mg/60 mL (1s, 7s)

**hydrocortisone sodium succinate** *see* hydrocortisone (systemic) *on this page*

## hydrocortisone (systemic) (hye droe KOR ti sone sis TEM ik)

**Sound-Alike/Look-Alike Issues**

hydrocortisone may be confused with hydrocodone, hydroxychloroquine, hydrochlorothiazide

Cortef® may be confused with Lortab®

Cortizone® may be confused with cortisone

HCT (occasional abbreviation for hydrocortisone) is an error-prone abbreviation (mistaken as hydrochlorothiazide)

**Synonyms** compound F; cortisol; hydrocortisone acetate; hydrocortisone sodium succinate

**U.S./Canadian Brand Names** Cortef® [US/Can]; Solu-Cortef® [US/Can]

**Therapeutic Category** Adrenal Corticosteroid

**Use** Management of adrenocortical insufficiency

**Usual Dosage** Dose should be based on severity of disease and patient response

Acute adrenal insufficiency: I.M., I.V.:

Infants and young Children: Succinate: 1-2 mg/kg/dose bolus, then 25-150 mg/day in divided doses every 6-8 hours

Older Children: Succinate: 1-2 mg/kg bolus then 150-250 mg/day in divided doses every 6-8 hours

Adults: Succinate: 100 mg I.V. bolus, then 300 mg/day in divided doses every 8 hours or as a continuous infusion for 48 hours; once patient is stable change to oral, 50 mg every 8 hours for 6 doses, then taper to 30-50 mg/day in divided doses

Chronic adrenal corticoid insufficiency: Adults: Oral: 20-30 mg/day

Anti-inflammatory or immunosuppressive:

Infants and Children:

Oral: 2.5-10 mg/kg/day **or** 75-300 mg/m$^2$/day every 6-8 hours

I.M., I.V.: Succinate: 1-5 mg/kg/day **or** 30-150 mg/m$^2$/day divided every 12-24 hours

Adolescents and Adults: Oral, I.M., I.V.: Succinate: 15-240 mg every 12 hours

Congenital adrenal hyperplasia: Oral: Initial: 10-20 mg/m$^2$/day in 3 divided doses; a variety of dosing schedules have been used. **Note:** Inconsistencies have occurred with liquid formulations; tablets may provide more reliable levels. Doses must be individualized by monitoring growth, bone age, and hormonal levels. Mineralocorticoid and sodium supplementation may be required based upon electrolyte regulation and plasma renin activity.

Physiologic replacement: Children:

Oral: 0.5-0.75 mg/kg/day **or** 20-25 mg/m$^2$/day every 8 hours

I.M.: Succinate: 0.25-0.35 mg/kg/day **or** 12-15 mg/m$^2$/day once daily

Shock: I.M., I.V.: Succinate:

Children: Initial: 50 mg/kg, then repeated in 4 hours and/or every 24 hours as needed

Adolescents and Adults: 500 mg to 2 g every 2-6 hours

Status asthmaticus: Children and Adults: I.V.: Succinate: 1-2 mg/kg/dose every 6 hours for 24 hours, then maintenance of 0.5-1 mg/kg every 6 hours

Adults:

Rheumatic diseases:

Intralesional, intra-articular, soft tissue injection: Acetate:

Large joints: 25 mg (up to 37.5 mg)

Small joints: 10-25 mg

Tendon sheaths: 5-12.5 mg

Soft tissue infiltration: 25-50 mg (up to 75 mg)

Bursae: 25-37.5 mg

Ganglia: 12.5-25 mg

Stress dosing (surgery) in patients known to be adrenally-suppressed or on chronic systemic steroids: I.V.:

Minor stress (ie, inguinal herniorrhaphy): 25 mg/day for 1 day

Moderate stress (ie, joint replacement, cholecystectomy): 50-75 mg/day (25 mg every 8-12 hours) for 1-2 days

Major stress (pancreatoduodenectomy, esophagogastrectomy, cardiac surgery): 100-150 mg/day (50 mg every 8-12 hours) for 2-3 days

**Dosage Forms**

Injection, powder for reconstitution, as sodium succinate (Solu-Cortef®): 100 mg, 250 mg, 500 mg, 1 g [diluent contains benzyl alcohol; strength expressed as base]

Tablet, as base: 20 mg

Cortef®: 5 mg, 10 mg, 20 mg

# hydrocortisone (topical) (hye droe KOR ti sone TOP i kal)

### Sound-Alike/Look-Alike Issues

hydrocortisone may be confused with hydrocodone, hydroxychloroquine, hydrochlorothiazide

Cortef® may be confused with Lortab®

Cortizone® may be confused with cortisone

HCT (occasional abbreviation for hydrocortisone) is an error-prone abbreviation (mistaken as hydrochlorothiazide)

Hytone® may be confused with Vytone®

**Synonyms** hydrocortisone butyrate; hydrocortisone valerate

**U.S./Canadian Brand Names** Aquacort® [Can]; Aquanil™ HC [US-OTC]; Beta-HC® [US]; Caldecort® [US-OTC]; Cetacort® [US]; Cortaid® Intensive Therapy [US-OTC]; Cortaid® Maximum Strength [US-OTC]; Cortaid® Sensitive Skin [US-OTC]; Cortamed® [Can]; Corticool® [US-OTC]; Cortizone®-10 Maximum Strength [US-OTC]; Cortizone®-10 Plus Maximum Strength [US-OTC]; Cortizone®-10 Quick Shot [US-OTC]; Dermarest Dricort® [US-OTC]; Dermtex® HC [US-OTC]; Hemril®-30 [US]; Hycort™ [Can]; Hyderm [Can]; HydroZone Plus [US-OTC]; Hytone® [US]; IvySoothe® [US-OTC]; Locoid Lipocream® [US]; Locoid® [US/Can]; Nupercainal® Hydrocortisone Cream [US-OTC]; Nutracort® [US]; Pandel® [US]; Post Peel Healing Balm [US-OTC]; Prevex® HC [Can]; Sarna® HC [Can]; Sarnol®-HC [US-OTC]; Summer's Eve® SpecialCare™ Medicated Anti-Itch Cream [US-OTC]; Texacort® [US]; Tucks® Anti-Itch [US-OTC]; Westcort® [US/Can]

**Therapeutic Category** Corticosteroid, Topical

**Use** Relief of inflammation of corticosteroid-responsive dermatoses (low and medium potency topical corticosteroid)

**Usual Dosage** Dermatosis: Children >2 years and Adults: Topical: Apply to affected area 2-4 times/day (Buteprate: Apply once or twice daily). Therapy should be discontinued when control is achieved; if no improvement is seen, reassessment of diagnosis may be necessary.

**Dosage Forms** [DSC] = Discontinued product

Cream, topical, as acetate: 0.5% (9 g, 30 g, 60 g) [available with aloe]; 1% (30 g, 454 g) [available with aloe]

Cream, topical, as base: 0.5% (30 g); 1% (1.5 g, 30 g, 114 g, 454 g); 2.5% (20 g, 30 g, 454 g)

Anusol-HC®: 2.5% (30 g) [contains benzyl alcohol]

(Continued)

## hydrocortisone (topical) *(Continued)*

Caldecort®: 1% (30 g) [contains aloe vera gel]
Cortaid® Intensive Therapy: 1% (60 g)
Cortaid® Maximum Strength: 1% (15 g, 30 g, 40 g, 60 g) [contains aloe vera gel and benzyl alcohol]
Cortaid® Sensitive Skin: 0.5% (15 g) [contains aloe vera gel]
Cortizone®-10 Maximum Strength: 1% (15 g, 30 g, 60 g) [contains aloe]
Cortizone®-10 Plus Maximum Strength: 1% (30 g, 60 g) [contains vitamins A, D, E and aloe]
Dermarest® Dricort®: 1% (15 g, 30 g)
HydroZone Plus, Proctocort®, Procto-Pak™: 1% (30 g)
Hytone®: 2.5% (30 g, 60 g)
IvySoothe®: 1% (30 g) [contains aloe]
Post Peel Healing Balm: 1% (23 g)
ProctoCream® HC: 2.5% (30 g) [contains benzyl alcohol]
Procto-Kit™: 1% (30 g) [packaged with applicator tips and finger cots]; 2.5% (30 g) [packaged with applicator tips and finger cots]
Proctosol-HC®, Proctozone-HC™: 2.5% (30 g)
Summer's Eve® SpecialCare™ Medicated Anti-Itch Cream: 1% (30 g)
Cream, topical, as butyrate (Locoid®, Locoid Lipocream®): 0.1% (15 g, 45 g)
Cream, topical, as probutate (Pandel®): 0.1% (15 g, 45 g, 80 g)
Cream, topical, as valerate (Westcort®): 0.2% (15 g, 45 g, 60 g)
Gel, topical, as base (Corticool®): 1% (45 g)
Lotion, topical, as base: 1% (120 mL); 2.5% (60 mL)
Aquanil™ HC: 1% (120 mL)
Beta-HC®, Cetacort®, Sarnol®-HC: 1% (60 mL)
HydroZone Plus: 1% (120 mL)
Hytone®: 2.5% (60 mL)
Nutracort®: 1% (60 mL, 120 mL); 2.5% (60 mL, 120 mL)
Ointment, topical, as acetate: 1% (30 g) [strength expressed as base; available with aloe]
Anusol® HC-1: 1% (21 g) [strength expressed as base]
Cortaid® Maximum Strength: 1% (15 g, 30 g) [strength expressed as base]
Ointment, topical, as base: 0.5% (30 g); 1% (30 g, 454 g); 2.5% (20 g, 30 g, 454 g)
Cortizone®-10 Maximum Strength: 1% (30 g, 60 g)
Hytone®: 2.5% (30 g)
Ointment, topical, as butyrate (Locoid®): 0.1% (15 g, 45 g)
Ointment, topical, as valerate (Westcort®): 0.2% (15 g, 45 g, 60 g)
Solution, otic, as base (EarSol® HC): 1% (30 mL) [contains alcohol 44%, benzyl benzoate, yerba santa]
Solution, topical, as base (Texacort®): 2.5% (30 mL) [contains alcohol]
Solution, topical, as butyrate (Locoid®): 0.1% (20 mL, 60 mL) [contains alcohol 50%]
Solution, topical spray, as base:
Cortaid® Intensive Therapy: 1% (60 mL) [contains alcohol]
Cortizone®-10 Quick Shot: 1% (44 mL) [contains benzyl alcohol]
Dermtex® HC: 1% (52 mL) [contains menthol 1%]

**hydrocortisone valerate** *see* hydrocortisone (topical) *on previous page*

**HydroDIURIL® *(Discontinued)*** *see* hydrochlorothiazide *on page 409*

**Hydro DP [US]** *see* hydrocodone, phenylephrine, and diphenhydramine *on page 414*

**Hydrogesic® *(Discontinued)*** *see* hydrocodone and acetaminophen *on page 411*

**Hydromet® [US]** *see* hydrocodone and homatropine *on page 413*

**Hydromorph Contin® [Can]** *see* hydromorphone *on this page*

**Hydromorph-IR® [Can]** *see* hydromorphone *on this page*

## hydromorphone (hye droe MOR fone)
### Sound-Alike/Look-Alike Issues
hydromorphone may be confused with morphine; significant overdoses have occurred when hydromorphone products have been inadvertently administered instead of morphine sulfate. Commercially available prefilled syringes of both products looks similar and are often stored in close proximity to each other. **Note:** Hydromorphone 1 mg oral is approximately equal to morphine 4 mg oral; hydromorphone 1 mg I.V. is approximately equal to morphine 5 mg I.V.
Dilaudid® may be confused with Demerol®, Dilantin®

Dilaudid®, Dilaudid-HP®: Extreme caution should be taken to avoid confusing the highly-concentrated (Dilaudid-HP®) injection with the less-concentrated (Dilaudid®) injectable product.

**Synonyms** dihydromorphinone; hydromorphone hydrochloride

**U.S./Canadian Brand Names** Dilaudid-HP-Plus® [Can]; Dilaudid-HP® [US/Can]; Dilaudid-XP® [Can]; Dilaudid® Sterile Powder [Can]; Dilaudid® [US/Can]; Hydromorph Contin® [Can]; Hydromorph-IR® [Can]; Hydromorphone HP [Can]; Palladone™ [US]; PMS-Hydromorphone [Can]

**Therapeutic Category** Analgesic, Narcotic

**Controlled Substance** C-II

**Use** Management of moderate-to-severe pain

**Usual Dosage**

Acute pain (moderate to severe): **Note:** These are guidelines and do not represent the maximum doses that may be required in all patients. Doses should be titrated to pain relief/prevention.

Young Children ≥6 months and <50 kg:

Oral: 0.03-0.08 mg/kg/dose every 3-4 hours as needed

I.V.: 0.015 mg/kg/dose every 3-6 hours as needed

Older Children >50 kg and Adults:

Oral: Initial: Opiate-naive: 2-4 mg every 3-4 hours as needed; patients with prior opiate exposure may require higher initial doses; usual dosage range: 2-8 mg every 3-4 hours as needed

I.V.: Initial: Opiate-naive: 0.2-0.6 mg every 2-3 hours as needed; patients with prior opiate exposure may tolerate higher initial doses

**Note:** More frequent dosing may be needed.

Mechanically-ventilated patients (based on 70 kg patient): 0.7-2 mg every 1-2 hours as needed; infusion (based on 70 kg patient): 0.5-1 mg/hour

Patient-controlled analgesia (PCA): (Opiate-naive: Consider lower end of dosing range)

Usual concentration: 0.2 mg/mL

Demand dose: Usual: 0.1-0.2 mg; range: 0.05-0.5 mg

Lockout interval: 5-15 minutes

4-hour limit: 4-6 mg

Epidural:

Bolus dose: 1-1.5 mg

Infusion concentration: 0.05-0.075 mg/mL

Infusion rate: 0.04-0.4 mg/hour

Demand dose: 0.15 mg

Lockout interval: 30 minutes

I.M., SubQ: **Note:** I.M. use may result in variable absorption and a lag time to peak effect.

Initial: Opiate-naive: 0.8-1 mg every 4-6 hours as needed; patients with prior opiate exposure may require higher initial doses; usual dosage range: 1-2 mg every 3-6 hours as needed

Rectal: 3 mg every 4-8 hours as needed

Chronic pain: Adults: Oral: **Note:** Patients taking opioids chronically may become tolerant and require doses higher than the usual dosage range to maintain the desired effect. Tolerance can be managed by appropriate dose titration. There is no optimal or maximal dose for hydromorphone in chronic pain. The appropriate dose is one that relieves pain throughout its dosing interval without causing unmanageable side effects.

Controlled release formulation (Hydromorph Contin®, not available in U.S.): 3-30 mg every 12 hours. **Note:** A patient's hydromorphone requirement should be established using prompt release formulations; conversion to long acting products may be considered when chronic, continuous treatment is required. Higher dosages should be reserved for use only in opioid-tolerant patients.

Extended release formulation (Palladone™): For use only in opioid-tolerant patients requiring extended treatment of pain. Initial Palladone™ dose should be calculated using standard conversion estimates based on previous total daily opioid dose, rounding off to the most appropriate strength available. Doses should be administered once every 24 hours. Discontinue all previous around-the-clock opioids when treatment is initiated. Dose may be adjusted every 2 days as needed.

Conversion from transdermal fentanyl to oral Palladone™ (limited clinical experience): Initiate Palladone™ 18 hours after removal of patch; substitute Palladone™ 12 mg/day for each fentanyl 50 mcg/hour patch; monitor closely

Conversion from opioid combination drugs: Initial dose: Palladone™ 12 mg/day in patients receiving around-the-clock fixed combination-opioid analgesics with a total dose greater than or equal to oxycodone 45 mg/day, hydrocodone 45 mg/day, or codeine 300 mg/day

**Dosage Forms** [CAN] = Canadian brand name

Capsule, controlled release (Hydromorph Contin®) [CAN]: 3 mg, 6 mg, 12 mg, 18 mg, 24 mg, 30 mg [not available in U.S.]

(Continued)

# hydromorphone *(Continued)*

Capsule, extended release, as hydrochloride (Palladone™): 12 mg, 16 mg, 24 mg, 32 mg *[withdrawn from market]*

Injection, powder for reconstitution, as hydrochloride (Dilaudid-HP®): 250 mg

Injection, solution, as hydrochloride: 1 mg/mL (1 mL); 2 mg/mL (1 mL, 20 mL); 4 mg/mL (1 mL); 10 mg/mL (1 mL, 5 mL, 10 mL)

Dilaudid®: 1 mg/mL (1 mL); 2 mg/mL (1 mL, 20 mL) [20 mL size contains edetate sodium; vial stopper contains latex]; 4 mg/mL (1 mL)

Dilaudid-HP®: 10 mg/mL (1 mL, 5 mL, 50 mL)

Liquid, oral, as hydrochloride (Dilaudid®): 1 mg/mL (480 mL) [may contain trace amounts of sodium bisulfite]

Suppository, rectal, as hydrochloride (Dilaudid®): 3 mg (6s)

Tablet, as hydrochloride (Dilaudid®): 2 mg, 4 mg, 8 mg (8 mg tablets may contain trace amounts of sodium bisulfite)

**Hydromorphone HP [Can]** *see* hydromorphone *on page 418*

**hydromorphone hydrochloride** *see* hydromorphone *on page 418*

**Hydromox® *(Discontinued)***

**Hydron CP [US]** *see* phenylephrine, hydrocodone, and chlorpheniramine *on page 643*

**Hydron PSC [US]** *see* pseudoephedrine, hydrocodone, and chlorpheniramine *on page 695*

**Hydropane® [US]** *see* hydrocodone and homatropine *on page 413*

**Hydro-Par® *(Discontinued)*** *see* hydrochlorothiazide *on page 409*

**Hydro-PC II [US]** *see* phenylephrine, hydrocodone, and chlorpheniramine *on page 643*

**Hydro PC II Plus [US]** *see* phenylephrine, hydrocodone, and chlorpheniramine *on page 643*

**hydroquinol** *see* hydroquinone *on this page*

# hydroquinone *(HYE droe kwin one)*

**Sound-Alike/Look-Alike Issues**

Eldopaque® may be confused with Eldoquin®

Eldoquin® may be confused with Eldopaque®

Eldopaque Forte® may be confused with Eldoquin Forte®

Eldoquin Forte® may be confused with Eldopaque Forte®

**Synonyms** hydroquinol; quinol

**U.S./Canadian Brand Names** Alphaquin HP [US]; Claripel™ [US]; Dermarest® Skin Correction Cream Plus [US-OTC]; Eldopaque Forte® [US]; Eldopaque® [US-OTC/Can]; Eldoquin Forte® [US]; Eldoquin® [US-OTC/Can]; EpiQuin™ Micro [US]; Esoterica® Regular [US-OTC]; Glyquin-XM™ [US]; Glyquin® XM [Can]; Glyquin® [US]; Lustra-AF™ [US]; Lustra® [US/Can]; Melanex® [US]; Melpaque HP® [US]; Melquin HP® [US]; Melquin-3® [US]; NeoStrata AHA [US-OTC]; NeoStrata® HQ [Can]; Nuquin HP® [US]; Palmer's® Skin Success Eventone® Fade Cream [US-OTC]; Solaquin Forte® [US/Can]; Solaquin® [US-OTC/Can]; Ultraquin™ [Can]

**Therapeutic Category** Topical Skin Product

**Use** Gradual bleaching of hyperpigmented skin conditions

**Usual Dosage** Children >12 years and Adults: Topical: Apply thin layer and rub in twice daily

**Dosage Forms**

Cream, topical: 4% (30 g) [may contain sodium metabisulfite]

Alphaquin HP: 4% (30 g, 60 g)

Eldoquin®: 2% (15 g, 30 g)

Eldoquin Forte®: 4% (30 g) [contains sodium metabisulfite]

EpiQuin™ Micro: 4% (30 g) [contains benzyl alcohol and sodium metabisulfite]

Esoterica® Regular: 2% (85 g) [contains sodium bisulfite]

Lustra®: 4% (30 g) [contains sodium metabisulfite]

Melquin HP®: 4% (15 g, 30 g) [contains sodium metabisulfite]

Cream, topical [with sunscreen]: 4% (30 g) [may contain sodium metabisulfite]

Claripel™: 4% (30 g, 45 g) [contains sodium metabisulfite]

Dermarest® Skin Correcting Cream Plus: 2% (85 g) [contains aloe vera, sodium bisulfite]

Eldopaque®: 2% (15 g, 30 g)

Eldopaque Forte®: 4% (30 g) [contains sodium metabisulfite]

Glyquin®: 4% (30 g)

Glyquin-XM™: 4% (30 g)
Lustra-AF™: 4% (30 g, 60 g) [contains sodium metabisulfite]
Melpaque HP®: 4% (15 g, 30 g) [contains sodium metabisulfite; sunblocking cream base]
Nuquin HP®: 4% (15 g, 30 g, 60 g) [contains sodium metabisulfite]
Palmer's® Skin Success Eventone® Fade Cream: 2% (81 g, 132 g) [contains sodium sulfite; available in regular, oily skin, and dry skin formulas]
Solaquin®: 2% (30 g)
Solaquin Forte®: 4% (30 g) [contains sodium metabisulfite]
Gel, topical (NeoStrata AHA): 2% (45 g) [contains glycolic acid 10%, sodium bisulfite, and sodium sulfite]
Gel, topical [with sunscreen]: 4% (30 g)
Nuquin HP: 4% (15 g, 30 g) [contains sodium bisulfite]
Solaquin Forte®: 4% (30 g) [contains sodium metabisulfite]
Solution, topical (Melanex®, Melquin-3®): 3% (30 mL) [contains alcohol]

**hydroquinone, fluocinolone acetonide, and tretinoin** *see* fluocinolone, hydroquinone, and tretinoin *on page 345*

**Hydrotropine®** *(Discontinued)* *see* hydrocodone and homatropine *on page 413*

**Hydro-Tussin™-CBX [US]** *see* carbinoxamine and pseudoephedrine *on page 144*

**Hydro-Tussin™ DM [US]** *see* guaifenesin and dextromethorphan *on page 385*

**Hydro-Tussin™ HC [US]** *see* pseudoephedrine, hydrocodone, and chlorpheniramine *on page 695*

**Hydro-Tussin™ HD [US]** *see* hydrocodone, pseudoephedrine, and guaifenesin *on page 415*

**Hydro-Tussin™ XP [US]** *see* hydrocodone, pseudoephedrine, and guaifenesin *on page 415*

**4-hydroxybutyrate** *see* sodium oxybate *on page 755*

**hydroxycarbamide** *see* hydroxyurea *on next page*

# hydroxychloroquine (hye droks ee KLOR oh kwin)

**Sound-Alike/Look-Alike Issues**
hydroxychloroquine may be confused with hydrocortisone
Plaquenil® may be confused with Platinol®

**Synonyms** hydroxychloroquine sulfate

**U.S./Canadian Brand Names** Apo-Hydroxyquine® [Can]; Gen-Hydroxychloroquine [Can]; Plaquenil® [US/Can]

**Therapeutic Category** Aminoquinoline (Antimalarial)

**Use** Suppression and treatment of acute attacks of malaria; treatment of systemic lupus erythematosus and rheumatoid arthritis

**Usual Dosage Note:** Hydroxychloroquine sulfate 200 mg is equivalent to 155 mg hydroxychloroquine base and 250 mg chloroquine phosphate. Oral:
Children:
Chemoprophylaxis of malaria: 5 mg/kg (base) once weekly; should not exceed the recommended adult dose; begin 2 weeks before exposure; continue for 4-6 weeks after leaving endemic area; if suppressive therapy is not begun prior to the exposure, double the initial dose and give in 2 doses, 6 hours apart
Acute attack: 10 mg/kg (base) initial dose; followed by 5 mg/kg at 6, 24, and 48 hours
JRA or SLE: 3-5 mg/kg/day divided 1-2 times/day; avoid exceeding 7 mg/kg/day
Adults:
Chemoprophylaxis of malaria: 310 mg base weekly on same day each week; begin 2 weeks before exposure; continue for 4-6 weeks after leaving endemic area; if suppressive therapy is not begun prior to the exposure, double the initial dose and give in 2 doses, 6 hours apart
Acute attack: 620 mg first dose day 1; 310 mg in 6 hours day 1; 310 mg in 1 dose day 2; and 310 mg in 1 dose on day 3
Rheumatoid arthritis: 310-465 mg/day to start taken with food or milk; increase dose until optimum response level is reached; usually after 4-12 weeks dose should be reduced by $1/2$ and a maintenance dose of 155-310 mg/day given
Lupus erythematosus: 310 mg every day or twice daily for several weeks depending on response; 155-310 mg/day for prolonged maintenance therapy

**Dosage Forms** Tablet, as sulfate: 200 mg [equivalent to 155 mg base]

**hydroxychloroquine sulfate** *see* hydroxychloroquine *on this page*

**hydroxydaunomycin hydrochloride** *see* doxorubicin *on page 270*

**1α-hydroxyergocalciferol** *see* doxercalciferol *on page 269*

**hydroxyethylcellulose** *see* artificial tears *on page 71*

**hydroxyethyl starch** *see* hetastarch *on page 403*

**hydroxyldaunorubicin hydrochloride** *see* doxorubicin *on page 270*

## hydroxyprogesterone caproate (hye droks ee proe JES te rone KAP roe ate)

**U.S./Canadian Brand Names** Hylutin® [US]; Prodrox® [US]

**Therapeutic Category** Progestin

**Use** Treatment of amenorrhea, abnormal uterine bleeding, submucous fibroids, endometriosis, uterine carcinoma, and testing of estrogen production

**Usual Dosage** Adults: I.M.:

Amenorrhea: 375 mg; if no bleeding, begin cyclic treatment with estradiol valerate

Endometriosis: Start cyclic therapy with estradiol valerate

Uterine carcinoma: 1 g one or more times/day (1-7 g/week) for up to 12 weeks

Test for endogenous estrogen production: 250 mg anytime; bleeding 7-14 days after injection indicate positive test

**Dosage Forms** Injection, as caproate (Hylutin®, Prodrox®): 250 mg/mL (5 mL)

## hydroxypropyl cellulose (hye droks ee PROE pil SEL yoo lose)

**U.S./Canadian Brand Names** Lacrisert® [US/Can]

**Therapeutic Category** Ophthalmic Agent, Miscellaneous

**Use** Dry eyes (moderate to severe)

**Usual Dosage** Adults: Ophthalmic: Apply once daily into the inferior cul-de-sac beneath the base of tarsus, not in apposition to the cornea nor beneath the eyelid at the level of the tarsal plate

**Dosage Forms** Insert, ophthalmic [preservative free]: 5 mg

## hydroxypropyl methylcellulose (hye droks ee PROE pil meth il SEL yoo lose)

**Sound-Alike/Look-Alike Issues**

Isopto® Tears may be confused with Isoptin®

**Synonyms** gonioscopic ophthalmic solution; hypromellose

**U.S./Canadian Brand Names** Cellugel® [US]; GenTeal® Mild [US-OTC]; Genteal® [Can]; GenTeal® [US-OTC]; Gonak™ [US-OTC]; Goniosoft™ [US]; Isopto® Tears [US-OTC/Can]; Tearisol® [US-OTC]; Tears Again® MC [US-OTC]

**Therapeutic Category** Ophthalmic Agent, Miscellaneous

**Use** Relief of burning and minor irritation due to dry eyes; diagnostic agent in gonioscopic examination

**Usual Dosage** Adults: Dry eyes: Ophthalmic: Instill 1-2 drops in affected eye(s) as needed

**Dosage Forms** [DSC] = Discontinued product

Gel, ophthalmic (GenTeal®): 0.3% (10 mL)

Solution, ophthalmic: 0.4% (15 mL)

GenTeal®: 0.3% (15 mL, 25 mL)

GenTeal® Mild: 0.2% (15 mL, 25 mL)

Gonak™: 2.5% (15 mL)

Goniosoft™: 2.5% (15 mL)

Goniosol®: 2.5% (15 mL) [contains benzalkonium chloride] [DSC]

Isopto® Tears: 0.5% (15 mL) [contains benzalkonium chloride]

Tearisol®: 0.5% (15 mL) [contains benzalkonium chloride]

Tears Again® MC: 0.3% (15 mL)

Solution, ophthalmic [for injection] (Cellugel®): 2% (1 mL)

## hydroxyurea (hye droks ee yoor EE a)

**Sound-Alike/Look-Alike Issues**

hydroxyurea may be confused with hydrOXYzine

**Synonyms** hydroxycarbamide

**U.S./Canadian Brand Names** Apo-Hydroxyurea® [Can]; Droxia™ [US]; Gen-Hydroxyurea [Can]; Hydrea® [US/Can]; Mylocel™ [US]

**Therapeutic Category** Antineoplastic Agent

**Use** CML in chronic phase; radiosensitizing agent in the treatment of primary brain tumors, head and neck tumors, uterine cervix and nonsmall cell lung cancer, and psoriasis; treatment of hematologic conditions such as essential thrombocythemia, polycythemia vera, hypereosinophilia, and hyperleuko-cytosis due to acute leukemia. Has shown activity against renal cell cancer, melanoma, ovarian cancer, head and neck cancer (excluding lip cancer), and prostate cancer.

**Orphan drug:** Droxia™: Sickle cell anemia: Specifically for patients >18 years of age who have had at least three "painful crises" in the previous year - to reduce frequency of these crises and the need for blood transfusions

**Usual Dosage** Oral (refer to individual protocols): All dosage should be based on ideal or actual body weight, whichever is less:

Children:

No FDA-approved dosage regimens have been established; dosages of 1500-3000 mg/m$^2$ as a single dose in combination with other agents every 4-6 weeks have been used in the treatment of pediatric astrocytoma, medulloblastoma, and primitive neuroectodermal tumors

CML: Initial: 10-20 mg/kg/day once daily; adjust dose according to hematologic response

Adults: Dose should always be titrated to patient response and WBC counts; usual oral doses range from 10-30 mg/kg/day or 500-3000 mg/day; if WBC count falls to <2500 cells/mm$^3$, or the platelet count to <100,000/mm$^3$, therapy should be stopped for at least 3 days and resumed when values rise toward normal

Solid tumors:
Intermittent therapy: 80 mg/kg as a single dose every third day
Continuous therapy: 20-30 mg/kg/day given as a single dose/day
Concomitant therapy with irradiation: 80 mg/kg as a single dose every third day starting at least 7 days before initiation of irradiation
Resistant chronic myelocytic leukemia: Continuous therapy: 20-30 mg/kg as a single daily dose
Sickle cell anemia (moderate/severe disease): Initial: 15 mg/kg/day, increased by 5 mg/kg every 12 weeks if blood counts are in an acceptable range until the maximum tolerated dose of 35 mg/kg/day is achieved or the dose that does not produce toxic effects

*Acceptable range:*
Neutrophils ≥2500 cells/mm$^3$
Platelets ≥95,000/mm$^3$
Hemoglobin >5.3 g/dL, and
Reticulocytes ≥95,000/mm$^3$ if the hemoglobin concentration is <9 g/dL
*Toxic range:*
Neutrophils <2000 cells/mm$^3$
Platelets <80,000/mm$^3$
Hemoglobin <4.5 g/dL
Reticulocytes <80,000/mm$^3$ if the hemoglobin concentration is <9 g/dL
Monitor for toxicity every 2 weeks; if toxicity occurs, stop treatment until the bone marrow recovers; restart at 2.5 mg/kg/day less than the dose at which toxicity occurs; if no toxicity occurs over the next 12 weeks, then the subsequent dose should be increased by 2.5 mg/kg/day; reduced dosage of hydroxyurea alternating with erythropoietin may decrease myelotoxicity and increase levels of fetal hemoglobin in patients who have not been helped by hydroxyurea alone

**Dosage Forms**
Capsule: 500 mg
Droxia™: 200 mg, 300 mg, 400 mg
Hydrea®: 500 mg
Tablet (Mylocel™): 1000 mg

# hydroxyzine (hye DROKS i zeen)

**Sound-Alike/Look-Alike Issues**
hydrOXYzine may be confused with hydrALAZINE, hydroxyurea
Atarax® may be confused with amoxicillin, Ativan®
Vistaril® may be confused with Restoril®, Versed, Zestril®

**Synonyms** hydroxyzine hydrochloride; hydroxyzine pamoate

**Tall-Man** hydroOXYzine

**U.S./Canadian Brand Names** Apo-Hydroxyzine® [Can]; Atarax® [US/Can]; Novo-Hydroxyzin [Can]; PMS-Hydroxyzine [Can]; Vistaril® [US/Can]

**Therapeutic Category** Antiemetic; Antihistamine

**Use** Treatment of anxiety; preoperative sedative; antipruritic
(Continued)

## hydroxyzine *(Continued)*

### Usual Dosage
Children:
Preoperative sedation:
Oral: 0.6 mg/kg/dose every 6 hours
I.M.: 0.5-1.1 mg/kg/dose every 4-6 hours as needed
Manufacturer labeling: Pruritus, anxiety:
<6 years: 50 mg daily in divided doses
≥6 years: 50-100 mg daily in divided doses
Adults:
Antiemetic: I.M.: 25-100 mg/dose every 4-6 hours as needed
Anxiety: Oral: 25-100 mg 4 times/day; maximum dose: 600 mg/day
Preoperative sedation:
Oral: 50-100 mg
I.M.: 25-100 mg
Management of pruritus: Oral: 25 mg 3-4 times/day

### Dosage Forms [DSC] = Discontinued product
Capsule, as pamoate (Vistaril®): 25 mg, 50 mg, 100 mg
Injection, solution, as hydrochloride: 25 mg/mL (1 mL); 50 mg/mL (1 mL, 2 mL, 10 mL)
Suspension, oral, as pamoate (Vistaril®): 25 mg/5 mL (120 mL, 480 mL) [lemon flavor]
Syrup, as hydrochloride: 10 mg/5 mL (120 mL, 480 mL)
Atarax®: 10 mg/5 mL (480 mL) [contains alcohol, sodium benzoate; mint flavor] [DSC]
Tablet, as hydrochloride: 10 mg, 25 mg, 50 mg
Atarax®: 10 mg, 25 mg, 50 mg, 100 mg [DSC]

**hydroxyzine hydrochloride** *see* hydroxyzine *on previous page*

**hydroxyzine pamoate** *see* hydroxyzine *on previous page*

**HydroZone Plus [US-OTC]** *see* hydrocortisone (topical) *on page 417*

**Hygroton® *(Discontinued)*** *see* chlorthalidone *on page 179*

**Hylaform® [US]** *see* hyaluronate and derivatives *on page 406*

**Hylaform® Plus [US]** *see* hyaluronate and derivatives *on page 406*

**hylan polymers** *see* hyaluronate and derivatives *on page 406*

**Hylutin® [US]** *see* hydroxyprogesterone caproate *on page 422*

**hyoscine butylbromide** *see* scopolamine derivatives *on page 740*

**hyoscine hydrobromide** *see* scopolamine derivatives *on page 740*

## hyoscyamine *(hye oh SYE a meen)*

### Sound-Alike/Look-Alike Issues
Anaspaz® may be confused with Anaprox®, Antispas®
Levbid® may be confused with Lithobid®, Lopid®, Lorabid®
Levsinex® may be confused with Lanoxin®

**Synonyms** *l*-hyoscyamine sulfate; hyoscyamine sulfate

**U.S./Canadian Brand Names** Anaspaz® [US]; Cystospaz® [US/Can]; Hyosine [US]; Levbid® [US]; Levsin/SL® [US]; Levsinex® [US]; Levsin® [US/Can]; NuLev™ [US]; Symax SL [US]; Symax SR [US]

**Therapeutic Category** Anticholinergic Agent

### Use
Oral: Adjunctive therapy for peptic ulcers, irritable bowel, neurogenic bladder/bowel; treatment of infant colic, GI tract disorders caused by spasm; to reduce rigidity, tremors, sialorrhea, and hyperhidrosis associated with parkinsonism; as a drying agent in acute rhinitis

Injection: Preoperative antimuscarinic to reduce secretions and block cardiac vagal inhibitory reflexes; to improve radiologic visibility of the kidneys; symptomatic relief of biliary and renal colic; reduce GI motility to facilitate diagnostic procedures (ie, endoscopy, hypotonic duodenography); reduce pain and hypersecretion in pancreatitis, certain cases of partial heart block associated with vagal activity; reversal of neuromuscular blockade

## Usual Dosage

Oral: Children: Gastrointestinal disorders: Dose as listed, based on age and weight (kg) using 0.125 mg/mL drops; repeat dose every 4 hours as needed:

Children <2 years:

3.4 kg: 4 drops; maximum: 24 drops/24 hours

5 kg: 5 drops; maximum: 30 drops/24 hours

7 kg: 6 drops; maximum: 36 drops/24 hours

10 kg: 8 drops; maximum: 48 drops/24 hours

Oral, S.L.:

Children 2-12 years: Gastrointestinal disorders: Dose as listed, based on age and weight (kg); repeat dose every 4 hours as needed:

10 kg: 0.031-0.033 mg; maximum: 0.75 mg/24 hours

20 kg: 0.0625 mg; maximum: 0.75 mg/24 hours

40 kg: 0.0938 mg; maximum: 0.75 mg/24 hours

50 kg: 0.125 mg; maximum: 0.75 mg/24 hours

Children >12 years and Adults: Gastrointestinal disorders: 0.125-0.25 mg every 4 hours or as needed (before meals or food); maximum: 1.5 mg/24 hours

Cystospaz®: 0.15-0.3 mg up to 4 times/day

Oral (timed release): Children >12 years and Adults: Gastrointestinal disorders: 0.375-0.75 mg every 12 hours; maximum: 1.5 mg/24 hours

I.M., I.V., SubQ: Children >12 years and Adults: Gastrointestinal disorders: 0.25-0.5 mg; may repeat as needed up to 4 times/day, at 4-hour intervals

I.V.: Children >2 year and Adults: I.V.: Preanesthesia: 5 mcg/kg given 30-60 minutes prior to induction of anesthesia or at the time preoperative narcotics or sedatives are administered

I.V.: Adults: Diagnostic procedures: 0.25-0.5 mg given 5-10 minutes prior to procedure

To reduce drug-induced bradycardia during surgery: 0.125 mg; repeat as needed

To reverse neuromuscular blockade: 0.2 mg for every 1 mg neostigmine (or the physostigmine/pyridostigmine equivalent)

## Dosage Forms [DSC] = Discontinued product

Capsule, timed release, as sulfate (Cystospaz-M® [DSC], Levsinex®): 0.375 mg

Elixir, as sulfate: 0.125 mg/5 mL (480 mL)

Hyosine: 0.125 mg/5 mL (480 mL) [contains alcohol 20% and sodium benzoate; orange flavor]

Levsin®: 0.125 mg/5 mL (480 mL) [contains alcohol 20%; orange flavor]

Injection, solution, as sulfate (Levsin®): 0.5 mg/mL (1 mL)

Liquid, as sulfate (Spacol [DSC]): 0.125 mg/5 mL (120 mL) [sugar free, alcohol free, simethicone based, bubble gum flavor]

Solution, oral drops, as sulfate: 0.125 mg/mL (15 mL)

Hyosine: 0.125 mg/mL (15 mL) [contains alcohol 5% and sodium benzoate; orange flavor]

Levsin®: 0.125 mg/mL (15 mL) [contains alcohol 5%; orange flavor]

Tablet (Cystospaz®): 0.15 mg

Tablet, as sulfate (Anaspaz®, Levsin®, Spacol [DSC]): 0.125 mg

Tablet, extended release, as sulfate (Levbid®, Symax SR, Spacol T/S [DSC]): 0.375 mg

Tablet, orally-disintegrating, as sulfate (NuLev™): 0.125 mg [contains phenylalanine 1.7 mg/tablet, mint flavor]

Tablet, sublingual, as sulfate: 0.125 mg

Levsin/SL®: 0.125 mg [peppermint flavor]

Symax SL: 0.125 mg

# hyoscyamine, atropine, scopolamine, and phenobarbital

(hye oh SYE a meen, A troe peen, skoe POL a meen, & fee noe BAR bi tal)

## Sound-Alike/Look-Alike Issues

Donnatal® may be confused with Donnagel®

**Synonyms** atropine, hyoscyamine, scopolamine, and phenobarbital; belladonna alkaloids with phenobarbital; phenobarbital, hyoscyamine, atropine, and scopolamine; scopolamine, hyoscyamine, atropine, and phenobarbital

**U.S./Canadian Brand Names** Donnatal Extentabs® [US]; Donnatal® [US]

**Therapeutic Category** Anticholinergic Agent

**Use** Adjunct in treatment of irritable bowel syndrome, acute enterocolitis, duodenal ulcer

**Usual Dosage** Oral:

Children: Donnatal® elixir: To be given every 4-6 hours; initial dose based on weight:

4.5 kg: 0.5 mL every 4 hours **or** 0.75 mL every 6 hours

10 kg: 1 mL every 4 hours **or** 1.5 mL every 6 hours

(Continued)

## hyoscyamine, atropine, scopolamine, and phenobarbital *(Continued)*

14 kg: 1.5 mL every 4 hours **or** 2 mL every 6 hours
23 kg: 2.5 mL every 4 hours **or** 3.8 mL every 6 hours
34 kg: 3.8 mL every 4 hours **or** 5 mL every 6 hours
≥45 kg: 5 mL every 4 hours **or** 7.5 mL every 6 hours
Adults:
Donnatal®: 1-2 tablets or 5-10 mL of elixir 3-4 times/day
Donnatal Extentabs®: 1 tablet every 12 hours; may increase to 1 tablet every 8 hours if needed
**Dosage Forms**
Elixir (Donnatal®): Hyoscyamine sulfate 0.1037 mg, atropine sulfate 0.0194 mg, scopolamine hydrobromide 0.0065 mg, and phenobarbital 16.2 mg per 5 mL (120 mL, 480 mL) [contains alcohol 95%; grape flavor]
Tablet (Donnatal®): Hyoscyamine sulfate 0.1037 mg, atropine sulfate 0.0194 mg, scopolamine hydrobromide 0.0065 mg, and phenobarbital 16.2 mg
Tablet, extended release (Donnatal Extentabs®): Hyoscyamine sulfate 0.3111 mg, atropine sulfate 0.0582 mg, scopolamine hydrobromide 0.0195 mg, and phenobarbital 48.6 mg

**hyoscyamine sulfate** *see* hyoscyamine *on page 424*

**Hyosine [US]** *see* hyoscyamine *on page 424*

**Hy-Pam® Oral *(Discontinued)*** *see* hydroxyzine *on page 423*

**Hypaque-Cysto® [US]** *see* radiological/contrast media (ionic) *on page 707*

**Hypaque® Meglumine [US]** *see* radiological/contrast media (ionic) *on page 707*

**Hypaque® Sodium [US]** *see* radiological/contrast media (ionic) *on page 707*

**Hyperab® *(Discontinued)*** *see* rabies immune globulin (human) *on page 707*

**Hyperstat® [US]** *see* diazoxide *on page 242*

**Hyper-Tet® *(Discontinued)*** *see* tetanus immune globulin (human) *on page 790*

**Hyphed [US]** *see* pseudoephedrine, hydrocodone, and chlorpheniramine *on page 695*

**Hy-Phen® *(Discontinued)*** *see* hydrocodone and acetaminophen *on page 411*

**HypoTears [US-OTC]** *see* artificial tears *on page 71*

**HypoTears PF [US-OTC]** *see* artificial tears *on page 71*

**HypRho®-D *(Discontinued)***

**HypRho®-D Mini-Dose *(Discontinued)***

**Hyprogest® 250 *(Discontinued)***

**hypromellose** *see* hydroxypropyl methylcellulose *on page 422*

**Hytakerol® [US/Can]** *see* dihydrotachysterol *on page 250*

**Hytinic® [US-OTC]** *see* polysaccharide-iron complex *on page 660*

**Hytone® [US]** *see* hydrocortisone (topical) *on page 417*

**Hytrin® [US/Can]** *see* terazosin *on page 786*

**Hyzaar® [US/Can]** *see* losartan and hydrochlorothiazide *on page 493*

**Hyzaar® DS [Can]** *see* losartan and hydrochlorothiazide *on page 493*

**Hyzine® *(Discontinued)*** *see* hydroxyzine *on page 423*

## ibandronate *(eye BAN droh nate)*
**Synonyms** ibandronate sodium
**U.S./Canadian Brand Names** Bondronat® [Can]; Boniva® [US]
**Therapeutic Category** Bisphosphonate Derivative
**Use** Treatment and prevention of osteoporosis in postmenopausal females
**Usual Dosage** Oral: Adults:
Treatment of postmenopausal osteoporosis: 2.5 mg/day or 150 mg once a month
Prevention of postmenopausal osteoporosis: 2.5 mg/day; 150 mg once a month may be considered
**Dosage Forms** Tablet: 2.5 mg [once-daily formulation]; 150 mg [once-monthly formulation]

**131 I anti-B1 antibody** *see* tositumomab and iodine I 131 tositumomab *on page 812*

**131 I-anti-B1 monoclonal antibody** *see* tositumomab and iodine I 131 tositumomab *on page 812*

**ibandronate sodium** *see* ibandronate *on this page*

**Iberet® [US-OTC]** *see* vitamins (multiple/oral) *on page 852*

**Iberet®-500 [US-OTC]** *see* vitamins (multiple/oral) *on page 852*

**ibidomide hydrochloride** *see* labetalol *on page 460*

## ibritumomab (ib ri TYOO mo mab)

**Synonyms** ibritumomab tiuxetan; In-111 zevalin; Y-90 zevalin

**U.S./Canadian Brand Names** Zevalin™ [US]

**Therapeutic Category** Antineoplastic Agent, Monoclonal Antibody;  Radiopharmaceutical

**Use** Treatment of relapsed or refractory low-grade, follicular, or transformed B-cell non-Hodgkin lymphoma (including rituximab-refractory follicular non-Hodgkin lymphoma) as part of a therapeutic regimen with rituximab (Zevalin™ therapeutic regimen); **not to be used as single-agent therapy**; must be radiolabeled prior to use

**Usual Dosage** I.V.: Adults: Ibritumomab is administered **only** as part of the Zevalin™ therapeutic regimen (a combined treatment regimen with rituximab). The regimen consists of two steps:

**Step 1:**
Rituximab infusion: 250 mg/m$^2$ at an initial rate of 50 mg/hour. If hypersensitivity or infusion-related events do not occur, increase infusion in increments of 50 mg/hour every 30 minutes, to a maximum of 400 mg/hour. Infusions should be temporarily slowed or interrupted if hypersensitivity or infusion-related events occur. The infusion may be resumed at one-half the previous rate upon improvement of symptoms.

In-111 ibritumomab infusion: Within 4 hours of the completion of rituximab infusion, inject 5 mCi (1.6 mg total antibody dose) over 10 minutes.

Biodistribution of In-111 ibritumomab should be assessed by imaging at 2-24 hours and at 48-72 hours postinjection. An optional third imaging may be performed 90-120 hours following injection. If biodistribution is not acceptable, the patient should not proceed to Step 2.

**Step 2 (initiated 7-9 days following Step 1):**
Rituximab infusion: 250 mg/m$^2$ at an initial rate of 100 mg/hour (50 mg/hour if infusion-related events occurred with the first infusion). If hypersensitivity or infusion-related events do not occur, increase infusion in increments of 100 mg/hour every 30 minutes, to a maximum of 400 mg/hour, as tolerated.

Y-90 ibritumomab infusion: Within 4 hours of the completion of rituximab infusion:
Platelet count >150,000 cells/mm$^3$: Inject 0.4 mCi/kg (14.8 MBq/kg actual body weight) over 10 minutes

Platelet count between 100,000-149,000 cells/mm$^3$: Inject 0.3 mCi/kg (11.1 MBq/kg actual body weight) over 10 minutes

Platelet count <100,000 cells/mm$^3$: Do **not** administer

**Maximum dose:** The prescribed, measured, and administered dose of Y-90 ibritumomab must not exceed 32 mCi (1184 MBq), regardless of the patient's body weight

**Dosage Forms** Each kit contains 4 vials for preparation of either In-111 or Y-90 conjugate (as indicated on container label)

Injection, solution: 1.6 mg/mL (2 mL) [supplied with sodium acetate solution, formulation buffer vial (includes albumin 750 mg), and an empty reaction vial]

**ibritumomab tiuxetan** *see* ibritumomab *on this page*

**Ibu-200 [US-OTC]** *see* ibuprofen *on this page*

**Ibuprin® *(Discontinued)*** *see* ibuprofen *on this page*

## ibuprofen (eye byoo PROE fen)

**Sound-Alike/Look-Alike Issues**
Haltran® may be confused with Halfprin®

**Synonyms** p-isobutylhydratropic acid

**U.S./Canadian Brand Names** Advil® Children's [US-OTC]; Advil® Infants' [US-OTC]; Advil® Junior [US-OTC]; Advil® Migraine [US-OTC]; Advil® [US-OTC/Can]; Apo-Ibuprofen® [Can]; ElixSure™ IB [US-OTC]; Genpril® [US-OTC]; I-Prin [US-OTC]; Ibu-200 [US-OTC]; Midol® Cramp and Body Aches [US-OTC]; Motrin® Children's [US-OTC/Can]; Motrin® IB [US-OTC/Can]; Motrin® Infants' [US-OTC]; Motrin® Junior Strength [US-OTC]; Motrin® [US]; Novo-Profen [Can]; Nu-Ibuprofen [Can]; Proprinal [US-OTC]; Ultraprin [US-OTC]

**Therapeutic Category** Analgesic, Nonnarcotic;  Antipyretic;  Nonsteroidal Antiinflammatory Drug (NSAID)

**Use** Inflammatory diseases and rheumatoid disorders including juvenile rheumatoid arthritis, mild to moderate pain, fever, dysmenorrhea

(Continued)

# ibuprofen *(Continued)*

**Usual Dosage** Oral:

Children:

Antipyretic: 6 months to 12 years: Temperature <102.5°F (39°C): 5 mg/kg/dose; temperature >102.5°F: 10 mg/kg/dose given every 6-8 hours (maximum daily dose: 40 mg/kg/day)

Juvenile rheumatoid arthritis: 30-50 mg/kg/24 hours divided every 8 hours; start at lower end of dosing range and titrate upward (maximum: 2.4 g/day)

Analgesic: 4-10 mg/kg/dose every 6-8 hours

OTC labeling (analgesic, antipyretic):

Children 6 months to 11 years: Use of weight to select dose is preferred; doses may be repeated every 6-8 hours (maximum: 4 doses/day) :

Weight 12-17 lbs (6-11 months of age): 50 mg

Weight 18-23 lbs (12-23 months of age): 75 mg

Weight 24-35 lbs (2-3 years of age): 100 mg

Weight 35-47 lbs (4-5 years of age): 150 mg

Weight 48-59 lbs (6-8 years of age): 200 mg

Weight 60-71 lbs (9-10 years of age): 250 mg

Weight 72-95 lbs (11 years of age): 300 mg

Children ≥12 years: 200 mg every 4-6 hours as needed (maximum: 1200 mg/24 hours)

Adults:

Inflammatory disease: 400-800 mg/dose 3-4 times/day (maximum dose: 3.2 g/day)

Analgesia/pain/fever/dysmenorrhea: 200-400 mg/dose every 4-6 hours (maximum daily dose: 1.2 g, unless directed by physician)

OTC labeling (analgesic, antipyretic): 200 mg every 4-6 hours as needed (maximum: 1200 mg/24 hours)

**Dosage Forms** [DSC] = Discontinued product

Caplet: 200 mg [OTC]

Advil®: 200 mg [contains sodium benzoate]

Ibu-200, Menadol® [DSC], Motrin® IB: 200 mg

Motrin® Junior Strength: 100 mg

Capsule, liqui-gel:

Advil®: 200 mg

Advil® Migraine: 200 mg [solubilized ibuprofen; contains potassium 20 mg]

Gelcap:

Advil®: 200 mg [contains coconut oil]

Motrin® IB: 200 mg [contains benzyl alcohol]

Suspension, oral: 100 mg/5 mL (5 mL, 120 mL, 480 mL)

Advil® Children's: 100 mg/5 mL (60 mL, 120 mL) [contains sodium benzoate; blue raspberry, fruit, and grape flavors]

ElixSure™ IB: 100 mg/5 mL (120 mL) [berry flavor]

Motrin® Children's: 100 mg/5 mL (60 mL, 120 mL) [contains sodium benzoate; berry, dye free berry, bubble gum, and grape flavors]

Suspension, oral drops: 40 mg/mL (15 mL)

Advil® Infants': 40 mg/mL (15 mL) [contains sodium benzoate; fruit and grape flavors]

Motrin® Infants': 40 mg/mL (15 mL, 30 mL) [contains sodium benzoate; berry and dye-free berry flavors]

Tablet: 200 mg [OTC], 400 mg, 600 mg, 800 mg

Advil®: 200 mg [contains sodium benzoate]

Advil® Junior: 100 mg [contains sodium benzoate; coated tablets]

Genpril®, I-Prin, Midol® Cramp and Body Aches, Motrin® IB, Proprinal, Ultraprin: 200 mg

Motrin®: 400 mg, 600 mg, 800 mg

Tablet, chewable:

Advil® Children's: 50 mg [contains phenylalanine 2.1 mg; grape flavors]

Advil® Junior: 100 mg [contains phenylalanine 4.2 mg; grape flavors]

Motrin® Children's: 50 mg [contains phenylalanine 1.4 mg; grape and orange flavor]

Motrin® Junior Strength: 100 mg [contains phenylalanine 2.1 mg; grape and orange flavors]

**ibuprofen and hydrocodone** *see* hydrocodone and ibuprofen *on page 413*

**ibuprofen and pseudoephedrine** *see* pseudoephedrine and ibuprofen *on page 694*

## ibutilide (i BYOO ti lide)

**Synonyms** ibutilide fumarate

**U.S./Canadian Brand Names** Corvert® [US]

**Therapeutic Category** Antiarrhythmic Agent, Class III

**Use** Acute termination of atrial fibrillation or flutter of recent onset; the effectiveness of ibutilide has not been determined in patients with arrhythmias >90 days in duration

**Usual Dosage** I.V.: Initial: Adults:
<60 kg: 0.01 mg/kg over 10 minutes
≥60 kg: 1 mg over 10 minutes
If the arrhythmia does not terminate within 10 minutes after the end of the initial infusion, a second infusion of equal strength may be infused over a 10-minute period

**Dosage Forms** Injection, solution, as fumarate: 0.1 mg/mL (10 mL)

**ibutilide fumarate** *see* ibutilide *on this page*

**IC-Green® [US]** *see* indocyanine green *on page 435*

**ICI-182,780** *see* fulvestrant *on page 363*

**ICI-204,219** *see* zafirlukast *on page 857*

**ICI-118630** *see* goserelin *on page 381*

**ICI-176334** *see* bicalutamide *on page 106*

**ICI-46474** *see* tamoxifen *on page 780*

**ICI-D1033** *see* anastrozole *on page 53*

**ICI-D1694** *see* raltitrexed *(Canada only)* *on page 710*

**ICRF-187** *see* dexrazoxane *on page 236*

**Idamycin® [Can]** *see* idarubicin *on this page*

**Idamycin® (Discontinued)** *see* idarubicin *on this page*

**Idamycin PFS® [US]** *see* idarubicin *on this page*

**Idarac® [Can]** *see* floctafenine *(Canada only)* *on page 341*

## idarubicin (eye da ROO bi sin)

**Sound-Alike/Look-Alike Issues**
idarubicin may be confused with DOXOrubicin, DAUNOrubicin
Idamycin PFS® may be confused with Adriamycin

**Synonyms** 4-demethoxydaunorubicin; 4-DMDR; idarubicin hydrochloride; IDR; IMI 30; NSC-256439; SC 33428

**U.S./Canadian Brand Names** Idamycin PFS® [US]; Idamycin® [Can]

**Therapeutic Category** Antineoplastic Agent

**Use** Treatment of acute leukemias (AML, ANLL, ALL), accelerated phase or blast crisis of chronic myelogenous leukemia (CML), breast cancer

**Usual Dosage** Refer to individual protocols. I.V.:
Children:
Leukemia: 10-12 mg/m$^2$/day for 3 days every 3 weeks
Solid tumors: 5 mg/m$^2$/day for 3 days every 3 weeks
Adults:
Leukemia induction: 12 mg/m$^2$/day for 3 days
Leukemia consolidation: 10-12 mg/m$^2$/day for 2 days

**Dosage Forms** Injection, solution, as hydrochloride [preservative free] (Idamycin PFS®): 1 mg/mL (5 mL, 10 mL, 20 mL)

**idarubicin hydrochloride** *see* idarubicin *on this page*

**IDEC-C2B8** *see* rituximab *on page 726*

**IDR** *see* idarubicin *on this page*

**Ifex® [US/Can]** *see* ifosfamide *on next page*

**IFLrA** *see* interferon alfa-2a *on page 440*

## ifosfamide (eye FOSS fa mide)
**Sound-Alike/Look-Alike Issues**
ifosfamide may be confused with cyclophosphamide
**Synonyms** isophosphamide; NSC-109724; Z4942
**U.S./Canadian Brand Names** Ifex® [US/Can]
**Therapeutic Category** Antineoplastic Agent
**Use** Treatment of lung cancer, Hodgkin's and non-Hodgkin's lymphoma, breast cancer, acute and chronic lymphocytic leukemias, ovarian cancer, sarcomas, pancreatic and gastric carcinomas
**Orphan drug:** Treatment of testicular cancer
**Usual Dosage** Refer to individual protocols. To prevent bladder toxicity, ifosfamide should be given with the urinary protector mesna and hydration of at least 2 L of oral or I.V. fluid per day. I.V.:
Children:
1200-1800 mg/m$^2$/day for 3-5 days every 21-28 days **or**
5 g/m$^2$ once every 21-28 days **or**
3 g/m$^2$/day for 2 days every 21-28 days
Adults:
50 mg/kg/day or 700-2000 mg/m$^2$ for 5 days every 3-4 weeks
Alternatives: 2400 mg/m$^2$/day for 3 days or 5000 mg/m$^2$ as a single dose every 3-4 weeks
**Dosage Forms**
Injection, powder for reconstitution: 1 g
Ifex®: 1 g, 3 g

**IG** *see* immune globulin (intramuscular) *on page 432*

**IGIM** *see* immune globulin (intramuscular) *on page 432*

**IL-1Ra** *see* anakinra *on page 52*

**IL-2** *see* aldesleukin *on page 25*

**IL-11** *see* oprelvekin *on page 601*

**Iletin® II Pork [Can]** *see* insulin preparations *on page 438*

**Ilopan-Choline® Oral *(Discontinued)*** *see* dexpanthenol *on page 235*

**Ilopan® Injection *(Discontinued)*** *see* dexpanthenol *on page 235*

**Ilosone® Pulvules® *(Discontinued)***

**Ilozyme® *(Discontinued)*** *see* pancrelipase *on page 615*

## imatinib (eye MAT eh nib)
**Synonyms** CGP 57148B; glivec; imatinib mesylate; STI571
**U.S./Canadian Brand Names** Gleevec® [US/Can]
**Therapeutic Category** Antineoplastic, Tyrosine Kinase Inhibitor
**Use** Treatment of adult patients with Philadelphia chromosome-positive (Ph+) chronic myeloid leukemia (CML); treatment of pediatric patients with Ph+ CML (chronic phase) recurring following stem cell transplant or who are resistant to interferon-alpha therapy; treatment of Kit-positive (CD117) unresectable and/or (metastatic) malignant gastrointestinal stromal tumors (GIST)
**Usual Dosage** Oral:
Children ≥3 years: CML (chronic phase): 260 mg/m$^2$/day; may be increased to 340 mg/m$^2$/day
Adults:
CML:
Chronic phase: 400 mg once daily; may be increased to 600 mg daily
Accelerated phase or blast crisis: 600 mg once daily; may be increased to 800 mg daily (400 mg twice daily)
Gastrointestinal stromal tumors: 400-600 mg/day
**Note:** Dosage should be increased by at least 50% when used concurrently with a potent enzyme-inducing agent (ie, rifampin, phenytoin).
**Dosage Forms** Tablet: 100 mg; 400 mg

**imatinib mesylate** *see* imatinib *on this page*

**IMC-C225** *see* cetuximab *on page 163*

**Imdur® [US/Can]** *see* isosorbide mononitrate *on page 452*

**IMI 30** *see* idarubicin *on previous page*

**imidazole carboxamide** *see* dacarbazine *on page 220*

**imidazole carboxamide dimethyltriazene** *see* dacarbazine *on page 220*

# imiglucerase (i mi GLOO ser ace)
**Sound-Alike/Look-Alike Issues**
 Cerezyme® may be confused with Cerebyx®, Ceredase®
**U.S./Canadian Brand Names** Cerezyme® [US/Can]
**Therapeutic Category** Enzyme
**Use** Long-term enzyme replacement therapy for patients with Type 1 Gaucher disease
**Usual Dosage** I.V.: Children ≥2 years and Adults: Initial: 30-60 units/kg every 2 weeks; dosing is individualized based on disease severity. Dosing range: 2.5 units/kg 3 times/week up to as much as 60 units/kg administered as frequently as once a week or as infrequently as every 4 weeks. Average dose: 60 units/kg administered every 2 weeks
**Dosage Forms** Injection, powder for reconstitution [preservative free]: 200 units, 400 units

**imipemide** *see* imipenem and cilastatin *on this page*

# imipenem and cilastatin (i mi PEN em & sye la STAT in)
**Sound-Alike/Look-Alike Issues**
 Primaxin® may be confused with Premarin®, Primacor®
**Synonyms** imipemide
**U.S./Canadian Brand Names** Primaxin® [US/Can]
**Therapeutic Category** Carbapenem (Antibiotic)
**Use** Treatment of respiratory tract, urinary tract, intra-abdominal, gynecologic, bone and joint, skin structure, and polymicrobic infections as well as bacterial septicemia and endocarditis. Antibacterial activity includes resistant gram-negative bacilli (*Pseudomonas aeruginosa* and *Enterobacter* sp), gram-positive bacteria (methicillin-sensitive *Staphylococcus aureus* and *Streptococcus* sp) and anaerobes.
 **Note:** I.M. administration is not intended for severe or life-threatening infections (eg, septicemia, endocarditis, shock)
**Usual Dosage** Dosage based on **imipenem** content:
Neonates: Non-CNS infections: I.V.:
 <1 week: 25 mg/kg every 12 hours
 1-4 weeks: 25 mg/kg every 8 hours
 4 weeks to 3 months: 25 mg/kg every 6 hours
Children: >3 months: Non-CNS infections: I.V.: 15-25 mg/kg every 6 hours
 Maximum dosage: Susceptible infections: 2 g/day; moderately susceptible organisms: 4 g/day
Children: Cystic fibrosis: I.V.: Doses up to 90 mg/kg/day have been used
Adults:
 Moderate infections:
 I.M.: 750 mg every 12 hours
 I.V.:
 Fully-susceptible organisms: 500 mg every 6-8 hours (1.5-2 g/day)
 Moderately-susceptible organisms: 500 mg every 6 hours or 1 g every 8 hours (2-3 g/day)
 Severe infections: I.V.: **Note:** I.M. administration is not intended for severe or life-threatening infections (eg, septicemia, endocarditis, shock):
 Fully-susceptible organisms: 500 mg every 6 hours (2 g/day)
 Moderately-susceptible organisms: 1 g every 6-8 hours (3-4 g/day)
 Maximum daily dose should not exceed 50 mg/kg or 4 g/day, whichever is lower
 Urinary tract infection, uncomplicated: I.V.: 250 mg every 6 hours (1 g/day)
 Urinary tract infection, complicated: I.V.: 500 mg every 6 hours (2 g/day)
 Mild infections: **Note:** Rarely a suitable option in mild infections; normally reserved for moderate-severe cases:
 I.M.: 500 mg every 12 hours; intra-abdominal infections: 750 mg every 12 hours
 I.V.:
 Fully-susceptible organisms: 250 mg every 6 hours (1g/day)
 Moderately-susceptible organisms: 500 mg every 6 hours (2 g/day)
**Dosage Forms**
 Injection, powder for reconstitution [I.M.]: Imipenem 500 mg and cilastatin 500 mg [contains sodium 32 mg (1.4 mEq)]
 Injection, powder for reconstitution [I.V.]: Imipenem 250 mg and cilastatin 250 mg [contains sodium 18.8 mg (0.8 mEq)]; imipenem 500 mg and cilastatin 500 mg [contains sodium 37.5 mg (1.6 mEq)]

# imipramine (im IP ra meen)

**Sound-Alike/Look-Alike Issues**
imipramine may be confused with amitriptyline, desipramine, Norpramin®

**Synonyms** imipramine hydrochloride; imipramine pamoate

**U.S./Canadian Brand Names** Apo-Imipramine® [Can]; Novo-Pramine [Can]; Tofranil-PM® [US]; Tofranil® [US/Can]

**Therapeutic Category** Antidepressant, Tricyclic (Tertiary Amine)

**Use** Treatment of depression; treatment of nocturnal enuresis in children

**Usual Dosage** Oral:
Children: Enuresis: ≥6 years: Initial: 25 mg at bedtime, if inadequate response still seen after 1 week of therapy, increase by 25 mg/day; dose should not exceed 2.5 mg/kg/day or 50 mg at bedtime if 6-12 years of age or 75 mg at bedtime if ≥12 years of age

Adolescents: Depression: Initial: 30-40 mg/day; increase gradually; maximum: 100 mg/day in single or divided doses

Adults: Depression: Initial: 25 mg 3-4 times/day, increase dose gradually, total dose may be given at bedtime; maximum: 300 mg/day

**Dosage Forms**
Capsule, as pamoate (Tofranil-PM®): 75 mg, 100 mg, 125 mg, 150 mg
Tablet, as hydrochloride (Tofranil®): 10 mg, 25 mg, 50 mg [generic tablets may contain sodium benzoate]

**imipramine hydrochloride** *see* imipramine *on this page*

**imipramine pamoate** *see* imipramine *on this page*

# imiquimod (i mi KWI mod)

**Sound-Alike/Look-Alike Issues**
Aldara™ may be confused with Alora®

**U.S./Canadian Brand Names** Aldara™ [US/Can]

**Therapeutic Category** Immune Response Modifier

**Use** Treatment of external genital and perianal warts/condyloma acuminata; nonhyperkeratotic, nonhypertrophic actinic keratosis on face or scalp; superficial basal cell carcinoma (sBCC) with a maximum tumor diameter of 2 cm located on the trunk, neck, or extremities (excluding hands or feet)

**Usual Dosage** Topical:
Children ≥12 years and Adults: Perianal warts/condyloma acuminata: Apply 3 times/week prior to bedtime and leave on skin for 6-10 hours. Remove with mild soap and water. Examples of 3 times/week application schedules are: Monday, Wednesday, Friday; or Tuesday, Thursday, Saturday. Continue imiquimod treatment until there is total clearance of the genital/perianal warts for ≤16 weeks. A rest period of several days may be taken if required by the patient's discomfort or severity of the local skin reaction. Treatment may resume once the reaction subsides.
Adults:
Actinic keratosis: Apply twice weekly for 16 weeks to a treatment area on face or scalp; apply prior to bedtime and leave on skin for 8 hours. Remove with mild soap and water.
Common oral worts (dental use): Apply once daily prior to bedtime
Superficial basal cell carcinoma: Apply once daily prior to bedtime, 5 days/week for 6 weeks. Treatment area should include a 1 cm margin of skin around the tumor. Leave on skin for 8 hours.

**Dosage Forms** Cream: 5% (12s) [contains benzyl alcohol; single-dose packets]

**Imitrex® [US]** *see* sumatriptan succinate *on page 776*

**Imitrex® DF [Can]** *see* sumatriptan succinate *on page 776*

**ImmuCyst® [Can]** *see* BCG vaccine *on page 90*

# immune globulin (intramuscular) (i MYUN GLOB yoo lin, IN tra MUS kyoo ler)

**Synonyms** gamma globulin; IG; IGIM; immune serum globulin; ISG

**U.S./Canadian Brand Names** BayGam® [US/Can]

**Therapeutic Category** Immune Globulin

**Use** Household and sexual contacts of persons with hepatitis A, measles, varicella, and possibly rubella; travelers to high-risk areas outside tourist routes; staff, attendees, and parents of diapered attendees in day-care center outbreaks

For travelers, IG is not an alternative to careful selection of foods and water; immune globulin can interfere with the antibody response to parenterally administered live virus vaccines. Frequent travelers should be tested for hepatitis A antibody, immune hemolytic anemia, and neutropenia (with ITP, I.V. route is usually used).

**Usual Dosage** I.M.:

Hepatitis A:

Pre-exposure prophylaxis upon travel into endemic areas (hepatitis A vaccine preferred):

0.02 mL/kg for anticipated risk 1-3 months

0.06 mL/kg for anticipated risk >3 months

Repeat approximate dose every 4-6 months if exposure continues

Postexposure prophylaxis: 0.02 mL/kg given within 7 days of exposure

Measles:

Prophylaxis: 0.25 mL/kg/dose (maximum dose: 15 mL) given within 6 days of exposure followed by live attenuated measles vaccine in 3 months or at 15 months of age (whichever is later)

For patients with leukemia, lymphoma, immunodeficiency disorders, generalized malignancy, or receiving immunosuppressive therapy: 0.5 mL/kg (maximum dose: 15 mL)

Poliomyelitis: Prophylaxis: 0.3 mL/kg/dose as a single dose

Rubella: Prophylaxis: 0.55 mL/kg/dose within 72 hours of exposure

Varicella: Prophylaxis: 0.6-1.2 mL/kg (varicella zoster immune globulin preferred) within 72 hours of exposure

IgG deficiency: 1.3 mL/kg, then 0.66 ml /kg in 3-4 weeks

Hepatitis B: Prophylaxis: 0.06 mL/kg/dose (HBIG preferred)

**Dosage Forms** Injection, solution [preservative free]: 15% to 18% (2 mL, 10 mL)

# immune globulin (intravenous) (i MYUN GLOB yoo lin, IN tra VEE nus)

## Sound-Alike/Look-Alike Issues

Gamimune® N may be confused with CytoGam®

## Synonyms IVIG

**U.S./Canadian Brand Names** Carimune™ NF [US]; Gamimune® N [US/Can]; Gammagard® Liquid [US]; Gammagard® S/D [US/Can]; Gammar®-P I.V. [US]; Gamunex® [US/Can]; Iveegam EN [US]; Iveegam Immuno® [Can]; Octagam® [US]; Panglobulin® NF [US]; Polygam® S/D [US]

**Therapeutic Category** Immune Globulin

## Use

Treatment of primary immunodeficiency syndromes (congenital agammaglobulinemia, severe combined immunodeficiency syndromes [SCIDS], common variable immunodeficiency, X-linked immunodeficiency, Wiskott-Aldrich syndrome); idiopathic thrombocytopenic purpura (ITP); Kawasaki disease (in combination with aspirin)

Prevention of bacterial infection in B-cell chronic lymphocytic leukemia (CLL); pediatric HIV infection; bone marrow transplant (BMT)

**Usual Dosage** Approved doses and regimens may vary between brands; check manufacturer guidelines. **Note:** Some clinicians dose IVIG on ideal body weight or an adjusted ideal body weight in morbidly obese patients. The volume of distribution of IVIG preparations in healthy subjects is similar to that observed with endogenous IgG. IVIG remains primarily in the intravascular space. Patients with congenital humoral immunodeficiencies appear to have about 70% of the IVIG available in the intravascular space.

Children: I.V.: Pediatric HIV: 400 mg/kg every 28 days

Children and Adults: I.V.:

Primary immunodeficiency disorders: 200-400 mg/kg every 4 weeks or as per monitored serum IgG concentrations

Gammagard® Liquid, Gamunex®, Octagam®: 300-600 mg/kg every 3-4 weeks; adjusted based on dosage and interval in conjunction with monitored serum IgG concentrations.

B-cell chronic lymphocytic leukemia (CLL): 400 mg/kg/dose every 3 weeks

Idiopathic thrombocytopenic purpura (ITP):

Acute: 400 mg/kg/day for 5 days or 1000 mg/kg/day for 1-2 days

Chronic: 400 mg/kg as needed to maintain platelet count >30,000/mm$^3$; may increase dose to 800 mg/kg (1000 mg/kg if needed)

Kawasaki disease: Initiate therapy within 10 days of disease onset: 2 g/kg as a single dose administered over 10 hours, or 400 mg/kg/day for 4 days. **Note:** Must be used in combination with aspirin: 80-100 mg/kg/day in 4 divided doses for 14 days, when fever subsides, dose aspirin at 3-5 mg/kg once daily for ≥6-8 weeks

Bone marrow transplant: 500 mg/kg beginning on days 7 and 2 pretransplant, then 500 mg/kg/week for 90 days post-transplant

(Continued)

# immune globulin (intravenous) *(Continued)*

### Dosage Forms

Injection, powder for reconstitution [preservative free]:
Gammar®-P I.V.: 5 g, 10 g [stabilized with human albumin and sucrose]
Iveegam EN: 5 g [stabilized with glucose]
Injection, powder for reconstitution [preservative free, nanofiltered]:
Carimune™ NF: 3 g, 6 g, 12 g [contains sucrose]
Panglobulin® NF: 6 g, 12 g [contains sucrose]
Injection, powder for reconstitution [preservative free, solvent detergent treated]
Gammagard® S/D: 2.5 g, 5 g, 10 g [stabilized with human albumin, glycine, glucose, and polyethylene glycol]
Polygam® S/D: 5 g, 10 g [stabilized with human albumin, glycine, glucose, and polyethylene glycol]
Injection, solution [preservative free; solvent detergent-treated]:
Gammagard® Liquid: 10% [100 mg/mL] (10 mL, 25 mL, 50 mL, 100 mL, 200 mL) [latex free, sucrose free; stabilized with glycine]
Octagam®: 5% [50 mg/mL] (20 mL, 50 mL, 100 mL, 200 mL) [sucrose free; contains sodium 30 mmol/L and maltose]
Injection, solution [preservative free] (Gamunex®): 10% (10 mL, 25 mL, 50 mL, 100 mL, 200 mL) [caprylate/chromatography purified]

**immune serum globulin** *see* immune globulin (intramuscular) *on page 432*

**Immunine® VH [Can]** *see* factor IX *on page 325*

**Imodium® [Can]** *see* loperamide *on page 489*

**Imodium® A-D [US-OTC]** *see* loperamide *on page 489*

**Imogam® Rabies-HT [US]** *see* rabies immune globulin (human) *on page 707*

**Imogam® Rabies Pasteurized [Can]** *see* rabies immune globulin (human) *on page 707*

**Imovane® [Can]** *see* zopiclone *(Canada only) on page 864*

**Imovax® Rabies [US/Can]** *see* rabies virus vaccine *on page 707*

**Imuran® [US/Can]** *see* azathioprine *on page 83*

**In-111 zevalin** *see* ibritumomab *on page 427*

# inamrinone *(eye NAM ri none)*

**Sound-Alike/Look-Alike Issues**
amrinone may be confused with amiloride, amiodarone
**Synonyms** amrinone lactate
**Therapeutic Category** Adrenergic Agonist Agent
**Use** Infrequently used as a last resort, short-term therapy in patients with intractable heart failure
**Usual Dosage** Dosage is based on clinical response (**Note:** Dose should not exceed 10 mg/kg/24 hours).
Infants, Children, and Adults: 0.75 mg/kg I.V. bolus over 2-3 minutes followed by maintenance infusion of 5-10 mcg/kg/minute; I.V. bolus may need to be repeated in 30 minutes.
**Dosage Forms** Injection, solution, as lactate: 5 mg/mL (20 mL) [contains sodium metabisulfite]

**I-Naphline® Ophthalmic *(Discontinued)*** *see* naphazoline *on page 561*

**Inapsine® [US]** *see* droperidol *on page 274*

# indapamide *(in DAP a mide)*

**Sound-Alike/Look-Alike Issues**
indapamide may be confused with Iopidine®
**U.S./Canadian Brand Names** Apo-Indapamide® [Can]; Gen-Indapamide [Can]; Lozide® [Can]; Lozol® [US/Can]; Novo-Indapamide [Can]; Nu-Indapamide [Can]; PMS-Indapamide [Can]
**Therapeutic Category** Diuretic, Miscellaneous
**Use** Management of mild to moderate hypertension; treatment of edema in congestive heart failure and nephrotic syndrome
**Usual Dosage** Adults: Oral:
Edema: 2.5-5 mg/day. **Note:** There is little therapeutic benefit to increasing the dose >5 mg/day; there is, however, an increased risk of electrolyte disturbances

Hypertension: 1.25 mg in the morning, may increase to 5 mg/day by increments of 1.25-2.5 mg; consider adding another antihypertensive and decreasing the dose if response is not adequate

**Dosage Forms**
Tablet: 1.25 mg, 2.5 mg
Lozol®: 1.25 mg

**Inderal® [US/Can]** *see propranolol on page 688*

**Inderal® LA [US/Can]** *see propranolol on page 688*

**Inderide® [US]** *see propranolol and hydrochlorothiazide on page 689*

## indinavir (in DIN a veer)
**Sound-Alike/Look-Alike Issues**
indinavir may be confused with Denavir™
**Synonyms** indinavir sulfate
**U.S./Canadian Brand Names** Crixivan® [US/Can]
**Therapeutic Category** Antiviral Agent
**Use** Treatment of HIV infection; should always be used as part of a multidrug regimen (at least three antiretroviral agents)
**Usual Dosage** Adults: Oral:
Unboosted regimen: 800 mg every 8 hours
Ritonavir-boosted regimens:
Ritonavir 100-200 mg twice daily plus indinavir 800 mg twice daily **or**
Ritonavir 400 mg twice daily plus indinavir 400 mg twice daily
**Dosage adjustments for indinavir when administered in combination therapy:**
Delavirdine, itraconazole, or ketoconazole: Reduce indinavir dose to 600 mg every 8 hours
Efavirenz: Increase indinavir dose to 1000 mg every 8 hours
Lopinavir and ritonavir (Kaletra™): Indinavir 600 mg twice daily
Nelfinavir: Increase indinavir dose to 1200 mg twice daily
Nevirapine: Increase indinavir dose to 1000 mg every 8 hours
Rifabutin: Reduce rifabutin to $1/2$ the standard dose plus increase indinavir to 1000 mg every 8 hours
**Dosage Forms** Capsule: 100 mg, 200 mg, 333 mg, 400 mg

**indinavir sulfate** *see indinavir on this page*

**Indocid® P.D.A. [Can]** *see indomethacin on next page*

**Indocin® [US/Can]** *see indomethacin on next page*

**Indocin® I.V. [US]** *see indomethacin on next page*

**Indocin® SR [US]** *see indomethacin on next page*

## indocyanine green (in doe SYE a neen green)
**U.S./Canadian Brand Names** IC-Green® [US]
**Therapeutic Category** Diagnostic Agent
**Use** Determining hepatic function, cardiac output and liver blood flow and for ophthalmic angiography
**Usual Dosage**
Angiography: Use 40 mg of dye in 2 mL of aqueous solvent, in some patients, half the volume (1 mL) has been found to produce angiograms of comparable resolution; immediately following the bolus dose of dye, a bolus of sodium chloride 0.9% is given; this regimen will deliver a spatially limited dye bolus of optimal concentration to the choroidal vasculature following I.V. injection
Determination of cardiac output: Dye is injected as rapidly as possible into the right atrium, right ventricle, or pulmonary artery through a cardiac catheter; the usual dose is 1.25 mg for infants, 2.5 mg for children, and 5 mg for adults; total dose should not exceed 2 mg/kg; the dye is diluted with sterile water for injection or sodium chloride 0.9% to make a final volume of 1 mL; doses are repeated periodically to obtain several dilution curves; the dye should be flushed from the catheter with sodium chloride 0.9% to prevent hemolysis
**Dosage Forms** Injection, powder for reconstitution: 25 mg [supplied with diluent]

**Indo-Lemmon [Can]** *see indomethacin on next page*

**indometacin** *see indomethacin on next page*

## indomethacin (in doe METH a sin)
**Sound-Alike/Look-Alike Issues**
Indocin® may be confused with Imodium®, Lincocin®, Minocin®, Vicodin®
**Synonyms** indometacin; indomethacin sodium trihydrate
**U.S./Canadian Brand Names** Apo-Indomethacin® [Can]; Indo-Lemmon [Can]; Indocid® P.D.A. [Can]; Indocin® I.V. [US]; Indocin® SR [US]; Indocin® [US/Can]; Indotec [Can]; Novo-Methacin [Can]; Nu-Indo [Can]; Rhodacine® [Can]
**Therapeutic Category** Analgesic, Nonnarcotic; Nonsteroidal Antiinflammatory Drug (NSAID)
**Use** Acute gouty arthritis, acute bursitis/tendonitis, moderate to severe osteoarthritis, rheumatoid arthritis, ankylosing spondylitis; I.V. form used as alternative to surgery for closure of patent ductus arteriosus in neonates
**Usual Dosage**
Patent ductus arteriosus:
Neonates: I.V.: Initial: 0.2 mg/kg, followed by 2 doses depending on postnatal age (PNA):
PNA **at time of first dose** <48 hours: 0.1 mg/kg at 12- to 24-hour intervals
PNA **at time of first dose** 2-7 days: 0.2 mg/kg at 12- to 24-hour intervals
PNA **at time of first dose** >7 days: 0.25 mg/kg at 12- to 24-hour intervals
In general, may use 12-hour dosing interval if urine output >1 mL/kg/hour after prior dose; use 24-hour dosing interval if urine output is <1 mL/kg/hour but >0.6 mL/kg/hour; doses should be withheld if patient has oliguria (urine output <0.6 mL/kg/hour) or anuria
Inflammatory/rheumatoid disorders: Oral:
Children: 1-2 mg/kg/day in 2-4 divided doses; maximum dose: 4 mg/kg/day; not to exceed 150-200 mg/day
Adults: 25-50 mg/dose 2-3 times/day; maximum dose: 200 mg/day; extended release capsule should be given on a 1-2 times/day schedule; maximum dose for sustained release is 150 mg/day
**Dosage Forms**
Capsule (Indocin®): 25 mg, 50 mg
Capsule, sustained release (Indocin® SR): 75 mg
Injection, powder for reconstitution, as sodium trihydrate (Indocin® I.V.): 1 mg
Suspension, oral (Indocin®): 25 mg/5 mL (237 mL) [contains alcohol 1%; pineapple-coconut-mint flavor]

**indomethacin sodium trihydrate** see indomethacin on this page

**Indotec [Can]** see indomethacin on this page

**INF-alpha 2** see interferon alfa-2b on page 440

**Infanrix® [US]** see diphtheria, tetanus toxoids, and acellular pertussis vaccine on page 259

**Infantaire Gas Drops [US-OTC]** see simethicone on page 748

**Infants' Tylenol® Cold Plus Cough Concentrated Drops [US-OTC]** see acetaminophen, dextromethorphan, and pseudoephedrine on page 11

**Infasurf® [US]** see calfactant on page 136

**INFeD® [US]** see iron dextran complex on page 448

**Infergen® [US]** see interferon alfacon-1 on page 442

**Inflamase® Mild [Can]** see prednisolone (ophthalmic) on page 673

## infliximab (in FLIKS e mab)
**Sound-Alike/Look-Alike Issues**
Remicade® may be confused with Renacidin®, Rituxan®
**Synonyms** infliximab, recombinant
**U.S./Canadian Brand Names** Remicade® [US/Can]
**Therapeutic Category** Monoclonal Antibody
**Use**
Ankylosing spondylitis: Improving signs and symptoms of disease
Crohn disease: Induction and maintenance of remission in patients with moderate to severe disease who have an inadequate response to conventional therapy; to reduce the number of draining enterocutaneous and rectovaginal fistulas and to maintain fistula closure
Psoriatic arthritis: Improving signs and symptoms of active arthritis in patients with psoriatic arthritis
Rheumatoid arthritis: Inhibits the progression of structural damage and improves physical function in patients with moderate to severe disease; used with methotrexate

Ulcerative colitis (UC): To reduce signs and symptoms, achieve clinical remission and mucosal healing and eliminate corticosteroid use in moderately to severely active UC inadequately responsive to conventional therapy

**Usual Dosage** I.V.: Adults:

Crohn disease:

Induction regimen: 5 mg/kg at 0, 2, and 6 weeks, followed by 5 mg/kg every 8 weeks thereafter; dose may be increased to 10 mg/kg in patients who respond but then lose their response. If no response by week 14, consider discontinuing therapy.

Psoriatic arthritis (with or without methotrexate): 5 mg/kg at 0, 2, and 6 weeks, then every 8 weeks

Rheumatoid arthritis (in combination with methotrexate therapy): 3 mg/kg at 0, 2, and 6 weeks, then every 8 weeks thereafter; doses have ranged from 3-10 mg/kg intravenous infusion repeated at 4- to 8-week intervals

Ankylosing spondylitis: 5 mg/kg at 0, 2, and 6 weeks, followed by 5 mg/kg every 6 weeks thereafter

**Dosage Forms** Injection, powder for reconstitution [preservative free]: 100 mg

**infliximab, recombinant** *see* infliximab *on previous page*

# influenza virus vaccine (in floo EN za VYE rus vak SEEN)

**Sound-Alike/Look-Alike Issues**

Influenza virus vaccine may be confused with tetanus toxoid and tuberculin products. Medication errors have occurred when tuberculin skin tests (PPD) have been inadvertently administered instead of tetanus toxoid products and influenza virus vaccine. These products are refrigerated and often stored in close proximity to each other.

**Synonyms** influenza virus vaccine (purified surface antigen); influenza virus vaccine (split-virus); influenza virus vaccine (trivalent, live); live attenuated influenza vaccine (LAIV); trivalent inactivated influenza vaccine (TIV)

**U.S./Canadian Brand Names** Fluarix™ [US]; fluMist® [US]; Fluviral S/F® [Can]; Fluvirin® [US]; Fluzone® [US]; Vaxigrip® [Can]

**Therapeutic Category** Vaccine, Inactivated Virus

**Use** Provide active immunity to influenza virus strains contained in the vaccine

Groups at Increased Risk for Influenza-Related Complications: Recommendations for vaccination:
- Persons ≥65 years of age
- Residents of nursing homes and other chronic-care facilities that house persons of any age with chronic medical conditions
- Adults and children with chronic disorders of the pulmonary or cardiovascular systems, including children with asthma
- Adults and children who have required regular medical follow-up or hospitalization during the preceding year because of chronic metabolic diseases (including diabetes mellitus), renal dysfunction, hemoglobinopathies, or immunosuppression (including immunosuppression caused by medications or HIV)
- Adults and children with conditions which may compromise respiratory function, the handling of respiratory secretions, or that can increase the risk of aspiration (eg, cognitive dysfunction, spinal; cord injuries, seizure disorders, other neuromuscular disorders)
- Children and adolescents (6 months to 18 years of age) who are receiving long-term aspirin therapy and therefore, may be at risk for developing Reye syndrome after influenza
- Women who will be pregnant during the influenza season
- Children 6-23 months of age

Vaccination is also recommended for persons 50-64 years of age, close contacts of children 0-23 months of age, healthy persons who may transmit influenza to those at risk, all healthcare workers, and persons who smoke.

**Usual Dosage** Optimal time to receive vaccine is October-November, prior to exposure to influenza; however, vaccination can continue into December and later as long as vaccine is available.

I.M.:

Fluzone®:

Children 6-35 months: 0.25 mL/dose (1 or 2 doses per season; see **Note**)

Children 3-8 years: 0.5 mL/dose (1 or 2 doses per season; see **Note**)

Children ≥9 years and Adults: 0.5 mL/dose (1 dose per season)

Fluvirin®:

Children 4-8 years: 0.5 mL/dose (1 or 2 doses per season; see **Note**)

Children ≥9 years and Adults: 0.5 mL/dose (1 dose per season)

**Note:** Previously unvaccinated children <9 years should receive 2 doses, given >1 month apart in order to achieve satisfactory antibody response.

(Continued)

## influenza virus vaccine *(Continued)*

Fluarix™: Adults: 0.5 mL/dose (1 dose per season)

Intranasal (fluMist®):

Children 5-8 years, previously **not vaccinated** with influenza vaccine: Initial season: Two 0.5 mL doses separated by 6-10 weeks

Children 5-8 years, previously **vaccinated** with influenza vaccine: 0.5 mL/dose (1 dose per season)

Children ≥9 years and Adults ≤49 years: 0.5 mL/dose (1 dose per season)

### Dosage Forms

Injection, solution, purified split-virus surface antigen [preservative free] (Fluvirin®): (0.5 mL) [prefilled syringe; contains thimerosal (trace amounts); manufactured using neomycin and polymyxin]; (5 mL) [multidose vial; contains thimerosal; manufactured using neomycin and polymyxin]

Injection, suspension, purified split-virus [produced in chick embryo cell culture]:

Fluarix™ [preservative free]: (0.5 mL) [prefilled syringe; syringe cap and rubber plunger contain natural latex rubber; may contain residual amounts of thimerosal, hydrocortisone, gentamicin, and ovalbumin]

Fluzone®: (5 mL) [vial; contains thimerosal]

Fluzone® [preservative free]: (0.25 mL) [prefilled syringe]; (0.5 mL) [vial]

Solution, nasal spray, trivalent, live virus [preservative free] (fluMist®): (0.5 mL) [manufactured using eggs and gentamicin]

**influenza virus vaccine (purified surface antigen)** *see* influenza virus vaccine *on previous page*

**influenza virus vaccine (split-virus)** *see* influenza virus vaccine *on previous page*

**influenza virus vaccine (trivalent, live)** *see* influenza virus vaccine *on previous page*

**Infufer® [Can]** *see* iron dextran complex *on page 448*

**Infumorph® [US]** *see* morphine sulfate *on page 549*

**Infuvite® Adult [US]** *see* vitamins (multiple/injectable) *on page 851*

**Infuvite® Pediatric [US]** *see* vitamins (multiple/injectable) *on page 851*

**INH** *see* isoniazid *on page 450*

## inhalation devices *(in hal LAY shun deh VYE sez)*

**U.S./Canadian Brand Names** AeroChamber™ [US]; InspirEase™ [US]

**Therapeutic Category** Inhalation, Miscellaneous

**Use** Improves the distribution and deposition in the lungs of aerosolized medication from metered dose inhalers (MDIs)

**Usual Dosage** Children and Adults: 0.3-0.6 mL (1 dose = 0.3 mL)

**Dosage Forms**

AeroChamber™, AeroChamber™ with mask (small, medium)

Inhalation kit (InspirEase™)

Replacement bags (InspirEase™)

**Inhibace® [Can]** *see* cilazapril *(Canada only) on page 182*

**Innohep® [US/Can]** *see* tinzaparin *on page 805*

**InnoPran XL™ [US]** *see* propranolol *on page 688*

**Inocor® *(Discontinued)***

**INOmax® [US/Can]** *see* nitric oxide *on page 577*

**insect sting kit** *see* epinephrine and chlorpheniramine *on page 289*

**insoluble prussian blue** *see* ferric hexacyanoferrate *on page 334*

**InspirEase™ [US]** *see* inhalation devices *on this page*

**Inspra™ [US]** *see* eplerenone *on page 290*

**Insta-Glucose® [US-OTC]** *see* glucose (instant) *on page 377*

**Instat™ [US]** *see* collagen hemostat *on page 206*

**Instat™ MCH [US]** *see* collagen hemostat *on page 206*

## insulin preparations *(IN su lin prep a RAY shuns)*

### Sound-Alike/Look-Alike Issues

Humalog® may be confused with Humulin®

Humalog® Mix 75/25™ may be confused with Humulin® 70/30

Humulin® may be confused with Humalog®, Humira®
Lantus® may be confused with Lente®
Lente® may be confused with Lantus®
Novolin® may be confused with NovoLog®
Novolin® 70/30 may be confused with NovoLog® Mix 70/30
NovoLog® may be confused with Novolin®
NovoLog® Mix 70/30 may be confused with Novolin® 70/30

**Synonyms** aspart, insulin; glargine, insulin; glulisine, insulin; lispro, insulin; NPH, insulin; regular, insulin

**U.S./Canadian Brand Names** Apidra™ [US]; Humalog® Mix 25™ [Can]; Humalog® Mix 75/25™ [US]; Humalog® [US/Can]; Humulin® 50/50 [US]; Humulin® 70/30 [US]; Humulin® N [US]; Humulin® R (Concentrated) U-500 [US]; Humulin® R [US]; Humulin® [Can]; Iletin® II Pork [Can]; Lantus® [US/Can]; Novolin® 70/30 [US]; Novolin® ge [Can]; Novolin® N [US]; Novolin® R [US]; NovoLog® Mix 70/30 [US]; NovoLog® [US]; NovoRapid [Can]

**Therapeutic Category** Antidiabetic Agent, Parenteral

**Use** Treatment of type 1 diabetes mellitus (insulin dependent, IDDM); type 2 diabetes mellitus (noninsulin dependent, NIDDM) unresponsive to treatment with diet and/or oral hypoglycemics; adjunct to parenteral nutrition; diabetic ketoacidosis (DKA)

**Usual Dosage** Dose requires continuous medical supervision; may administer I.M., or SubQ; regular insulin may also be administered I.V.

Diabetes mellitus: The number and size of daily doses, time of administration, and diet and exercise require continuous medical supervision. In addition, specific formulations may require distinct administration procedures.

Children and Adults: 0.5-1 unit/kg/day in divided doses

Adolescents (growth spurts): 0.8-1.2 units/kg/day in divided doses

Adjust dose to maintain premeal and bedtime blood glucose of 80-140 mg/dL (children <5 years: 100-200 mg/dL)

Insulin glargine (Lantus®): SubQ:

Type 2 diabetes (patient not already on insulin): 10 units once daily, adjusted according to patient response (range in clinical study 2-100 units/day)

Patients already receiving insulin: In clinical studies, when changing to insulin glargine from once-daily NPH or Ultralente® insulin, the initial dose was not changed; when changing from twice-daily NPH to once-daily insulin glargine, the total daily dose was reduced by 20% and adjusted according to patient response

Diabetic ketoacidosis: Children and Adults: Regular insulin: I.V. loading dose: 0.1 unit/kg, then maintenance continuous infusion: 0.1 unit/kg/hour (range: 0.05-0.2 units/kg/hour depending upon the rate of decrease of serum glucose - too rapid decrease of serum glucose may lead to cerebral edema).

Optimum rate of decrease (serum glucose): 80-100 mg/dL/hour

**Note:** Newly-diagnosed patients with IDDM presenting in DKA and patients with blood sugars <800 mg/dL may be relatively "sensitive" to insulin and should receive loading and initial maintenance doses approximately 1/2 of those indicated above.

**Dosage Forms** [DSC] = Discontinued product
RAPID-ACTING:
Injection, solution, aspart [human] (NovoLog®): 100 units/mL (3 mL) [FlexPen® prefilled syringe or PenFill® prefilled cartridge]; (10 mL) [vial]
Injection, solution, lispro [human] (Humalog®): 100 units/mL (3 mL) [prefilled cartridge or prefilled disposable pen]; (10 mL) [vial]
Injection, solution, glulisine [human] (Apidra™): 100 units/mL (10 mL) [vial]

SHORT-ACTING:
Injection, solution, regular [human]:
Humulin® R: 100 units/mL (10 mL) [vial]
Novolin® R: 100 units/mL (3 mL) [InnoLet® prefilled syringe or PenFill® prefilled cartridge]; (10 mL) [vial]
Injection, solution, regular [human concentrate] (Humulin® R U-500): 500 units/mL (20 mL vial)
Injection, solution, regular [purified pork] (Regular Iletin® II): 100 units/mL (10 mL) [vial] [DSC]

INTERMEDIATE-ACTING:
Injection, suspension, zinc, [human, lente] (Humulin® L): 100 units/mL (10 mL) [vial] [DSC]
Injection, suspension, isophane [human, NPH]:
Humulin® N: 100 units/mL (3 mL) [disposable pen]; (10 mL) [vial]
Novolin® N: 100 units/mL (3 mL) [InnoLet® prefilled syringe or PenFill® prefilled cartridge]; (10 mL) [vial]
Injection, suspension, isophane [purified pork, NPH] (NPH Iletin® II): 100 units/mL (10 mL) [vial] [DSC]
(Continued)

## insulin preparations *(Continued)*

LONG-ACTING:
Injection, suspension, extended zinc [human, Ultralente®] (Humulin®) 100 units/mL (10 mL) [vial] [DSC]
Injection, solution, glargine [human] (Lantus®): 100 unit/mL (3 mL) [cartridge]; (10 mL) [vial]

COMBINATION PRODUCT, INTERMEDIATE-ACTING:  Injection, suspension:
Humalog® Mix 75/25™: Lispro protamine human suspension 75% [intermediate acting] and lispro human solution 25% [rapid acting]: 100 units/mL (3 mL) [disposable pen]; (10 mL) [vial]
Humulin® 50/50: Isophane (NPH) human insulin suspension 50% [intermediate acting] and regular human insulin solution 50% [short acting]: 100 units/mL (10 mL) [vial]
Humulin® 70/30: Isophane (NPH) human insulin suspension 70% [intermediate acting] and regular human insulin solution 30% [short acting]: 100 units/mL (3 mL) [disposable pen]; (10 mL) [vial]
Novolin® 70/30: Isophane (NPH) human insulin suspension 70% [intermediate acting] and regular human insulin solution 30% [short acting]: 100 units/mL (3 mL) [InnoLet® prefilled syringe or PenFill® prefilled cartridge]; (10 mL) [vial]
NovoLog® Mix 70/30: Aspart protamine human suspension 70% [intermediate acting] and aspart human solution 30% [rapid acting]: 100 units/mL (3 mL) [PenFill® prefilled cartridge or FlexPen® prefilled syringe]; (10 mL) [vial]

**Intal®** **[US/Can]** *see* cromolyn sodium *on page 211*

**Integrilin®** **[US/Can]** *see* eptifibatide *on page 292*

**Intensol® Solution** *(Discontinued)* *see* metoclopramide *on page 533*

α-2-interferon *see* interferon alfa-2b *on this page*

## interferon alfa-2a (in ter FEER on AL fa too aye)

**Sound-Alike/Look-Alike Issues**
interferon alfa-2a may be confused with interferon alfa-2b
Roferon-A® may be confused with Rocephin®

**Synonyms** IFLrA; rIFN-A

**U.S./Canadian Brand Names** Roferon-A® [US/Can]

**Therapeutic Category** Biological Response Modulator

**Use**
Patients >18 years of age: Hairy cell leukemia, AIDS-related Kaposi sarcoma, chronic hepatitis C
Children and Adults: Chronic myelogenous leukemia (CML), Philadelphia chromosome positive, within 1 year of diagnosis (limited experience in children)

**Usual Dosage** Refer to individual protocols
Children (limited data): Chronic myelogenous leukemia (CML): I.M.: 2.5-5 million units/m$^2$/day; **Note:** In juveniles, higher dosages (30 million units/m$^2$/day) have been associated with severe adverse events, including death
Adults:
Hairy cell leukemia: SubQ, I.M.: 3 million units/day for 16-24 weeks, then 3 million units 3 times/week for up to 6-24 months
Chronic myelogenous leukemia (CML): SubQ, I.M.: 9 million units/day, continue treatment until disease progression
AIDS-related Kaposi sarcoma: SubQ, I.M.: 36 million units/day for 10-12 weeks, then 36 million units 3 times/week; to minimize adverse reactions, can use escalating dose (3-, 9-, then 18 million units each day for 3 days, then 36 million units daily thereafter).
Hepatitis C: SubQ, I.M.: 3 million units 3 times/week for 12 months

**Dosage Forms** Injection, solution, [single-dose prefilled syringe; SubQ use only]: 3 million units/0.5 mL (0.5 mL); 6 million units/0.5 mL (0.5 mL); 9 million units/0.5 mL (0.5 mL) [contains benzyl alcohol]

**interferon alfa-2a (PEG conjugate)** *see* peginterferon alfa-2a *on page 624*

## interferon alfa-2b (in ter FEER on AL fa too bee)

**Sound-Alike/Look-Alike Issues**
interferon alfa-2b may be confused with interferon alfa-2a

**Synonyms** INF-alpha 2; rLFN-α2; α-2-interferon

**U.S./Canadian Brand Names** Intron® A [US/Can]

**Therapeutic Category** Biological Response Modulator

**Use**
Patients ≥1 year of age: Chronic hepatitis B

Patients ≥18 years of age: Condyloma acuminata, chronic hepatitis C, hairy cell leukemia, malignant melanoma, AIDS-related Kaposi sarcoma, follicular non-Hodgkin lymphoma

**Usual Dosage** Refer to individual protocols

Children 1-17 years: Chronic hepatitis B: SubQ: 3 million units/m$^2$ 3 times/week for 1 week; then 6 million units/m$^2$ 3 times/week; maximum: 10 million units 3 times/week; total duration of therapy 16-24 weeks

Adults:

Hairy cell leukemia: I.M., SubQ: 2 million units/m$^2$ 3 times/week for 2-6 months

Lymphoma (follicular): SubQ: 5 million units 3 times/week for up to 18 months

Malignant melanoma: 20 million units/m$^2$ I.V. for 5 consecutive days per week for 4 weeks, then 10 million units/m$^2$ SubQ 3 times/week for 48 weeks

AIDS-related Kaposi's sarcoma: I.M., SubQ: 30 million units/m$^2$ 3 times/week

Chronic hepatitis B: I.M., SubQ: 5 million units/day or 10 million units 3 times/week for 16 weeks

Chronic hepatitis C: I.M., SubQ: 3 million units 3 times/week for 16 weeks. In patients with normalization of ALT at 16 weeks, continue treatment for 18-24 months; consider discontinuation if normalization does not occur at 16 weeks. **Note:** May be used in combination therapy with ribavirin in previously untreated patients or in patients who relapse following alpha interferon therapy; refer to interferon alfa-2b and ribavirin.

Condyloma acuminata: Intralesionally: 1 million units/lesion (maximum: 5 lesions/treatment) 3 times/week (on alternate days) for 3 weeks; may administer a second course at 12-16 weeks

**Dosage Forms**

Injection, powder for reconstitution: 10 million units; 18 million units; 50 million units [contains human albumin]

Injection, solution [multidose prefilled pen]:

Delivers 3 million units/0.2 mL (1.5 mL) [delivers 6 doses; 18 million units]

Delivers 5 million units/0.2 mL (1.5 mL) [delivers 6 doses; 30 million units]

Delivers 10 million units/0.2 mL (1.5 mL) [delivers 6 doses; 60 million units]

Injection, solution [multidose vial]: 6 million units/mL (3 mL); 10 million units/mL (2.5 mL)

Injection, solution [single-dose vial]: 10 million units/ mL (1 mL)

See also Interferon Alfa-2b and Ribavirin Combination Pack monograph.

# interferon alfa-2b and ribavirin (in ter FEER on AL fa too bee & rye ba VYE rin)

**Synonyms** interferon alfa-2b and ribavirin combination pack; ribavirin and interferon alfa-2b combination pack

**U.S./Canadian Brand Names** Rebetron® [US]

**Therapeutic Category** Antiviral Agent; Biological Response Modulator

**Use** Combination therapy for the treatment of chronic hepatitis C in patients with compensated liver disease previously untreated with alpha interferon or who have relapsed after alpha interferon therapy

**Usual Dosage**

Children ≥3 years: Chronic hepatitis C: **Note:** Duration of therapy: genotype 1: 48 weeks; genotype 2 or 3: 24 weeks. Discontinue treatment in any patient if HCV-RNA is not below the limits of detection of the assay after 24 weeks of therapy. Combination therapy:

Intron® A: SubQ:

25-61 kg: 3 million int. units/m$^2$ 3 times/week

>61 kg: Refer to Adults dosing

Rebetol®: Oral: **Note:** Oral solution should be used in children 3-5 years of age, children ≤25 kg, or those unable to swallow capsules.

Capsule/solution: 15 mg/kg/day in 2 divided doses (morning and evening)

Capsule dosing recommendations:

25-36 kg: 400 mg/day (200 mg morning and evening)

37-49 kg: 600 mg/day (200 mg in the morning and two 200 mg capsules in the evening)

50-61 kg: 800 mg/day (two 200 mg capsules morning and evening)

>61 kg: Refer to Adults dosing

Adults: Chronic hepatitis C: Recommended dosage of combination therapy:

Intron® A: SubQ: 3 million int. units 3 times/week **and**

Rebetol® capsule: Oral:

≤75 kg (165 lb): 1000 mg/day (two 200 mg capsules In the morning and three 200 mg capsules in the evening)

>75 kg: 1200 mg/day (three 200 mg capsules in the morning and three 200 mg capsules in the evening)

(Continued)

## interferon alfa-2b and ribavirin *(Continued)*

Treatment duration recommendations:

Following relapse after alpha interferon monotherapy: 24 weeks

Previously untreated: 24-48 weeks (individualized based on response, tolerance, and baseline characteristics)

Consider discontinuing therapy in any patient not achieving HCV-RNA below the limit of assay detection by 24 weeks.

**Dosage Forms Combination package:**

**For patients ≤75 kg [contains single-dose vials]:**

Injection, solution: Interferon alfa-2b (Intron® A): 3 million int. units/0.5 mL (0.5 mL) [6 vials (3 million int. units/vial), 6 syringes, and alcohol swabs]

Capsule: Ribavirin (Rebetol®): 200 mg (70s)

**For patients ≤75 kg [contains multidose vials]:**

Injection, solution: Interferon alfa-2b (Intron® A): 3 million int. units/0.5 mL (3.8 mL) [1 multidose vial (18 million int. units/vial), 6 syringes, and alcohol swabs]

Capsule: Ribavirin (Rebetol®): 200 mg (70s)

**For patients ≤75 kg [contains multidose pen]:**

Injection, solution: Interferon alfa-2b (Intron® A): 3 million int. units/0.2 mL (1.5 mL) [1 multidose pen (18 million int. units/pen), 6 needles, and alcohol swabs]

Capsule: Ribavirin (Rebetol®): 200 mg (70s)

**For patients >75 kg [contains single-dose vials]:**

Injection, solution: Interferon alfa-2b (Intron® A): 3 million int. units/0.5 mL (0.5 mL) [6 vials (3 million int. units/vial), 6 syringes, and alcohol swabs]

Capsule: Ribavirin (Rebetol®): 200 mg (84s)

**For patients >75 kg [contains multidose vials]:**

Injection, solution: Interferon alfa-2b (Intron® A): 3 million int. units/0.5 mL (3.8 mL) [1 multidose vial (18 million int. units/vial), 6 syringes, and alcohol swabs]

Capsule: Ribavirin (Rebetol®): 200 mg (84s)

**For patients >75 kg [contains multidose pen]:**

Injection, solution: Interferon alfa-2b (Intron® A): 3 million int. units/0.2 mL (1.5 mL) [1 multidose pen (18 million int. units/pen), 6 needles, and alcohol swabs]

Capsule: Ribavirin (Rebetol®): 200 mg (84s)

**For Rebetol® dose reduction [contains single-dose vials]:**

Injection, solution: Interferon alfa-2b (Intron® A): 3 million int. units/0.5 mL (0.5 mL) [6 vials (3 million int. units/vial), 6 syringes, and alcohol swabs]

Capsule: Ribavirin (Rebetol®): 200 mg (42s)

**For Rebetol® dose reduction [contains multidose vials]:**

Injection, solution: Interferon alfa-2b (Intron® A): 3 million int. units/0.5 mL (3.8 mL) [1 multidose vial (18 million int. units/vial), 6 syringes, and alcohol swabs]

Capsule: Ribavirin (Rebetol®): 200 mg (42s)

**For Rebetol® dose reduction [contains multidose pen]:**

Injection, solution: Interferon alfa-2b (Intron® A): 3 million int. units/0.2 mL (1.5 mL) [1 multidose pen (18 million int. units/pen), 6 needles, and alcohol swabs]

Capsule: Ribavirin (Rebetol®): 200 mg (42s)

**interferon alfa-2b and ribavirin combination pack** *see* interferon alfa-2b and ribavirin *on* *previous page*

**interferon alfa-2b (PEG conjugate)** *see* peginterferon alfa-2b *on page 624*

## interferon alfacon-1 (in ter FEER on AL fa con one)

**U.S./Canadian Brand Names** Infergen® [US]

**Therapeutic Category** Interferon

**Use** Treatment of chronic hepatitis C virus (HCV) infection in patients ≥18 years of age with compensated liver disease and anti-HCV serum antibodies or HCV RNA.

**Usual Dosage** Adults ≥18 years: SubQ:

Chronic HCV infection: 9 mcg 3 times/week for 24 weeks; allow 48 hours between doses

Patients who have previously tolerated interferon therapy but did not respond or relapsed: 15 mcg 3 times/week for 6 months

Dose reduction for toxicity: Dose should be held in patients who experience a severe adverse reaction, and treatment should be stopped or decreased if the reaction does not become tolerable.

Doses were reduced from 9 mcg to 7.5 mcg in the pivotal study.

For patients receiving 15 mcg/dose, doses were reduced in 3 mcg increments. Efficacy is decreased with doses <7.5 mcg

**Dosage Forms** Injection, solution [preservative free]: 30 mcg/mL (0.3 mL, 0.5 mL)

## interferon alfa-n3 (in ter FEER on AL fa en three)
**Sound-Alike/Look-Alike Issues**
Alferon® may be confused with Alkeran®
**U.S./Canadian Brand Names** Alferon® N [US/Can]
**Therapeutic Category** Biological Response Modulator
**Use** Patients ≥18 years of age: Intralesional treatment of refractory or recurring genital or venereal warts (condylomata acuminata)
**Usual Dosage** Adults: Inject 250,000 units (0.05 mL) in each wart twice weekly for a maximum of 8 weeks; therapy should not be repeated for at least 3 months after the initial 8-week course of therapy
**Dosage Forms** Injection, solution: 5 million int. units (1 mL) [contains albumin]

## interferon beta-1a (in ter FEER on BAY ta won aye)
**Sound-Alike/Look-Alike Issues**
Avonex® may be confused with Avelox®
**Synonyms** rIFN beta-1a
**U.S./Canadian Brand Names** Avonex® [US/Can]; Rebif® [US/Can]
**Therapeutic Category** Biological Response Modulator
**Use** Treatment of relapsing forms of multiple sclerosis (MS)
**Usual Dosage** Adults: **Note:** Analgesics and/or antipyretics may help decrease flu-like symptoms on treatment days:
I.M. (Avonex®): 30 mcg once weekly
SubQ (Rebif®): Doses should be separated by at least 48 hours:
**Target dose 44 mcg 3 times/week:** 11
Initial: 8.8 mcg (20 % of final dose) 3 times/week for 8 weeks
Titration: 22 mcg (50% of final dose) 3 times/week for 8 weeks
Final dose: 44 mcg 3 times/week
**Target dose 22 mcg 3 times/week:**
Initial: 4.4 mcg (20 % of final dose) 3 times/week for 8 weeks
Titration: 11 mcg (50% of final dose) 3 times/week for 8 weeks
Final dose: 22 mcg 3 times/week
**Dosage Forms**
Combination package [preservative free] (Rebif® Titration Pack):
Injection, solution: 8.8 mcg/0.2 mL (0.2 mL) [6 prefilled syringes; contains albumin]
Injection, solution: 22 mcg/0.5 mL (0.5 mL) [6 prefilled syringes; contains albumin]
Injection, powder for reconstitution (Avonex®): 33 mcg [6.6 million units; provides 30 mcg/mL following reconstitution] [contains albumin; packaged with SWFI, alcohol wipes, and access pin and needle]
Injection, solution (Avonex®): 30 mcg/0.5 mL (0.5 mL) [albumin free; prefilled syringe; syringe cap contains latex; packaged with alcohol wipes, gauze pad, and adhesive bandages]
Injection, solution [preservative free] (Rebif®): 22 mcg/0.5 mL (0.5 mL) [prefilled syringe; contains albumin]; 44 mcg/0.5 mL (0.5 mL) [prefilled syringe; contains albumin]

## interferon beta-1b (in ter FEER on BAY ta won bee)
**Synonyms** rIFN beta-1b
**U.S./Canadian Brand Names** Betaseron® [US/Can]
**Therapeutic Category** Biological Response Modulator
**Use** Treatment of relapsing forms of multiple sclerosis (MS)
**Usual Dosage** SubQ:
Children <18 years: Not recommended
Adults: 0.25 mg (8 million units) every other day
**Dosage Forms** Injection, powder for reconstitution [preservative free]: 0.3 mg [9.6 million units] [contains albumin; packaged with prefilled syringe containing diluent]

## interferon gamma-1b (in ter FEER on GAM ah won bee)
**U.S./Canadian Brand Names** Actimmune® [US/Can]
**Therapeutic Category** Biological Response Modulator
**Use** Reduce frequency and severity of serious infections associated with chronic granulomatous disease; delay time to disease progression in patients with severe, malignant osteopetrosis
**Usual Dosage** If severe reactions occur, modify dose (50% reduction) or therapy should be discontinued until adverse reactions abate.

Chronic granulomatous disease: Children >1 year and Adults: SubQ:
BSA ≤0.5 m$^2$: 1.5 mcg/kg/dose 3 times/week
BSA >0.5 m$^2$: 50 mcg/m$^2$ (1 million int. units/m$^2$) 3 times/week

Severe, malignant osteopetrosis: Children >1 year: SubQ:
BSA ≤0.5 m$^2$: 1.5 mcg/kg/dose 3 times/week
BSA >0.5 m$^2$: 50 mcg/m$^2$ (1 million int. units/m$^2$) 3 times/week

**Note:** Previously expressed as 1.5 million units/m$^2$; 50 mcg is equivalent to 1 million int. units/m$^2$.
**Dosage Forms** Injection, solution [preservative free]: 100 mcg [2 million int. units] (0.5 mL)
*Previously, 100 mcg was expressed as 3 million units. This is equivalent to 2 million int. units.*

**interleukin-1 receptor antagonist** *see* anakinra *on page 52*

**interleukin-2** *see* aldesleukin *on page 25*

**interleukin-11** *see* oprelvekin *on page 601*

**Intralipid® [US/Can]** *see* fat emulsion *on page 328*

**intravenous fat emulsion** *see* fat emulsion *on page 328*

**intrifiban** *see* eptifibatide *on page 292*

**Intron® A [US/Can]** *see* interferon alfa-2b *on page 440*

**Intropin® *(Discontinued)*** *see* dopamine *on page 266*

**Invanz® [US/Can]** *see* ertapenem *on page 294*

**Inversine® [US/Can]** *see* mecamylamine *on page 505*

**Invirase® [US/Can]** *see* saquinavir *on page 738*

**iocetamic acid** *see* radiological/contrast media (ionic) *on page 707*

**iodamide meglumine** *see* radiological/contrast media (ionic) *on page 707*

**Iodex [US-OTC]** *see* iodine *on this page*

**Iodex-p® *(Discontinued)*** *see* povidone-iodine *on page 668*

## iodine (EYE oh dyne)
**Sound-Alike/Look-Alike Issues**
iodine may be confused with codeine, Iopidine®, Lodine®
**U.S./Canadian Brand Names** Iodex [US-OTC]; Iodoflex™ [US]; Iodosorb® [US]
**Therapeutic Category** Topical Skin Product
**Use** Used topically as an antiseptic in the management of minor, superficial skin wounds and has been used to disinfect the skin preoperatively
**Usual Dosage** Apply topically as necessary to affected areas of skin
**Dosage Forms**
Dressing, topical [gel pad] (Iodoflex™): 0.9% (5 g, 10 g)
Gel, topical (Iodosorb®): 0.9% (40 g)
Ointment (Iodex): 4.7% (30 g, 720 g)
Tincture, topical: 2% (30 mL, 480 mL); 7% (30 mL, 480 mL)

**iodine I 131 tositumomab and tositumomab** *see* tositumomab and iodine I 131 tositumomab *on page 812*

**iodipamide meglumine** *see* radiological/contrast media (ionic) *on page 707*

**iodochlorhydroxyquin** *see* clioquinol *on page 193*

**iodochlorhydroxyquin and flumethasone** *see* clioquinol and flumethasone *(Canada only)* on page 193

**Iodoflex™ [US]** *see* iodine *on this page*

**Iodopen® [US]** *see* trace metals *on page 813*

## iodoquinol (eye oh doe KWIN ole)
**Synonyms** diiodohydroxyquin
**U.S./Canadian Brand Names** Diodoquin® [Can]; Yodoxin® [US]
**Therapeutic Category** Amebicide
**Use** Treatment of acute and chronic intestinal amebiasis; asymptomatic cyst passers; *Blastocystis hominis* infections; ineffective for amebic hepatitis or hepatic abscess
**Usual Dosage** Oral:
Children: 30-40 mg/kg/day (maximum: 650 mg/dose) in 3 divided doses for 20 days; not to exceed 1.95 g/day
Adults: 650 mg 3 times/day after meals for 20 days; not to exceed 1.95 g/day
**Dosage Forms** Tablet: 210 mg, 650 mg

## iodoquinol and hydrocortisone (eye oh doe KWIN ole & hye droe KOR ti sone)
**Sound-Alike/Look-Alike Issues**
Vytone® may be confused with Hytone®, Zydone®
**Synonyms** hydrocortisone and iodoquinol
**U.S./Canadian Brand Names** Dermazene® [US]; Vytone® [US]
**Therapeutic Category** Antifungal/Corticosteroid
**Use** Treatment of eczema; infectious dermatitis; chronic eczematoid otitis externa; mycotic dermatoses
**Usual Dosage** Apply 3-4 times/day
**Dosage Forms**
Cream: Iodoquinol 1% and hydrocortisone acetate 1% (30 g)
Dermazene®: Iodoquinol 1% and hydrocortisone acetate 1% (30 g, 45 g)
Vytone®: Iodoquinol 1% and hydrocortisone acetate 1% (30 g)

**Iodosorb® [US]** *see* iodine *on previous page*

**iohexol** *see* radiological/contrast media (nonionic) *on page 709*

**Ionamin® [US/Can]** *see* phentermine *on page 639*

**Ionil® [US-OTC]** *see* salicylic acid *on page 734*

**Ionil® Plus [US-OTC]** *see* salicylic acid *on page 734*

**Ionil T® [US-OTC]** *see* coal tar *on page 201*

**Ionil T® Plus [US-OTC]** *see* coal tar *on page 201*

**iopamidol** *see* radiological/contrast media (nonionic) *on page 709*

**iopanoic acid** *see* radiological/contrast media (ionic) *on page 707*

**Iophen-C NR [US]** *see* guaifenesin and codeine *on page 384*

**Iophen DM NR [US]** *see* guaifenesin and dextromethorphan *on page 385*

**Iophen NR [US]** *see* guaifenesin *on page 383*

**Iopidine® [US/Can]** *see* apraclonidine *on page 67*

**Iosat™ [US-OTC]** *see* potassium iodide *on page 665*

**iothalamate meglumine and iothalamate sodium** *see* radiological/contrast media (ionic) *on page 707*

**iothalamate sodium** *see* radiological/contrast media (ionic) *on page 707*

**ioversol** *see* radiological/contrast media (nonionic) *on page 709*

## ipecac syrup (IP e kak SIR up)
**Synonyms** syrup of ipecac
**Therapeutic Category** Antidote
**Use** Treatment of acute oral drug overdosage and in certain poisonings
**Usual Dosage** Oral:
Children:
6-12 months: 5-10 mL followed by 10-20 mL/kg of water; repeat dose one time if vomiting does not occur within 20 minutes
1-12 years: 15 mL followed by 10-20 mL/kg of water; repeat dose one time if vomiting does not occur within 20 minutes
If emesis does not occur within 30 minutes after second dose, ipecac must be removed from stomach by gastric lavage
(Continued)

445

## ipecac syrup *(Continued)*

Adults: 15-30 mL followed by 200-300 mL of water; repeat dose one time if vomiting does not occur within 20 minutes

**Dosage Forms** Syrup: 70 mg/mL (30 mL) [contains alcohol]

**I-Pentolate® *(Discontinued)*** *see* cyclopentolate *on page 214*

**I-Phrine® Ophthalmic Solution *(Discontinued)*** *see* phenylephrine *on page 640*

**I-Picamide® *(Discontinued)*** *see* tropicamide *on page 829*

**IPM Wound Gel™ [US-OTC]** *see* hyaluronate and derivatives *on page 406*

**ipodate calcium** *see* radiological/contrast media (ionic) *on page 707*

**ipodate sodium** *see* radiological/contrast media (ionic) *on page 707*

**IPOL® [US/Can]** *see* poliovirus vaccine (inactivated) *on page 657*

## ipratropium (i pra TROE pee um)

**Sound-Alike/Look-Alike Issues**

Atrovent® may be confused with Alupent®

**Synonyms** ipratropium bromide

**U.S./Canadian Brand Names** Alti-Ipratropium [Can]; Apo-Ipravent® [Can]; Atrovent® HFA [US/Can]; Atrovent® [US/Can]; Gen-Ipratropium [Can]; Novo-Ipramide [Can]; Nu-Ipratropium [Can]; PMS-Ipratropium [Can]

**Therapeutic Category** Anticholinergic Agent

**Use** Anticholinergic bronchodilator used in bronchospasm associated with COPD, bronchitis, and emphysema; symptomatic relief of rhinorrhea associated with the common cold and allergic and nonallergic rhinitis

**Usual Dosage**

Nebulization:

Infants and Children ≤12 years: 125-250 mcg 3 times/day

Children >12 years and Adults: 500 mcg (one unit-dose vial) 3-4 times/day with doses 6-8 hours apart

Oral inhalation: MDI:

Children 3-12 years: 1-2 inhalations 3 times/day, up to 6 inhalations/24 hours

Children >12 years and Adults: 2 inhalations 4 times/day, up to 12 inhalations/24 hours

Intranasal: Nasal spray:

Symptomatic relief of rhinorrhea associated with the common cold (safety and efficacy of use beyond 4 days in patients with the common cold have not been established):

Children 5-11 years: 0.06%: 2 sprays in each nostril 3 times/day

Children ≥5 years and Adults: 0.06%: 2 sprays in each nostril 3-4 times/day

Symptomatic relief of rhinorrhea associated with allergic/nonallergic rhinitis: Children ≥6 years and Adults: 0.03%: 2 sprays in each nostril 2-3 times/day

**Dosage Forms**

Solution for nebulization, as bromide: 0.02% (2.5 mL)

Solution for oral inhalation, as bromide (Atrovent®): 18 mcg/actuation (14 g) [contains soya lecithin and chlorofluorocarbons]

Solution for oral inhalation, as bromide (Atrovent® HFA): 17 mcg/actuation (12.9 g)

Solution, intranasal spray, as bromide (Atrovent®): 0.03% (30 mL); 0.06% (15 mL)

## ipratropium and albuterol (i pra TROE pee um & al BYOO ter ole)

**Sound-Alike/Look-Alike Issues**

Combivent® may be confused with Combivir®

**Synonyms** albuterol and ipratropium

**U.S./Canadian Brand Names** Combivent® [US/Can]; DuoNeb™ [US]

**Therapeutic Category** Bronchodilator

**Use** Treatment of COPD in those patients that are currently on a regular bronchodilator who continue to have bronchospasms and require a second bronchodilator

**Usual Dosage** Adults:

Inhalation: 2 inhalations 4 times/day (maximum: 12 inhalations/24 hours)

Inhalation via nebulization: Initial: 3 mL every 6 hours (maximum: 3 mL every 4 hours)

Dosage Forms
Aerosol for oral inhalation (Combivent®): Ipratropium bromide 18 mcg and albuterol sulfate 103 mcg per actuation [200 doses] (14.7 g) [contains soya lecithin]
Solution for oral inhalation (DuoNeb™): Ipratropium bromide 0.5 mg [0.017%] and albuterol base 2.5 mg [0.083%] per 3 mL vial (30s, 60s)

**ipratropium bromide** *see* ipratropium *on previous page*

**I-Prin [US-OTC]** *see* ibuprofen *on page 427*

**iproveratril hydrochloride** *see* verapamil *on page 843*

**IPV** *see* poliovirus vaccine (inactivated) *on page 657*

**Iquix® [US]** *see* levofloxacin *on page 475*

## irbesartan (ir be SAR tan)
Sound-Alike/Look-Alike Issues
Avapro® may be confused with Anaprox®
U.S./Canadian Brand Names Avapro® [US/Can]
Therapeutic Category Angiotensin II Receptor Antagonist
Use Treatment of hypertension alone or in combination with other antihypertensives; treatment of diabetic nephropathy in patients with type 2 diabetes mellitus (noninsulin dependent, NIDDM) and hypertension
Usual Dosage Oral:
Hypertension:
Children:
<6 years: Safety and efficacy have not been established.
≥6-12 years: Initial: 75 mg once daily; may be titrated to a maximum of 150 mg once daily
Children ≥13 years and Adults: 150 mg once daily; patients may be titrated to 300 mg once daily
**Note:** Starting dose in volume-depleted patients should be 75 mg
Nephropathy in patients with type 2 diabetes and hypertension: Adults: Target dose: 300 mg once daily
Dosage Forms Tablet: 75 mg, 150 mg, 300 mg

## irbesartan and hydrochlorothiazide (ir be SAR tan & hye droe klor oh THYE a zide)
Sound-Alike/Look-Alike Issues
Avalide® may be confused with Avandia®
Synonyms Avapro® HCT; hydrochlorothiazide and irbesartan
U.S./Canadian Brand Names Avalide® [US/Can]
Therapeutic Category Antihypertensive Agent, Combination
Use Combination therapy for the management of hypertension
Usual Dosage Dose must be individualized. A patient who is not controlled with either agent alone may be switched to the combination product. Mean effect increases with the dose of each component. The lowest dosage available is irbesartan 150 mg/hydrochlorothiazide 12.5 mg. Dose increases should be made not more frequently than every 2-4 weeks.
Dosage Forms Tablet:
Irbesartan 150 mg and hydrochlorothiazide 12.5 mg
Irbesartan 300 mg and hydrochlorothiazide 12.5 mg
Irbesartan 300 mg and hydrochlorothiazide 25 mg

**Ircon® [US-OTC]** *see* ferrous fumarate *on page 334*

**IRESSA® [US]** *see* gefitinib *on page 368*

## irinotecan (eye rye no TEE kan)
Synonyms camptothecin-11; CPT-11; NSC-616348
U.S./Canadian Brand Names Camptosar® [US/Can]
Therapeutic Category Antineoplastic Agent
Use Treatment of metastatic carcinoma of the colon or rectum
Usual Dosage I.V. (Refer to individual protocols): **Note:** A reduction in the starting dose by one dose level should be considered for patients ≥65 years of age, prior pelvic/abdominal radiotherapy, performance status of 2, homozygosity for UGT1A1*28 allele, or increased bilirubin (dosing for patients with a bilirubin >2 mg/dL cannot be recommended based on lack of data per manufacturer).
**Single-agent therapy:**
125 mg/m$^2$ over 90 minutes on days 1, 8, 15, and 22, followed by a 2-week rest
Adjusted dose level -1: 100 mg/m$^2$
(Continued)

# irinotecan *(Continued)*

Adjusted dose level -2: 75 mg/m$^2$

Once-every-3-week regimen: 350 mg/m$^2$ over 90 minutes, once every 3 weeks

Adjusted dose level -1: 300 mg/m$^2$

Adjusted dose level -2: 250 mg/m$^2$

Depending on the patient's ability to tolerate therapy, doses should be adjusted in increments of 25-50 mg/m$^2$. Irinotecan doses may range from 50-150 mg/m$^2$ for the weekly regimen. Patients may be dosed as low as 200 mg/m$^2$ (in 50 mg/m$^2$ decrements) for the once-every-3-week regimen.

**Combination therapy with fluorouracil and leucovorin:** Six-week (42-day) cycle:

Regimen 1: 125 mg/m$^2$ over 90 minutes on days 1, 8, 15, and 22; to be given in combination with bolus leucovorin and fluorouracil (leucovorin administered immediately following irinotecan; fluorouracil immediately following leucovorin)

Adjusted dose level -1: 100 mg/m$^2$

Adjusted dose level -2: 75 mg/m$^2$

Regimen 2: 180 mg/m$^2$ over 90 minutes on days 1, 15, and 29; to be given in combination with infusional leucovorin and bolus/infusion fluorouracil (leucovorin administered immediately following irinotecan; fluorouracil immediately following leucovorin)

Adjusted dose level -1: 150 mg/m$^2$

Adjusted dose level -2: 120 mg/m$^2$

**Note: For all regimens:** It is recommended that new courses begin only after the granulocyte count recovers to ≥1500/mm$^3$, the platelet count recovers to ≥100,000/mm$^3$, and treatment-related diarrhea has fully resolved. Treatment should be delayed 1-2 weeks to allow for recovery from treatment-related toxicities. If the patient has not recovered after a 2-week delay, consideration should be given to discontinuing irinotecan.

**Dosage Forms** Injection, solution, as hydrochloride: 20 mg/mL (2 mL, 5 mL)

# iron dextran complex (EYE ern DEKS tran KOM pleks)

**Sound-Alike/Look-Alike Issues**

Dexferrum® may be confused with Desferal®

**U.S./Canadian Brand Names** Dexferrum® [US]; Dexiron™ [Can]; INFeD® [US]; Infufer® [Can]

**Therapeutic Category** Electrolyte Supplement, Oral

**Use** Treatment of microcytic hypochromic anemia resulting from iron deficiency in patients in whom oral administration is infeasible or ineffective

**Usual Dosage** I.M. (Z-track method should be used for I.M. injection), I.V.:

A 0.5 mL test dose (0.25 mL in infants) should be given prior to starting iron dextran therapy; total dose should be divided into a daily schedule for I.M., total dose may be given as a single continuous infusion

Iron-deficiency anemia: Dose (mL) = 0.0476 x LBW (kg) x (normal hemoglobin - observed hemoglobin) + (1 mL/5 kg of LBW to maximum of 14 mL for iron stores)

LBW = Lean Body Weight

Iron replacement therapy for blood loss: Replacement iron (mg) = blood loss (mL) x hematocrit

Maximum daily dosage:

Manufacturer's labeling: **Note:** Replacement of larger estimated iron deficits may be achieved by serial administration of smaller incremental dosages. Daily dosages should be limited to:

Children:

5-15 kg: 50 mg iron (1 mL)

15-50 kg: 100 mg iron (2 mL)

Adults >50 kg: 100 mg iron (2 mL)

**Dosage Forms Note:** Strength expressed as elemental iron

Injection, solution:

Dexferrum®: 50 mg/mL (1 mL, 2 mL)

INFeD®: 50 mg/mL (2 mL)

**iron fumarate** *see* ferrous fumarate *on page 334*

**iron gluconate** *see* ferrous gluconate *on page 335*

**iron-polysaccharide complex** *see* polysaccharide-iron complex *on page 660*

## iron sucrose (EYE ern SOO krose)

**U.S./Canadian Brand Names** Venofer® [US/Can]

**Therapeutic Category** Iron Salt

**Use** Treatment of iron-deficiency anemia in chronic renal failure, including nondialysis-dependent patients (either receiving or not receiving erythropoietin therapy) and patients undergoing chronic hemodialysis receiving supplemental erythropoietin therapy

**Usual Dosage** Doses expressed in mg of **elemental** iron

I.V.: Adults: Iron-deficiency anemia in chronic renal disease:

Hemodialysis-dependent patient: 100 mg (5 mL of iron sucrose injection) administered 1-3 times/week during dialysis, to a total dose of 1000 mg (10 doses); administer no more than 3 times/week; may continue to administer at lowest dose necessary to maintain target hemoglobin, hematocrit, and iron storage parameters

Test dose: Product labeling does not indicate need for a test dose in product-naive patients; test doses were administered in some clinical trials as 50 mg (2.5 mL) in 50 mL 0.9% NaCl administered over 3-10 minutes

Nondialysis-dependent patient: 200 mg slow injection (over 2-5 minutes) on 5 different occasions within a 14-day period. Total cumulative dose: 1000 mg in 14-day period. **Note:** Dosage has also been administered as two infusions of 500 mg in 250 mL NS infused over 3.5-4 hours on day 1 and day 14 (limited experience)

**Dosage Forms** Injection, solution [preservative free]: 20 mg of elemental iron/mL (5 mL)

**iron sulfate** *see* ferrous sulfate *on page 335*

**iron sulfate and vitamin C** *see* ferrous sulfate and ascorbic acid *on page 335*

**ISD** *see* isosorbide dinitrate *on page 451*

**ISDN** *see* isosorbide dinitrate *on page 451*

**ISG** *see* immune globulin (intramuscular) *on page 432*

**ISMN** *see* isosorbide mononitrate *on page 452*

**Ismo® [US]** *see* isosorbide mononitrate *on page 452*

**isoamyl nitrite** *see* amyl nitrite *on page 52*

**isobamate** *see* carisoprodol *on page 148*

**Isocal® [US-OTC]** *see* nutritional formula, enteral/oral *on page 591*

## isocarboxazid (eye soe kar BOKS a zid)

**U.S./Canadian Brand Names** Marplan® [US]

**Therapeutic Category** Antidepressant, Monoamine Oxidase Inhibitor

**Use** Treatment of depression

**Usual Dosage** Adults: Oral: 10 mg 2-3 times/day; reduce to 10-20 mg/day in divided doses when condition improves

**Dosage Forms** Tablet: 10 mg

**Isochron™ [US]** *see* isosorbide dinitrate *on page 451*

## isoflurane (eye soe FLURE ane)

**Sound-Alike/Look-Alike Issues**

isoflurane may be confused with enflurane, isoflurophate

**U.S./Canadian Brand Names** Forane® [US/Can]

**Therapeutic Category** General Anesthetic

**Use** Maintenance of general anesthesia

**Usual Dosage** Minimum alveolar concentration (MAC), the concentration at which 50% of patients do not respond to surgical incision, is 1.2% for isoflurane. The concentration at which amnesia and loss of awareness occur (MAC - awake) is 0.4%. Surgical levels of anesthesia are achieved with concentrations between 1% to 2.5%.

**Dosage Forms** Solution: 100 mL, 250 mL

## Isollyl® Improved *(Discontinued)*

**isometheptene, acetaminophen, and dichloralphenazone** *see* acetaminophen, isometheptene, and dichloralphenazone *on page 12*

**isometheptene, dichloralphenazone, and acetaminophen** *see* acetaminophen, isomethep-tene, and dichloralphenazone *on page 12*

## isoniazid (eye soe NYE a zid)
**Synonyms** INH; isonicotinic acid hydrazide
**U.S./Canadian Brand Names** Isotamine® [Can]; PMS-Isoniazid [Can]
**Therapeutic Category** Antitubercular Agent
**Use** Treatment of susceptible tuberculosis infections; treatment of latent tuberculosis infection (LTBI)
**Usual Dosage** Recommendations often change due to resistant strains and newly-developed informa-tion; consult *MMWR* for current CDC recommendations:
Oral (injectable is available for patients who are unable to either take or absorb oral therapy):
**Infants and Children:**
Treatment of latent TB infection (LTBI): 10-20 mg/kg/day in 1-2 divided doses (maximum: 300 mg/day) or 20-40 mg/kg (maximum: 900 mg/dose) twice weekly for 9 months
Treatment of active TB infection:
Daily therapy: 10-15 mg/kg/day in 1-2 divided doses (maximum: 300 mg/day)
Twice weekly directly observed therapy (DOT): 20-30 mg/kg (maximum: 900 mg)
**Adults:**
Treatment of latent tuberculosis infection (LTBI): 300 mg/day or 900 mg twice weekly for 6-9 months in patients who do not have HIV infection (9 months is optimal, 6 months may be considered to reduce costs of therapy) and 9 months in patients who have HIV infection. Extend to 12 months of therapy if interruptions in treatment occur.
Treatment of active TB infection (drug susceptible):
Daily therapy: 5 mg/kg/day given daily (usual dose: 300 mg/day); 10 mg/kg/day in 1-2 divided doses in patients with disseminated disease
Twice weekly directly observed therapy (DOT): 15 mg/kg (maximum: 900 mg); 3 times/week therapy: 15 mg/kg (maximum: 900 mg)
**Note:** Treatment may be defined by the number of doses administered (eg, "six-month" therapy involves 192 doses of INH and rifampin, and 56 doses of pyrazinamide). Six months is the shortest interval of time over which these doses may be administered, assuming no interruption of therapy.
**Note:** Concomitant administration of 6-50 mg/day pyridoxine is recommended in malnourished patients or those prone to neuropathy (eg, alcoholics, diabetics)
**Dosage Forms**
Injection, solution (Nydrazid®): 100 mg/mL (10 mL) [DSC]
Syrup: 50 mg/5 mL (473 mL) [orange flavor]
Tablet: 100 mg, 300 mg

**isoniazid and rifampin** *see* rifampin and isoniazid *on page 722*

**isoniazid, rifampin, and pyrazinamide** *see* rifampin, isoniazid, and pyrazinamide *on page 723*

**isonicotinic acid hydrazide** *see* isoniazid *on this page*

**isonipecaine hydrochloride** *see* meperidine *on page 512*

**isophosphamide** *see* ifosfamide *on page 430*

## isoproterenol (eye soe proe TER e nole)
**Sound-Alike/Look-Alike Issues**
Isuprel® may be confused with Disophrol®, Ismelin®, Isordil®
**Synonyms** isoproterenol hydrochloride
**U.S./Canadian Brand Names** Isuprel® [US]
**Therapeutic Category** Adrenergic Agonist Agent
**Use** Ventricular arrhythmias due to AV nodal block; hemodynamically compromised bradyarrhythmias or atropine- and dopamine-resistant bradyarrhythmias (when transcutaneous/venous pacing is not avail-able); temporary use in third-degree AV block until pacemaker insertion
**Usual Dosage** I.V.: Cardiac arrhythmias:
Children: Initial: 0.1 mcg/kg/minute (usual effective dose 0.2-2 mcg/kg/minute)
Adults: Initial: 2 mcg/minute; titrate to patient response (2-10 mcg/minute)
**Dosage Forms** Injection, solution, as hydrochloride: 0.02 mg/mL (10 mL); 0.2 mg/mL (1:5000) (1 mL, 5 mL) [contains sodium metabisulfite]

**isoproterenol hydrochloride** *see* isoproterenol *on this page*

**Isoptin**® *(Discontinued)* *see* verapamil *on page 843*

**Isoptin**® **SR [US/Can]** *see* verapamil *on page 843*

**Isopto**® **Atropine [US/Can]** *see* atropine *on page 79*

**Isopto**® **Carbachol [US/Can]** *see* carbachol *on page 140*

**Isopto**® **Carpine [US/Can]** *see* pilocarpine *on page 647*

**Isopto**® **Cetapred**® *(Discontinued)*

**Isopto**® **Eserine [Can]** *see* physostigmine *on page 646*

**Isopto**® **Eserine** *(Discontinued)* *see* physostigmine *on page 646*

**Isopto**® **Frin Ophthalmic Solution** *(Discontinued)* *see* phenylephrine *on page 640*

**Isopto**® **Homatropine [US]** *see* homatropine *on page 405*

**Isopto**® **Hyoscine [US]** *see* scopolamine derivatives *on page 740*

**Isopto**® **Plain Solution** *(Discontinued)* *see* artificial tears *on page 71*

**Isopto**® **Tears [US-OTC]** *see* artificial tears *on page 71*

**Isordil**® **[US]** *see* isosorbide dinitrate *on this page*

## isosorbide dinitrate (eye soe SOR bide dye NYE trate)

**Sound-Alike/Look-Alike Issues**
Isordil® may be confused with Inderal®, Isuprel®

**Synonyms** ISD; ISDN

**U.S./Canadian Brand Names** Apo-ISDN® [Can]; Cedocard®-SR [Can]; Coronex® [Can]; Dilatrate®-SR [US]; Isochron™ [US]; Isordil® [US]; Novo-Sorbide [Can]; PMS-Isosorbide [Can]

**Therapeutic Category** Vasodilator

**Use** Prevention and treatment of angina pectoris; for congestive heart failure; to relieve pain, dysphagia, and spasm in esophageal spasm with GE reflux

**Usual Dosage** Adults Oral:
Angina: 5-40 mg 4 times/day or 40 mg every 8-12 hours in sustained-release dosage form
Congestive heart failure:
  Initial dose: 10 mg 3 times/day
  Target dose: 40 mg 3 times/day
  Maximum dose: 80 mg 3 times/day
Sublingual: 2.5-10 mg every 4-6 hours
Chewable tablet: 5-10 mg every 2-3 hours
**Tolerance to nitrate effects develops with chronic exposure:** Dose escalation does not overcome this effect. Tolerance can only be overcome by short periods of nitrate absence from the body. Short periods (10-12 hours) of nitrate withdrawal help minimize tolerance. General recommendations are to take the last dose of short-acting agents no later than 7 PM; administer 2-3 times/day rather than 4 times/day. Sustained release preparations could be administered at times to allow a 15- to 17-hour interval between first and last daily dose. Example: Administer sustained release at 8 AM and 2 PM for a twice daily regimen.

**Dosage Forms** [DSC] = Discontinued product
Capsule, sustained release (Dilatrate®-SR): 40 mg
Tablet: 5 mg, 10 mg, 20 mg, 30 mg,
  Isordil®: 5 mg, 10 mg [DSC], 20 mg [DSC], 30 mg [DSC], 40 mg
Tablet, extended release (Isochron™): 40 mg
Tablet, sublingual: 2.5 mg, 5 mg
  Isordil®: 2.5 mg, 5 mg, 10 mg [DSC]

## isosorbide dinitrate and hydralazine
(eye soe SOR bide dye NYE trate & hye DRAL a zeen)

**Synonyms** hydralazine and isosorbide dinitrate

**U.S./Canadian Brand Names** BiDil® [US]

**Therapeutic Category** Vasodilator

**Use** Treatment of heart failure, adjunct to standard therapy, in self identified African-Americans

**Usual Dosage** Oral: Adults: Initial: 1 tablet 3 times/day; titrate to a maximum dose of 2 tablets 3 times/day

**Dosage Forms** Tablet: Isosorbide dinitrate 20 mg and hydralazine 37.5 mg

# isosorbide mononitrate (eye soe SOR bide mon oh NYE trate)

**Sound-Alike/Look-Alike Issues**
Imdur® may be confused with Imuran®, Inderal LA®, K-Dur®
Monoket® may be confused with Monopril®

**Synonyms** ISMN

**U.S./Canadian Brand Names** Imdur® [US/Can]; Ismo® [US]; Monoket® [US]

**Therapeutic Category** Vasodilator

**Use** Long-acting metabolite of the vasodilator isosorbide dinitrate used for the prophylactic treatment of angina pectoris

**Usual Dosage** Adults and Geriatrics (start with lowest recommended dose): Oral:
Regular tablet: 5-10 mg twice daily with the two doses given 7 hours apart (eg, 8 AM and 3 PM) to decrease tolerance development; then titrate to 10 mg twice daily in first 2-3 days.
Extended release tablet: Initial: 30-60 mg given in morning as a single dose; titrate upward as needed, giving at least 3 days between increases; maximum daily single dose: 240 mg

**Dosage Forms**
Tablet: 10 mg, 20 mg
Ismo®: 20 mg
Monoket®: 10 mg, 20 mg
Tablet, extended release (Imdur®): 30 mg, 60 mg, 120 mg

**isosulfan blue** *see* radiological/contrast media (ionic) *on page 707*

**Isotamine® [Can]** *see* isoniazid *on page 450*

# isotretinoin (eye soe TRET i noyn)

**Sound-Alike/Look-Alike Issues**
Accutane® may be confused with Accolate®, Accupril®

**Synonyms** 13-*cis*-retinoic acid

**U.S./Canadian Brand Names** Accutane® [US/Can]; Amnesteem™ [US]; Claravis™ [US]; Isotrex® [Can]; Sotret® [US]

**Therapeutic Category** Retinoic Acid Derivative

**Use** Treatment of severe recalcitrant nodular acne unresponsive to conventional therapy

**Usual Dosage** Oral:
Children: Maintenance therapy for neuroblastoma (investigational): 100-250 mg/m$^2$/day in 2 divided doses
Children and Adults: Severe recalcitrant nodular acne: 0.5-2 mg/kg/day in 2 divided doses (dosages as low as 0.05 mg/kg/day have been reported to be beneficial) for 15-20 weeks or until the total cyst count decreases by 70%, whichever is sooner. A second course of therapy may be initiated after a period of ≥2 months off therapy.

**Dosage Forms** Capsule:
Accutane®: 10 mg, 20 mg, 40 mg [contains soybean oil and parabens]
Amnesteem™: 10 mg, 20 mg, 40 mg [contains soybean oil]
Claravis™: 10 mg, 20 mg, 40 mg
Sotret®: 10 mg, 20 mg, 30 mg, 40 mg [contains soybean oil]

**Isotrex® [Can]** *see* isotretinoin *on this page*

**Isovue® [US]** *see* radiological/contrast media (nonionic) *on page 709*

# isoxsuprine (eye SOKS syoo preen)

**Sound-Alike/Look-Alike Issues**
Vasodilan® may be confused with Vasocidin®

**Synonyms** isoxsuprine hydrochloride

**Therapeutic Category** Vasodilator

**Use** Treatment of peripheral vascular diseases, such as arteriosclerosis obliterans and Raynaud disease

**Usual Dosage** Oral: Adults: 10-20 mg 3-4 times/day

**Dosage Forms** Tablet, as hydrochloride: 10 mg, 20 mg

**isoxsuprine hydrochloride** *see* isoxsuprine *on this page*

# isradipine (iz RA di peen)

**Sound-Alike/Look-Alike Issues**

DynaCirc® may be confused with Dynabac®, Dynacin®

**U.S./Canadian Brand Names** DynaCirc® CR [US]; DynaCirc® [US/Can]

**Therapeutic Category** Calcium Channel Blocker

**Use** Treatment of hypertension

**Usual Dosage** Oral: Adults: 2.5 mg twice daily; antihypertensive response occurs in 2-3 hours; maximal response in 2-4 weeks; increase dose at 2- to 4-week intervals at 2.5-5 mg increments; usual dose range (JNC 7): 2.5-10 mg/day in 2 divided doses. **Note:** Most patients show no improvement with doses >10 mg/day except adverse reaction rate increases; therefore, maximal dose in older adults should be 10 mg/day.

**Dosage Forms**

Capsule (DynaCirc®): 2.5 mg, 5 mg

Tablet, controlled release (DynaCirc® CR): 5 mg, 10 mg

**Istalol™ [US]** *see* timolol *on page 803*

**Isuprel® [US]** *see* isoproterenol *on page 450*

**Itch-X® [US-OTC]** *see* pramoxine *on page 670*

# itraconazole (i tra KOE na zole)

**Sound-Alike/Look-Alike Issues**

Sporanox® may be confused with Suprax®

**U.S./Canadian Brand Names** Sporanox® [US/Can]

**Therapeutic Category** Antifungal Agent

**Use** Treatment of susceptible fungal infections in immunocompromised and immunocompetent patients including blastomycosis and histoplasmosis; indicated for aspergillosis, and onychomycosis of the toenail; treatment of onychomycosis of the fingernail without concomitant toenail infection via a pulse-type dosing regimen; has activity against *Aspergillus*, *Candida*, *Coccidioides*, *Cryptococcus*, *Sporothrix*, tinea unguium

Oral: Useful in superficial mycoses including dermatophytoses (eg, tinea capitis), pityriasis versicolor, sebopsoriasis, vaginal and chronic mucocutaneous candidiases; systemic mycoses including candidiasis, meningeal and disseminated cryptococcal infections, paracoccidioidomycosis, coccidioidomycoses; miscellaneous mycoses such as sporotrichosis, chromomycosis, leishmaniasis, fungal keratitis, alternariosis, zygomycosis

Oral solution: Treatment of oral and esophageal candidiasis

Intravenous solution: Indicated in the treatment of blastomycosis, histoplasmosis (nonmeningeal), and aspergillosis (in patients intolerant or refractory to amphotericin B therapy); empiric therapy of febrile neutropenic fever

**Usual Dosage Note:** Capsule: Absorption is best if taken with food, therefore, it is best to administer itraconazole after meals; Solution: Should be taken on an empty stomach.

Children: Efficacy and safety have not been established; a small number of patients 3-16 years of age have been treated with 100 mg/day for systemic fungal infections with no serious adverse effects reported. A dose of 5 mg/kg once daily was used in a pharmacokinetic study using the oral solution in patients 6 months to 12 years; duration of study was 2 weeks.

Adults:

Oral:

Blastomycosis/histoplasmosis: 200 mg once daily, if no obvious improvement or there is evidence of progressive fungal disease, increase the dose in 100 mg increments to a maximum of 400 mg/day; doses >200 mg/day are given in 2 divided doses; length of therapy varies from 1 day to >6 months depending on the condition and mycological response

Aspergillosis: 200-400 mg/day

Onychomycosis: 200 mg once daily for 12 consecutive weeks

Life-threatening infections: Loading dose: 200 mg 3 times/day (600 mg/day) should be given for the first 3 days of therapy

Oropharyngeal candidiasis: Oral solution: 200 mg once daily for 1-2 weeks; in patients unresponsive or refractory to fluconazole: 100 mg twice daily (clinical response expected in 1-2 weeks)

Esophageal candidiasis: Oral solution: 100-200 mg once daily for a minimum of 3 weeks; continue dosing for 2 weeks after resolution of symptoms

I.V.: 200 mg twice daily for 4 doses, followed by 200 mg daily

(Continued)

## itraconazole (Continued)

**Dosage Forms**
Capsule: 100 mg
Injection, solution: 10 mg/mL (25 mL) [packaged in a kit containing sodium chloride 0.9% (50 mL); filtered infusion set (1)]
Solution, oral: 100 mg/10 mL (150 mL) [cherry flavor]

**I-Tropine® *(Discontinued)*** see atropine *on page 79*

**Iveegam EN [US]** see immune globulin (intravenous) *on page 433*

**Iveegam Immuno® [Can]** see immune globulin (intravenous) *on page 433*

## ivermectin (eye ver MEK tin)

**U.S./Canadian Brand Names** Stromectol® [US]

**Therapeutic Category** Antibiotic, Miscellaneous

**Use** Treatment of the following infections: Strongyloidiasis of the intestinal tract due to the nematode parasite *Strongyloides stercoralis*. Onchocerciasis due to the nematode parasite *Onchocerca volvulus*. Ivermectin is only active against the immature form of *Onchocerca volvulus*, and the intestinal forms of *Strongyloides stercoralis*.

**Usual Dosage** Oral: Children ≥15 kg and Adults:
Strongyloidiasis: 200 mcg/kg as a single dose; follow-up stool examinations
Onchocerciasis: 150 mcg/kg as a single dose; retreatment may be required every 3-12 months until the adult worms die

**Dosage Forms** Tablet [scored]: 3 mg

**IVIG** see immune globulin (intravenous) *on page 433*

**IvyBlock® [US-OTC]** see bentoquatam *on page 94*

**Ivy-Rid® [US-OTC]** see benzocaine *on page 95*

**IvySoothe® [US-OTC]** see hydrocortisone (topical) *on page 417*

**Janimine® *(Discontinued)*** see imipramine *on page 432*

**Jantoven™ [US]** see warfarin *on page 854*

## Japanese encephalitis virus vaccine (inactivated)

(jap a NEESE en sef a LYE tis VYE rus vak SEEN, in ak ti VAY ted)

**U.S./Canadian Brand Names** JE-VAX® [US/Can]

**Therapeutic Category** Vaccine, Inactivated Virus

**Use** Active immunization against Japanese encephalitis for persons 1 year of age and older who plan to spend 1 month or more in endemic areas in Asia, especially persons traveling during the transmission season or visiting rural areas; consider vaccination for shorter trips to epidemic areas or extensive outdoor activities in rural endemic areas; elderly (>55 years of age) individuals should be considered for vaccination, since they have increased risk of developing symptomatic illness after infection; those planning travel to or residence in endemic areas should consult the Travel Advisory Service (Central Campus) for specific advice

**Usual Dosage** U.S. recommended primary immunization schedule:
Children 1-3 years: SubQ: Three 0.5 mL doses given on days 0, 7, and 30; abbreviated schedules should be used only when necessary due to time constraints
Children >3 years and Adults: SubQ: Three 1 mL doses given on days 0, 7, and 30. Give third dose on day 14 when time does not permit waiting; 2 doses a week apart produce immunity in about 80% of recipients; the longest regimen yields highest titers after 6 months.
Booster dose: Give after 2 years, or according to current recommendation
**Note:** Travel should not commence for at least 10 days after the last dose of vaccine, to allow adequate antibody formation and recognition of any delayed adverse reaction
Advise concurrent use of other means to reduce the risk of mosquito exposure when possible, including bed nets, insect repellents, protective clothing, avoidance of travel in endemic areas, and avoidance of outdoor activity during twilight and evening periods

**Dosage Forms** Injection, powder for reconstitution: 1 mL, 10 mL

**Jenamicin® *(Discontinued)*** see gentamicin *on page 372*

**Jenest™-28 *(Discontinued)*** see ethinyl estradiol and norethindrone *on page 314*

**JE-VAX® [US/Can]** see Japanese encephalitis virus vaccine (inactivated) *on this page*

**Jolivette**™ **[US]** *see* norethindrone *on page 582*

**Junel**™ **[US]** *see* ethinyl estradiol and norethindrone *on page 314*

**Junel**™ **Fe [US]** *see* ethinyl estradiol and norethindrone *on page 314*

**Just Tears**® **Solution** *(Discontinued) see* artificial tears *on page 71*

**K-10**® **[Can]** *see* potassium chloride *on page 663*

**Kabikinase**® *(Discontinued) see* streptokinase *on page 766*

**Kadian**® **[US/Can]** *see* morphine sulfate *on page 549*

**Kala**® **[US-OTC]** *see* Lactobacillus *on page 462*

**Kalcinate**® *(Discontinued) see* calcium gluconate *on page 134*

**Kaletra**® **[US/Can]** *see* lopinavir and ritonavir *on page 490*

**Kalmz [US-OTC]** *see* fructose, dextrose, and phosphoric acid *on page 362*

## kanamycin (kan a MYE sin)

**Sound-Alike/Look-Alike Issues**
  kanamycin may be confused with Garamycin®, gentamicin
**Synonyms** kanamycin sulfate
**U.S./Canadian Brand Names** Kantrex® [US/Can]
**Therapeutic Category** Aminoglycoside (Antibiotic)
**Use** Treatment of serious infections caused by susceptible strains of *E. coli*, *Proteus* species, *Entero-bacter aerogenes*, *Klebsiella pneumoniae*, *Serratia marcescens*, and *Acinetobacter* species; second-line treatment of *Mycobacterium tuberculosis*
**Usual Dosage Note:** Dosing should be based on ideal body weight
  Children: Infections: I.M., I.V.: 15 mg/kg/day in divided doses every 8-12 hours
  Adults:
    Infections: I.M., I.V.: 5-7.5 mg/kg/dose in divided doses every 8-12 hours (<15 mg/kg/day)
    Intraperitoneal: After contamination in surgery: 500 mg
    Irrigating solution: 0.25%; maximum 1.5 g/day (via all administration routes)
    Aerosol: 250 mg 2-4 times/day
**Dosage Forms** Injection, solution, as sulfate: 1 g/3 mL (3 mL) [contains sodium bisulfate]

**kanamycin sulfate** *see* kanamycin *on this page*

**Kank-A**® **[Can]** *see* cetylpyridinium and benzocaine *on page 164*

**Kanka**® **Soft Brush**™ **[US-OTC]** *see* benzocaine *on page 95*

**Kantrex**® **[US/Can]** *see* kanamycin *on this page*

**Kaochlor-Eff**® *(Discontinued)*

**Kaochlor**® **SF** *(Discontinued) see* potassium chloride *on page 663*

**Kaodene**® *(Discontinued) see* kaolin and pectin *on this page*

**Kaodene**® **NN** *(Discontinued) see* kaolin and pectin *on this page*

## kaolin and pectin (KAY oh lin & PEK tin)

**Synonyms** pectin and kaolin
**Therapeutic Category** Antidiarrheal
**Use** Treatment of uncomplicated diarrhea
**Usual Dosage** Oral:
  Children:
    <6 years: Do not use
    6-12 years: 30-60 mL after each loose stool
  Adults: 60-120 mL after each loose stool
**Dosage Forms** [DSC] = Discontinued product
  Suspension, oral:
    Kaodene® NN: Kaolin 650 mg and pectin 32.4 mg per 5 mL (120 mL) [contains bismuth subsalicylate 2.8 mg/5 mL] [DSC]
    Kao-Spen®: Kaolin 860 mg and pectin 43 mg per 5 mL (3840 mL) [DSC]
    Kapectolin®: Kaolin 15 g and pectin 33 mg per 5 mL (480 mL) [DSC]

**Kaon-Cl-10**® **[US]** *see* potassium chloride *on page 663*

Kaon-Cl® 20 [US] *see* potassium chloride *on page 663*

Kao-Paverin® [US-OTC] *see* loperamide *on page 489*

Kaopectate® [OTC] *see* bismuth subsalicylate *on page 108*

Kaopectate® II *(Discontinued) see* loperamide *on page 489*

Kaopectate® Advanced Formula *(Discontinued) see* attapulgite *on page 81*

Kaopectate® Extra Strength [OTC] *see* bismuth subsalicylate *on page 108*

Kaopectate® Maximum Strength Caplets *(Discontinued) see* attapulgite *on page 81*

Kao-Spen® *(Discontinued) see* kaolin and pectin *on previous page*

Kapectolin® *(Discontinued) see* kaolin and pectin *on previous page*

Karidium® *(Discontinued) see* fluoride *on page 347*

Karigel® *(Discontinued) see* fluoride *on page 347*

Karigel®-N *(Discontinued) see* fluoride *on page 347*

Kariva™ [US] *see* ethinyl estradiol and desogestrel *on page 309*

Kasof® *(Discontinued) see* docusate *on page 263*

Kaybovite-1000® *(Discontinued) see* cyanocobalamin *on page 212*

Kay Ciel® [US] *see* potassium chloride *on page 663*

Kayexalate® [US/Can] *see* sodium polystyrene sulfonate *on page 758*

K-Citra® [Can] *see* potassium citrate *on page 664*

KCl *see* potassium chloride *on page 663*

K-Dur® [Can] *see* potassium chloride *on page 663*

K-Dur® 10 [US] *see* potassium chloride *on page 663*

K-Dur® 20 [US] *see* potassium chloride *on page 663*

Keflex® [US] *see* cephalexin *on page 161*

Keftab® [Can] *see* cephalexin *on page 161*

Kefurox® Injection *(Discontinued) see* cefuroxime *on page 158*

Kefzol® *(Discontinued) see* cefazolin *on page 153*

K-Electrolyte® Effervescent *(Discontinued) see* potassium bicarbonate *on page 662*

Kemadrin® [US] *see* procyclidine *on page 681*

Kemsol® [Can] *see* dimethyl sulfoxide *on page 253*

Kenacort® Oral *(Discontinued)*

Kenaject® Injection *(Discontinued)*

Kenalog® [US/Can] *see* triamcinolone (systemic) *on page 819*

Kenalog-10® [US] *see* triamcinolone (systemic) *on page 819*

Kenalog-40® [US] *see* triamcinolone (systemic) *on page 819*

Kenalog® in Orabase [Can] *see* triamcinolone (topical) *on page 820*

Kenonel® Topical *(Discontinued)*

keoxifene hydrochloride *see* raloxifene *on page 710*

Kepivance™ [US] *see* palifermin *on page 613*

Keppra® [US/Can] *see* levetiracetam *on page 472*

Keralyt® [Can] *see* salicylic acid and propylene glycol *on page 736*

Kerlac® [US] *see* urea *on page 834*

Kerlone® [US] *see* betaxolol *on page 104*

Kerr Insta-Char® [US-OTC] *see* charcoal *on page 165*

Ketalar® [US/Can] *see* ketamine *on this page*

## ketamine (KEET a meen)

### Sound-Alike/Look-Alike Issues

Ketalar® may be confused with Kenalog®

**Synonyms** ketamine hydrochloride
**U.S./Canadian Brand Names** Ketalar® [US/Can]
**Therapeutic Category** General Anesthetic
**Controlled Substance** C-III
**Use** Induction and maintenance of general anesthesia, especially when cardiovascular depression must be avoided (ie, hypotension, hypovolemia, cardiomyopathy, constrictive pericarditis); sedation; analgesia
**Usual Dosage** Used in combination with anticholinergic agents to decrease hypersalivation
Children:
Oral: 6-10 mg/kg for 1 dose (mixed in 0.2-0.3 mL/kg of cola or other beverage) given 30 minutes before the procedure
I.M.: 3-7 mg/kg
I.V.: Range: 0.5-2 mg/kg, use smaller doses (0.5-1 mg/kg) for sedation for minor procedures; usual induction dosage: 1-2 mg/kg
Continuous I.V. infusion: Sedation: 5-20 mcg/kg/minute
Adults:
I.M.: 3-8 mg/kg
I.V.: Range: 1-4.5 mg/kg; usual induction dosage: 1-2 mg/kg
Children and Adults: Maintenance: Supplemental doses of $^1/_3$ to $^1/_2$ of initial dose
**Dosage Forms**
Injection, solution: 50 mg/mL (10 mL); 100 mg/mL (5 mL)
Ketalar®: 10 mg/mL (20 mL); 50 mg/mL (10 mL); 100 mg/mL (5 mL)

**ketamine hydrochloride** *see* ketamine *on previous page*

**Ketek® [US/Can]** *see* telithromycin *on page 783*

# ketoconazole (kee toe KOE na zole)
**Sound-Alike/Look-Alike Issues**
Nizoral® may be confused with Nasarel®, Neoral®, Nitrol®
**U.S./Canadian Brand Names** Apo-Ketoconazole® [Can]; Ketoderm® [Can]; Nizoral® A-D [US-OTC]; Nizoral® [US]; Novo-Ketoconazole [Can]
**Therapeutic Category** Antifungal Agent
**Use** Treatment of susceptible fungal infections, including candidiasis, oral thrush, blastomycosis, histoplasmosis, paracoccidioidomycosis, coccidioidomycosis, chromomycosis, candiduria, chronic mucocutaneous candidiasis, as well as certain recalcitrant cutaneous dermatophytoses; used topically for treatment of tinea corporis, tinea cruris, tinea versicolor, and cutaneous candidiasis, seborrheic dermatitis
**Usual Dosage** Fungal infections:
Oral:
Children ≥2 years: 3.3-6.6 mg/kg/day as a single dose for 1-2 weeks for candidiasis, for at least 4 weeks in recalcitrant dermatophyte infections, and for up to 6 months for other systemic mycoses
Adults: 200-400 mg/day as a single daily dose for durations as stated above
Shampoo: Apply twice weekly for 4 weeks with at least 3 days between each shampoo
Topical: Rub gently into the affected area once daily to twice daily
**Dosage Forms**
Cream, topical: 2% (15 g, 30 g, 60 g)
Shampoo, topical (Nizoral® A-D): 1% (6 mL, 120 mL, 210 mL)
Tablet (Nizoral®): 200 mg

**Ketoderm® [Can]** *see* ketoconazole *on this page*

# ketoprofen (kee toe PROE fen)
**Sound-Alike/Look-Alike Issues**
Oruvail® may be confused with Clinoril®, Elavil®
**U.S./Canadian Brand Names** Apo-Keto SR® [Can]; Apo-Keto-E® [Can]; Apo-Keto® [Can]; Novo-Keto [Can]; Novo-Keto-EC [Can]; Nu-Ketoprofen [Can]; Nu-Ketoprofen-E [Can]; Oruvail® [Can]; Rhodis SR™ [Can]; Rhodis-EC™ [Can]; Rhodis™ [Can]
**Therapeutic Category** Analgesic, Nonnarcotic; Nonsteroidal Antiinflammatory Drug (NSAID)
**Use** Acute and long-term treatment of rheumatoid arthritis and osteoarthritis; primary dysmenorrhea; mild to moderate pain
(Continued)

# ketoprofen *(Continued)*

**Usual Dosage** Oral: Children ≥16 years and Adults:

Rheumatoid arthritis or osteoarthritis:
  Capsule: 50-75 mg 3-4 times/day up to a maximum of 300 mg/day
  Capsule, extended release: 200 mg once daily
  Mild to moderate pain: Capsule: 25-50 mg every 6-8 hours up to a maximum of 300 mg/day
  OTC labeling: 12.5 mg every 4-6 hours, up to a maximum of 6 tablets/24 hours
**Dosage Forms** [DSC] = Discontinued product
  Capsule: 50 mg, 75 mg
  Capsule, extended release: 200 mg
  Tablet (Orudis® KT): 12.5 mg [contains tartrazine and sodium benzoate] [DSC]

# ketorolac (KEE toe role ak)

**Sound-Alike/Look-Alike Issues**
  Acular® may be confused with Acthar®, Ocular®
  Toradol® may be confused with Foradil®, Inderal®, Tegretol®, Torecan®, tramadol
**Synonyms** ketorolac tromethamine
**U.S./Canadian Brand Names** Acular LS™ [US/Can]; Acular® PF [US]; Acular® [US/Can]; Apo-Ketorolac Injectable® [Can]; Apo-Ketorolac® [Can]; Novo-Ketorolac [Can]; ratio-Ketorolac [Can]; Toradol® IM [Can]; Toradol® [US/Can]
**Therapeutic Category** Analgesic, Nonnarcotic; Nonsteroidal Antiinflammatory Drug (NSAID)
**Use**

Oral, injection: Short-term (≤5 days) management of moderately-severe acute pain requiring analgesia at the opioid level
Ophthalmic: Temporary relief of ocular itching due to seasonal allergic conjunctivitis; postoperative inflammation following cataract extraction; reduction of ocular pain and photophobia following incisional refractive surgery, reduction of ocular pain, burning and stinging following corneal refractive surgery

**Usual Dosage**

Children 2-16 years: **Do not exceed adult doses**
  Single-dose treatment:
    I.M.: 1 mg/kg (maximum: 30 mg)
    I.V.: 0.5 mg/kg (maximum: 15 mg)

Adults (pain relief usually begins within 10 minutes with parenteral forms): **Note:** The maximum combined duration of treatment (for parenteral and oral) is 5 days; do not increase dose or frequency; supplement with low-dose opioids if needed for breakthrough pain.
  I.M.: 60 mg as a single dose or 30 mg every 6 hours (maximum daily dose: 120 mg)
  I.V.: 30 mg as a single dose or 30 mg every 6 hours (maximum daily dose: 120 mg)
  Oral: 20 mg, followed by 10 mg every 4-6 hours; do not exceed 40 mg/day; oral dosing is intended to be a continuation of I.M. or I.V. therapy only
Ophthalmic: Children ≥3 years and Adults:
  Allergic conjunctivitis (relief of ocular itching) (Acular®): Instill 1 drop (0.25 mg) 4 times/day for seasonal allergic conjunctivitis
  Inflammation following cataract extraction (Acular®): Instill 1 drop (0.25 mg) to affected eye(s) 4 times/day beginning 24 hours after surgery; continue for 2 weeks
  Pain and photophobia following incisional refractive surgery (Acular® PF): Instill 1 drop (0.25 mg) 4 times/day to affected eye for up to 3 days
  Pain following corneal refractive surgery (Acular LS™): Instill 1 drop 4 times/day as needed to affected eye for up to 4 days

**Dosage Forms**
  Injection, solution, as tromethamine: 15 mg/mL (1 mL); 30 mg/mL (1 mL, 2 mL, 10 mL) [contains alcohol]
  Solution, ophthalmic, as tromethamine:
    Acular®: 0.5% (3 mL, 5 mL, 10 mL) [contains benzalkonium chloride]
    Acular LS™: 0.4% (5 mL) [contains benzalkonium chloride]
    Acular® P.F. [preservative free]: 0.5% (0.4 mL)
  Tablet, as tromethamine (Toradol®): 10 mg

**ketorolac tromethamine** *see ketorolac on this page*

# ketotifen (kee toe TYE fen)

**Synonyms** ketotifen fumarate
**U.S./Canadian Brand Names** Apo-Ketotifen® [Can]; Novo-Ketotifen [Can]; Zaditen® [Can]; Zaditor™ [US/Can]

**Therapeutic Category** Antihistamine, $H_1$ Blocker, Ophthalmic

**Use** Temporary prevention of eye itching due to allergic conjunctivitis

**Usual Dosage** Children ≥3 years and Adults: Ophthalmic: Instill 1 drop into the affected eye(s) twice daily, every 8-12 hours

**Dosage Forms** Solution, ophthalmic, as fumarate: 0.025% (5 mL) [contains benzalkonium chloride]

**ketotifen fumarate** *see* ketotifen *on previous page*

**Key-E® [US-OTC]** *see* vitamin E *on page 850*

**Key-E® Kaps [US-OTC]** *see* vitamin E *on page 850*

**Keygesic [US-OTC]** *see* magnesium salicylate *on page 499*

**Key-Pred®** *(Discontinued)*

**Key-Pred-SP®** *(Discontinued)*

**K-G®** *(Discontinued) see* potassium gluconate *on page 665*

**K-Gen® Effervescent** *(Discontinued) see* potassium bicarbonate *on page 662*

**KI** *see* potassium iodide *on page 665*

**K-Ide®** *(Discontinued)*

**Kidkare Cough and Cold [US-OTC]** *see* chlorpheniramine, pseudoephedrine, and dextromethorphan *on page 177*

**Kidkare Decongestant [US-OTC]** *see* pseudoephedrine *on page 692*

**Kidrolase® [Can]** *see* asparaginase *on page 72*

**Kinerase®** *(Discontinued) see* hyaluronidase *on page 407*

**Kineret® [US/Can]** *see* anakinra *on page 52*

**Kinesed®** *(Discontinued) see* hyoscyamine, atropine, scopolamine, and phenobarbital *on page 425*

**Kinevac® [US]** *see* sincalide *on page 749*

**Kionex™ [US]** *see* sodium polystyrene sulfonate *on page 758*

**Klaron® [US]** *see* sulfacetamide *on page 771*

**Klean-Prep® [Can]** *see* polyethylene glycol-electrolyte solution *on page 658*

**K-Lease®** *(Discontinued) see* potassium chloride *on page 663*

**Klerist-D® Tablet** *(Discontinued) see* chlorpheniramine and pseudoephedrine *on page 172*

**Klonopin® [US/Can]** *see* clonazepam *on page 197*

**K-Lor® [US/Can]** *see* potassium chloride *on page 663*

**Klor-Con® [US]** *see* potassium chloride *on page 663*

**Klor-Con® 8 [US]** *see* potassium chloride *on page 663*

**Klor-Con® 10 [US]** *see* potassium chloride *on page 663*

**Klor-Con®/25 [US]** *see* potassium chloride *on page 663*

**Klor-Con® M [US]** *see* potassium chloride *on page 663*

**Klor-Con®/EF [US]** *see* potassium bicarbonate and potassium citrate, effervescent *on page 663*

**Klorominr® Oral** *(Discontinued) see* chlorpheniramine *on page 171*

**Klorvess®** *(Discontinued) see* potassium chloride *on page 663*

**Klorvess® Effervescent** *(Discontinued)*

**K-Lyte® [Can]** *see* potassium citrate *on page 664*

**K-Lyte/Cl® [US]** *see* potassium bicarbonate and potassium chloride, effervescent *on page 662*

**K-Lyte/Cl® 50 [US]** *see* potassium bicarbonate and potassium chloride, effervescent *on page 662*

**K-Lyte® DS [US]** *see* potassium bicarbonate and potassium citrate, effervescent *on page 663*

**K-Lyte® Effervescent** *(Discontinued) see* potassium bicarbonate *on page 662*

**K-Norm®** *(Discontinued) see* potassium chloride *on page 663*

**Koate®-HP** *(Discontinued) see* antihemophilic factor (human) *on page 55*

**Kodet SE [US-OTC]** *see* pseudoephedrine *on page 692*

**Koffex DM-D [Can]** *see* pseudoephedrine and dextromethorphan *on page 693*

**Koffex DM + Decongestant + Expectorant [Can]** *see* guaifenesin, pseudoephedrine, and dextromethorphan *on page 391*

**Koffex DM-Expectorant [Can]** *see* guaifenesin and dextromethorphan *on page 385*

**Koffex Expectorant [Can]** *see* guaifenesin *on page 383*

**Kogenate® [Can]** *see* antihemophilic factor (recombinant) *on page 57*

**Kogenate® *(Discontinued)*** *see* antihemophilic factor (recombinant) *on page 57*

**Kogenate® FS [US/Can]** *see* antihemophilic factor (recombinant) *on page 57*

**Kolephrin® #1 [US]** *see* guaifenesin and codeine *on page 384*

**Kolephrin® GG/DM [US-OTC]** *see* guaifenesin and dextromethorphan *on page 385*

**Konakion [Can]** *see* phytonadione *on page 646*

**Konakion® Injection *(Discontinued)*** *see* phytonadione *on page 646*

**Kondon's Nasal® *(Discontinued)*** *see* ephedrine *on page 287*

**Konsyl® [US-OTC]** *see* psyllium *on page 697*

**Konsyl-D® [US-OTC]** *see* psyllium *on page 697*

**Konsyl® Easy Mix [US-OTC]** *see* psyllium *on page 697*

**Konsyl® Fiber Tablets [US-OTC]** *see* polycarbophil *on page 657*

**Konsyl® Orange [US-OTC]** *see* psyllium *on page 697*

**Koāte®-DVI [US]** *see* antihemophilic factor (human) *on page 55*

**K-Pek II [US-OTC]** *see* loperamide *on page 489*

**K-Pek® *(Discontinued)*** *see* attapulgite *on page 81*

**K-Phos® MF [US]** *see* potassium phosphate and sodium phosphate *on page 667*

**K-Phos® Neutral [US]** *see* potassium phosphate and sodium phosphate *on page 667*

**K-Phos® No. 2 [US]** *see* potassium phosphate and sodium phosphate *on page 667*

**K-Phos® Original [US]** *see* potassium acid phosphate *on page 662*

**KPN Prenatal [US]** *see* vitamins (multiple/prenatal) *on page 852*

**K+ Potassium [US]** *see* potassium chloride *on page 663*

**Kristalose™ [US]** *see* lactulose *on page 464*

**Kronofed-A® [US]** *see* chlorpheniramine and pseudoephedrine *on page 172*

**Kronofed-A®-Jr [US]** *see* chlorpheniramine and pseudoephedrine *on page 172*

**K-Tab® [US]** *see* potassium chloride *on page 663*

**kutrase® [US]** *see* pancrelipase *on page 615*

**ku-zyme® [US]** *see* pancrelipase *on page 615*

**ku-zyme® HP [US]** *see* pancrelipase *on page 615*

**Kwelcof® [US]** *see* hydrocodone and guaifenesin *on page 412*

**Kwellada-P™ [Can]** *see* permethrin *on page 635*

**Kytril® [US/Can]** *see* granisetron *on page 382*

**L-749,345** *see* ertapenem *on page 294*

**L-M-X™ 4 [US-OTC]** *see* lidocaine *on page 479*

**L-M-X™ 5 [US-OTC]** *see* lidocaine *on page 479*

**L 754030** *see* aprepitant *on page 67*

**LA 20304a** *see* gemifloxacin *on page 370*

# labetalol (la BET a lole)

## Sound-Alike/Look-Alike Issues

labetalol may be confused with betaxolol, Hexadrol®, lamotrigine

Trandate® may be confused with tramadol, Trendar®, Trental®, Tridrate®

**Synonyms** ibidomide hydrochloride; labetalol hydrochloride

**U.S./Canadian Brand Names** Apo-Labetalol® [Can]; Normodyne® [Can]; Trandate® [US/Can]

**Therapeutic Category** Alpha-/Beta- Adrenergic Blocker

**Use** Treatment of mild to severe hypertension; I.V. for hypertensive emergencies

**Usual Dosage** Due to limited documentation of its use, labetalol should be initiated cautiously in pediatric patients with careful dosage adjustment and blood pressure monitoring.

Children:

Oral: Limited information regarding labetalol use in pediatric patients is currently available in literature. Some centers recommend initial oral doses of 4 mg/kg/day in 2 divided doses. Reported oral doses have started at 3 mg/kg/day and 20 mg/kg/day and have increased up to 40 mg/kg/day.

I.V., intermittent bolus doses of 0.3-1 mg/kg/dose have been reported.

For treatment of pediatric hypertensive emergencies, initial continuous infusions of 0.4-1 mg/kg/hour with a maximum of 3 mg/kg/hour have been used. Administration requires the use of an infusion pump.

Adults:

Oral: Initial: 100 mg twice daily, may increase as needed every 2-3 days by 100 mg until desired response is obtained; usual dose: 200-400 mg twice daily; may require up to 2.4 g/day.

Usual dose range (JNC 7): 200-800 mg/day in 2 divided doses

I.V.: 20 mg (0.25 mg/kg for an 80 kg patient) IVP over 2 minutes; may administer 40-80 mg at 10-minute intervals, up to 300 mg total dose.

I.V. infusion: Initial: 2 mg/minute; titrate to response up to 300 mg total dose, if needed. Administration requires the use of an infusion pump.

I.V. infusion (500 mg/250 mL $D_5W$) rates:

1 mg/minute: 30 mL/hour

2 mg/minute: 60 mL/hour

3 mg/minute: 90 mL/hour

4 mg/minute: 120 mL/hour

5 mg/minute: 150 mL/hour

6 mg/minute: 180 mL/hour

**Dosage Forms**

Injection, solution, as hydrochloride: 5 mg/mL (4 mL, 20 mL, 40 mL)

Trandate®: 5 mg/mL (20 mL, 40 mL)

Tablet, as hydrochloride: 100 mg, 200 mg, 300 mg

Trandate®: 100 mg, 200 mg [contains sodium benzoate], 300 mg

**labetalol hydrochloride** *see* labetalol *on previous page*

**Lac-Hydrin® [US]** *see* lactic acid and ammonium hydroxide *on next page*

**Lac-Hydrin® Five [US-OTC]** *see* lactic acid and ammonium hydroxide *on next page*

**LAClotion™ [US]** *see* lactic acid and ammonium hydroxide *on next page*

**Lacril® Ophthalmic Solution (Discontinued)** *see* artificial tears *on page 71*

**Lacrinorm [Can]** *see* carbopol 940 *(Canada only) on page 147*

**Lacrisert® [US/Can]** *see* hydroxypropyl cellulose *on page 422*

**Lactaid® Extra Strength (Discontinued)** *see* lactase *on this page*

**Lactaid® Fast Act [US-OTC]** *see* lactase *on this page*

**Lactaid® Original [US-OTC]** *see* lactase *on this page*

**Lactaid® Ultra (Discontinued)** *see* lactase *on this page*

# lactase (LAK tase)

**U.S./Canadian Brand Names** Dairyaid® [Can]; Lactaid® Fast Act [US-OTC]; Lactaid® Original [US-OTC]; Lactrase® [US-OTC]

**Therapeutic Category** Nutritional Supplement

**Use** Help digest lactose in milk for patients with lactose intolerance

**Usual Dosage** Oral:

Capsule: 1-2 capsules taken with milk or meal; pretreat milk with 1-2 capsules/quart of milk

Liquid: 5-15 drops/quart of milk

Tablet: 1-3 tablets with meals

(Continued)

# lactase *(Continued)*

**Dosage Forms**
Caplet:
Lactaid® Original: 3000 FCC lactase units [contains sodium 5 mg per 3 caplets]
Lactaid® Extra Strength: 4500 FCC lactase units [DSC]
Lactaid® Fast Act: 9000 FCC lactase units [contains sodium 5 mg]
Lactaid® Ultra: 9000 FCC lactase units [DSC]
Capsule (Lactrase®): 250 mg standardized enzyme lactase
Tablet, chewable:
Lactaid® Fast Act: 9000 FCC lactase units [contains sodium 5 mg; vanilla twist flavor]
Lactaid® Ultra: 9000 FCC lactase units [vanilla twist flavor] [DSC]

# lactic acid *(LAK tik AS id)*

**Synonyms** sodium-PCA and lactic acid
**U.S./Canadian Brand Names** LactiCare® [US-OTC]; Lactinol-E® [US]; Lactinol® [US]
**Therapeutic Category** Topical Skin Product
**Use** Lubricate and moisturize the skin counteracting dryness and itching
**Usual Dosage** Adults: Lubricant/moisturizer: Topical: Apply twice daily
**Dosage Forms**
Cream: 10% (120 g) [contains vitamin E]
Lactinol-E®: 10% (120 g, 240 g) [contains vitamin E 3500 int. units/ounce]
Lotion: 10% (360 mL)
LactiCare®: 5% (222 mL, 340 mL) [contains sodium PCA]
Lactinol®: 10% (360 mL, 480 mL)

# lactic acid and ammonium hydroxide

*(LAK tik AS id with a MOE nee um hye DROKS ide)*
**Synonyms** ammonium lactate
**U.S./Canadian Brand Names** AmLactin® [US-OTC]; Geri-Hydrolac™ [US-OTC]; Geri-Hydrolac™-12 [US-OTC]; Lac-Hydrin® Five [US-OTC]; Lac-Hydrin® [US]; LAClotion™ [US]
**Therapeutic Category** Topical Skin Product
**Use** Treatment of moderate to severe xerosis and ichthyosis vulgaris
**Usual Dosage** Children ≥2 years and Adults: Topical: Apply twice daily to affected area; rub in well
**Dosage Forms**
Cream, topical: Lactic acid 12% with ammonium hydroxide (140 g, 280 g, 385 g)
AmLactin®: Lactic acid 12% with ammonium hydroxide (140 g)
Lac-Hydrin®: Lactic acid 12% with ammonium hydroxide (280 g, 385 g)
Lotion, topical (AmLactin®, Lac-Hydrin®, LAClotion™): Lactic acid 12% with ammonium hydroxide (225 g, 400 g)
Geri-Hydrolac™, Lac-Hydrin® Five: Lactic acid 5% with ammonium hydroxide (120 mL, 240 mL)
Geri-Hydrolac™-12: Lactic acid 12% with ammonium hydroxide (120 mL, 240 mL)

**LactiCare® [US-OTC]** *see* lactic acid *on this page*

**Lactinex™ [US-OTC]** *see* Lactobacillus *on this page*

**Lactinol® [US]** *see* lactic acid *on this page*

**Lactinol-E® [US]** *see* lactic acid *on this page*

# Lactobacillus *(lak toe ba SIL us)*

**Synonyms** *Lactobacillus acidophilus; Lactobacillus bifidus; Lactobacillus bulgaricus; Lactobacillus casei; Lactobacillus paracasei; Lactobacillus reuteri; Lactobacillus rhamnosus* GG
**U.S./Canadian Brand Names** Bacid® [US-OTC/Can]; Culturelle® [US-OTC]; Dofus [US-OTC]; Fermalac [Can]; Flora-Q™ [US-OTC]; Kala® [US-OTC]; Lactinex™ [US-OTC]; Lacto-Bifidus [US-OTC]; Lacto-Key [US-OTC]; Lacto-Pectin [US-OTC]; Lacto-TriBlend [US-OTC]; Megadophilus® [US-OTC]; MoreDophilus® [US-OTC]; Superdophilus® [US-OTC]
**Therapeutic Category** Gastrointestinal Agent, Miscellaneous
**Use** Promote normal bacterial flora of the intestinal tract
**Usual Dosage**
Dietary supplement: Oral: Dosing varies by manufacturer; consult product labeling
Children (Culturelle®): 1 capsule daily

Adults:
Bacid®: 2 caplets/day
Culturelle®: 1 capsule daily; may increase to twice daily
Flora-Q™: 1 capsule/day
Lacto-Key 100 or 600: 1-2 capsules/day
Lactinex™: 1 packet or 4 tablets 3-4 times/day

## Dosage Forms

Capsule:
Culturelle®: *L. rhamnosus* GG 10 billion colony forming units [contains casein and whey]
Dofus: *L. acidophilus* and *L. bifidus* 10:1 ratio [beet root powder base]
Flora-Q™: *L. acidophilus* and *L. paracasei* ≥8 billion colony-forming units [also contains *Bifidobacterium* and *S. thermophilus*]
Lacto-Key:
100: *L. acidophilus* 1 billion colony-forming units [milk, soy, and yeast free; rice derived]
600: *L. acidophilus* 6 billion colony-forming units [milk, soy, and yeast free; rice derived]
Lacto-Bifidus:
100: *L. bifidus* 1 billion colony-forming units [milk, soy, and yeast free; rice derived]
600: *L. bifidus* 6 billion colony-forming units [milk, soy, and yeast free; rice derived]
Lacto-Pectin: *L. acidophilus* and *L. casei* ≥5 billion colony-forming units [also contains *Bifidobacterium lactis* and citrus pectin cellulose complex]
Lact-TriBlend:
100: *L. acidophilus, L. bifidus,* and *L. bulgaricus* 1 billion colony-forming units [milk, soy and yeast free; rice derived]
600: *L. acidophilus, L. bifidus,* and *L. bulgaricus* 6 billion colony-forming units [milk, soy and yeast free; rice derived]
Megadophilus®, Superdophilus®: *L. acidophilus* 2 billion units [available in dairy based or dairy free formulations]

Capsule, softgel: *L. acidophilus* 100 active units

Caplet (Bacid®): *L. acidophilus* 80% and *L. bulgaricus* 10% [also contains *Bifidobacterium biffidum* 5% and *S. thermophilus* 5%]

Granules (Lactinex™): *L. acidophilus* and *L. bulgaricus* 100 million live cells per 1 g packet (12s) [contains whey, evaporated milk, soy peptone, lactose, and beef extract]

Powder:
Lact-TriBlend: *L. acidophilus, L. bifidus,* and *L. bulgaricus* 10 billion colony-forming units per 1/4 teaspoon (60 g) [milk, soy, and yeast free; rice derived]
Megadophilus®, Superdophilus®: *L. acidophilus* 2 billion units per half-teaspoon (49 g, 70 g, 84 g, 126 g) [available in dairy based or dairy free (garbanzo bean) formulations]
MoreDophilus®: *L. acidophilus* 12.4 billion units per teaspoon (30 g, 120 g) [dairy free, yeast free; soy and carrot derived]

Tablet:
Kala®: *L. acidophilus* 200 million units [dairy free, yeast free; soy based]
Lactinex™: *L. acidophilus* and *L. bulgaricus* 1 million live cells [contains whey, evaporated milk, soy peptone, lactose, and beef extract; contains sodium 5.6 mg/4 tablets]

Tablet, chewable: *L. reuteri* 100 million organisms

Wafer: *L. acidophilus* 90 mg and *L. bifidus* 25 mg (100s) [provides 1 billion organisms/wafer at time of manufacture; milk free]

**Lactobacillus acidophilus** *see* Lactobacillus *on previous page*

**Lactobacillus bifidus** *see* Lactobacillus *on previous page*

**Lactobacillus bulgaricus** *see* Lactobacillus *on previous page*

**Lactobacillus casei** *see* Lactobacillus *on previous page*

**Lactobacillus paracasei** *see* Lactobacillus *on previous page*

**Lactobacillus reuteri** *see* Lactobacillus *on previous page*

**Lactobacillus rhamnosus GG** *see* Lactobacillus *on previous page*

**Lacto-Bifidus [US-OTC]** *see* Lactobacillus *on previous page*

**lactoflavin** *see* riboflavin *on page 721*

**Lacto-Key [US-OTC]** *see* Lactobacillus *on previous page*

**Lacto-Pectin [US-OTC]** *see* Lactobacillus *on page 462*

**Lacto-TriBlend [US-OTC]** *see* Lactobacillus *on page 462*

**Lactrase® [US-OTC]** *see* lactase *on page 461*

## lactulose (LAK tyoo lose)

**Sound-Alike/Look-Alike Issues**
lactulose may be confused with lactose

**U.S./Canadian Brand Names** Acilac [Can]; Apo-Lactulose® [Can]; Constulose® [US]; Enulose® [US]; Generlac [US]; Kristalose™ [US]; Laxilose [Can]; PMS-Lactulose [Can]

**Therapeutic Category** Ammonium Detoxicant; Laxative

**Use** Adjunct in the prevention and treatment of portal-systemic encephalopathy; treatment of chronic constipation

**Usual Dosage** Diarrhea may indicate overdosage and responds to dose reduction

Prevention of portal systemic encephalopathy (PSE): Oral:
Infants: 2.5-10 mL/day divided 3-4 times/day; adjust dosage to produce 2-3 stools/day
Older Children: Daily dose of 40-90 mL divided 3-4 times/day; if initial dose causes diarrhea, then reduce it immediately; adjust dosage to produce 2-3 stools/day

Constipation: Oral:
Children: 5 g/day (7.5 mL) after breakfast
Adults: 15-30 mL/day increased to 60 mL/day in 1-2 divided doses if necessary

Acute PSE: Adults:
Oral: 20-30 g (30-45 mL) every 1-2 hours to induce rapid laxation; adjust dosage daily to produce 2-3 soft stools; doses of 30-45 mL may be given hourly to cause rapid laxation, then reduce to recommended dose; usual daily dose: 60-100 g (90-150 mL) daily
Rectal administration: 200 g (300 mL) diluted with 700 mL of $H_2O$ or NS; administer rectally via rectal balloon catheter and retain 30-60 minutes every 4-6 hours

**Dosage Forms**
Crystals for reconstitution (Kristalose™): 10 g/packet (30s), 20 g/packet (30s)
Syrup: 10 g/15 mL (15 mL, 30 mL, 237 mL, 473 mL, 946 mL, 1890 mL)
Constulose®: 10 g/15 mL (240 mL, 960 mL)
Enulose®: 10 g/15 mL (480 mL)
Generlac: 10 g/15 mL (480 mL, 1920 mL)

**Lactulose PSE®** *(Discontinued)* *see* lactulose *on this page*

**ladakamycin** *see* azacitidine *on page 82*

**L-AmB** *see* amphotericin B liposomal *on page 50*

**Lamictal® [US/Can]** *see* lamotrigine *on next page*

**Lamisil® Oral [US/Can]** *see* terbinafine (oral) *on page 786*

**Lamisil® Topical [US/Can]** *see* terbinafine (topical) *on page 786*

## lamivudine (la MI vyoo deen)

**Sound-Alike/Look-Alike Issues**
lamivudine may be confused with lamotrigine
Epivir® may be confused with Combivir®

**Synonyms** 3TC

**U.S./Canadian Brand Names** 3TC® [Can]; Epivir-HBV® [US]; Epivir® [US]; Heptovir® [Can]

**Therapeutic Category** Antiviral Agent

**Use**
Epivir®: Treatment of HIV infection when antiretroviral therapy is warranted; should always be used as part of a multidrug regimen (at least three antiretroviral agents)
Epivir-HBV®: Treatment of chronic hepatitis B associated with evidence of hepatitis B viral replication and active liver inflammation

**Usual Dosage Note:** The formulation and dosage of Epivir-HBV® are not appropriate for patients infected with both HBV and HIV. Use with at least two other antiretroviral agents when treating HIV
Oral:
Children 3 months to 16 years: HIV: 4 mg/kg twice daily (maximum: 150 mg twice daily)
Children 2-17 years: Treatment of hepatitis B (Epivir-HBV®): 3 mg/kg once daily (maximum: 100 mg/day)

Adults:
HIV: 150 mg twice daily **or** 300 mg once daily
<50 kg: 4 mg/kg twice daily  (maximum: 150 mg twice daily)
Treatment of hepatitis B (Epivir-HBV®): 100 mg/day
**Dosage Forms**
Solution, oral:
Epivir®: 10 mg/mL (240 mL) [strawberry-banana flavor]
Epivir-HBV®: 5 mg/mL (240 mL) [strawberry-banana flavor]
Tablet:
Epivir®: 150 mg, 300 mg
Epivir-HBV®: 100 mg

**lamivudine, abacavir, and zidovudine** *see* abacavir, lamivudine, and zidovudine *on page 2*

**lamivudine and abacavir** *see* abacavir and lamivudine *on page 2*

**lamivudine and zidovudine** *see* zidovudine and lamivudine *on page 860*

# lamotrigine (la MOE tri jeen)
**Sound-Alike/Look-Alike Issues**
lamotrigine may be confused with labetalol, Lamisil®, lamivudine, Lomotil®, ludiomil
Lamictal® may be confused with Lamisil®, Lomotil®, ludiomil
**Synonyms** BW-430C; LTG
**U.S./Canadian Brand Names** Apo-Lamotrigine® [Can]; Lamictal® [US/Can]; Novo-Lamotrigine [Can]; PMS-Lamotrigine [Can]; ratio-Lamotrigine [Can]
**Therapeutic Category** Anticonvulsant
**Use** Adjunctive therapy in the treatment of generalized seizures of Lennox-Gastaut syndrome and partial seizures in adults and children ≥2 years of age; conversion to monotherapy in adults with partial seizures who are receiving treatment with valproate or a single enzyme-inducing antiepileptic drug; maintenance treatment of bipolar disorder
**Usual Dosage Note:** Only whole tablets should be used for dosing, round calculated dose down to the nearest whole tablet: Oral:
Children 2-12 years: Lennox-Gastaut (adjunctive) or partial seizures (adjunctive): **Note:** Children 2-6 years will likely require maintenance doses at the higher end of recommended range:
Patients receiving AED regimens containing valproic acid:
Weeks 1 and 2: 0.15 mg/kg/day in 1-2 divided doses; round dose down to the nearest whole tablet. For patients >6.7 kg and <14 kg, dosing should be 2 mg every other day.
Weeks 3 and 4: 0.3 mg/kg/day in 1-2 divided doses; round dose down to the nearest whole tablet; may use combinations of 2 mg and 5 mg tablets. For patients >6.7 kg and <14 kg, dosing should be 2 mg/day.
Maintenance dose: Titrate dose to effect; after week 4, increase dose every 1-2 weeks by a calculated increment; calculate increment as 0.3 mg/kg/day rounded down to the nearest whole tablet; add this amount to the previously administered daily dose; usual maintenance: 1-5 mg/kg/day in 1-2 divided doses; maximum: 200 mg/day given in 1-2 divided doses
Patients receiving enzyme-inducing AED regimens without valproic acid:
Weeks 1 and 2: 0.6 mg/kg/day in 2 divided doses; round dose down to the nearest whole tablet
Weeks 3 and 4: 1.2 mg/kg/day in 2 divided doses; round dose down to the nearest whole tablet
Maintenance dose: Titrate dose to effect; after week 4, increase dose every 1-2 weeks by a calculated increment; calculate increment as 1.2 mg/kg/day rounded down to the nearest whole tablet; add this amount to the previously administered daily dose; usual maintenance: 5-15 mg/kg/day in 2 divided doses; maximum: 400 mg/day
Children >12 years: Lennox-Gastaut (adjunctive) or partial seizures (adjunctive): Refer to Adults dosing
Children ≥16 years: Conversion from single enzyme-inducing AED regimen to monotherapy: Refer to Adults dosing

Adults:
Lennox-Gastaut (adjunctive) or treatment of partial seizures (adjunctive):
Patients receiving AED regimens containing valproic acid: Initial dose: 25 mg every other day for 2 weeks, then 25 mg every day for 2 weeks. Dose may be increased by 25-50 mg every day for 1-2 weeks in order to achieve maintenance dose. Maintenance dose: 100-400 mg/day in 1-2 divided doses (usual range 100-200 mg/day).
Patients receiving enzyme-inducing AED regimens without valproic acid: Initial dose: 50 mg/day for 2 weeks, then 100 mg in 2 doses for 2 weeks; thereafter, daily dose can be increased by 100 mg every
(Continued)

# lamotrigine *(Continued)*

1-2 weeks to be given in 2 divided doses. Usual maintenance dose: 300-500 mg/day in 2 divided doses; doses as high as 700 mg/day have been reported

Conversion to monotherapy (partial seizures in patients ≥16 years of age):

Adjunctive therapy with valproate: Initiate and titrate as per recommendations to a lamotrigine dose of 200 mg/day. Then taper valproate dose in decrements of not more than 500 mg/day at intervals of one week (or longer) to a valproate dosage of 500 mg/day; this dosage should be maintained for one week. The lamotrigine dosage should then be increased to 300 mg/day while valproate is decreased to 250 mg/day; this dosage should be maintained for one week. Valproate may then be discontinued, while the lamotrigine dose is increased by 100 mg/day at weekly intervals to achieve a lamotrigine maintenance dose of 500 mg/day.

Adjunctive therapy with enzyme-inducing AED: Initiate and titrate as per recommendations to a lamotrigine dose of 500 mg/day. Concomitant enzyme-inducing AED should then be withdrawn by 20% decrements each week over a 4-week period. Patients should be monitored for rash.

Adjunctive therapy with nonenzyme-inducing AED: No specific guidelines available

Bipolar disorder: 25 mg/day for 2 weeks, followed by 50 mg/day for 2 weeks, followed by 100 mg/day for 1 week; thereafter, daily dosage may be increased to 200 mg/day

Patients receiving valproic acid: Initial: 25 mg every other day for 2 weeks, followed by 25 mg/day for 2 weeks, followed by 50 mg/day for 1 week, followed by 100 mg/day (target dose) thereafter. **Note:** If valproate is discontinued, increase daily lamotrigine dose in 50 mg increments at weekly intervals until daily dosage of 200 mg is attained.

Patients receiving enzyme-inducing drugs (eg, carbamazepine): Initial: 50 mg/day for 2 weeks, followed by 100 mg/day (in divided doses) for 2 weeks, followed by 200 mg/day (in divided doses) for 1 week, followed by 300 mg/day (in divided doses) for 1 week. May increase to 400 mg/day (in divided doses) during week 7 and thereafter. **Note:** If carbamazepine (or other enzyme-inducing drug) is discontinued, decrease daily lamotrigine dose in 100 mg increments at weekly intervals until daily dosage of 200 mg is attained.

**Discontinuing therapy:** Children and Adults: Decrease dose by ~50% per week, over at least 2 weeks unless safety concerns require a more rapid withdrawal.

**Restarting therapy after discontinuation:** If lamotrigine has been withheld for >5 half-lives, consider restarting according to initial dosing recommendations.

## Dosage Forms

Tablet: 25 mg, 100 mg, 150 mg, 200 mg [contains lactose]

Tablet, combination package [each unit-dose starter kit contains]:

Lamictal® (blue kit; for patients taking valproate):

Tablet: Lamotrigine 25 mg (35s)

Lamictal® (green kit; for patients taking carbamazepine, phenytoin, phenobarbital, primidone or rifampin and **not** taking valproate):

Tablet: Lamotrigine 25 mg (84s)

Tablet: Lamotrigine 100 mg (14s)

Lamictal® (orange kit; for patients **not** taking carbamazepine, phenytoin, phenobarbital, primidone, rifampin, or valproate; for use in bipolar patients only):

Tablet: Lamotrigine 25 mg (42s)

Tablet: Lamotrigine 100 mg (7s)

Tablet, dispersible/chewable: 2 mg, 5 mg, 25 mg [black currant flavor]

**Lamprene® [Can]** *see* clofazimine *on page 195*

**Lamprene® *(Discontinued)*** *see* clofazimine *on page 195*

**Lanacane® [US-OTC]** *see* benzocaine *on page 95*

**Lanacane® Maximum Strength [US-OTC]** *see* benzocaine *on page 95*

**Lanaphilic® [US-OTC]** *see* urea *on page 834*

# lanolin, cetyl alcohol, glycerin, petrolatum, and mineral oil

(LAN oh lin, SEE til AL koe hol, GLIS er in, pe troe LAY tum, & MIN er al oyl)

**Synonyms** mineral oil, petrolatum, lanolin, cetyl alcohol, and glycerin

**U.S./Canadian Brand Names** Lubriderm® Fragrance Free [US-OTC]; Lubriderm® [US-OTC]

**Therapeutic Category** Topical Skin Product

**Use** Treatment of dry skin

**Usual Dosage** Topical: Apply to skin as necessary

**Dosage Forms**
Lotion, topical [bottle]: 180 mL, 300 mL, 480 mL
Lotion, topical [tube]: 100 mL

**lanolin, coal tar, and mineral oil** *see* coal tar, lanolin, and mineral oil *on page 202*

**lanolin, mineral oil, and coal tar** *see* coal tar, lanolin, and mineral oil *on page 202*

**Lanorinal**® *(Discontinued)*

**Lanoxicaps**® **[US/Can]** *see* digoxin *on page 247*

**Lanoxin**® **[US/Can]** *see* digoxin *on page 247*

# lansoprazole (lan SOE pra zole)

**Sound-Alike/Look-Alike Issues**
Prevacid® may be confused with Pravachol®, Prevpac®, Prilosec®, Prinivil®

**U.S./Canadian Brand Names** Prevacid® SoluTab™ [US]; Prevacid® [US/Can]

**Therapeutic Category** Gastric Acid Secretion Inhibitor

**Use**
Oral: Short-term treatment of active duodenal ulcers; maintenance treatment of healed duodenal ulcers; as part of a multidrug regimen for *H. pylori* eradication to reduce the risk of duodenal ulcer recurrence; short-term treatment of active benign gastric ulcer; treatment of NSAID-associated gastric ulcer; to reduce the risk of NSAID-associated gastric ulcer in patients with a history of gastric ulcer who require an NSAID; short-term treatment of symptomatic GERD; short-term treatment for all grades of erosive esophagitis; to maintain healing of erosive esophagitis; long-term treatment of pathological hypersecretory conditions, including Zollinger-Ellison syndrome
I.V.: Short-term treatment (≤7 days) of erosive esophagitis in adults unable to take oral medications

**Usual Dosage**
Children 1-11 years: GERD, erosive esophagitis: Oral:
≤30 kg: 15 mg once daily
>30 kg: 30 mg once daily
**Note:** Doses were increased in some pediatric patients if still symptomatic after 2 or more weeks of treatment (maximum dose: 30 mg twice daily)
Children 12-17 years: Oral:
Nonerosive GERD: 15 mg once daily for up to 8 weeks
Erosive esophagitis: 30 mg once daily for up to 8 weeks
Adults:
Duodenal ulcer: Oral: Short-term treatment: 15 mg once daily for 4 weeks; maintenance therapy: 15 mg once daily
Gastric ulcer: Oral: Short-term treatment: 30 mg once daily for up to 8 weeks
NSAID-associated gastric ulcer (healing): Oral: 30 mg once daily for 8 weeks; controlled studies did not extend past 8 weeks of therapy
NSAID-associated gastric ulcer (to reduce risk): Oral: 15 mg once daily for up to 12 weeks; controlled studies did not extend past 12 weeks of therapy
Symptomatic GERD: Oral: Short-term treatment: 15 mg once daily for up to 8 weeks
Erosive esophagitis:
Oral: Short-term treatment: 30 mg once daily for up to 8 weeks; continued treatment for an additional 8 weeks may be considered for recurrence or for patients that do not heal after the first 8 weeks of therapy; maintenance therapy: 15 mg once daily
I.V.: 30 mg once daily for up to 7 days; patients should be switched to an oral formulation as soon as they can take oral medications
Hypersecretory conditions: Oral: Initial: 60 mg once daily; adjust dose based upon patient response and to reduce acid secretion to <10 mEq/hour (5 mEq/hour in patients with prior gastric surgery); doses of 90 mg twice daily have been used; administer doses >120 mg/day in divided doses
*Helicobacter pylori* eradication: Oral: Currently accepted recommendations (may differ from product labeling): Dose varies with regimen: 30 mg once daily or 60 mg/day in 2 divided doses; requires combination therapy with antibiotics

**Dosage Forms**
Capsule, delayed release (Prevacid®): 15 mg, 30 mg
Granules, for oral suspension, delayed release (Prevacid®): 15 mg/packet (30s), 30 mg/packet (30s) [strawberry flavor]
Injection, powder for reconstitution (Prevacid®): 30 mg
Tablet, orally-disintegrating (Prevacid® SoluTab™): 15 mg [contains phenylalanine 2.5 mg; strawberry flavor]; 30 mg [contains phenylalanine 5.1 mg; strawberry flavor]

## lansoprazole, amoxicillin, and clarithromycin
(lan SOE pra zole, a moks i SIL in, & kla RITH roe mye sin)
**Sound-Alike/Look-Alike Issues**
Prevpac® may be confused with Prevacid®
**Synonyms** amoxicillin, lansoprazole, and clarithromycin; clarithromycin, lansoprazole, and amoxicillin
**U.S./Canadian Brand Names** Hp-PAC® [Can]; Prevpac® [US/Can]
**Therapeutic Category** Antibiotic, Macrolide Combination; Antibiotic, Penicillin; Gastrointestinal Agent, Miscellaneous
**Use** Eradication of *H. pylori* to reduce the risk of recurrent duodenal ulcer
**Usual Dosage** Oral: Adults: Lansoprazole 30 mg, amoxicillin 1 g, and clarithromycin 500 mg taken together twice daily for 10 or 14 days
**Dosage Forms** Combination package (Prevpac®) [each administration card contains]:
Capsule (Trimox®): Amoxicillin 500 mg (4 capsules/day)
Capsule, delayed release (Prevacid®): Lansoprazole 30 mg (2 capsules/day)
Tablet (Biaxin®): Clarithromycin 500 mg (2 tablets/day)

## lansoprazole and naproxen (lan SOE pra zole & na PROKS en)
**Sound-Alike/Look-Alike Issues**
Prevacid® may be confused with Pravachol®, Prevpac®, Prilosec®, Prinivil®
**Synonyms** NapraPAC™; naproxen and lansoprazole
**U.S./Canadian Brand Names** Prevacid® NapraPAC™ [US]
**Therapeutic Category** Gastric Acid Secretion Inhibitor; Nonsteroidal Antiinflammatory Drug (NSAID)
**Use** Reduction of the risk of NSAID-associated gastric ulcers in patients with history of gastric ulcer who require an NSAID for the treatment of rheumatoid arthritis, osteoarthritis, and ankylosing spondylitis
**Usual Dosage** Oral: Adults: Reduce NSAID-associated gastric ulcers during treatment for arthritis: Lansoprazole 15 mg once daily in the morning; naproxen 375 mg or 500 mg twice daily
**Dosage Forms** Combination package:
Prevacid® NapraPAC™ 375 [each administration card contains]:
Capsule, delayed release (Prevacid®): Lansoprazole 15 mg (7 capsules per card)
Tablet (Naprosyn®): Naproxen 375 mg (14 tablets per card)
Prevacid® NapraPAC™ 500 [each administration card contains]:
Capsule, delayed release (Prevacid®): Lansoprazole 15 mg (7 capsules per card)
Tablet (Naprosyn®): Naproxen 500 mg (14 tablets per card)

## lanthanum (LAN tha num)
**Synonyms** lanthanum carbonate
**U.S./Canadian Brand Names** Fosrenol™ [US]
**Therapeutic Category** Phosphate Binder
**Use** Reduction of serum phosphate in patients with end-stage renal disease (ESRD)
**Usual Dosage** Oral: Adults: Initial: 750-1500 mg/day divided and taken with meals; typical increases of 750 mg/day every 2-3 weeks are suggested as needed to bring the serum phosphate level <6 mg/dL; usual dosage range: 1500-3000 mg; doses of up to 3750 mg have been used
**Dosage Forms** Tablet, chewable: 250 mg, 500 mg

**lanthanum carbonate** *see* lanthanum *on this page*

**Lantus® [US/Can]** *see* insulin preparations *on page 438*

**Lanvis® [Can]** *see* thioguanine *on page 797*

**Lapase [US]** *see* pancrelipase *on page 615*

**Largactil® [Can]** *see* chlorpromazine *on page 178*

**Lariam® [US/Can]** *see* mefloquine *on page 508*

## laronidase (lair OH ni days)
**Synonyms** recombinant α-L-iduronidase (glycosaminoglycan α-L-iduronohydrolase)
**U.S./Canadian Brand Names** Aldurazyme® [US/Can]
**Therapeutic Category** Enzyme
**Use** Treatment of Hurler and Hurler-Scheie forms of mucopolysaccharidosis I (MPS I); treatment of Scheie form of MPS I in patients with moderate to severe symptoms
**Usual Dosage** I.V.: Children ≥5 years and Adults: 0.58 mg/kg once weekly; dose should be rounded up to the nearest whole vial
**Dosage Forms** Injection, solution [preservative free]: 2.9 mg/5 mL (5 mL)

**Lasix®** **[US/Can]** *see* furosemide *on page 364*

**Lasix®** **Special [Can]** *see* furosemide *on page 364*

**L-asparaginase** *see* asparaginase *on page 72*

**lassar's zinc paste** *see* zinc oxide *on page 861*

## latanoprost (la TA noe prost)

**Sound-Alike/Look-Alike Issues**
Xalatan® may be confused with Travatan®, Zarontin®

**U.S./Canadian Brand Names** Xalatan® [US/Can]

**Therapeutic Category** Prostaglandin

**Use** Reduction of elevated intraocular pressure in patients with open-angle glaucoma or ocular hypertension

**Usual Dosage** Adults: Ophthalmic: 1 drop (1.5 mcg) in the affected eye(s) once daily in the evening; do not exceed the once daily dosage because it has been shown that more frequent administration may decrease the IOP lowering effect

**Note:** A medication delivery device (Xal-Ease™) is available for use with Xalatan®.

**Dosage Forms** Solution, ophthalmic: 0.005% (2.5 mL) [contains benzalkonium chloride]

**Lavacol®** **[US-OTC]** *see* alcohol (ethyl) *on page 24*

**Laxilose [Can]** *see* lactulose *on page 464*

***l*-bunolol hydrochloride** *see* levobunolol *on page 472*

**L-carnitine** *see* levocarnitine *on page 474*

**LCD** *see* coal tar *on page 201*

**LCR** *see* vincristine *on page 846*

**L-deprenyl** *see* selegiline *on page 742*

**LDP-341** *see* bortezomib *on page 110*

**Lectopam®** **[Can]** *see* bromazepam *(Canada only) on page 114*

## leflunomide (le FLOO noh mide)

**U.S./Canadian Brand Names** Apo-Leflunomide® [Can]; Arava® [US/Can]; Novo-Leflunomide [Can]

**Therapeutic Category** Antiinflammatory Agent

**Use** Treatment of active rheumatoid arthritis; indicated to reduce signs and symptoms, and to retard structural damage and improve physical function

**Orphan drug:** Prevention of acute and chronic rejection in recipients of solid organ tranplants

**Usual Dosage** Oral: Adults: Rheumatoid arthritis: Initial: 100 mg/day for 3 days, followed by 20 mg/day; dosage may be decreased to 10 mg/day in patients who have difficulty tolerating the 20 mg dose. Due to the long half-life of the active metabolite, plasma levels may require a prolonged period to decline after dosage reduction.

**Dosage Forms**
Tablet (Arava®): 10 mg, 20 mg

**Legatrin PM®** **[US-OTC]** *see* acetaminophen and diphenhydramine *on page 7*

**Lente®** **L** *(Discontinued)* *see* insulin preparations *on page 438*

**Lente®** **Iletin®** **II** *(Discontinued)* *see* insulin preparations *on page 438*

**Lente®** **Insulin** *(Discontinued)* *see* insulin preparations *on page 438*

## lepirudin (leh puh ROO din)

**Synonyms** lepirudin (rDNA); recombinant hirudin

**U.S./Canadian Brand Names** Refludan® [US/Can]

**Therapeutic Category** Anticoagulant (Other)

**Use** Indicated for anticoagulation in patients with heparin-induced thrombocytopenia (HIT) and associated thromboembolic disease in order to prevent further thromboembolic complications

**Usual Dosage** Adults: Maximum dose: Do not exceed 0.21 mg/kg/hour unless an evaluation of coagulation abnormalities limiting response has been completed. **Dosing is weight-based, however, patients**
(Continued)

## lepirudin *(Continued)*

**weighing >110 kg should not receive doses greater than the recommended dose for a patient weighing 110 kg (44 mg bolus and initial maximal infusion rate of 16.5 mg/hour).**

Heparin-induced thrombocytopenia: Bolus dose: 0.4 mg/kg IVP (over 15-20 seconds), followed by continuous infusion at 0.15 mg/kg/hour; bolus and infusion must be reduced in renal insufficiency

Concomitant use with thrombolytic therapy: Bolus dose: 0.2 mg/kg IVP (over 15-20 seconds), followed by continuous infusion at 0.1 mg/kg/hour

Dosing adjustments during infusions: Monitor first aPTT 4 hours after the start of the infusion. Subsequent determinations of aPTT should be obtained at least once daily during treatment. More frequent monitoring is recommended in renally impaired patients. Any aPTT ratio measurement out of range (1.5-2.5) should be confirmed prior to adjusting dose, unless a clinical need for immediate reaction exists. If the aPTT is below target range, increase infusion by 20%. If the aPTT is in excess of the target range, decrease infusion rate by 50%. A repeat aPTT should be obtained 4 hours after any dosing change.

Use in patients scheduled for switch to oral anticoagulants: Reduce lepirudin dose gradually to reach aPTT ratio just above 1.5 before starting warfarin therapy; as soon as INR reaches 2.0, lepirudin therapy should be discontinued.

**Dosage Forms** Injection, powder for reconstitution: 50 mg

**lepirudin (rDNA)** *see lepirudin on previous page*

**Lescol® [US/Can]** *see fluvastatin on page 355*

**Lescol® XL [US]** *see fluvastatin on page 355*

**Lessina™ [US]** *see ethinyl estradiol and levonorgestrel on page 312*

## letrozole *(LET roe zole)*

**Sound-Alike/Look-Alike Issues**
Femara® may be confused with femhrt®

**U.S./Canadian Brand Names** Femara® [US/Can]

**Therapeutic Category** Antineoplastic Agent, Hormone (Antiestrogen)

**Use** First-line treatment of hormone receptor positive or hormone receptor unknown, locally advanced, or metastatic breast cancer in postmenopausal women; treatment of advanced breast cancer in postmenopausal women with disease progression following antiestrogen therapy; extended adjuvant treatment of early breast cancer in postmenopausal women who have received 5 years of adjuvant tamoxifen therapy

**Usual Dosage** Oral (refer to individual protocols): Adults: Breast cancer: 2.5 mg once daily

**Dosage Forms** Tablet: 2.5 mg

## leucovorin *(loo koe VOR in)*

**Sound-Alike/Look-Alike Issues**
leucovorin may be confused with Leukeran®, Leukine®
folinic acid may be confused with folic acid

**Synonyms** 5-formyl tetrahydrofolate; calcium leucovorin; citrovorum factor; folinic acid; leucovorin calcium

**Therapeutic Category** Folic Acid Derivative

**Use** Antidote for folic acid antagonists (methotrexate, trimethoprim, pyrimethamine); treatment of megaloblastic anemias when folate is deficient as in infancy, sprue, pregnancy, and nutritional deficiency when oral folate therapy is not possible; in combination with fluorouracil in the treatment of colon cancer

**Usual Dosage** Children and Adults:
Treatment of folic acid antagonist overdosage: Oral: 2-15 mg/day for 3 days or until blood counts are normal, **or** 5 mg every 3 days; doses of 6 mg/day are needed for patients with platelet counts <100,000/mm$^3$

Folate-deficient megaloblastic anemia: I.M.: 1 mg/day

Megaloblastic anemia secondary to congenital deficiency of dihydrofolate reductase: I.M.: 3-6 mg/day

Rescue dose: Initial: I.V.: 10 mg/m$^2$, then:
Oral, I.M., I.V., SubQ: 10-15 mg/m$^2$ every 6 hours until methotrexate level <0.05 micromole/L; if methotrexate level remains >5 micromole/L at 48-72 hours after the end of the methotrexate infusion, increase to 20-100 mg/m$^2$ every 6 hours until methotrexate level <0.05 micromole/L

**Dosage Forms**
Injection, powder for reconstitution, as calcium: 50 mg, 100 mg, 200 mg, 350 mg, 500 mg

Injection, solution, as calcium: 10 mg/mL (50 mL)
Tablet, as calcium: 5 mg, 10 mg, 15 mg, 25 mg

**leucovorin calcium** *see* leucovorin *on previous page*

**Leukeran® [US/Can]** *see* chlorambucil *on page 166*

**Leukine® [US/Can]** *see* sargramostim *on page 739*

# leuprolide acetate (loo PROE lide AS e tate)

**Sound-Alike/Look-Alike Issues**
Lupron® may be confused with Nuprin®

**Synonyms** abbott-43818; leuprorelin acetate; NSC-377526; TAP-144

**U.S./Canadian Brand Names** Eligard® [US/Can]; Lupron Depot-Ped® [US]; Lupron Depot® [US/Can]; Lupron® [US/Can]; Viadur® [US/Can]

**Therapeutic Category** Antineoplastic Agent; Luteinizing Hormone-Releasing Hormone Analog

**Use** Palliative treatment of advanced prostate carcinoma; management of endometriosis as initial treatment and/or treatment of recurrent symptoms; preoperative treatment of anemia caused by uterine leiomyomata (fibroids); central precocious puberty

**Usual Dosage**
Children: Precocious puberty (consider discontinuing by age 11 for females and by age 12 for males):
SubQ (Lupron®): 20-45 mcg/kg/day; titrate dose upward by 10 mcg/kg/day if down-regulation is not achieved
I.M. (Lupron Depot-Ped®): 0.3 mg/kg/dose given every 28 days (minimum dose: 7.5 mg)
≤25 kg: 7.5 mg
>25-37.5 kg: 11.25 mg
>37.5 kg: 15 mg
Titrate dose upward in 3.75 mg every 4 weeks if down-regulation is not achieved.
Adults:
Advanced prostatic carcinoma:
SubQ:
Eligard®: 7.5 mg monthly **or** 22.5 mg every 3 months **or** 30 mg every 4 months **or** 45 mg every 6 months
Lupron®: 1 mg/day
Viadur®: 65 mg implanted subcutaneously every 12 months
I.M.:
Lupron Depot®: 7.5 mg/dose given monthly (every 28-33 days) **or**
Lupron Depot-3®: 22.5 mg every 3 months **or**
Lupron Depot-4®: 30 mg every 4 months
Endometriosis: I.M.: Initial therapy may be with leuprolide alone or in combination with norethindrone; if retreatment for an additional 6 months is necessary, norethindrone should be used. Retreatment is not recommended for longer than one additional 6-month course.
Lupron Depot®: 3.75 mg/month for up to 6 months **or**
Lupron Depot-3®: 11.25 mg every 3 months for up to 2 doses (6 months total duration of treatment)
Uterine leiomyomata (fibroids): I.M. (in combination with iron):
Lupron Depot®: 3.75 mg/month for up to 3 months **or**
Lupron Depot-3®: 11.25 mg as a single injection

**Dosage Forms**
Implant (Viadur®): 65 mg [released over 12 months; packaged with administration kit]
Injection, solution, as acetate (Lupron®): 5 mg/mL (2.8 mL) [contains benzyl alcohol; packaged with syringes and alcohol swabs]
Injection, powder for reconstitution, as acetate [depot formulation; prefilled syringe]:
Eligard®:
7.5 mg [released over 1 month]
22.5 mg [released over 3 months]
30 mg [released over 4 months]
45 mg [released over 6 months]
Lupron Depot®: 3.75 mg, 7.5 mg [released over 1 month; contains polysorbate 80]
Lupron Depot®-3 Month: 11.25 mg, 22.5 mg [released over 3 months; contains polysorbate 80]
Lupron Depot®-4 Month: 30 mg [released over 4 months; contains polysorbate 80]
Lupron Depot-Ped®: 7.5 mg, 11.25 mg, 15 mg [released over 1 month; contains polysorbate 80]

**leuprorelin acetate** *see* leuprolide acetate *on this page*

**leurocristine sulfate** *see* vincristine *on page 846*

**Leustatin**® **[US/Can]** *see* cladribine *on page 189*

## levalbuterol (leve al BYOO ter ole)

**Sound-Alike/Look-Alike Issues**

Xopenex® may be confused with Xanax®

**Synonyms** levalbuterol hydrochloride; levalbuterol tartrate; R-albuterol

**U.S./Canadian Brand Names** Xopenex HFA™ [US]; Xopenex® [US/Can]

**Therapeutic Category** Adrenergic Agonist Agent; Beta$_2$-Adrenergic Agonist Agent; Bronchodilator

**Use** Treatment or prevention of bronchospasm in children and adults with reversible obstructive airway disease

**Usual Dosage**

Metered-dose inhalation: Aerosol: Children ≥4 years and Adults: 1-2 puffs every 4-6 hours

Nebulization:

Children 6-11 years: 0.31 mg 3 times/day (maximum dose: 0.63 mg 3 times/day)

Children >12 years and Adults: 0.63 mg 3 times/day at intervals of 6-8 hours; dosage may be increased to 1.25 mg 3 times/day with close monitoring for adverse effects. Most patients gain optimal benefit from regular use

**Dosage Forms Note:** Strength expressed as base.

Aerosol, oral, as tartrate: 45 mcg/actuation (15 g) [200 doses; chlorofluorocarbon free]

Solution for nebulization, as hydrochloride: 0.31 mg/3 mL (24s); 0.63 mg/3 mL (24s); 1.25 mg/3 mL (24s)

Solution for nebulization, concentrate, as hydrochloride: 1.25 mg/0.5 mL (30s)

**levalbuterol hydrochloride** *see* levalbuterol *on this page*

**levalbuterol tartrate** *see* levalbuterol *on this page*

**Levall G [US]** *see* guaifenesin and pseudoephedrine *on page 388*

**Levaquin**® **[US/Can]** *see* levofloxacin *on page 475*

**levarterenol bitartrate** *see* norepinephrine *on page 581*

**Levate**® **[Can]** *see* amitriptyline *on page 42*

**Levatol**® **[US/Can]** *see* penbutolol *on page 626*

**Levbid**® **[US]** *see* hyoscyamine *on page 424*

## levetiracetam (lee va tye RA se tam)

**Sound-Alike/Look-Alike Issues**

Potential for dispensing errors between Keppra® and Kaletra™ (lopinavir/ritonavir)

**U.S./Canadian Brand Names** Keppra® [US/Can]

**Therapeutic Category** Anticonvulsant, Miscellaneous

**Use** Adjunctive therapy in the treatment of partial onset seizures

**Usual Dosage** Oral:

Children 4-15 years: Partial onset seizures: 10 mg/kg/dose given twice daily; may increase every 2 weeks by 10 mg/kg/dose to a maximum of 30 mg/kg/dose twice daily

Children ≥16 years and Adults: Partial onset seizure: Initial: 500 mg twice daily; may increase every 2 weeks by 500 mg/dose to a maximum of 1500 mg twice daily. Doses >3000 mg/day have been used in trials; however, there is no evidence of increased benefit.

**Dosage Forms**

Solution, oral: 100 mg/mL (480 mL) [dye free; grape flavor]

Tablet: 250 mg, 500 mg, 750 mg

**Levitra**® **[US/Can]** *see* vardenafil *on page 840*

**Levlen**® **[US]** *see* ethinyl estradiol and levonorgestrel *on page 312*

**Levlite**™ **[US]** *see* ethinyl estradiol and levonorgestrel *on page 312*

## levobunolol (lee voe BYOO noe lole)

**Sound-Alike/Look-Alike Issues**

levobunolol may be confused with levocabastine

Betagan® may be confused with Betadine®

**Synonyms** *l*-bunolol hydrochloride; levobunolol hydrochloride

**U.S./Canadian Brand Names** Apo-Levobunolol® [Can]; Betagan® [US/Can]; Novo-Levobunolol [Can]; Optho-Bunolol® [Can]; PMS-Levobunolol [Can]

**Therapeutic Category** Beta-Adrenergic Blocker

**Use** To lower intraocular pressure in chronic open-angle glaucoma or ocular hypertension

**Usual Dosage** Adults: Ophthalmic: Instill 1 drop in the affected eye(s) 1-2 times/day

**Dosage Forms**

Solution, ophthalmic, as hydrochloride: 0.25% (5 mL, 10 mL); 0.5% (5 mL, 10 mL, 15 mL) [contains benzalkonium chloride and sodium metabisulfite]

Betagan®: 0.25% (5 mL, 10 mL); 0.5% (2 mL, 5 mL, 10 mL, 15 mL) [contains benzalkonium chloride and sodium metabisulfite]

**levobunolol hydrochloride** *see* levobunolol *on previous page*

## levobupivacaine (LEE voe byoo PIV a kane)

**U.S./Canadian Brand Names** Chirocaine® [Can]

**Therapeutic Category** Local Anesthetic, Amide Derivative; Local Anesthetic, Injectable

**Use** Production of local or regional anesthesia for surgery and obstetrics, and for postoperative pain management

**Usual Dosage** Adults: **Note:** Rapid injection of a large volume of local anesthetic solution should be avoided. Fractional (incremental) doses are recommended.

**Surgical Anesthesia:**

Epidural for surgery: Concentration: 0.5% to 0.75%; volume: 10-20 mL; dose: 50-150 mg; moderate to complete motor block

Epidural for C-section: Concentration: 0.5%; volume: 20-30 mL; dose: 100-150 mg; moderate to complete motor block

Peripheral nerve: Concentration: 0.25% to 0.5%; volume: 0.4 mL/kg (30 mL); dose: 1-2 mg/kg (75-150 mg); moderate to complete motor block

Ophthalmic: Concentration: 0.75%; volume: 5-15 mL; dose: 37.5-112.5 mg; moderate to complete motor block

Local infiltration: Concentration: 0.25%; volume: 60 mL; dose: 150 mg; motor block - not applicable

**Pain Management:** Levobupivacaine can be used epidurally with fentanyl or clonidine; dilutions for epidural administration should be made with preservative free 0.9% saline according to standard hospital procedures for sterility

Labor analgesia (epidural bolus): Concentration: 0.25%; volume: 10-20 mL; dose: 25-50 mg; minimal to moderate motor block

Postoperative pain (epidural infusion): Concentration: 0.125% to 0.25%; volume: 4-10 mL/hour; dose:5-25 mg/hour; minimal to moderate motor block. **Note:** 0.125% concentration is to be used only as adjunct therapy in combination with fentanyl or clonidine.

**Maximum dosage:** Epidural doses up to 375 mg have been administered incrementally to patients during a surgical procedure.

Intraoperative block and postoperative pain: 695 mg in 24 hours

Postoperative epidural infusion over 24 hours: 570 mg

Single-fractionated injection for brachial plexus block: 300 mg

**Dosage Forms** [DSC] = Discontinued product

Injection, solution [preservative free]: 2.5 mg/mL (10 mL, 30 mL); 5 mg/mL (10 mL, 30 mL); 7.5 mg/mL (10 mL, 30 mL) [DSC]

## levocabastine (LEE voe kab as teen)

**Sound-Alike/Look-Alike Issues**

levocabastine may be confused with levobunolol, levocarnitine

Livostin® may be confused with lovastatin

**Synonyms** levocabastine hydrochloride

**U.S./Canadian Brand Names** Livostin® [Can]

**Therapeutic Category** Antihistamine

**Use** Treatment of allergic conjunctivitis

**Usual Dosage** Children ≥12 years and Adults: Instill 1 drop in affected eye(s) 4 times/day for up to 2 weeks

**Dosage Forms** [DSC] = Discontinued product

Suspension, ophthalmic: 0.05% (5 mL, 10 mL) [contains benzalkonium chloride] [DSC]

**levocabastine hydrochloride** *see* levocabastine *on previous page*

# levocarnitine (lee voe KAR ni teen)

**Sound-Alike/Look-Alike Issues**
levocarnitine may be confused with levocabastine

**Synonyms** L-carnitine

**U.S./Canadian Brand Names** Carnitor® [US/Can]

**Therapeutic Category** Dietary Supplement

**Use** *Orphan drug:*
Oral: Primary systemic carnitine deficiency; acute and chronic treatment of patients with an inborn error of metabolism which results in secondary carnitine deficiency

I.V.: Acute and chronic treatment of patients with an inborn error of metabolism which results in secondary carnitine deficiency; prevention and treatment of carnitine deficiency in patients with end-stage renal disease (ESRD) who are undergoing hemodialysis.

**Usual Dosage**
Oral:
Infants/Children: Initial: 50 mg/kg/day; titrate to 50-100 mg/kg/day in divided doses with a maximum dose of 3 g/day
Adults: 990 mg (oral tablets) 2-3 times/day or 1-3 g/day (oral solution)
I.V.:
Metabolic disorders: 50 mg/kg as a slow 2- to 3-minute I.V. bolus or by I.V. infusion
Severe metabolic crisis:
A loading dose of 50 mg/kg over 2-3 minutes followed by an equivalent dose over the following 24 hours administered as every 3 hours or every 4 hours (never less than every 6 hours either by infusion or by intravenous injection)
All subsequent daily doses are recommended to be in the range of 50 mg/kg or as therapy may require
The highest dose administered has been 300 mg/kg
It is recommended that a plasma carnitine concentration be obtained prior to beginning parenteral therapy accompanied by weekly and monthly monitoring
ESRD patients on hemodialysis:
Predialysis levocarnitine concentrations below normal (40-50 µmol/L): 10-20 mg/kg dry body weight as a slow 2- to 3-minute bolus after each dialysis session
Dosage adjustments should be guided by predialysis trough levocarnitine concentrations and downward dose adjustments (to 5 mg/kg after dialysis) may be made as early as every 3rd or 4th week of therapy
**Note:** Safety and efficacy of oral carnitine have not been established in ESRD. Chronic administration of high oral doses to patients with severely compromised renal function or ESRD patients on dialysis may result in accumulation of metabolites.

**Dosage Forms**
Capsule: 250 mg
Injection, solution (Carnitor®): 200 mg/mL (5 mL)
Solution, oral (Carnitor®): 100 mg/mL (118 mL) [cherry flavor]
Tablet: 500 mg
Carnitor®: 330 mg

**levodopa and benserazide** *see* benserazide and levodopa *(Canada only)* on page 94

# levodopa and carbidopa (lee voe DOE pa & kar bi DOE pa)

**Synonyms** carbidopa and levodopa

**U.S./Canadian Brand Names** Apo-Levocarb® [Can]; Endo®-Levodopa/Carbidopa [Can]; Novo-Levo-carbidopa [Can]; Nu-Levocarb [Can]; Parcopa™ [US]; Sinemet® CR [US/Can]; Sinemet® [US/Can]

**Therapeutic Category** Anti-Parkinson Agent; Dopaminergic Agent (Anti-Parkinson)

**Use** Idiopathic Parkinson's disease; postencephalitic parkinsonism; symptomatic parkinsonism

**Usual Dosage** Oral: Adults: Parkinson's disease:
Immediate release tablet:
Initial: Carbidopa 25 mg/levodopa 100 mg 3 times/day
Dosage adjustment: Alternate tablet strengths may be substituted according to individual carbidopa/levodopa requirements. Increase by 1 tablet every other day as necessary, except when using the carbidopa 25 mg/levodopa 250 mg tablets where increases should be made using 1/2-1 tablet every 1-2 days. Use of more than 1 dosage strength or dosing 4 times/day may be required (maximum: 8 tablets of any strength/day or 200 mg of carbidopa and 2000 mg of levodopa)

Sustained release tablet:
Initial: Carbidopa 50 mg/levodopa 200 mg 2 times/day, at intervals not <6 hours
Dosage adjustment: May adjust every 3 days; intervals should be between 4-8 hours during the waking day (maximum: 8 tablets/day)

### Dosage Forms
Tablet immediate release (Sinemet®):
10/100: Carbidopa 10 mg and levodopa 100 mg
25/100: Carbidopa 25 mg and levodopa 100 mg
25/250: Carbidopa 25 mg and levodopa 250 mg
Tablet, immediate release, orally-disintegrating (Parcopa™):
10/100: Carbidopa 10 mg and levodopa 100 mg [contains phenylalanine 3.4 mg/tablet; mint flavor]
25/100: Carbidopa 25 mg and levodopa 100 mg [contains phenylalanine 3.4 mg/tablet; mint flavor]
25/250: Carbidopa 25 mg and levodopa 250 mg [contains phenylalanine 8.4 mg/tablet; mint flavor]
Tablet, sustained release (Sinemet® CR):
Carbidopa 25 mg and levodopa 100 mg
Carbidopa 50 mg and levodopa 200 mg

# levodopa, carbidopa, and entacapone
(lee voe DOE pa, kar bi DOE pa, & en TA ka pone)

**Synonyms** carbidopa, levodopa, and entacapone; entacapone, carbidopa, and levodopa

**U.S./Canadian Brand Names** Stalevo™ [US]

**Therapeutic Category** Anti-Parkinson Agent (Dopamine Agonist); Anti-Parkinson Agent, COMT Inhibitor

**Use** Treatment of idiopathic Parkinson's disease

**Usual Dosage** Oral: Adults: Parkinson's disease:
**Note:** All strengths of Stalevo™ contain a carbidopa/levodopa ratio of 1:4 plus entacapone 200 mg.
Dose should be individualized based on therapeutic response; doses may be adjusted by changing strength or adjusting interval. Fractionated doses are not recommended and only 1 tablet should be given at each dosing interval; maximum dose: 8 tablets/day (equivalent to entacapone 1600 mg/day)
Patients previously treated with carbidopa/levodopa immediate release tablets (ratio of 1:4):
With current entacapone therapy: May switch directly to corresponding strength of combination tablet. No data available on transferring patients from controlled release preparations or products with a 1:10 ratio of carbidopa/levodopa.
Without entacapone therapy:
If current levodopa dose is >600 mg/day: Levodopa dose reduction may be required when adding entacapone to therapy; therefore, titrate dose using individual products first (carbidopa/levodopa immediate release with a ratio of 1:4 plus entacapone 200 mg); then transfer to combination product once stabilized.
If current levodopa dose is <600 mg without dyskinesias: May transfer to corresponding dose of combination product; monitor, dose reduction of levodopa may be required.

**Dosage Forms** Tablet [film coated]:
50: Carbidopa 12.5 mg, levodopa 50 mg, and entacapone 200 mg
100: Carbidopa 25 mg, levodopa 100 mg, and entacapone 200 mg
150: Carbidopa 37.5 mg, levodopa 150 mg, and entacapone 200 mg

**Levo-Dromoran® [US]** see levorphanol on page 477

# levofloxacin (lee voe FLOKS a sin)

**U.S./Canadian Brand Names** Iquix® [US]; Levaquin® [US/Can]; Novo-Levofloxacin [Can]; Quixin™ [US]

**Therapeutic Category** Antibiotic, Ophthalmic; Antibiotic, Quinolone

**Use**
Systemic: Treatment of mild, moderate, or severe infections caused by susceptible organisms. Includes the treatment of community-acquired pneumonia, including multidrug resistant strains of *S. pneumoniae* (MDRSP); nosocomial pneumonia; chronic bronchitis (acute bacterial exacerbation); acute bacterial sinusitis; urinary tract infection (uncomplicated or complicated), including acute pyelonephritis caused by *E. coli*; prostatitis (chronic bacterial); skin or skin structure infections (uncomplicated or complicated); prevention of inhalational anthrax (postexposure)
Ophthalmic: Treatment of bacterial conjunctivitis caused by susceptible organisms (Quixin™ 0.5% ophthalmic solution); treatment of corneal ulcer caused by susceptible organisms (Iquix® 1.5% ophthalmic solution)
(Continued)

# levofloxacin (Continued)

## Usual Dosage
Oral, I.V.: Adults:

**Note:** Sequential therapy (intravenous to oral) may be instituted based on prescriber's discretion.

Bacterial sinusitis (acute): 500 mg every 24 hours for 10-14 days or 750 mg every 24 hours for 5 days

Chronic bronchitis (acute bacterial exacerbation): 500 mg every 24 hours for at least 7 days

Inhalational anthrax: 500 mg every 24 hours for 60 days, beginning as soon as possible after exposure

Pneumonia:

Community-acquired: 500 mg every 24 hours for 7-14 days or 750 mg every 24 hours for 5 days (efficacy of 5-day regimen for MDRSP not established)

Nosocomial: 750 mg every 24 hours for 7-14 days

Prostatitis (chronic bacterial): 500 mg every 24 hours for 28 days

Skin infections:

Uncomplicated: 500 mg every 24 hours for 7-10 days

Complicated: 750 mg every 24 hours for 7-14 days

Urinary tract infections:

Uncomplicated: 250 mg once daily for 3 days

Complicated, including acute pyelonephritis: 250 mg every 24 hours for 10 days

Ophthalmic:

Conjunctivitis (0.5% ophthalmic solution): Children ≥1 year and Adults:

Treatment day 1 and day 2: Instill 1-2 drops into affected eye(s) every 2 hours while awake, up to 8 times/day

Treatment day 3 through day 7: Instill 1-2 drops into affected eye(s) every 4 hours while awake, up to 4 times/day

Corneal ulceration (1.5% ophthalmic solution): Children ≥6 years and Adults:

Treatment day 1 through day 3: Instill 1-2 drops into affected eye(s) every 30 minutes to 2 hours while awake and ~4-6 hours after retiring.

Treatment day 4 to treatment completion: Instill 1-2 drops into affected eye(s) every 1-4 hours while awake.

## Dosage Forms
Infusion [premixed in $D_5W$] (Levaquin®): 250 mg (50 mL); 500 mg (100 mL); 750 mg (150 mL)

Injection, solution [preservative free] (Levaquin®): 25 mg/mL (20 mL, 30 mL)

Solution, ophthalmic:

Iquix®: 1.5% (5 mL)

Quixin™: 0.5% (5 mL) [contains benzalkonium chloride]

Solution, oral (Levaquin®): 25 mg/mL (480 mL) [contains benzyl alcohol]

Tablet (Levaquin®): 250 mg, 500 mg, 750 mg

Levaquin® Leva-Pak: 750 mg (5s)

**levomepromazine** *see* methotrimeprazine *(Canada only)* on page 526

# levonorgestrel (LEE voe nor jes trel)

**Synonyms** LNg 20

**U.S./Canadian Brand Names** Mirena® [US/Can]; Norplant® Implant [Can]; Plan B® [US/Can]

**Therapeutic Category** Contraceptive, Implant (Progestin); Contraceptive, Progestin Only

**Use** Prevention of pregnancy

**Usual Dosage** Adults: Females:

**Long-term prevention of pregnancy:** Intrauterine system: To be inserted into uterine cavity; should be inserted within 7 days of onset of menstruation or immediately after 1st trimester abortion; releases 20 mcg levonorgestrel/day over 5 years. May be removed and replaced with a new unit at anytime during menstrual cycle; do not leave any one system in place for >5 years

**Emergency contraception:** Oral tablet: One 0.75 mg tablet as soon as possible within 72 hours of unprotected sexual intercourse; a second 0.75 mg tablet should be taken 12 hours after the first dose; may be used at any time during menstrual cycle

**Dosage Forms**

Intrauterine device (Mirena®): 52 mg levonorgestrel/unit [releases levonorgestrel 20 mcg/day]

Tablet (Plan B®): 0.75 mg

**levonorgestrel and estradiol** *see* estradiol and levonorgestrel on page 301

**levonorgestrel and ethinyl estradiol** *see* ethinyl estradiol and levonorgestrel on page 312

**Levophed® [US/Can]** *see* norepinephrine on page 581

**Levora**® **[US]** *see* ethinyl estradiol and levonorgestrel *on page 312*

# levorphanol (lee VOR fa nole)
**Synonyms** levorphan tartrate; levorphanol tartrate
**U.S./Canadian Brand Names** Levo-Dromoran® [US]
**Therapeutic Category** Analgesic, Narcotic
**Controlled Substance** C-II
**Use** Relief of moderate to severe pain; also used parenterally for preoperative sedation and an adjunct to nitrous oxide/oxygen anesthesia; 2 mg levorphanol produces analgesia comparable to that produced by 10 mg of morphine
**Usual Dosage** Adults: **Note:** These are guidelines and do not represent the maximum doses that may be required in all patients. Doses should be titrated to pain relief/prevention.
Acute pain (moderate to severe):
Oral: Initial: Opiate-naive: 2 mg every 6-8 hours as needed; patients with prior opiate exposure may require higher initial doses; usual dosage range: 2-4 mg every 6-8 hours as needed
I.M., SubQ: Initial: Opiate-naive: 1 mg every 6-8 hours as needed; patients with prior opiate exposure may require higher initial doses; usual dosage range: 1-2 mg every 6-8 hours as needed
Slow I.V.: Initial: Opiate-naive: Up to 1 mg/dose every 3-6 hours as needed; patients with prior opiate exposure may require higher initial doses
Chronic pain: Patients taking opioids chronically may become tolerant and require doses higher than the usual dosage range to maintain the desired effect. Tolerance can be managed by appropriate dose titration. There is no optimal or maximal dose for levorphanol in chronic pain. The appropriate dose is one that relieves pain throughout its dosing interval without causing unmanageable side effects.
Premedication: I.M., SubQ: 1-2 mg/dose 60-90 minutes prior to surgery; older or debilitated patients usually require less drug
**Dosage Forms**
Injection, solution, as tartrate: 2 mg/mL (1 mL, 10 mL)
Tablet, as tartrate: 2 mg

**levorphanol tartrate** *see* levorphanol *on this page*

**levorphan tartrate** *see* levorphanol *on this page*

**Levo-T**™ *(Discontinued)* *see* levothyroxine *on this page*

**Levothroid**® **[US]** *see* levothyroxine *on this page*

# levothyroxine (lee voe thye ROKS een)
**Sound-Alike/Look-Alike Issues**
levothyroxine may be confused with liothyronine
Levoxyl® may be confused with Lanoxin®, Luvox®
Synthroid® may be confused with Symmetrel®
**Synonyms** *L*-thyroxine sodium; levothyroxine sodium; $T_4$
**U.S./Canadian Brand Names** Eltroxin® [Can]; Levothroid® [US]; Levoxyl® [US]; Synthroid® [US/Can]; Unithroid® [US]
**Therapeutic Category** Thyroid Product
**Use** Replacement or supplemental therapy in hypothyroidism; pituitary TSH suppression
**Usual Dosage** Doses should be adjusted based on clinical response and laboratory parameters.
Oral:
Children: Hypothyroidism:
Newborns: Initial: 10-15 mcg/kg/day. Lower doses of 25 mcg/day should be considered in newborns at risk for cardiac failure. Newborns with $T_4$ levels <5 mcg/dL should be started at 50 mcg/day. Adjust dose at 4- to 6-week intervals.
Infants and Children: Dose based on body weight and age as listed below. Children with severe or chronic hypothyroidism should be started at 25 mcg/day; adjust dose by 25 mcg every 2-4 weeks. In older children, hyperactivity may be decreased by starting with $1/4$ of the recommended dose and increasing by $1/4$ dose each week until the full replacement dose is reached. Refer to adult dosing once growth and puberty are complete.
0-3 months: 10-15 mcg/kg/day
3-6 months: 8-10 mcg/kg/day
6-12 months: 6-8 mcg/kg/day
1-5 years: 5-6 mcg/kg/day
6-12 years: 4-5 mcg/kg/day
>12 years: 2-3 mcg/kg/day
(Continued)

# levothyroxine *(Continued)*

Adults:

Hypothyroidism: 1.7 mcg/kg/day in otherwise healthy adults <50 years old, children in whom growth and puberty are complete, and older adults who have been recently treated for hyperthyroidism or who have been hypothyroid for only a few months. Titrate dose every 6 weeks. Average starting dose ~100 mcg; usual doses are ≤200 mcg/day; doses ≥300 mcg/day are rare (consider poor compliance, malabsorption, and/or drug interactions).

Severe hypothyroidism: Initial: 12.5-25 mcg/day; adjust dose by 25 mcg/day every 2-4 weeks as appropriate; **Note:** Oral agents are not recommended for myxedema (see I.V. dosing).

Subclinical hypothyroidism (if treated): 1 mcg/kg/day

TSH suppression:

Well-differentiated thyroid cancer: Highly individualized; Doses >2 mcg/kg/day may be needed to suppress TSH to <0.1 mU/L.

Benign nodules and nontoxic multinodular goiter: Goal TSH suppression: 0.1-0.3 mU/L

I.M., I.V.: Children, Adults: Hypothyroidism: 50% of the oral dose

I.V.: Adults: Myxedema coma or stupor: 200-500 mcg, then 100-300 mcg the next day if necessary; smaller doses should be considered in patients with cardiovascular disease

## Dosage Forms

Injection, powder for reconstitution, as sodium: 0.2 mg, 0.5 mg

Tablet, as sodium: 25 mcg, 50 mcg, 75 mcg, 88 mcg, 100 mcg, 112 mcg, 125 mcg, 150 mcg, 175 mcg, 200 mcg, 300 mcg

Levothroid®: 25 mcg, 50 mcg, 75 mcg, 88 mcg, 100 mcg, 112 mcg, 125 mcg, 150 mcg, 175 mcg, 200 mcg, 300 mcg

Levoxyl®, Synthroid®: 25 mcg, 50 mcg, 75 mcg, 88 mcg, 100 mcg, 112 mcg, 125 mcg, 137 mcg, 150 mcg, 175 mcg, 200 mcg, 300 mcg

Unithroid®: 25 mcg, 50 mcg, 75 mcg, 88 mcg, 100 mcg, 112 mcg, 125 mcg, 150 mcg, 175 mcg, 200 mcg, 300 mcg

**levothyroxine sodium** *see* levothyroxine *on previous page*

**Levoxyl® [US]** *see* levothyroxine *on previous page*

**Levsin® [US/Can]** *see* hyoscyamine *on page 424*

**Levsinex® [US]** *see* hyoscyamine *on page 424*

**Levsin/SL® [US]** *see* hyoscyamine *on page 424*

**Levulan® [Can]** *see* aminolevulinic acid *on page 40*

**Levulan® Kerastick® [US]** *see* aminolevulinic acid *on page 40*

**levulose, dextrose and phosphoric acid** *see* fructose, dextrose, and phosphoric acid *on page 362*

**Lexapro™ [US]** *see* escitalopram *on page 297*

**Lexiva™ [US]** *see* fosamprenavir *on page 360*

**Lexxel® [US/Can]** *see* enalapril and felodipine *on page 284*

**LFA-3/IgG(1) fusion protein, human** *see* alefacept *on page 25*

**LHRH** *see* gonadorelin *on page 381*

**l-hyoscyamine sulfate** *see* hyoscyamine *on page 424*

**Librax® [Can]** *see* clidinium and chlordiazepoxide *on page 191*

**Librax® [original formulation] *(Discontinued)*** *see* clidinium and chlordiazepoxide *on page 191*

**Librium® [US]** *see* chlordiazepoxide *on page 167*

**Lice-Aid [US-OTC]** *see* pyrethrins and piperonyl butoxide *on page 699*

**Lice-Enz® Shampoo *(Discontinued)***

**Licide® [US-OTC]** *see* pyrethrins and piperonyl butoxide *on page 699*

**LidaMantle® [US]** *see* lidocaine *on next page*

**Lida-Mantle® HC [US]** *see* lidocaine and hydrocortisone *on page 482*

**Lidemol® [Can]** *see* fluocinonide *on page 345*

**Lidex® [US/Can]** *see* fluocinonide *on page 345*

**Lidex-E**® **[US]** *see* fluocinonide *on page 345*

# lidocaine (LYE doe kane)

**Synonyms** lidocaine hydrochloride; lignocaine hydrochloride

**U.S./Canadian Brand Names** Anestacon® [US]; Band-Aid® Hurt-Free™ Antiseptic Wash [US-OTC]; Betacaine® [Can]; Burn Jel [US-OTC]; Burn-O-Jel [US-OTC]; Burnamycin [US-OTC]; L-M-X™ 4 [US-OTC]; L-M-X™ 5 [US-OTC]; LidaMantle® [US]; Lidodan™ [Can]; Lidoderm® [US/Can]; LTA® 360 [US]; Premjact® [US-OTC]; Solarcaine® Aloe Extra Burn Relief [US-OTC]; Topicaine® [US-OTC]; Xylocaine® MPF [US]; Xylocaine® Viscous [US]; Xylocaine® [US/Can]; Xylocard® [Can]; Zilactin® [Can]; Zilactin-L® [US-OTC]

**Therapeutic Category** Analgesic, Topical; Antiarrhythmic Agent, Class I-B; Local Anesthetic

**Use** Local anesthetic and acute treatment of ventricular arrhythmias from myocardial infarction, cardiac manipulation, digitalis intoxication; drug of choice for ventricular ectopy, ventricular tachycardia (VT), ventricular fibrillation (VF); for pulseless VT or VF preferably administer **after** defibrillation and epinephrine; control of premature ventricular contractions, wide-complex paroxysmal supraventricular tachycardia (PSVT); control of hemodynamically compromising PVCs; hemodynamically stable VT

Rectal: Temporary relief of pain and itching due to anorectal disorders

Topical: Local anesthetic for use in laser, cosmetic, and outpatient surgeries; minor burns, cuts, and abrasions of the skin

**Orphan drug:** Lidoderm® Patch: Relief of allodynia (painful hypersensitivity) and chronic pain in postherpetic neuralgia

## Usual Dosage

**Antiarrhythmic:**

Children:

I.V., I.O.: (**Note:** For use in pulseless VT or VF, give after defibrillation and epinephrine): Loading dose: 1 mg/kg; follow with continuous infusion; may administer second bolus of 0.5-1 mg/kg if delay between bolus and start of infusion is >15 minutes; continuous infusion: 20-50 mcg/kg/minute. Use 20 mcg/kg/minute in patients with shock, hepatic disease, cardiac arrest, mild CHF; moderate-to-severe CHF may require $^1/_2$ loading dose and lower infusion rates to avoid toxicity.

E.T. (loading dose only): 2-10 times the I.V. bolus dose; dilute with NS to a volume of 3-5 mL and follow with several positive-pressure ventilations

Adults:

Ventricular fibrillation or pulseless ventricular tachycardia (after defibrillation and epinephrine): I.V.: Initial: 1-1.5 mg/kg. Refractory ventricular tachycardia or ventricular fibrillation, a repeat 0.5-0.75 mg/kg bolus may be given over 3-5 minutes after initial dose. Total dose should not exceed 200-300 mg during a 1-hour period or 3 mg/kg total dose. Follow with continuous infusion (1-4 mg/minute) after return of perfusion. Reappearance of arrhythmia during constant infusion: 0.5 mg/kg bolus and reassessment of infusion.

**Infusion rates:** 2 g/250 mL D$_5$W (infusion pump should be used):

1 mg/minute: 7.5 mL/hour
2 mg/minute: 15 mL/hour
3 mg/minute: 22.5 mL/hour
4 mg/minute: 30 mL/hour

**E.T. (loading dose only):** 2-2.5 times the recommended I.V. dose; dilute in 10 mL NS or distilled water. **Note:** Absorption is greater with distilled water, but causes more adverse effects on PaO$_2$.

Hemodynamically stable VT: 0.5-0.75 mg/kg followed by synchronized cardioversion

**Note:** Decrease dose in patients with CHF, shock, or hepatic disease.

**Anesthesia, topical:**

Cream:

LidaMantle®: Skin irritation: Children and Adults: Apply to affected area 2-3 times/day as needed

L-M-X™ 4: Children ≥2 years and Adults: Apply $^1/_4$ inch thick layer to intact skin. Leave on until adequate anesthetic effect is obtained. Remove cream and cleanse area before beginning procedure.

L-M-X™ 5: Relief of anorectal pain and itching: Children ≥12 years and Adults: Rectal: Apply topically to clean, dry area **or** using applicator, insert rectally, up to 6 times/day

Gel, ointment, solution: Adults: Apply to affected area ≤3 times/day as needed (maximum dose: 4.5 mg/kg, not to exceed 300 mg)

Jelly:

Children ≥10 years: Dose varies with age and weight (maximum dose: 4.5 mg/kg)

Adults (maximum dose: 30 mL [600 mg] in any 12-hour period):

Anesthesia of male urethra: 5-30 mL

Anesthesia of female urethra: 3-5 mL

(Continued)

## lidocaine *(Continued)*

Lubrication of endotracheal tube: Apply a moderate amount to external surface only

Liquid: Cold sores and fever blisters: Children ≥5 years and Adults: Apply to affected area every 6 hours as needed

Patch: Postherpetic neuralgia: Adults: Apply patch to most painful area. Up to 3 patches may be applied in a single application. Patch may remain in place for up to 12 hours in any 24-hour period.

**Anesthetic, local injectable:** Children and Adults: Varies with procedure, degree of anesthesia needed, vascularity of tissue, duration of anesthesia required, and physical condition of patient; maximum: 4.5 mg/kg/dose; do not repeat within 2 hours.

**Dosage Forms** [DSC] = Discontinued product

Cream, rectal (L-M-X™ 5): 5% (15 g) [contains benzyl alcohol; packaged with applicator]; (30 g) [contains benzyl alcohol]

Cream, topical (L-M-X™ 4): 4% (5 g) [contains benzyl alcohol; packaged with Tegaderm™ dressing]; (15 g, 30 g) [contains benzyl alcohol]

Cream, topical, as hydrochloride: 3% (30 g)

LidaMantle®: 3% (30 g, 85 g)

Gel, topical:

Burn-O-Jel: 0.5% (90 g)

Topicaine®: 4% (10 g, 30 g, 113 g) [contains alcohol 35%, benzyl alcohol, aloe vera, and jojoba]

Gel, topical, as hydrochloride:

Burn Jel: 2% (3.5 g, 120 g)

Solarcaine® Aloe Extra Burn Relief: 0.5% (113 g, 226 g) [contains aloe vera gel and tartrazine]

Infusion, as hydrochloride [premixed in $D_5W$]: 0.4% [4 mg/mL] (250 mL, 500 mL); 0.8% [8 mg/mL] (250 mL, 500 mL)

Injection, solution, as hydrochloride: 0.5% [5 mg/mL] (50 mL); 1% [10 mg/mL] (2 mL, 10 mL, 20 mL, 30 mL, 50 mL); 2% [20 mg/mL] (2 mL, 5 mL, 20 mL, 50 mL)

Xylocaine®: 0.5% [5 mg/mL] (50 mL); 1% [10 mg/mL] (10 mL, 20 mL, 50 mL); 2% [20 mg/mL] (1.8 mL, 10 mL, 20 mL, 50 mL)

Injection, solution, as hydrochloride [preservative free]: 0.5% [5 mg/mL] (50 mL); 1% [10 mg/mL] (2 mL, 5 mL, 30 mL); 1.5% [15 mg/mL] (20 mL); 2% [20 mg/mL] (2 mL, 5 mL, 10 mL); 4% [40 mg/mL] (5 mL)

Xylocaine®: 10% [100 mg/mL] (5 mL) [for ventricular arrhythmias]

Xylocaine® MPF: 0.5% [5 mg/mL] (50 mL); 1% [10 mg/mL] (2 mL, 5 mL, 10 mL, 30 mL); 1.5% [15 mg/mL] (10 mL, 20 mL); 2% [20 mg/mL] (2 mL, 5 mL, 10 mL); 4% [40 mg/mL] (5 mL)

Injection, solution, as hydrochloride [premixed in $D_{7.5}W$, preservative free]: 5% (2 mL)

Xylocaine® MPF: 1.5% (2 mL) [DSC]

Jelly, topical, as hydrochloride: 2% (5 mL, 30 mL)

Anestacon®: 2% (15 mL) [contains benzalkonium chloride]

Xylocaine®: 2% (5 mL, 30 mL)

Liquid, topical (Zilactin®-L): 2.5% (7.5 mL)

Lotion, topical, as hydrochloride (LidaMantle®): 3% (177 mL)

Ointment, topical: 5% (37 g, 50 g)

Solution, topical, as hydrochloride: 4% [40 mg/mL] (50 mL)

Band-Aid® Hurt-Free™ Antiseptic Wash: 2% (180 mL)

LTA® 360: 4% [40 mg/mL] (4 mL) [packaged with cannula for laryngotracheal administration

Xylocaine®: 4% [40 mg/mL] (50 mL)

Solution, viscous, as hydrochloride: 2% [20 mg/mL] (20 mL, 100 mL)

Xylocaine® Viscous: 2% [20 mg/mL] (100 mL, 450 mL)

Spray, topical:

Burnamycin: 0.5% (60 mL) [contains aloe vera gel and menthol]

Premjact®: 9.6% (13 mL)

Solarcaine® Aloe Extra Burn Relief: 0.5% (127 g) [contains aloe vera]

Transdermal system, topical (Lidoderm®): 5% (30s)

## lidocaine and epinephrine *(LYE doe kane & ep i NEF rin)*

**Synonyms** epinephrine and lidocaine

**U.S./Canadian Brand Names** LidoSite™ [US]; Xylocaine® MPF With Epinephrine [US]; Xylocaine® With Epinephrine [US/Can]

**Therapeutic Category** Local Anesthetic

**Use** Local infiltration anesthesia; AVS for nerve block; topical local analgesia for superficial dermatologic procedures

**Usual Dosage** Dosage varies with the anesthetic procedure, degree of anesthesia needed, vascularity of tissue, duration of anesthesia required, and physical condition of patient.

Dental anesthesia, infiltration, or conduction block:

Children <10 years: 20-30 mg (1-1.5 mL) of lidocaine hydrochloride as a 2% solution with epinephrine 1:100,000; maximum: 4-5 mg of lidocaine hydrochloride/kg of body weight or 100-150 mg as a single dose

Children >10 years and Adults: Do not exceed 6.6 mg/kg body weight or 300 mg of lidocaine hydrochloride and 3 mcg (0.003 mg) of epinephrine/kg of body weight or 0.2 mg epinephrine per dental appointment. The effective anesthetic dose varies with procedure, intensity of anesthesia needed, duration of anesthesia required, and physical condition of the patient. Always use the lowest effective dose along with careful aspiration.

The following numbers of dental carpules (1.8 mL) provide the indicated amounts of lidocaine hydrochloride 2% and epinephrine 1:100,000:

**1 Cartridge:** 36 mg lidocaine HCl 2% and 0.018 mg epinephrine 1:100,000
**2 Cartridges:** 72 mg lidocaine HCl 2% and 0.036 mg epinephrine 1:100,000
**3 Cartridges:** 108 mg lidocaine HCl 2% and 0.054 mg epinephrine 1:100,000
**4 Cartridges:** 144 mg lidocaine HCl 2% and 0.072 mg epinephrine 1:100,000
**5 Cartridges:** 180 mg lidocaine HCl 2% and 0.090 mg epinephrine 1:100,000
**6 Cartridges:** 216 mg lidocaine HCl 2% and 0.108 mg epinephrine 1:100,000
**7 Cartridges:** 252 mg lidocaine HCl 2% and 0.126 mg epinephrine 1:100,000
**8 Cartridges:** 288 mg lidocaine HCl 2% and 0.144 mg epinephrine 1:100,000
**9 Cartridges:** 324 mg lidocaine HCl 2% and 0.162 mg epinephrine 1:100,000
**10 Cartridges:** 360 mg lidocaine HCl 2% and 0.180 mg epinephrine 1:100,000

For most routine dental procedures, lidocaine hydrochloride 2% with epinephrine 1:100,000 is preferred. When a more pronounced hemostasis is required, a 1:50,000 epinephrine concentration should be used. The following numbers of dental carpules (1.8 mL) provide the indicated amounts of lidocaine hydrochloride 2% and epinephrine 1:50,000:

**1 Cartridge:** 36 mg lidocaine HCl 2% and 0.036 mg epinephrine 1:50,000
**2 Cartridges:** 72 mg lidocaine HCl 2% and 0.072 mg epinephrine 1:50,000
**3 Cartridges:** 108 mg lidocaine HCl 2% and 0.108 mg epinephrine 1:50,000
**4 Cartridges:** 144 mg lidocaine HCl 2% and 0.144 mg epinephrine 1:50,000
**5 Cartridges:** 180 mg lidocaine HCl 2% and 0.180 mg epinephrine 1:50,000
**6 Cartridges:** 216 mg lidocaine HCl 2% and 0.216 mg epinephrine 1:50,000

Dermatologic procedure: Children ≥5 and Adults: Topical: Place 1 transdermal patch over area requiring analgesia; attach patch to iontophoretic controller and leave on for 10 minutes. Remove patch and perform procedure within 10-20 minutes of patch removal. Do not use another patch for 30 minutes.

**Dosage Forms**

**Injection, solution:**

0.5% / 1:200,000: Lidocaine hydrochloride 0.5% and epinephrine 1:200,000 (50 mL)

1% / 1:100,000: Lidocaine hydrochloride 1% and epinephrine 1:100,000 (20 mL, 30 mL, 50 mL)

1% / 1:200,000: Lidocaine hydrochloride 1% and epinephrine 1:200,000 (30 mL)

1.5% / 1:200,000: Lidocaine hydrochloride 1.5% and epinephrine 1:200,000 (30 mL)

2% / 1:100,000: Lidocaine hydrochloride 2% and epinephrine 1:100,000 (30 mL, 50 mL)

2% / 1:200,000: Lidocaine hydrochloride 2% and epinephrine 1:200,000 (20 mL)

*Xylocaine®  with Epinephrine:*

0.5% / 1:200,000: Lidocaine hydrochloride 0.5% and epinephrine 1:200,000 (50 mL) [contains methylparaben]

1% / 1:100,000: Lidocaine hydrochloride 1% and epinephrine 1:100,000 (10 mL, 20 mL, 50 mL) [contains methylparaben]

2% / 1:50,000: Lidocaine hydrochloride 2% and epinephrine 1:50,000 (1.8 mL) [contains sodium metabisulfite]

2% / 1:100,000: Lidocaine hydrochloride 2% and epinephrine 1:100,000 (1.8 mL) [contains sodium metabisulfite]; (10 mL, 20 mL, 50 mL) [contains methylparaben]

*Xylocaine®-MPF with Epinephrine:*

1% / 1:200,000: Lidocaine hydrochloride 1% and epinephrine 1:200,000 (5 mL, 10 mL, 30 mL) [contains sodium metabisulfite]

1.5% / 1:200,000: Lidocaine hydrochloride 1.5% and epinephrine 1:200,000 (5 mL, 10 mL, 30 mL) [contains sodium metabisulfite]

2% / 1:200,000: Lidocaine hydrochloride 2% and epinephrine 1:200,000 (5 mL, 10 mL, 20 mL) [contains sodium metabisulfite]

(Continued)

## lidocaine and epinephrine *(Continued)*

**Transdermal system (LidoSite™):** Lidocaine hydrochloride 10% and epinephrine 0.1% (25s) [contains sodium metabisulfite; for use only with LidoSite™ controller]

## lidocaine and hydrocortisone *(LYE doe kane & hye droe KOR ti sone)*

**Synonyms** hydrocortisone and lidocaine

**U.S./Canadian Brand Names** AnaMantle® HC [US]; Lida-Mantle® HC [US]

**Therapeutic Category** Anesthetic/Corticosteroid

**Use** Topical anti-inflammatory and anesthetic for skin disorders; rectal for the treatment of hemorrhoids, anal fissures, pruritus ani, or similar conditions

**Usual Dosage** Adults:
Topical: Apply 2-3 times/day
Rectal: One applicatorful twice daily

**Dosage Forms**
Cream, rectal (AnaMantle® HC): Lidocaine hydrochloride 3% and hydrocortisone acetate 0.5% (7 g) [kit contains 14 single-use tubes (7 g each) and 14 applicators]
Cream, topical: Lidocaine hydrochloride 3% and hydrocortisone acetate 0.5% (30 g)
Lida-Mantle® HC: Lidocaine hydrochloride 3% and hydrocortisone acetate 0.5% (30 g, 85 g)
Lotion, topical (Lida-Mantle® HC): Lidocaine hydrochloride 3% and hydrocortisone acetate 0.5% (177 mL)

## lidocaine and prilocaine *(LYE doe kane & PRIL oh kane)*

**Synonyms** prilocaine and lidocaine

**U.S./Canadian Brand Names** EMLA® [US/Can]

**Therapeutic Category** Analgesic, Topical

**Use** Topical anesthetic for use on normal intact skin to provide local analgesia for minor procedures such as I.V. cannulation or venipuncture; has also been used for painful procedures such as lumbar puncture and skin graft harvesting; for superficial minor surgery of genital mucous membranes and as an adjunct for local infiltration anesthesia in genital mucous membranes.

**Usual Dosage** Although the incidence of systemic adverse effects with EMLA® is very low, caution should be exercised, particularly when applying over large areas and leaving on for >2 hours
Children (intact skin): EMLA® should **not** be used in neonates with a gestation age <37 weeks nor in infants <12 months of age who are receiving treatment with methemoglobin-inducing agents
Dosing is based on child's age and weight:
Age 0-3 months or <5 kg: Apply a maximum of 1 g over no more than 10 cm$^2$ of skin; leave on for no longer than 1 hour
Age 3 months to 12 months and >5 kg: Apply no more than a maximum 2 g total over no more than 20 cm$^2$ of skin; leave on for no longer than 4 hours
Age 1-6 years and >10 kg: Apply no more than a maximum of 10 g total over no more than 100 cm$^2$ of skin; leave on for no longer than 4 hours.
Age 7-12 years and >20 kg: Apply no more than a maximum 20 g total over no more than 200 cm$^2$ of skin; leave on for no longer than 4 hours.
**Note:** If a patient greater than 3 months old does not meet the minimum weight requirement, the maximum total dose should be restricted to the corresponding maximum based on patient weight.

Adults (intact skin):
EMLA® cream and EMLA® anesthetic disc: A thick layer of EMLA® cream is applied to intact skin and covered with an occlusive dressing, or alternatively, an EMLA® anesthetic disc is applied to intact skin
Minor dermal procedures (eg, I.V. cannulation or venipuncture): Apply 2.5 g of cream (1/2 of the 5 g tube) over 20-25 cm of skin surface area, or 1 anesthetic disc (1 g over 10 cm$^2$) for at least 1 hour.
**Note:** In clinical trials, 2 sites were usually prepared in case there was a technical problem with cannulation or venipuncture at the first site.
Major dermal procedures (eg, more painful dermatological procedures involving a larger skin area such as split thickness skin graft harvesting): Apply 2 g of cream per 10 cm$^2$ of skin and allow to remain in contact with the skin for at least 2 hours.
Adult male genital skin (eg, pretreatment prior to local anesthetic infiltration): Apply a thick layer of cream (1 g/10 cm$^2$) to the skin surface for 15 minutes. Local anesthetic infiltration should be performed immediately after removal of EMLA® cream.
**Note:** Dermal analgesia can be expected to increase for up to 3 hours under occlusive dressing and persist for 1-2 hours after removal of the cream
Adult females: Genital mucous membranes: Minor procedures (eg, removal of condylomata acuminata, pretreatment for local anesthetic infiltration): Apply 5-10 g (thick layer) of cream for 5-10 minutes

**Dosage Forms**
Cream, topical: Lidocaine 2.5% and prilocaine 2.5% (5 g, 30 g)
EMLA®: Lidocaine 2.5% and prilocaine 2.5% (5 g, 30 g) [each packaged with Tegaderm® dressings]
Disc, topical: Lidocaine 2.5% and prilocaine 2.5% per disc (2s, 10s) [each 1 g disc is 10 cm$^2$]

**lidocaine hydrochloride** *see* lidocaine *on page 479*

**Lidodan™ [Can]** *see* lidocaine *on page 479*

**Lidoderm® [US/Can]** *see* lidocaine *on page 479*

**LidoPen® I.M. Injection Auto-Injector *(Discontinued)*** *see* lidocaine *on page 479*

**LidoSite™ [US]** *see* lidocaine and epinephrine *on page 480*

**LID-Pack® [Can]** *see* bacitracin and polymyxin B *on page 86*

**lignocaine hydrochloride** *see* lidocaine *on page 479*

**Limbitrol® [US/Can]** *see* amitriptyline and chlordiazepoxide *on page 43*

**Limbitrol® DS [US]** *see* amitriptyline and chlordiazepoxide *on page 43*

**Lin-Amox [Can]** *see* amoxicillin *on page 46*

**Lin-Buspirone [Can]** *see* buspirone *on page 123*

# lindane (LIN dane)
**Synonyms** benzene hexachloride; gamma benzene hexachloride; hexachlorocyclohexane
**U.S./Canadian Brand Names** Hexit™ [Can]; PMS-Lindane [Can]
**Therapeutic Category** Scabicides/Pediculicides
**Use** Treatment of *Sarcoptes scabiei* (scabies), *Pediculus capitis* (head lice), and *Phthirus pubis* (crab lice); FDA recommends reserving lindane as a second-line agent or with inadequate response to other therapies
**Usual Dosage** Children and Adults: Topical:
Scabies: Apply a thin layer of lotion and massage it on skin from the neck to the toes; after 8-12 hours, bathe and remove the drug
Head lice, crab lice: Apply shampoo to dry hair and massage into hair for 4 minutes; add small quantities of water to hair until lather forms, then rinse hair thoroughly and comb with a fine tooth comb to remove nits. Amount of shampoo needed is based on length and density of hair; most patients will require 30 mL (maximum: 60 mL).
**Dosage Forms**
Lotion, topical: 1% (60 mL)
Shampoo, topical: 1% (60 mL) [contains alcohol 0.5%]

# linezolid (li NE zoh lid)
**Sound-Alike/Look-Alike Issues**
Zyvox™ may be confused with Vioxx®, Zosyn®, Zovirax®
**U.S./Canadian Brand Names** Zyvoxam® [Can]; Zyvox™ [US]
**Therapeutic Category** Antibiotic, Oxazolidinone
**Use** Treatment of vancomycin-resistant *Enterococcus faecium* (VRE) infections, nosocomial pneumonia caused by *Staphylococcus aureus* including MRSA or *Streptococcus pneumoniae* (including multidrug-resistant strains [MDRSP]), complicated and uncomplicated skin and skin structure infections (including diabetic foot infections without concomitant osteomyelitis), and community-acquired pneumonia caused by susceptible gram-positive organisms
**Usual Dosage**
VRE infections: Oral, I.V.:
Preterm neonates (<34 weeks gestational age): 10 mg/kg every 12 hours; neonates with a suboptimal clinical response can be advanced to 10 mg/kg every 8 hours. By day 7 of life, all neonates should receive 10 mg/kg every 8 hours.
Infants (excluding preterm neonates <1 week) and Children ≤11 years: 10 mg/kg every 8 hours for 14-28 days
Children ≥12 years and Adults: 600 mg every 12 hours for 14-28 days
Nosocomial pneumonia, complicated skin and skin structure infections, community acquired pneumonia including concurrent bacteremia: Oral, I.V.:
Infants (excluding preterm neonates <1 week) and Children ≤11 years: 10 mg/kg every 8 hours for 10-14 days
Children ≥12 years and Adults: 600 mg every 12 hours for 10-14 days
(Continued)

## linezolid *(Continued)*

Uncomplicated skin and skin structure infections: Oral:

Infants (excluding preterm neonates <1 week) and Children <5 years: 10 mg/kg every 8 hours for 10-14 days

Children 5-11 years: 10 mg/kg every 12 hours for 10-14 days

Children ≥12-18 years: 600 mg every 12 hours for 10-14 days

Adults: 400 mg every 12 hours for 10-14 days

**Dosage Forms**

Infusion [premixed]: 200 mg (100 mL) [contains sodium 1.7 mEq]; 400 mg (200 mL) [contains sodium 3.3 mEq]; 600 mg (300 mL) [contains sodium 5 mEq]

Powder for oral suspension: 20 mg/mL (150 mL) [contains phenylalanine 20 mg/5 mL, sodium benzoate, and sodium 0.4 mEq/5 mL; orange flavor]

Tablet: 600 mg [contains sodium 0.1 mEq/tablet]

**Lin-Sotalol [Can]** *see* sotalol *on page 762*

**Lioresal® [US/Can]** *see* baclofen *on page 88*

**Liotec [Can]** *see* baclofen *on page 88*

## liothyronine *(lye oh THYE roe neen)*

**Sound-Alike/Look-Alike Issues**

liothyronine may be confused with levothyroxine

$T_3$ sodium is an error-prone abbreviation

**Synonyms** liothyronine sodium; sodium *L*-triiodothyronine

**U.S./Canadian Brand Names** Cytomel® [US/Can]; Triostat® [US]

**Therapeutic Category** Thyroid Product

**Use**

Oral: Replacement or supplemental therapy in hypothyroidism; management of nontoxic goiter; a diagnostic aid

I.V.: Treatment of myxedema coma/precoma

**Usual Dosage** Doses should be adjusted based on clinical response and laboratory parameters.

Children: Congenital hypothyroidism: Oral: 5 mcg/day increase by 5 mcg every 3-4 days until the desired response is achieved. Usual maintenance dose: 20 mcg/day for infants, 50 mcg/day for children 1-3 years of age, and adult dose for children >3 years.

Adults:

Hypothyroidism: Oral: 25 mcg/day increase by increments of 12.5-25 mcg/day every 1-2 weeks to a maximum of 100 mcg/day; usual maintenance dose: 25-75 mcg/day.

Patients with cardiovascular disease: Oral: 5 mcg/day; increase by 5 mcg/day every 2 weeks

$T_3$ suppression test: Oral: 75-100 mcg/day for 7 days

Myxedema: Oral: Initial: 5 mcg/day; increase in increments of 5-10 mcg/day every 1-2 weeks. When 25 mcg/day is reached, dosage may be increased at intervals of 5-25 mcg/day every 1-2 weeks. Usual maintenance dose: 50-100 mcg/day.

Myxedema coma: I.V.: 25-50 mcg

Patients with known or suspected cardiovascular disease: 10-20 mcg

**Note:** Normally, at least 4 hours should be allowed between doses to adequately assess therapeutic response and no more than 12 hours should elapse between doses to avoid fluctuations in hormone levels. Oral therapy should be resumed as soon as the clinical situation has been stabilized and the patient is able to take oral medication. If levothyroxine rather than liothyronine sodium is used in initiating oral therapy, the physician should bear in mind that there is a delay of several days in the onset of levothyroxine activity and that I.V. therapy should be discontinued gradually.

Simple (nontoxic) goiter: Oral: Initial: 5 mcg/day; increase by 5-10 mcg every 1-2 weeks; after 25 mcg/day is reached, may increase dose by 12.5-25 mcg. Usual maintenance dose: 75 mcg/day

**Dosage Forms**

Injection, solution, as sodium (Triostat®): 10 mcg/mL (1 mL) [contains alcohol 6.8%]

Tablet, as sodium (Cytomel®): 5 mcg, 25 mcg, 50 mcg

**liothyronine sodium** *see* liothyronine *on this page*

## liotrix *(LYE oh triks)*

**Sound-Alike/Look-Alike Issues**

liotrix may be confused with Klotrix®

Thyrolar® may be confused with Theolair™, Thyrogen®, Thytropar®

**Synonyms** T$_3$/T$_4$ liotrix

**U.S./Canadian Brand Names** Thyrolar® [US/Can]

**Therapeutic Category** Thyroid Product

**Use** Replacement or supplemental therapy in hypothyroidism (uniform mixture of T$_4$:T$_3$ in 4:1 ratio by weight); little advantage to this product exists and cost is not justified

**Usual Dosage** Oral:

Congenital hypothyroidism:

Children (dose of T$_4$ or levothyroxine/day):

0-6 months: 8-10 mcg/kg or 25-50 mcg/day

6-12 months: 6-8 mcg/kg or 50-75 mcg/day

1-5 years: 5-6 mcg/kg or 75-100 mcg/day

6-12 years: 4-5 mcg/kg or 100-150 mcg/day

>12 years: 2-3 mcg/kg or >150 mcg/day

Hypothyroidism (dose of thyroid equivalent): Adults: 30 mg/day (15 mg/day if cardiovascular impairment), increasing by increments of 15 mg/day at 2- to 3-week intervals to a maximum of 180 mg/day (usual maintenance dose: 60-120 mg/day)

**Dosage Forms** Tablet:

$^1/_4$ [levothyroxine sodium 12.5 mcg and liothyronine sodium 3.1 mcg]

$^1/_2$ [levothyroxine sodium 25 mcg and liothyronine sodium 6.25 mcg]

1 [levothyroxine sodium 50 mcg and liothyronine sodium 12.5 mcg]

2 [levothyroxine sodium 100 mcg and liothyronine sodium 25 mcg]

3 [levothyroxine sodium 150 mcg and liothyronine sodium 37.5 mcg]

**lipancreatin** *see* pancrelipase *on page 615*

**Lipidil EZ® [Can]** *see* fenofibrate *on page 330*

**Lipidil Micro® [Can]** *see* fenofibrate *on page 330*

**Lipidil Supra® [Can]** *see* fenofibrate *on page 330*

**Lipitor® [US/Can]** *see* atorvastatin *on page 78*

**Liposyn® III [US]** *see* fat emulsion *on page 328*

**Lipram 4500 [US]** *see* pancrelipase *on page 615*

**Lipram-CR [US]** *see* pancrelipase *on page 615*

**Lipram-PN [US]** *see* pancrelipase *on page 615*

**Lipram-UL [US]** *see* pancrelipase *on page 615*

**Liquaemin® *(Discontinued)*** *see* heparin *on page 398*

**Liquibid-D [US]** *see* guaifenesin and phenylephrine *on page 387*

**Liquibid® 1200 *(Discontinued)*** *see* guaifenesin *on page 383*

**Liquibid® *(Discontinued)*** *see* guaifenesin *on page 383*

**Liquibid-PD [US]** *see* guaifenesin and phenylephrine *on page 387*

**Liqui-Char® *(Discontinued)*** *see* charcoal *on page 165*

**liquid antidote** *see* charcoal *on page 165*

**Liquid Barosperse® [US]** *see* radiological/contrast media (ionic) *on page 707*

**Liquid Pred® *(Discontinued)*** *see* prednisone *on page 674*

**Liquifilm® Forte Solution *(Discontinued)*** *see* artificial tears *on page 71*

**Liquifilm® Tears [US-OTC]** *see* artificial tears *on page 71*

**Liquifilm® Tears Solution *(Discontinued)*** *see* artificial tears *on page 71*

**Liquipake® [US]** *see* radiological/contrast media (ionic) *on page 707*

# lisinopril (lyse IN oh pril)

**Sound-Alike/Look-Alike Issues**

lisinopril may be confused with fosinopril, Lioresal®, Risperdal®

Prinivil® may be confused with Plendil®, Pravachol®, Prevacid®, Prilosec®, Proventil®

Zestril® may be confused with Desyrel®, Restoril®, Vistaril®, Zetia™, Zostrix®

(Continued)

# lisinopril *(Continued)*

**U.S./Canadian Brand Names** Apo-Lisinopril® [Can]; Prinivil® [US/Can]; Zestril® [US/Can]

**Therapeutic Category** Angiotensin-Converting Enzyme (ACE) Inhibitor

**Use** Treatment of hypertension, either alone or in combination with other antihypertensive agents; adjunctive therapy in treatment of CHF (afterload reduction); treatment of acute myocardial infarction within 24 hours in hemodynamically-stable patients to improve survival; treatment of left ventricular dysfunction after myocardial infarction

**Usual Dosage** Oral:

Hypertension:

Children ≥6 years: Initial: 0.07 mg/kg once daily (up to 5 mg); increase dose at 1- to 2-week intervals; doses >0.61 mg/kg or >40 mg have not been evaluated.

Adults: Usual dosage range(JNC 7): 10-40 mg/day

*Not maintained on diuretic:* Initial: 10 mg/day

*Maintained on diuretic:* Initial: 5 mg/day

**Note:** Antihypertensive effect may diminish toward the end of the dosing interval especially with doses of 10 mg/day. An increased dose may aid in extending the duration of antihypertensive effect. Doses up to 80 mg/day have been used, but do not appear to give greater effect (Zestril® Product Information, 12/04).

Patients taking diuretics should have them discontinued 2-3 days prior to initiating lisinopril if possible. Restart diuretic after blood pressure is stable if needed. If diuretic cannot be discontinued prior to therapy, begin with 5 mg with close supervision until stable blood pressure. In patients with hyponatremia (<130 mEq/L), start dose at 2.5 mg/day

Congestive heart failure: Adults: Initial: 5 mg; then increase by no more than 10 mg increments at intervals no less than 2 weeks to a maximum daily dose of 40 mg. Usual maintenance: 5-40 mg/day as a single dose. Patients should start/continue standard therapy, including diuretics, beta-blockers, and digoxin, as indicated.

**Note:** If patient has hyponatremia (serum sodium <130 meq/L) or renal impairment ($Cl_{cr}$ <30 mL/minute or creatinine >3 mg/dL), then initial dose should be 2.5 mg/day

Acute myocardial infarction (within 24 hours in hemodynamically stable patients): Oral: 5 mg immediately, then 5 mg at 24 hours, 10 mg at 48 hours, and 10 mg every day thereafter for 6 weeks. Patients should continue to receive standard treatments such as thrombolytics, aspirin, and beta-blockers.

**Dosage Forms** [DSC] = Discontinued product

Tablet: 2.5 mg, 5 mg, 10 mg, 20 mg, 30 mg, 40 mg

Prinivil®: 2.5 mg [DSC], 5 mg, 10 mg, 20 mg, 30 mg, 40 mg

Zestril®: 2.5 mg, 5 mg, 10 mg, 20 mg, 30 mg, 40 mg

# lisinopril and hydrochlorothiazide *(lyse IN oh pril & hye droe klor oh THYE a zide)*

**Synonyms** hydrochlorothiazide and lisinopril

**U.S./Canadian Brand Names** Prinzide® [US/Can]; Zestoretic® [US/Can]

**Therapeutic Category** Antihypertensive Agent, Combination

**Use** Treatment of hypertension

**Usual Dosage** Adults: Oral: Dosage is individualized; see each component for appropriate dosing suggestions; doses >80 mg/day lisinopril or >50 mg/day hydrochlorothiazide are not recommended.

**Dosage Forms** Tablet:

Lisinopril 10 mg and hydrochlorothiazide 12.5 mg

Lisinopril 20 mg and hydrochlorothiazide 12.5 mg

Lisinopril 20 mg and hydrochlorothiazide 25 mg

**lispro, insulin** *see* insulin preparations *on page 438*

**Listermint® With Fluoride *(Discontinued)*** *see* fluoride *on page 347*

**Lithane™ [Can]** *see* lithium *on this page*

**Lithane® *(Discontinued)*** *see* lithium *on this page*

# lithium *(LITH ee um)*

**Sound-Alike/Look-Alike Issues**

Eskalith® may be confused with Estratest®

Lithobid® may be confused with Levbid®, Lithostat®

**Synonyms** lithium carbonate; lithium citrate

**U.S./Canadian Brand Names** Apo-Lithium® [Can]; Carbolith™ [Can]; Duralith® [Can]; Eskalith CR® [US]; Eskalith® [US]; Lithane™ [Can]; Lithobid® [US]; PMS-Lithium Carbonate [Can]; PMS-Lithium Citrate [Can]

**Therapeutic Category** Antimanic Agent

**Use** Management of bipolar disorders; treatment of mania in individuals with bipolar disorder (maintenance treatment prevents or diminishes intensity of subsequent episodes)

**Usual Dosage** Oral: Monitor serum concentrations and clinical response (efficacy and toxicity) to determine proper dose

Children 6-12 years: Bipolar disorder: 15-60 mg/kg/day in 3-4 divided doses; dose not to exceed usual adult dosage

Adults: Bipolar disorder: 900-2400 mg/day in 3-4 divided doses or 900-1800 mg/day (sustained release) in 2 divided doses

**Dosage Forms** [DSC] = Discontinued product

Capsule, as carbonate: 150 mg, 300 mg, 600 mg

Eskalith®: 300 mg [contains benzyl alcohol] [DSC]

Syrup, as citrate: 300 mg/5 mL (5 mL, 10 mL, 480 mL) [contains alcohol]

Tablet, as carbonate: 300 mg

Tablet, controlled release, as carbonate (Eskalith CR®): 450 mg

Tablet, slow release, as carbonate (Lithobid®): 300 mg

**lithium carbonate** *see* lithium *on previous page*

**lithium citrate** *see* lithium *on previous page*

**Lithobid® [US]** *see* lithium *on previous page*

**Lithonate® (Discontinued)** *see* lithium *on previous page*

**Lithostat® [US/Can]** *see* acetohydroxamic acid *on page 14*

**Lithotabs® (Discontinued)** *see* lithium *on previous page*

**live attenuated influenza vaccine (LAIV)** *see* influenza virus vaccine *on page 437*

**Livostin® [Can]** *see* levocabastine *on page 473*

**Livostin® (Discontinued)** *see* levocabastine *on page 473*

**l-lysine** (el LYE seen)

**Synonyms** l-lysine hydrochloride

**U.S./Canadian Brand Names** Lysinyl [US-OTC]

**Therapeutic Category** Dietary Supplement

**Use** Improves utilization of vegetable proteins

**Usual Dosage**

Oral: Adults: 334-1500 mg/day

Recurrent herpes simplex infection (dental use): 2000 mg every 4 hours until symptoms subside. Begin treatment during early stage of recurrence.

**Dosage Forms**

Capsule (Lysinyl): 500 mg

Tablet: 500 mg, 1000 mg

**l-lysine hydrochloride** *see* l-lysine *on this page*

**LMD® [US]** *see* dextran *on page 236*

**LNg 20** *see* levonorgestrel *on page 476*

**Locacorten® Vioform® [Can]** *see* clioquinol and flumethasone *(Canada only) on page 193*

**LoCHOLEST® (Discontinued)** *see* cholestyramine resin *on page 180*

**LoCHOLEST® Light (Discontinued)** *see* cholestyramine resin *on page 180*

**Locoid® [US/Can]** *see* hydrocortisone (topical) *on page 417*

**Locoid Lipocream® [US]** *see* hydrocortisone (topical) *on page 417*

**Lodine® [US/Can]** *see* etodolac *on page 321*

**Lodine® XL (Discontinued)** *see* etodolac *on page 321*

**Lodosyn® [US]** *see* carbidopa *on page 143*

## Iodoxamide tromethamine (loe DOKS a mide troe METH a meen)
**U.S./Canadian Brand Names** Alomide® [US/Can]
**Therapeutic Category** Mast Cell Stabilizer
**Use** Treatment of vernal keratoconjunctivitis, vernal conjunctivitis, and vernal keratitis
**Usual Dosage** Ophthalmic: Instill 1-2 drops in eye(s) 4 times/day for up to 3 months
**Dosage Forms** Solution, ophthalmic: 0.1% (10 mL) [contains benzalkonium chloride]

**Lodrane® [US]** *see* brompheniramine and pseudoephedrine *on page 115*

**Lodrane® 12D [US]** *see* brompheniramine and pseudoephedrine *on page 115*

**Lodrane® 12 Hour [US-OTC]** *see* brompheniramine *on page 115*

**Lodrane® LD [US]** *see* brompheniramine and pseudoephedrine *on page 115*

**Loestrin® [US]** *see* ethinyl estradiol and norethindrone *on page 314*

**Loestrin™ 1.5.30 [Can]** *see* ethinyl estradiol and norethindrone *on page 314*

**Loestrin® Fe [US]** *see* ethinyl estradiol and norethindrone *on page 314*

**Lofibra™ [US]** *see* fenofibrate *on page 330*

**Logen® (Discontinued)** *see* diphenoxylate and atropine *on page 257*

**LoHist-D [US]** *see* chlorpheniramine and pseudoephedrine *on page 172*

**L-OHP** *see* oxaliplatin *on page 605*

**LoKara™ [US]** *see* desonide *on page 231*

**Lomanate® (Discontinued)** *see* diphenoxylate and atropine *on page 257*

## Iomefloxacin (loe me FLOKS a sin)
**Synonyms** lomefloxacin hydrochloride
**U.S./Canadian Brand Names** Maxaquin® [US]
**Therapeutic Category** Quinolone
**Use** Acute bacterial exacerbation of chronic bronchitis caused by susceptible gram-negative organisms; urinary tract infections (uncomplicated and complicated) caused by susceptible organisms; surgical prophylaxis (transrectal prostate biopsy or transurethral procedures)
**Usual Dosage** Oral: Adults:
  Acute bacterial exacerbation of chronic bronchitis: 400 mg once daily for 10 days
  Urinary tract infection (UTI) due to susceptible organisms:
   Uncomplicated cystitis caused by *Escherichia coli*: 400 mg once daily for 3 successive days
   Uncomplicated cystitis caused by *Klebsiella pneumoniae*, *Proteus mirabilis*, or *Staphylococcus saprophyticus*: 400 mg once daily for 10 successive days
   Complicated UTI caused by *Escherichia coli*, *Klebsiella pneumoniae*, *Proteus mirabilis*, or *Pseudomonas aeruginosa*: 400 mg once daily for 14 successive days
  Urologic surgical prophylaxis:
   Transrectal prostate biopsy: 400 mg as a single dose, 1-6 hours before procedure
   Transurethral surgical procedure: 400 mg as a single dose, 2-6 hours before procedure
**Dosage Forms** [DSC] = Discontinued product
  Tablet: 400 mg [DSC]

**Iomefloxacin hydrochloride** *see* lomefloxacin *on this page*

**Lomine [Can]** *see* dicyclomine *on page 245*

**Lomotil® [US/Can]** *see* diphenoxylate and atropine *on page 257*

## Iomustine (loe MUS teen)
**Sound-Alike/Look-Alike Issues**
  lomustine may be confused with carmustine
**Synonyms** CCNU
**U.S./Canadian Brand Names** CeeNU® [US/Can]
**Therapeutic Category** Antineoplastic Agent
**Use** Treatment of brain tumors and Hodgkin's disease, non-Hodgkin's lymphoma, melanoma, renal carcinoma, lung cancer, colon cancer
**Usual Dosage** Oral (refer to individual protocols):
  Children: 75-150 mg/m$^2$ as a single dose every 6 weeks; subsequent doses are readjusted after initial treatment according to platelet and leukocyte counts

Adults: 100-130 mg/m$^2$ as a single dose every 6 weeks; readjust after initial treatment according to platelet and leukocyte counts

With compromised marrow function: Initial dose: 100 mg/m$^2$ as a single dose every 6 weeks

Repeat courses should only be administered after adequate recovery: WBC >4000 and platelet counts >100,000

**Subsequent dosing adjustment based on nadir**:

Leukocytes 2000-2900/mm$^3$, platelets 25,000-74,999/mm$^3$: Administer 70% of prior dose

Leukocytes <2000/mm$^3$, platelets <25,000/mm$^3$: Administer 50% of prior dose

**Dosage Forms**

Capsule: 10 mg, 40 mg, 100 mg

Capsule [dose pack]: 10 mg (2s); 40 mg (2s); 100 mg (2s)

**Loniten**® **[US]** *see* minoxidil *on page 543*

**Lonox**® **[US]** *see* diphenoxylate and atropine *on page 257*

**Lo/Ovral**® **[US]** *see* ethinyl estradiol and norgestrel *on page 318*

**Loperacap [Can]** *see* loperamide *on this page*

# loperamide (loe PER a mide)

**Sound-Alike/Look-Alike Issues**

Imodium® A-D may be confused with Indocin®, Ionamin®

**Synonyms** loperamide hydrochloride

**U.S./Canadian Brand Names** Apo-Loperamide® [Can]; Diamode [US-OTC]; Diarr-Eze [Can]; Imodium® A-D [US-OTC]; Imodium® [Can]; K-Pek II [US-OTC]; Kao-Paverin® [US-OTC]; Loperacap [Can]; Novo-Loperamide [Can]; PMS-Loperamine [Can]; Rho®-Loperamine [Can]; Riva-Loperamine [Can]

**Therapeutic Category** Antidiarrheal

**Use** Treatment of acute diarrhea and chronic diarrhea associated with inflammatory bowel disease; chronic functional diarrhea (idiopathic), chronic diarrhea caused by bowel resection or organic lesions; to decrease the volume of ileostomy discharge

**Usual Dosage** Oral:

Children:

Acute diarrhea: Initial doses (in first 24 hours):

2-6 years: 1 mg 3 times/day

6-8 years: 2 mg twice daily

8-12 years: 2 mg 3 times/day

Maintenance: After initial dosing, 0.1 mg/kg doses after each loose stool, but not exceeding initial dosage

Chronic diarrhea: 0.08-0.24 mg/kg/day divided 2-3 times/day, maximum: 2 mg/dose

Adults:

Acute diarrhea: Initial: 4 mg (2 capsules), followed by 2 mg after each loose stool, up to 16 mg/day (8 capsules)

Chronic diarrhea: Initial: Follow acute diarrhea; maintenance dose should be slowly titrated downward to minimum required to control symptoms (typically, 4-8 mg/day in divided doses)

Traveler's diarrhea: Treat for no more than 2 days

6-8 years: 1 mg after first loose stool followed by 1 mg after each subsequent stool; maximum dose: 4 mg/day

9-11 years: 2 mg after first loose stool followed by 1 mg after each subsequent stool; maximum dose: 6 mg/day

12 years to Adults: 4 mg after first loose stool followed by 2 mg after each subsequent stool; maximum dose: 8 mg/day

**Dosage Forms**

Caplet, as hydrochloride: 2 mg

Diamode, Imodium® A-D, Kao-Paverin®: 2 mg

Capsule, as hydrochloride: 2 mg

Liquid, oral, as hydrochloride: 1 mg/5 mL (5 mL, 10 mL, 120 mL)

Imodium® A-D: 1 mg/5 mL (60 mL, 120 mL) [contains alcohol, sodium benzoate, benzoic acid; cherry mint flavor]

Imodium® A-D [new formulation]: 1 mg/7.5 mL (60 mL, 120 mL, 360 mL) [contains sodium 10 mg/30 mL, sodium benzoate; creamy mint flavor]

Tablet, as hydrochloride: 2 mg

K-Pek II: 2 mg

**loperamide hydrochloride** *see loperamide* *on previous page*

**Lopid**® **[US/Can]** *see gemfibrozil* *on page 370*

## lopinavir and ritonavir (loe PIN a veer & rit ON uh veer)

**Sound-Alike/Look-Alike Issues**
Potential for dispensing errors between Kaletra™ and Keppra® (levetiracetam)
**Synonyms** ritonavir and lopinavir
**U.S./Canadian Brand Names** Kaletra® [US/Can]
**Therapeutic Category** Antiretroviral Agent, Non-nucleoside Reverse Transcriptase Inhibitor (NNRTI)
**Use** Treatment of HIV infection in combination with other antiretroviral agents
**Usual Dosage** Oral (take with food):
  Children 6 months to 12 years: Dosage based on weight, presented based on mg of lopinavir (maximum dose: Lopinavir 400 mg/ritonavir 100 mg)
    7-<15 kg: 12 mg/kg twice daily
    15-40 kg: 10 mg/kg twice daily
    >40 kg: Refer to adult dosing. **Note:** Once-daily dosing regimen has not been evaluated in pediatric patients.
  Children >12 years and Adults:
    Therapy-naive: Lopinavir 800 mg/ritonavir 200 mg once daily **or** lopinavir 400 mg/ritonavir 100 mg twice daily
    Therapy-experienced: Lopinavir 400 mg/ritonavir 100 mg twice daily
    **Note:** Once-daily dosing regimen has not been evaluated with concurrent indinavir or saquinavir and should not be used with concomitant phenytoin, carbamazepine, or phenobarbital therapy.
  **Dosage adjustment when taken with amprenavir, efavirenz, nelfinavir, or nevirapine:**
    **Note:** Once-daily dosing regimen should not be used when concomitantly taking amprenavir, efavirenz, nelfinavir, or nevirapine therapy.
    Children 6 months to 12 years:
      7-<15 kg: 13 mg/kg twice daily
      15-45 kg: 11 mg/kg twice daily
      >45 kg: Refer to adult dosing
      **Note:** In the USHHS guidelines, the cutoff for adult dosing is 50 kg. (Pediatric Guidelines - March 24, 2005, are available at http://www.aidsinfo.nih.gov)
    Children >12 years and Adults: Lopinavir 533 mg/ritonavir 133 mg twice daily
**Dosage Forms**
  Capsule: Lopinavir 133.3 mg and ritonavir 33.3 mg
  Solution, oral: Lopinavir 80 mg and ritonavir 20 mg per mL (160 mL) [contains alcohol 42.4%]

**Lopressor**® **[US/Can]** *see metoprolol* *on page 534*

**Loprox**® **[US/Can]** *see ciclopirox* *on page 182*

**Lorabid**® **[US/Can]** *see loracarbef* *on this page*

## loracarbef (lor a KAR bef)

**Sound-Alike/Look-Alike Issues**
Lorabid® may be confused with Levbid®, Lopid®, Lortab®, Slo-bid™
**U.S./Canadian Brand Names** Lorabid® [US/Can]
**Therapeutic Category** Antibiotic, Carbacephem
**Use** Infections caused by susceptible organisms involving the respiratory tract, acute otitis media, sinusitis, skin and skin structure, bone and joint, and urinary tract and gynecologic
**Usual Dosage** Oral:
  Children:
    Acute otitis media: 15 mg/kg twice daily for 10 days
    Pharyngitis and impetigo: 7.5-15 mg/kg twice daily for 10 days
  Adults:
    Uncomplicated urinary tract infections: 200 mg once daily for 7 days
    Skin and soft tissue: 200-400 mg every 12-24 hours
    Uncomplicated pyelonephritis: 400 mg every 12 hours for 14 days
    Upper/lower respiratory tract infection: 200-400 mg every 12-24 hours for 7-14 days
**Dosage Forms**
  Capsule: 200 mg, 400 mg

Powder for oral suspension: 100 mg/5 mL (100 mL); 200 mg/5 mL (100 mL) [strawberry bubble gum flavor]

## loratadine (lor AT a deen)
**Sound-Alike/Look-Alike Issues**
Dimetapp® may be confused with Dermatop®, Dimetabs®, Dimetane®
**U.S./Canadian Brand Names** Alavert™ [US-OTC]; Apo-Loratadine® [Can]; Claritin® Hives Relief [US-OTC]; Claritin® Kids [Can]; Claritin® [US-OTC/Can]; Dimetapp® Children's ND [US-OTC]; Tavist® ND [US-OTC]
**Therapeutic Category** Antihistamine
**Use** Relief of nasal and non-nasal symptoms of seasonal allergic rhinitis; treatment of chronic idiopathic urticaria
**Usual Dosage** Oral: Seasonal allergic rhinitis, chronic idiopathic urticaria:
Children 2-5 years: 5 mg once daily
Children ≥6 years and Adults: 10 mg once daily
**Dosage Forms**
Syrup (Claritin®): 1 mg/mL (120 mL) [contains sodium benzoate; fruit flavor]
Tablet (Alavert™, Claritin®, Claritin® Hives Relief; Tavist® ND): 10 mg
Tablet, rapidly-disintegrating: 10 mg
Alavert™: 10 mg [contains phenylalanine 8.4 mg/tablet]
Claritin® RediTabs®: 10 mg [mint flavor]
Dimetapp® Children's ND: 10 mg [contains phenylalanine 8.4 mg/tablet]

## loratadine and pseudoephedrine (lor AT a deen & soo doe e FED rin)
**Synonyms** pseudoephedrine and loratadine
**U.S./Canadian Brand Names** Alavert™ Allergy and Sinus [US-OTC]; Chlor-Tripolon ND® [Can]; Claritin-D® 12-Hour [US-OTC]; Claritin-D® 24-Hour [US-OTC]; Claritin® Extra [Can]; Claritin® Liberator [Can]
**Therapeutic Category** Antihistamine/Decongestant Combination
**Use** Temporary relief of symptoms of seasonal allergic rhinitis, other upper respiratory allergies, or the common cold
**Usual Dosage** Children ≥12 years and Adults: Oral:
Claritin-D® 12-Hour: 1 tablet every 12 hours
Alavert™ Allergy and Sinus, Claritin-D® 24-Hour: 1 tablet daily
**Dosage Forms**
Tablet, extended release: Loratadine 10 mg and pseudoephedrine sulfate 240 mg
Alavert™ Allergy and Sinus, Claritin-D® 12-hour: Loratadine 5 mg and pseudoephedrine sulfate 120 mg
Claritin-D® 24-hour: Loratadine 10 mg and pseudoephedrine sulfate 240 mg

## lorazepam (lor A ze pam)
**Sound-Alike/Look-Alike Issues**
lorazepam may be confused with alprazolam, clonazepam, diazepam, temazepam
Ativan® may be confused with Atarax®, Atgam®, Avitene®
**U.S./Canadian Brand Names** Apo-Lorazepam® [Can]; Ativan® [US/Can]; Lorazepam Intensol® [US]; Novo-Lorazepam [Can]; Nu-Loraz [Can]; PMS-Lorazepam [Can]; Riva-Lorazepam [Can]
**Therapeutic Category** Benzodiazepine
**Controlled Substance** C-IV
**Use**
Oral: Management of anxiety disorders or short-term relief of the symptoms of anxiety or anxiety associated with depressive symptoms
I.V.: Status epilepticus, preanesthesia for desired amnesia, antiemetic adjunct
**Usual Dosage**
Antiemetic:
Children 2-15 years: I.V.: 0.05 mg/kg (up to 2 mg/dose) prior to chemotherapy
Adults: Oral, I.V. (**Note:** May be administered sublingually; not a labeled route): 0.5-2 mg every 4-6 hours as needed
Anxiety and sedation:
Infants and Children: Oral, I.M., I.V.: Usual: 0.05 mg/kg/dose (range: 0.02-0.09 mg/kg) every 4-8 hours
I.V.: May use smaller doses (eg, 0.01-0.03 mg/kg) and repeat every 20 minutes, as needed to titrate to effect
Adults: Oral: 1-10 mg/day in 2-3 divided doses; usual dose: 2-6 mg/day in divided doses
(Continued)

# lorazepam *(Continued)*

Insomnia: Adults: Oral: 2-4 mg at bedtime

Preoperative: Adults:

I.M.: 0.05 mg/kg administered 2 hours before surgery (maximum: 4 mg/dose)

I.V.: 0.044 mg/kg 15-20 minutes before surgery (usual maximum: 2 mg/dose)

Preprocedural anxiety (dental use): Adults: Oral: 1-2 mg 1 hour before procedure

Operative amnesia: Adults: I.V.: Up to 0.05 mg/kg (maximum: 4 mg/dose)

Sedation (preprocedure): Infants and Children:

Oral, I.M., I.V.: Usual: 0.05 mg/kg (range: 0.02-0.09 mg/kg);

I.V.: May use smaller doses (eg, 0.01-0.03 mg/kg) and repeat every 20 minutes, as needed to titrate to effect

Status epilepticus: I.V.:

Infants and Children: 0.1 mg/kg slow I.V. over 2-5 minutes; do not exceed 4 mg/single dose; may repeat second dose of 0.05 mg/kg slow I.V. in 10-15 minutes if needed

Adolescents: 0.07 mg/kg slow I.V. over 2-5 minutes; maximum: 4 mg/dose; may repeat in 10-15 minutes

Adults: 4 mg/dose slow I.V. over 2-5 minutes; may repeat in 10-15 minutes; usual maximum dose: 8 mg

Rapid tranquilization of agitated patient (administer every 30-60 minutes):

Oral: 1-2 mg

I.M.: 0.5-1 mg

Average total dose for tranquilization: Oral, I.M.: 4-8 mg

**Dosage Forms**

Injection, solution (Ativan®): 2 mg/mL (1 mL, 10 mL); 4 mg/mL (1 mL, 10 mL) [contains benzyl alcohol]

Solution, oral concentrate (Lorazepam Intensol®): 2 mg/mL (30 mL) [alcohol free, dye free]

Tablet (Ativan®): 0.5 mg, 1 mg, 2 mg

**Lorazepam Intensol® [US]** *see* lorazepam *on previous page*

**Lorcet® 10/650 [US]** *see* hydrocodone and acetaminophen *on page 411*

**Lorcet®-HD *(Discontinued)*** *see* hydrocodone and acetaminophen *on page 411*

**Lorcet® Plus [US]** *see* hydrocodone and acetaminophen *on page 411*

**Loroxide® [US-OTC]** *see* benzoyl peroxide *on page 98*

**Lorsin® *(Discontinued)*** *see* acetaminophen, chlorpheniramine, and pseudoephedrine *on page 10*

**Lortab® [US]** *see* hydrocodone and acetaminophen *on page 411*

**Lortab® ASA *(Discontinued)*** *see* hydrocodone and aspirin *on page 412*

# losartan *(loe SAR tan)*

**Sound-Alike/Look-Alike Issues**

losartan may be confused with valsartan

Cozaar® may be confused with Hyzaar®, Zocor®

**Synonyms** DuP 753; losartan potassium; MK594

**U.S./Canadian Brand Names** Cozaar® [US/Can]

**Therapeutic Category** Angiotensin II Receptor Antagonist

**Use** Treatment of hypertension (HTN); treatment of diabetic nephropathy in patients with type 2 diabetes mellitus (noninsulin dependent, NIDDM) and a history of hypertension; stroke risk reduction in patients with HTN and left ventricular hypertrophy (LVH)

**Usual Dosage** Oral:

Hypertension:

Children 6-16 years: 0.7 mg/kg once daily (maximum: 50 mg/day); adjust dose based on response; doses >1.4 mg/kg (maximum: 100 mg) have not been studied

Adults: Usual starting dose: 50 mg once daily; can be administered once or twice daily with total daily doses ranging from 25-100 mg

Patients receiving diuretics or with intravascular volume depletion: Usual initial dose: 25 mg

Nephropathy in patients with type 2 diabetes and hypertension: Adults: Initial: 50 mg once daily; can be increased to 100 mg once daily based on blood pressure response

Stroke reduction (HTN with LVH): Adults: 50 mg once daily (maximum daily dose: 100 mg); may be used in combination with a thiazide diuretic

**Dosage Forms** Tablet [film coated], as potassium: 25 mg, 50 mg, 100 mg

## losartan and hydrochlorothiazide (loe SAR tan & hye droe klor oh THYE a zide)

**Sound-Alike/Look-Alike Issues**
Hyzaar® may be confused with Cozaar®

**Synonyms** hydrochlorothiazide and losartan

**U.S./Canadian Brand Names** Hyzaar® DS [Can]; Hyzaar® [US/Can]

**Therapeutic Category** Antihypertensive Agent, Combination

**Use** Treatment of hypertension; stroke risk reduction in patients with HTN and left ventricular hypertrophy (LVH)

**Usual Dosage**
Oral: Adults: Dose is individualized (combination substituted for individual components); dose may be titrated after 2-4 weeks of therapy
Hypertension/stroke reduction in hypertension (with LVH): Usual recommended starting dose of losartan: 50 mg once daily when used as monotherapy in patients who are not volume depleted

**Dosage Forms** Tablet [film coated]:
50-12.5: Losartan potassium 50 mg and hydrochlorothiazide 12.5 mg
100-25: Losartan potassium 100 mg and hydrochlorothiazide 25 mg

**losartan potassium** *see* losartan *on previous page*

**Losec® [Can]** *see* omeprazole *on page 598*

**Losec MUPS® [Can]** *see* omeprazole *on page 598*

**Losopan®** *(Discontinued)* *see* magaldrate and simethicone *on page 496*

**Lotemax® [US/Can]** *see* loteprednol *on this page*

**Lotensin® [US/Can]** *see* benazepril *on page 93*

**Lotensin® HCT [US]** *see* benazepril and hydrochlorothiazide *on page 93*

## loteprednol (loe te PRED nol)

**Synonyms** loteprednol etabonate

**U.S./Canadian Brand Names** Alrex® [US/Can]; Lotemax® [US/Can]

**Therapeutic Category** Corticosteroid, Ophthalmic

**Use**
Suspension, 0.2% (Alrex®): Temporary relief of signs and symptoms of seasonal allergic conjunctivitis
Suspension, 0.5% (Lotemax®): Inflammatory conditions (treatment of steroid-responsive inflammatory conditions of the palpebral and bulbar conjunctiva, cornea, and anterior segment of the globe such as allergic conjunctivitis, acne rosacea, superficial punctate keratitis, herpes zoster keratitis, iritis, cyclitis, selected infective conjunctivitis, when the inherent hazard of steroid use is accepted to obtain an advisable diminution in edema and inflammation) and treatment of postoperative inflammation following ocular surgery

**Usual Dosage** Adults: Ophthalmic:
Suspension, 0.2% (Alrex®): Instill 1 drop into affected eye(s) 4 times/day
Suspension, 0.5% (Lotemax®):
Inflammatory conditions: Apply 1-2 drops into the conjunctival sac of the affected eye(s) 4 times/day. During the initial treatment within the first week, the dosing may be increased up to 1 drop every hour. Advise patients not to discontinue therapy prematurely. If signs and symptoms fail to improve after 2 days, re-evaluate the patient.
Postoperative inflammation: Apply 1-2 drops into the conjunctival sac of the operated eye(s) 4 times/day beginning 24 hours after surgery and continuing throughout the first 2 weeks of the postoperative period

**Dosage Forms** Suspension, ophthalmic, as etabonate:
Alrex®: 0.2% (5 mL, 10 mL) [contains benzalkonium chloride]
Lotemax®: 0.5% (2.5 mL, 5 mL, 10 mL, 15 mL) [contains benzalkonium chloride]

**loteprednol etabonate** *see* loteprednol *on this page*

**Lotrel® [US]** *see* amlodipine and benazepril *on page 44*

**Lotriderm® [Can]** *see* betamethasone and clotrimazole *on page 102*

**Lotrimin® AF Athlete's Foot Cream [US-OTC]** *see* clotrimazole *on page 199*

**Lotrimin® AF Athlete's Foot Solution [US-OTC]** *see* clotrimazole *on page 199*

**Lotrimin® AF Cream** *(Discontinued)* *see* clotrimazole *on page 199*

**Lotrimin® AF Jock Itch Cream [US-OTC]** *see* clotrimazole *on page 199*

**Lotrimin® AF Jock Itch Powder Spray [US-OTC]** *see* miconazole *on page 537*

**Lotrimin® AF Lotion *(Discontinued)*** *see* clotrimazole *on page 199*

**Lotrimin® AF Powder/Spray [US-OTC]** *see* miconazole *on page 537*

**Lotrimin® AF Solution *(Discontinued)*** *see* clotrimazole *on page 199*

**Lotrimin® Ultra™ [US-OTC]** *see* butenafine *on page 125*

**Lotrisone® [US]** *see* betamethasone and clotrimazole *on page 102*

**Lotronex® [US]** *see* alosetron *on page 30*

# lovastatin (LOE va sta tin)
**Sound-Alike/Look-Alike Issues**
lovastatin may be confused with Leustatin®, Livostin®, Lotensin®
Mevacor® may be confused with Mivacron®
**Synonyms** mevinolin; monacolin K
**U.S./Canadian Brand Names** Altoprev™ [US]; Apo-Lovastatin® [Can]; CO Lovastatin [Can]; Gen-Lovastatin [Can]; Mevacor® [US/Can]; Novo-Lovastatin [Can]; Nu-Lovastatin [Can]; PMS-Lovastatin [Can]; ratio-Lovastatin [Can]
**Therapeutic Category** HMG-CoA Reductase Inhibitor
**Use**
Adjunct to dietary therapy to decrease elevated serum total and LDL-cholesterol concentrations in primary hypercholesterolemia
Primary prevention of coronary artery disease (patients without symptomatic disease with average to moderately elevated total and LDL-cholesterol and below average HDL-cholesterol); slow progression of coronary atherosclerosis in patients with coronary heart disease
Adjunct to dietary therapy in adolescent patients (10-17 years of age, females >1 year postmenarche) with heterozygous familial hypercholesterolemia having LDL >189 mg/dL, **or** LDL >160 mg/dL with positive family history of premature cardiovascular disease (CVD), **or** LDL >160 mg/dL with the presence of at least two other CVD risk factors
**Usual Dosage** Oral:
Adolescents 10-17 years: Immediate release tablet:
LDL reduction <20%: Initial: 10 mg/day with evening meal
LDL reduction ≥20%: Initial: 20 mg/day with evening meal
Usual range: 10-40 mg with evening meal, then adjust dose at 4-week intervals
Adults: Initial: 20 mg with evening meal, then adjust at 4-week intervals; maximum dose: 80 mg/day immediate release tablet **or** 60 mg/day extended release tablet
**Dosage modification/limits based on concurrent therapy:**
Cyclosporine and other immunosuppressant drugs: Initial dose: 10 mg/day with a maximum recommended dose of 20 mg/day
Concurrent therapy with fibrates and/or lipid-lowering doses of niacin (>1 g/day): Maximum recommended dose: 20 mg/day. Concurrent use with fibrates should be avoided unless risk to benefit favors use.
Concurrent therapy with amiodarone or verapamil: Maximum recommended dose: 40 mg/day of regular release or 20 mg/day with extended release.
**Dosage Forms**
Tablet: 10 mg, 20 mg, 40 mg
Mevacor®: 20 mg, 40 mg
Tablet, extended release (Altoprev™): 10 mg, 20 mg, 40 mg, 60 mg

**lovastatin and niacin** *see* niacin and lovastatin *on page 573*

**Lovenox® [US/Can]** *see* enoxaparin *on page 285*

**Lovenox® HP [Can]** *see* enoxaparin *on page 285*

**Low-Ogestrel® [US]** *see* ethinyl estradiol and norgestrel *on page 318*

# loxapine (LOKS a peen)
**Sound-Alike/Look-Alike Issues**
Loxitane® may be confused with Soriatane®
**Synonyms** loxapine succinate; oxilapine succinate
**U.S./Canadian Brand Names** Apo-Loxapine® [Can]; Loxitane® [US]; Nu-Loxapine [Can]; PMS-Loxapine [Can]

**Therapeutic Category** Antipsychotic Agent, Dibenzoxazepine

**Use** Management of psychotic disorders

**Usual Dosage** Oral: Adults: 10 mg twice daily, increase dose until psychotic symptoms are controlled; usual dose range: 20-100 mg/day in divided doses 2-4 times/day; dosages >250 mg/day are not recommended

**Dosage Forms** Capsule, as succinate: 5 mg, 10 mg, 25 mg, 50 mg

**loxapine succinate** *see* loxapine *on previous page*

**Loxitane**® **[US]** *see* loxapine *on previous page*

**Loxitane**® **I.M.** *(Discontinued)* *see* loxapine *on previous page*

**Lozide**® **[Can]** *see* indapamide *on page 434*

**Lozi-Flur**™ **[US]** *see* fluoride *on page 347*

**Lozi-Tab**® *(Discontinued)* *see* fluoride *on page 347*

**Lozol**® **[US/Can]** *see* indapamide *on page 434*

**L-PAM** *see* melphalan *on page 509*

**LRH** *see* gonadorelin *on page 381*

**L-sarcolysin** *see* melphalan *on page 509*

**LTA**® **360 [US]** *see* lidocaine *on page 479*

**LTG** *see* lamotrigine *on page 465*

**Lu-26-054** *see* escitalopram *on page 297*

**Lubriderm**® **[US-OTC]** *see* lanolin, cetyl alcohol, glycerin, petrolatum, and mineral oil *on page 466*

**Lubriderm**® **Fragrance Free [US-OTC]** *see* lanolin, cetyl alcohol, glycerin, petrolatum, and mineral oil *on page 466*

**LubriTears**® **Solution** *(Discontinued)* *see* artificial tears *on page 71*

**Ludiomil**® *(Discontinued)* *see* maprotiline *on page 503*

**Lufyllin**® **[US/Can]** *see* dyphylline *on page 277*

**Lumigan**® **[US/Can]** *see* bimatoprost *on page 106*

**Luminal**® **Sodium [US]** *see* phenobarbital *on page 638*

**Lumitene**™ **[US]** *see* beta-carotene *on page 101*

**Lunelle**™ **[US]** *see* estradiol cypionate and medroxyprogesterone acetate *on page 303*

**Lunesta**™ **[US]** *see* eszopiclone *on page 307*

**LupiCare**™ **II Psoriasis [US-OTC]** *see* salicylic acid *on page 734*

**LupiCare**™ **Dandruff [US-OTC]** *see* salicylic acid *on page 734*

**LupiCare**™ **Psoriasis [US-OTC]** *see* salicylic acid *on page 734*

**Lupron**® **[US/Can]** *see* leuprolide acetate *on page 471*

**Lupron Depot**® **[US/Can]** *see* leuprolide acetate *on page 471*

**Lupron Depot-Ped**® **[US]** *see* leuprolide acetate *on page 471*

**Luride**® **[US]** *see* fluoride *on page 347*

**Luride**® **Lozi-Tab**® **[US]** *see* fluoride *on page 347*

**Luride**®**-SF** *(Discontinued)* *see* fluoride *on page 347*

**Lustra**® **[US/Can]** *see* hydroquinone *on page 420*

**Lustra-AF**™ **[US]** *see* hydroquinone *on page 420*

**luteinizing hormone releasing hormone** *see* gonadorelin *on page 381*

**Lutera**™ **[US]** *see* ethinyl estradiol and levonorgestrel *on page 312*

**Lutrepulse**™ **[Can]** *see* gonadorelin *on page 381*

**Luvox**® *(Discontinued)* *see* fluvoxamine *on page 356*

**Luxiq**® **[US]** *see* betamethasone (topical) *on page 103*

**LY139603** *see* atomoxetine *on page 77*

**LY146032** *see* daptomycin *on page 224*

**LY170053** *see* olanzapine *on page 595*

**LY2148568** *see* exenatide *on page 324*

**LY231514** *see* pemetrexed *on page 626*

**LY248686** *see* duloxetine *on page 275*

**Lycolan® Elixir *(Discontinued)*** *see* l-lysine *on page 487*

**Lyderm® [Can]** *see* fluocinonide *on page 345*

**LYMErix™ *(Discontinued)***

**Lymphazurin® [US/Can]** *see* radiological/contrast media (ionic) *on page 707*

**lymphocyte immune globulin** *see* antithymocyte globulin (equine) *on page 59*

**lymphocyte mitogenic factor** *see* aldesleukin *on page 25*

**Lyphocin® Injection *(Discontinued)*** *see* vancomycin *on page 839*

**Lysinyl [US-OTC]** *see* l-lysine *on page 487*

**Lysodren® [US/Can]** *see* mitotane *on page 544*

**M-M-R® II [US/Can]** *see* measles, mumps, and rubella vaccines, combined *on page 504*

**Maalox® [US-OTC]** *see* aluminum hydroxide, magnesium hydroxide, and simethicone *on page 35*

**Maalox® Anti-Gas *(Discontinued)*** *see* aluminum hydroxide, magnesium hydroxide, and simethicone *on page 35*

**Maalox® Anti-Gas Extra Strength *(Discontinued)*** *see* aluminum hydroxide, magnesium hydroxide, and simethicone *on page 35*

**Maalox® Extra Strength *(Discontinued)*** *see* aluminum hydroxide and magnesium hydroxide *on page 35*

**Maalox® Max [US-OTC]** *see* aluminum hydroxide, magnesium hydroxide, and simethicone *on page 35*

**Maalox® Plus *(Discontinued)*** *see* aluminum hydroxide, magnesium hydroxide, and simethicone *on page 35*

**Maalox® TC (Therapeutic Concentrate) *(Discontinued)*** *see* aluminum hydroxide and magnesium hydroxide *on page 35*

**Macrobid® [US/Can]** *see* nitrofurantoin *on page 577*

**Macrodantin® [US/Can]** *see* nitrofurantoin *on page 577*

**Macrodex® *(Discontinued)*** *see* dextran *on page 236*

**Macugen® [US]** *see* pegaptanib *on page 623*

## mafenide (MA fe nide)

**Synonyms** mafenide acetate
**U.S./Canadian Brand Names** Sulfamylon® [US]
**Therapeutic Category** Antibacterial, Topical
**Use** Adjunct in the treatment of second- and third-degree burns to prevent septicemia caused by susceptible organisms such as *Pseudomonas aeruginosa*
  **Orphan drug:** Prevention of graft loss of meshed autografts on excised burn wounds
**Usual Dosage** Children and Adults: Topical: Apply once or twice daily with a sterile gloved hand; apply to a thickness of approximately 16 mm; the burned area should be covered with cream at all times
**Dosage Forms**
  Cream, topical, as acetate: 85 mg/g (60 g, 120 g, 454 g) [contains sodium metabisulfite]
  Powder, for topical solution: 5% (5s) [50 g/packet]

**mafenide acetate** *see* mafenide *on this page*

## magaldrate and simethicone (MAG al drate & sye METH i kone)

**Sound-Alike/Look-Alike Issues**
  Riopan Plus® may be confused with Repan®

**Synonyms** simethicone and magaldrate

**Therapeutic Category** Antacid; Antiflatulent

**Use** Relief of hyperacidity associated with peptic ulcer, gastritis, peptic esophagitis and hiatal hernia which are accompanied by symptoms of gas

**Usual Dosage** Adults: Oral: 540-1080 mg magaldrate between meals and at bedtime

**Dosage Forms** [DSC] = Discontinued product

Suspension, oral: Magaldrate 540 mg and simethicone 20 mg per 5 mL (360 mL)

Riopan Plus®: Magaldrate 540 mg and simethicone 20 mg per 5 mL (360 mL) [DSC]

Riopan Plus® Double Strength: Magaldrate 1080 mg and simethicone 40 mg per 5 mL (360 mL) [DSC]

**Magalox Plus®** *(Discontinued)* *see* aluminum hydroxide, magnesium hydroxide, and simethicone *on page 35*

**Magan®** *(Discontinued)* *see* magnesium salicylate *on page 499*

**Mag Delay® [US-OTC]** *see* magnesium chloride *on this page*

**Mag G® [US-OTC]** *see* magnesium gluconate *on next page*

**Maginex™ [US-OTC]** *see* magnesium L-aspartate hydrochloride *on this page*

**Maginex™ DS [US-OTC]** *see* magnesium L-aspartate hydrochloride *on this page*

**Magnacal® [US-OTC]** *see* nutritional formula, enteral/oral *on page 591*

**magnesia magma** *see* magnesium hydroxide *on next page*

# magnesium L-aspartate hydrochloride
(mag NEE zhum el as PAR tate hye droe KLOR ide)

**Synonyms** MAH

**U.S./Canadian Brand Names** Maginex™ DS [US-OTC]; Maginex™ [US-OTC]

**Therapeutic Category** Electrolyte Supplement, Oral

**Use** Dietary supplement

**Usual Dosage** Adults:

Recommended dietary allowance (RDA) of magnesium:

Male: 400-420 mg

Female: 310-320 mg

During pregnancy: 360 mg

During lactation: 320 mg

Dietary supplement: Oral: Magnesium-L-aspartate 1230 mg (magnesium 122 mg) up to 3 times/day

**Dosage Forms**

Granules (Maginex™ DS): 1230 mg [magnesium 10 mEq; equivalent to magnesium 122 mg; lemon flavor]

Tablet (Maginex™): 615 mg [magnesium 5 mEq; equivalent to magnesium 61 mg]

**magnesium carbonate and aluminum hydroxide** *see* aluminum hydroxide and magnesium carbonate *on page 35*

# magnesium chloride (mag NEE zhum KLOR ide)

**U.S./Canadian Brand Names** Chloromag® [US]; Mag Delay® [US-OTC]; Mag-SR® [US-OTC]; Slow-Mag® [US-OTC]

**Therapeutic Category** Electrolyte Supplement, Oral

**Use** Correction or prevention of hypomagnesemia

**Usual Dosage** Dietary supplement:

Oral: Adults: 54-483 mg/day in divided doses; refer to product labeling. The recommended dietary allowance (RDA) of magnesium is 4.5 mg/kg which is a total daily allowance of 350-400 mg for adult men and 280-300 mg for adult women. During pregnancy the RDA is 300 mg and during lactation the RDA is 355 mg.

I.V. in TPN:

Children: 2-10 mEq/day

The usual recommended pediatric maintenance intake of magnesium ranges from 0.2-0.6 mEq/kg/day. The dose of magnesium may also be based on the caloric intake; on that basis, 3-10 mEq/day of magnesium are needed; maximum maintenance dose: 8-16 mEq/day

Adults: 8-24 mEq/day

**Dosage Forms**

Injection, solution (Chloromag®): 200 mg/mL [1.97 mEq/mL] (50 mL)

(Continued)

## magnesium chloride *(Continued)*

Tablet [enteric coated] (Slow-Mag®): Elemental magnesium 64 mg [contains elemental calcium 106 mg]
Tablet, extended release (Mag Delay®, Mag-SR®): Magnesium chloride hexahydrate 535 mg [equivalent to elemental magnesium 64 mg]

## magnesium citrate (mag NEE zhum SIT rate)

**Synonyms** citrate of magnesia
**U.S./Canadian Brand Names** Citro-Mag® [Can]
**Therapeutic Category** Laxative
**Use** Evacuation of bowel prior to certain surgical and diagnostic procedures or overdose situations
**Usual Dosage** Cathartic: Oral:
Children:
<6 years: 0.5 mL/kg up to a maximum of 200 mL repeated every 4-6 hours until stools are clear
6-12 years: 100-150 mL
Children ≥12 years and Adults: 1/2 to 1 full bottle (120-300 mL)
**Dosage Forms**
Solution, oral: 290 mg/5 mL (300 mL) [cherry and lemon flavors]
Tablet: 100 mg [as elemental magnesium]

## magnesium gluconate (mag NEE zhum GLOO koe nate)

**U.S./Canadian Brand Names** Almora® [US-OTC]; Mag G® [US-OTC]; Magonate® [US-OTC]; Magtrate® [US-OTC]
**Therapeutic Category** Electrolyte Supplement, Oral
**Use** Dietary supplement for treatment of magnesium deficiencies
**Usual Dosage** The recommended dietary allowance (RDA) of magnesium is 4.5 mg/kg which is a total daily allowance of 350-400 mg for adult men and 280-300 mg for adult women. During pregnancy the RDA is 300 mg and during lactation the RDA is 355 mg.

Dietary supplement: Oral:
Children: 3-6 mg/kg/day in divided doses 3-4 times/day; maximum: 400 mg/day
Adults: 54-483 mg/day in divided doses; refer to product labeling
**Dosage Forms** [DSC] = Discontinued product
Solution:
Magonate®: 1000 mg/5 mL (480 mL) [magnesium 4.8 mEq/5 mL; equivalent to elemental magnesium 54 mg/5 mL; contains sodium benzoate]
Magonate® Sport: 1000 mg/5 mL (30 mL) [magnesium 4.8 mEq/5 mL; equivalent to elemental magnesium 54 mg/5 mL; contains sodium benzoate; fruit flavor] [DSC]
Tablet (Almora®, Mag G®, Magonate®, Magtrate®): 500 mg [magnesium 2.4 mEq; equivalent to elemental magnesium 27 mg]

## magnesium hydroxide (mag NEE zhum hye DROKS ide)

**Synonyms** magnesia magma; milk of magnesia; MOM
**U.S./Canadian Brand Names** Dulcolax® Milk of Magnesia [US-OTC]; Phillips'® Milk of Magnesia [US-OTC]
**Therapeutic Category** Antacid; Electrolyte Supplement, Oral; Laxative
**Use** Short-term treatment of occasional constipation and symptoms of hyperacidity, magnesium replacement therapy
**Usual Dosage** Oral:
Average daily intakes of dietary magnesium have declined in recent years due to processing of food; the latest estimate of the average American dietary intake was 349 mg/day
Laxative:
Liquid:
Children
<2 years: 0.5 mL/kg/dose
2-5 years: 5-15 mL/day (2.5-7.5 mL/day of liquid concentrate) or in divided doses
6-12 years: 15-30 mL/day (7.5-15 mL/day of liquid concentrate) or in divided doses
Children ≥12 years and Adults: 30-60 mL/day (15-30 mL/day of liquid concentrate) or in divided doses
Tablet:
Children:
2-5 years: 1-2 tablets before bedtime
6-11 years: 3-4 tablets before bedtime

Children ≥12 years and Adults: 6-8 tablets before bedtime
Antacid:
Liquid:
Children: 2.5-5 mL as needed up to 4 times/day
Adults: 5-15 mL (2.5-7.5 mL of liquid concentrate) as needed up to 4 times/day
Tablet:
Children 7-14 years: 1 tablet up to 4 times/day
Adults: 2-4 tablets up to 4 times/day

**Dosage Forms**
Liquid, oral: 400 mg/5 mL (360 mL, 480 mL, 960 mL, 3780 mL)
Dulcolax® Milk of Magnesia: 400 mg/5 mL (360 mL, 780 mL) [regular and mint flavors]
Phillips'® Milk of Magnesia: 400 mg/5 mL (120 mL, 360 mL, 780 mL) [original, French vanilla, cherry, and mint flavors]
Liquid, oral concentrate: 800 mg/5 mL (100 mL, 400 mL)
Phillips'® Milk of Magnesia [concentrate]: 800 mg/5 mL (240 mL) [strawberry créme flavor]
Tablet, chewable (Phillips'® Milk of Magnesia): 311 mg [mint flavor]

**magnesium hydroxide, aluminum hydroxide, and simethicone** *see* aluminum hydroxide, magnesium hydroxide, and simethicone *on page 35*

**magnesium hydroxide and aluminum hydroxide** *see* aluminum hydroxide and magnesium hydroxide *on page 35*

**magnesium hydroxide and calcium carbonate** *see* calcium carbonate and magnesium hydroxide *on page 132*

# magnesium hydroxide and mineral oil emulsion
(mag NEE zhum hye DROKS ide & MIN er al oyl)
**Synonyms** Haley's M-O; MOM/mineral oil emulsion
**U.S./Canadian Brand Names** Phillips'® M-O [US-OTC]
**Therapeutic Category** Laxative
**Use** Short-term treatment of occasional constipation
**Usual Dosage**
Children 6-11 years: 5-15 mL at bedtime or upon rising
Children ≥12 years and Adults: 30-60 mL at bedtime or upon rising
**Dosage Forms** Suspension, oral: Magnesium hydroxide 300 mg and mineral oil 1.25 mL per 5 mL (360 mL, 780 mL) [original and mint flavors]

**magnesium hydroxide, famotidine, and calcium carbonate** *see* famotidine, calcium carbonate, and magnesium hydroxide *on page 328*

# magnesium oxide (mag NEE zhum OKS ide)
**U.S./Canadian Brand Names** Mag-Ox® 400 [US-OTC]; Uro-Mag® [US-OTC]
**Therapeutic Category** Antacid; Electrolyte Supplement, Oral; Laxative
**Use** Electrolyte replacement
**Usual Dosage** The recommended dietary allowance (RDA) of magnesium is 4.5 mg/kg which is a total daily allowance of 350-400 mg for adult men and 280-300 mg for adult women. During pregnancy the RDA is 300 mg and during lactation the RDA is 355 mg.
Adults: Oral: Dietary supplement: 20-40 mEq (1-2 tablets) 2-3 times
**Product labeling:**
Mag-Ox 400®: 1-2 tablets daily with food
Uro-Mag®: 1-2 tablets 3 times/day with food
**Dosage Forms**
Capsule (Uro-Mag®): 140 mg [magnesium 7 mEq; equivalent to elemental magnesium 84 mg]
Tablet (Mag-Ox® 400): 400 mg [magnesium 20 mEq; equivalent to elemental magnesium 242 mg]

# magnesium salicylate (mag NEE zhum sa LIS i late)
**U.S./Canadian Brand Names** Doan's® Extra Strength [US-OTC]; Doan's® [US-OTC]; Keygesic [US-OTC], Momentum® [US-OTC]
**Therapeutic Category** Nonsteroidal Antiinflammatory Drug (NSAID)
**Use** Mild to moderate pain, fever, various inflammatory conditions
**Usual Dosage** Oral: Children ≥12 years and Adults:
Doan's®: Two caplets every 4 hours as needed (maximum: 12 caplets/24 hours)
(Continued)

## magnesium salicylate *(Continued)*

Doan's® Extra Strength, Momentum®: Two caplets every 6 hours (maximum: 8 caplets/24 hours)

Keygesic: One caplet every 4 hours as needed (maximum 4 caplets/24 hours)

**Dosage Forms**

Caplet, as anhydrous magnesium salicylate: 467 mg
Doan's®: 304 mg
Doan's® Extra Strength: 467 mg
Keygesic: 650 mg
Momentum®: 467 mg

## magnesium sulfate (mag NEE zhum SUL fate)

**Sound-Alike/Look-Alike Issues**

magnesium sulfate may be confused with manganese sulfate, morphine sulfate

$MgSO_4$ is an error-prone abbreviation (mistaken as morphine sulfate)

**Synonyms** epsom salts

**Therapeutic Category** Anticonvulsant; Electrolyte Supplement, Oral; Laxative

**Use** Treatment and prevention of hypomagnesemia; seizure prevention in severe pre-eclampsia or eclampsia, pediatric acute nephritis; short-term treatment torsade de pointes; treatment of cardiac arrhythmias (VT/VF) caused by hypomagnesemia; short-term treatment of constipation or soaking aid

**Usual Dosage** The recommended dietary allowance (RDA) of magnesium is 4.5 mg/kg which is a total daily allowance of 350-400 mg for adult men and 280-300 mg for adult women. During pregnancy the RDA is 300 mg and during lactation the RDA is 355 mg. Average daily intakes of dietary magnesium have declined in recent years due to processing of food. The latest estimate of the average American dietary intake was 349 mg/day. Dose represented as magnesium sulfate unless stated otherwise.

**Note:** Serum magnesium is poor reflection of repletional status as the majority of magnesium is intracellular; serum levels may be transiently normal for a few hours after a dose is given, therefore, aim for consistently high normal serum levels in patients with normal renal function for most efficient repletion

Hypomagnesemia:

Children: I.M., I.V.: 25-50 mg/kg/dose (0.2-0.4 mEq/kg/dose) every 4-6 hours for 3-4 doses, maximum single dose: 2000 mg (16 mEq), may repeat if hypomagnesemia persists (higher dosage up to 100 mg/kg/dose magnesium sulfate I.V. has been used); maintenance: I.V.: 30-60 mg/kg/day (0.25-0.5 mEq/kg/day)

Adults:

Oral: 3 g every 6 hours for 4 doses as needed

I.M., I.V.: 1 g every 6 hours for 4 doses; for severe hypomagnesemia: 8-12 g magnesium sulfate/day in divided doses has been used

Management of seizures and hypertension: Children: I.M., I.V.: 20-100 mg/kg/dose every 4-6 hours as needed; in severe cases doses as high as 200 mg/kg/dose have been used

Eclampsia, pre-eclampsia: Adults:

I.M.: 1-4 g every 4 hours

I.V.: Initial: 4 g, then switch to I.M. or 1-4 g/hour by continuous infusion

**Note:** Maximum dose not to exceed 30-40 g/day; maximum rate of infusion: 1-2 g/hour

Life-threatening arrhythmia: I.V.: 1-2 g (8-16 mEq) in 100 mL $D_5W$, administered over 5-60 minutes followed by an infusion of 0.5-1 g/hour, **or**

1-6 g administered over several minutes, followed by (in some cases) I.V. infusion of 3-20 mg/minute for 5-48 hours (depending on patient response and serum magnesium levels)

Maintenance electrolyte requirements:

Daily requirements: 0.2-0.5 mEq/kg/24 hours or 3-10 mEq/1000 kcal/24 hours

Maximum: 8-16 mEq/24 hours

Cathartic: Oral:

Children:

2-5 years: 2.5-5 g/kg/day in a single or divided doses

6-11 years: 5-10 g/day in a single or divided doses

Children ≥12 years and Adults: 10-30 g/day in a single or divided doses

Soaking aid: Topical: Adults: Dissolve 2 capfuls of powder per gallon of warm water

**Dosage Forms**

Infusion [premixed in $D_5W$]: 10 mg/mL (100 mL); 20 mg/mL (500 mL, 1000 mL)

Infusion [premixed in water for injection]: 40 mg/mL (100 mL, 500 mL, 1000 mL); 80 mg/mL (50 mL)

Injection, solution: 125 mg/mL (8 mL); 500 mg/mL (2 mL, 5 mL, 10 mL, 20 mL, 50 mL)

Powder: Magnesium sulfate USP (480 g, 1810 g, 1920 g)

**Magnevist**® **[US/Can]** *see* radiological/contrast media (ionic) *on page 707*

**Magonate**® **[US-OTC]** *see* magnesium gluconate *on page 498*

**Magonate**® **Sport** *(Discontinued)* *see* magnesium gluconate *on page 498*

**Mag-Ox**® **400 [US-OTC]** *see* magnesium oxide *on page 499*

**Magsal**® *(Discontinued)* *see* magnesium salicylate *on page 499*

**Mag-SR**® **[US-OTC]** *see* magnesium chloride *on page 497*

**Magtrate**® **[US-OTC]** *see* magnesium gluconate *on page 498*

**MAH** *see* magnesium L-aspartate hydrochloride *on page 497*

**Majeptil**® **[Can]** *see* thioproperazine *(Canada only) on page 798*

**Malarone**® **[US/Can]** *see* atovaquone and proguanil *on page 78*

## malathion (mal a THYE on)

**U.S./Canadian Brand Names** Ovide® [US]

**Therapeutic Category** Scabicides/Pediculicides

**Use** Treatment of head lice and their ova

**Usual Dosage** Sprinkle Ovide® lotion on dry hair and rub gently until the scalp is thoroughly moistened; pay special attention to the back of the head and neck. Allow to dry naturally - use no heat and leave uncovered. After 8-12 hours, the hair should be washed with a nonmedicated shampoo; rinse and use a fine-toothed comb to remove dead lice and eggs. If required, repeat with second application in 7-9 days. Further treatment is generally not necessary. Other family members should be evaluated to determine if infested and if so, receive treatment.

**Dosage Forms** Lotion: 0.5% (59 mL) [contains isopropyl alcohol 78%]

**Mallisol**® *(Discontinued)* *see* povidone-iodine *on page 668*

## maltodextrin (mal toe DEK strin)

**U.S./Canadian Brand Names** Gelclair® [US]; Multidex® [US-OTC]; OraRinse™ [US-OTC]

**Therapeutic Category** Skin and Mucous Membrane Agent

**Use** Topical: Treatment of infected or noninfected wounds

**Usual Dosage** Adults:

Oral: Management of pain due to oral lesions:

Gelclair®: Using contents of 1 reconstituted packet, rinse around mouth for ~1 minute, 3 times/day or more if needed; gargle and expectorate. May be used undiluted or with less dilution if adequate pain relief is not achieved.

OraRinse™: 1 tablespoonful, swish or gargle for ~1 minute, 4 times/day or more if needed

Topical: Wound dressing: Multidex®: After debridement and irrigation of wound, apply and cover with a nonadherent, nonocclusive dressing. May be applied to moist or dry, infected or noninfected wounds.

**Dosage Forms**

Gel, oral [concentrate] (Gelclair®): 15 mL/packet (21s) [contains benzalkonium chloride and sodium benzoate]

Gel, topical dressing (Multidex®): (4 mL, 7 mL, 14 mL, 85 mL)

Powder, for oral suspension (OraRinse™): (19 g) [contains phenylalanine; also contains aloe vera, fructose, and sodium benzoate; vanilla flavor]

Powder, topical dressing (Multidex®): (6 g, 12 g, 25 g, 45 g)

## malt soup extract (malt soop EKS trakt)

**Therapeutic Category** Laxative

**Use** Short-term treatment of constipation

**Usual Dosage** Oral:

Infants >1 month:

Breast-fed:

Liquid: 1-2 teaspoonfuls In 2-4 oz of water or fruit juice 1-2 times/day for 3-4 days

Powder: 4 g in 2-4 oz of water or fruit juice daily for 3-4 days

Bottle-fed:

Liquid: $\frac{1}{2}$ to 2 tablespoonfuls/day in formula for 3-4 days, then 1-2 teaspoonfuls/day

Powder: 8-16 g/day in formula for 3-4 days, then 4-8 g/day

(Continued)

# malt soup extract *(Continued)*

Children:
2-6 years:
Liquid: 7.5 mL 1-2 times/day for 3-4 days
Powder: 8 g twice daily for 3-4 days
6-12 years:
Liquid: 15-30 mL 1-2 times/day for 3-4 days
Powder: Up to 16 g/day for 3-4 days
Children ≥12 years and Adults:
Liquid: 30 mL twice daily for 3-4 days, then 15-30 mL at bedtime
Powder: Up to 32 g twice daily for 3-4 days, then 16-32 g at bedtime
Tablet: 4 tablets 4 times/day (maximum dose: 64 g/day)
**Dosage Forms** [DSC] = Discontinued product
Liquid: Nondiastatic barley malt extract 16 g/15 mL (240 mL, 480 mL) [DSC]
Powder: Nondiastatic barley malt extract 8 g/tablespoonful (240 g, 480 g) [DSC]
Tablet: Nondiastatic barley malt extract 750 mg [DSC]

**Maltsupex®** *(Discontinued)* see malt soup extract *on previous page*

**Mandelamine® [US/Can]** see methenamine *on page 522*

**mandrake** see podophyllum resin *on page 656*

**Manerix® [Can]** see moclobemide *(Canada only) on page 546*

**manganese** see trace metals *on page 813*

# mannitol (MAN i tole)

**Sound-Alike/Look-Alike Issues**
Osmitrol® may be confused with esmolol
**Synonyms** *D*-mannitol
**U.S./Canadian Brand Names** Osmitrol® [US/Can]; Resectisol® [US]
**Therapeutic Category** Diuretic, Osmotic
**Use** Reduction of increased intracranial pressure associated with cerebral edema; promotion of diuresis in the prevention and/or treatment of oliguria or anuria due to acute renal failure; reduction of increased intraocular pressure; promoting urinary excretion of toxic substances; genitourinary irrigant in transurethral prostatic resection or other transurethral surgical procedures
**Usual Dosage**
Children: I.V.:
Test dose (to assess adequate renal function): 200 mg/kg over 3-5 minutes to produce a urine flow of at least 1 mL/kg for 1-3 hours
Initial: 0.25-1 g/kg
Maintenance: 0.25-0.5 g/kg given every 4-6 hours
Adults:
I.V.:
Test dose (to assess adequate renal function): 12.5 g (200 mg/kg) over 3-5 minutes to produce a urine flow of at least 30-50 mL of urine per hour. If urine flow does not increase, a second test dose may be given. If test dose does not produce an acceptable urine output, then need to reassess management.
Initial: 0.5-1 g/kg
Maintenance: 0.25-0.5 g/kg every 4-6 hours; usual daily dose: 20-200 g/24 hours
Intracranial pressure: Cerebral edema: 0.25-1.5 g/kg/dose I.V. as a 15% to 20% solution over ≥30 minutes; maintain serum osmolality 310 to <320 mOsm/kg
Prevention of acute renal failure (oliguria): 50-100 g dose
Treatment of oliguria: 100 g dose
Preoperative for neurosurgery: 1.5-2 g/kg administered 1-1.5 hours prior to surgery
Reduction of intraocular pressure: 1.5-2 g/kg as a 15% to 20% solution; administer over 30 minutes
Topical: Transurethral irrigation: Use urogenital solution as required for irrigation
**Dosage Forms**
Injection, solution: 5% [50 mg/mL] (1000 mL); 10% [100 mg/mL] (500 mL, 1000 mL); 15% [150 mg/mL] (500 mL); 20% [200 mg/mL] (150 mL, 250 mL, 500 mL); 25% [250 mg/mL] (50 mL)
Osmitrol®: 5% [50 mg/mL] (1000 mL); 10% [100 mg/mL] (500 mL, 1000 mL); 15% [150 mg/mL] (500 mL); 20% [200 mg/mL] (250 mL, 500 mL)
Solution, urogenital (Resectisol®): 5% [50 mg/mL] (2000 mL, 4000 mL)

*D*-**mannitol** *see* mannitol *on previous page*

**mantoux** *see* tuberculin tests *on page 830*

**Maox**® *(Discontinued)* *see* magnesium oxide *on page 499*

**Mapap**® **[US-OTC]** *see* acetaminophen *on page 4*

**Mapap**® **Arthritis [US-OTC]** *see* acetaminophen *on page 4*

**Mapap**® **Children's [US-OTC]** *see* acetaminophen *on page 4*

**Mapap**® **Extra Strength [US-OTC]** *see* acetaminophen *on page 4*

**Mapap**® **Infants [US-OTC]** *see* acetaminophen *on page 4*

**Mapap Sinus Maximum Strength [US-OTC]** *see* acetaminophen and pseudoephedrine *on page 8*

**maprotiline** (ma PROE ti leen)
  Sound-Alike/Look-Alike Issues
    Ludiomil® may be confused with Lamictal®, lamotrigine, Lomotil®
  Synonyms maprotiline hydrochloride
  U.S./Canadian Brand Names Novo-Maprotiline [Can]
  Therapeutic Category Antidepressant, Tetracyclic
  Use Treatment of depression and anxiety associated with depression
  Usual Dosage Oral: Adults: Depression/anxiety: 75 mg/day to start, increase by 25 mg every 2 weeks up to 150-225 mg/day; given in 3 divided doses or in a single daily dose
  Dosage Forms Tablet, as hydrochloride: 25 mg, 50 mg, 75 mg

**maprotiline hydrochloride** *see* maprotiline *on this page*

**Marcaine**® **[US/Can]** *see* bupivacaine *on page 120*

**Marcaine**® **Spinal [US]** *see* bupivacaine *on page 120*

**Margesic**® **H [US]** *see* hydrocodone and acetaminophen *on page 411*

**Marinol**® **[US/Can]** *see* dronabinol *on page 274*

**Marmine**® **Injection** *(Discontinued)* *see* dimenhydrinate *on page 252*

**Marmine**® **Oral** *(Discontinued)* *see* dimenhydrinate *on page 252*

**Marplan**® **[US]** *see* isocarboxazid *on page 449*

**Marthritic**® *(Discontinued)* *see* salsalate *on page 738*

**Marvelon**® **[Can]** *see* ethinyl estradiol and desogestrel *on page 309*

**Matulane**® **[US/Can]** *see* procarbazine *on page 680*

**3M**™ **Avagard**® *(Discontinued)* *see* chlorhexidine gluconate *on page 168*

**Mavik**® **[US/Can]** *see* trandolapril *on page 815*

**Maxair**™ **Autohaler**™ **[US]** *see* pirbuterol *on page 650*

**Maxalt**® **[US/Can]** *see* rizatriptan *on page 727*

**Maxalt-MLT**® **[US]** *see* rizatriptan *on page 727*

**Maxalt RPD**™ **[Can]** *see* rizatriptan *on page 727*

**Maxaquin**® **[US]** *see* lomefloxacin *on page 488*

**Maxidex**® **[US/Can]** *see* dexamethasone (ophthalmic) *on page 232*

**Maxidone**™ **[US]** *see* hydrocodone and acetaminophen *on page 411*

**Maxifed**® **[US]** *see* guaifenesin and pseudoephedrine *on page 388*

**Maxifed**® **DM [US]** *see* guaifenesin, pseudoephedrine, and dextromethorphan *on page 391*

**Maxifed-G**® **[US]** *see* guaifenesin and pseudoephedrine *on page 388*

**Maxiflor**® *(Discontinued)* *see* diflorasone *on page 247*

**Maximum Strength Desenex**® **Antifungal Cream** *(Discontinued)* *see* miconazole *on page 537*

**Maximum Strength Dex-A-Diet**® *(Discontinued)*

**Maximum Strength Dexatrim**® *(Discontinued)*

**Maxipime**® **[US/Can]** *see* cefepime *on page 154*

**Maxitrol**® **[US/Can]** *see* neomycin, polymyxin B, and dexamethasone *on page 567*

**Maxi-Tuss HC**® **[US]** *see* phenylephrine, hydrocodone, and chlorpheniramine *on page 643*

**Maxi-Tuss HCG [US]** *see* hydrocodone and guaifenesin *on page 412*

**Maxi-Tuss HCX [US]** *see* phenylephrine, hydrocodone, and chlorpheniramine *on page 643*

**Maxivate**® **[US]** *see* betamethasone (topical) *on page 103*

**Maxolon**® *(Discontinued) see* metoclopramide *on page 533*

**Maxzide**® **[US]** *see* hydrochlorothiazide and triamterene *on page 410*

**Maxzide**®**-25 [US]** *see* hydrochlorothiazide and triamterene *on page 410*

**may apple** *see* podophyllum resin *on page 656*

**3M**™ **Cavilon**™ **Skin Cleanser [US-OTC]** *see* benzalkonium chloride *on page 95*

**MCH** *see* collagen hemostat *on page 206*

## m-cresyl acetate (em-KREE sil AS e tate)
U.S./Canadian Brand Names Cresylate® [US]
Therapeutic Category Otic Agent, Antiinfective
Use Provides an acid medium; for external otitis infections caused by susceptible bacteria or fungus
Usual Dosage Otic: Instill 2-4 drops as required
Dosage Forms Solution, otic: 25% (15 mL) [with isopropanol 25%, chlorobutanol 1%, benzyl alcohol 1%, and castor oil 5% in propylene glycol]

**MCT** *see* medium chain triglycerides *on page 507*

**MCT Oil**® **[US-OTC/Can]** *see* medium chain triglycerides *on page 507*

**MCV4** *see* meningococcal polysaccharide (Groups A / C / Y and W-135) diphtheria toxoid conjugate vaccine *on page 510*

**MD-Gastroview**® **[US]** *see* radiological/contrast media (ionic) *on page 707*

**MDL 73,147EF** *see* dolasetron *on page 265*

**ME-500**® **[US]** *see* methionine *on page 523*

## measles, mumps, and rubella vaccines, combined
(MEE zels, mumpz & roo BEL a vak SEENS, kom BINED)
Synonyms MMR; mumps, measles and rubella vaccines, combined; rubella, measles and mumps vaccines, combined
U.S./Canadian Brand Names M-M-R® II [US/Can]; Priorix™ [Can]
Therapeutic Category Vaccine, Live Virus
Use Measles, mumps, and rubella prophylaxis
Usual Dosage SubQ:
Infants <12 months: If there is risk of exposure to measles, single-antigen measles vaccine should be administered at 6-11 months of age with a second dose (of MMR) at >12 months of age.
Children ≥12 months: 0.5 mL at 12 months and then repeated at 4-6 years of age. If the second dose was not received, the schedule should be completed by the 11- to 12-year old visit. Administer in outer aspect of the upper arm. Recommended age of primary immunization is 12-15 months; revaccination is recommended prior to elementary school.
Dosage Forms Injection, powder for reconstitution [preservative free]: Measles virus 1000 $TCID_{50}$, rubella virus 1000 $TCID_{50}$, and mumps virus 20,000 $TCID_{50}$ [contains neomycin 25 mcg, gelatin, human albumin, and bovine serum; produced in chick embryo cell culture]

## measles virus vaccine (live) (MEE zels VYE rus vak SEEN, live)
Sound-Alike/Look-Alike Issues
Attenuvax® may be confused with Meruvax®
Synonyms more attenuated enders strain; rubeola vaccine
U.S./Canadian Brand Names Attenuvax® [US]
Therapeutic Category Vaccine, Live Virus
Use Adults born before 1957 are generally considered to be immune. All those born in or after 1957 without documentation of live vaccine on or after first birthday, physician-diagnosed measles, or laboratory evidence of immunity should be vaccinated, ideally with two doses of vaccine separated by no less than 1 month. For those previously vaccinated with one dose of measles vaccine, revaccination is

recommended for students entering colleges and other institutions of higher education, for healthcare workers at the time of employment, and for international travelers who visit endemic areas.

**MMR is the vaccine of choice if recipients are likely to be susceptible to rubella and/or mumps as well as to measles. Persons vaccinated between 1963 and 1967 with a killed measles vaccine, followed by live vaccine within 3 months, or with a vaccine of unknown type should be revaccinated with live measles virus vaccine.**

Usual Dosage Children ≥15 months and Adults: SubQ: 0.5 mL in outer aspect of the upper arm, no routine boosters

Dosage Forms Injection, powder for reconstitution [preservative free]: 1000 $TCID_{50}$ [contains human albumin, bovine serum, and neomycin; produced in chick embryo cell culture]

**Measurin**® *(Discontinued)* *see* aspirin *on page 73*

**Mebaral**® **[US/Can]** *see* mephobarbital *on page 513*

# mebendazole (me BEN da zole)

U.S./Canadian Brand Names Vermox® [Can]

Therapeutic Category Anthelmintic

Use Treatment of pinworms (*Enterobius vermicularis*), whipworms (*Trichuris trichiura*), roundworms (*Ascaris lumbricoides*), and hookworms (*Ancylostoma duodenale*)

Usual Dosage Children and Adults: Oral:
Pinworms: 100 mg as a single dose; may need to repeat after 2 weeks; treatment should include family members in close contact with patient
Whipworms, roundworms, hookworms: One tablet twice daily, morning and evening on 3 consecutive days; if patient is not cured within 3-4 weeks, a second course of treatment may be administered
Capillariasis: 200 mg twice daily for 20 days

Dosage Forms Tablet, chewable: 100 mg

# mecamylamine (mek a MIL a meen)

Sound-Alike/Look-Alike Issues
mecamylamine may be confused with mesalamine

Synonyms mecamylamine hydrochloride

U.S./Canadian Brand Names Inversine® [US/Can]

Therapeutic Category Ganglionic Blocking Agent

Use Treatment of moderately severe to severe hypertension and in uncomplicated malignant hypertension

Usual Dosage Adults: Oral: 2.5 mg twice daily after meals for 2 days; increased by increments of 2.5 mg at intervals ≥2 days until desired blood pressure response is achieved; average daily dose: 25 mg (usually in 3 divided doses)

**Note:** Reduce dosage of other antihypertensives when combined with mecamylamine with exception of thiazide diuretics which may be maintained at usual dose while decreasing mecamylamine by 50%

Dosage Forms Tablet, as hydrochloride: 2.5 mg

**mecamylamine hydrochloride** *see* mecamylamine *on this page*

# mechlorethamine (me klor ETH a meen)

Synonyms chlorethazine mustard; chlorethazine; $HN_2$; mechlorethamine hydrochloride; mustine; nitrogen mustard; NSC-762

U.S./Canadian Brand Names Mustargen® [US/Can]

Therapeutic Category Antineoplastic Agent

Use Combination therapy of Hodgkin disease and malignant lymphomas; non-Hodgkin lymphoma; may be used by intracavitary injection for treatment of metastatic tumors; pleural and other malignant effusions; topical treatment of mycosis fungoides

Usual Dosage Refer to individual protocols.
Children and Adults: I.V.: 6 mg/m² on days 1 and 8 of a 28-day cycle (MOPP regimen)
Adults:
I.V.: 0.4 mg/kg **or** 12-16 mg/m² for one dose **or** divided into 0.1 mg/kg/day for 4 days, repeated at 4- to 6-week intervals
Intracavitary: 0.2-0.4 mg/kg (10-20 mg) as a single dose; may be repeated if fluid continues to accumulate.
Intrapericardially: 0.2-0.4 mg/kg as a single dose; may be repeated if fluid continues to accumulate.
(Continued)

# mechlorethamine *(Continued)*

Topical: 0.01% to 0.02% solution, lotion, or ointment

**Dosage Forms** Injection, powder for reconstitution, as hydrochloride: 10 mg

**mechlorethamine hydrochloride** *see* mechlorethamine *on previous page*

**Meclan**® **Topical** *(Discontinued)*

# meclizine (MEK li zeen)

**Sound-Alike/Look-Alike Issues**

Antivert® may be confused with Axert™

**Synonyms** meclizine hydrochloride; meclozine hydrochloride

**U.S./Canadian Brand Names** Antivert® [US]; Bonamine™ [Can]; Bonine® [US-OTC/Can]; Dramamine® Less Drowsy Formula [US-OTC]

**Therapeutic Category** Antihistamine

**Use** Prevention and treatment of symptoms of motion sickness; management of vertigo with diseases affecting the vestibular system

**Usual Dosage** Children >12 years and Adults: Oral:

Motion sickness: 12.5-25 mg 1 hour before travel, repeat dose every 12-24 hours if needed; doses up to 50 mg may be needed

Vertigo: 25-100 mg/day in divided doses

**Dosage Forms**

Tablet, as hydrochloride: 12.5 mg, 25 mg

Antivert®: 12.5 mg, 25 mg, 50 mg

Dramamine® Less Drowsy Formula: 25 mg

Tablet, chewable, as hydrochloride (Bonine®): 25 mg

**meclizine hydrochloride** *see* meclizine *on this page*

# meclofenamate (me kloe fen AM ate)

**Synonyms** meclofenamate sodium

**U.S./Canadian Brand Names** Meclomen® [Can]

**Therapeutic Category** Analgesic, Nonnarcotic; Nonsteroidal Antiinflammatory Drug (NSAID)

**Use** Treatment of inflammatory disorders, arthritis, mild to moderate pain, dysmenorrhea

**Usual Dosage** Children >14 years and Adults: Oral:

Mild to moderate pain: 50 mg every 4-6 hours; increases to 100 mg may be required; maximum dose: 400 mg

Rheumatoid arthritis and osteoarthritis: 50 mg every 4-6 hours; increase, over weeks, to 200-400 mg/day in 3-4 divided doses; do not exceed 400 mg/day; maximal benefit for any dose may not be seen for 2-3 weeks

**Dosage Forms** Capsule, as sodium: 50 mg, 100 mg

**meclofenamate sodium** *see* meclofenamate *on this page*

**Meclomen**® **[Can]** *see* meclofenamate *on this page*

**meclozine hydrochloride** *see* meclizine *on this page*

**Med-Diltiazem [Can]** *see* diltiazem *on page 251*

**medicinal carbon** *see* charcoal *on page 165*

**medicinal charcoal** *see* charcoal *on page 165*

**Medicone**® **[US-OTC]** *see* phenylephrine *on page 640*

**Medidin**® **Liquid** *(Discontinued) see* hydrocodone and guaifenesin *on page 412*

**Medigesic**® **[US]** *see* butalbital, acetaminophen, and caffeine *on page 124*

**Medihaler-Iso**® *(Discontinued) see* isoproterenol *on page 450*

**Medipain 5**® *(Discontinued) see* hydrocodone and acetaminophen *on page 411*

**Mediplast**® **[US-OTC]** *see* salicylic acid *on page 734*

**Medipren**® *(Discontinued) see* ibuprofen *on page 427*

**Medi-Quick**® **Topical Ointment** *(Discontinued) see* bacitracin, neomycin, and polymyxin B *on page 87*

**Medi-Sleep**® **[US-OTC]** *see* doxylamine *on page 273*

**Medispaz**® *(Discontinued)* *see* hyoscyamine *on page 424*

**Medi-Synal [US-OTC]** *see* acetaminophen and pseudoephedrine *on page 8*

**Medi-Tuss**® *(Discontinued)* *see* guaifenesin *on page 383*

## medium chain triglycerides (mee DEE um chane trye GLIS er ides)

**Synonyms** MCT; triglycerides, medium chain

**U.S./Canadian Brand Names** MCT Oil® [US-OTC/Can]

**Therapeutic Category** Nutritional Supplement

**Use** Dietary supplement for those who cannot digest long chain fats; malabsorption associated with disorders such as pancreatic insufficiency, bile salt deficiency, short bowel syndrome, and bacterial overgrowth of the small bowel; induce ketosis as a prevention for seizures

**Usual Dosage** Oral:

Infants: Initial: 0.5 mL every other feeding, then advance to every feeding, then increase in increments of 0.25-0.5 mL/feeding at intervals of 2-3 days as tolerated

Seizures: About 39 mL with each meal or 50% to 70% (800-1120 kcal) of total calories (1600 kcal) as the oil will induce ketosis necessary for seizure control

Cystic fibrosis: 3 tablespoons/day is tolerated without adverse symptoms by most children

Adults: 15 mL 3-4 times/day

**Dosage Forms** Oil: 14 g/15 mL (960 mL) [115 calories/15 mL; derived from coconut oil]

**Medralone**® **Injection** *(Discontinued)* *see* methylprednisolone *on page 531*

**Medrol**® **[US/Can]** *see* methylprednisolone *on page 531*

## medroxyprogesterone acetate (me DROKS ee proe JES te rone)

**Sound-Alike/Look-Alike Issues**

medroxyPROGESTERone may be confused with hydroxyprogesterone, methylPREDNISolone, meth-ylTESTOSTERone

Provera® may be confused with Covera®, Parlodel®, Premarin®

**Synonyms** acetoxymethylprogesterone; medroxyprogesterone acetate; methylacetoxyprogesterone; MPA

**Tall-Man** medroxyPROGESTERone acetate

**U.S./Canadian Brand Names** Alti-MPA [Can]; Apo-Medroxy® [Can]; Depo-Prevera® [Can]; Depo-Provera® Contraceptive [US]; Depo-Provera® [US]; depo-subQ provera 104™ [US]; Gen-Medroxy [Can]; Novo-Medrone [Can]; Provera® [US/Can]

**Therapeutic Category** Contraceptive, Progestin Only; Progestin

**Use** Endometrial carcinoma or renal carcinoma; secondary amenorrhea or abnormal uterine bleeding due to hormonal imbalance; reduction of endometrial hyperplasia in nonhysterectomized postmenopausal women receiving conjugated estrogens; prevention of pregnancy; management of endometriosis-associated pain

**Usual Dosage**

Adolescents and Adults:

Amenorrhea: Oral: 5-10 mg/day for 5-10 days

Abnormal uterine bleeding: Oral: 5-10 mg for 5-10 days starting on day 16 or 21 of cycle

Contraception:

Depo-Provera® Contraceptive: I.M.: 150 mg every 3 months

depo-subQ provera 104™: SubQ: 104 mg every 3 months (every 12-14 weeks)

Endometriosis: depo-subQ provera 104™: SubQ: 104 mg every 3 months (every 12-14 weeks)

Adults:

Endometrial or renal carcinoma (Depo-Provera®): I.M.: 400-1000 mg/week

Accompanying cyclic estrogen therapy, postmenopausal: Oral: 5-10 mg for 12-14 consecutive days each month, starting on day 1 or day 16 of the cycle; lower doses may be used if given with estrogen continuously throughout the cycle

**Dosage Forms**

Injection, suspension, as acetate: 150 mg/mL (1 mL)

Depo-Provera®: 400 mg/mL (2.5 mL)

Depo-Provera® Contraceptive: 150 mg/mL (1 mL) [prefilled syringe or vial]

depo-subQ provera 104™: 104 mg/0.65 mL (0.65 mL) [prefilled syringe]

Tablet, as acetate (Provera®): 2.5 mg, 5 mg, 10 mg

## medroxyprogesterone acetate and estradiol cypionate *see* estradiol cypionate and medroxyprogesterone acetate *on page 303*

**medroxyprogesterone and estrogens (conjugated)** *see* estrogens (conjugated/equine) and medroxyprogesterone *on page 304*

## medrysone (ME dri sone)
**Therapeutic Category** Adrenal Corticosteroid
**Use** Treatment of allergic conjunctivitis, vernal conjunctivitis, episcleritis, ophthalmic epinephrine sensitivity reaction
**Usual Dosage** Children ≥3 years and Adults: Ophthalmic: Instill 1 drop in conjunctival sac 2-4 times/day up to every 4 hours; may use every 1-2 hours during first 1-2 days
**Dosage Forms** [DSC] = Discontinued product
Solution, ophthalmic: 1% (5 mL, 10 mL) [contains benzalkonium chloride] [DSC]

## mefenamic acid (me fe NAM ik AS id)
**Sound-Alike/Look-Alike Issues**
Ponstel® may be confused with Pronestyl®
**U.S./Canadian Brand Names** Apo-Mefenamic® [Can]; Nu-Mefenamic [Can]; PMS-Mefenamic Acid [Can]; Ponstel® [US/Can]
**Therapeutic Category** Analgesic, Nonnarcotic; Nonsteroidal Antiinflammatory Drug (NSAID)
**Use** Short-term relief of mild to moderate pain including primary dysmenorrhea
**Usual Dosage** Children >14 years and Adults: Oral: 500 mg to start then 250 mg every 4 hours as needed; maximum therapy: 1 week
**Dosage Forms** Capsule: 250 mg

## mefloquine (ME floe kwin)
**Synonyms** mefloquine hydrochloride
**U.S./Canadian Brand Names** Apo-Mefloquine® [Can]; Lariam® [US/Can]
**Therapeutic Category** Antimalarial Agent
**Use** Treatment of acute malarial infections and prevention of malaria
**Usual Dosage** Oral (dose expressed as mg of mefloquine hydrochloride):
Children ≥6 months and >5 kg:
Malaria treatment: 20-25 mg/kg in 2 divided doses, taken 6-8 hours apart (maximum: 1250 mg) Take with food and an ample amount of water. If clinical improvement is not seen within 48-72 hours, an alternative therapy should be used for retreatment.
Malaria prophylaxis: 5 mg/kg/once weekly (maximum dose: 250 mg) starting 1 week before, arrival in endemic area, continuing weekly during travel and for 4 weeks after leaving endemic area. Take with food and an ample amount of water.
Adults:
Malaria treatment (mild to moderate infection): 5 tablets (1250 mg) as a single dose. Take with food and at least 8 oz of water. If clinical improvement is not seen within 48-72 hours, an alternative therapy should be used for retreatment.
Malaria prophylaxis: 1 tablet (250 mg) weekly starting 1 week before, arrival in endemic area, continuing weekly during travel and for 4 weeks after leaving endemic area. Take with food and at least 8 oz of water.
**Dosage Forms** Tablet, as hydrochloride: 250 mg [equivalent to 228 mg base]

**mefloquine hydrochloride** *see* mefloquine *on this page*

**Mefoxin® [US]** *see* cefoxitin *on page 155*

**Megace® [US/Can]** *see* megestrol acetate *on this page*

**Megace® ES [US]** *see* megestrol acetate *on this page*

**Megace® OS [Can]** *see* megestrol acetate *on this page*

**Megadophilus® [US-OTC]** *see* Lactobacillus *on page 462*

## megestrol acetate (me JES trole AS e tate)
**Sound-Alike/Look-Alike Issues**
Megace® may be confused with Reglan®
**Synonyms** 5071-1DL(6); NSC-10363
**U.S./Canadian Brand Names** Apo-Megestrol® [Can]; Megace® ES [US]; Megace® OS [Can]; Megace® [US/Can]; Nu-Megestrol [Can]

**Therapeutic Category** Antineoplastic Agent; Progestin

**Use** Palliative treatment of breast and endometrial carcinoma; treatment of anorexia, cachexia, or unexplained significant weight loss in patients with AIDS

**Usual Dosage** Adults: Oral:

Female (refer to individual protocols):

Breast carcinoma: 40 mg 4 times/day

Endometrial carcinoma: 40-320 mg/day in divided doses; use for 2 months to determine efficacy; maximum doses used have been up to 800 mg/day

Male/Female: HIV-related cachexia:

Megace®: Initial dose: 800 mg/day; daily doses of 400 and 800 mg/day were found to be clinically effective

Megace ES®: 625 mg/day

**Dosage Forms**

Suspension, oral, as acetate: 40 mg/mL (240 mL, 480 mL)

Megace®: 40 mg/mL (240 mL) [contains alcohol 0.06% and sodium benzoate; lemon-lime flavor]

Megace® ES: 125 mg/mL (150 mL) [contains alcohol 0.06% and sodium benzoate; lemon-lime flavor]

Tablet, as acetate: 20 mg, 40 mg

**Melanex®** [US] *see* hydroquinone *on page 420*

**Melfiat®** [US] *see* phendimetrazine *on page 637*

**Mellaril®** [Can] *see* thioridazine *on page 798*

**Mellaril®** (all products) *(Discontinued)* *see* thioridazine *on page 798*

**Mellaril-S®** *(Discontinued)* *see* thioridazine *on page 798*

## meloxicam (mel OKS i kam)

**U.S./Canadian Brand Names** Apo-Meloxicam® [Can]; CO Meloxicam [Can]; Gen-Meloxicam [Can]; Mobicox® [Can]; Mobic® [US/Can]; Novo-Meloxicam [Can]; PMS-Meloxicam [Can]

**Therapeutic Category** Nonsteroidal Antiinflammatory Drug (NSAID)

**Use** Relief of signs and symptoms of osteoarthritis, rheumatoid arthritis, and juvenile rheumatoid arthritis (JRA)

**Usual Dosage** Oral:

Children ≥2 years: JRA: 0.125 mg/kg/day; maximum dose: 7.5 mg/day

Adults: Osteoarthritis, rheumatoid arthritis: Initial: 7.5 mg once daily; some patients may receive additional benefit from an increased dose of 15 mg once daily; maximum dose: 15 mg/day

**Dosage Forms**

Suspension: 7.5 mg/5 mL (100 mL) [contains sodium benzoate; raspberry flavor]

Tablet: 7.5 mg, 15 mg

**Melpaque HP®** [US] *see* hydroquinone *on page 420*

## melphalan (MEL fa lan)

**Sound-Alike/Look-Alike Issues**

melphalan may be confused with Mephyton®, Myleran®

Alkeran® may be confused with Alferon®, Leukeran®

**Synonyms** L-PAM; L-sarcolysin; phenylalanine mustard

**U.S./Canadian Brand Names** Alkeran® [US/Can]

**Therapeutic Category** Antineoplastic Agent

**Use** Palliative treatment of multiple myeloma and nonresectable epithelial ovarian carcinoma; neuroblastoma, rhabdomyosarcoma, breast cancer

**Usual Dosage** Refer to individual protocols.

Oral: Dose should always be adjusted to patient response and weekly blood counts:

Children: 4-20 mg/m$^2$/day for 1-21 days

Adults:

Multiple myeloma: 6 mg/day initially adjusted as indicated **or** 0.15 mg/kg/day for 7 days **or** 0.25 mg/kg/day for 4 days; repeat at 4- to 6-week intervals.

Ovarian carcinoma: 0.2 mg/kg/day for 5 days, repeat every 4-5 weeks.

I.V.:

Children:

Pediatric rhabdomyosarcoma: 10-35 mg/m$^2$/dose every 21-28 days

(Continued)

## melphalan (Continued)

High-dose melphalan with bone marrow transplantation for neuroblastoma: I.V.: 100-220 mg/m$^2$ as a single dose or divided into 2-5 daily doses. Infuse over 20-60 minutes.

Adults: Multiple myeloma: 16 mg/m$^2$ administered at 2-week intervals for 4 doses, then repeat monthly as per protocol for multiple myeloma.

**Dosage Forms**

Injection, powder for reconstitution: 50 mg [diluent contains ethanol and propylene glycol]

Tablet: 2 mg

**Melquin-3**® **[US]** *see* hydroquinone *on page 420*

**Melquin HP**® **[US]** *see* hydroquinone *on page 420*

## memantine (me MAN teen)

**Synonyms** memantine hydrochloride

**U.S./Canadian Brand Names** Ebixa® [Can]; Namenda™ [US]

**Therapeutic Category** N-Methyl-D-Aspartate Receptor Antagonist

**Use** Treatment of moderate-to-severe dementia of the Alzheimer type

**Usual Dosage** Oral: Adults:

Alzheimer's disease: Initial: 5 mg/day; increase dose by 5 mg/day to a target dose of 20 mg/day; wait at least 1 week between dosage changes. Doses >5 mg/day should be given in 2 divided doses.

Suggested titration: 5 mg/day for ≥1 week; 5 mg twice daily for ≥1 week; 15 mg/day given in 5 mg and 10 mg separated doses for ≥1 week; then 10 mg twice daily

**Dosage Forms**

Solution, oral: 2 mg/mL (360 mL) [alcohol free, dye free, sugar free; peppermint flavor]

Tablet, as hydrochloride: 5 mg, 10 mg

Combination package [titration pack contains two separate tablet formulations]: Memantine hydrochloride 5 mg (28s) and memantine hydrochloride 10 mg (21s)

**memantine hydrochloride** *see* memantine *on this page*

**Menactra**™ **[US]** *see* meningococcal polysaccharide (Groups A / C / Y and W-135) diphtheria toxoid conjugate vaccine *on this page*

**Menest**® **[US/Can]** *see* estrogens (esterified) *on page 305*

**Meni-D**® **(Discontinued)** *see* meclizine *on page 506*

**Meningitec**® **[Can]** *see* meningococcal polysaccharide (Groups A / C / Y and W-135) diphtheria toxoid conjugate vaccine *on this page*

## meningococcal polysaccharide (Groups A / C / Y and W-135) diphtheria toxoid conjugate vaccine

(me NIN joe kok al pol i SAK a ride groops aye, see, why & dubl yoo won thur tee fyve dif THEER ee a TOKS oyds KON joo gate vak SEEN)

**Synonyms** MCV4

**U.S./Canadian Brand Names** Menactra™ [US]; Meningitec® [Can]

**Therapeutic Category** Vaccine

**Use** Provide active immunization of adolescents and adults (11-55 years of age) against invasive meningococcal disease caused by *N. meningitidis* serogroups A, C, Y and W-135

The ACIP recommends routine vaccination of all adolescents at age 11-12 years. For adolescents not previously vaccinated, vaccine should be administered prior to high school entry (~15 years of age).

The ACIP also recommends routine vaccination for persons at increased risk for meningococcal disease. (MCV4 is preferred for persons aged 11-55 years; MPSV4 may be used if MCV4 is not available). Persons at increased risk include:

College freshmen living in dormitories

Microbiologists routinely exposed to isolates of *N. meningitides*

Military recruits

Persons traveling to or who reside in countries where *N. meningitides* is hyperendemic or epidemic, particularly if contact with local population will be prolonged

Persons with terminal complement component deficiencies

Persons with anatomic or functional asplenia

Use is also recommended during meningococcal outbreaks caused by vaccine preventable serogroups.

**Usual Dosage** I.M.: Adolescents 11-18 years and Adults ≤55 years: 0.5 mL

NOTE: Revaccination: May be indicated in patients previously vaccinated with MPSV4 who remain at increased risk for infection. The ACIP recommends the use of MCV4 for revaccination in patients 11-55 years, however use of MPSV4 is also acceptable. Consider revaccination after 3-5 years. The need for revaccination in patients previously vaccinated with MCV4 is currently under study.

**Dosage Forms** Injection, solution: 4 mcg each of polysaccharide antigen groups A, C, Y and W-135 per 0.5 mL [conjugated to 48 mcg diphtheria toxoid protein; adjuvant and preservative free; vial stopper contains dry, natural latex rubber]

# meningococcal polysaccharide vaccine (groups A / C / Y and W-135)
(me NIN joe kok al pol i SAK a ride vak SEEN groops aye, see, why & dubl yoo won thur tee fyve)

**Synonyms** MPSV4

**U.S./Canadian Brand Names** Menomune®-A/C/Y/W-135 [US]

**Therapeutic Category** Vaccine, Live Bacteria

**Use** Provide active immunity to meningococcal serogroups contained in the vaccine

The ACIP recommends routine vaccination for persons at increased risk for meningococcal disease. (Use of MPSV4 is recommended in children 2-10 years and adults > 55 years. MCV4 is preferred for persons aged 11-55 years; MPSV4 may be used if MCV4 is not available). Persons at increased risk include:
College freshmen living in dormitories
Microbiologists routinely exposed to isolates of *N. meningitides*
Military recruits
Persons traveling to or who reside in countries where *N. meningitides* is hyperendemic or epidemic, particularly if contact with local population will be prolonged
Persons with terminal complement component deficiencies
Persons with anatomic or functional asplenia
Use is also recommended during meningococcal outbreaks caused by vaccine preventable serogroups.

**Usual Dosage** SubQ:
Children <2 years: Not usually recommended. Two doses (0.5 mL/dose), 3 months apart, may be considered in children 3-18 months to elicit short-term protection against serogroup A disease. A single dose may be considered in children 19-23 months.
Children ≥2 years and Adults: 0.5 mL
**Note:** Revaccination: May be indicated in patients previously vaccinated with MPSV4 who remain at increased risk for infection. The ACIP recommends the use of MCV4 for revaccination in patients 11-55 years, however use of MPSV4 is also acceptable.
Children first vaccinated at <4 years: Revaccinate after 2-3 years.
Adults: Not determined, consider revaccination after 3-5 years.

**Dosage Forms** Injection, powder for reconstitution: 50 mcg each of polysaccharide antigen groups A, C, Y, and W-135 [contains lactose; packaged with 0.78 mL preservative free diluent or 6 mL diluent containing thimerosal; vial stoppers contain dry, natural latex rubber]

**Menomune®-A/C/Y/W-135 [US]** *see* meningococcal polysaccharide vaccine (groups A / C / Y and W-135) *on this page*

**Menopur® [US]** *see* menotropins *on this page*

**Menostar™ [US]** *see* estradiol *on page 299*

# menotropins (men oh TROE pins)
**Sound-Alike/Look-Alike Issues**
Repronex® may be confused with Regranex®

**U.S./Canadian Brand Names** Menopur® [US]; Repronex® [US/Can]

**Therapeutic Category** Gonadotropin

**Use**
Female:
In conjunction with hCG to induce ovulation and pregnancy in infertile females experiencing oligoa-novulation or anovulation when the cause of anovulation is functional and not caused by primary ovarlan failure (Pergonal®, Repronex®)
Stimulation of multiple follicle development in ovulatory patients as part of an assisted reproductive technology (ART) (Menopur®, Pergonal®, Repronex®)
Male: Stimulation of spermatogenesis in primary or secondary hypogonadotropic hypogonadism (Pergonal®)
(Continued)

## menotropins *(Continued)*

**Usual Dosage** Adults:

**Pergonal®:** I.M.

*Spermatogenesis (Male):* Following pretreatment with hCG: 75 int. units 3 times/week and hCG 2000 units twice weekly until sperm is detected in the ejaculate (4-6 months); may then be increased to menotropins 150 int. units 3 times/week

*Induction of ovulation (Female):* 75 int. units for 7-12 days, followed by 10,000 units hCG one day after the last dose; repeated at least twice at same level before increasing dosage to 150 int. units

**Repronex®:** I.M., SubQ:

*Induction of ovulation in patients with oligoanovulation (Female):* Initial: 150 int. units daily for the first 5 days of treatment. Adjustments should not be made more frequently than once every 2 days and should not exceed 75-150 int. units per adjustment. Maximum daily dose should not exceed 450 int. units and dosing beyond 12 days is not recommended. If patient's response is appropriate, hCG 5000-10,000 units should be given one day following the last dose of Repronex®. Hold dose if serum estradiol is >2000 pg/mL, if the ovaries are abnormally enlarged, or if abdominal pain occurs; the patient should also be advised to refrain from intercourse. May repeat process if follicular development is inadequate or if pregnancy does not occur.

*Assisted reproductive technologies (Female):* Initial (in patients who have received GnRH agonist or antagonist pituitary suppression): 225 int. units; adjustments in dose should not be made more frequently than once every 2 days and should not exceed more than 75-150 int. units per adjustment. The maximum daily doses of Repronex® given should not exceed 450 int. units and dosing beyond 12 days is not recommended. Once adequate follicular development is evident, hCG (5000-10,000 units) should be administered to induce final follicular maturation in preparation for oocyte retrieval. Withhold treatment when ovaries are abnormally enlarged on last day of therapy (to reduce chance of developing OHSS).

**Menopur®:** SubQ:

*Assisted reproductive technologies (ART):* Initial (in patients who have received GnRH agonist for pituitary suppression): 225 int. units; adjustments in dose should not be made more frequently than once every 2 days and should not exceed more than 150 int. units per adjustment. The maximum daily dose given should not exceed 450 int. units and dosing beyond 20 days is not recommended. Once adequate follicular development is evident, hCG should be administered to induce final follicular maturation in preparation for oocyte retrieval. Withhold treatment when ovaries are abnormally enlarged on last day of therapy (to reduce chance of developing OHSS).

**Dosage Forms** [DSC] = Discontinued product

Injection, powder for reconstitution:

Menopur®: Follicle stimulating hormone activity 75 int. units and luteinizing hormone activity 75 int. units [packaged with diluent; contains lactose 21 mg]

Pergonal®: Follicle stimulating hormone activity 75 int. units and luteinizing hormone activity 75 int. units [packaged with diluent; contains lactose 10 mg] [DSC]

Repronex®: Follicle stimulating hormone activity 75 int. units and luteinizing hormone activity 75 int. units [packaged with diluent]

**Mentax® [US]** *see* butenafine *on page 125*

**292 MEP® [Can]** *see* aspirin and meprobamate *on page 75*

## mepenzolate *(me PEN zoe late)*

**Sound-Alike/Look-Alike Issues**

Cantil® may be confused with Bentyl®

**Synonyms** mepenzolate bromide

**U.S./Canadian Brand Names** Cantil® [Can]

**Therapeutic Category** Anticholinergic Agent

**Use** Adjunctive treatment of peptic ulcer disease

**Usual Dosage** Adults: Oral: 25-50 mg 4 times/day with meals and at bedtime

**Dosage Forms** [DSC] = Discontinued product

Tablet, as bromide: 25 mg [contains tartrazine] [DSC]

**mepenzolate bromide** *see* mepenzolate *on this page*

**mepergan** *see* meperidine and promethazine *on next page*

## meperidine *(me PER i deen)*

**Sound-Alike/Look-Alike Issues**

meperidine may be confused with meprobamate

Demerol® may be confused with Demulen®, Desyrel®, dicumarol, Dilaudid®, Dymelor®, Pamelor®

**Synonyms** isonipecaine hydrochloride; meperidine hydrochloride; pethidine hydrochloride

**U.S./Canadian Brand Names** Demerol® [US/Can]; Meperitab® [US]

**Therapeutic Category** Analgesic, Narcotic

**Controlled Substance** C-II

**Use** Management of moderate to severe pain; adjunct to anesthesia and preoperative sedation

**Usual Dosage Note:** Doses should be titrated to necessary analgesic effect. When changing route of administration, note that oral doses are about half as effective as parenteral dose. Not recommended for chronic pain. These are guidelines and do not represent the maximum doses that may be required in all patients. In patients with normal renal function, doses of ≤600 mg/24 hours and use for ≤48 hours are recommended.

Children: Pain: Oral, I.M., I.V., SubQ: 1-1.5 mg/kg/dose every 3-4 hours as needed; 1-2 mg/kg as a single dose preoperative medication may be used; maximum 100 mg/dose (Note: Oral route is not recommended for acute pain.)

Adults: Pain:

Oral: Initial: Opiate-naive: 50 mg every 3-4 hours as needed; usual dosage range: 50-150 mg every 2-4 hours as needed (manufacturers recommendation; oral route is not recommended for acute pain)

I.M., SubQ: Initial: Opiate-naive: 50-75 mg every 3-4 hours as needed; patients with prior opiate exposure may require higher initial doses

Preoperatively: 50-100 mg given 30-90 minutes before the beginning of anesthesia

Slow I.V.: Initial: 5-10 mg every 5 minutes as needed

Patient-controlled analgesia (PCA): Usual concentration: 10 mg/mL

Initial dose: 10 mg

Demand dose: 1-5 mg (manufacturer recommendations); range 5-25 mg (American Pain Society, 1999).

Lockout interval: 5-10 minutes

**Dosage Forms**

Injection, solution, as hydrochloride [ampul]: 25 mg/0.5 mL (0.5 mL); 25 mg/mL (1 mL); 50 mg/mL (1 mL, 1.5 mL, 2 mL); 75 mg/mL (1 mL); 100 mg/mL (1 mL)

Injection, solution, as hydrochloride [prefilled syringe]: 25 mg/mL (1 mL); 50 mg/mL (1 mL); 75 mg/mL (1 mL); 100 mg/mL (1 mL)

Injection, solution, as hydrochloride [for PCA pump]: 10 mg/mL (30 mL, 50 mL, 60 mL)

Injection, solution, as hydrochloride [vial]: 25 mg/mL (1 mL); 50 mg/mL (1 mL, 30 mL); 75 mg/mL (1 mL); 100 mg/mL (1 mL, 20 mL) [may contain sodium metabisulfite]

Syrup, as hydrochloride: 50 mg/5 mL (500 mL) [contains sodium benzoate]

Demerol®: 50 mg/5 mL (480 mL) [contains benzoic acid; banana flavor]

Tablet, as hydrochloride (Demerol®, Meperitab®): 50 mg, 100 mg

## meperidine and promethazine (me PER i deen & proe METH a zeen)

**Sound-Alike/Look-Alike Issues**

mepergan may be confused with meprobamate

**Synonyms** mepergan; promethazine and meperidine

**Therapeutic Category** Analgesic, Narcotic

**Controlled Substance** C-II

**Use** Management of moderate to severe pain

**Usual Dosage** Adults: Oral: One (1) capsule every 4-6 hours as needed

**Dosage Forms** Capsule: Meperidine hydrochloride 50 mg and promethazine hydrochloride 25 mg

## meperidine hydrochloride see meperidine on previous page

## Meperitab® [US] see meperidine on previous page

## mephobarbital (me foe BAR bi tal)

**Sound-Alike/Look-Alike Issues**

mephobarbital may be confused with methocarbamol

Mebaral® may be confused with Medrol®, Mellaril®, Tegretol®

**Synonyms** methylphenobarbital

**U.S./Canadian Brand Names** Mebaral® [US/Can]

**Therapeutic Category** Barbiturate

**Controlled Substance** C-IV

**Use** Sedative; treatment of grand mal and petit mal epilepsy

(Continued)

## mephobarbital *(Continued)*

Usual Dosage Oral:
Epilepsy:
Children: 6-12 mg/kg/day in 2-4 divided doses
Adults: 200-600 mg/day in 2-4 divided doses
Sedation:
Children:
<5 years: 16-32 mg 3-4 times/day
>5 years: 32-64 mg 3-4 times/day
Adults: 32-100 mg 3-4 times/day
Dosage Forms Tablet: 32 mg, 50 mg, 100 mg

**Mephyton**® **[US/Can]** *see* phytonadione *on page 646*

## mepivacaine *(me PIV a kane)*

Sound-Alike/Look-Alike Issues
mepivacaine may be confused with bupivacaine
Polocaine® may be confused with prilocaine
Synonyms mepivacaine hydrochloride
U.S./Canadian Brand Names Carbocaine® [US/Can]; Polocaine® MPF [US]; Polocaine® [US/Can]
Therapeutic Category Local Anesthetic
Use Not for use in spinal anesthesia
Usual Dosage Children and Adults: Injectable local anesthetic: Varies with procedure, degree of anesthesia needed, vascularity of tissue, duration of anesthesia required, and physical condition of patient
Dosage Forms
Injection, solution, as hydrochloride:
Carbocaine®: 1% (50 mL); 2% (50 mL)
Polocaine®: 1% (50 mL); 2% (50 mL)
Injection, solution, as hydrochloride [preservative free]:
Carbocaine®: 1% (30 mL); 1.5% (30 mL); 2% (20 mL)
Polocaine® MPF: 1% (30 mL); 1.5% (30 mL); 2% (20 mL)

**mepivacaine hydrochloride** *see* mepivacaine *on this page*

## meprobamate *(me proe BA mate)*

Sound-Alike/Look-Alike Issues
meprobamate may be confused with Mepergan, meperidine
Equanil® may be confused with Elavil®
U.S./Canadian Brand Names Miltown® [US]; Novo-Mepro [Can]
Therapeutic Category Antianxiety Agent, Miscellaneous
Controlled Substance C-IV
Use Management of anxiety disorders
Usual Dosage Oral:
Children 6-12 years: Anxiety: 100-200 mg 2-3 times/day
Adults: Anxiety: 400 mg 3-4 times/day, up to 2400 mg/day
Dosage Forms Tablet: 200 mg, 400 mg

**meprobamate and aspirin** *see* aspirin and meprobamate *on page 75*

**Mepron**® **[US/Can]** *see* atovaquone *on page 78*

## mequinol and tretinoin *(ME kwi nole & TRET i noyn)*

Synonyms tretinoin and mequinol
U.S./Canadian Brand Names Solagé™ [US/Can]
Therapeutic Category Retinoic Acid Derivative; Vitamin A Derivative; Vitamin, Topical
Use Treatment of solar lentigines; the efficacy of using Solagé™ daily for >24 weeks has not been established. The local cutaneous safety of Solagé™ in non-Caucasians has not been adequately established.
Usual Dosage Solar lentigines: Topical: Apply twice daily to solar lentigines using the applicator tip while avoiding application to the surrounding skin. Separate application by at least 8 hours or as directed by physician.

**Dosage Forms** Liquid, topical: Mequinol 2% and tretinoin 0.01% (30 mL) [contains alcohol 78%; dispensed in applicator bottle]

# merbromin (mer BROE min)
**U.S./Canadian Brand Names** Mercurochrome® [US]
**Therapeutic Category** Topical Skin Product
**Use** Topical antiseptic
**Usual Dosage** Apply freely, until injury has healed
**Dosage Forms** Solution, topical: 2% (30 mL)

# mercaptopurine (mer kap toe PYOOR een)
**Sound-Alike/Look-Alike Issues**
Purinethol® may be confused with propylthiouracil
**Synonyms** 6-mercaptopurine; 6-MP; NSC-755
**U.S./Canadian Brand Names** Purinethol® [US/Can]
**Therapeutic Category** Antineoplastic Agent
**Use** Treatment (maintenance and induction) of acute lymphoblastic leukemia (ALL)
**Usual Dosage** Oral (refer to individual protocols):
Children:
Induction: 2.5-5 mg/kg/day **or** 70-100 mg/m²/day given once daily
Maintenance: 1.5-2.5 mg/kg/day **or** 50-75 mg/m²/day given once daily
Adults:
Induction: 2.5-5 mg/kg/day (100-200 mg)
Maintenance: 1.5-2.5 mg/kg/day **or** 80-100 mg/m²/day given once daily
Dosage adjustment with concurrent allopurinol: Reduce mercaptopurine dosage to $^1/_3$ to $^1/_2$ the usual dose.
Dosage adjustment in TPMT-deficiency: Not established; substantial reductions are generally required only in homozygous deficiency.
**Dosage Forms** Tablet [scored]: 50 mg

**6-mercaptopurine** *see* mercaptopurine *on this page*

**mercapturic acid** *see* acetylcysteine *on page 15*

# mercuric oxide (mer KYOOR ik OKS ide)
**Synonyms** yellow mercuric oxide
**Therapeutic Category** Antibiotic, Ophthalmic
**Use** Treatment of irritation and minor infections of the eyelids
**Usual Dosage** Apply small amount to inner surface of lower eyelid once or twice daily
**Dosage Forms** Ointment, ophthalmic: 1%, 2% [OTC]

**Mercurochrome® [US]** *see* merbromin *on this page*

**Meridia® [US/Can]** *see* sibutramine *on page 746*

# meropenem (mer oh PEN em)
**U.S./Canadian Brand Names** Merrem® I.V. [US]; Merrem® [Can]
**Therapeutic Category** Carbapenem (Antibiotic)
**Use** Treatment of intra-abdominal infections (complicated appendicitis and peritonitis); treatment of bacterial meningitis in pediatric patients ≥3 months of age caused by *S. pneumoniae*, *H. influenzae*, and *N. meningitidis*; treatment of complicated skin and skin structure infections caused by susceptible organisms
**Usual Dosage** I.V.:
Children >3 months (<50 kg):
Complicated skin and skin structure infections: 10 mg/kg every 8 hours (maximum dose: 500 mg every 8 hours)
Intra-abdominal infections: 20 mg/kg every 8 hours (maximum dose: 1 g every 8 hours)
Meningitis: 40 mg/kg every 8 hours (maximum dose: 2 g every 8 hours)
Children >50 kg and Adults:
Complicated skin and skin structure infections: 500 mg every 8 hours
Intra-abdominal infections: 1 g every 8 hours
Meningitis: 2 g every 8 hours
(Continued)

# meropenem *(Continued)*

**Dosage Forms** Injection, powder for reconstitution: 500 mg [contains sodium 45.1 mg as sodium carbonate (1.96 mEq)]; 1 g [contains sodium 90.2 mg as sodium carbonate (3.92 mEq)]

**Merrem**® **[Can]** *see* meropenem *on previous page*

**Merrem**® **I.V. [US]** *see* meropenem *on previous page*

**Mersol**® **[US-OTC]** *see* thimerosal *on page 797*

**Merthiolate**® **[US-OTC]** *see* thimerosal *on page 797*

**Meruvax**® **II [US]** *see* rubella virus vaccine (live) *on page 733*

# mesalamine *(me SAL a meen)*

**Sound-Alike/Look-Alike Issues**

mesalamine may be confused with mecamylamine

Asacol® may be confused with Ansaid®, Os-Cal®

**Synonyms** 5-aminosalicylic acid; 5-ASA; fisalamine; mesalazine

**U.S./Canadian Brand Names** Asacol® [US/Can]; Canasa™ [US]; Mesasal® [Can]; Novo-5 ASA [Can]; Pentasa® [US/Can]; Quintasa® [Can]; Rowasa® [US/Can]; Salofalk® [Can]

**Therapeutic Category** 5-Aminosalicylic Acid Derivative

**Use**

Oral: Treatment and maintenance of remission of mildly to moderately active ulcerative colitis

Rectal: Treatment of active mild to moderate distal ulcerative colitis, proctosigmoiditis, or proctitis

**Usual Dosage** Adults (usual course of therapy is 3-8 weeks):

Oral:

Treatment of ulcerative colitis:

Capsule: 1 g 4 times/day

Tablet: Initial: 800 mg (2 tablets) 3 times/day for 6 weeks

Maintenance of remission of ulcerative colitis:

Capsule: 1 g 4 times/day

Tablet: 1.6 g/day in divided doses

Rectal:

Retention enema: 60 mL (4 g) at bedtime, retained overnight, approximately 8 hours

Rectal suppository (Canasa™):

500 mg: Insert 1 suppository in rectum twice daily; may increase to 3 times/day if inadequate response is seen after 2 weeks

1000 mg: Insert 1 suppository in rectum daily at bedtime

**Note:** Suppositories should be retained for at least 1-3 hours to achieve maximum benefit.

**Note:** Some patients may require rectal and oral therapy concurrently.

**Dosage Forms**

Capsule, controlled release (Pentasa®): 250 mg, 500 mg

Suppository, rectal (Canasa™): 500 mg [DSC], 1000 mg [contains saturated vegetable fatty acid esters]

Suspension, rectal: 4 g/60 mL (7s, 28s) [contains potassium metabisulfite and sodium benzoate]

Rowasa®: 4 g/60 mL (7s, 28s) [contains potassium metabisulfite and sodium benzoate]

Tablet, delayed release [enteric coated] (Asacol®): 400 mg

**mesalazine** *see* mesalamine *on this page*

**Mesasal**® **[Can]** *see* mesalamine *on this page*

**M-Eslon**® **[Can]** *see* morphine sulfate *on page 549*

# mesna *(MES na)*

**Synonyms** sodium 2-mercaptoethane sulfonate

**U.S./Canadian Brand Names** Mesnex® [US/Can]; Uromitexan [Can]

**Therapeutic Category** Antidote

**Use Orphan drug:** Prevention of hemorrhagic cystitis induced by ifosfamide

**Usual Dosage** Children and Adults (refer to individual protocols):

I.V.: Recommended dose is 60% of the ifosfamide dose given in 3 divided doses (0, 4, and 8 hours after the start of ifosfamide)

Alternative I.V. regimens include 80% of the ifosfamide dose given in 4 divided doses (0, 3, 6, and 9 hours after the start of ifosfamide) and continuous infusions

I.V./Oral: Recommended dose is 100% of the ifosfamide dose, given as 20% of the ifosfamide dose I.V. at hour 0, followed by 40% of the ifosfamide dose given orally 2 and 6 hours after start of ifosfamide

**Dosage Forms**

Injection, solution: 100 mg/mL (10 mL) [contains benzyl alcohol]

Tablet: 400 mg

**Mesnex® [US/Can]** *see mesna on previous page*

## mesoridazine (mez oh RID a zeen)

**Sound-Alike/Look-Alike Issues**

Serentil® may be confused with selegiline, Serevent®, Seroquel®, sertraline, Serzone®, Sinequan®, Surgicel®

**Synonyms** mesoridazine besylate

**U.S./Canadian Brand Names** Serentil® [Can]

**Therapeutic Category** Phenothiazine Derivative

**Use** Management of schizophrenic patients who fail to respond adequately to treatment with other antipsychotic drugs, either because of insufficient effectiveness or the inability to achieve an effective dose due to intolerable adverse effects from these drugs

**Usual Dosage** Concentrate may be diluted just prior to administration with distilled water, acidified tap water, orange or grape juice; do not prepare and store bulk dilutions

Adults: Schizophrenia/psychoses:

Oral: 25-50 mg 3 times/day; maximum: 100-400 mg/day

I.M.: Initial: 25 mg, repeat in 30-60 minutes as needed; optimal dosage range: 25-200 mg/day

**Dosage Forms** [DSC] = Discontinued product

Injection, solution, as besylate [DSC]: 25 mg/mL (1 mL)

Liquid, oral, as besylate [DSC]: 25 mg/mL (118 mL) [contains alcohol 0.61%]

Tablet, as besylate [DSC]: 10 mg, 25 mg, 50 mg, 100 mg

**mesoridazine besylate** *see mesoridazine on this page*

**Mestinon® [US/Can]** *see pyridostigmine on page 700*

**Mestinon® Injection (Discontinued)** *see pyridostigmine on page 700*

**Mestinon®-SR [Can]** *see pyridostigmine on page 700*

**Mestinon® Timespan® [US]** *see pyridostigmine on page 700*

## mestranol and norethindrone (MES tra nole & nor eth IN drone)

**Sound-Alike/Look-Alike Issues**

Norinyl® may be confused with Nardil®

**Synonyms** norethindrone and mestranol

**U.S./Canadian Brand Names** Necon® 1/50 [US]; Norinyl® 1+50 [US]; Ortho-Novum® 1/50 [US/Can]

**Therapeutic Category** Contraceptive, Oral

**Use** Prevention of pregnancy

**Usual Dosage** Oral: Adults: Female: Contraception:

Schedule 1 (Sunday starter): Dose begins on first Sunday after onset of menstruation; if the menstrual period starts on Sunday, take first tablet that very same day. **With a Sunday start, an additional method of contraception should be used until after the first 7 days of consecutive administration.**

For 21-tablet package: Dosage is 1 tablet daily for 21 consecutive days, followed by 7 days off of the medication; a new course begins on the 8th day after the last tablet is taken.

For 28-tablet package: Dosage is 1 tablet daily without interruption.

Schedule 2 (Day 1 starter): Dose starts on first day of menstrual cycle taking 1 tablet daily.

For 21-tablet package: Dosage is 1 tablet daily for 21 consecutive days, followed by 7 days off of the medication; a new course begins on the 8th day after the last tablet is taken.

For 28-tablet package: Dosage is 1 tablet daily without interruption.

If all doses have been taken on schedule and one menstrual period is missed, continue dosing cycle. If two consecutive menstrual periods are missed, pregnancy test is required before new dosing cycle is started.

Missed doses **monophasic formulations** (refer to package insert for complete information):

One dose missed: Take as soon as remembered or take 2 tablets next day

(Continued)

## mestranol and norethindrone (Continued)

Two consecutive doses missed in the first 2 weeks: Take 2 tablets as soon as remembered or 2 tablets next 2 days. **An additional method of contraception should be used for 7 days after missed dose.**

Two consecutive doses missed in week 3 or three consecutive doses missed at any time: **An additional method of contraception must be used for 7 days after a missed dose:**

Schedule 1 (Sunday starter): Continue dose of 1 tablet daily until Sunday, then discard the rest of the pack, and a new pack should be started that same day.

Schedule 2 (Day 1 starter): Current pack should be discarded, and a new pack should be started that same day.

**Dosage Forms** Tablet, monophasic formulations:

Necon® 1/50: Norethindrone 1 mg and mestranol 0.05 mg [21 light blue tablets and 7 white inactive tablets] (28s)

Norinyl® 1+50: Norethindrone 1 mg and mestranol 0.05 mg [21 white tablets and 7 orange inactive tablets] (28s)

Ortho-Novum® 1/50: Norethindrone 1 mg and mestranol 0.05 mg [21 yellow tablets and 7 green inactive tablets] (28s)

**metacortandralone** see prednisolone (systemic) on page 674

**Metadate® CD [US]** see methylphenidate on page 530

**Metadate® ER [US]** see methylphenidate on page 530

**Metadol™ [Can]** see methadone on page 521

**Metaglip™ [US]** see glipizide and metformin on page 376

**Metahydrin® [Can]** see trichlormethiazide on page 822

**Metahydrin® (Discontinued)** see trichlormethiazide on page 822

**Metamucil® [US-OTC/Can]** see psyllium on page 697

**Metamucil® Plus Calcium [US-OTC]** see psyllium on page 697

**Metamucil® Smooth Texture [US-OTC]** see psyllium on page 697

**Metaprel® Tablet (Discontinued)**

## metaproterenol (met a proe TER e nol)

**Sound-Alike/Look-Alike Issues**
metaproterenol may be confused with metipranolol, metoprolol
Alupent® may be confused with Atrovent®

**Synonyms** metaproterenol sulfate; orciprenaline sulfate

**U.S./Canadian Brand Names** Alupent® [US]

**Therapeutic Category** Adrenergic Agonist Agent

**Use** Bronchodilator in reversible airway obstruction due to asthma or COPD; because of its delayed onset of action (1 hour) and prolonged effect (4 or more hours), this may not be the drug of choice for assessing response to a bronchodilator

**Usual Dosage**

Oral:

Children:

<2 years: 0.4 mg/kg/dose given 3-4 times/day; in infants, the dose can be given every 8-12 hours

2-6 years: 1-2.6 mg/kg/day divided every 6 hours

6-9 years: 10 mg/dose 3-4 times/day

Children >9 years and Adults: 20 mg 3-4 times/day

Inhalation: Children >12 years and Adults: 2-3 inhalations every 3-4 hours, up to 12 inhalations in 24 hours

Nebulizer:

Infants and Children: 0.01-0.02 mL/kg of 5% solution; minimum dose: 0.1 mL; maximum dose: 0.3 mL diluted in 2-3 mL normal saline every 4-6 hours (may be given more frequently according to need)

Adolescents and Adults: 5-20 breaths of full strength 5% metaproterenol **or** 0.2 to 0.3 mL 5% metaproterenol in 2.5-3 mL normal saline until nebulized every 4-6 hours (can be given more frequently according to need)

**Dosage Forms**

Aerosol for oral inhalation, as sulfate (Alupent®): 0.65 mg/inhalation (14 g) [200 doses]

Solution for oral inhalation, as sulfate [preservative free]: 0.4% [4 mg/mL] (2.5 mL); 0.6% [6 mg/mL] (2.5 mL)

Syrup, as sulfate: 10 mg/5 mL (480 mL) [may contain sodium benzoate]

Tablet, as sulfate: 10 mg, 20 mg

**metaproterenol sulfate** *see* metaproterenol *on previous page*

## metaraminol (met a RAM i nole)

**Sound-Alike/Look-Alike Issues**
Aramine® may be confused with Artane®

**Synonyms** metaraminol bitartrate

**U.S./Canadian Brand Names** Aramine® [Can]

**Therapeutic Category** Adrenergic Agonist Agent

**Use** Acute hypotensive crisis in the treatment of shock

**Usual Dosage**
Children:
I.M.: 0.01 mg/kg as a single dose
I.V.: 0.01 mg/kg as a single dose or intravenous infusion of 5 mcg/kg/minute
Adults:
Prevention of hypotension: I.M., SubQ: 2-10 mg
Adjunctive treatment of hypotension: I.V.: 15-100 mg in 250-500 mL NS or 5% dextrose in water
Severe shock: I.V.: 0.5-5 mg direct I.V. injection followed by intravenous infusion of 15-100 mg in 250-500 mL NS or D$_5$W; may also be administered endotracheally

**Dosage Forms** [DSC] = Discontinued product
Injection, solution, as bitartrate [DSC]: 10 mg/mL (10 mL) [contains sodium bisulfite]

**metaraminol bitartrate** *see* metaraminol *on this page*

**Metasep®** *(Discontinued)*

**Metastron®** **[US/Can]** *see* strontium-89 *on page 768*

**Metatensin®** **[Can]** *see* trichlormethiazide *on page 822*

## metaxalone (me TAKS a lone)

**Sound-Alike/Look-Alike Issues**
metaxalone may be confused with metolazone

**U.S./Canadian Brand Names** Skelaxin® [US/Can]

**Therapeutic Category** Skeletal Muscle Relaxant

**Use** Relief of discomfort associated with acute, painful musculoskeletal conditions

**Usual Dosage** Children >12 years and Adults: Oral: 800 mg 3-4 times/day

**Dosage Forms** [DSC] = Discontinued product
Tablet: 400 mg [DSC], 800 mg

## metformin (met FOR min)

**Sound-Alike/Look-Alike Issues**
metformin may be confused with metronidazole
Glucophage® may be confused with Glucotrol®, Glutofac®

**Synonyms** metformin hydrochloride

**U.S./Canadian Brand Names** Alti-Metformin [Can]; Apo-Metformin® [Can]; Fortamet™ [US]; Gen-Metformin [Can]; Glucophage® XR [US]; Glucophage® [US/Can]; Glycon [Can]; Novo-Metformin [Can]; Nu-Metformin [Can]; PMS-Metformin [Can]; Rho®-Metformin [Can]; Riomet™ [US]

**Therapeutic Category** Antidiabetic Agent, Oral

**Use** Management of type 2 diabetes mellitus (noninsulin dependent, NIDDM) as monotherapy when hyperglycemia cannot be managed on diet alone. May be used concomitantly with a sulfonylurea or insulin to improve glycemic control.

**Usual Dosage Note:** Allow 1-2 weeks between dose titrations: Generally, clinically significant responses are not seen at doses <1500 mg daily; however, a lower recommended starting dose and gradual increased dosage is recommended to minimize gastrointestinal symptoms

Children 10-16 years: Management of type 2 diabetes mellitus: Oral (500 mg tablet or oral solution): Initial: 500 mg twice daily (given with the morning and evening meals); increases in daily dosage should be made in increments of 500 mg at weekly intervals, given in divided doses, up to a maximum of 2000 mg/day

(Continued)

# metformin *(Continued)*

Adults ≥17 years: Management of type 2 diabetes mellitus: Oral:

Immediate release tablet or oral solution: Initial: 500 mg twice daily (give with the morning and evening meals) **or** 850 mg once daily; increase dosage incrementally.

Incremental dosing recommendations based on dosage form:

500 mg tablet: One tablet/day at weekly intervals

850 mg tablet: One tablet/day every other week

Oral solution: 500 mg twice daily every other week

Doses of up to 2000 mg/day may be given twice daily. If a dose >2000 mg/day is required, it may be better tolerated in three divided doses. Maximum recommended dose 2550 mg/day.

Extended release tablet: Initial: 500 mg once daily (with the evening meal); dosage may be increased by 500 mg weekly; maximum dose: 2000 mg once daily. If glycemic control is not achieved at maximum dose, may divide dose to 1000 mg twice daily. If doses >2000 mg/day are needed, switch to regular release tablets and titrate to maximum dose of 2550 mg/day.

**Transfer from other antidiabetic agents:** No transition period is generally necessary except when transferring from chlorpropamide. When transferring from chlorpropamide, care should be exercised during the first 2 weeks because of the prolonged retention of chlorpropamide in the body, leading to overlapping drug effects and possible hypoglycemia.

**Concomitant metformin and oral sulfonylurea therapy:** If patients have not responded to 4 weeks of the maximum dose of metformin monotherapy, consider a gradual addition of an oral sulfonylurea, even if prior primary or secondary failure to a sulfonylurea has occurred. Continue metformin at the maximum dose.

**Failed sulfonylurea therapy:** Patients with prior failure on glyburide may be treated by gradual addition of metformin. Initiate with glyburide 20 mg and metformin 500 mg daily. Metformin dosage may be increased by 500 mg/day at weekly intervals, up to a maximum of 2500 mg/day (dosage of glyburide maintained at 20 mg/day).

**Concomitant metformin and insulin therapy:** Initial: 500 mg metformin once daily, continue current insulin dose; increase by 500 mg metformin weekly until adequate glycemic control is achieved

Maximum dose: 2500 mg metformin; 2000 mg metformin extended release

Decrease insulin dose 10% to 25% when FPG <120 mg/dL; monitor and make further adjustments as needed

**Dosage Forms**

Solution, oral, as hydrochloride (Riomet™): 100 mg/mL (118 mL, 473 mL) [contains saccharin; cherry flavor]

Tablet, as hydrochloride (Glucophage®): 500 mg, 850 mg, 1000 mg

Tablet, extended release, as hydrochloride: 500 mg

Fortamet™: 500 mg, 1000 mg

Glucophage® XR: 500 mg, 750 mg

**metformin and glipizide** *see* glipizide and metformin *on page 376*

**metformin and glyburide** *see* glyburide and metformin *on page 378*

**metformin and rosiglitazone** *see* rosiglitazone and metformin *on page 731*

**metformin hydrochloride** *see* metformin *on previous page*

**metformin hydrochloride and rosiglitazone maleate** *see* rosiglitazone and metformin *on page 731*

# methacholine *(meth a KOLE leen)*

**Synonyms** methacholine chloride

**U.S./Canadian Brand Names** Provocholine® [US/Can]

**Therapeutic Category** Diagnostic Agent

**Use** Diagnosis of bronchial airway hyperactivity

**Usual Dosage** Before inhalation challenge, perform baseline pulmonary function tests; the patient must have an $FEV_1$ of at least 70% of the predicted value. The following is a suggested schedule for administration of methacholine challenge. Calculate cumulative units by multiplying number of breaths by concentration given. Total cumulative units is the sum of cumulative units for each concentration given. See table on next page.

**Dosage Forms** Powder for oral inhalation, as chloride: 100 mg

**Methacholine**

| Vial | Serial Concentration (mg/mL) | No. of Breaths | Cumulative Units per Concentration | Total Cumulative Units |
|------|------------------------------|----------------|------------------------------------|------------------------|
| E | 0.025 | 5 | 0.125 | 0.125 |
| D | 0.25 | 5 | 1.25 | 1.375 |
| C | 2.5 | 5 | 12.5 | 13.88 |
| B | 10 | 5 | 50 | 63.88 |
| A | 25 | 5 | 125 | 188.88 |

**methacholine chloride** *see* methacholine *on previous page*

**Methadex [US]** *see* neomycin, polymyxin B, and dexamethasone *on page 567*

# methadone (METH a done)

**Sound-Alike/Look-Alike Issues**
methadone may be confused with Mephyton®, methylphenidate

**Synonyms** methadone hydrochloride

**U.S./Canadian Brand Names** Dolophine® [US/Can]; Metadol™ [Can]; Methadone Diskets® [US]; Methadone Intensol™ [US]; Methadose® [US/Can]

**Therapeutic Category** Analgesic, Narcotic

**Controlled Substance** C-II

**Use** Management of severe pain; detoxification and maintenance treatment of narcotic addiction (if used for detoxification and maintenance treatment of narcotic addiction, it must be part of an FDA-approved program)

**Usual Dosage Note:** These are guidelines and do not represent the maximum doses that may be required in all patients. Methadone accumulates with repeated doses and dosage may need reduction after 3-5 days to prevent CNS depressant effects. Some patients may benefit from every 8-12 hour dosing interval for chronic pain management. Doses should be titrated to appropriate effects.

Adults:
Pain (analgesia):
Oral: Initial: 5-10 mg; dosing interval may range from 4-12 hours during initial therapy; decrease in dose or frequency may be required (~days 2-5) due to accumulation with repeated doses
Manufacturer's labeling: 2.5-10 mg every 3-4 hours as needed
I.V.: Manufacturers labeling: Initial: 2.5-10 mg every 8-12 hours in opioid-naive patients; titrate slowly to effect; may also be administered by SubQ or I.M. injection
**Conversion from oral to parenteral dose:** Initial dose: Oral: parenteral: 2:1 ratio
Detoxification: Oral:
Initial: 20-30 mg; lower doses should be considered in patients with low tolerance at initiation (eg, absence of opioids ≥5 days); an additional 5-10 mg of methadone may be provided if withdrawal symptoms have not been suppressed or if symptoms reappear after 2-4 hours; total daily dose on the first day should not exceed 40 mg
Maintenance: Usual range: 80-120 mg/day (titration should occur cautiously)
Withdrawal: Dose reductions should be <10% of the maintenance dose, every 10-14 days
Detoxification (short-term): Oral:
Initial: Titrate to 40 mg/day in 2 divided doses
Maintenance: Continue 40 mg dose for 2-3 days
Withdrawal: Decrease daily or every other day, keeping withdrawal symptoms tolerable; hospitalized patients may tolerate a 20% reduction/day; ambulatory patients may require a slower reduction
**Dosage adjustment during pregnancy:** Methadone dose may need to be increased, or the dosing interval decreased; use should be reserved for cases where the benefits clearly outweigh the risks

**Dosage Forms**
Injection, solution, as hydrochloride: 10 mg/mL (20 mL)
Solution, oral, as hydrochloride: 5 mg/5 mL (500 mL); 10 mg/5 mL (500 mL) [contains alcohol 8%; citrus flavor]
Solution, oral concentrate, as hydrochloride: 10 mg/mL (946 mL)
Methadone Intensol™: 10 mg/mL (30 mL)
Methadose®: 10 mg/mL (1000 mL) [cherry flavor]
Methadose®: 10 mg/mL (1000 mL) [dye free, sugar free, unflavored]
Tablet, as hydrochloride (Dolophine®, Methadose®): 5 mg, 10 mg
(Continued)

# methadone *(Continued)*

Tablet, dispersible, as hydrochloride:
Methadose®: 40 mg
Methadone Diskets®: 40 mg [orange-pineapple flavor]

**Methadone Diskets® [US]** *see* methadone *on previous page*

**methadone hydrochloride** *see* methadone *on previous page*

**Methadone Intensol™ [US]** *see* methadone *on previous page*

**Methadose® [US/Can]** *see* methadone *on previous page*

**methaminodiazepoxide hydrochloride** *see* chlordiazepoxide *on page 167*

# methamphetamine *(meth am FET a meen)*

**Sound-Alike/Look-Alike Issues**
Desoxyn® may be confused with digoxin
**Synonyms** desoxyephedrine hydrochloride; methamphetamine hydrochloride
**U.S./Canadian Brand Names** Desoxyn® [US/Can]
**Therapeutic Category** Amphetamine
**Controlled Substance** C-II
**Use** Treatment of attention-deficit/hyperactivity disorder (ADHD); exogenous obesity (short-term adjunct)
**Usual Dosage** Oral:
Children >6 years and Adults: ADHD: 2.5-5 mg 1-2 times/day; may increase by 5 mg increments at weekly intervals until optimum response is achieved, usually 20-25 mg/day
Children >12 years and Adults: Exogenous obesity: 5 mg 30 minutes before each meal; treatment duration should not exceed a few weeks
**Dosage Forms** Tablet, as hydrochloride: 5 mg

**methamphetamine hydrochloride** *see* methamphetamine *on this page*

# methazolamide *(meth a ZOE la mide)*

**Sound-Alike/Look-Alike Issues**
methazolamide may be confused with methenamine, metolazone
Neptazane® may be confused with Nesacaine®
**U.S./Canadian Brand Names** Apo-Methazolamide® [Can]
**Therapeutic Category** Carbonic Anhydrase Inhibitor
**Use** Adjunctive treatment of open-angle or secondary glaucoma; short-term therapy of narrow-angle glaucoma when delay of surgery is desired
**Usual Dosage** Adults: Oral: 50-100 mg 2-3 times/day
**Dosage Forms** Tablet: 25 mg, 50 mg

# methenamine *(meth EN a meen)*

**Sound-Alike/Look-Alike Issues**
methenamine may be confused with methazolamide, methionine
Urex® may be confused with Eurax®, Serax®
**Synonyms** hexamethylenetetramine; methenamine hippurate; methenamine mandelate
**U.S./Canadian Brand Names** Dehydral® [Can]; Hiprex® [US/Can]; Mandelamine® [US/Can]; Urasal® [Can]; Urex® [US/Can]
**Therapeutic Category** Antibiotic, Miscellaneous
**Use** Prophylaxis or suppression of recurrent urinary tract infections; urinary tract discomfort secondary to hypermotility
**Usual Dosage** Oral:
Children:
>2-6 years: *Mandelate:* 50-75 mg/kg/day in 3-4 doses or 0.25 g/30 lb 4 times/day
6-12 years:
*Hippurate:* 0.5-1 g twice daily
*Mandelate:* 50-75 mg/kg/day in 3-4 doses or 0.5 g 4 times/day
Children >12 years and Adults:
*Hippurate:* 0.5-1 g twice daily
*Mandelate:* 1 g 4 times/day after meals and at bedtime

**Dosage Forms**
Tablet, as hippurate (Hiprex®, Urex®): 1 g [Hiprex® contains tartrazine dye]
Tablet, enteric coated, as mandelate (Mandelamine®): 500 mg, 1 g

## methenamine hippurate *see* methenamine *on previous page*

## methenamine mandelate *see* methenamine *on previous page*

# methenamine, phenyl salicylate, atropine, hyoscyamine, benzoic acid, and methylene blue
(meth EN a meen, fen nil sa LIS i late, A troe peen, hye oh SYE a meen, ben ZOE ik AS id, & METH i leen bloo)
**U.S./Canadian Brand Names** Atrosept® [US]; Dolsed® [US]; UAA® [US]; Uridon Modified® [US]; Urised® [US]; Uritin® [US]
**Therapeutic Category** Antibiotic, Urinary Antiinfective; Urinary Tract Product
**Use** Urinary tract infections
**Usual Dosage** Adults: Oral: Two tablets 4 times/day
**Dosage Forms** Tablet: Methenamine 40.8 mg, phenyl salicylate 18.1 mg, atropine sulfate 0.03 mg, hyoscyamine sulfate 0.03 mg, benzoic acid 4.5 mg, and methylene blue 5.4 mg

## Methergine® [US/Can] *see* methylergonovine *on page 530*

# methimazole (meth IM a zole)
**Sound-Alike/Look-Alike Issues**
methimazole may be confused with metolazone
**Synonyms** thiamazole
**U.S./Canadian Brand Names** Tapazole® [US/Can]
**Therapeutic Category** Antithyroid Agent
**Use** Palliative treatment of hyperthyroidism, return the hyperthyroid patient to a normal metabolic state prior to thyroidectomy, and to control thyrotoxic crisis that may accompany thyroidectomy. The use of antithyroid thioamides is as effective in elderly as they are in younger adults; however, the expense, potential adverse effects, and inconvenience (compliance, monitoring) make them undesirable. The use of radioiodine due to ease of administration and less concern for long-term side effects and reproduction problems (some older males) makes it a more appropriate therapy.
**Usual Dosage** Oral: Administer in 3 equally divided doses at approximately 8-hour intervals
Children: Initial: 0.4 mg/kg/day in 3 divided doses; maintenance: 0.2 mg/kg/day in 3 divided doses up to 30 mg/24 hours maximum
Alternatively: Initial: 0.5-0.7 mg/kg/day **or** 15-20 mg/m$^2$/day in 3 divided doses
Maintenance: $1/3$ to $2/3$ of the initial dose beginning when the patient is euthyroid
Maximum: 30 mg/24 hours
Adults: Initial: 15 mg/day for mild hyperthyroidism; 30-40 mg/day in moderately severe hyperthyroidism; 60 mg/day in severe hyperthyroidism; maintenance: 5-15 mg/day
Adjust dosage as required to achieve and maintain serum $T_3$, $T_4$, and TSH levels in the normal range. An elevated $T_3$ may be the sole indicator of inadequate treatment. An elevated TSH indicates excessive antithyroid treatment.
**Dosage Forms**
Tablet: 5 mg, 10 mg, 20 mg
Tapazole® 5 mg, 10 mg

# methionine (me THYE oh neen)
**Sound-Alike/Look-Alike Issues**
methionine may be confused with methenamine
**U.S./Canadian Brand Names** ME-500® [US]; Pedameth® [US]
**Therapeutic Category** Dietary Supplement
**Use** Treatment of diaper rash and control of odor, dermatitis and ulceration caused by ammoniacal urine
**Usual Dosage** Oral:
Children: Control of diaper rash: 75 mg in formula or other liquid 3-4 times/day for 3-5 days
Adults:
Control of odor in incontinent adults: 200-400 mg 3-4 times/day
Dietary supplement: 500 mg/day
**Dosage Forms**
Capsule (ME-500®): 500 mg
(Continued)

# methionine *(Continued)*

Liquid (Pedameth®): 75 mg/5 mL (480 mL)
Tablet: 500 mg

**Methitest**™ **[US]** *see* methyltestosterone *on page 533*

# methocarbamol *(meth oh KAR ba mole)*

**Sound-Alike/Look-Alike Issues**
methocarbamol may be confused with mephobarbital
Robaxin® may be confused with Rubex®

**U.S./Canadian Brand Names** Robaxin® [US/Can]

**Therapeutic Category** Skeletal Muscle Relaxant

**Use** Treatment of muscle spasm associated with acute painful musculoskeletal conditions; supportive therapy in tetanus

**Usual Dosage**

Tetanus: I.V.:

Children: Recommended **only** for use in tetanus: 15 mg/kg/dose or 500 mg/m$^2$/dose, may repeat every 6 hours if needed; maximum dose: 1.8 g/m$^2$/day for 3 days only

Adults: Initial dose: 1-3 g; may repeat dose every 6 hours until oral dosing is possible; injection should not be used for more than 3 consecutive days

Muscle spasm: Children ≥16 years and Adults:

Oral: 1.5 g 4 times/day for 2-3 days (up to 8 g/day may be given in severe conditions), then decrease to 4-4.5 g/day in 3-6 divided doses

I.M., I.V.: 1 g every 8 hours if oral not possible; injection should not be used for more than 3 consecutive days. If condition persists, may repeat course of therapy after a drug-free interval of 48 hours.

**Dosage Forms**

Injection, solution: 100 mg/mL (10 mL) [in polyethylene glycol; vial stopper contains latex]
Tablet: 500 mg, 750 mg

# methohexital *(meth oh HEKS i tal)*

**Sound-Alike/Look-Alike Issues**
Brevital® may be confused with Brevibloc®

**Synonyms** methohexital sodium

**U.S./Canadian Brand Names** Brevital® Sodium [US]; Brevital® [Can]

**Therapeutic Category** Barbiturate

**Controlled Substance** C-IV

**Use** Induction and maintenance of general anesthesia for short procedures

**Can be used in pediatric patients ≥1 month of age as follows:** For rectal or intramuscular induction of anesthesia prior to the use of other general anesthetic agents, as an adjunct to subpotent inhalational anesthetic agents for short surgical procedures, or for short surgical, diagnostic, or therapeutic procedures associated with minimal painful stimuli

**Usual Dosage** Doses must be titrated to effect

Manufacturer's recommendations:

Infants <1 month: Safety and efficacy not established

Infants ≥1 month and Children:

I.M.: Induction: 6.6-10 mg/kg of a 5% solution

Rectal: Induction: Usual: 25 mg/kg of a 1% solution

Alternative pediatric dosing:

Children 3-12 years:

I.M.: Preoperative: 5-10 mg/kg/dose

I.V.: Induction: 1-2 mg/kg/dose

Rectal: Preoperative/induction: 20-35 mg/kg/dose; usual: 25 mg/kg/dose; maximum dose: 500 mg/dose; give as 10% aqueous solution

Adults: I.V.: Induction: 50-120 mg to start; 20-40 mg every 4-7 minutes

**Dosage Forms** Injection, powder for reconstitution, as sodium: 500 mg, 2.5 g, 5 g

**methohexital sodium** *see* methohexital *on this page*

# methotrexate *(meth oh TREKS ate)*

**Sound-Alike/Look-Alike Issues**
methotrexate may be confused with metolazone, mitoxantrone

MTX is an error-prone abbreviation (mistaken as mitoxantrone)

**Synonyms** amethopterin; methotrexate sodium; NSC-740

**U.S./Canadian Brand Names** Apo-Methotrexate® [Can]; ratio-Methotrexate [Can]; Rheumatrex® [US]; Trexall™ [US]

**Therapeutic Category** Antineoplastic Agent

**Use** Treatment of trophoblastic neoplasms; leukemias; psoriasis; rheumatoid arthritis (RA), including polyarticular-course juvenile rheumatoid arthritis (JRA); breast, head and neck, and lung carcinomas; osteosarcoma; soft-tissue sarcomas; carcinoma of gastrointestinal tract, esophagus, testes; lymphomas

**Usual Dosage** Refer to individual protocols.

**Note:** Doses between 100-500 mg/m$^2$ **may require** leucovorin rescue. Doses >500 mg/m$^2$ **require** leucovorin rescue: Oral, I.M., I.V.: Leucovorin 10-15 mg/m$^2$ every 6 hours for 8 or 10 doses, starting 24 hours after the start of methotrexate infusion. Continue until the methotrexate level is ≤0.1 micromolar ($10^{-7}$M). Some clinicians continue leucovorin until the methotrexate level is <0.05 micromolar (5 x 10$^{-8}$M) or 0.01 micromolar ($10^{-8}$M).

If the 48-hour methotrexate level is >1 micromolar ($10^{-7}$M) or the 72-hour methotrexate level is >0.2 micromolar (2 x $10^{-7}$M): I.V., I.M, Oral: Leucovorin 100 mg/m$^2$ every 6 hours until the methotrexate level is ≤0.1 micromolar ($10^{-7}$M). Some clinicians continue leucovorin until the methotrexate level is <0.05 micromolar (5 x $10^{-8}$M) or 0.01 micromolar ($10^{-8}$M).

Children:

Dermatomyositis: Oral: 15-20 mg/m$^2$/week as a single dose once weekly **or** 0.3-1 mg/kg/dose once weekly

Juvenile rheumatoid arthritis: Oral, I.M.: 10 mg/m$^2$ once weekly, then 5-15 mg/m$^2$/week as a single dose **or** as 3 divided doses given 12 hours apart

Antineoplastic dosage range:

Oral, I.M.: 7.5-30 mg/m$^2$/week **or** every 2 weeks

I.V.: 10-18,000 mg/m$^2$ bolus dosing **or** continuous infusion over 6-42 hours

Dosing schedule: **Note:** Doses between 100-500 mg/m$^2$ may require leucovorin rescue in some patients:

Conventional dose:

15-20 mg/m$^2$ oral twice weekly

30-50 mg/m$^2$ oral, I.V. weekly

15 mg/day for 5 days oral, I.M. every 2-3 weeks

Intermediate dose:

50-150 mg/m$^2$ I.V. push every 2-3 weeks

240 mg/m$^2$ I.V. infusion every 4-7 days

0.5-1 g/m$^2$ (followed with leucovorin rescue - refer to Leucovorin monograph) I.V. infusion every 2-3 weeks

High dose: 1-25 g/m$^2$ I.V. infusion every 1-3 weeks

Pediatric solid tumors (high-dose): I.V.:

<12 years: 12-25 g/m$^2$

≥12 years: 8 g/m$^2$

Acute lymphocytic leukemia (intermediate-dose): I.V.: Loading: 100 mg/m$^2$ bolus dose, followed by 900 mg/m$^2$/day infusion over 23-41 hours.

Meningeal leukemia: I.T.: 10-15 mg/m$^2$ (maximum dose: 15 mg) **or** an age-based dosing regimen; one possible system is:

≤3 months: 3 mg/dose

4-11 months: 6 mg/dose

1 year: 8 mg/dose

2 years: 10 mg/dose

≥3 years: 12 mg/dose

Adults: I.V.: Range is wide from 30-40 mg/m$^2$/week to 100-12,000 mg/m$^2$ with leucovorin rescue

Trophoblastic neoplasms:

Oral, I.M.: 15-30 mg/day for 5 days; repeat in 7 days for 3-5 courses

I.V.: 11 mg/m$^2$ days 1 through 5 every 3 weeks

Head and neck cancer: Oral, I.M., I.V.: 25-50 mg/m$^2$ once weekly

Mycosis fungoides (cutaneous I-cell lymphoma): Oral, I.M.: Inltlal (early stages):

5-50 mg once weekly **or**

15-37.5 mg twice weekly

Bladder cancer: I.V.:

30 mg/m$^2$ day 1 and 8 every 3 weeks **or**

(Continued)

# methotrexate *(Continued)*

30 mg/m$^2$ day 1, 15, and 22 every 4 weeks

Breast cancer: I.V.: 30-60 mg/m$^2$ days 1 and 8 every 3-4 weeks

Gastric cancer: I.V.:1500 mg/m$^2$ every 4 weeks

Lymphoma, non-Hodgkin's: I.V.:

30 mg/m$^2$ days 3 and 10 every 3 weeks **or**

120 mg/m$^2$ day 8 and 15 every 3-4 weeks **or**

200 mg/m$^2$ day 8 and 15 every 3 weeks **or**

400 mg/m$^2$ every 4 weeks for 3 cycles **or**

1 g/m$^2$ every 3 weeks **or**

1.5 g/m$^2$ every 4 weeks

Sarcoma: I.V.: 8-12 g/m$^2$ weekly for 2-4 weeks

Rheumatoid arthritis: Oral: 7.5 mg once weekly **or** 2.5 mg every 12 hours for 3 doses/week, not to exceed 20 mg/week

Psoriasis:

Oral: 2.5-5 mg/dose every 12 hours for 3 doses given weekly **or**

Oral, I.M.: 10-25 mg/dose given once weekly

Ectopic pregnancy: I.M., I.V.: 50 mg/m$^2$ as a single dose

## Dosage Forms

Injection, powder for reconstitution [preservative free]: 20 mg, 1 g

Injection, solution: 25 mg/mL (2 mL, 10 mL) [contains benzyl alcohol]

Injection, solution [preservative free]: 25 mg/mL (2 mL, 4 mL, 8 mL, 10 mL)

Tablet: 2.5 mg

Trexall™: 5 mg, 7.5 mg, 10 mg, 15 mg

Tablet, as sodium [dose pack] (Rheumatrex® Dose Pack): 2.5 mg (4 cards with 2, 3, 4, 5, or 6 tablets each)

**methotrexate sodium** *see* methotrexate *on page 524*

# methotrexate *(Canada only)* (meth oh trye MEP ra zeen)

**Synonyms** levomepromazine; methotrimeprazine hydrochloride

**U.S./Canadian Brand Names** Apo-Methoprazine® [Can]; Nozinan® [Can]

**Therapeutic Category** Neuroleptic Agent

**Use** Treatment of schizophrenia or psychosis; management of pain, including pain caused by neuralgia or cancer; adjunct to general anesthesia; management of nausea and vomiting; sedation

## Usual Dosage

Children >2 years:

Oral: 0.25 mg/kg/day in 2-3 divided doses; may increase gradually based on response.

Maximum dose: 40 mg/day in children <12 years

I.M.: 0.06-0.125 mg/kg/day in 1-3 divided doses

Adults:

Oral:

Anxiety, mild-moderate pain: 6-25 mg/day in 3 divided doses

Psychoses, severe pain: 50-75 mg/day in 2-3 divided doses; titrate to effect (doses up to 1000 mg/day or greater have been used in treatment of some patients with psychoses). If higher dosages are used to initiate therapy (100-200 mg/day), patients should be restricted to bed for the first few days of therapy.

Sedative: 10-25 mg at bedtime

I.M.:

Psychoses, severe pain: 75-100 mg (administered in 3-4 deep I.M. injections)

Analgesia (postoperative): 10-25 mg every 8 hours (2.5-7.5 mg every 4-6 hours is suggested postoperatively if residual effects of anesthetic may be present)

Premedication: 10-25 mg every 8 hours (final preoperative dose may be 25-50 mg administered ~1 hour prior to surgery)

I.V.: During surgical procedures/labor: 20-50 mcg/minute (some patients may require up to 100 mcg/minute)

SubQ (continuous infusion): Palliative care: 25-200 mcg/day (via syringe driver)

## Dosage Forms

Injection, solution, as hydrochloride: 25 mg/mL (1 mL)

Solution, oral: 5 mg/mL (500 mL) [contains ethanol 2%]

Solution, oral drops: 40 mg/mL (100 mL) [contains ethanol 16.5%]

Tablet, as maleate: 2 mg, 5 mg, 25 mg, 50 mg

**methotrimeprazine hydrochloride** *see* methotrimeprazine *(Canada only)* on previous page

# methoxsalen (meth OKS a len)

**Synonyms** 8-methoxypsoralen; 8-MOP; methoxypsoralen

**U.S./Canadian Brand Names** 8-MOP® [US/Can]; Oxsoralen-Ultra® [US/Can]; Oxsoralen® [US/Can]; Ultramop™ [Can]; Uvadex® [US/Can]

**Therapeutic Category** Psoralen

**Use**

Oral: Symptomatic control of severe, recalcitrant disabling psoriasis; repigmentation of idiopathic vitiligo; palliative treatment of skin manifestations of cutaneous T-cell lymphoma (CTCL)

Topical: Repigmentation of idiopathic vitiligo

Extracorporeal: Palliative treatment of skin manifestations of CTCL

**Usual Dosage Note:** Refer to treatment protocols for UVA exposure guidelines.

Children >12 years and Adults: Vitiligo: Topical: Apply lotion 1-2 hours before exposure to UVA light, no more than once weekly

Adults:

Psoriasis: Oral: 10-70 mg 11/2-2 hours before exposure to UVA light; dose may be repeated 2-3 times per week, based on UVA exposure; doses must be given at least 48 hours apart; dosage is based upon patient's body weight and skin type:

<30 kg: 10 mg

30-50 kg: 20 mg

51-65 kg: 30 mg

66-80 kg: 40 mg

81-90 kg: 50 mg

91-115 kg: 60 mg

>115 kg: 70 mg

Vitiligo: (8-MOP®): Oral: 20 mg 2-4 hours before exposure to UVA light; dose may be repeated based on erythema and tenderness of skin; do not give on 2 consecutive days

CTCL: Extracorporeal (Uvadex®): 200 mcg injected into the photoactivation bag during the collection cycle using the UVAR® photopheresis system (consult user's guide). Treatment schedule: Two consecutive days every 4 weeks for a minimum of 7 treatment cycles

**Dosage Forms**

Capsule:

8-MOP®: 10 mg [hard-gelatin capsule]

Oxsoralen-Ultra®: 10 mg [soft-gelatin capsule]

Lotion (Oxsoralen®): 1% (30 mL) [contains alcohol 71%]

Solution, for extracorporeal administration (Uvadex®): 20 mcg/mL (10 mL) **[not for injection]**

# methoxycinnamate and oxybenzone (meth OKS ee SIN a mate & oks i BEN zone)

**Synonyms** sunscreen (paba-free)

**U.S./Canadian Brand Names** PreSun® 29 [US-OTC]; Ti-Screen® [US-OTC]

**Therapeutic Category** Sunscreen

**Use** Reduce the chance of premature aging of the skin and skin cancer from overexposure to the sun

**Usual Dosage** Adults: Topical: Apply liberally to all exposed areas at least 30 minutes prior to sun exposure

**Dosage Forms** Lotion:

SPF 15: 120 mL

SPF 29: 120 mL

**methoxypsoralen** *see* methoxsalen *on this page*

**8-methoxypsoralen** *see* methoxsalen *on this page*

# methscopolamine (meth skoe POL a meen)

**Synonyms** methscopolamine bromide

**U.S./Canadian Brand Names** Pamine® Forte [US]; Pamine® [US/Can]

**Therapeutic Category** Anticholinergic Agent

**Use** Adjunctive therapy in the treatment of peptic ulcer

**Usual Dosage** Adults: Oral: 2.5 mg 30 minutes before meals or food and 2.5-5 mg at bedtime; may increase dose to 5 mg twice daily

(Continued)

## methscopolamine *(Continued)*

**Dosage Forms** Tablet, as bromide:
Pamine®: 2.5 mg [lactose free]
Pamine® Forte: 5 mg [lactose free; dosepak]

**methscopolamine bromide** *see* methscopolamine *on previous page*

**methscopolamine, chlorpheniramine, and phenylephrine** *see* chlorpheniramine, phenylephrine, and methscopolamine *on page 175*

## methsuximide (meth SUKS i mide)

**Sound-Alike/Look-Alike Issues**
methsuximide may be confused with ethosuximide
**U.S./Canadian Brand Names** Celontin® [US/Can]
**Therapeutic Category** Anticonvulsant
**Use** Control of absence (petit mal) seizures that are refractory to other drugs
**Usual Dosage** Oral:
Children: Anticonvulsant: Initial: 10-15 mg/kg/day in 3-4 divided doses; increase weekly up to maximum of 30 mg/kg/day
Adults: Anticonvulsant: 300 mg/day for the first week; may increase by 300 mg/day at weekly intervals up to 1.2 g/day in 2-4 divided doses/day
**Dosage Forms** Capsule: 150 mg, 300 mg

## methyclothiazide (meth i kloe THYE a zide)

**Sound-Alike/Look-Alike Issues**
Enduron® may be confused with Empirin®, Imuran®, Inderal®
**U.S./Canadian Brand Names** Aquatensen® [Can]; Enduron® [Can]
**Therapeutic Category** Diuretic, Thiazide
**Use** Management of mild to moderate hypertension; treatment of edema in congestive heart failure and nephrotic syndrome
**Usual Dosage** Adults: Oral:
Edema: 2.5-10 mg/day
Hypertension: 2.5-5 mg/day; may add another antihypertensive if 5 mg is not adequate after a trial of 8-12 weeks of therapy
**Dosage Forms** Tablet: 5 mg

## methyclothiazide and deserpidine (meth i kloe THYE a zide & de SER pi deen)

**Sound-Alike/Look-Alike Issues**
Enduronyl® may be confused with Inderal®
Enduronyl® Forte may be confused with Inderal® 40
**Synonyms** deserpidine and methyclothiazide
**U.S./Canadian Brand Names** Enduronyl® Forte [US/Can]; Enduronyl® [Can]
**Therapeutic Category** Antihypertensive Agent, Combination
**Use** Management of mild to moderately severe hypertension
**Usual Dosage** Oral: Individualized, normally 1-4 tablets/day
**Dosage Forms** Tablet:
Enduronyl®: Methyclothiazide 5 mg and deserpidine 0.25 mg
Enduronyl® Forte: Methyclothiazide 5 mg and deserpidine 0.5 mg

**methylacetoxyprogesterone** *see* medroxyprogesterone acetate *on page 507*

## methylbenzethonium chloride (meth il ben ze THOE nee um KLOR ide)

**U.S./Canadian Brand Names** Diaparene® [US-OTC]; Puri-Clens™ [US-OTC]
**Therapeutic Category** Topical Skin Product
**Use** Treatment of diaper rash and ammonia dermatitis
**Usual Dosage** Topical: Apply to area as needed
**Dosage Forms**
Cream, topical: 0.1% (30 g, 60 g, 120 g)
Ointment, topical: 0.1% (30 g, 60 g, 120 g)
Powder, topical: 0.055% (120 g, 270 g, 420 g)

## methylcellulose (meth il SEL yoo lose)

**Sound-Alike/Look-Alike Issues**
Citrucel® may be confused with Citracal®
**U.S./Canadian Brand Names** Citrucel® [US-OTC]; FiberEase™ [US-OTC]
**Therapeutic Category** Laxative
**Use** Adjunct in treatment of constipation
**Usual Dosage** Oral:
Children 6-12 years:
Citrucel® caplet: 1 caplet up to 6 times/day; follow each dose with 8 oz of water
Citrucel® powder: Half the adult dose in 4 oz of cold water, 1-3 times/day
Children ≥12 years and Adults:
Citrucel® caplet: 2-4 caplets 1-3 times/day; follow each dose with 8 oz of water
Citrucel® powder: 1 heaping tablespoon (19 g) in 8 oz of cold water, 1-3 times/day
FiberEase™: 2 tablespoonsful mixed in 7 oz of water, 1-3 times/day
**Dosage Forms**
Caplet (Citrucel®): 500 mg
Liquid (FiberEase™): 4 g/30 mL (414 mL) [available in regular or dietetic formulations; orange and apple-raspberry flavors]
Powder:
Citrucel® [clear mix formulation]: 2 g/level scoop (275 g, 539 g)
Citrucel® [regular formulation]: 2 g/level scoop (448 g, 840 g); 2 g/packet (20s) [orange flavor]
Citrucel® [sugar free formulation]: 2 g/level scoop (241 g, 473 g) [contains phenylalanine 52 mg/level scoop; orange flavor]; 2 g/packet (20s) [contains phenylalanine 52 mg/packet; orange flavor]

**methylcellulose, gelatin, and pectin** *see* gelatin, pectin, and methylcellulose *on page 369*

## methyldopa (meth il DOE pa)

**Sound-Alike/Look-Alike Issues**
methyldopa may be confused with L-dopa, levodopa
**Synonyms** methyldopate hydrochloride
**U.S./Canadian Brand Names** Apo-Methyldopa® [Can]; Nu-Medopa [Can]
**Therapeutic Category** Alpha-Adrenergic Blocking Agent
**Use** Management of moderate to severe hypertension
**Usual Dosage**
Children:
Oral: Initial: 10 mg/kg/day in 2-4 divided doses; increase every 2 days as needed to maximum dose of 65 mg/kg/day; do not exceed 3 g/day.
I.V.: 5-10 mg/kg/dose every 6-8 hours up to a total dose of 65 mg/kg/24 hours or 3 g/24 hours
Adults:
Oral: Initial: 250 mg 2-3 times/day; increase every 2 days as needed (maximum dose: 3 g/day): usual dose range (JNC 7): 250-1000 mg/day in 2 divided doses
I.V.: 250-500 mg every 6-8 hours; maximum dose: 1 g every 6 hours
**Dosage Forms**
Injection, solution, as methyldopate hydrochloride: 50 mg/mL (5 mL) [contains sodium bisulfite]
Tablet: 250 mg, 500 mg

## methyldopa and hydrochlorothiazide (meth il DOE pa & hye droe klor oh THYE a zide)

**Sound-Alike/Look-Alike Issues**
Aldoril® may be confused with Aldoclor®, Aldomet®, Elavil®
**Synonyms** hydrochlorothiazide and methyldopa
**U.S./Canadian Brand Names** Aldoril® [US]; Apo-Methazide® [Can]
**Therapeutic Category** Antihypertensive Agent, Combination
**Use** Management of moderate to severe hypertension
**Usual Dosage** Oral: Dosage titrated on individual components, then switch to combination product; no more than methyldopa 3 g/day and/or hydrochlorothiazide 50 mg/day; maintain initial dose for first 48 hours, then decrease or increase at intervals of not less than 2 days until an adequate response is achieved
Methyldopa 250 mg and hydrochlorothiazide 15 mg: 2-3 times/day
Methyldopa 250 mg and hydrochlorothiazide 25 mg: Twice daily
Methyldopa 500 mg and hydrochlorothiazide 30 mg: Once daily
(Continued)

# methyldopa and hydrochlorothiazide *(Continued)*
Dosage Forms
Tablet:
Methyldopa 250 mg and hydrochlorothiazide 15 mg
Methyldopa 250 mg and hydrochlorothiazide 25 mg
Aldoril® 25: Methyldopa 250 mg and hydrochlorothiazide 25 mg

**methyldopate hydrochloride** *see* methyldopa *on previous page*

# methylene blue (METH i leen bloo)
U.S./Canadian Brand Names Urolene Blue® [US]
Therapeutic Category Antidote
Use Antidote for cyanide poisoning and drug-induced methemoglobinemia, indicator dye
Usual Dosage
Children: NADPH-methemoglobin reductase deficiency: Oral: 1-1.5 mg/kg/day (maximum: 300 mg/day) given with 5-8 mg/kg/day of ascorbic acid
Children and Adults: Methemoglobinemia: I.V.: 1-2 mg/kg or 25-50 mg/m$^2$ over several minutes; may be repeated in 1 hour if necessary
Adults: Genitourinary antiseptic: Oral: 65-130 mg 3 times/day with a full glass of water (maximum: 390 mg/day)
Dosage Forms
Injection, solution: 10 mg/mL (1 mL, 10 mL)
Tablet (Urolene Blue®): 65 mg

**methylergometrine maleate** *see* methylergonovine *on this page*

# methylergonovine (meth il er goe NOE veen)
Sound-Alike/Look-Alike Issues
methylergonovine and terbutaline parenteral dosage forms look similar. Due to their contrasting indications, use care when administering these agents.
Synonyms methylergometrine maleate; methylergonovine maleate
U.S./Canadian Brand Names Methergine® [US/Can]
Therapeutic Category Ergot Alkaloid and Derivative
Use Prevention and treatment of postpartum and postabortion hemorrhage caused by uterine atony or subinvolution
Usual Dosage Adults:
Oral: 0.2 mg 3-4 times/day for 2-7 days
I.M., I.V.: 0.2 mg after delivery of anterior shoulder, after delivery of placenta, or during puerperium; may be repeated as required at intervals of 2-4 hours
Dosage Forms
Injection, solution, as maleate: 0.2 mg/mL (1 mL)
Tablet, as maleate: 0.2 mg

**methylergonovine maleate** *see* methylergonovine *on this page*

**Methylin® [US]** *see* methylphenidate *on this page*

**Methylin® ER [US]** *see* methylphenidate *on this page*

**methylmorphine** *see* codeine *on page 203*

# methylphenidate (meth il FEN i date)
Sound-Alike/Look-Alike Issues
methylphenidate may be confused with methadone
Ritalin® may be confused with Ismelin®, Rifadin®
Synonyms methylphenidate hydrochloride
U.S./Canadian Brand Names Concerta® [US/Can]; Metadate® CD [US]; Metadate® ER [US]; Methylin® ER [US]; Methylin® [US]; PMS-Methylphenidate [Can]; Riphenidate [Can]; Ritalin-SR® [US/Can]; Ritalin® LA [US]; Ritalin® [US/Can]
Therapeutic Category Central Nervous System Stimulant, Nonamphetamine
Controlled Substance C-II
Use Treatment of attention-deficit/hyperactivity disorder (ADHD); symptomatic management of narcolepsy

**Usual Dosage** Oral (discontinue periodically to re-evaluate or if no improvement occurs within 1 month):

Children ≥6 years and Adults: ADHD: Initial: 0.3 mg/kg/dose or 2.5-5 mg/dose given before breakfast and lunch; increase by 0.1 mg/kg/dose or by 5-10 mg/day at weekly intervals; usual dose: 0.5-1 mg/kg/day; maximum dose: 2 mg/kg/day or 90 mg/day

**Extended release products:**

*Metadate® ER, Methylin® ER, Ritalin® SR:* Duration of action is 8 hours. May be given in place of regular tablets, once the daily dose is titrated using the regular tablets and the titrated 8-hour dosage corresponds to sustained release tablet size.

*Metadate® CD, Ritalin® LA:* Initial: 20 mg once daily; may be adjusted in 10-20 mg increments at weekly intervals; maximum: 60 mg/day

*Concerta®:* Duration of action is 12 hours:

Initial dose:

Children not currently taking methylphenidate: 18 mg once daily in the morning

Children currently taking methylphenidate: **Note:** Dosing based on current regimen and clinical judgment; suggested dosing listed below:

Patients taking methylphenidate 5 mg 2-3 times/day or 20 mg/day sustained release formulation: 18 mg once every morning

Patients taking methylphenidate 10 mg 2-3 times/day or 40 mg/day sustained release formulation: 36 mg once every morning

Patients taking methylphenidate 15 mg 2-3 times/day or 60 mg/day sustained release formulation: 54 mg once every morning

Dose adjustment: May increase dose in increments of 18 mg; dose may be adjusted at weekly intervals. A dosage strength of 27 mg is available for situations in which a dosage between 18-36 mg is desired. Maximum dose should not exceed 2 mg/kg/day **or** 54 mg/day in children 6-12 years or 72 mg/day in children 13-17 years.

Adults: Narcolepsy: 10 mg 2-3 times/day, up to 60 mg/day

**Dosage Forms**

Capsule, extended release, as hydrochloride:

Metadate® CD: 10 mg, 20 mg, 30 mg

Ritalin® LA: 10 mg, 20 mg, 30 mg, 40 mg

Solution, oral, as hydrochloride:

Methylin®: 5 mg/5 mL (500 mL) [grape flavor]; 10 mg/5 mL (500 mL) [grape flavor]

Tablet, as hydrochloride: 5 mg, 10 mg, 20 mg

Methylin®, Ritalin®: 5 mg, 10 mg, 20 mg

Tablet, chewable, as hydrochloride:

Methylin®: 2.5 mg [contains phenylalanine 0.42 mg; grape flavor]; 5 mg [contains phenylalanine 0.84 mg; grape flavor]; 10 mg [contains phenylalanine 1.68 mg; grape flavor]

Tablet, extended release, as hydrochloride: 20 mg

Concerta®: 18 mg, 27 mg, 36 mg, 54 mg [osmotic controlled release]

Metadate® ER, Methylin® ER: 10 mg, 20 mg

Tablet, sustained release, as hydrochloride (Ritalin-SR®): 20 mg

**methylphenidate hydrochloride** *see* methylphenidate *on previous page*

**methylphenobarbital** *see* mephobarbital *on page 513*

**methylphenoxy-benzene propanamine** *see* atomoxetine *on page 77*

**methylphenyl isoxazolyl penicillin** *see* oxacillin *on page 604*

**methylphytyl napthoquinone** *see* phytonadione *on page 646*

# methylprednisolone (meth il pred NIS oh lone)

**Sound-Alike/Look-Alike Issues**

methylPREDNISolone may be confused with medroxyPROGESTERone, predniSONE

Depo-Medrol® may be confused with Solu-Medrol®

Medrol® may be confused with Mebaral®

Solu-Medrol® may be confused with Depo-Medrol®

**Synonyms** 6-α-methylprednisolone; A-methapred; methylprednisolone acetate; methylprednisolone sodium succinate

**Tall-Man** methyl**PREDNIS**olone

(Continued)

# methylprednisolone *(Continued)*

**U.S./Canadian Brand Names** Depo-Medrol® [US/Can]; Medrol® [US/Can]; Solu-Medrol® [US/Can]

**Therapeutic Category** Adrenal Corticosteroid

**Use** Primarily as an anti-inflammatory or immunosuppressant agent in the treatment of a variety of diseases including those of hematologic, allergic, inflammatory, neoplastic, and autoimmune origin. Prevention and treatment of graft-versus-host disease following allogeneic bone marrow transplantation.

**Usual Dosage** Dosing should be based on the lesser of ideal body weight or actual body weight

**Only sodium succinate may be given I.V.;** methylprednisolone sodium succinate is highly soluble and has a rapid effect by I.M. and I.V. routes. Methylprednisolone acetate has a low solubility and has a sustained I.M. effect.

Children:

Antiinflammatory or immunosuppressive: Oral, I.M., I.V. (sodium succinate): 0.5-1.7 mg/kg/day **or** 5-25 mg/m$^2$/day in divided doses every 6-12 hours; "Pulse" therapy: 15-30 mg/kg/dose over ≥30 minutes given once daily for 3 days

Status asthmaticus: I.V. (sodium succinate): Loading dose: 2 mg/kg/dose, then 0.5-1 mg/kg/dose every 6 hours for up to 5 days

Acute spinal cord injury: I.V. (sodium succinate): 30 mg/kg over 15 minutes, followed in 45 minutes by a continuous infusion of 5.4 mg/kg/hour for 23 hours

Lupus nephritis: I.V. (sodium succinate): 30 mg/kg over ≥30 minutes every other day for 6 doses

Adults: **Only sodium succinate may be given I.V.;** methylprednisolone sodium succinate is highly soluble and has a rapid effect by I.M. and I.V. routes. Methylprednisolone acetate has a low solubility and has a sustained I.M. effect.

Acute spinal cord injury: I.V. (sodium succinate): 30 mg/kg over 15 minutes, followed in 45 minutes by a continuous infusion of 5.4 mg/kg/hour for 23 hours

Antiinflammatory or immunosuppressive:

Oral: 2-60 mg/day in 1-4 divided doses to start, followed by gradual reduction in dosage to the lowest possible level consistent with maintaining an adequate clinical response.

I.M. (sodium succinate): 10-80 mg/day once daily

I.M. (acetate): 10-80 mg every 1-2 weeks

I.V. (sodium succinate): 10-40 mg over a period of several minutes and repeated I.V. or I.M. at intervals depending on clinical response; when high dosages are needed, give 30 mg/kg over a period ≥30 minutes and may be repeated every 4-6 hours for 48 hours.

Status asthmaticus: I.V. (sodium succinate): Loading dose: 2 mg/kg/dose, then 0.5-1 mg/kg/dose every 6 hours for up to 5 days

Lupus nephritis: High-dose "pulse" therapy: I.V. (sodium succinate): 1 g/day for 3 days

Aplastic anemia: I.V. (sodium succinate): 1 mg/kg/day or 40 mg/day (whichever dose is higher), for 4 days. After 4 days, change to oral and continue until day 10 or until symptoms of serum sickness resolve, then rapidly reduce over approximately 2 weeks.

*Pneumocystis* pneumonia in AIDs patients: I.V.: 40-60 mg every 6 hours for 7-10 days

Intra-articular (acetate): Administer every 1-5 weeks.

Large joints: 20-80 mg

Small joints: 4-10 mg

Intralesional (acetate): 20-60 mg every 1-5 weeks

**Dosage Forms**

Injection, powder for reconstitution, as sodium succinate: 125 mg [strength expressed as base]

Solu-Medrol®: 40 mg, 125 mg, 500 mg, 1 g, 2 g [packaged with diluent; diluent contains benzyl alcohol; strength expressed as base]

Solu-Medrol®: 500 mg, 1 g

Injection, suspension, as acetate (Depo-Medrol®): 20 mg/mL (5 mL); 40 mg/mL (5 mL); 80 mg/mL (5 mL) [contains benzyl alcohol; strength expressed as base]

Injection, suspension, as acetate [single-dose vial] (Depo-Medrol®): 40 mg/mL (1 mL, 10 mL); 80 mg/mL (1 mL)

Tablet: 4 mg

Medrol®: 2 mg, 4 mg, 8 mg, 16 mg, 32 mg

Tablet, dose-pack: 4 mg (21s)

Medrol® Dosepack™: 4 mg (21s)

**6-α-methylprednisolone** *see* methylprednisolone *on previous page*

**methylprednisolone acetate** *see* methylprednisolone *on previous page*

**methylprednisolone sodium succinate** *see* methylprednisolone *on previous page*

**4-methylpyrazole** *see* fomepizole *on page 358*

## methyltestosterone (meth il tes TOS te rone)
**Sound-Alike/Look-Alike Issues**
methylTESTOSTERone may be confused with medroxyPROGESTERone
Virilon® may be confused with Verelan®
**Tall-Man** methyl**TESTOSTER**one
**U.S./Canadian Brand Names** Android® [US]; Methitest™ [US]; Testred® [US]; Virilon® [US]
**Therapeutic Category** Androgen
**Controlled Substance** C-III
**Use**
Male: Hypogonadism; delayed puberty; impotence and climacteric symptoms
Female: Palliative treatment of metastatic breast cancer
**Usual Dosage** Adults (buccal absorption produces twice the androgenic activity of oral tablets):
Male:
Hypogonadism, male climacteric and impotence: Oral: 10-40 mg/day
Androgen deficiency:
Oral: 10-50 mg/day
Buccal: 5-25 mg/day
Postpubertal cryptorchidism: Oral: 30 mg/day
Female:
Breast pain/engorgement:
Oral: 80 mg/day for 3-5 days
Buccal: 40 mg/day for 3-5 days
Breast cancer:
Oral: 50-200 mg/day
Buccal: 25-100 mg/day
**Dosage Forms**
Capsule (Android®, Testred®, Virilon®): 10 mg
Tablet (Methitest™): 10 mg

**Meticorten®** *(Discontinued)* *see* prednisone *on page 674*

## metipranolol (met i PRAN oh lol)
**Sound-Alike/Look-Alike Issues**
metipranolol may be confused with metaproterenol
**Synonyms** metipranolol hydrochloride
**U.S./Canadian Brand Names** OptiPranolol® [US/Can]
**Therapeutic Category** Beta-Adrenergic Blocker
**Use** Agent for lowering intraocular pressure in patients with chronic open-angle glaucoma
**Usual Dosage** Ophthalmic: Adults: Instill 1 drop in the affected eye(s) twice daily
**Dosage Forms** Solution, ophthalmic: 0.3% (5 mL, 10 mL) [contains benzalkonium chloride]

**metipranolol hydrochloride** *see* metipranolol *on this page*

## metoclopramide (met oh kloe PRA mide)
**Sound-Alike/Look-Alike Issues**
metoclopramide may be confused with metolazone
Reglan® may be confused with Megace®, Regonol®, Renagel®
**U.S./Canadian Brand Names** Apo-Metoclop® [Can]; Nu-Metoclopramide [Can]; Reglan® [US]
**Therapeutic Category** Gastrointestinal Agent, Prokinetic
**Use**
Oral: Symptomatic treatment of diabetic gastric stasis; gastroesophageal reflux
I.V., I.M.: Symptomatic treatment of diabetic gastric stasis; postpyloric placement of enteral feeding tubes; prevention and/or treatment of nausea and vomiting associated with chemotherapy, or post-surgery; to stimulate gastric emptying and intestinal transit of barium during radiological examination
**Usual Dosage**
Children:
Gastroesophageal reflux: Oral: 0.1-0.2 mg/kg/dose up to 4 times/day; efficacy of continuing metoclopramide beyond 12 weeks in reflux has not been determined; total daily dose should not exceed 0.5 mg/kg/day
(Continued)

## metoclopramide *(Continued)*

Gastrointestinal hypomotility (gastroparesis): Oral, I.M., I.V.: 0.1 mg/kg/dose up to 4 times/day, not to exceed 0.5 mg/kg/day

Adults:

Gastroesophageal reflux: Oral: 10-15 mg/dose up to 4 times/day 30 minutes before meals or food and at bedtime; single doses of 20 mg are occasionally needed for provoking situations

Gastrointestinal hypomotility (gastroparesis):

Oral: 10 mg 30 minutes before each meal and at bedtime for 2-8 weeks

I.V. (for severe symptoms): 10 mg over 1-2 minutes; 10 days of I.V. therapy may be necessary for best response

**Dosage Forms**

Injection, solution (Reglan®): 5 mg/mL (2 mL, 10 mL, 30 mL)

Syrup: 5 mg/5 mL (10 mL, 480 mL)

Tablet (Reglan®): 5 mg, 10 mg

## metolazone (me TOLE a zone)

**Sound-Alike/Look-Alike Issues**

metolazone may be confused with metaxalone, methazolamide, methimazole, methotrexate, metoclopramide, metoprolol, minoxidil

Zaroxolyn® may be confused with Zarontin®

**U.S./Canadian Brand Names** Mykrox® [Can]; Zaroxolyn® [US/Can]

**Therapeutic Category** Diuretic, Miscellaneous

**Use** Management of mild to moderate hypertension; treatment of edema in congestive heart failure and nephrotic syndrome, impaired renal function

**Usual Dosage** Adults: Oral:

Edema: 5-20 mg/dose every 24 hours

Hypertension (Zaroxolyn®): 2.5-5 mg/dose every 24 hours

Hypertension (Mykrox®): 0.5 mg/day; if response is not adequate, increase dose to maximum of 1 mg/day

**Dosage Forms** Tablet, slow acting: 2.5 mg, 5 mg, 10 mg

**Metopirone® [US]** *see metyrapone on page 536*

## metoprolol (me toe PROE lole)

**Sound-Alike/Look-Alike Issues**

metoprolol may be confused with metaproterenol, metolazone, misoprostol

Toprol-XL® may be confused with Topamax®

**Synonyms** metoprolol succinate; metoprolol tartrate

**U.S./Canadian Brand Names** Apo-Metoprolol® [Can]; Betaloc® Durules® [Can]; Betaloc® [Can]; Lopressor® [US/Can]; Novo-Metoprolol [Can]; Nu-Metop [Can]; PMS-Metoprolol [Can]; Toprol-XL® [US/Can]

**Therapeutic Category** Beta-Adrenergic Blocker

**Use** Treatment of hypertension and angina pectoris; prevention of myocardial infarction, atrial fibrillation, flutter, symptomatic treatment of hypertrophic subaortic stenosis; to reduce mortality/hospitalization in patients with congestive heart failure (stable NYHA Class II or III) in patients already receiving ACE inhibitors, diuretics, and/or digoxin (sustained-release only)

**Usual Dosage**

Children: Oral: 1-5 mg/kg/24 hours divided twice daily; allow 3 days between dose adjustments

Adults:

Hypertension: Oral: 100-450 mg/day in 2-3 divided doses, begin with 50 mg twice daily and increase doses at weekly intervals to desired effect; usual dosage range (JNC 7): 50-100 mg/day

Extended release: Initial: 25-100 mg/day (maximum: 400 mg/day)

Angina, SVT, MI prophylaxis: Oral: 100-450 mg/day in 2-3 divided doses, begin with 50 mg twice daily and increase doses at weekly intervals to desired effect

Extended release: Initial: 100 mg/day (maximum: 400 mg/day)

Hypertension/ventricular rate control: I.V. (in patients having nonfunctioning GI tract): Initial: 1.25-5 mg every 6-12 hours; titrate initial dose to response. Initially, low doses may be appropriate to establish response; however, up to 15 mg every 3-6 hours has been employed.

Congestive heart failure: Oral (extended release): Initial: 25 mg once daily (reduce to 12.5 mg once daily in NYHA class higher than class II); may double dosage every 2 weeks as tolerated, up to 200 mg/day

Myocardial infarction (acute): I.V.: 5 mg every 2 minutes for 3 doses in early treatment of myocardial infarction; thereafter give 50 mg orally every 6 hours 15 minutes after last I.V. dose and continue for 48 hours; then administer a maintenance dose of 100 mg twice daily.

### Dosage Forms

Injection, solution, as tartrate (Lopressor®): 1 mg/mL (5 mL)

Tablet, as tartrate 25 mg, 50 mg, 100 mg

Lopressor®: 50 mg, 100 mg

Tablet, extended release, as succinate (Toprol-XL®): 25 mg, 50 mg, 100 mg, 200 mg [expressed as mg equivalent to tartrate]

**metoprolol succinate** *see* metoprolol *on previous page*

**metoprolol tartrate** *see* metoprolol *on previous page*

**Metreton® *(Discontinued)***

**metrizamide** *see* radiological/contrast media (nonionic) *on page 709*

**MetroCream® [US/Can]** *see* metronidazole *on this page*

**Metrodin® *(Discontinued)*** *see* urofollitropin *on page 835*

**MetroGel® [US/Can]** *see* metronidazole *on this page*

**MetroGel-Vaginal® [US]** *see* metronidazole *on this page*

**Metro I.V.® Injection *(Discontinued)*** *see* metronidazole *on this page*

**MetroLotion® [US]** *see* metronidazole *on this page*

# metronidazole (me troe NI da zole)

### Sound-Alike/Look-Alike Issues

metronidazole may be confused with metformin.

### Synonyms metronidazole hydrochloride

### U.S./Canadian Brand Names Apo-Metronidazole® [Can]; Flagyl ER® [US]; Flagyl® I.V. RTU™ [US]; Flagyl® [US/Can]; Florazole® ER [Can]; MetroCream® [US/Can]; MetroGel-Vaginal® [US]; MetroGel® [US/Can]; MetroLotion® [US]; Nidagel™ [Can]; Noritate® [US/Can]; Trikacide [Can]

### Therapeutic Category Amebicide; Antibiotic, Miscellaneous; Antibiotic, Topical; Antiprotozoal

Use Treatment of susceptible anaerobic bacterial and protozoal infections in the following conditions: Amebiasis, symptomatic and asymptomatic trichomoniasis; skin and skin structure infections; CNS infections; intra-abdominal infections (as part of combination regimen); systemic anaerobic infections; treatment of antibiotic-associated pseudomembranous colitis (AAPC), bacterial vaginosis; as part of a multidrug regimen for *H. pylori* eradication to reduce the risk of duodenal ulcer recurrence

Topical: Treatment of inflammatory lesions and erythema of rosacea

### Usual Dosage

Infants and Children:

Amebiasis: Oral: 35-50 mg/kg/day in divided doses every 8 hours for 10 days

Trichomoniasis: Oral: 15-30 mg/kg/day in divided doses every 8 hours for 7 days

Anaerobic infections:

Oral: 15-35 mg/kg/day in divided doses every 8 hours

I.V.: 30 mg/kg/day in divided doses every 6 hours

*Clostridium difficile* (antibiotic-associated colitis): Oral: 20 mg/kg/day divided every 6 hours

Maximum dose: 2 g/day

Adults:

Amebiasis: Oral: 500-750 mg every 8 hours for 5-10 days

Trichomoniasis: Oral: 250 mg every 8 hours for 7 days **or** 375 mg twice daily for 7 days **or** 2 g as a single dose

Anaerobic infections: Oral, I.V.: 500 mg every 6-8 hours, not to exceed 4 g/day

Antibiotic-associated pseudomembranous colitis: Oral: 250-500 mg 3-4 times/day for 10-14 days

*Helicobacter pylori* eradication: Oral: 250-500 mg with meals and at bedtime for 14 days; requires combination therapy with at least one other antibiotic and an acid-suppressing agent (proton pump inhibitor or $H_2$ blocker)

Bacterial vaginosis:

Oral: 750 mg (extended release tablet) once daily for 7 days

Vaginal: 1 applicatorful (~37.5 mg metronidazole) intravaginally once or twice daily for 5 days; apply once in morning and evening if using twice daily, if daily, use at bedtime

(Continued)

# metronidazole *(Continued)*

Acne rosacea: Topical:

0.75%: Apply and rub a thin film twice daily, morning and evening, to entire affected areas after washing. Significant therapeutic results should be noticed within 3 weeks. Clinical studies have demonstrated continuing improvement through 9 weeks of therapy.

1%: Apply thin film to affected area once daily

**Dosage Forms**

Capsule (Flagyl®): 375 mg

Cream, topical: 0.75% (45 g)

MetroCream®: 0.75% (45 g) [contains benzyl alcohol]

Noritate®: 1% (60 g)

Gel, topical (MetroGel®): 0.75% (45 g), 1% (45 g)

Gel, vaginal (MetroGel-Vaginal®, Vandazole™): 0.75% (70 g)

Infusion (Flagyl® I.V. RTU™) [premixed iso-osmotic sodium chloride solution]: 500 mg (100 mL) [contains sodium 14 mEq]

Lotion, topical (MetroLotion®): 0.75% (60 mL) [contains benzyl alcohol]

Tablet (Flagyl®): 250 mg, 500 mg

Tablet, extended release (Flagyl® ER): 750 mg

**metronidazole, bismuth subsalicylate, and tetracycline** *see* bismuth subsalicylate, metronidazole, and tetracycline *on page 108*

**metronidazole hydrochloride** *see* metronidazole *on previous page*

**metronidazole, tetracycline, and bismuth subsalicylate** *see* bismuth subsalicylate, metronidazole, and tetracycline *on page 108*

# metyrapone (me TEER a pone)

**Sound-Alike/Look-Alike Issues**

metyrapone may be confused with metyrosine

**U.S./Canadian Brand Names** Metopirone® [US]

**Therapeutic Category** Diagnostic Agent

**Use** Diagnostic test for hypothalamic-pituitary ACTH function

**Usual Dosage** Oral:

Children: 15 mg/kg every 4 hours for 6 doses; minimum dose: 250 mg

Adults: 750 mg every 4 hours for 6 doses

**Dosage Forms** Capsule: 250 mg

# metyrosine (me TYE roe seen)

**Sound-Alike/Look-Alike Issues**

metyrosine may be confused with metyrapone

**Synonyms** AMPT; OGMT

**U.S./Canadian Brand Names** Demser® [US/Can]

**Therapeutic Category** Tyrosine Hydroxylase Inhibitor

**Use** Short-term management of pheochromocytoma before surgery, long-term management when surgery is contraindicated or when chronic malignant pheochromocytoma exists

**Usual Dosage** Children >12 years and Adults: Oral: Initial: 250 mg 4 times/day, increased by 250-500 mg/day up to 4 g/day; maintenance: 2-3 g/day in 4 divided doses; for preoperative preparation, administer optimum effective dosage for 5-7 days

**Dosage Forms** Capsule: 250 mg

**Mevacor® [US/Can]** *see* lovastatin *on page 494*

**mevinolin** *see* lovastatin *on page 494*

# mexiletine (MEKS i le teen)

**U.S./Canadian Brand Names** Novo-Mexiletine [Can]

**Therapeutic Category** Antiarrhythmic Agent, Class I-B

**Use** Management of serious ventricular arrhythmias; suppression of PVCs

**Usual Dosage** Adults: Oral: Initial: 200 mg every 8 hours (may load with 400 mg if necessary); adjust dose every 2-3 days; usual dose: 200-300 mg every 8 hours; maximum dose: 1.2 g/day (some patients respond to every 12-hour dosing). When switching from another antiarrhythmic, initiate a 200 mg dose 6-12 hours after stopping former agents, 3-6 hours after stopping procainamide.

Dosage Forms [DSC] = Discontinued product
Capsule, as hydrochloride: 150 mg, 200 mg, 250 mg
Mexitil®: 150 mg, 200 mg, 250 mg [DSC]

**Mexitil® *(Discontinued)*** *see* mexiletine *on previous page*

**MG 217® [US-OTC]** *see* coal tar *on page 201*

**MG 217® Medicated Tar [US-OTC]** *see* coal tar *on page 201*

**MG217 Sal-Acid® [US-OTC]** *see* salicylic acid *on page 734*

**Miacalcin® [US]** *see* calcitonin *on page 129*

**Miacalcin® NS [Can]** *see* calcitonin *on page 129*

**Mi-Acid™ [US-OTC]** *see* aluminum hydroxide, magnesium hydroxide, and simethicone *on page 35*

**Mi-Acid™ Double Strength [US-OTC]** *see* calcium carbonate and magnesium hydroxide *on page 132*

**Mi-Acid™ Maximum Strength [US-OTC]** *see* aluminum hydroxide, magnesium hydroxide, and simethicone *on page 35*

**Micaderm® [US-OTC]** *see* miconazole *on this page*

## micafungin (mi ka FUN gin)

**Synonyms** micafungin sodium
**U.S./Canadian Brand Names** Mycamine™ [US]
**Therapeutic Category** Antifungal Agent, Parental; Drug-induced Neuritis, Treatment Agent
**Use** Esophageal candidiasis; *Candida* prophylaxis in patients undergoing hematopoietic stem cell transplant
**Usual Dosage** I.V.: Adults:
Esophageal candidiasis: 150 mg daily; median duration of therapy (from clinical trials) was 14 days
Prophylaxis of *Candida* infection in hematopoietic stem cell transplantation: 50 mg daily; median duration of therapy (from clinical trials) was 18 days
**Dosage Forms** Injection, powder for reconstitution, as sodium [preservative-free]: Micafungin 50 mg [contains lactose]

**micafungin sodium** *see* micafungin *on this page*

**Micanol® [Can]** *see* anthralin *on page 54*

**Micardis® [US/Can]** *see* telmisartan *on page 783*

**Micardis® HCT [US]** *see* telmisartan and hydrochlorothiazide *on page 783*

**Micardis® Plus [Can]** *see* telmisartan and hydrochlorothiazide *on page 783*

**Micatin® [Can]** *see* miconazole *on this page*

**Micatin® Athlete's Foot [US-OTC]** *see* miconazole *on this page*

**Micatin® Jock Itch [US-OTC]** *see* miconazole *on this page*

## miconazole (mi KON a zole)

**Sound-Alike/Look-Alike Issues**
miconazole may be confused with Micronase®, Micronor®
Lotrimin® may be confused with Lotrisone®, Otrivin®
Micatin® may be confused with Miacalcin®
**Synonyms** miconazole nitrate
**U.S./Canadian Brand Names** Aloe Vesta® 2-n-1 Antifungal [US-OTC]; Baza® Antifungal [US-OTC]; Carrington Antifungal [US-OTC]; DermaFungal [US-OTC]; Dermagran® AF [US-OTC]; Dermazole [Can]; DiabetAid™ Antifungal Foot Bath [US-OTC]; Fungoid® Tincture [US-OTC]; Lotrimin® AF Jock Itch Powder Spray [US-OTC]; Lotrimin® AF Powder/Spray [US-OTC]; Micaderm® [US-OTC]; Micatin® Athlete's Foot [US-OTC]; Micatin® Jock Itch [US-OTC]; Micatin® [Can]; Micozole [Can]; Micro-Guard® [US-OTC]; Mitrazol™ [US-OTC]; Monistat-Derm® [US]; Monistat® 1 Combination Pack [US-OTC]; Monistat® 3 [US-OTC/Can]; Monistat® 7 [US-OTC]; Monistat® [Can]; Neosporin® AF [US-OTC]; Podactin Cream [US-OTC]; Secura® Antifungal [US-OTC]; Zeasorb®-AF [US-OTC]
**Therapeutic Category** Antifungal Agent
**Use** Treatment of vulvovaginal candidiasis and a variety of skin and mucous membrane fungal infections
(Continued)

# miconazole *(Continued)*

## Usual Dosage
Topical: Children and Adults: **Note:** Not for OTC use in children <2 years:
Tinea corporis: Apply twice daily for 4 weeks
Tinea pedis: Apply twice daily for 4 weeks
  Effervescent tablet: Dissolve 1 tablet in ~1 gallon of water; soak feet for 15-30 minutes; pat dry
Tinea cruris: Apply twice daily for 2 weeks
Vaginal: Adults: Vulvovaginal candidiasis:
Cream, 2%: Insert 1 applicatorful at bedtime for 7 days
Cream, 4%: Insert 1 applicatorful at bedtime for 3 days
Suppository, 100 mg: Insert 1 suppository at bedtime for 7 days
Suppository, 200 mg: Insert 1 suppository at bedtime for 3 days
Suppository, 1200 mg: Insert 1 suppository (a one-time dose); may be used at bedtime or during the day

**Note:** Many products are available as a combination pack, with a suppository for vaginal instillation and cream to relieve external symptoms. External cream may be used twice daily, as needed, for up to 7 days.

## Dosage Forms [DSC] = Discontinued product
Combination products: Miconazole nitrate vaginal suppository 200 mg (3s) and miconazole nitrate external cream 2%
Monistat® 1 Combination Pack: Miconazole nitrate vaginal insert 1200 mg (1) and miconazole external cream 2% (5 g) [Note: Do not confuse with 1-Day™ (formerly Monistat® 1) which contains tioconazole]
Monistat® 3 Combination Pack:
  Miconazole nitrate vaginal suppository 200 mg (3s) and miconazole nitrate external cream 2%
  Miconazole nitrate vaginal cream 4% and miconazole nitrate external cream 2%
Monistat® 7 Combination Pack:
  Miconazole nitrate vaginal suppository 100 mg (7s) and miconazole nitrate external cream 2%
  Miconazole nitrate vaginal cream 2% (7 prefilled applicators) and miconazole nitrate external cream 2%
Cream, topical, as nitrate: 2% (15 g, 30 g, 45 g)
  Baza® Antifungal: 2% (4 g, 57 g, 142 g) [zinc oxide based formula]
  Carrington Antifungal: 2% (150 g)
  Micaderm®, Neosporin® AF, Podactin: 2% (30 g)
  Micatin® Athlete's Foot, Micatin® Jock Itch: 2% (15 g)
  Micro-Guard®, Mitrazol™: 2% (60 g)
  Monistat-Derm®: 2% (15 g, 30 g, 85 g)
  Secura® Antifungal: 2% (60 g, 98 g)
Cream, vaginal, as nitrate [prefilled or refillable applicator]: 2% (45 g)
  Monistat® 3: 4% (15 g, 25 g)
  Monistat® 7: 2% (45 g)
Liquid, spray, topical, as nitrate:
Micatin® Athlete's Foot:: 2% (90 mL) [contains alcohol]
Neosporin AF®: 2% (105 mL)
Lotion, powder, as nitrate (Zeasorb®-AF): 2% (56 g) [contains alcohol 36%]
Ointment, topical, as nitrate:
  Aloe Vesta® 2-n-1 Antifungal: 2% (60 g, 150 g)
  DermaFungal: 2% (113 g)
  Dermagran® AF: (113 g ) [contains vitamin A and zinc]
Powder, topical, as nitrate:
  Lotrimin® AF: 2% (160 g)
  Micro-Guard®: 2% (90 g)
  Mitrazol™: 2% (30 g)
  Zeasorb®-AF: 2% (70 g)
Powder spray, topical, as nitrate:
  Lotrimin® AF, Lotrimin® AF Jock Itch: 2% (140 g)
  Micatin® Athlete's Foot, Micatin® Jock Itch: 2% (90 g) [contains alcohol]
  Neosporin® AF: 2% (85 g)
Suppository, vaginal, as nitrate: 100 mg (7s); 200 mg (3s)
  Monistat® 3: 200 mg (3s)
  Monistat® 7: 100 mg (7s)
Tablet, effervescent, topical, as nitrate (DiabetAid™ Antifungal Foot Bath): 2% (10s)

Tincture, topical, as nitrate (Fungoid®): 2% (30 mL, 473 mL) [contains isopropyl alcohol 30%]; 30 mL size also available in a treatment kit which contains nail scrub and nail brush]

**miconazole nitrate** *see* miconazole *on page 537*

**Micozole [Can]** *see* miconazole *on page 537*

**MICRhoGAM® [US]** *see* Rh₀(D) immune globulin *on page 717*

**microfibrillar collagen hemostat** *see* collagen hemostat *on page 206*

**Microgestin™ [US]** *see* ethinyl estradiol and norethindrone *on page 314*

**Microgestin™ Fe [US]** *see* ethinyl estradiol and norethindrone *on page 314*

**Micro-Guard® [US-OTC]** *see* miconazole *on page 537*

**microK® [US]** *see* potassium chloride *on page 663*

**microK® 10 [US]** *see* potassium chloride *on page 663*

**Micro-K Extencaps® [Can]** *see* potassium chloride *on page 663*

**Micro-K® LS *(Discontinued)*** *see* potassium chloride *on page 663*

**Microlipid™ [US-OTC]** *see* nutritional formula, enteral/oral *on page 591*

**Micronase® [US]** *see* glyburide *on page 378*

**microNefrin® *(Discontinued)*** *see* epinephrine *on page 287*

**Micronor® [US/Can]** *see* norethindrone *on page 582*

**Microzide™ [US]** *see* hydrochlorothiazide *on page 409*

**Midamor® *(Discontinued)*** *see* amiloride *on page 39*

## midazolam (MID aye zoe lam)

**Sound-Alike/Look-Alike Issues**
Versed® may be confused with VePesid®, Vistaril®

**Synonyms** midazolam hydrochloride

**U.S./Canadian Brand Names** Apo-Midazolam® [Can]

**Therapeutic Category** Benzodiazepine

**Controlled Substance** C-IV

**Use** Preoperative sedation and provides conscious sedation prior to diagnostic or radiographic procedures; ICU sedation (continuous infusion); intravenous anesthesia (induction); intravenous anesthesia (maintenance)

**Usual Dosage** The dose of midazolam needs to be individualized based on the patient's age, underlying diseases, and concurrent medications. Decrease dose (by ~30%) if narcotics or other CNS depressants are administered concomitantly. **Personnel and equipment needed for standard respiratory resuscitation should be immediately available during midazolam administration.**

Children <6 years may require higher doses and closer monitoring than older children; calculate dose on ideal body weight

Conscious sedation for procedures or preoperative sedation:

Oral: 0.25-0.5 mg/kg as a single dose preprocedure, up to a maximum of 20 mg; administer 30-45 minutes prior to procedure. Children <6 years or less cooperative patients may require as much as 1 mg/kg as a single dose; 0.25 mg/kg may suffice for children 6-16 years of age.

Intranasal (not an approved route): 0.2 mg/kg (up to 0.4 mg/kg in some studies), to a maximum of 15 mg; may be administered 30-45 minutes prior to procedure

I.M.: 0.1-0.15 mg/kg 30-60 minutes before surgery or procedure; range 0.05-0.15 mg/kg; doses up to 0.5 mg/kg have been used in more anxious patients; maximum total dose: 10 mg

I.V.:

Infants <6 months: Limited information is available in nonintubated infants; dosing recommendations not clear; infants <6 months are at higher risk for airway obstruction and hypoventilation; titrate dose in small increments to desired effect; monitor carefully

Infants 6 months to Children 5 years: Initial: 0.05-0.1 mg/kg; titrate dose carefully; total dose of 0.6 mg/kg may be required; usual maximum total dose: 6 mg

Children 6-12 years: Initial: 0.025-0.05 mg/kg; titrate dose carefully; total doses of 0.4 mg/kg may be required; usual maximum total dose: 10 mg

Children 12-16 years: Dose as adults; usual maximum total dose: 10 mg

(Continued)

## midazolam *(Continued)*

Conscious sedation during mechanical ventilation: Children: Loading dose: 0.05-0.2 mg/kg, followed by initial continuous infusion: 0.06-0.12 mg/kg/hour (1-2 mcg/kg/minute); titrate to the desired effect; usual range: 0.4-6 mcg/kg/minute

Adults:

Preoperative sedation:

I.M.: 0.07-0.08 mg/kg 30-60 minutes prior to surgery/procedure; usual dose: 5 mg; **Note:** Reduce dose in patients with COPD, high-risk patients, patients ≥60 years of age, and patients receiving other narcotics or CNS depressants

I.V.: 0.02-0.04 mg/kg; repeat every 5 minutes as needed to desired effect or up to 0.1-0.2 mg/kg

Intranasal (not an approved route): 0.2 mg/kg (up to 0.4 mg/kg in some studies); administer 30-45 minutes prior to surgery/procedure

Conscious sedation: I.V.: Initial: 0.5-2 mg slow I.V. over at least 2 minutes; slowly titrate to effect by repeating doses every 2-3 minutes if needed; usual total dose: 2.5-5 mg

Healthy Adults <60 years: Some patients respond to doses as low as 1 mg; no more than 2.5 mg should be administered over a period of 2 minutes. Additional doses of midazolam may be administered after a 2-minute waiting period and evaluation of sedation after each dose increment. A total dose >5 mg is generally not needed. If narcotics or other CNS depressants are administered concomitantly, the midazolam dose should be reduced by 30%.

Anesthesia: I.V.:

Induction:

Unpremedicated patients: 0.3-0.35 mg/kg (up to 0.6 mg/kg in resistant cases)

Premedicated patients: 0.15-0.35 mg/kg

Maintenance: 0.05-0.3 mg/kg as needed, or continuous infusion 0.25-1.5 mcg/kg/minute

Sedation in mechanically-ventilated patients: I.V. continuous infusion: 100 mg in 250 mL $D_5W$ or NS (if patient is fluid-restricted, may concentrate up to a maximum of 0.5 mg/mL); initial dose: 0.02-0.08 mg/kg (~1 mg to 5 mg in 70 kg adult) initially and either repeated at 5-15 minute intervals until adequate sedation is achieved or continuous infusion rates of 0.04-0.2 mg/kg/hour and titrate to reach desired level of sedation

**Dosage Forms**

Injection, solution: 1 mg/mL (2 mL, 5 mL, 10 mL); 5 mg/mL (1 mL, 2 mL, 5 mL, 10 mL) [contains benzyl alcohol 1%]

Injection, solution [preservative free]: 1 mg/mL (2 mL, 5 mL); 5 mg/mL (1 mL, 2 mL)

Syrup: 2 mg/mL (118 mL) [contains sodium benzoate; cherry flavor]

**midazolam hydrochloride** *see* midazolam *on previous page*

## midodrine *(MI doe dreen)*

**Sound-Alike/Look-Alike Issues**

ProAmatine® may be confused with protamine

**Synonyms** midodrine hydrochloride

**U.S./Canadian Brand Names** Amatine® [Can]; Orvaten™ [US]; ProAmatine® [US]

**Therapeutic Category** Alpha-Adrenergic Agonist

**Use Orphan drug:** Treatment of symptomatic orthostatic hypotension

**Usual Dosage** Adults: Oral: 10 mg 3 times/day during daytime hours (every 3-4 hours) when patient is upright (maximum: 40 mg/day)

**Dosage Forms** Tablet, as hydrochloride: 2.5 mg, 5 mg, 10 mg

**midodrine hydrochloride** *see* midodrine *on this page*

**Midol® Cramp and Body Aches [US-OTC]** *see* ibuprofen *on page 427*

**Midrin® [US]** *see* acetaminophen, isometheptene, and dichloralphenazone *on page 12*

**Mifeprex® [US]** *see* mifepristone *on this page*

## mifepristone *(mi FE pris tone)*

**Sound-Alike/Look-Alike Issues**

Mifeprex® may be confused with Mirapex®

Synonyms RU-38486; RU-486

U.S./Canadian Brand Names Mifeprex® [US]

Therapeutic Category Abortifacient; Antineoplastic Agent, Hormone Antagonist; Antiprogestin

Use Medical termination of intrauterine pregnancy, through day 49 of pregnancy. Patients may need treatment with misoprostol and possibly surgery to complete therapy

Usual Dosage Oral: Adults:

Termination of pregnancy: Treatment consists of three office visits by the patient; the patient must read medication guide and sign patient agreement prior to treatment:

Day 1: 600 mg (three 200 mg tablets) taken as a single dose under physician supervision

Day 3: Patient must return to the healthcare provider 2 days following administration of mifepristone; if termination of pregnancy cannot be confirmed using ultrasound or clinical examination: 400 mcg (two 200 mcg tablets) of misoprostol; patient may need treatment for cramps or gastrointestinal symptoms at this time

Day 14: Patient must return to the healthcare provider ~14 days after administration of mifepristone; confirm complete termination of pregnancy by ultrasound or clinical exam. Surgical termination is recommended to manage treatment failures.

Dosage Forms Tablet: 200 mg

## miglitol (MIG li tol)

U.S./Canadian Brand Names Glyset® [US/Can]

Therapeutic Category Antidiabetic Agent, Oral

Use Type 2 diabetes mellitus (noninsulin-dependent, NIDDM):

Monotherapy adjunct to diet to improve glycemic control in patients with type 2 diabetes mellitus (noninsulin-dependent, NIDDM) whose hyperglycemia cannot be managed with diet alone

Combination therapy with a sulfonylurea when diet plus either miglitol or a sulfonylurea alone do not result in adequate glycemic control. The effect of miglitol to enhance glycemic control is additive to that of sulfonylureas when used in combination.

Usual Dosage Adults: Oral: 25 mg 3 times/day with the first bite of food at each meal; the dose may be increased to 50 mg 3 times/day after 4-8 weeks; maximum recommended dose: 100 mg 3 times/day

Dosage Forms Tablet: 25 mg, 50 mg, 100 mg

## miglustat (MIG loo stat)

Synonyms OGT-918

U.S./Canadian Brand Names Zavesca® [US/Can]

Therapeutic Category Enzyme Inhibitor

Use Treatment of mild-to-moderate type 1 Gaucher disease when enzyme replacement therapy is not a therapeutic option

Usual Dosage Oral: Adults: Type 1 Gaucher disease: 100 mg 3 times/day; dose may be reduced to 100 mg 1-2 times/day in patients with adverse effects (ie, tremor, GI distress)

Dosage Forms Capsule: 100 mg

**Migranal® [US/Can]** see dihydroergotamine on page 250

**Migrapap® (Discontinued)** see acetaminophen, isometheptene, and dichloralphenazone on page 12

**Migratine® (Discontinued)** see acetaminophen, isometheptene, and dichloralphenazone on page 12

**Migrin-A [US]** see acetaminophen, isometheptene, and dichloralphenazone on page 12

**milk of magnesia** see magnesium hydroxide on page 498

**Milontin® (Discontinued)**

**Milophene® [Can]** see clomiphene on page 196

**Milophene® (Discontinued)** see clomiphene on page 196

## milrinone (MIL ri none)

Sound-Alike/Look-Alike Issues

Primacor® may be confused with Primaxin®

Synonyms milrinone lactate

U.S./Canadian Brand Names Primacor® [US/Can]

Therapeutic Category Cardiovascular Agent, Other

Use Short-term I.V. therapy of congestive heart failure; calcium antagonist intoxication

(Continued)

# milrinone *(Continued)*

**Usual Dosage** Adults: I.V.: Loading dose: 50 mcg/kg administered over 10 minutes followed by a maintenance dose titrated according to the hemodynamic and clinical response

**Dosage Forms** [DSC] = Discontinued product
Infusion [premixed in D$_5$W] (Primacor®): 200 mcg/mL (100 mL, 200 mL)
Injection, solution: 1 mg/mL (10 mL, 20 mL, 50 mL)
 Primacor®: 1 mg/mL (10 mL, 20 mL; 50 mL [DSC])

**milrinone lactate** *see* milrinone *on previous page*

**Miltown® [US]** *see* meprobamate *on page 514*

**Mindal DM [US]** *see* guaifenesin and dextromethorphan *on page 385*

**mineral oil, coal tar, and lanolin** *see* coal tar, lanolin, and mineral oil *on page 202*

**mineral oil, lanolin, and coal tar** *see* coal tar, lanolin, and mineral oil *on page 202*

**mineral oil, petrolatum, lanolin, cetyl alcohol, and glycerin** *see* lanolin, cetyl alcohol, glycerin, petrolatum, and mineral oil *on page 466*

**Minestrin™ 1/20 [Can]** *see* ethinyl estradiol and norethindrone *on page 314*

**Minidyne® [US-OTC]** *see* povidone-iodine *on page 668*

**Mini-Gamulin® Rh** *(Discontinued)*

**Minipress® [US/Can]** *see* prazosin *on page 672*

**Minirin® [Can]** *see* desmopressin acetate *on page 230*

**Minitran™ [US/Can]** *see* nitroglycerin *on page 578*

**Minizide® [US]** *see* prazosin and polythiazide *on page 672*

**Minocin® [US/Can]** *see* minocycline *on this page*

## minocycline *(mi noe SYE kleen)*

**Sound-Alike/Look-Alike Issues**
Dynacin® may be confused with Dyazide®, Dynabac®, DynaCirc®, Dynapen®
Minocin® may be confused with Indocin®, Lincocin®, Minizide®, Mithracin®, niacin

**Synonyms** minocycline hydrochloride

**U.S./Canadian Brand Names** Alti-Minocycline [Can]; Apo-Minocycline® [Can]; Dynacin® [US]; Gen-Minocycline [Can]; Minocin® [US/Can]; myrac™ [US]; Novo-Minocycline [Can]; PMS-Minocycline [Can]; Rhoxal-minocycline [Can]

**Therapeutic Category** Tetracycline Derivative

**Use** Treatment of susceptible bacterial infections of both gram-negative and gram-positive organisms; treatment of anthrax (inhalational, cutaneous, and gastrointestinal); acne; meningococcal carrier state; Rickettsial diseases (including Rocky Mountain spotted fever, Q fever); nongonococcal urethritis, gonorrhea; acute intestinal amebiasis

**Usual Dosage** Oral:
Children >8 years: Initial: 4 mg/kg followed by 2 mg/kg/dose every 12 hours
Adults:
Susceptible infections: 200 mg initially, followed by 100 mg every 12 hours, not to exceed 400 mg/24 hours
Acne: 50-100 mg daily
Chlamydial or *Ureaplasma urealyticum* infection, uncomplicated: Urethral, endocervical, or rectal: 100 mg every 12 hours for at least 7 days
Gonococcal infection, uncomplicated (males): Without urethritis or anorectal infection: 200 mg initially, followed by 100 mg every 12 hours for at least 4 days (cultures 2-3 days post-therapy)
Gonococcal infection, uncomplicated urethritis: 100 mg every 12 hours for 5 days
Meningococcal carrier state: 100 mg every 12 hours for 5 days
*Mycobacterium marinum*: 100 mg every 12 hours for 6-8 weeks (**Note:** Optimal doses have not been established)
Syphilis: 200 mg initially, followed by 100 mg every 12 hours for 10-15 days

**Dosage Forms** [DSC] = Discontinued product
Capsule: 50 mg, 75 mg, 100 mg
 Dynacin®: 50 mg [DSC], 75 mg, 100 mg
Capsule, pellet-filled (Minocin®): 50 mg, 100 mg
Tablet (Dynacin®, myrac™): 50 mg, 75 mg, 100 mg

**minocycline hydrochloride** *see* minocycline *on previous page*

**Min-Ovral® [Can]** *see* ethinyl estradiol and levonorgestrel *on page 312*

**Minox [Can]** *see* minoxidil *on this page*

## minoxidil (mi NOKS i dil)

### Sound-Alike/Look-Alike Issues
minoxidil may be confused with metolazone, Monopril®
Loniten® may be confused with clonidine, Lioresal®, Lotensin®

**U.S./Canadian Brand Names** Apo-Gain® [Can]; Loniten® [US]; Minox [Can]; Rogaine® Extra Strength for Men [US-OTC]; Rogaine® for Men [US-OTC]; Rogaine® for Women [US-OTC]; Rogaine® [Can]

**Therapeutic Category** Topical Skin Product; Vasodilator

**Use** Management of severe hypertension (usually in combination with a diuretic and beta-blocker); treatment (topical formulation) of alopecia androgenetica in males and females

### Usual Dosage
Children <12 years: Hypertension: Oral: Initial: 0.1-0.2 mg/kg once daily; maximum: 5 mg/day; increase gradually every 3 days; usual dosage: 0.25-1 mg/kg/day in 1-2 divided doses; maximum: 50 mg/day
Children >12 years and Adults: Hypertension: Oral: Initial: 5 mg once daily, increase gradually every 3 days (maximum: 100 mg/day); usual dose range (JNC 7): 2.5-80 mg/day in 1-2 divided doses
Adults: Alopecia: Topical: Apply twice daily; 4 months of therapy may be necessary for hair growth.

### Dosage Forms [DSC] = Discontinued product
Solution, topical: 2% [20 mg/metered dose] (60 mL); 5% [50 mg/metered dose] (60 mL)
 Rogaine® for Men, Rogaine® for Women: 2% [20 mg/metered dose] (60 mL)
 Rogaine® Extra Strength for Men: 5% [50 mg/metered dose] (60 mL)
 Tablet: 2.5 mg, 10 mg
 Loniten®: 2.5 mg [DSC], 10 mg

**Mintab DM [US]** *see* guaifenesin and dextromethorphan *on page 385*

**Mintezol® [US]** *see* thiabendazole *on page 796*

**Mintox Extra Strength [US-OTC]** *see* aluminum hydroxide, magnesium hydroxide, and simethicone *on page 35*

**Mintox Plus [US-OTC]** *see* aluminum hydroxide, magnesium hydroxide, and simethicone *on page 35*

**Mintuss HC [US]** *see* phenylephrine, hydrocodone, and chlorpheniramine *on page 643*

**Mintuss HD [US]** *see* phenylephrine, hydrocodone, and chlorpheniramine *on page 643*

**Mintuss MS [US]** *see* phenylephrine, hydrocodone, and chlorpheniramine *on page 643*

**Minute-Gel® *(Discontinued)*** *see* fluoride *on page 347*

**Miochol-E® [US/Can]** *see* acetylcholine *on page 14*

**Miostat® [US/Can]** *see* carbachol *on page 140*

**MiraLax™ [US]** *see* polyethylene glycol-electrolyte solution *on page 658*

**Mirapex® [US/Can]** *see* pramipexole *on page 669*

**Miraphen PSE [US]** *see* guaifenesin and pseudoephedrine *on page 388*

**Mircette® [US]** *see* ethinyl estradiol and desogestrel *on page 309*

**Mirena® [US/Can]** *see* levonorgestrel *on page 476*

## mirtazapine (mir TAZ a peen)

### Sound-Alike/Look-Alike Issues
Remeron® may be confused with Premarin®, Zemuron®

**U.S./Canadian Brand Names** Gen-Mirtazapine [Can]; Novo-Mirtazapine [Can]; PMS-Mirtazapine [Can]; Remeron SolTab® [US]; Remeron® RD [Can]; Remeron® [US/Can]; Rhoxal-mirtazapine [Can]

**Therapeutic Category** Antidepressant, Alpha-2 Antagonist

**Use** Treatment of depression

### Usual Dosage
Children: Safety and efficacy in children have not been established
Treatment of depression: Adults: Oral: Initial: 15 mg nightly, titrate up to 15-45 mg/day with dose increases made no more frequently than every 1-2 weeks; there is an inverse relationship between dose and sedation
(Continued)

# mirtazapine *(Continued)*

**Dosage Forms**
Tablet (Remeron®): 15 mg, 30 mg, 45 mg
Tablet, orally-disintegrating: 15 mg, 30 mg
Remeron SolTab®:
15 mg [contains phenylalanine 2.6 mg/tablet; orange flavor]
30 mg [contains phenylalanine 5.2 mg/tablet; orange flavor]
45 mg [contains phenylalanine 7.8 mg/tablet; orange flavor]

# misoprostol *(mye soe PROST ole)*

**Sound-Alike/Look-Alike Issues**
misoprostol may be confused with metoprolol
Cytotec® may be confused with Cytoxan®, Sytobex®
**U.S./Canadian Brand Names** Apo-Misoprostol® [Can]; Cytotec® [US]; Novo-Misoprostol [Can]
**Therapeutic Category** Prostaglandin
**Use** Prevention of NSAID-induced gastric ulcers; medical termination of pregnancy of ≤49 days (in conjunction with mifepristone)
**Usual Dosage** Oral: Adults:
Prevention of NSAID-induced gastric ulcers: 200 mcg 4 times/day with food; if not tolerated, may decrease dose to 100 mcg 4 times/day with food or 200 mcg twice daily with food; last dose of the day should be taken at bedtime
Medical termination of pregnancy: Refer to mifepristone monograph.
**Dosage Forms** Tablet: 100 mcg, 200 mcg

**misoprostol and diclofenac** *see diclofenac and misoprostol on page 244*

**Mito-Carn®** *(Discontinued) see levocarnitine on page 474*

# mitomycin *(mye toe MYE sin)*

**Sound-Alike/Look-Alike Issues**
mitomycin may be confused with mithramycin, mitotane, mitoxantrone, Mutamycin®
Mutamycin® may be confused with mitomycin
**Synonyms** mitomycin-C; mitomycin-X; MTC; NSC-26980
**U.S./Canadian Brand Names** Mutamycin® [US/Can]
**Therapeutic Category** Antineoplastic Agent
**Use** Treatment of adenocarcinoma of stomach or pancreas, bladder cancer, breast cancer, or colorectal cancer
**Usual Dosage** Refer to individual protocols. Children and Adults:
Single agent therapy: I.V.: 20 mg/m$^2$ every 6-8 weeks
Combination therapy: I.V.: 10 mg/m$^2$ every 6-8 weeks
Bladder carcinoma: Intravesicular instillation (unapproved route): 20-40 mg/dose instilled into the bladder for 3 hours repeated up to 3 times/week for up to 20 procedures per course
**Dosage Forms** Injection, powder for reconstitution: 5 mg, 20 mg, 40 mg

**mitomycin-X** *see mitomycin on this page*

**mitomycin-C** *see mitomycin on this page*

# mitotane *(MYE toe tane)*

**Sound-Alike/Look-Alike Issues**
mitotane may be confused with mitomycin
**Synonyms** NSC-38721; o,p'-DDD
**U.S./Canadian Brand Names** Lysodren® [US/Can]
**Therapeutic Category** Antineoplastic Agent
**Use** Treatment of adrenocortical carcinoma
**Usual Dosage** Oral:
Children: 0.1-0.5 mg/kg or 1-2 g/day in divided doses increasing gradually to a maximum of 5-7 g/day
Adults: Start at 1-6 g/day in divided doses, then increase incrementally to 8-10 g/day in 3-4 divided doses (maximum daily dose: 18 g)
**Dosage Forms** Tablet [scored]: 500 mg

# mitoxantrone (mye toe ZAN trone)

**Sound-Alike/Look-Alike Issues**
mitoxantrone may be confused with methotrexate, mitomycin

**Synonyms** DAD; DHAD; DHAQ; dihydroxyanthracenedione dihydrochloride; mitoxantrone hydrochloride CL-232315; mitozantrone; NSC-301739

**U.S./Canadian Brand Names** Novantrone® [US/Can]

**Therapeutic Category** Antineoplastic Agent

**Use** Treatment of acute leukemias, lymphoma, breast cancer, pediatric sarcoma, progressive or relapsing-remitting multiple sclerosis, prostate cancer

**Usual Dosage** Refer to individual protocols. I.V. (dilute in $D_5W$ or NS):
Acute leukemias:
Children ≤2 years: 0.4 mg/kg/day once daily for 3-5 days
Children >2 years and Adults: 8-12 mg/m$^2$/day once daily for 4-5 days
Solid tumors:
Children: 18-20 mg/m$^2$ every 3-4 weeks **or** 5-8 mg/m$^2$ every week
Adults: 12-14 mg/m$^2$ every 3-4 weeks **or** 2-4 mg/m$^2$/day for 5 days every 4 weeks
Hormone-refractory prostate cancer: Adults: 12-14 mg/m$^2$
Multiple sclerosis: Adults: 12 mg/m$^2$ every 3 months (maximum lifetime cumulative dose: 140 mg/m$^2$

**Dosage Forms** Injection, solution: 2 mg/mL (10 mL, 12.5 mL, 15 mL)

**mitoxantrone hydrochloride CL-232315** *see* mitoxantrone *on this page*

**mitozantrone** *see* mitoxantrone *on this page*

**Mitran® Oral *(Discontinued)*** *see* chlordiazepoxide *on page 167*

**Mitrazol™ [US-OTC]** *see* miconazole *on page 537*

**Mivacron® [US/Can]** *see* mivacurium *on this page*

# mivacurium (mye va KYOO ree um)

**Sound-Alike/Look-Alike Issues**
Mivacron® may be confused with Mevacor®

**Synonyms** mivacurium chloride

**U.S./Canadian Brand Names** Mivacron® [US/Can]

**Therapeutic Category** Skeletal Muscle Relaxant

**Use** Adjunct to general anesthesia to facilitate endotracheal intubation and to relax skeletal muscles during surgery; to facilitate mechanical ventilation in ICU patients; does not relieve pain or produce sedation

**Usual Dosage** Continuous infusion requires an infusion pump; dose to effect; doses will vary due to interpatient variability; use ideal body weight for obese patients

Children 2-12 years (duration of action is shorter and dosage requirements are higher): 0.2 mg/kg I.V. followed by average infusion rate of 14 mcg/kg/minute (range: 5-31 mcg/kg/minute) upon evidence of spontaneous recovery from initial dose

Adults: Initial: I.V.: 0.15-0.25 mg/kg bolus followed by maintenance doses of 0.1 mg/kg at approximately 15-minute intervals; for prolonged neuromuscular block, initial infusion of 9-10 mcg/kg/minute is used upon evidence of spontaneous recovery from initial dose, usual infusion rate of 6-7 mcg/kg/minute (1-15 mcg/kg/minute) under balanced anesthesia; initial dose after succinylcholine for intubation (balanced anesthesia): Adults: 0.1 mg/kg
Pretreatment/priming: 10% of intubating dose given 3-5 minutes before initial dose

**Dosage Forms**
Injection, solution [preservative free]: 2 mg/mL (5 mL, 10 mL)
Injection, solution: 2 mg/mL (20 mL, 50 mL) [with benzyl alcohol]

**mivacurium chloride** *see* mivacurium *on this page*

**MK383** *see* tirofiban *on page 806*

**MK462** *see* rizatriptan *on page 727*

**MK594** *see* losartan *on page 492*

**MK0826** *see* ertapenem *on page 294*

**MK 869** *see* aprepitant *on page 67*

**MLN341** *see* bortezomib *on page 110*

**MMF** *see* mycophenolate *on page 554*

**MMR** *see* measles, mumps, and rubella vaccines, combined *on page 504*

**Moban**® **[US/Can]** *see* molindone *on next page*

**Mobic**® **[US/Can]** *see* meloxicam *on page 509*

**Mobicox**® **[Can]** *see* meloxicam *on page 509*

**Mobidin**® *(Discontinued) see* magnesium salicylate *on page 499*

**Mobisyl**® **[US-OTC]** *see* triethanolamine salicylate *on page 823*

## moclobemide *(Canada only)* (moe KLOE be mide)

**U.S./Canadian Brand Names** Alti-Moclobemide [Can]; Apo-Moclobemide® [Can]; Manerix® [Can]; Novo-Moclobemide [Can]; Nu-Moclobemide [Can]; PMS-Moclobemide [Can]

**Therapeutic Category** Antidepressant, Monoamine Oxidase Inhibitor

**Use** Symptomatic relief of depressive illness

**Usual Dosage** Oral: Adults: Initial: 300 mg/day in 2 divided doses; increase gradually to maximum of 600 mg/day; **Note:** Individual patient response may allow a reduction in daily dose in long-term therapy.

**Dosage Forms** Tablet: 150 mg, 300 mg

## modafinil (moe DAF i nil)

**U.S./Canadian Brand Names** Alertec® [Can]; Provigil® [US/Can]

**Therapeutic Category** Central Nervous System Stimulant, Nonamphetamine

**Controlled Substance** C-IV

**Use** Improve wakefulness in patients with excessive daytime sleepiness associated with narcolepsy and shift work sleep disorder (SWSD); adjunctive therapy for obstructive sleep apnea/hypopnea syndrome (OSAHS)

**Usual Dosage** Oral: Adults:

Narcolepsy, OSAHS: Initial: 200 mg as a single daily dose in the morning

SWSD: Initial: 200 mg as a single dose taken ~1 hour prior to start of work shift

**Note:** Doses of 400 mg/day, given as a single dose, have been well tolerated, but there is no consistent evidence that this dose confers additional benefit

**Dosage Forms** Tablet: 100 mg, 200 mg

**Modane**® **Bulk [US-OTC]** *see* psyllium *on page 697*

**Modane**® **Soft** *(Discontinued) see* docusate *on page 263*

**Modane Tablets**® **[US-OTC]** *see* bisacodyl *on page 107*

**Modecate**® **[Can]** *see* fluphenazine *on page 351*

**Modicon**® **[US]** *see* ethinyl estradiol and norethindrone *on page 314*

**modified Dakin's solution** *see* sodium hypochlorite solution *on page 754*

**Moducal**® **[US-OTC]** *see* glucose polymers *on page 377*

**Modulon**® **[Can]** *see* trimebutine *(Canada only) on page 824*

**Moduretic**® **[Can]** *see* amiloride and hydrochlorothiazide *on page 40*

**Moduretic**® *(Discontinued) see* amiloride and hydrochlorothiazide *on page 40*

## moexipril (mo EKS i pril)

**Sound-Alike/Look-Alike Issues**

moexipril may be confused with Monopril®

**Synonyms** moexipril hydrochloride

**U.S./Canadian Brand Names** Univasc® [US]

**Therapeutic Category** Angiotensin-Converting Enzyme (ACE) Inhibitor

**Use** Treatment of hypertension, alone or in combination with thiazide diuretics; treatment of left ventricular dysfunction after myocardial infarction

**Usual Dosage** Adults: Oral: Initial: 7.5 mg once daily (in patients **not** receiving diuretics), 1 hour prior to a meal **or** 3.75 mg once daily (when combined with thiazide diuretics); maintenance dose: 7.5-30 mg/day in 1 or 2 divided doses 1 hour before meals

**Dosage Forms** Tablet, as hydrochloride [film coated, scored]: 7.5 mg, 15 mg

## moexipril and hydrochlorothiazide (mo EKS i pril & hye droe klor oh THYE a zide)
**Synonyms** hydrochlorothiazide and moexipril
**U.S./Canadian Brand Names** Uniretic® [US/Can]
**Therapeutic Category** Angiotensin-Converting Enzyme (ACE) Inhibitor; Diuretic, Thiazide
**Use** Combination therapy for hypertension, however, not indicated for initial treatment of hypertension; replacement therapy in patients receiving separate dosage forms (for patient convenience); when monotherapy with one component fails to achieve desired antihypertensive effect, or when dose-limiting adverse effects limit upward titration of monotherapy
**Usual Dosage** Adults: Oral: 7.5-30 mg of moexipril, taken either in a single or divided dose one hour before meals; hydrochlorothiazide dose should be ≤50 mg/day
**Dosage Forms** Tablet [film coated, scored]:
7.5/12.5: Moexipril hydrochloride 7.5 mg and hydrochlorothiazide 12.5 mg
15/12.5: Moexipril hydrochloride 15 mg and hydrochlorothiazide 12.5 mg
15/25: Moexipril hydrochloride 15 mg and hydrochlorothiazide 25 mg

**moexipril hydrochloride** *see* moexipril *on previous page*

**Moi-Stir® [US-OTC]** *see* saliva substitute *on page 737*

**Moisture® Eyes [US-OTC]** *see* artificial tears *on page 71*

**Moisture® Eyes PM [US-OTC]** *see* artificial tears *on page 71*

## molindone (moe LIN done)
**Sound-Alike/Look-Alike Issues**
molindone may be confused with Mobidin®
Moban® may be confused with Mobidin®, Modane®
**Synonyms** molindone hydrochloride
**U.S./Canadian Brand Names** Moban® [US/Can]
**Therapeutic Category** Antipsychotic Agent, Dihydroindoline
**Use** Management of schizophrenia
**Usual Dosage** Oral:
Children: Schizophrenia/psychoses:
3-5 years: 1-2.5 mg/day in 4 divided doses
5-12 years: 0.5-1 mg/kg/day in 4 divided doses
Adults: Schizophrenia/psychoses: 50-75 mg/day increase at 3- to 4-day intervals up to 225 mg/day
**Dosage Forms** Tablet, as hydrochloride: 5 mg, 10 mg, 25 mg, 50 mg

**molindone hydrochloride** *see* molindone *on this page*

**molybdenum** *see* trace metals *on page 813*

**Molypen® [US]** *see* trace metals *on page 813*

**MOM** *see* magnesium hydroxide *on page 498*

**Momentum® [US-OTC]** *see* magnesium salicylate *on page 499*

## mometasone furoate (moe MET a sone FYOOR oh ate)
**U.S./Canadian Brand Names** Asmanex® Twisthaler® [US]; Elocom® [Can]; Elocon® [US]; Nasonex® [US/Can]; ratio-Mometasone [Can]
**Therapeutic Category** Corticosteroid, Intranasal; Corticosteroid, Topical
**Use** Relief of the inflammatory and pruritic manifestations of corticosteroid-responsive dermatoses (medium potency topical corticosteroid); treatment of nasal symptoms of seasonal and perennial allergic rhinitis; prevention of nasal symptoms associated with seasonal allergic rhinitis; treatment of nasal polyps in adults; maintenance treatment of asthma as prophylactic therapy or as a supplement in asthma patients requiring oral corticosteroids for the purpose of decreasing or eliminating the oral corticosteroid requirement
**Usual Dosage**
Oral inhalation: Children ≥12 years and Adults: Previous therapy:
Bronchodilators or inhaled corticosteroids: Initial: 1 inhalation (220 mcg) daily (maximum 2 inhalations or 440 mcg/day); may be given in the evening or in divided doses twice daily
Oral corticosteroids: Initial: 440 mcg twice daily (maximum 880 mcg/day); prednisone should be reduced no faster than 2.5 mg/day on a weekly basis, beginning after at least 1 week of mometasone furoate use
(Continued)

## mometasone furoate *(Continued)*

**Note:** Maximum effects may not be evident for 1-2 weeks or longer; dose should be titrated to effect, using the lowest possible dose

Nasal spray:

Allergic rhinitis:

Children 2-11 years: 1 spray (50 mcg) in each nostril daily

Children ≥12 years and Adults: 2 sprays (100 mcg) in each nostril daily; when used for the prevention of allergic rhinitis, treatment should begin 2-4 weeks prior to pollen season

Nasal polyps: Adults: 2 sprays (100 mcg) in each nostril twice daily; 2 sprays (100 mcg) once daily may be effective in some patients

Topical: Apply sparingly, do not use occlusive dressings. Therapy should be discontinued when control is achieved; if no improvement is seen in 2 weeks, reassessment of diagnosis may be necessary.

Cream, ointment: Children ≥2 years and Adults: Apply a thin film to affected area once daily; do not use in pediatric patients for longer than 3 weeks

Lotion: Children ≥12 years and Adults: Apply a few drops to affected area once daily

**Dosage Forms**

Cream, topical (Elocon®): 0.1% (15 g, 45 g)

Lotion, topical (Elocon®): 0.1% (30 mL, 60 mL) [contains isopropyl alcohol 40%]

Ointment, topical (Elocon®): 0.1% (15 g, 45 g)

Powder for oral inhalation (Asmanex® Twisthaler®): 220 mcg (30 units, 60 units, 120 units) [contains lactose]

Suspension, intranasal spray (Nasonex®): 50 mcg/spray (17 g) [delivers 120 sprays; contains benzalkonium chloride]

**MOM/mineral oil emulsion** *see* magnesium hydroxide and mineral oil emulsion *on page 499*

**monacolin K** *see* lovastatin *on page 494*

**Monafed® *(Discontinued)*** *see* guaifenesin *on page 383*

**Monafed® DM *(Discontinued)*** *see* guaifenesin and dextromethorphan *on page 385*

**Monarc® M [US]** *see* antihemophilic factor (human) *on page 55*

**Monilia skin test** *see* Candida albicans (Monilia) *on page 137*

**Monistat® [Can]** *see* miconazole *on page 537*

**Monistat® 1 Combination Pack [US-OTC]** *see* miconazole *on page 537*

**Monistat® 3 [US-OTC/Can]** *see* miconazole *on page 537*

**Monistat® 7 [US-OTC]** *see* miconazole *on page 537*

**Monistat-Derm® [US]** *see* miconazole *on page 537*

**Monistat i.v.™ Injection *(Discontinued)*** *see* miconazole *on page 537*

**Monitan® [Can]** *see* acebutolol *on page 4*

## monobenzone *(mon oh BEN zone)*

**U.S./Canadian Brand Names** Benoquin® [US]

**Therapeutic Category** Topical Skin Product

**Use** Final depigmentation in extensive vitiligo

**Usual Dosage** Children ≥12 years and Adults: Topical: Apply 2-3 times daily; once desired degree of pigmentation is obtained, may apply as needed (usually 2 times/week)

**Dosage Forms** Cream, topical: 20% (35 g)

**Monocaps [US-OTC]** *see* vitamins (multiple/oral) *on page 852*

**Monoclate-P® [US]** *see* antihemophilic factor (human) *on page 55*

**monoclonal antibody** *see* muromonab-CD3 *on page 554*

**Monocor® [Can]** *see* bisoprolol *on page 108*

**Monodox® [US]** *see* doxycycline *on page 271*

**monoethanolamine** *see* ethanolamine oleate *on page 308*

**Monoket® [US]** *see* isosorbide mononitrate *on page 452*

**MonoNessa™ [US]** *see* ethinyl estradiol and norgestimate *on page 317*

**Mononine® [US/Can]** *see* factor IX *on page 325*

**Monopril**® **[US/Can]** *see* fosinopril *on page 361*

**Monopril-HCT**® **[US/Can]** *see* fosinopril and hydrochlorothiazide *on page 361*

## montelukast (mon te LOO kast)
**Sound-Alike/Look-Alike Issues**
Singulair® may be confused with Sinequan®
**Synonyms** montelukast sodium
**U.S./Canadian Brand Names** Singulair® [US/Can]
**Therapeutic Category** Leukotriene Receptor Antagonist
**Use** Prophylaxis and chronic treatment of asthma; relief of symptoms of seasonal allergic rhinitis and perennial allergic rhinitis
**Usual Dosage** Oral:
Children:
6-23 months: Perennial allergic rhinitis: 4 mg (oral granules) once daily
12-23 months: Asthma: 4 mg (oral granules) once daily, taken in the evening
2-5 years: Asthma, seasonal or perennial allergic rhinitis: 4 mg (chewable tablet or oral granules) once daily, taken in the evening
6-14 years: Asthma, seasonal or perennial allergic rhinitis: Chew one 5 mg chewable tablet/day, taken in the evening
Children ≥15 years and Adults: Asthma, seasonal or perennial allergic rhinitis: 10 mg/day, taken in the evening
**Dosage Forms**
Granules: 4 mg/packet
Tablet: 10 mg
Tablet, chewable: 4 mg [contains phenylalanine 0.674 mg; cherry flavor]; 5 mg [contains phenylalanine 0.842 mg; cherry flavor]

**montelukast sodium** *see* montelukast *on this page*

**Monurol**™ **[US/Can]** *see* fosfomycin *on page 360*

**8-MOP** *see* methoxsalen *on page 527*

**more attenuated enders strain** *see* measles virus vaccine (live) *on page 504*

**MoreDophilus**® **[US-OTC]** *see* Lactobacillus *on page 462*

## moricizine (mor I siz een)
**Sound-Alike/Look-Alike Issues**
Ethmozine® may be confused with Erythrocin®, erythromycin
**Synonyms** moricizine hydrochloride
**U.S./Canadian Brand Names** Ethmozine® [US/Can]
**Therapeutic Category** Antiarrhythmic Agent, Class I
**Use** Treatment of ventricular tachycardia and life-threatening ventricular arrhythmias
**Usual Dosage** Adults: Oral: 200-300 mg every 8 hours, adjust dosage at 150 mg/day at 3-day intervals.
**Dosage Forms** Tablet, as hydrochloride: 200 mg, 250 mg, 300 mg

**moricizine hydrochloride** *see* moricizine *on this page*

**morning after pill** *see* ethinyl estradiol and norgestrel *on page 318*

**Morphine HP**® **[Can]** *see* morphine sulfate *on this page*

**Morphine LP**® **Epidural [Can]** *see* morphine sulfate *on this page*

## morphine sulfate (MOR feen SUL fate)
**Sound-Alike/Look-Alike Issues**
morphine may be confused with hydromorphone
morphine sulfate may be confused with magnesium sulfate
$MSO_4$ is an error-prone abbreviation (mistaken as magnesium sulfate)
Avinza™ may be confused with Evista®, Invanz®
Roxanol™ may be confused with OxyFast®, Roxicet™
**U.S./Canadian Brand Names** Astramorph/PF™ [US]; Avinza™ [US]; DepoDur™ [US]; Duramorph® [US]; Infumorph® [US]; Kadian® [US/Can]; M-Eslon® [Can]; M.O.S.-Sulfate® [Can]; Morphine HP® [Can]; Morphine LP® Epidural [Can]; MS Contin® [US/Can]; MS-IR® [Can]; Oramorph SR® [US]; PMS- (Continued)

# morphine sulfate *(Continued)*

Morphine Sulfate SR [Can]; ratio-Morphine SR [Can]; RMS® [US]; Roxanol 100™ [US]; Roxanol™ [US]; Roxanol™-T [US]; Statex® [Can]

**Therapeutic Category** Analgesic, Narcotic

**Controlled Substance** C-II

**Use** Relief of moderate to severe acute and chronic pain; relief of pain of myocardial infarction; relief of dyspnea of acute left ventricular failure and pulmonary edema; preanesthetic medication

DepoDur™: Epidural (lumbar) single-dose management of surgical pain

Infumorph®: Used in microinfusion devices for intraspinal administration in treatment of intractable chronic pain

**Usual Dosage Note:** These are guidelines and do not represent the doses that may be required in all patients. Doses should be titrated to pain relief/prevention.

**Children >6 months and <50 kg: Acute pain (moderate-to-severe):**
Oral (prompt release): 0.15-0.3 mg/kg every 3-4 hours as needed
I.M.: 0.1 mg/kg every 3-4 hours as needed
I.V.: 0.05-0.1 mg/kg every 3-4 hours as needed
I.V. infusion: Range: 10-30 mcg/kg/hour

**Adolescents >12 years: Sedation/analgesia for procedures:** I.V.: 3-4 mg and repeat in 5 minutes if necessary

**Adults:**

**Acute pain (moderate-to-severe):**
Oral: Prompt release formulations: Opiate-naive: Initial: 10 mg every 3-4 hours as needed; patients with prior opiate exposure may require higher initial doses: usual dosage range: 10-30 mg every 3-4 hours as needed

I.M., SubQ: **Note:** Repeated SubQ administration causes local tissue irritation, pain, and induration.
Initial: Opiate-naive: 5-10 mg every 3-4 hours as needed; patients with prior opiate exposure may require higher initial doses; usual dosage range: 5-20 mg every 3-4 hours as needed

Rectal: 10-20 mg every 3-4 hours

I.V.: Initial: Opiate-naive: 2.5-5 mg every 3-4 hours; patients with prior opiate exposure may require higher initial doses. **Note:** Repeated doses (up to every 5 minutes if needed) in small increments (eg, 1-4 mg) may be preferred to larger and less frequent doses.

I.V., SubQ continuous infusion: 0.8-10 mg/hour; usual range: Up to 80 mg/hour

Mechanically-ventilated patients (based on 70 kg patient): 0.7-10 mg every 1-2 hours as needed; infusion: 5-35 mg/hour

Patient-controlled analgesia (PCA): (Opiate-naive: Consider lower end of dosing range):
Usual concentration: 1 mg/mL
Demand dose: Usual: 1 mg; range: 0.5-2.5 mg
Lockout interval: 5-10 minutes

Intrathecal (I.T.): **Note:** Administer with extreme caution and in reduced dosage to geriatric or debilitated patients.
Opioid-naive: 0.2-0.25 mg/dose (may provide adequate relief for 24 hours); repeat doses are **not** recommended.

Epidural: **Note:** Administer with extreme caution and in reduced dosage to geriatric or debilitated patients. Vigilant monitoring is particularly important in these patients.
Pain management:
Single-dose (Duramorph®): Intial: 3-5 mg
Infusion:
Bolus dose: 1-6 mg
Infusion rate: 0.1-0.2 mg/hour
Maximum dose: 10 mg/24 hours

**Surgical anesthesia:** Epidural: Single-dose (extended release, Depo-Dur™): Lumbar epidural only; not recommended in patients <18 years of age:
Cesarean section: 10 mg
Lower abdominal/pelvic surgery: 10-15 mg
Major orthopedic surgery of lower extremity: 15 mg

For Depo-Dur™: To minimize the pharmacokinetic interaction resulting in higher peak serum concentrations of morphine, administer the test dose of the local anesthetic at least 15 minutes prior to Depo-Dur™ administration. Use of Depo-Dur™ with epidural local anesthetics has not been studied.

**Note:** Some patients may benefit from a 20 mg dose, however, the incidence of adverse effects may be increased.

**Chronic pain: Note:** Patients taking opioids chronically may become tolerant and require doses higher than the usual dosage range to maintain the desired effect. Tolerance can be managed by appropriate dose titration. There is no optimal or maximal dose for morphine in chronic pain. The appropriate dose is one that relieves pain throughout its dosing interval without causing unmanageable side effects.

Oral: Controlled-, extended-, or sustained-release formulations: A patient's morphine requirement should be established using prompt-release formulations. Conversion to long-acting products may be considered when chronic, continuous treatment is required. Higher dosages should be reserved for use only in opioid-tolerant patients.

Capsules, extended release (Avinza™): Daily dose administered once daily (for best results, administer at same time each day)

Capsules, sustained release (Kadian®): Daily dose administered once daily or in 2 divided doses daily (every 12 hours)

Tablets, controlled release (MS Contin®), sustained release (Oramorph SR®), or extended release: Daily dose divided and administered every 8 or every 12 hours

**Dosage Forms**

Capsule, extended release (Avinza™): 30 mg, 60 mg, 90 mg, 120 mg

Capsule, sustained release (Kadian®): 20 mg, 30 mg, 50 mg, 60 mg, 100 mg

Infusion [premixed in $D_5W$]: 1 mg/mL (100 mL, 250 mL)

Injection, extended release liposomal suspension [lumbar epidural injection, preservative free] (DepoDur™): 10 mg/mL (1 mL, 1.5 mL, 2 mL)

Injection, solution: 2 mg/mL (1 mL); 4 mg/mL (1 mL); 5 mg/mL (1 mL); 8 mg/mL (1 mL); 10 mg/mL (1 mL, 10 mL); 15 mg/mL (1 mL, 20 mL); 25 mg/mL (4 mL, 10 mL, 20 mL, 40 mL, 50 mL, 100 mL, 250 mL); 50 mg/mL (20 mL, 40 mL) [some preparations contain sodium metabisulfite]

Injection, solution [epidural, intrathecal, or I.V. infusion; preservative free]:

Astramorph/PF™: 0.5 mg/mL (2 mL, 10 mL); 1 mg/mL (2 mL, 10 mL)

Duramorph®: 0.5 mg/mL (10 mL); 1 mg/mL (10 mL)

Injection, solution [epidural or intrathecal infusion via microinfusion device; preservative free] (Infumorph®): 10 mg/mL (20 mL); 25 mg/mL (20 mL)

Injection, solution [I.V. infusion via PCA pump]: 0.5 mg/mL (30 mL); 1 mg/mL (30 mL, 50 mL); 2 mg/mL (30 mL); 5 mg/mL (30 mL, 50 mL)

Injection, solution [preservative free]: 0.5 mg/mL (10 mL); 1 mg/mL (10 mL); 25 mg/mL (4 mL, 10 mL, 20 mL)

Solution, oral: 10 mg/5 mL (5 mL, 10 mL, 100 mL, 500 mL); 20 mg/5 mL (100 mL, 500 mL); 20 mg/mL (30 mL, 120 mL, 240 mL)

Roxanol™: 20 mg/mL (30 mL, 120 mL)

Roxanol 100™: 100 mg/5 mL (240 mL) [with calibrated spoon]

Roxanol™-T: 20 mg/mL (30 mL, 120 mL) [tinted, flavored]

Suppository, rectal (RMS®): 5 mg (12s), 10 mg (12s), 20 mg (12s), 30 mg (12s)

Tablet: 15 mg, 30 mg

Tablet, controlled release (MS Contin®): 15 mg, 30 mg, 60 mg, 100 mg, 200 mg

Tablet, extended release: 15 mg, 30 mg, 60 mg, 100 mg, 200 mg

Tablet, sustained release (Oramorph SR®): 15 mg, 30 mg, 60 mg, 100 mg

## morrhuate sodium (MOR yoo ate SOW dee um)

**U.S./Canadian Brand Names** Scleromate® [US]

**Therapeutic Category** Sclerosing Agent

**Use** Treatment of small, uncomplicated varicose veins of the lower extremities

**Usual Dosage** Adults: I.V.: 50-250 mg, repeated at 5- to 7-day intervals (50-100 mg for small veins, 150-250 mg for large veins)

**Dosage Forms** Injection, solution: 50 mg/mL (30 mL)

**Mosco® Corn and Callus Remover [US-OTC]** see salicylic acid on page 734

**M.O.S.-Sulfate® [Can]** see morphine sulfate on page 549

**Motilium® [Can]** see domperidone (Canada only) on page 266

**Motofen® [US]** see difenoxin and atropine on page 247

**Motrin® [US]** see ibuprofen on page 427

**Motrin® Children's [US-OTC/Can]** see ibuprofen on page 427

**Motrin® Cold and Sinus [US-OTC]** see pseudoephedrine and ibuprofen on page 694

**Motrin® Cold, Children's [US-OTC]** see pseudoephedrine and ibuprofen on page 694

**Motrin® IB [US-OTC/Can]** see ibuprofen on page 427

**Motrin® IB Sinus (Discontinued)** see pseudoephedrine and ibuprofen on page 694

**Motrin® Infants' [US-OTC]** *see* ibuprofen *on page 427*

**Motrin® Junior Strength [US-OTC]** *see* ibuprofen *on page 427*

**Mouthkote® [US-OTC]** *see* saliva substitute *on page 737*

**moxifloxacin** (moxs i FLOKS a sin)

  **Sound-Alike/Look-Alike Issues**
    Avelox® may be confused with Avonex®
  **Synonyms** moxifloxacin hydrochloride
  **U.S./Canadian Brand Names** Avelox® I.V. [US]; Avelox® [US/Can]; Vigamox™ [US/Can]
  **Therapeutic Category** Antibiotic, Quinolone
  **Use** Treatment of mild-to-moderate community-acquired pneumonia, including multidrug-resistant *Streptococcus pneumoniae* (MDRSP); acute bacterial exacerbation of chronic bronchitis; acute bacterial sinusitis; complicated and uncomplicated skin and skin structure infections; bacterial conjunctivitis (ophthalmic formulation)
  **Usual Dosage**
    Ophthalmic: Children ≥1 year and Adults: Instill 1 drop into affected eye(s) 3 times/day for 7 days
    Oral, I.V.: Adults:
      Acute bacterial sinusitis: 400 mg every 24 hours for 10 days
      Chronic bronchitis, acute bacterial exacerbation: 400 mg every 24 hours for 5 days
      **Note:** Avelox® ABC Pack™ (Avelox® Bronchitis Course) contains five tablets of 400 mg each.
      Community-acquired pneumonia (including MDRSP): 400 mg every 24 hours for 7-14 days
      Complicated skin and skin structure infections: 400 mg every 24 hours for 7-21 days
      Uncomplicated skin and skin structure infections: 400 mg every 24 hours for 7 days
  **Dosage Forms**
    Infusion [premixed in sodium chloride 0.8%] (Avelox® I.V.): 400 mg (250 mL)
    Solution, ophthalmic (Vigamox™): 0.5% (3 mL)
    Tablet [film coated]:
      Avelox®: 400 mg
      Avelox® ABC Pack [unit-dose pack]: 400 mg (5s)

**moxifloxacin hydrochloride** *see* moxifloxacin *on this page*

**Moxilin® [US]** *see* amoxicillin *on page 46*

**4-MP** *see* fomepizole *on page 358*

**6-MP** *see* mercaptopurine *on page 515*

**MPA** *see* medroxyprogesterone acetate *on page 507*

**MPA and estrogens (conjugated)** *see* estrogens (conjugated/equine) and medroxyprogesterone *on page 304*

**M-Prednisol® Injection *(Discontinued)*** *see* methylprednisolone *on page 531*

**MPSV4** *see* meningococcal polysaccharide vaccine (groups A / C / Y and W-135) *on page 511*

**MS Contin® [US/Can]** *see* morphine sulfate *on page 549*

**MS-IR® [Can]** *see* morphine sulfate *on page 549*

**MTA** *see* pemetrexed *on page 626*

**MTC** *see* mitomycin *on page 544*

**M.T.E.-4® [US]** *see* trace metals *on page 813*

**M.T.E.-5® [US]** *see* trace metals *on page 813*

**M.T.E.-6® [US]** *see* trace metals *on page 813*

**M.T.E.-7® [US]** *see* trace metals *on page 813*

**Mucinex® [US-OTC]** *see* guaifenesin *on page 383*

**Mucinex®-D [US-OTC]** *see* guaifenesin and pseudoephedrine *on page 388*

**Mucinex® DM [US-OTC]** *see* guaifenesin and dextromethorphan *on page 385*

**Mucomyst® [US/Can]** *see* acetylcysteine *on page 15*

**Mucosil™ *(Discontinued)*** *see* acetylcysteine *on page 15*

**Multidex® [US-OTC]** *see* maltodextrin *on page 501*

**multiple vitamins** *see* vitamins (multiple/oral) *on page 852*

**Multiret Folic 500 [US]** *see* vitamins (multiple/oral) *on page 852*

**multitargeted antifolate** *see* pemetrexed *on page 626*

**Multitest CMI**® *(Discontinued)*

**Multitrace™-4 [US]** *see* trace metals *on page 813*

**Multitrace™-4 Neonatal [US]** *see* trace metals *on page 813*

**Multitrace™-4 Pediatric [US]** *see* trace metals *on page 813*

**Multitrace™-5 [US]** *see* trace metals *on page 813*

**multivitamins/fluoride** *see* vitamins (multiple/pediatric) *on page 852*

**mumps, measles and rubella vaccines, combined** *see* measles, mumps, and rubella vaccines, combined *on page 504*

**Mumpsvax**® **[US]** *see* mumps virus vaccine, live, attenuated *on this page*

# mumps virus vaccine, live, attenuated
(mumpz VYE rus vak SEEN, live, a ten YOO ate ed)
**U.S./Canadian Brand Names** Mumpsvax® [US]
**Therapeutic Category** Vaccine, Live Virus
**Use** Mumps prophylaxis by promoting active immunity
**Note:** Trivalent measles-mumps-rubella (MMR) vaccine is the preferred agent for most children and many adults; persons born prior to 1957 are generally considered immune and need not be vaccinated
**Usual Dosage** Children ≥12-15 months and Adults: SubQ: 0.5 mL as a single dose
**Dosage Forms** Injection, powder for reconstitution [preservative free]: 20,000 $TCID_{50}$ [contains human albumin, bovine serum, gelatin, neomycin; packaged with diluent]

# mupirocin (myoo PEER oh sin)
**Sound-Alike/Look-Alike Issues**
Bactroban® may be confused with bacitracin, baclofen
**Synonyms** mupirocin calcium; pseudomonic acid A
**U.S./Canadian Brand Names** Bactroban® Nasal [US]; Bactroban® [US/Can]; Centany™ [US]
**Therapeutic Category** Antibiotic, Topical
**Use**
Intranasal: Eradication of nasal colonization with MRSA in adult patients and healthcare workers
Topical treatment of impetigo due to *Staphylococcus aureus*, beta-hemolytic *Streptococcus*, and *S. pyogenes*
**Usual Dosage**
Children ≥12 years and Adults: Intranasal: Approximately one-half of the ointment from the single-use tube should be applied into one nostril and the other half into the other nostril twice daily for 5 days
Children ≥3 months and Adults: Topical: Apply small amount to affected area 2-5 times/day for 5-14 days
**Dosage Forms**
Cream, topical, as calcium (Bactroban®): 2% (15 g, 30 g) [contains benzyl alcohol]
Ointment, intranasal, topical, as calcium (Bactroban® Nasal): 2% (1 g) [single-use tube]
Ointment, topical: 2% (22 g)
Bactroban®: 2% (22 g)
Centany™: 2% (15 g, 30 g)

**mupirocin calcium** *see* mupirocin *on this page*

**Murine**® **Ear Wax Removal System [US-OTC]** *see* carbamide peroxide *on page 141*

**Murine**® **Tears [US-OTC]** *see* artificial tears *on page 71*

**Murine**® **Tears Plus [US-OTC]** *see* tetrahydrozoline *on page 792*

**Muro 128**® **[US-OTC]** *see* sodium chloride *on page 752*

**Murocel**® **[US-OTC]** *see* artificial tears *on page 71*

**Murocoll-2**® **[US]** *see* phenylephrine and scopolamine *on page 642*

## muromonab-CD3 (myoo roe MOE nab see dee three)

**Synonyms** monoclonal antibody; OKT3
**U.S./Canadian Brand Names** Orthoclone OKT® 3 [US/Can]
**Therapeutic Category** Immunosuppressant Agent
**Use** Treatment of acute allograft rejection in renal transplant patients; treatment of acute hepatic, kidney, and pancreas rejection episodes resistant to conventional treatment. Acute graft-versus-host disease following bone marrow transplantation resistant to conventional treatment.
**Usual Dosage** I.V. (refer to individual protocols):
Children <30 kg: 2.5 mg/day once daily for 7-14 days
Children >30 kg: 5 mg/day once daily for 7-14 days
**OR**
Children <12 years: 0.1 mg/kg/day once daily for 10-14 days
Children ≥12 years and Adults: 5 mg/day once daily for 10-14 days
**Dosage Forms** Injection, solution: 1 mg/mL (5 mL) [contains sodium 43 mg/5 mL]

**Muroptic-5® *(Discontinued)*** see sodium chloride on page 752

**Muse® [US]** see alprostadil on page 31

**Muse® Pellet [Can]** see alprostadil on page 31

**Mustargen® [US/Can]** see mechlorethamine on page 505

**mustine** see mechlorethamine on page 505

**Mutamycin® [US/Can]** see mitomycin on page 544

**M.V.I.®-12 *(Discontinued)*** see vitamins (multiple/injectable) on page 851

**M.V.I. Adult™ [US]** see vitamins (multiple/injectable) on page 851

**M.V.I® Pediatric [US]** see vitamins (multiple/injectable) on page 851

**Myambutol® [US]** see ethambutol on page 308

**Mycamine™ [US]** see micafungin on page 537

**Mycelex® [US]** see clotrimazole on page 199

**Mycelex®-3 [US-OTC]** see butoconazole on page 126

**Mycelex®-7 [US-OTC]** see clotrimazole on page 199

**Mycelex®-G *(Discontinued)*** see clotrimazole on page 199

**Mycelex® Twin Pack [US-OTC]** see clotrimazole on page 199

**Mycifradin® Sulfate *(Discontinued)*** see neomycin on page 566

**Mycinettes® [US-OTC]** see benzocaine on page 95

**Mycobutin® [US/Can]** see rifabutin on page 721

**Mycolog®-II *(Discontinued)*** see nystatin and triamcinolone on page 592

**Myco-Nail [US-OTC]** see triacetin on page 818

**Myconel® Topical *(Discontinued)*** see nystatin and triamcinolone on page 592

## mycophenolate (mye koe FEN oh late)

**Synonyms** MMF; MPA; mycophenolate mofetil; mycophenolate sodium; mycophenolic acid
**U.S./Canadian Brand Names** CellCept® [US/Can]; Myfortic® [US/Can]
**Therapeutic Category** Immunosuppressant Agent
**Use** Prophylaxis of organ rejection concomitantly with cyclosporine and corticosteroids in patients receiving allogenic renal (CellCept®, Myfortic®), cardiac (CellCept®), or hepatic (CellCept®) transplants
**Usual Dosage**
Children: Renal transplant: Oral:
CellCept® suspension: 600 mg/m²/dose twice daily; maximum dose: 1 g twice daily
Alternatively, may use solid dosage forms according to BSA as follows:
BSA 1.25-1.5 m²: 750 mg capsule twice daily
BSA >1.5 m²: 1 g capsule or tablet twice daily
Myfortic®:
BSA <1.19 m²: Use of this formulation is not recommended
BSA 1.19-1.58 m²: 400 mg/m² twice daily (maximum: 1080 mg/day)
BSA >1.58 m²: 400 mg/m² twice daily (maximum: 1440 mg/day)

Adults: The initial dose should be given as soon as possible following transplantation; intravenous solution may be given until the oral medication can be tolerated (up to 14 days)

Renal transplant:

CellCept®:

Oral: 1 g twice daily. Although a dose of 1.5 g twice daily was used in clinical trials and shown to be effective, no efficacy advantage was established. Patients receiving 2 g/day demonstrated an overall better safety profile than patients receiving 3 g/day. Doses >2 g/day are not recommended in these patients because of the possibility for enhanced immunosuppression as well as toxicities.

I.V.: 1 g twice daily

Myfortic®: Oral: 720 mg twice daily (1440 mg/day)

Cardiac transplantation:

Oral (CellCept®): 1.5 g twice daily

I.V. (CellCept®): 1.5 g twice daily

Hepatic transplantation:

Oral (CellCept®): 1.5 g twice daily

I.V. (CellCept®): 1 g twice daily

**Dosage Forms**

Capsule, as mofetil (CellCept®): 250 mg

Injection, powder for reconstitution, as mofetil hydrochloride (CellCept®): 500 mg [contains polysorbate 80]

Powder for oral suspension, as mofetil (CellCept®): 200 mg/mL (225 mL) [provides 175 mL suspension following reconstitution; contains phenylalanine 0.56 mg/mL; mixed fruit flavor]

Tablet, as mofetil [film coated] (CellCept®): 500 mg [may contain ethyl alcohol]

Tablet, delayed release, as mycophenolic acid [film coated] (Myfortic®): 180 mg, 360 mg [formulated as a sodium salt]

**mycophenolate mofetil** *see* mycophenolate *on previous page*

**mycophenolate sodium** *see* mycophenolate *on previous page*

**mycophenolic acid** *see* mycophenolate *on previous page*

**Mycostatin®** **[US]** *see* nystatin *on page 592*

**Mydfrin®** **[US/Can]** *see* phenylephrine *on page 640*

**Mydral™** **[US]** *see* tropicamide *on page 829*

**Mydriacyl®** **[US/Can]** *see* tropicamide *on page 829*

**My First Flintstones®** **[US-OTC]** *see* vitamins (multiple/pediatric) *on page 852*

**Myfortic®** **[US/Can]** *see* mycophenolate *on previous page*

**Mykrox®** **[Can]** *see* metolazone *on page 534*

**Mykrox®** *(Discontinued)* *see* metolazone *on page 534*

**Mylanta™** **[Can]** *see* aluminum hydroxide and magnesium hydroxide *on page 35*

**Mylanta®-II** *(Discontinued)* *see* aluminum hydroxide, magnesium hydroxide, and simethicone *on page 35*

**Mylanta AR®** *(Discontinued)* *see* famotidine *on page 327*

**Mylanta®** **Children's [US-OTC]** *see* calcium carbonate *on page 130*

**Mylanta®** **Double Strength [Can]** *see* aluminum hydroxide, magnesium hydroxide, and simethicone *on page 35*

**Mylanta®** **Extra Strength [Can]** *see* aluminum hydroxide, magnesium hydroxide, and simethicone *on page 35*

**Mylanta®** **Gas [US-OTC]** *see* simethicone *on page 748*

**Mylanta®** **Gas Maximum Strength [US-OTC]** *see* simethicone *on page 748*

**Mylanta®** **Gelcaps®** **[US-OTC]** *see* calcium carbonate and magnesium hydroxide *on page 132*

**Mylanta®** **Liquid [US-OTC]** *see* aluminum hydroxide, magnesium hydroxide, and simethicone *on page 35*

**Mylanta®** **Maximum Strength Liquid [US-OTC]** *see* aluminum hydroxide, magnesium hydroxide, and simethicone *on page 35*

**Mylanta®** **Regular Strength [Can]** *see* aluminum hydroxide, magnesium hydroxide, and simethicone *on page 35*

**Mylanta**® **Supreme [US-OTC]** *see* calcium carbonate and magnesium hydroxide *on page 132*

**Mylanta**® **Ultra [US-OTC]** *see* calcium carbonate and magnesium hydroxide *on page 132*

**Myleran**® **[US/Can]** *see* busulfan *on page 123*

**Mylicon**® **Infants [US-OTC]** *see* simethicone *on page 748*

**Mylocel**™ **[US]** *see* hydroxyurea *on page 422*

**Mylotarg**® **[US/Can]** *see* gemtuzumab ozogamicin *on page 370*

**Myminic**® **Expectorant** *(Discontinued)*

**Myobloc**® **[US]** *see* botulinum toxin type B *on page 112*

**Myochrysine**® **[Can]** *see* gold sodium thiomalate *on page 380*

**Myoflex**® **[US-OTC/Can]** *see* triethanolamine salicylate *on page 823*

**Myotonachol**® **[Can]** *see* bethanechol *on page 104*

**Myotonachol**™ *(Discontinued)* *see* bethanechol *on page 104*

**myrac**™ **[US]** *see* minocycline *on page 542*

**Mysoline**® **[US]** *see* primidone *on page 678*

**Mytelase**® **[US/Can]** *see* ambenonium *on page 37*

**Mytussin**® **AC [US]** *see* guaifenesin and codeine *on page 384*

**Mytussin**® **DAC [US]** *see* guaifenesin, pseudoephedrine, and codeine *on page 391*

**N-9** *see* nonoxynol 9 *on page 580*

**Nabi-HB**® **[US]** *see* hepatitis B immune globulin *on page 401*

**NAB-paclitaxel** *see* paclitaxel (protein bound) *on page 613*

## nabumetone (na BYOO me tone)

**U.S./Canadian Brand Names** Apo-Nabumetone® [Can]; Gen-Nabumetone [Can]; Novo-Nabumetone [Can]; Relafen® [US/Can]; Rhoxal-nabumetone [Can]

**Therapeutic Category** Analgesic, Nonnarcotic;  Nonsteroidal Antiinflammatory Drug (NSAID)

**Use** Management of osteoarthritis and rheumatoid arthritis

**Usual Dosage** Adults: Oral: 1000 mg/day; an additional 500-1000 mg may be needed in some patients to obtain more symptomatic relief; may be administered once or twice daily

**Dosage Forms** Tablet: 500 mg, 750 mg

**NAC** *see* acetylcysteine *on page 15*

***n*-acetyl-L-cysteine** *see* acetylcysteine *on page 15*

***n*-acetylcysteine** *see* acetylcysteine *on page 15*

**n-acetyl-p-aminophenol** *see* acetaminophen *on page 4*

**NaCl** *see* sodium chloride *on page 752*

## nadolol (nay DOE lole)

**Sound-Alike/Look-Alike Issues**

nadolol may be confused with Mandol®

Corgard® may be confused with Cognex®

**U.S./Canadian Brand Names** Alti-Nadolol [Can]; Apo-Nadol® [Can]; Corgard® [US/Can]; Novo-Nadolol [Can]

**Therapeutic Category** Beta-Adrenergic Blocker

**Use** Treatment of hypertension and angina pectoris; prophylaxis of migraine headaches

**Usual Dosage** Oral: Adults: Initial: 40 mg/day, increase dosage gradually by 40-80 mg increments at 3- to 7-day intervals until optimum clinical response is obtained with profound slowing of heart rate; doses up to 160-240 mg/day in angina and 240-320 mg/day in hypertension may be necessary.

Hypertension: Usual dosage range (JNC 7): 40-120 mg once daily

**Dosage Forms** Tablet: 20 mg, 40 mg, 80 mg, 120 mg, 160 mg

**nadroparin calcium** *see* nadroparin *(Canada only)* *on next page*

## nadroparin *(Canada only)* (nad roe PA rin)
**Synonyms** nadroparin calcium
**U.S./Canadian Brand Names** Fraxiparine™ Forte [Can]; Fraxiparine™ [Can]
**Therapeutic Category** Low Molecular Weight Heparin
**Use** Prophylaxis of thromboembolic disorders (particularly deep venous thrombosis and pulmonary embolism) in general and orthopedic surgery; treatment of deep venous thrombosis; prevention of clotting during hemodialysis
**Usual Dosage** SubQ: Adults:
Prophylaxis of thromboembolic disorders in general surgery: 2850 anti-Xa int. units once daily; begin 2-4 hours before surgery and continue for 7 days
Prophylaxis of thromboembolic disorders in hip replacement: 38 anti-Xa int. units/kg 12 hours before and 12 hours after surgery, **followed by** 38 anti-Xa int. units/kg/day up to and including day 3, **then** 57 anti-Xa int. units/kg/day for up to 10 days total therapy
Treatment of thromboembolic disorders: 171 anti-Xa int. units/kg/day to a maximum of 17,100 int. units; plasma anti-Xa levels should be 1.2-1.8 anti-Xa int. units/mL 3-4 hours postinjection
Patients at increased risk of bleeding: 86 anti-Xa int. units/kg twice daily; plasma anti-Xa levels should be 0.5-1.1 anti-Xa int. units/mL 3-4 hours postinjection
Prevention of clotting during hemodialysis: Single dose of 65 anti-Xa int. units/kg into arterial line at start of each dialysis session; may give additional dose if session lasts longer than 4 hours
Patients at risk of hemorrhage: Administer 50% of dose
**Dosage Forms** Injection, solution, as calcium:
Fraxiparine™:
9500 anti-Xa int. units/mL (0.2 mL, 0.3 mL, 0.4 mL) [ungraduated prefilled syringe]
9500 anti-Xa int. units/mL (0.6 mL, 0.8 mL, 1 mL) [graduated prefilled syringe]
Fraxiparine™ Forte: 19,000 anti-Xa int. units/mL (0.6 mL, 0.8 mL, 1 mL) [graduated prefilled syringe]

## nafarelin (NAF a re lin)
**Sound-Alike/Look-Alike Issues**
nafarelin may be confused with Anafranil®, enalapril
**Synonyms** nafarelin acetate
**U.S./Canadian Brand Names** Synarel® [US/Can]
**Therapeutic Category** Hormone, Posterior Pituitary
**Use** Treatment of endometriosis, including pain and reduction of lesions; treatment of central precocious puberty (gonadotropin-dependent precocious puberty) in children of both sexes
**Usual Dosage**
Endometriosis: Adults: Female: 1 spray (200 mcg) in 1 nostril each morning and the other nostril each evening starting on days 2-4 of menstrual cycle for 6 months
Central precocious puberty: Children: Males/Females: 2 sprays (400 mcg) into each nostril in the morning 2 sprays (400 mcg) into each nostril in the evening. If inadequate suppression, may increase dose to 3 sprays (600 mcg) into alternating nostrils 3 times/day.
**Dosage Forms** Solution, intranasal spray: 2 mg/mL (8 mL) [200 mcg/spray: 60 metered doses; contains benzalkonium chloride]

**nafarelin acetate** *see* nafarelin *on this page*

**Nafazair® Ophthalmic *(Discontinued)*** *see* naphazoline *on page 561*

## nafcillin (naf SIL in)
**Synonyms** ethoxynaphthamido penicillin sodium; nafcillin sodium; sodium nafcillin
**U.S./Canadian Brand Names** Nallpen® [Can]; Unipen® [Can]
**Therapeutic Category** Penicillin
**Use** Treatment of infections such as osteomyelitis, septicemia, endocarditis, and CNS infections caused by susceptible strains of staphylococci species
**Usual Dosage**
Neonates:
<2000 g, <7 days: 50 mg/kg/day divided every 12 hours
<2000 g, >7 days: 75 mg/kg/day divided every 8 hours
>2000 g, <7 days: 50 mg/kg/day divided every 8 hours
>2000 g, >7 days: 75 mg/kg/day divided every 6 hours
Children:
I.M.: 25 mg/kg twice daily
(Continued)

## nafcillin *(Continued)*

I.V.:
 Mild to moderate infections: 50-100 mg/kg/day in divided doses every 6 hours
 Severe infections: 100-200 mg/kg/day in divided doses every 4-6 hours
 Maximum dose: 12 g/day
Adults:
 I.M.: 500 mg every 4-6 hours
 I.V.: 500-2000 mg every 4-6 hours

**Dosage Forms**
 Infusion [premixed iso-osmotic dextrose solution]: 1 g (50 mL); 2 g (100 mL)
 Injection, powder for reconstitution, as sodium: 1 g, 2 g, 10 g

**nafcillin sodium** *see* nafcillin *on previous page*

## naftifine *(NAF ti feen)*

**Synonyms** naftifine hydrochloride
**U.S./Canadian Brand Names** Naftin® [US]
**Therapeutic Category** Antifungal Agent
**Use** Topical treatment of tinea cruris (jock itch), tinea corporis (ringworm), and tinea pedis (athlete's foot)
**Usual Dosage** Adults: Topical: Apply cream once daily and gel twice daily (morning and evening) for up to 4 weeks
**Dosage Forms**
 Cream, as hydrochloride: 1% (15 g, 30 g, 60 g) [contains benzyl alcohol]
 Gel, as hydrochloride: 1% (20 g, 40 g, 60 g) [contains alcohol 52%]

**naftifine hydrochloride** *see* naftifine *on this page*

**Naftin® [US]** *see* naftifine *on this page*

**Naglazyme™ [US]** *see* galsulfase *on page 366*

**NaHCO₃** *see* sodium bicarbonate *on page 752*

## nalbuphine *(NAL byoo feen)*

**Sound-Alike/Look-Alike Issues**
 Nubain® may be confused with Navane®, Nebcin®
**Synonyms** nalbuphine hydrochloride
**U.S./Canadian Brand Names** Nubain® [US]
**Therapeutic Category** Analgesic, Narcotic
**Use** Relief of moderate to severe pain; preoperative analgesia, postoperative and surgical anesthesia, and obstetrical analgesia during labor and delivery
**Usual Dosage** Adults:
 Pain management: I.M., I.V., SubQ: 10 mg/70 kg every 3-6 hours; maximum single dose in nonopioid-tolerant patients: 20 mg; maximum daily dose: 160 mg
 Surgical anesthesia supplement: I.V.: Induction: 0.3-3 mg/kg over 10-15 minutes; maintenance doses of 0.25-0.5 mg/kg may be given as required
**Dosage Forms** [DSC] = Discontinued product
 Injection, solution, as hydrochloride: 10 mg/mL (10 mL); 20 mg/mL (10 mL)
 Nubain®: 10 mg/mL (10 mL) [DSC]; 20 mg/mL (10 mL)
 Injection, solution, as hydrochloride [preservative free]: 10 mg/mL (1 mL); 20 mg/mL (1 mL)
 Nubain®: 10 mg/mL (1 mL); 20 mg/mL (1 mL)

**nalbuphine hydrochloride** *see* nalbuphine *on this page*

**Nalcrom® [Can]** *see* cromolyn sodium *on page 211*

**Naldecon® DX Adult Liquid** *(Discontinued)*

**Naldecon-EX® Children's Syrup** *(Discontinued)*

**Naldecon Senior EX® [US-OTC]** *see* guaifenesin *on page 383*

**Nalex®-A [US]** *see* chlorpheniramine, phenylephrine, and phenyltoloxamine *on page 176*

**Nalfon® [US/Can]** *see* fenoprofen *on page 331*

# nalidixic acid (nal i DIKS ik AS id)
**Synonyms** nalidixinic acid
**U.S./Canadian Brand Names** NegGram® [US/Can]
**Therapeutic Category** Quinolone
**Use** Treatment of urinary tract infections
**Usual Dosage** Oral:
Children 3 months to 12 years: 55 mg/kg/day divided every 6 hours; suppressive therapy is 33 mg/kg/day divided every 6 hours
Adults: 1 g 4 times/day for 2 weeks; then suppressive therapy of 500 mg 4 times/day
**Dosage Forms** [DSC] = Discontinued product
Suspension, oral: 250 mg/5 mL (473 mL) [raspberry flavor]
Tablet: 250 mg [DSC], 500 mg, 1 g [DSC]

**nalidixinic acid** *see* nalidixic acid *on this page*

**Nallpen® [Can]** *see* nafcillin *on page 557*

**Nallpen® (Discontinued)** *see* nafcillin *on page 557*

**N-allylnoroxymorphine hydrochloride** *see* naloxone *on this page*

# nalmefene (NAL me feen)
**Sound-Alike/Look-Alike Issues**
Revex® may be confused with Nimbex®, ReVia®
**Synonyms** nalmefene hydrochloride
**U.S./Canadian Brand Names** Revex® [US]
**Therapeutic Category** Antidote
**Use** Complete or partial reversal of opioid drug effects, including respiratory depression induced by natural or synthetic opioids; reversal of postoperative opioid depression; management of known or suspected opioid overdose
**Usual Dosage**
Reversal of postoperative opioid depression: Blue labeled product (100 mcg/mL): Titrate to reverse the undesired effects of opioids; initial dose for nonopioid dependent patients: 0.25 mcg/kg followed by 0.25 mcg/kg incremental doses at 2- to 5-minute intervals; after a total dose >1 mcg/kg, further therapeutic response is unlikely
Management of known/suspected opioid overdose: Green labeled product (1000 mcg/mL): Initial dose: 0.5 mg/70 kg; may repeat with 1 mg/70 kg in 2-5 minutes; further increase beyond a total dose of 1.5 mg/70 kg will not likely result in improved response and may result in cardiovascular stress and precipitated withdrawal syndrome. (If opioid dependency is suspected, administer a challenge dose of 0.1 mg/70 kg; if no withdrawal symptoms are observed in 2 minutes, the recommended doses can be administered.)
**Note:** If recurrence of respiratory depression is noted, dose may again be titrated to clinical effect using incremental doses.
**Note:** If I.V. access is lost or not readily obtainable, a single SubQ or I.M. dose of 1 mg may be effective in 5-15 minutes.
**Dosage Forms** Injection, solution: 100 mcg/mL (1 mL) [blue label]; 1000 mcg/mL (2 mL) [green label]

**nalmefene hydrochloride** *see* nalmefene *on this page*

# naloxone (nal OKS one)
**Sound-Alike/Look-Alike Issues**
naloxone may be confused with naltrexone
Narcan® may be confused with Marcaine®, Norcuron®
**Synonyms** N-allylnoroxymorphine hydrochloride; naloxone hydrochloride
**Therapeutic Category** Antidote
**Use**
Complete or partial reversal of opioid depression, including respiratory depression, induced by natural and synthetic opioids, including propoxyphene, methadone, and certain mixed agonist-antagonist analgesics: nalbuphine, pentazocine, and butorphanol
Diagnosis of suspected opioid tolerance or acute opioid overdose
Adjunctive agent to increase blood pressure in the management of septic shock
(Continued)

# naloxone *(Continued)*

**Usual Dosage** I.M., I.V. (preferred), intratracheal, SubQ:

Postanesthesia narcotic reversal: Infants and Children: 0.01 mg/kg; may repeat every 2-3 minutes, as needed based on response

Opiate intoxication:

Children:

Birth (including premature infants) to 5 years or <20 kg: 0.1 mg/kg; repeat every 2-3 minutes if needed; may need to repeat doses every 20-60 minutes

>5 years or ≥20 kg: 2 mg/dose; if no response, repeat every 2-3 minutes; may need to repeat doses every 20-60 minutes

Children and Adults: Continuous infusion: I.V.: If continuous infusion is required, calculate dosage/hour based on effective intermittent dose used and duration of adequate response seen, titrate dose 0.04-0.16 mg/kg/hour for 2-5 days in children, adult dose typically 0.25-6.25 mg/hour (short-term infusions as high as 2.4 mg/kg/hour have been tolerated in adults during treatment for septic shock); alternatively, continuous infusion utilizes $2/3$ of the initial naloxone bolus on an hourly basis; add 10 times this dose to each liter of $D_5W$ and infuse at a rate of 100 mL/hour; $1/2$ of the initial bolus dose should be readministered 15 minutes after initiation of the continuous infusion to prevent a drop in naloxone levels; increase infusion rate as needed to assure adequate ventilation

Narcotic overdose: Adults: I.V.: 0.4-2 mg every 2-3 minutes as needed; may need to repeat doses every 20-60 minutes, if no response is observed after 10 mg, question the diagnosis. **Note:** Use 0.1-0.2 mg increments in patients who are opioid dependent and in postoperative patients to avoid large cardiovascular changes.

**Dosage Forms**

Injection, solution, as hydrochloride: 0.4 mg/mL (1 mL, 10 mL)

Narcan®: 0.4 mg/mL (1 mL) [DSC]

**naloxone and buprenorphine** *see* buprenorphine and naloxone *on page 122*

**naloxone hydrochloride** *see* naloxone *on previous page*

**naloxone hydrochloride and pentazocine hydrochloride** *see* pentazocine *on page 631*

**naloxone hydrochloride dihydrate and buprenorphine hydrochloride** *see* buprenorphine and naloxone *on page 122*

# naltrexone (nal TREKS one)

**Sound-Alike/Look-Alike Issues**

naltrexone may be confused with naloxone

ReVia® may be confused with Revex®

**Synonyms** naltrexone hydrochloride

**U.S./Canadian Brand Names** Depade® [US]; ReVia® [US/Can]

**Therapeutic Category** Antidote

**Use** Treatment of ethanol dependence; blockade of the effects of exogenously administered opioids

**Usual Dosage** Do not give until patient is opioid-free for 7-10 days as determined by urine analysis

Adults: Oral: 25 mg; if no withdrawal signs within 1 hour give another 25 mg; maintenance regimen is flexible, variable and individualized (50 mg/day to 100-150 mg 3 times/week for 12 weeks); up to 800 mg/day has been tolerated in adults without an adverse effect

**Dosage Forms**

Tablet, as hydrochloride: 50 mg

Depade®: 25 mg, 50 mg, 100 mg

ReVia®: 50 mg

**naltrexone hydrochloride** *see* naltrexone *on this page*

**Namenda™ [US]** *see* memantine *on page 510*

# nandrolone (NAN droe lone)

**Synonyms** nandrolone decanoate; nandrolone phenpropionate

**U.S./Canadian Brand Names** Deca-Durabolin® [Can]; Durabolin® [Can]

**Therapeutic Category** Androgen

**Controlled Substance** C-III

**Use** Control of metastatic breast cancer; management of anemia of renal insufficiency

**Usual Dosage** Deep I.M. (into gluteal muscle):

Children 2-13 years (decanoate): 25-50 mg every 3-4 weeks

Adults:
Male:
Breast cancer (phenpropionate): 50-100 mg/week
Anemia of renal insufficiency (decanoate): 100-200 mg/week
Female: 50-100 mg/week
Breast cancer (phenpropionate): 50-100 mg/week
Anemia of renal insufficiency (decanoate): 50-100 mg/week
**Dosage Forms** Injection, solution, as decanoate [in sesame oil]: 100 mg/mL (2 mL); 200 mg/mL (1 mL) [contains benzyl alcohol]

**nandrolone decanoate** *see* nandrolone *on previous page*

**nandrolone phenpropionate** *see* nandrolone *on previous page*

**NAPA and NABZ** *see* sodium phenylacetate and sodium benzoate *on page 755*

# naphazoline (naf AZ oh leen)

**Synonyms** naphazoline hydrochloride

**U.S./Canadian Brand Names** AK-Con™ [US]; Albalon® [US]; Allersol® [US]; Clear Eyes® ACR [US-OTC]; Clear Eyes® Extra Relief [US-OTC]; Naphcon Forte® [Can]; Naphcon® [US-OTC]; Privine® [US-OTC]; Vasocon® [Can]

**Therapeutic Category** Adrenergic Agonist Agent

**Use** Topical ocular vasoconstrictor; will temporarily relieve congestion, itching, and minor irritation, and to control hyperemia in patients with superficial corneal vascularity; treatment of nasal congestion; adjunct for sinusitis

**Usual Dosage**
Nasal:
Children:
<6 years: Intranasal: Not recommended (especially infants) due to CNS depression
6-12 years: 1 spray of 0.05% into each nostril every 6 hours if necessary; therapy should not exceed 3-5 days
Children >12 years and Adults: 0.05%, instill 1-2 drops or sprays every 6 hours if needed; therapy should not exceed 3-5 days
Ophthalmic:
Children <6 years: Not recommended for use due to CNS depression (especially in infants)
Children >6 years and Adults: Instill 1-2 drops into conjunctival sac of affected eye(s) every 3-4 hours; therapy generally should not exceed 3-4 days

**Dosage Forms** [DSC] = Discontinued product
Solution, intranasal drops, as hydrochloride (Privine®): 0.05% (25 mL)
Solution, intranasal spray, as hydrochloride (Privine®): 0.05% (20 mL)
Solution, ophthalmic, as hydrochloride: 0.1% (15 mL) [DSC]
AK-Con™, Albalon®, Allersol®: 0.1% (15 mL) [contains benzalkonium chloride]
Clear Eyes® ACR: 0.012% (15 mL, 30 mL) [contains glycerin 0.2%, zinc sulfate 0.25%, and benzalkonium chloride]
Clear Eyes® Extra Relief: 0.012% (6 mL, 15 mL, 30 mL) [contains glycerin 0.2% and benzalkonium chloride]
Naphcon®: 0.012% (15 mL) [contains benzalkonium chloride]

# naphazoline and antazoline (naf AZ oh leen & an TAZ oh leen)

**Synonyms** antazoline and naphazoline

**U.S./Canadian Brand Names** Albalon®-A Liquifilm [Can]; Vasocon®-A [Can]

**Therapeutic Category** Antihistamine/Decongestant Combination

**Use** Topical ocular congestion, irritation and itching

**Usual Dosage** Ophthalmic: 1-2 drops every 3-4 hours

**Dosage Forms** [DSC] = Discontinued product
Solution, ophthalmic: Naphazoline hydrochloride 0.05% and antazoline phosphate 0.5% (15 mL) [contains benzalkonium chloride] [DSC]

# naphazoline and pheniramine (naf AZ oh leen & fen NIR a meen)

**Sound-Alike/Look-Alike Issues**
Visine® may be confused with Visken®
(Continued)

## naphazoline and pheniramine *(Continued)*

**Synonyms** pheniramine and naphazoline

**U.S./Canadian Brand Names** Naphcon-A® [US-OTC/Can]; Opcon-A® [US-OTC]; Visine-A™ [US-OTC]; Visine® Advanced Allergy [Can]

**Therapeutic Category** Antihistamine/Decongestant Combination

**Use** Treatment of ocular congestion, irritation, and itching

**Usual Dosage** Ophthalmic: Children ≥6 years and Adults: 1-2 drops up to 4 times/day

**Dosage Forms**

Solution, ophthalmic: Naphazoline hydrochloride 0.025% and pheniramine 0.3% (15 mL) [contains benzalkonium chloride]

Naphcon-A®: Naphazoline hydrochloride 0.025% and pheniramine 0.3% (5 mL) [contains benzalkonium chloride; 2 bottles/box], (15 mL) [contains benzalkonium chloride]

Opcon-A®, Visine-A™: Naphazoline hydrochloride 0.025% and pheniramine 0.3% (15 mL) [contains benzalkonium chloride]

**naphazoline hydrochloride** *see* naphazoline *on previous page*

**Naphcon® [US-OTC]** *see* naphazoline *on previous page*

**Naphcon-A® [US-OTC/Can]** *see* naphazoline and pheniramine *on previous page*

**Naphcon Forte® [Can]** *see* naphazoline *on previous page*

**Naphcon Forte® Ophthalmic *(Discontinued)*** *see* naphazoline *on previous page*

**NapraPAC™** *see* lansoprazole and naproxen *on page 468*

**Naprelan® [US]** *see* naproxen *on this page*

**Naprosyn® [US/Can]** *see* naproxen *on this page*

## naproxen (na PROKS en)

**Sound-Alike/Look-Alike Issues**

naproxen may be confused with Naprosyn®

Aleve® may be confused with Alesse®

Anaprox® may be confused with Anaspaz®, Avapro®

Naprelan® may be confused with Naprosyn®

Naprosyn® may be confused with Naprelan®, naproxen, Natacyn®, Nebcin®

**Synonyms** naproxen sodium

**U.S./Canadian Brand Names** Aleve® [US-OTC]; Anaprox® DS [US/Can]; Anaprox® [US/Can]; Apo-Napro-Na DS® [Can]; Apo-Napro-Na® [Can]; Apo-Naproxen SR® [Can]; Apo-Naproxen® [Can]; EC-Naprosyn® [US]; Gen-Naproxen EC [Can]; Naprelan® [US]; Naprosyn® [US/Can]; Naxen® [Can]; Novo-Naproc EC [Can]; Novo-Naprox Sodium DS [Can]; Novo-Naprox Sodium [Can]; Novo-Naprox SR [Can]; Novo-Naprox [Can]; Nu-Naprox [Can]; Pamprin® Maximum Strength All Day Relief [US-OTC]; Riva-Naproxen [Can]

**Therapeutic Category** Analgesic, Nonnarcotic; Antipyretic; Nonsteroidal Antiinflammatory Drug (NSAID)

**Use** Management of ankylosing spondylitis, osteoarthritis, and rheumatoid disorders (including juvenile rheumatoid arthritis); acute gout; mild to moderate pain; tendonitis, bursitis; dysmenorrhea; fever, migraine headache

**Usual Dosage** Oral:

Children >2 years: Juvenile arthritis: 10 mg/kg/day in 2 divided doses

Adults:

Acute gout: Initial: 750 mg, followed by 250 mg every 8 hours until attack subsides; **Note:** EC-Naprosyn® is not recommended

Rheumatoid arthritis, osteoarthritis, and ankylosing spondylitis: 500-1000 mg/day in 2 divided doses; may increase to 1.5 g/day of naproxen base for limited time period

Mild-to-moderate pain, dysmenorrhea, acute tendonitis, bursitis: Initial: 500 mg, then 250 mg every 6-8 hours; maximum: 1250 mg/day naproxen base

**OTC labeling:** Pain/fever:

Children ≥12 years and Adults ≤65 years: 200 mg naproxen base every 8-12 hours; if needed, may take 400 mg naproxen base for the initial dose; maximum: 600 mg naproxen base/24 hours

Adults >65 years: 200 mg naproxen base every 12 hours

**Dosage Forms**

Caplet, as sodium (Aleve®, Midol® Extended Relief, Pamprin® Maximum Strength All Day Relief): 220 mg [equivalent to naproxen 200 mg and sodium 20 mg]

Gelcap, as sodium (Aleve®): 220 mg [equivalent to naproxen 200 mg and sodium 20 mg]

Suspension, oral (Naprosyn®): 125 mg/5 mL (480 mL) [contains sodium 0.3 mEq/mL; orange-pineapple flavor]

Tablet (Naprosyn®): 250 mg, 375 mg, 500 mg

Tablet, as sodium: 220 mg [equivalent to naproxen 200 mg and sodium 20 mg]; 275 mg [equivalent to naproxen 250 mg and sodium 25 mg]; 550 mg [equivalent to naproxen 500 mg and sodium 50 mg]
Aleve®: 220 mg [equivalent to naproxen 200 mg and sodium 20 mg]
Anaprox®: 275 mg [equivalent to naproxen 250 mg and sodium 25 mg]
Anaprox® DS: 550 mg [equivalent to naproxen 500 mg and sodium 50 mg]

Tablet, controlled release, as sodium: 550 mg [equivalent to naproxen 500 mg and sodium 50 mg]
Naprelan®: 421.5 mg [equivalent to naproxen 375 mg and sodium 37.5 mg]; 550 mg [equivalent to naproxen 500 mg and sodium 50 mg]

Tablet, delayed release (EC-Naprosyn®): 375 mg, 500 mg

**naproxen and lansoprazole** see lansoprazole and naproxen on page 468

**naproxen sodium** see naproxen on previous page

**Naqua® [Can]** see trichlormethiazide on page 822

## naratriptan (NAR a trip tan)

**Sound-Alike/Look-Alike Issues**
Amerge® may be confused with Altace®, Amaryl®
**Synonyms** naratriptan hydrochloride
**U.S./Canadian Brand Names** Amerge® [US/Can]
**Therapeutic Category** Antimigraine Agent; Serotonin Agonist
**Use** Treatment of acute migraine headache with or without aura
**Usual Dosage** Adults: Oral: 1-2.5 mg at the onset of headache; it is recommended to use the lowest possible dose to minimize adverse effects. If headache returns or does not fully resolve, the dose may be repeated after 4 hours; do not exceed 5 mg in 24 hours.
**Dosage Forms** Tablet: 1 mg, 2.5 mg

**naratriptan hydrochloride** see naratriptan on this page

**Narcan®** *(Discontinued)* see naloxone on page 559

**Nardil® [US/Can]** see phenelzine on page 637

**Naropin® [US/Can]** see ropivacaine on page 730

**Nasacort® AQ [US/Can]** see triamcinolone (inhalation, nasal) on page 819

**Nasacort® HFA [US]** see triamcinolone (inhalation, nasal) on page 819

**Nasahist B®** *(Discontinued)* see brompheniramine on page 115

**NaSal™ [US-OTC]** see sodium chloride on page 752

**NasalCrom® [US-OTC]** see cromolyn sodium on page 211

**Nasalide® [Can]** see flunisolide on page 344

**Nasal Moist® [US-OTC]** see sodium chloride on page 752

**Nasarel® [US]** see flunisolide on page 344

**Nasatab® LA [US]** see guaifenesin and pseudoephedrine on page 388

**Nascobal® [US]** see cyanocobalamin on page 212

**Nasonex® [US/Can]** see mometasone furoate on page 547

**Natabec®** *(Discontinued)*

**Natabec® FA** *(Discontinued)*

**Natabec® Rx** *(Discontinued)*

**NataChew™ [US]** see vitamins (multiple/prenatal) on page 852

**Natacyn® [US/Can]** see natamycin on next page

**NataFort® [US]** see vitamins (multiple/prenatal) on page 852

**NatalCare® CFe 60** *(Discontinued)* see vitamins (multiple/prenatal) on page 852

**NatalCare® GlossTabs™ [US]** see vitamins (multiple/prenatal) on page 852

**NatalCare® PIC [US]** see vitamins (multiple/prenatal) on page 852

**NatalCare® PIC Forte [US]** *see* vitamins (multiple/prenatal) *on page 852*

**NatalCare® Plus [US]** *see* vitamins (multiple/prenatal) *on page 852*

**NatalCare® Rx [US]** *see* vitamins (multiple/prenatal) *on page 852*

**NatalCare® Three [US]** *see* vitamins (multiple/prenatal) *on page 852*

**Natalins® Rx *(Discontinued)***

**natamycin** (na ta MYE sin)
  **Sound-Alike/Look-Alike Issues**
    Natacyn® may be confused with Naprosyn®
  **Synonyms** pimaricin
  **U.S./Canadian Brand Names** Natacyn® [US/Can]
  **Therapeutic Category** Antifungal Agent
  **Use** Treatment of blepharitis, conjunctivitis, and keratitis caused by susceptible fungi (*Aspergillus*, *Candida*), *Cephalosporium*, *Curvularia*, *Fusarium*, *Penicillium*, *Microsporum*, *Epidermophyton*, *Blastomyces dermatitidis*, *Coccidioides immitis*, *Cryptococcus neoformans*, *Histoplasma capsulatum*, *Sporothrix schenckii*, and *Trichomonas vaginalis*
  **Usual Dosage** Adults: Ophthalmic: Instill 1 drop in conjunctival sac every 1-2 hours, after 3-4 days reduce to one drop 6-8 times/day; usual course of therapy is 2-3 weeks.
  **Dosage Forms** Suspension, ophthalmic: 5% (15 mL) [contains benzalkonium chloride]

**NataTab™ CFe [US]** *see* vitamins (multiple/prenatal) *on page 852*

**NataTab™ FA [US]** *see* vitamins (multiple/prenatal) *on page 852*

**NataTab™ Rx [US]** *see* vitamins (multiple/prenatal) *on page 852*

**nateglinide** (na te GLYE nide)
  **U.S./Canadian Brand Names** Starlix® [US/Can]
  **Therapeutic Category** Antidiabetic Agent
  **Use** Management of type 2 diabetes mellitus (noninsulin dependent, NIDDM) as monotherapy when hyperglycemia cannot be managed by diet and exercise alone; in combination with metformin or a thiazolidinedione to lower blood glucose in patients whose hyperglycemia cannot be controlled by exercise, diet, or a single agent alone
  **Usual Dosage**
    Children: Safety and efficacy have not been established
    Adults: Management of type 2 diabetes mellitus: Oral: Initial and maintenance dose: 120 mg 3 times/day, 1-30 minutes before meals; may be given alone or in combination with metformin or a thiazolidinedione; patients close to Hb $A_{1c}$ goal may be started at 60 mg 3 times/day
  **Dosage Forms** Tablet: 60 mg, 120 mg

**Natrecor® [US]** *see* nesiritide *on page 570*

**natriuretic peptide** *see* nesiritide *on page 570*

**Natulan® [Can]** *see* procarbazine *on page 680*

**Natural Fiber Therapy [US-OTC]** *see* psyllium *on page 697*

**natural lung surfactant** *see* beractant *on page 101*

**Nature's Tears® [US-OTC]** *see* artificial tears *on page 71*

**Nature-Throid® NT [US]** *see* thyroid *on page 800*

**Naturetin® *(Discontinued)*** *see* bendroflumethiazide *on page 93*

**Naus-A-Way® *(Discontinued)***

**Nausea Relief [US-OTC]** *see* fructose, dextrose, and phosphoric acid *on page 362*

**Nausetrol® [US-OTC]** *see* fructose, dextrose, and phosphoric acid *on page 362*

**Navane® [US/Can]** *see* thiothixene *on page 799*

**Navelbine® [US/Can]** *see* vinorelbine *on page 847*

**Naxen® [Can]** *see* naproxen *on page 562*

**Na-Zone® [US-OTC]** *see* sodium chloride *on page 752*

***n*-docosanol** *see* docosanol *on page 263*

**ND-Stat**® **Solution [US-OTC]** *see* brompheniramine *on page 115*

**Nebcin**® *(Discontinued)* *see* tobramycin *on page 807*

**NebuPent**® **[US]** *see* pentamidine *on page 630*

**Necon**® **0.5/35 [US]** *see* ethinyl estradiol and norethindrone *on page 314*

**Necon**® **1/35 [US]** *see* ethinyl estradiol and norethindrone *on page 314*

**Necon**® **1/50 [US]** *see* mestranol and norethindrone *on page 517*

**Necon**® **7/7/7 [US]** *see* ethinyl estradiol and norethindrone *on page 314*

**Necon**® **10/11 [US]** *see* ethinyl estradiol and norethindrone *on page 314*

## nedocromil (inhalation) (ne doe KROE mil in hil LA shun)

**U.S./Canadian Brand Names** Tilade® [US/Can]

**Therapeutic Category** Mast Cell Stabilizer

**Use** Maintenance therapy in patients with mild to moderate bronchial asthma

**Usual Dosage** Children >6 years and Adults: 2 inhalations 4 times/day; may reduce dosage to 2-3 times/day once desired clinical response to initial dose is observed

**Dosage Forms** Aerosol for inhalation, as sodium (Tilade®): 1.75 mg/activation (16.2 g)

## nedocromil (ophthalmic) (ne doe KROE mil op THAL mik)

**U.S./Canadian Brand Names** Alocril® [US/Can]

**Therapeutic Category** Mast Cell Stabilizer

**Use** Treatment of itching associated with allergic conjunctivitis

**Usual Dosage** Adults: Ophthalmic: 1-2 drops in eye(s) twice daily

**Dosage Forms** Solution, ophthalmic, as sodium (Alocril®): 2% (5 mL) [contains benzalkonium chloride]

## nefazodone (nef AY zoe done)

**Sound-Alike/Look-Alike Issues**

Serzone® may be confused with selegiline, Serentil®, Seroquel®, sertraline

**Synonyms** nefazodone hydrochloride

**Therapeutic Category** Antidepressant, Miscellaneous

**Use** Treatment of depression

**Usual Dosage** Oral: Adults: Depression: 200 mg/day, administered in 2 divided doses initially, with a range of 300-600 mg/day in 2 divided doses thereafter

**Dosage Forms**

Tablet, as hydrochloride: 50 mg, 100 mg, 150 mg, 200 mg, 250 mg

Serzone® [DSC]: 50 mg, 100 mg, 150 mg, 200 mg, 250 mg

**nefazodone hydrochloride** *see* nefazodone *on this page*

**NegGram**® **[US/Can]** *see* nalidixic acid *on page 559*

## nelfinavir (nel FIN a veer)

**Sound-Alike/Look-Alike Issues**

nelfinavir may be confused with nevirapine

Viracept® may be confused with Viramune®

**Synonyms** NFV

**U.S./Canadian Brand Names** Viracept® [US/Can]

**Therapeutic Category** Antiviral Agent

**Use** In combination with other antiretroviral therapy in the treatment of HIV infection

**Usual Dosage** Oral:

Children 2-13 years: 45-55 mg/kg twice daily **or** 25-35 mg/kg 3 times/day (maximum: 2500 mg/day); all doses should be taken with a meal. If tablets are unable to be taken, use oral powder in small amount of water, milk, formula, or dietary supplements; do not use acidic food/juice or store for >6 hours.

Adults: 750 mg 3 times/day with meals or 1250 mg twice daily with meals in combination with other antiretroviral therapies

**Note:** Dosage adjustments for nelfinavir when administered in combination with ritonavir: Nelfinavir 500-750 mg twice daily plus ritonavir 400 mg twice daily

**Dosage Forms**

Powder, oral: 50 mg/g (144 g) [contains phenylalanine 11.2 mg/g]

Tablet [film coated]: 250 mg, 625 mg

**Nelova**™ **0.5/35E** *(Discontinued)* *see* ethinyl estradiol and norethindrone *on page 314*

**Nelova**™ **1/35E** *(Discontinued)* *see* ethinyl estradiol and norethindrone *on page 314*

**Nelova**™ **1/50M** *(Discontinued)* *see* mestranol and norethindrone *on page 517*

**Nelova**™ **10/11** *(Discontinued)* *see* ethinyl estradiol and norethindrone *on page 314*

**Nembutal**® **[US]** *see* pentobarbital *on page 631*

**Nembutal**® **Sodium [Can]** *see* pentobarbital *on page 631*

**Neo-Calglucon**® *(Discontinued)* *see* calcium glubionate *on page 133*

**NeoCeuticals**™ **Acne Spot Treatment [US-OTC]** *see* salicylic acid *on page 734*

**NeoDecadron**® **[US]** *see* neomycin and dexamethasone *on this page*

**Neo-Dexameth**® **Ophthalmic** *(Discontinued)* *see* neomycin and dexamethasone *on this page*

**Neo-Durabolic**® *(Discontinued)* *see* nandrolone *on page 560*

**Neofed**® *(Discontinued)* *see* pseudoephedrine *on page 692*

**Neo-Fradin**™ **[US]** *see* neomycin *on this page*

**Neomixin**® **Topical** *(Discontinued)* *see* bacitracin, neomycin, and polymyxin B *on page 87*

## neomycin (nee oh MYE sin)

**Synonyms** neomycin sulfate

**U.S./Canadian Brand Names** Neo-Fradin™ [US]; Neo-Rx [US]

**Therapeutic Category** Aminoglycoside (Antibiotic); Antibiotic, Topical

**Use** Orally to prepare GI tract for surgery; topically to treat minor skin infections; treatment of diarrhea caused by *E. coli*; adjunct in the treatment of hepatic encephalopathy; bladder irrigation; ocular infections

**Usual Dosage**

Children: Oral:

Preoperative intestinal antisepsis: 90 mg/kg/day divided every 4 hours for 2 days; or 25 mg/kg at 1 PM, 2 PM, and 11 PM on the day preceding surgery as an adjunct to mechanical cleansing of the intestine and in combination with erythromycin base

Hepatic encephalopathy: 50-100 mg/kg/day in divided doses every 6-8 hours or 2.5-7 g/m$^2$/day divided every 4-6 hours for 5-6 days not to exceed 12 g/day

Children and Adults: Topical: Topical solutions containing 0.1% to 1% neomycin have been used for irrigation

Adults: Oral:

Preoperative intestinal antisepsis: 1 g each hour for 4 doses then 1 g every 4 hours for 5 doses; or 1 g at 1 PM, 2 PM, and 11 PM on day preceding surgery as an adjunct to mechanical cleansing of the bowel and oral erythromycin; or 6 g/day divided every 4 hours for 2-3 days

Hepatic encephalopathy: 500-2000 mg every 6-8 hours or 4-12 g/day divided every 4-6 hours for 5-6 days

Chronic hepatic insufficiency: 4 g/day for an indefinite period

**Dosage Forms**

Powder, micronized, as sulfate [for prescription compounding] (Neo-Rx): (10 g, 100 g)

Solution, oral, as sulfate (Neo-Fradin™): 125 mg/5 mL (60 mL, 480 mL) [contains benzoic acid; cherry flavor]

Tablet, as sulfate: 500 mg

## neomycin and dexamethasone (nee oh MYE sin & deks a METH a sone)

**Synonyms** dexamethasone and neomycin

**U.S./Canadian Brand Names** NeoDecadron® [US]

**Therapeutic Category** Antibiotic/Corticosteroid, Ophthalmic; Antibiotic/Corticosteroid, Topical

**Use** Treatment of steroid responsive inflammatory conditions of the palpebral and bulbar conjunctiva, lid, cornea, and anterior segment of the globe

**Usual Dosage** Ophthalmic: Instill 1-2 drops in eye(s) every 3-4 hours

**Dosage Forms** Solution, ophthalmic: Neomycin sulfate 0.35% [3.5 mg/mL] and dexamethasone sodium phosphate 0.1% [1 mg/mL] (5 mL) [contains benzalkonium chloride and sodium bisulfite]

## neomycin and polymyxin B (nee oh MYE sin & pol i MIKS in bee)

**Synonyms** polymyxin B and neomycin

**U.S./Canadian Brand Names** Neosporin® G.U. Irrigant [US]; Neosporin® Irrigating Solution [Can]

**Therapeutic Category** Antibiotic, Topical; Genitourinary Irrigant

**Use** Short-term as a continuous irrigant or rinse in the urinary bladder to prevent bacteriuria and gram-negative rod septicemia associated with the use of indwelling catheters; to help prevent infection in minor cuts, scrapes, and burns

**Usual Dosage** Children and Adults: Bladder irrigation: **Not for injection**; add 1 mL irrigant to 1 liter isotonic saline solution and connect container to the inflow of lumen of 3-way catheter. Continuous irrigant or rinse in the urinary bladder for up to a maximum of 10 days with administration rate adjusted to patient's urine output; usually no more than 1 L of irrigant is used per day.

**Dosage Forms** Solution, irrigant: Neomycin 40 mg and polymyxin B sulfate 200,000 units per mL (1 mL, 20 mL)

**neomycin, bacitracin, and polymyxin B** *see* bacitracin, neomycin, and polymyxin B *on page 87*

**neomycin, bacitracin, polymyxin B, and hydrocortisone** *see* bacitracin, neomycin, polymyxin B, and hydrocortisone *on page 87*

## neomycin, colistin, hydrocortisone, and thonzonium
(nee oh MYE sin, koe LIS tin, hye droe KOR ti sone, & thon ZOE nee um)

**Synonyms** colistin, neomycin, hydrocortisone, and thonzonium; hydrocortisone, neomycin, colistin, and thonzonium; thonzonium, neomycin, colistin, and hydrocortisone

**U.S./Canadian Brand Names** Coly-Mycin® S [US]; Cortisporin®-TC [US]

**Therapeutic Category** Antibiotic/Corticosteroid, Otic

**Use** Treatment of superficial and susceptible bacterial infections of the external auditory canal; for treatment of susceptible bacterial infections of mastoidectomy and fenestration cavities

**Usual Dosage** Otic:
Calibrated dropper:
 Children: 4 drops in affected ear 3-4 times/day
 Adults: 5 drops in affected ear 3-4 times/day
Dropper bottle:
 Children: 3 drops in affected ear 3-4 times/day
 Adults: 4 drops in affected ear 3-4 times/day
**Note:** Alternatively, a cotton wick may be inserted in the ear canal and saturated with suspension every 4 hours; wick should be replaced at least every 24 hours

**Dosage Forms** Suspension, otic [drops]:
Coly-Mycin® S: Neomycin 0.33%, colistin 0.3%, hydrocortisone acetate 1%, and thonzonium bromide 0.05% (5 mL) [contains thimerosal; packaged with dropper]
Cortisporin®-TC: Neomycin 0.33%, colistin 0.3%, hydrocortisone acetate 1%, and thonzonium bromide 0.05% (10 mL) [contains thimerosal; packaged with dropper]

## neomycin, polymyxin B, and dexamethasone
(nee oh MYE sin, pol i MIKS in bee, & deks a METH a sone)

**Sound-Alike/Look-Alike Issues**
AK-Trol® may be confused with AKTob®

**Synonyms** dexamethasone, neomycin, and polymyxin B; polymyxin B, neomycin, and dexamethasone

**U.S./Canadian Brand Names** AK-Trol® [US]; Dexasporin [US]; Dioptrol® [Can]; Maxitrol® [US/Can]; Methadex [US]

**Therapeutic Category** Antibiotic/Corticosteroid, Ophthalmic

**Use** Steroid-responsive inflammatory ocular conditions in which a corticosteroid is indicated and where bacterial infection or a risk of bacterial infection exists

**Usual Dosage** Children and Adults: Ophthalmic:
Ointment: Place a small amount (~1/2") in the affected eye 3-4 times/day or apply at bedtime as an adjunct wsith drops
Suspension: Instill 1-2 drops into affected eye(s) every 3-4 hours; in severe disease, drops may be used hourly and tapered to discontinuation

**Dosage Forms** [DSC] = Discontinued product
Ointment, ophthalmic (Dexacine™ [DSC], Maxitrol®): Neomycin 3.5 mg, polymyxin B sulfate 10,000 units, and dexamethasone 0.1% per g (3.5 g)
(Continued)

## neomycin, polymyxin B, and dexamethasone *(Continued)*

Suspension, ophthalmic (AK-Trol®, Dexacidin® [DSC], Dexasporin, Maxitrol®, Methadex): Neomycin 3.5 mg, polymyxin B sulfate 10,000 units, and dexamethasone 0.1% per mL (5 mL) [contains benzalkonium chloride]

## neomycin, polymyxin B, and gramicidin

(nee oh MYE sin, pol i MIKS in bee, & gram i SYE din)

**Synonyms** gramicidin, neomycin, and polymyxin B; polymyxin B, neomycin, and gramicidin

**U.S./Canadian Brand Names** Neosporin® Ophthalmic Solution [US]; Neosporin® [Can]; Optimyxin Plus® [Can]

**Therapeutic Category** Antibiotic, Ophthalmic

**Use** Treatment of superficial ocular infection

**Usual Dosage** Children and Adults: Ophthalmic: Instill 1-2 drops 4-6 times/day or more frequently as required for severe infections

**Dosage Forms** Solution, ophthalmic: Neomycin 1.75 mg, polymyxin B 10,000 units, and gramicidin 0.025 mg per mL (10 mL) [contains alcohol 0.5% and thimerosal]

## neomycin, polymyxin B, and hydrocortisone

(nee oh MYE sin, pol i MIKS in bee, & hye droe KOR ti sone)

**Synonyms** hydrocortisone, neomycin, and polymyxin B; polymyxin B, neomycin, and hydrocortisone

**U.S./Canadian Brand Names** AntibiOtic® Ear [US]; Cortimyxin® [Can]; Cortisporin® Cream [US]; Cortisporin® Ophthalmic [US]; Cortisporin® Otic [US/Can]; PediOtic® [US]

**Therapeutic Category** Antibiotic/Corticosteroid, Ophthalmic; Antibiotic/Corticosteroid, Otic; Antibiotic/Corticosteroid, Topical

**Use** Steroid-responsive inflammatory condition for which a corticosteroid is indicated and where bacterial infection or a risk of bacterial infection exists

**Usual Dosage** Duration of use should be limited to 10 days unless otherwise directed by the physician

Otic solution is used **only** for swimmer's ear (infections of external auditory canal)

Otic:

Children: Instill 3 drops into affected ear 3-4 times/day

Adults: Instill 4 drops 3-4 times/day; otic suspension is the preferred otic preparation

Children and Adults:

Ophthalmic: Drops: Instill 1-2 drops 2-4 times/day, or more frequently as required for severe infections; in acute infections, instill 1-2 drops every 15-30 minutes gradually reducing the frequency of administration as the infection is controlled

Topical: Apply a thin layer 1-4 times/day. Therapy should be discontinued when control is achieved; if no improvement is seen, reassessment of diagnosis may be necessary.

**Dosage Forms**

Cream, topical (Cortisporin®): Neomycin 3.5 mg, polymyxin B 10,000 units, and hydrocortisone 5 mg per g (7.5 g)

Solution, otic (AntibiOtic® Ear; Cortisporin®): Neomycin 3.5 mg, polymyxin B 10,000 units, and hydrocortisone 10 mg per mL (10 mL) [contains potassium metabisulfite]

Suspension, ophthalmic (Cortisporin®): Neomycin 3.5 mg, polymyxin B 10,000 units, and hydrocortisone 10 mg per mL (7.5 mL) [contains thimerosal]

Suspension, otic: Neomycin 3.5 mg, polymyxin B 10,000 units, and hydrocortisone 10 mg per mL (10 mL)

AntibiOtic® Ear, Cortisporin®: Neomycin 3.5 mg, polymyxin B 10,000 units, and hydrocortisone 10 mg per mL (10 mL) [contains thimerosal]

PediOtic®: Neomycin 3.5 mg, polymyxin B 10,000 units, and hydrocortisone 10 mg per mL (7.5 mL) [contains thimerosal]

## neomycin, polymyxin B, and prednisolone

(nee oh MYE sin, pol i MIKS in bee, & pred NIS oh lone)

**Synonyms** polymyxin B, neomycin, and prednisolone; prednisolone, neomycin, and polymyxin B

**U.S./Canadian Brand Names** Poly-Pred® [US]

**Therapeutic Category** Antibiotic/Corticosteroid, Ophthalmic

**Use** Steroid-responsive inflammatory ocular condition in which bacterial infection or a risk of bacterial ocular infection exists

**Usual Dosage** Children and Adults: Ophthalmic: Instill 1-2 drops every 3-4 hours; acute infections may require every 30-minute instillation initially with frequency of administration reduced as the infection is brought under control. To treat the lids: Instill 1-2 drops every 3-4 hours, close the eye and rub the excess on the lids and lid margins.

**Dosage Forms** Suspension, ophthalmic: Neomycin 0.35%, polymyxin B 10,000 units per mL, and prednisolone acetate 0.5% (5 mL; 10 mL [DSC]) [contains thimerosal]

**neomycin sulfate** *see* neomycin *on page 566*

**neonatal trace metals** *see* trace metals *on page 813*

**Neoral**® **[US/Can]** *see* cyclosporine *on page 215*

**Neo-Rx [US]** *see* neomycin *on page 566*

**Neosporin**® **[Can]** *see* neomycin, polymyxin B, and gramicidin *on previous page*

**Neosporin**® **AF [US-OTC]** *see* miconazole *on page 537*

**Neosporin**® **G.U. Irrigant [US]** *see* neomycin and polymyxin B *on page 567*

**Neosporin**® **Irrigating Solution [Can]** *see* neomycin and polymyxin B *on page 567*

**Neosporin**® **Neo To Go**® **[US-OTC]** *see* bacitracin, neomycin, and polymyxin B *on page 87*

**Neosporin**® **Ophthalmic Ointment [US/Can]** *see* bacitracin, neomycin, and polymyxin B *on page 87*

**Neosporin**® **Ophthalmic Solution [US]** *see* neomycin, polymyxin B, and gramicidin *on previous page*

**Neosporin**® **Topical [US-OTC]** *see* bacitracin, neomycin, and polymyxin B *on page 87*

## neostigmine (nee oh STIG meen)

**Sound-Alike/Look-Alike Issues**
Prostigmin® may be confused with physostigmine

**Synonyms** neostigmine bromide; neostigmine methylsulfate

**U.S./Canadian Brand Names** Prostigmin® [US/Can]

**Therapeutic Category** Cholinergic Agent

**Use** Diagnosis and treatment of myasthenia gravis; prevention and treatment of postoperative bladder distention and urinary retention; reversal of the effects of nondepolarizing neuromuscular-blocking agents after surgery

**Usual Dosage**
Myasthenia gravis: Diagnosis: I.M.:
Children: 0.04 mg/kg as a single dose
Adults: 0.02 mg/kg as a single dose
Myasthenia gravis: Treatment:
Children:
Oral: 2 mg/kg/day divided every 3-4 hours
I.M., I.V., SubQ: 0.01-0.04 mg/kg every 2-4 hours
Adults:
Oral: 15 mg/dose every 3-4 hours up to 375 mg/day maximum; interval between doses must be individualized to maximal response
I.M., I.V., SubQ: 0.5-2.5 mg every 1-3 hours up to 10 mg/24 hours maximum
Reversal of nondepolarizing neuromuscular blockade after surgery in conjunction with atropine (must administer atropine several minutes prior to neostigmine): I.V.:
Infants: 0.025-0.1 mg/kg/dose
Children: 0.025-0.08 mg/kg/dose
Adults: 0.5-2.5 mg; total dose not to exceed 5 mg
Bladder atony: Adults: I.M., SubQ:
Prevention: 0.25 mg every 4-6 hours for 2-3 days
Treatment: 0.5-1 mg every 3 hours for 5 doses after bladder has emptied

**Dosage Forms**
Injection, solution, as methylsulfate: 0.5 mg/mL (1 mL, 10 mL); 1 mg/mL (10 mL)
Tablet, as bromide: 15 mg

**neostigmine bromide** *see* neostigmine *on this page*

**neostigmine methylsulfate** *see* neostigmine *on this page*

**NeoStrata AHA [US-OTC]** *see* hydroquinone *on page 420*

**NeoStrata**® **HQ [Can]** *see* hydroquinone *on page 420*

**Neo-Synephrine**® **[Can]** *see* phenylephrine *on page 640*

**Neo-Synephrine® 12 Hour [US-OTC]** *see* oxymetazoline *on page 610*

**Neo-Synephrine® 12 Hour Extra Moisturizing [US-OTC]** *see* oxymetazoline *on page 610*

**Neo-Synephrine® Extra Strength [US-OTC]** *see* phenylephrine *on page 640*

**Neo-Synephrine® Mild [US-OTC]** *see* phenylephrine *on page 640*

**Neo-Synephrine® Ophthalmic [US]** *see* phenylephrine *on page 640*

**Neo-Synephrine® Regular Strength [US-OTC]** *see* phenylephrine *on page 640*

**Neo-Tabs®** *(Discontinued) see* neomycin *on page 566*

**Neotrace-4® [US]** *see* trace metals *on page 813*

**NeoVadrin®** *(Discontinued)*

**NephPlex® Rx [US]** *see* vitamin B complex combinations *on page 849*

**Nephro-Calci® [US-OTC]** *see* calcium carbonate *on page 130*

**Nephrocaps® [US]** *see* vitamin B complex combinations *on page 849*

**Nephro-Fer® [US-OTC]** *see* ferrous fumarate *on page 334*

**Nephron FA® [US]** *see* vitamin B complex combinations *on page 849*

**Nephro-Vite® [US]** *see* vitamin B complex combinations *on page 849*

**Nephro-Vite® Rx [US]** *see* vitamin B complex combinations *on page 849*

**Nephrox Suspension** *(Discontinued) see* aluminum hydroxide *on page 34*

**Neptazane®** *(Discontinued) see* methazolamide *on page 522*

**Nervocaine® Injection** *(Discontinued) see* lidocaine *on page 479*

**Nesacaine® [US]** *see* chloroprocaine *on page 169*

**Nesacaine®-CE [Can]** *see* chloroprocaine *on page 169*

**Nesacaine®-MPF [US]** *see* chloroprocaine *on page 169*

**nesiritide** (ni SIR i tide)

**Synonyms** B-type natriuretic peptide (human); hBNP; natriuretic peptide

**U.S./Canadian Brand Names** Natrecor® [US]

**Therapeutic Category** Natriuretic Peptide, B-type, Human; Vasodilator

**Use** Treatment of acutely decompensated congestive heart failure (CHF) in patients with dyspnea at rest or with minimal activity

**Usual Dosage** Adults: I.V.: Initial: 2 mcg/kg (bolus); followed by continuous infusion at 0.01 mcg/kg/minute; **Note:** Should not be initiated at a dosage higher than initial recommended dose. At intervals of ≥3 hours, the dosage may be increased by 0.005 mcg/kg/minute (preceded by a bolus of 1 mcg/kg), up to a maximum of 0.03 mcg/kg/minute. Increases beyond the initial infusion rate should be limited to selected patients and accompanied by hemodynamic monitoring.

Patients experiencing hypotension during the infusion: Infusion should be interrupted. May attempt to restart at a lower dose (reduce initial infusion dose by 30% and omit bolus).

**Dosage Forms** Injection, powder for reconstitution: 1.5 mg

**Nestabs® CBF [US]** *see* vitamins (multiple/prenatal) *on page 852*

**Nestabs® FA [US]** *see* vitamins (multiple/prenatal) *on page 852*

**Nestabs® RX [US]** *see* vitamins (multiple/prenatal) *on page 852*

**Nestrex®** *(Discontinued) see* pyridoxine *on page 701*

**Netromycin®** *(Discontinued)*

**Neucalm-50® Injection** *(Discontinued) see* hydroxyzine *on page 423*

**Neulasta™ [US/Can]** *see* pegfilgrastim *on page 623*

**Neuleptil® [Can]** *see* pericyazine *(Canada only) on page 634*

**Neumega® [US]** *see* oprelvekin *on page 601*

**Neupogen® [US/Can]** *see* filgrastim *on page 338*

**Neuramate®** *(Discontinued) see* meprobamate *on page 514*

**Neurontin® [US/Can]** *see* gabapentin *on page 365*

**Neut® [US]** *see* sodium bicarbonate *on page 752*

**NeutraCare**® **[US]** *see* fluoride *on page 347*

**NeutraGard**® **[US-OTC]** *see* fluoride *on page 347*

**Neutra-Phos**® **[US-OTC]** *see* potassium phosphate and sodium phosphate *on page 667*

**Neutra-Phos**®**-K [US-OTC]** *see* potassium phosphate *on page 666*

**NeuTrexin**® **[US]** *see* trimetrexate glucuronate *on page 826*

**Neutrogena**® **Acne Mask [US-OTC]** *see* benzoyl peroxide *on page 98*

**Neutrogena**® **Acne Wash [US-OTC]** *see* salicylic acid *on page 734*

**Neutrogena**® **Body Clear**™ **[US-OTC]** *see* salicylic acid *on page 734*

**Neutrogena**® **Clear Pore [US-OTC]** *see* salicylic acid *on page 734*

**Neutrogena**® **Clear Pore Shine Control [US-OTC]** *see* salicylic acid *on page 734*

**Neutrogena**® **Healthy Scalp [US-OTC]** *see* salicylic acid *on page 734*

**Neutrogena**® **Maximum Strength T/Sal**® **[US-OTC]** *see* salicylic acid *on page 734*

**Neutrogena**® **On The Spot**® **Acne Patch [US-OTC]** *see* salicylic acid *on page 734*

**Neutrogena**® **On The Spot**® **Acne Treatment [US-OTC]** *see* benzoyl peroxide *on page 98*

**Neutrogena**® **T/Gel [US-OTC]** *see* coal tar *on page 201*

**Neutrogena**® **T/Gel Extra Strength [US-OTC]** *see* coal tar *on page 201*

## nevirapine (ne VYE ra peen)

**Sound-Alike/Look-Alike Issues**
nevirapine may be confused with nelfinavir
Viramune® may be confused with Viracept®

**Synonyms** NVP

**U.S./Canadian Brand Names** Viramune® [US/Can]

**Therapeutic Category** Antiviral Agent

**Use** In combination therapy with other antiretroviral agents for the treatment of HIV-1

**Usual Dosage** Oral:

Children 2 months to <8 years: Initial: 4 mg/kg/dose once daily for 14 days; increase dose to 7 mg/kg/dose every 12 hours if no rash or other adverse effects occur; maximum dose: 200 mg/dose every 12 hours

Children ≥8 years: Initial: 4 mg/kg/dose once daily for 14 days; increase dose to 4 mg/kg/dose every 12 hours if no rash or other adverse effects occur; maximum dose: 200 mg/dose every 12 hours

**Note:** Alternative pediatric dosing (AIDSinfo guidelines): 120-200 mg/m² every 12 hours; this dosing has been proposed due to the fact that dosing based on mg/kg may result in an abrupt decrease in dose at the 8th birthday, which may be inappropriate.

Adults: Initial: 200 mg once daily for 14 days; maintenance: 200 mg twice daily (in combination with an additional antiretroviral agent)

**Note:** If patient experiences a rash during the 14-day lead-in period, dose should not be increased until the rash has resolved. Discontinue if severe rash, or rash with constitutional symptoms, is noted. If therapy is interrupted for >7 days, restart with initial dose for 14 days. Use of prednisone to prevent nevirapine-associated rash is not recommended. Permanently discontinue if symptomatic hepatic events occur.

**Dosage Forms**
Suspension, oral: 50 mg/5 mL (240 mL)
Tablet: 200 mg

**Nexium**® **[US/Can]** *see* esomeprazole *on page 298*

**NFV** *see* nelfinavir *on page 565*

**N.G.A.**® **Topical *(Discontinued)*** *see* nystatin and triamcinolone *on page 592*

## niacin (NYE a sin)

**Sound-Alike/Look-Alike Issues**
niacin may be confused with Minocin®, Niaspan®, Nispan®
Niaspan® may be confused with niacin
Nicobid® may be confused with Nitro-Bid®

(Continued)

# niacin *(Continued)*

**Synonyms** nicotinic acid; vitamin B$_3$

**U.S./Canadian Brand Names** Niacor® [US]; Niaspan® [US/Can]; Slo-Niacin® [US-OTC]

**Therapeutic Category** Vitamin, Water Soluble

**Use** Adjunctive treatment of dyslipidemias (types IIa and IIb or primary hypercholesterolemia) to lower the risk of recurrent MI and/or slow progression of coronary artery disease, including combination therapy with other antidyslipidemic agents when additional triglyceride-lowering or HDL-increasing effects are desired; treatment of hypertriglyceridemia in patients at risk of pancreatitis; treatment of peripheral vascular disease and circulatory disorders; treatment of pellagra; dietary supplement

**Usual Dosage**

Children: Oral:

Pellagra: 50-100 mg/dose 3 times/day

Recommended daily allowances:

0-0.5 years: 5 mg/day

0.5-1 year: 6 mg/day

1-3 years: 9 mg/day

4-6 years: 12 mg/day

7-10 years: 13 mg/day

Children and Adolescents: Recommended daily allowances:

Male:

11-14 years: 17 mg/day

15-18 years: 20 mg/day

19-24 years: 19 mg/day

Female: 11-24 years: 15 mg/day

Adults: Oral:

Recommended daily allowances:

Male: 25-50 years: 19 mg/day; >51 years: 15 mg/day

Female: 25-50 years: 15 mg/day; >51 years: 13 mg/day

Hyperlipidemia: Usual target dose: 1.5-6 g/day in 3 divided doses with or after meals using a dosage titration schedule; extended release: 375 mg to 2 g once daily at bedtime

Regular release formulation (Niacor®): Initial: 250 mg once daily (with evening meal); increase frequency and/or dose every 4-7 days to desired response or first-level therapeutic dose (1.5-2 g/day in 2-3 divided doses); after 2 months, may increase at 2- to 4-week intervals to 3 g/day in 3 divided doses

Extended release formulation (Niaspan®): 500 mg at bedtime for 4 weeks, then 1 g at bedtime for 4 weeks; adjust dose to response and tolerance; can increase to a maximum of 2 g/day, but only at 500 mg/day at 4-week intervals

With lovastatin: Maximum lovastatin dose: 40 mg/day

Pellagra: 50-100 mg 3-4 times/day, maximum: 500 mg/day

Niacin deficiency: 10-20 mg/day, maximum: 100 mg/day

**Dosage Forms**

Capsule, extended release: 125 mg, 250 mg, 400 mg, 500 mg

Capsule, timed release: 250 mg

Tablet: 50 mg, 100 mg, 250 mg, 500 mg

Niacor®: 500 mg

Tablet, controlled release (Slo-Niacin®): 250 mg, 500 mg, 750 mg

Tablet, extended release (Niaspan®): 500 mg, 750 mg, 1000 mg

**Note:** 500 mg and 750 mg tablets are not interchangeable (eg, three 500 mg tablets are not equivalent to two 750 mg tablets)

Tablet, timed release: 250 mg, 500 mg, 750 mg, 1000 mg

# niacinamide *(nye a SIN a mide)*

**Sound-Alike/Look-Alike Issues**

niacinamide may be confused with niCARdipine

**Synonyms** nicotinamide; nicotinic acid amide; vitamin B$_3$

**U.S./Canadian Brand Names** Nicomide-T™ [US]

**Therapeutic Category** Vitamin, Water Soluble

**Use**

Oral: Prophylaxis and treatment of pellagra

Topical: Improve the appearance of acne and decrease visible inflammation and irritation caused by acne medications

**Usual Dosage**
  Pellagra: Oral:
    Children: 100-300 mg/day in divided doses
    Adults: 300-500 mg/day
  Acne: Topical: Adults: Apply to affected area on face twice daily
**Dosage Forms**
  Cream (Nicomide-T™): 4% (30 g) [contains benzyl alcohol]
  Gel (Nicomide-T™): 4% (30 g) [contains alcohol]
  Tablet: 100 mg, 250 mg, 500 mg

# niacin and lovastatin (NYE a sin & LOE va sta tin)

**Sound-Alike/Look-Alike Issues**
  Advicor® may be confused with Advair, Altocor™
**Synonyms** lovastatin and niacin
**U.S./Canadian Brand Names** Advicor® [US]
**Therapeutic Category** HMG-CoA Reductase Inhibitor; Vitamin, Water Soluble
**Use** Treatment of primary hypercholesterolemia (heterozygous familial and nonfamilial) and mixed dyslipidemia (Fredrickson types IIa and IIb) in patients previously treated with either agent alone (patients who require further lowering of triglycerides (TG) or increase in HDL-cholesterol (HDL-C) from addition of niacin or further lowering of LDL-cholesterol (LDL-C) from addition of lovastatin). Combination product; not intended for initial treatment.
**Usual Dosage** Dosage forms are a fixed combination of niacin and lovastatin.
  Oral: Adults: Lowest dose: Niacin 500 mg/lovastatin 20 mg; may increase by not more than 500 mg (niacin) at 4-week intervals (maximum dose: Niacin 2000 mg/lovastatin 40 mg daily); should be taken at bedtime with a low-fat snack
  Not for use as initial therapy of dyslipidemias. May be substituted for equivalent dose of Niaspan®, however, manufacturer does not recommend direct substitution with other niacin products.
**Dosage Forms** [DSC] = Discontinued product
  Tablet, variable release:
    500/20: Niacin 500 mg [extended release] and lovastatin 20 mg [immediate release]
    750/20: Niacin 750 mg [extended release] and lovastatin 20 mg [immediate release] [DSC]
    1000/20: Niacin 1000 mg [extended release] and lovastatin 20 mg [immediate release]

**Niacor® [US]** *see* niacin *on page 571*

**Niaspan® [US/Can]** *see* niacin *on page 571*

**Niastase® [Can]** *see* factor VIIa (recombinant) *on page 325*

# nicardipine (nye KAR de peen)

**Sound-Alike/Look-Alike Issues**
  niCARdipine may be confused with niacinamide, NIFEdipine, nimodipine
  Cardene® may be confused with Cardizem®, Cardura®, codeine
**Synonyms** nicardipine hydrochloride
**Tall-Man** niCARdipine
**U.S./Canadian Brand Names** Cardene® I.V. [US]; Cardene® SR [US]; Cardene® [US]
**Therapeutic Category** Calcium Channel Blocker
**Use** Chronic stable angina (immediate-release product only); management of essential hypertension (immediate and sustained release; parenteral only for short time that oral treatment is not feasible)
**Usual Dosage** Adults:
  Oral:
    Immediate release: Initial: 20 mg 3 times/day; usual: 20-40 mg 3 times/day (allow 3 days between dose increases)
    Sustained release: Initial: 30 mg twice daily, titrate up to 60 mg twice daily
    **Note:** The total daily dose of immediate-release product may not automatically be equivalent to the daily sustained-release dose; use caution in converting.
  I.V. (dilute to 0.1 mg/mL):
    Acute hypertension: Initial: 5 mg/hour increased by 2.5 mg/hour every 15 minutes to a maximum of 15 mg/hour; consider reduction to 3 mg/hour after response is achieved. Monitor and titrate to lowest dose necessary to maintain stable blood pressure.
    Substitution for oral therapy (approximate equivalents):
      20 mg every 8 hours oral, equivalent to 0.5 mg/hour I.V. infusion
      30 mg every 8 hours oral, equivalent to 1.2 mg/hour I.V. infusion
(Continued)

## nicardipine *(Continued)*

40 mg every 8 hours oral, equivalent to 2.2 mg/hour I.V. infusion

### Dosage Forms

Capsule (Cardene®): 20 mg, 30 mg
Capsule, sustained release (Cardene® SR): 30 mg, 45 mg, 60 mg
Injection, solution (Cardene® IV): 2.5 mg/mL (10 mL)

**nicardipine hydrochloride** *see nicardipine on previous page*

**N'ice® *(Discontinued)*** *see ascorbic acid on page 71*

**Nicobid® *(Discontinued)*** *see niacin on page 571*

**Nicoderm® [Can]** *see nicotine on this page*

**NicoDerm® CQ® [US-OTC]** *see nicotine on this page*

**Nicolar® *(Discontinued)*** *see niacin on page 571*

**Nicomide-T™ [US]** *see niacinamide on page 572*

**Nicorette® [US-OTC/Can]** *see nicotine on this page*

**Nicorette® Plus [Can]** *see nicotine on this page*

**nicotinamide** *see niacinamide on page 572*

## nicotine (nik oh TEEN)

### Sound-Alike/Look-Alike Issues

NicoDerm® may be confused with Nitroderm
Nicorette® may be confused with Nordette®

**U.S./Canadian Brand Names** Commit™ [US-OTC]; Habitrol® [Can]; NicoDerm® CQ® [US-OTC]; Nicoderm® [Can]; Nicorette® Plus [Can]; Nicorette® [US-OTC/Can]; Nicotrol® Inhaler [US]; Nicotrol® NS [US]; Nicotrol® Patch [US-OTC]; Nicotrol® [Can]

**Therapeutic Category** Smoking Deterrent

**Use** Treatment to aid smoking cessation for the relief of nicotine withdrawal symptoms (including nicotine craving)

### Usual Dosage

Smoking deterrent: Patients should be advised to completely stop smoking upon initiation of therapy.

Gum: Chew 1 piece of gum when urge to smoke, up to 30 pieces/day; most patients require 10-12 pieces of gum/day

Inhaler: Usually 6 to 16 cartridges per day; best effect was achieved by frequent continuous puffing (20 minutes); recommended duration of treatment is 3 months, after which patients may be weaned from the inhaler by gradual reduction of the daily dose over 6-12 weeks

Lozenge: Patients who smoke their first cigarette within 30 minutes of waking should use the 4 mg strength; otherwise the 2 mg strength is recommended.

Weeks 1-6: One lozenge every 1-2 hours
Weeks 7-9: One lozenge every 2-4 hours
Weeks 10-12: One lozenge every 4-8 hours

**Note:** Use at least 9 lozenges/day during first 6 weeks to improve chances of quitting; do not use more than one lozenge at a time (maximum: 5 lozenges every 6 hours, 20 lozenges/day)

Transdermal patch: Apply new patch every 24 hours to nonhairy, clean, dry skin on the upper body or upper outer arm; each patch should be applied to a different site. **Note:** Adjustment may be required during initial treatment (move to higher dose if experiencing withdrawal symptoms; lower dose if side effects are experienced).

Habitrol®, NicoDerm CQ®:

Patients smoking ≥10 cigarettes/day: Begin with **step 1** (21 mg/day) for 4-6 weeks, followed by **step 2** (14 mg/day) for 2 weeks; finish with **step 3** (7 mg/day) for 2 weeks

Patients smoking <10 cigarettes/day: Begin with **step 2** (14 mg/day) for 6 weeks, followed by **step 3** (7 mg/day) for 2 weeks

**Note:** Initial starting dose for patients <100 pounds, history of cardiovascular disease: 14 mg/day for 4-6 weeks, followed by 7 mg/day for 2-4 weeks

**Note:** Patients receiving >600 mg/day of cimetidine: Decrease to the next lower patch size

Nicotrol®: One patch daily for 6 weeks

**Note:** Benefits of use of nicotine transdermal patches beyond 3 months have not been demonstrated.

Spray: 1-2 sprays/hour; do not exceed more than 5 doses (10 sprays) per hour; each dose (2 sprays) contains 1 mg of nicotine. **Warning:** A dose of 40 mg can cause fatalities.

**Dosage Forms**
   Gum, chewing, as polacrilex: 2 mg (48s, 108s); 4 mg (48s, 108s)
     Nicorette®: 2 mg (48s, 50s, 108s, 110s, 168s, 170s, 192s, 200s, 216s); 4 mg (48s, 108s, 168s) [mint, fresh mint, orange, and original flavors]
   Lozenge, as polacrilex (Commit™): 2 mg (48s, 72s) [contains phenylalanine 3.4 mg/lozenge; mint flavor]; 4 mg (48s, 72s) [contains phenylalanine 3.4 mg/lozenge; mint flavor]
   Oral inhalation system (Nicotrol® Inhaler): 10 mg cartridge [delivering 4 mg nicotine] (168s) [each unit consists of 5 mouthpieces, 28 storage trays each containing 6 cartridges, and 1 storage case]
   Patch, transdermal: 7 mg/24 (30s); 14 mg/24 hours (30s); 21 mg/24 hours (30s)
     NicoDerm® CQ®: 7 mg/24 hours (14s); 14 mg/24 hours (14s); 21 mg/24 hours (14s) [available in tan or clear patch]
     Nicotrol®: 15 mg/16 hours (7s, 14s) [step 1]; 10 mg/16 hours (14s) [step 2]; 5 mg/16 hours (14s) [step 3]
   Solution, intranasal spray (Nicotrol® NS): 10 mg/mL (10 mL) [delivers 0.5 mg/spray; 200 sprays]

**nicotinic acid** *see niacin on page 571*

**nicotinic acid amide** *see niacinamide on page 572*

**Nicotrol® [Can]** *see nicotine on previous page*

**Nicotrol® Inhaler [US]** *see nicotine on previous page*

**Nicotrol® NS [US]** *scc nicotine on previous page*

**Nicotrol® Patch [US-OTC]** *see nicotine on previous page*

**Nico-Vert®** *(Discontinued) see meclizine on page 506*

**Nidagel™ [Can]** *see metronidazole on page 535*

**Nifediac™ CC [US]** *see nifedipine on this page*

**Nifedical™ XL [US]** *see nifedipine on this page*

## nifedipine (nye FED i peen)

**Sound-Alike/Look-Alike Issues**
   NIFEdipine may be confused with niCARdipine, nimodipine, nisoldipine
   Procardia XL® may be confused with Cartia® XT
**Tall-Man NIFE**dipine
**U.S./Canadian Brand Names** Adalat® CC [US]; Adalat® XL® [Can]; Afeditab™ CR [US]; Apo-Nifed PA® [Can]; Apo-Nifed® [Can]; Nifediac™ CC [US]; Nifedical™ XL [US]; Novo-Nifedin [Can]; Nu-Nifed [Can]; Procardia XL® [US]; Procardia® [US/Can]
**Therapeutic Category** Calcium Channel Blocker
**Use** Angina and hypertension (sustained release only), pulmonary hypertension
**Usual Dosage** Oral:
   Children: Hypertrophic cardiomyopathy: 0.6-0.9 mg/kg/24 hours in 3-4 divided doses
   Adolescents and Adults: (**Note:** When switching from immediate release to sustained release formulations, total daily dose will start the same)
     Initial: 30 mg once daily as sustained release formulation, or if indicated, 10 mg 3 times/day as capsules
     Usual dose: 10-30 mg 3 times/day as capsules or 30-60 mg once daily as sustained release
     Maximum dose: 120-180 mg/day
      *Increase sustained release at 7- to 14-day intervals*
**Dosage Forms**
   Capsule, softgel: 10 mg, 20 mg
     Procardia®: 10 mg
   Tablet, extended release: 30 mg, 60 mg, 90 mg
     Adalat® CC, Procardia XL®: 30 mg, 60 mg, 90 mg
     Afeditab™ CR, Nifedical™ XL: 30 mg, 60 mg
     Nifediac™ CC: 30 mg, 60 mg, 90 mg [90 mg tablet contains tartrazine]

**Niferex® [US-OTC]** *see polysaccharide-iron complex on page 660*

**Niferex® 150 [US-OTC]** *see polysaccharide-iron complex on page 660*

**Niferex®-PN [US]** *see vitamins (multiple/prenatal) on page 852*

**Niferex®-PN Forte [US]** *see vitamins (multiple/prenatal) on page 852*

**niftolid** *see flutamide on page 353*

**Night-Time Sleep Aid [US-OTC]** *see doxylamine on page 273*

**Nilandron**® **[US]** *see* nilutamide *on this page*

**Nilstat [Can]** *see* nystatin *on page 592*

**Nilstat**® *(Discontinued)* *see* nystatin *on page 592*

## nilutamide (ni LOO ta mide)

**Synonyms** RU-23908

**U.S./Canadian Brand Names** Anandron® [Can]; Nilandron® [US]

**Therapeutic Category** Antineoplastic Agent

**Use** Treatment of metastatic prostate cancer

**Usual Dosage** Refer to individual protocols.
  Adults: Oral: 300 mg daily for 30 days starting the same day or day after surgical castration, then 150 mg/day

**Dosage Forms** Tablet: 150 mg

**Nimbex**® **[US/Can]** *see* cisatracurium *on page 187*

## nimodipine (nye MOE di peen)

**Sound-Alike/Look-Alike Issues**
  nimodipine may be confused with niCARdipine, NIFEdipine

**U.S./Canadian Brand Names** Nimotop® [US/Can]

**Therapeutic Category** Calcium Channel Blocker

**Use** Spasm following subarachnoid hemorrhage from ruptured intracranial aneurysms regardless of the patients neurological condition postictus (Hunt and Hess grades I-V)

**Usual Dosage** Adults: Oral: 60 mg every 4 hours for 21 days, start therapy within 96 hours after subarachnoid hemorrhage.

**Dosage Forms** Capsule, liquid filled: 30 mg

**Nimotop**® **[US/Can]** *see* nimodipine *on this page*

**Nipent**® **[US/Can]** *see* pentostatin *on page 632*

**Niravam**™ **[US]** *see* alprazolam *on page 30*

## nisoldipine (NYE sole di peen)

**Sound-Alike/Look-Alike Issues**
  nisoldipine may be confused with NIFEdipine

**U.S./Canadian Brand Names** Sular® [US]

**Therapeutic Category** Calcium Channel Blocker

**Use** Management of hypertension, alone or in combination with other antihypertensive agents

**Usual Dosage** Adults: Oral: Initial: 20 mg once daily, then increase by 10 mg/week (or longer intervals) to attain adequate control of blood pressure; usual dose range (JNC 7): 10-40 mg once daily; doses >60 mg once daily are not recommended.

**Dosage Forms** Tablet, extended release: 10 mg, 20 mg, 30 mg, 40 mg

**nitalapram** *see* citalopram *on page 188*

## nitazoxanide (nye ta ZOX a nide)

**Synonyms** NTZ

**U.S./Canadian Brand Names** Alinia® [US]

**Therapeutic Category** Antiprotozoal

**Use** Treatment of diarrhea caused by *Cryptosporidium parvum* or *Giardia lamblia*

**Usual Dosage** Diarrhea caused by *Cryptosporidium parvum* or *Giardia lamblia*:
  Children 1-3 years: 100 mg every 12 hours for 3 days
  Children 4-11 years: 200 mg every 12 hours for 3 days
  Children ≥12 years and Adults: 500 mg every 12 hours for 3 days

**Dosage Forms**
  Powder for oral suspension: 100 mg/5 mL (60 mL) [contains sucrose 1.48 g/5 mL, sodium benzoate; strawberry flavor]
  Tablet: 500 mg
  Alinia® 3-Day Therapy Packs™ [unit-dose pack]: 500 mg (6s)

## nitisinone (ni TIS i known)

**U.S./Canadian Brand Names** Orfadin® [US]

**Therapeutic Category** 4-Hydroxyphenylpyruvate Dioxygenase Inhibitor

**Use** Treatment of hereditary tyrosinemia type 1 (HT-1); to be used with dietary restriction of tyrosine and phenylalanine

**Usual Dosage** Oral: **Note:** Must be used in conjunction with a low protein diet restricted in tyrosine and phenylalanine.

Infants: See dosing for Children and Adults; infants may require maximal dose once liver function has improved

Children and Adults: Initial: 1 mg/kg/day in divided doses, given in the morning and evening, 1 hour before meals; doses do not need to be divided evenly

**Dosage Forms** Capsule: 2 mg, 5 mg, 10 mg

**Nitoman**™ **[Can]** *see* tetrabenazine *(Canada only)* on page 790

## nitrazepam *(Canada only)* (nye TRA ze pam)

**Synonyms** nitrozepamum

**Therapeutic Category** Benzodiazepine

**Use Investigational**: Short-term management of insomnia; treatment of infantile spasm and seizures

**Usual Dosage** Oral:

Insomnia:

Children:

1-6 years: 2.5 mg

≥7 years: 5 mg

Adults: 5-10 mg at night

Epilepsy: Children and Adults: 1-6 mg/day; dosage should be decreased in elderly, hypothyroid patients, and cirrhosis

Children maximum dose: 60 mg

Adult maximum dose: 20 mg

**Dosage Forms**

Capsule: 5 mg

Tablet: 5 mg

**Nitrek**® **[US]** *see* nitroglycerin on next page

## nitric oxide (NYE trik OKS ide)

**U.S./Canadian Brand Names** INOmax® [US/Can]

**Therapeutic Category** Vasodilator, Pulmonary

**Use** Treatment of term and near-term (>34 weeks) neonates with hypoxic respiratory failure associated with pulmonary hypertension; used concurrently with ventilatory support and other agents

**Usual Dosage** Inhalation: Neonates (up to 14 days old): 20 ppm. Treatment should be maintained up to 14 days or until the underlying oxygen desaturation has resolved and the neonate is ready to be weaned from therapy. In the CINRGI trial, patients whose oxygenation improved had their dose reduced to 5 ppm at the end of 4 hours of treatment. Doses above 20 ppm should not be used because of the risk of methemoglobinemia and elevated $NO_2$.

**Dosage Forms** Gas, for inhalation:

100 ppm [nitric oxide 0.01% and nitrogen 99.99%] (353 L) [delivers 344 L], (1963 L) [delivers 1918 L]

800 ppm [nitric oxide 0.08% and nitrogen 99.92%] (353 L) [delivers 344 L], (1963 L) [delivers 1918 L]

**4′-nitro-3′-trifluoromethylisobutyrantide** *see* flutamide on page 353

**Nitro-Bid**® **[US]** *see* nitroglycerin on next page

**Nitrodisc**® **Patch** *(Discontinued)* *see* nitroglycerin on next page

**Nitro-Dur**® **[US/Can]** *see* nitroglycerin on next page

**nitrofural** *see* nitrofurazone on next page

## nitrofurantoin (nye troe fyoor AN toyn)

**U.S./Canadian Brand Names** Apo-Nitrofurantoin® [Can]; Furadantin® [US]; Macrobid® [US/Can]; Macrodantin® [US/Can]; Novo-Furantoin [Can]

(Continued)

## nitrofurantoin *(Continued)*

**Therapeutic Category** Antibiotic, Miscellaneous

**Use** Prevention and treatment of urinary tract infections caused by susceptible gram-negative and some gram-positive organisms; *Pseudomonas*, *Serratia*, and most species of *Proteus* are generally resistant to nitrofurantoin

**Usual Dosage** Oral:

Children >1 month: 5-7 mg/kg/day in divided doses every 6 hours; maximum: 400 mg/day

UTI prophylaxis (chronic): 1-2 mg/kg/day in divided doses every 12-24 hours; maximum: 100 mg/day

Adults: 50-100 mg/dose every 6 hours

Macrocrystal/monohydrate: 100 mg twice daily

UTI prophylaxis (chronic): 50-100 mg/dose at bedtime

**Dosage Forms**

Capsule, macrocrystal: 50 mg, 100 mg

Macrodantin®: 25 mg, 50 mg, 100 mg

Capsule, macrocrystal/monohydrate (Macrobid®): 100 mg

Suspension, oral (Furadantin®): 25 mg/5 mL (470 mL)

## nitrofurazone *(nye troe FYOOR a zone)*

**Synonyms** nitrofural

**Therapeutic Category** Antibacterial, Topical

**Use** Antibacterial agent used in second- and third-degree burns and skin grafting

**Usual Dosage** Children and Adults: Topical: Apply once daily or every few days to lesion or place on gauze

**Dosage Forms**

Cream: 0.2% (28 g)

Ointment, soluble dressing: 0.2% (28 g, 56 g, 454 g, 480 g)

Solution, topical: 0.2% (480 mL)

**nitrogen mustard** *see* mechlorethamine *on page 505*

## nitroglycerin *(nye troe GLI ser in)*

**Sound-Alike/Look-Alike Issues**

nitroglycerin may be confused with nitroprusside

Nitro-Bid® may be confused with Nicobid®

Nitroderm may be confused with NicoDerm®

Nitrol® may be confused with Nizoral®

Nitrostat® may be confused with Hyperstat®, Nilstat®, nystatin

**Synonyms** glyceryl trinitrate; nitroglycerol; NTG

**U.S./Canadian Brand Names** Gen-Nitro [Can]; Minitran™ [US/Can]; Nitrek® [US]; Nitro-Bid® [US]; Nitro-Dur® [US/Can]; Nitro-Tab® [US]; Nitrolingual® [US]; Nitrol® [Can]; NitroQuick® [US]; Nitrostat® [US/Can]; NitroTime® [US]; Rho-Nitro [Can]; Transderm-Nitro® [Can]

**Therapeutic Category** Vasodilator

**Use** Treatment of angina pectoris; I.V. for congestive heart failure (especially when associated with acute myocardial infarction); pulmonary hypertension; hypertensive emergencies occurring perioperatively (especially during cardiovascular surgery)

**Usual Dosage** **Note:** Hemodynamic and antianginal tolerance often develop within 24-48 hours of continuous nitrate administration. Nitrate-free interval (10-12 hours/day) is recommended to avoid tolerance development; gradually decrease dose in patients receiving NTG for prolonged period to avoid withdrawal reaction.

Children: Pulmonary hypertension: Continuous infusion: Start 0.25-0.5 mcg/kg/minute and titrate by 1 mcg/kg/minute at 20- to 60-minute intervals to desired effect; usual dose: 1-3 mcg/kg/minute; maximum: 5 mcg/kg/minute

Adults:

Oral: 2.5-9 mg 2-4 times/day (up to 26 mg 4 times/day)

I.V.: 5 mcg/minute, increase by 5 mcg/minute every 3-5 minutes to 20 mcg/minute; if no response at 20 mcg/minute increase by 10 mcg/minute every 3-5 minutes, up to 200 mcg/minute

Ointment: 1/2" upon rising and 1/2" 6 hours later; the dose may be doubled and even doubled again as needed

Patch, transdermal: Initial: 0.2-0.4 mg/hour, titrate to doses of 0.4-0.8 mg/hour; tolerance is minimized by using a patch-on period of 12-14 hours and patch-off period of 10-12 hours

Sublingual: 0.2-0.6 mg every 5 minutes for maximum of 3 doses in 15 minutes; may also use prophylactically 5-10 minutes prior to activities which may provoke an attack

Translingual: 1-2 sprays into mouth under tongue every 3-5 minutes for maximum of 3 doses in 15 minutes, may also be used 5-10 minutes prior to activities which may provoke an attack prophylactically

**Dosage Forms**

Capsule, extended release (Nitro-Time®): 2.5 mg, 6.5 mg, 9 mg

Infusion [premixed in $D_5W$]: 25 mg (250 mL) [0.1 mg/mL]; 50 mg (250 mL) [0.2 mg/mL]; 50 mg (500 mL) [0.1 mg/mL]; 100 mg (250 mL) [0.4 mg/mL]; 200 mg (500 mL) [0.4 mg/mL]

Injection, solution: 5 mg/mL (5 mL, 10 mL) [contains alcohol and propylene glycol]

Ointment, topical (Nitro-Bid®): 2% [20 mg/g] (1 g, 30 g, 60 g)

Solution, translingual spray (Nitrolingual®): 0.4 mg/metered spray (4.9 g) [contains alcohol 20%; 60 metered sprays]; (12 g) [contains alcohol 20%; 200 metered sprays]

Tablet, sublingual (NitroQuick®, Nitrostat®, Nitro-Tab®): 0.3 mg, 0.4 mg, 0.6 mg

Transdermal system [once daily patch]: 0.1 mg/hour (30s); 0.2 mg/hour (30s); 0.4 mg/hour (30s); 0.6 mg/hour (30s)

Minitran™: 0.1 mg/hour (30s); 0.2 mg/hour (30s); 0.4 mg/hour (30s); 0.6 mg/hour (30s)

Nitrek®: 0.2 mg/hour (30s); 0.4 mg/hour (30s); 0.6 mg/hour (30s)

Nitro-Dur®: 0.1 mg/hour (30s); 0.2 mg/hour (30s); 0.3 mg/hour (30s); 0.4 mg/hour (30s); 0.6 mg/hour (30s); 0.8 mg/hour (30s)

**nitroglycerol** *see* nitroglycerin *on previous page*

**Nitrol® [Can]** *see* nitroglycerin *on previous page*

**Nitrol® *(Discontinued)*** *see* nitroglycerin *on previous page*

**Nitrolingual® [US]** *see* nitroglycerin *on previous page*

**Nitrong® Oral Tablet *(Discontinued)*** *see* nitroglycerin *on previous page*

**Nitropress® [US]** *see* nitroprusside *on this page*

## nitroprusside (nye troe PRUS ide)

**Sound-Alike/Look-Alike Issues**

nitroprusside may be confused with nitroglycerin

**Synonyms** nitroprusside sodium; sodium nitroferricyanide; sodium nitroprusside

**U.S./Canadian Brand Names** Nitropress® [US]

**Therapeutic Category** Vasodilator

**Use** Management of hypertensive crises; congestive heart failure; used for controlled hypotension to reduce bleeding during surgery

**Usual Dosage** Administration requires the use of an infusion pump. Average dose: 5 mcg/kg/minute.

Children: Pulmonary hypertension: I.V.: Initial: 1 mcg/kg/minute by continuous I.V. infusion; increase in increments of 1 mcg/kg/minute at intervals of 20-60 minutes; titrating to the desired response; usual dose: 3 mcg/kg/minute, rarely need >4 mcg/kg/minute; maximum: 5 mcg/kg/minute.

Adults: I.V. Initial: 0.3-0.5 mcg/kg/minute; increase in increments of 0.5 mcg/kg/minute, titrating to the desired hemodynamic effect or the appearance of headache or nausea; usual dose: 3 mcg/kg/minute; rarely need >4 mcg/kg/minute; maximum: 10 mcg/kg/minute. When administered by prolonged infusion faster than 2 mcg/kg/minute, cyanide is generated faster than an unaided patient can handle.

**Dosage Forms** Injection, solution, as sodium: 25 mg/mL (2 mL)

**nitroprusside sodium** *see* nitroprusside *on this page*

**NitroQuick® [US]** *see* nitroglycerin *on previous page*

**Nitrostat® [US/Can]** *see* nitroglycerin *on previous page*

**Nitro-Tab® [US]** *see* nitroglycerin *on previous page*

**NitroTime® [US]** *see* nitroglycerin *on previous page*

## nitrous oxide (NYE trus OKS ide)

**Therapeutic Category** Anesthetic, Gas

**Use** Produces sedation and analgesia; principal adjunct to inhalation and intravenous general anesthesia

**Usual Dosage** Children and Adults:

Surgical: For sedation and analgesia: Concentrations of 25% to 50% nitrous oxide with oxygen. For general anesthesia, concentrations of 40% to 70% via mask or endotracheal tube. Minimal alveolar concentration (MAC), which can be considered the $ED_{50}$ of inhalational anesthetics, is 105%; therefore (Continued)

## nitrous oxide *(Continued)*

delivery in a hyperbaric chamber is necessary to use as a complete anesthetic. When administered at 70%, reduces the MAC of other anesthetics by half.

Dental: For sedation and analgesia: Concentrations of 25% to 50% nitrous oxide with oxygen

**Dosage Forms** Supplied in blue cylinders

**nitrozepamum** *see* nitrazepam *(Canada only) on page 577*

**Nix®** **[US-OTC/Can]** *see* permethrin *on page 635*

## nizatidine (ni ZA ti deen)

**Sound-Alike/Look-Alike Issues**

Axid® may be confused with Ansaid®

**U.S./Canadian Brand Names** Apo-Nizatidine® [Can]; Axid® AR [US-OTC]; Axid® [US/Can]; Gen-Nizatidine [Can]; Novo-Nizatidine [Can]; Nu-Nizatidine [Can]; PMS-Nizatidine [Can]

**Therapeutic Category** Histamine $H_2$ Antagonist

**Use** Treatment and maintenance of duodenal ulcer; treatment of benign gastric ulcer; treatment of gastroesophageal reflux disease (GERD); OTC tablet used for the prevention of meal-induced heartburn, acid indigestion, and sour stomach

**Usual Dosage** Oral:

Children ≥12 years:

GERD: Refer to Adults dosing

Meal-induced heartburn, acid indigestion and sour stomach: Refer to Adults dosing

Adults:

Duodenal ulcer:

Treatment of active ulcer: 300 mg at bedtime or 150 mg twice daily

Maintenance of healed ulcer: 150 mg/day at bedtime

Gastric ulcer: 150 mg twice daily or 300 mg at bedtime

GERD: 150 mg twice daily

Meal-induced heartburn, acid indigestion, and sour stomach: 75 mg tablet [OTC] twice daily, 30 to 60 minutes prior to consuming food or beverages

**Dosage Forms**

Capsule (Axid®): 150 mg, 300 mg

Solution, oral (Axid®): 15 mg/mL (120 mL, 480 mL) [bubble gum flavor]

Tablet (Axid® AR): 75 mg

**Nizoral®** **[US]** *see* ketoconazole *on page 457*

**Nizoral®** **A-D** **[US-OTC]** *see* ketoconazole *on page 457*

**N-methylhydrazine** *see* procarbazine *on page 680*

**Nocosyn™** **[US]** *see* sulfur and sulfacetamide *on page 776*

**Nolahist®** **[US-OTC/Can]** *see* phenindamine *on page 637*

**Nolex®** **LA** *(Discontinued)*

**Nolvadex®** **[US/Can]** *see* tamoxifen *on page 780*

**Nolvadex®-D** **[Can]** *see* tamoxifen *on page 780*

## nonoxynol 9 (non OKS i nole nine)

**Sound-Alike/Look-Alike Issues**

Delfen® may be confused with Delsym®

**Synonyms** N-9

**U.S./Canadian Brand Names** Advantage-S™ [US-OTC]; Conceptrol® [US-OTC]; Delfen® [US-OTC]; Encare® [US-OTC]; Gynol II® [US-OTC]; Today® Sponge [US-OTC]; VCF™ [US-OTC]

**Therapeutic Category** Spermicide

**Use** Prevention of pregnancy

**Usual Dosage Note:** Prior to use, refer to specific product labeling for complete instructions.

Prevention of pregnancy: Vaginal:

Advantage-S®, Conceptrol®: Insert 1 applicatorful vaginally up to 1 hour prior to intercourse

Encare®: Unwrap and insert 1 suppository vaginally at least 10 minutes prior to intercourse; effective for 1 hour

Today® Sponge: Insert 1 sponge vaginally prior to intercourse; allow to remain in place for 6 hours after intercourse before removing; effective for use up to 24 continuous hours. Do not leave in place for >30 hours.

VCF®:

Film: Insert 1 film vaginally at least 15 minutes, but no more than 3 hours, prior to intercourse. Insert new film for each act of intercourse or if more than 3 hours have elapsed.

Foam: Insert 1 applicatorful at least 15 minutes prior to intercourse; effective for up to 1 hour

**Dosage Forms** [DSC] = Discontinued product

Film, vaginal (VCF™): 28% (3s, 6s,12s)

Foam, vaginal:

Delfen®: 12.5% (18 g)

Emko®: 8% (40 g, 90 g) [DSC]

VCF™: 12.5% (40 g)

Gel, vaginal:

Advantage-S™: 3.5% (1.5 g) [packaged in 3s or with 6 prefilled applicators]; (30g) [packaged with reusable applicator]

Conceptrol®: 4% (2.7 g) [packaged in 6s and 10s with disposable applicators]

Gynol II®: 2% (85 g, 114 g)

Shur-Seal®: 2% (6 g) [packaged in 24s] [DSC]

Sponge, vaginal (Today®): 1 g (3s, 6s, 12s) [contains sodium metabisulfite]

Suppository, vaginal (Encare®): 100 mg (12s, 18s)

**No Pain-HP®** *(Discontinued)* see capsaicin *on page 138*

**Nora-BE™ [US]** see norethindrone *on next page*

**noradrenaline** see norepinephrine *on this page*

**noradrenaline acid tartrate** see norepinephrine *on this page*

**Norcet®** *(Discontinued)* see hydrocodone and acetaminophen *on page 411*

**Norco® [US]** see hydrocodone and acetaminophen *on page 411*

**Norcuron® [Can]** see vecuronium *on page 842*

**Norcuron®** *(Discontinued)* see vecuronium *on page 842*

**nordeoxyguanosine** see ganciclovir *on page 366*

**Nordette® [US]** see ethinyl estradiol and levonorgestrel *on page 312*

**Norditropin® [US]** see somatropin *on page 760*

**Norditropin® NordiFlex® [US]** see somatropin *on page 760*

**Nordryl® Injection** *(Discontinued)* see diphenhydramine *on page 254*

**Nordryl® Oral** *(Discontinued)* see diphenhydramine *on page 254*

**norelgestromin and ethinyl estradiol** see ethinyl estradiol and norelgestromin *on page 314*

**norepinephrine** (nor ep i NEF rin)

**Synonyms** levarterenol bitartrate; noradrenaline acid tartrate; noradrenaline; norepinephrine bitartrate

**U.S./Canadian Brand Names** Levophed® [US/Can]

**Therapeutic Category** Adrenergic Agonist Agent

**Use** Treatment of shock which persists after adequate fluid volume replacement

**Usual Dosage Administration requires the use of an infusion pump!**

**Note:** Norepinephrine dosage is stated in terms of norepinephrine base and intravenous formulation is norepinephrine bitartrate

Norepinephrine bitartrate 2 mg = Norepinephrine base 1 mg

Continuous I.V. infusion:

Children: Initial: 0.05-0.1 mcg/kg/minute; titrate to desired effect; maximum dose: 1-2 mcg/kg/minute

Adults: Initial: 0.5-1 mcg/minute and titrate to desired response; 8-30 mcg/minute is usual range; range used in clinical trials: 0.01-3 mcg/kg/minute; ACLS dosage range: 0.5-30 mcg/minute

**Dosage Forms** Injection, solution, as bitartrate: 1 mg/mL (4 mL) [contains sodium metabisulfite]

**norepinephrine bitartrate** see norepinephrine *on this page*

**Norethin™ 1/35E** *(Discontinued)* see ethinyl estradiol and norethindrone *on page 314*

## norethindrone (nor eth IN drone)

**Sound-Alike/Look-Alike Issues**
Micronor® may be confused with miconazole, Micronase®

**Synonyms** norethindrone acetate; norethisterone

**U.S./Canadian Brand Names** Aygestin® [US]; Camila™ [US]; Errin™ [US]; Jolivette™ [US]; Micronor® [US/Can]; Nor-QD® [US]; Nora-BE™ [US]

**Therapeutic Category** Contraceptive, Progestin Only; Progestin

**Use** Treatment of amenorrhea; abnormal uterine bleeding; endometriosis, oral contraceptive; **higher rate of failure with progestin only contraceptives**

**Usual Dosage** Oral: Adolescents and Adults: Female:
Contraception: Progesterone only: Norethindrone 0.35 mg every day of the year starting on first day of menstruation; if one dose is missed, discontinue and use an alternative method of contraception
Amenorrhea and abnormal uterine bleeding:
Norethindrone: 5-20 mg/day for 5-10 days during the second half of the menstrual cycle
Acetate salt: 2.5-10 mg/day for 5-10 days during the second half of the menstrual cycle
Endometriosis:
Norethindrone: 10 mg/day for 2 weeks; increase at increments of 5 mg/day every 2 weeks until 30 mg/day; continue for 6-9 months or until breakthrough bleeding demands temporary termination
Acetate salt: 5 mg/day for 14 days; increase at increments of 2.5 mg/day every 2 weeks up to 15 mg/day; continue for 6-9 months or until breakthrough bleeding demands temporary termination

**Dosage Forms**
Tablet (Camila™, Errin™, Jolivette™, Micronor®, Nora-BE™, Nor-QD®): 0.35 mg
Tablet, as acetate (Aygestin®): 5 mg

**norethindrone acetate** *see* norethindrone *on this page*

**norethindrone acetate and ethinyl estradiol** *see* ethinyl estradiol and norethindrone *on page 314*

**norethindrone and estradiol** *see* estradiol and norethindrone *on page 302*

**norethindrone and mestranol** *see* mestranol and norethindrone *on page 517*

**norethisterone** *see* norethindrone *on this page*

**Norflex™ [US/Can]** *see* orphenadrine *on page 602*

## norfloxacin (nor FLOKS a sin)

**Sound-Alike/Look-Alike Issues**
norfloxacin may be confused with Norflex™, Noroxin®
Noroxin® may be confused with Neurontin®, Norflex™, norfloxacin

**U.S./Canadian Brand Names** Apo-Norflox® [Can]; Norfloxacine® [Can]; Noroxin® [US]; Novo-Norfloxacin [Can]; PMS-Norfloxacin [Can]; Riva-Norfloxacin [Can]

**Therapeutic Category** Quinolone

**Use** Uncomplicated urinary tract infections and cystitis caused by susceptible gram-negative and gram-positive bacteria; sexually-transmitted disease (eg, uncomplicated urethral and cervical gonorrhea) caused by *N. gonorrhoeae*; prostatitis due to *E. coli*

**Usual Dosage** Oral: Adults:
Urinary tract infections: 400 mg twice daily for 3-21 days depending on severity of infection or organism sensitivity; maximum: 800 mg/day
Uncomplicated gonorrhea: 800 mg as a single dose (CDC recommends as an alternative regimen to ciprofloxacin or ofloxacin)
Prostatitis: 400 mg every 12 hours for 4 weeks

**Dosage Forms** Tablet: 400 mg

**Norfloxacine® [Can]** *see* norfloxacin *on this page*

**Norgesic™ [US/Can]** *see* orphenadrine, aspirin, and caffeine *on page 603*

**Norgesic™ Forte [US/Can]** *see* orphenadrine, aspirin, and caffeine *on page 603*

**norgestimate and estradiol** *see* estradiol and norgestimate *on page 302*

**norgestimate and ethinyl estradiol** *see* ethinyl estradiol and norgestimate *on page 317*

## norgestrel (nor JES trel)

**U.S./Canadian Brand Names** Ovrette® [Can]

**Therapeutic Category** Contraceptive, Progestin Only

**Use** Prevention of pregnancy; **progestin only products have higher risk of failure in contraceptive use**

**Usual Dosage** Oral: Administer daily, starting the first day of menstruation, take 1 tablet at the same time each day, every day of the year. If one dose is missed, take as soon as remembered, then next tablet at regular time; if two doses are missed, take 1 tablet as soon as it is remembered, followed by an additional dose that same day at the usual time. When one or two doses are missed, additional contraceptive measures should be used until 14 consecutive tablets have been taken. If three doses are missed, discontinue norgestrel and use an additional form of birth control until menses or pregnancy is ruled out.

**Dosage Forms** [DSC] = Discontinued product

Tablet: 0.075 mg [contains tartrazine] [DSC]

**norgestrel and ethinyl estradiol** *see* ethinyl estradiol and norgestrel *on page 318*

**Norinyl® 1+35 [US]** *see* ethinyl estradiol and norethindrone *on page 314*

**Norinyl® 1+50 [US]** *see* mestranol and norethindrone *on page 517*

**Noritate® [US/Can]** *see* metronidazole *on page 535*

**normal human serum albumin** *see* albumin *on page 22*

**normal saline** *see* sodium chloride *on page 752*

**normal serum albumin (human)** *see* albumin *on page 22*

**Normiflo® *(Discontinued)***

**Normodyne® [Can]** *see* labetalol *on page 460*

**Noroxin® [US]** *see* norfloxacin *on previous page*

**Norpace® [US/Can]** *see* disopyramide *on page 261*

**Norpace® CR [US]** *see* disopyramide *on page 261*

**Norplant® Implant [Can]** *see* levonorgestrel *on page 476*

**Norplant® Implant *(Discontinued)*** *see* levonorgestrel *on page 476*

**Norpramin® [US/Can]** *see* desipramine *on page 230*

**Nor-QD® [US]** *see* norethindrone *on previous page*

**North American coral snake antivenin** *see* antivenin *(Micrurus fulvius) on page 61*

**North and South American antisnake-bite serum** *see* antivenin *(Crotalidae)* polyvalent *on page 60*

**Nortrel™ [US]** *see* ethinyl estradiol and norethindrone *on page 314*

**Nortrel™ 7/7/7 [US]** *see* ethinyl estradiol and norethindrone *on page 314*

## nortriptyline (nor TRIP ti leen)

**Sound-Alike/Look-Alike Issues**

nortriptyline may be confused with amitriptyline, desipramine, Norpramin®

Aventyl® HCl may be confused with Bentyl®

Pamelor® may be confused with Demerol®, Dymelor®

**Synonyms** nortriptyline hydrochloride

**U.S./Canadian Brand Names** Alti-Nortriptyline [Can]; Apo-Nortriptyline® [Can]; Aventyl® [Can]; Gen-Nortriptyline [Can]; Norventyl [Can]; Novo-Nortriptyline [Can]; Nu-Nortriptyline [Can]; Pamelor® [US]; PMS-Nortriptyline [Can]

**Therapeutic Category** Antidepressant, Tricyclic (Secondary Amine)

**Use** Treatment of symptoms of depression

**Usual Dosage** Oral:

Depression:

Adults: 25 mg 3-4 times/day up to 150 mg/day

Initial: 10-25 mg at bedtime

Dosage can be increased by 25 mg every 3 days for inpatients and weekly for outpatients if tolerated

Usual maintenance dose: 75 mg as a single bedtime dose or 2 divided doses; however, lower or higher doses may be required to stay within the therapeutic window

(Continued)

## nortriptyline *(Continued)*

Myofascial pain, neuralgia, burning mouth syndrome (dental use): Initial: 10-25 mg at bedtime; dosage may be increased by 25 mg/day weekly, if tolerated; usual maintenance dose: 75 mg as a single bedtime dose or 2 divided doses

**Dosage Forms**

Capsule, as hydrochloride: 10 mg, 25 mg, 50 mg, 75 mg

Pamelor®: 10 mg, 25 mg, 50 mg, 75 mg [may contain benzyl alcohol; 50 mg may also contain sodium bisulfite]

Solution, as hydrochloride (Pamelor®): 10 mg/5 mL (473 mL) [contains alcohol 4% and benzoic acid]

**nortriptyline hydrochloride** *see* nortriptyline *on previous page*

**Norvasc® [US/Can]** *see* amlodipine *on page 43*

**Norventyl [Can]** *see* nortriptyline *on previous page*

**Norvir® [US/Can]** *see* ritonavir *on page 725*

**Norvir® SEC [Can]** *see* ritonavir *on page 725*

**Nostril® [US-OTC]** *see* phenylephrine *on page 640*

**Novacet® *(Discontinued)*** *see* sulfur and sulfacetamide *on page 776*

**Novafed® A *(Discontinued)*** *see* chlorpheniramine and pseudoephedrine *on page 172*

**Novahistex® DM Decongestant [Can]** *see* pseudoephedrine and dextromethorphan *on page 693*

**Novahistex® DM Decongestant Expectorant [Can]** *see* guaifenesin, pseudoephedrine, and dextromethorphan *on page 391*

**Novahistex® Expectorant with Decongestant [Can]** *see* guaifenesin and pseudoephedrine *on page 388*

**Novahistine® DM Decongestant [Can]** *see* pseudoephedrine and dextromethorphan *on page 693*

**Novahistine® DM Decongestant Expectorant [Can]** *see* guaifenesin, pseudoephedrine, and dextromethorphan *on page 391*

**Novamilor [Can]** *see* amiloride and hydrochlorothiazide *on page 40*

**Novamoxin® [Can]** *see* amoxicillin *on page 46*

**Novantrone® [US/Can]** *see* mitoxantrone *on page 545*

**Novarel™ [US]** *see* chorionic gonadotropin (human) *on page 181*

**Novasen [Can]** *see* aspirin *on page 73*

**Novo-5 ASA [Can]** *see* mesalamine *on page 516*

**Novo-Acebutolol [Can]** *see* acebutolol *on page 4*

**Novo-Alendronate [Can]** *see* alendronate *on page 26*

**Novo-Alprazol [Can]** *see* alprazolam *on page 30*

**Novo-Amiodarone [Can]** *see* amiodarone *on page 41*

**Novo-Ampicillin [Can]** *see* ampicillin *on page 50*

**Novo-Atenol [Can]** *see* atenolol *on page 76*

**Novo-Azathioprine [Can]** *see* azathioprine *on page 83*

**Novo-Benzydamine [Can]** *see* benzydamine *(Canada only) on page 100*

**Novo-Bromazepam [Can]** *see* bromazepam *(Canada only) on page 114*

**Novo-Bupropion SR [Can]** *see* bupropion *on page 122*

**Novo-Buspirone [Can]** *see* buspirone *on page 123*

**Novocain® [US]** *see* procaine *on page 679*

**Novo-Captopril [Can]** *see* captopril *on page 139*

**Novo-Carbamaz [Can]** *see* carbamazepine *on page 140*

**Novo-Carvedilol [Can]** *see* carvedilol *on page 150*

**Novo-Cefaclor [Can]** *see* cefaclor *on page 152*

**Novo-Cefadroxil [Can]** *see* cefadroxil *on page 152*

Novo-Chloroquine [Can] *see* chloroquine phosphate *on page 170*

Novo-Chlorpromazine [Can] *see* chlorpromazine *on page 178*

Novo-Cholamine [Can] *see* cholestyramine resin *on page 180*

Novo-Cholamine Light [Can] *see* cholestyramine resin *on page 180*

Novo-Cilazapril [Can] *see* cilazapril *(Canada only) on page 182*

Novo-Cimetidine [Can] *see* cimetidine *on page 183*

Novo-Ciprofloxacin [Can] *see* ciprofloxacin *on page 184*

Novo-Citalopram [Can] *see* citalopram *on page 188*

Novo-Clavamoxin [Can] *see* amoxicillin and clavulanate potassium *on page 47*

Novo-Clindamycin [Can] *see* clindamycin *on page 192*

Novo-Clobazam [Can] *see* clobazam *(Canada only) on page 194*

Novo-Clobetasol [Can] *see* clobetasol *on page 194*

Novo-Clonazepam [Can] *see* clonazepam *on page 197*

Novo-Clonidine [Can] *see* clonidine *on page 197*

Novo-Clopate [Can] *see* clorazepate *on page 199*

Novo-Cloxin [Can] *see* cloxacillin *on page 200*

Novo-Cycloprine [Can] *see* cyclobenzaprine *on page 213*

Novo-Difenac [Can] *see* diclofenac *on page 243*

Novo-Difenac K [Can] *see* diclofenac *on page 243*

Novo-Difenac-SR [Can] *see* diclofenac *on page 243*

Novo-Diflunisal [Can] *see* diflunisal *on page 247*

Novo-Digoxin [Can] *see* digoxin *on page 247*

Novo-Diltazem [Can] *see* diltiazem *on page 251*

Novo-Diltazem-CD [Can] *see* diltiazem *on page 251*

Novo-Dimenate [Can] *see* dimenhydrinate *on page 252*

Novo-Dipam [Can] *see* diazepam *on page 241*

Novo-Divalproex [Can] *see* valproic acid and derivatives *on page 837*

Novo-Docusate Calcium [Can] *see* docusate *on page 263*

Novo-Docusate Sodium [Can] *see* docusate *on page 263*

Novo-Domperidone [Can] *see* domperidone *(Canada only) on page 266*

Novo-Doxazosin [Can] *see* doxazosin *on page 268*

Novo-Doxepin [Can] *see* doxepin *on page 269*

Novo-Doxylin [Can] *see* doxycycline *on page 271*

Novo-Famotidine [Can] *see* famotidine *on page 327*

Novo-Fenofibrate [Can] *see* fenofibrate *on page 330*

Novo-Ferrogluc [Can] *see* ferrous gluconate *on page 335*

Novo-Fluconazole [Can] *see* fluconazole *on page 341*

Novo-Fluoxetine [Can] *see* fluoxetine *on page 349*

Novo-Flurprofen [Can] *see* flurbiprofen *on page 352*

Novo-Flutamide [Can] *see* flutamide *on page 353*

Novo-Fluvoxamine [Can] *see* fluvoxamine *on page 356*

Novo-Fosinopril [Can] *see* fosinopril *on page 361*

Novo-Furantoin [Can] *see* nitrofurantoin *on page 577*

Novo-Gabapentin [Can] *see* gabapentin *on page 365*

Novo-Gemfibrozil [Can] *see* gemfibrozil *on page 370*

Novo-Gesic [Can] *see* acetaminophen *on page 4*

Novo-Gliclazide [Can] *see* gliclazide *(Canada only) on page 375*

**Novo-Glyburide [Can]** *see* glyburide *on page 378*

**Novo-Hydrazide [Can]** *see* hydrochlorothiazide *on page 409*

**Novo-Hydroxyzin [Can]** *see* hydroxyzine *on page 423*

**Novo-Hylazin [Can]** *see* hydralazine *on page 408*

**Novo-Indapamide [Can]** *see* indapamide *on page 434*

**Novo-Ipramide [Can]** *see* ipratropium *on page 446*

**Novo-Keto [Can]** *see* ketoprofen *on page 457*

**Novo-Ketoconazole [Can]** *see* ketoconazole *on page 457*

**Novo-Keto-EC [Can]** *see* ketoprofen *on page 457*

**Novo-Ketorolac [Can]** *see* ketorolac *on page 458*

**Novo-Ketotifen [Can]** *see* ketotifen *on page 458*

**Novo-Lamotrigine [Can]** *see* lamotrigine *on page 465*

**Novo-Leflunomide [Can]** *see* leflunomide *on page 469*

**Novo-Levobunolol [Can]** *see* levobunolol *on page 472*

**Novo-Levocarbidopa [Can]** *see* levodopa and carbidopa *on page 474*

**Novo-Levofloxacin [Can]** *see* levofloxacin *on page 475*

**Novo-Lexin [Can]** *see* cephalexin *on page 161*

**Novolin® L Insulin** *(Discontinued)*

**Novolin® 70/30 [US]** *see* insulin preparations *on page 438*

**Novolin® ge [Can]** *see* insulin preparations *on page 438*

**Novolin® N [US]** *see* insulin preparations *on page 438*

**Novolin® R [US]** *see* insulin preparations *on page 438*

**NovoLog® [US]** *see* insulin preparations *on page 438*

**NovoLog® Mix 70/30 [US]** *see* insulin preparations *on page 438*

**Novo-Loperamide [Can]** *see* loperamide *on page 489*

**Novo-Lorazepam [Can]** *see* lorazepam *on page 491*

**Novo-Lovastatin [Can]** *see* lovastatin *on page 494*

**Novo-Maprotiline [Can]** *see* maprotiline *on page 503*

**Novo-Medrone [Can]** *see* medroxyprogesterone acetate *on page 507*

**Novo-Meloxicam [Can]** *see* meloxicam *on page 509*

**Novo-Mepro [Can]** *see* meprobamate *on page 514*

**Novo-Metformin [Can]** *see* metformin *on page 519*

**Novo-Methacin [Can]** *see* indomethacin *on page 436*

**Novo-Metoprolol [Can]** *see* metoprolol *on page 534*

**Novo-Mexiletine [Can]** *see* mexiletine *on page 536*

**Novo-Minocycline [Can]** *see* minocycline *on page 542*

**Novo-Mirtazapine [Can]** *see* mirtazapine *on page 543*

**Novo-Misoprostol [Can]** *see* misoprostol *on page 544*

**Novo-Moclobemide [Can]** *see* moclobemide *(Canada only)* *on page 546*

**Novo-Nabumetone [Can]** *see* nabumetone *on page 556*

**Novo-Nadolol [Can]** *see* nadolol *on page 556*

**Novo-Naproc EC [Can]** *see* naproxen *on page 562*

**Novo-Naprox [Can]** *see* naproxen *on page 562*

**Novo-Naprox Sodium [Can]** *see* naproxen *on page 562*

**Novo-Naprox Sodium DS [Can]** *see* naproxen *on page 562*

**Novo-Naprox SR [Can]** *see* naproxen *on page 562*

**Novo-Nifedin [Can]** *see* nifedipine *on page 575*

**Novo-Nizatidine [Can]** *see* nizatidine *on page 580*
**Novo Nordisk®  (all products)** *(Discontinued)*
**Novo-Norfloxacin [Can]** *see* norfloxacin *on page 582*
**Novo-Nortriptyline [Can]** *see* nortriptyline *on page 583*
**Novo-Ofloxacin [Can]** *see* ofloxacin *on page 594*
**Novo-Oxybutynin [Can]** *see* oxybutynin *on page 607*
**Novo-Paroxetine [Can]** *see* paroxetine *on page 620*
**Novo-Pen-VK [Can]** *see* penicillin V potassium *on page 627*
**Novo-Peridol [Can]** *see* haloperidol *on page 396*
**Novo-Pheniram [Can]** *see* chlorpheniramine *on page 171*
**Novo-Pindol [Can]** *see* pindolol *on page 648*
**Novo-Pirocam [Can]** *see* piroxicam *on page 650*
**Novo-Pramine [Can]** *see* imipramine *on page 432*
**Novo-Pranol [Can]** *see* propranolol *on page 688*
**Novo-Pravastatin [Can]** *see* pravastatin *on page 671*
**Novo-Prazin [Can]** *see* prazosin *on page 672*
**Novo-Prednisolone [Can]** *see* prednisolone (systemic) *on page 674*
**Novo-Prednisone [Can]** *see* prednisone *on page 674*
**Novo-Profen [Can]** *see* ibuprofen *on page 427*
**Novo-Propamide [Can]** *see* chlorpropamide *on page 179*
**Novo-Purol [Can]** *see* allopurinol *on page 28*
**Novo-Quinidin [Can]** *see* quinidine *on page 705*
**Novo-Quinine [Can]** *see* quinine *on page 705*
**Novo-Ranidine [Can]** *see* ranitidine hydrochloride *on page 710*
**NovoRapid [Can]** *see* insulin preparations *on page 438*
**Novo-Rythro Estolate [Can]** *see* erythromycin *on page 295*
**Novo-Rythro Ethylsuccinate [Can]** *see* erythromycin *on page 295*
**Novo-Selegiline [Can]** *see* selegiline *on page 742*
**Novo-Semide [Can]** *see* furosemide *on page 364*
**Novo-Sertraline [Can]** *see* sertraline *on page 744*
**NovoSeven® [US]** *see* factor VIIa (recombinant) *on page 325*
**Novo-Simvastatin [Can]** *see* simvastatin *on page 748*
**Novo-Sorbide [Can]** *see* isosorbide dinitrate *on page 451*
**Novo-Sotalol [Can]** *see* sotalol *on page 762*
**Novo-Soxazole [Can]** *see* sulfisoxazole *on page 775*
**Novo-Spiroton [Can]** *see* spironolactone *on page 764*
**Novo-Spirozine [Can]** *see* hydrochlorothiazide and spironolactone *on page 410*
**Novo-Sucralate [Can]** *see* sucralfate *on page 769*
**Novo-Sundac [Can]** *see* sulindac *on page 776*
**Novo-Tamoxifen [Can]** *see* tamoxifen *on page 780*
**Novo-Temazepam [Can]** *see* temazepam *on page 784*
**Novo-Terazosin [Can]** *see* terazosin *on page 786*
**Novo-Theophyl SR [Can]** *see* theophylline *on page 793*
**Novo-Tiaprofenic [Can]** *see* tiaprofenic acid *(Canada only)* *on page 801*
**Novo-Ticlopidlne [Can]** *see* ticlopidine *on page 802*
**Novo-Trazodone [Can]** *see* trazodone *on page 817*
**Novo-Triamzide [Can]** *see* hydrochlorothiazide and triamterene *on page 410*

**Novo-Trifluzine [Can]** *see* trifluoperazine *on page 823*

**Novo-Trimel [Can]** *see* sulfamethoxazole and trimethoprim *on page 773*

**Novo-Trimel D.S. [Can]** *see* sulfamethoxazole and trimethoprim *on page 773*

**Novo-Triptyn [Can]** *see* amitriptyline *on page 42*

**Novo-Veramil SR [Can]** *see* verapamil *on page 843*

**Novoxapram® [Can]** *see* oxazepam *on page 606*

**Novo-Zopiclone [Can]** *see* zopiclone *(Canada only) on page 864*

**Nozinan® [Can]** *see* methotrimeprazine *(Canada only) on page 526*

**NP-27® *(Discontinued)*** *see* tolnaftate *on page 809*

**NPH Iletin® II *(Discontinued)*** *see* insulin preparations *on page 438*

**NPH Iletin® Insulin *(Discontinued)***

**NPH, insulin** *see* insulin preparations *on page 438*

**NRS® [US-OTC]** *see* oxymetazoline *on page 610*

**NSC-740** *see* methotrexate *on page 524*

**NSC-752** *see* thioguanine *on page 797*

**NSC-755** *see* mercaptopurine *on page 515*

**NSC-762** *see* mechlorethamine *on page 505*

**NSC-102816** *see* azacitidine *on page 82*

**NSC-10363** *see* megestrol acetate *on page 508*

**NSC-106977 (*Erwinia*)** *see* asparaginase *on page 72*

**NSC-109229 (*E. coli*)** *see* asparaginase *on page 72*

**NSC-109724** *see* ifosfamide *on page 430*

**NSC-122758** *see* tretinoin (oral) *on page 817*

**NSC-123127** *see* doxorubicin *on page 270*

**NSC-125066** *see* bleomycin *on page 109*

**NSC-125973** *see* paclitaxel *on page 612*

**NSC-13875** *see* altretamine *on page 34*

**NSC-147834** *see* flutamide *on page 353*

**NSC-180973** *see* tamoxifen *on page 780*

**NSC-218321** *see* pentostatin *on page 632*

**NSC-256439** *see* idarubicin *on page 429*

**NSC-26271** *see* cyclophosphamide *on page 214*

**NSC-266046** *see* oxaliplatin *on page 605*

**NSC-26980** *see* mitomycin *on page 544*

**NSC-27640** *see* floxuridine *on page 341*

**NSC-301739** *see* mitoxantrone *on page 545*

**NSC-3053** *see* dactinomycin *on page 221*

**NSC-3088** *see* chlorambucil *on page 166*

**NSC-352122** *see* trimetrexate glucuronate *on page 826*

**NSC-362856** *see* temozolomide *on page 784*

**NSC-373364** *see* aldesleukin *on page 25*

**NSC-377526** *see* leuprolide acetate *on page 471*

**NSC-38721** *see* mitotane *on page 544*

**NSC-409962** *see* carmustine *on page 149*

**NSC-49842** *see* vinblastine *on page 846*

**NSC-606864** *see* goserelin *on page 381*

**NSC606869** *see* clofarabine *on page 195*

**NSC-609699** *see* topotecan *on page 811*

**NSC-616348** *see* irinotecan *on page 447*

**NSC-628503** *see* docetaxel *on page 263*

**NSC-63878** *see* cytarabine *on page 219*

**NSC-639186** *see* raltitrexed *(Canada only) on page 710*

**NSC-644954** *see* pegaspargase *on page 623*

**NSC-67574** *see* vincristine *on page 846*

**NSC-698037** *see* pemetrexed *on page 626*

**NSC-706363** *see* arsenic trioxide *on page 70*

**NSC-715055** *see* gefitinib *on page 368*

**NSC-718781** *see* erlotinib *on page 294*

**NSC-77213** *see* procarbazine *on page 680*

**NSC-82151** *see* daunorubicin hydrochloride *on page 225*

**NSC-85998** *see* streptozocin *on page 767*

**NSC-89199** *see* estramustine *on page 303*

**NTG** *see* nitroglycerin *on page 578*

**NTZ** *see* nitazoxanide *on page 576*

**NTZ® Long Acting Nasal Solution *(Discontinued)*** *see* oxymetazoline *on page 610*

**Nu-Acebutolol [Can]** *see* acebutolol *on page 4*

**Nu-Acyclovir [Can]** *see* acyclovir *on page 17*

**Nu-Alprax [Can]** *see* alprazolam *on page 30*

**Nu-Amilzide [Can]** *see* amiloride and hydrochlorothiazide *on page 40*

**Nu-Amoxi [Can]** *see* amoxicillin *on page 46*

**Nu-Ampi [Can]** *see* ampicillin *on page 50*

**Nu-Atenol [Can]** *see* atenolol *on page 76*

**Nu-Baclo [Can]** *see* baclofen *on page 88*

**Nubain® [US]** *see* nalbuphine *on page 558*

**Nu-Beclomethasone [Can]** *see* beclomethasone *on page 91*

**Nu-Bromazepam [Can]** *see* bromazepam *(Canada only) on page 114*

**Nu-Buspirone [Can]** *see* buspirone *on page 123*

**Nu-Capto [Can]** *see* captopril *on page 139*

**Nu-Carbamazepine [Can]** *see* carbamazepine *on page 140*

**Nu-Cefaclor [Can]** *see* cefaclor *on page 152*

**Nu-Cephalex [Can]** *see* cephalexin *on page 161*

**Nu-Cimet [Can]** *see* cimetidine *on page 183*

**Nu-Clonazepam [Can]** *see* clonazepam *on page 197*

**Nu-Clonidine [Can]** *see* clonidine *on page 197*

**Nu-Cloxi [Can]** *see* cloxacillin *on page 200*

**Nucofed® Expectorant [US]** *see* guaifenesin, pseudoephedrine, and codeine *on page 391*

**Nucofed® Pediatric Expectorant [US]** *see* guaifenesin, pseudoephedrine, and codeine *on page 391*

**Nu-Cotrimox [Can]** *see* sulfamethoxazole and trimethoprim *on page 773*

**Nu-Cromolyn [Can]** *see* cromolyn sodium *on page 211*

**Nu-Cyclobenzaprine [Can]** *see* cyclobenzaprine *on page 213*

**Nu-Desipramine [Can]** *see* desipramine *on page 230*

**Nu-Diclo [Can]** *see* diclofenac *on page 243*

**Nu-Diclo-SR [Can]** *see* diclofenac *on page 243*

**Nu-Diflunisal [Can]** *see* diflunisal *on page 247*

**Nu-Diltiaz [Can]** *see* diltiazem *on page 251*

**Nu-Diltiaz-CD [Can]** *see* diltiazem *on page 251*

**Nu-Divalproex [Can]** *see* valproic acid and derivatives *on page 837*

**Nu-Domperidone [Can]** *see* domperidone *(Canada only) on page 266*

**Nu-Doxycycline [Can]** *see* doxycycline *on page 271*

**Nu-Erythromycin-S [Can]** *see* erythromycin *on page 295*

**Nu-Famotidine [Can]** *see* famotidine *on page 327*

**Nu-Fenofibrate [Can]** *see* fenofibrate *on page 330*

**Nu-Fluoxetine [Can]** *see* fluoxetine *on page 349*

**Nu-Flurprofen [Can]** *see* flurbiprofen *on page 352*

**Nu-Fluvoxamine [Can]** *see* fluvoxamine *on page 356*

**Nu-Gabapentin [Can]** *see* gabapentin *on page 365*

**Nu-Gemfibrozil [Can]** *see* gemfibrozil *on page 370*

**Nu-Glyburide [Can]** *see* glyburide *on page 378*

**Nu-Hydral [Can]** *see* hydralazine *on page 408*

**Nu-Ibuprofen [Can]** *see* ibuprofen *on page 427*

**Nu-Indapamide [Can]** *see* indapamide *on page 434*

**Nu-Indo [Can]** *see* indomethacin *on page 436*

**Nu-Ipratropium [Can]** *see* ipratropium *on page 446*

**Nu-Iron® 150 [US-OTC]** *see* polysaccharide-iron complex *on page 660*

**Nu-Ketoprofen [Can]** *see* ketoprofen *on page 457*

**Nu-Ketoprofen-E [Can]** *see* ketoprofen *on page 457*

**NuLev™ [US]** *see* hyoscyamine *on page 424*

**Nu-Levocarb [Can]** *see* levodopa and carbidopa *on page 474*

**Nullo® [US-OTC]** *see* chlorophyll *on page 169*

**Nu-Loraz [Can]** *see* lorazepam *on page 491*

**Nu-Lovastatin [Can]** *see* lovastatin *on page 494*

**Nu-Loxapine [Can]** *see* loxapine *on page 494*

**NuLYTELY® [US]** *see* polyethylene glycol-electrolyte solution *on page 658*

**Nu-Medopa [Can]** *see* methyldopa *on page 529*

**Nu-Mefenamic [Can]** *see* mefenamic acid *on page 508*

**Nu-Megestrol [Can]** *see* megestrol acetate *on page 508*

**Nu-Metformin [Can]** *see* metformin *on page 519*

**Nu-Metoclopramide [Can]** *see* metoclopramide *on page 533*

**Nu-Metop [Can]** *see* metoprolol *on page 534*

**Nu-Moclobemide [Can]** *see* moclobemide *(Canada only) on page 546*

**Numorphan® [US]** *see* oxymorphone *on page 611*

**Numzident® *(Discontinued)*** *see* benzocaine *on page 95*

**Nu-Naprox [Can]** *see* naproxen *on page 562*

**Nu-Nifed [Can]** *see* nifedipine *on page 575*

**Nu-Nizatidine [Can]** *see* nizatidine *on page 580*

**Nu-Nortriptyline [Can]** *see* nortriptyline *on page 583*

**Nu-Oxybutyn [Can]** *see* oxybutynin *on page 607*

**Nu-Pentoxifylline SR [Can]** *see* pentoxifylline *on page 632*

**Nu-Pen-VK [Can]** *see* penicillin V potassium *on page 627*

**Nupercainal® [US-OTC]** *see* dibucaine *on page 242*

**Nupercainal® Hydrocortisone Cream [US-OTC]** *see* hydrocortisone (topical) *on page 417*

**Nu-Pindol [Can]** *see* pindolol *on page 648*

**Nu-Pirox [Can]** *see* piroxicam *on page 650*

**Nu-Prazo [Can]** *see* prazosin *on page 672*

**Nuprin® *(Discontinued)*** *see* ibuprofen *on page 427*

**Nu-Prochlor [Can]** *see* prochlorperazine *on page 680*

**Nu-Propranolol [Can]** *see* propranolol *on page 688*

**Nuquin HP® [US]** *see* hydroquinone *on page 420*

**Nu-Ranit [Can]** *see* ranitidine hydrochloride *on page 710*

**Nuromax® [US]** *see* doxacurium *on page 267*

**Nu-Selegiline [Can]** *see* selegiline *on page 742*

**Nu-Sertraline [Can]** *see* sertraline *on page 744*

**Nu-Sotalol [Can]** *see* sotalol *on page 762*

**Nu-Sucralate [Can]** *see* sucralfate *on page 769*

**Nu-Sulfinpyrazone [Can]** *see* sulfinpyrazone *on page 775*

**Nu-Sundac [Can]** *see* sulindac *on page 776*

**Nu-Tears® [US-OTC]** *see* artificial tears *on page 71*

**Nu-Tears® II [US-OTC]** *see* artificial tears *on page 71*

**Nu-Temazepam [Can]** *see* temazepam *on page 784*

**Nu-Terazosin [Can]** *see* terazosin *on page 786*

**Nu-Tetra [Can]** *see* tetracycline *on page 791*

**Nu-Tiaprofenic [Can]** *see* tiaprofenic acid *(Canada only) on page 801*

**Nu-Ticlopidine [Can]** *see* ticlopidine *on page 802*

**Nu-Timolol [Can]** *see* timolol *on page 803*

**Nutracort® [US]** *see* hydrocortisone (topical) *on page 417*

**Nutraplus® [US-OTC]** *see* urea *on page 834*

**Nu-Trazodone [Can]** *see* trazodone *on page 817*

**Nu-Triazide [Can]** *see* hydrochlorothiazide and triamterene *on page 410*

**Nu-Trimipramine [Can]** *see* trimipramine *on page 826*

**NutriNate® [US]** *see* vitamins (multiple/prenatal) *on page 852*

## nutritional formula, enteral/oral (noo TRISH un al FOR myoo la, EN ter al/OR al)

**Synonyms** dietary supplements

**U.S./Canadian Brand Names** Carnation Instant Breakfast® [US-OTC]; Citrotein® [US-OTC]; Criticare HN® [US-OTC]; Ensure Plus® [US-OTC]; Ensure® [US-OTC]; Isocal® [US-OTC]; Magnacal® [US-OTC]; Microlipid™ [US-OTC]; Osmolite® HN [US-OTC]; Pedialyte® [US-OTC]; Portagen® [US-OTC]; Pregestimil® [US-OTC]; Propac™ [US-OTC]; Soyalac® [US-OTC]; Vital HN® [US-OTC]; Vitaneed™ [US-OTC]; Vivonex® T.E.N. [US-OTC]; Vivonex® [US-OTC]

**Therapeutic Category** Nutritional Supplement

**Dosage Forms**

Liquid: Calcium and sodium caseinate, maltodextrin, sucrose, partially hydrogenated soy oil, soy lecithin

Powder: Amino acids, predigested carbohydrates, safflower oil

**Nutropin® [US]** *see* somatropin *on page 760*

**Nutropin AQ® [US]** *see* somatropin *on page 760*

**Nutropine® [Can]** *see* somatropin *on page 760*

**NuvaRing® [US/Can]** *see* ethinyl estradiol and etonogestrel *on page 311*

**Nu-Verap [Can]** *see* verapamil *on page 843*

**Nu-Zopiclone [Can]** *see* zopiclone *(Canada only) on page 864*

**NVB** *see* vinorelbine *on page 847*

**NVP** *see* nevirapine *on page 571*

**Nyaderm [Can]** *see* nystatin *on this page*

**Nyamyc™ [US]** *see* nystatin *on this page*

**Nydrazid®** *(Discontinued)* *see* isoniazid *on page 450*

## nystatin (nye STAT in)

**Sound-Alike/Look-Alike Issues**
nystatin may be confused with Nilstat®, Nitrostat®
Nilstat® may be confused with Nitrostat®, nystatin

**U.S./Canadian Brand Names** Bio-Statin® [US]; Candistatin® [Can]; Mycostatin® [US]; Nilstat [Can]; Nyaderm [Can]; Nyamyc™ [US]; Nystat-Rx® [US]; Nystop® [US]; Pedi-Dri® [US]; PMS-Nystatin [Can]

**Therapeutic Category** Antifungal Agent

**Use** Treatment of susceptible cutaneous, mucocutaneous, and oral cavity fungal infections normally caused by the *Candida* species

**Usual Dosage**
Oral candidiasis:
Suspension (swish and swallow orally):
Premature infants: 100,000 units 4 times/day
Infants: 200,000 units 4 times/day or 100,000 units to each side of mouth 4 times/day
Children and Adults: 400,000-600,000 units 4 times/day
Powder for compounding: Children and Adults: 1/8 teaspoon (500,000 units) to equal approximately 1/2 cup of water; give 4 times/day
Mucocutaneous infections: Children and Adults: Topical: Apply 2-3 times/day to affected areas; very moist topical lesions are treated best with powder
Intestinal infections: Adults: Oral: 500,000-1,000,000 units every 8 hours
Vaginal infections: Adults: Vaginal tablets: Insert 1 tablet/day at bedtime for 2 weeks

**Dosage Forms**
Capsule (Bio-Statin®): 500,000 units, 1 million units
Cream: 100,000 units/g (15 g, 30 g)
Mycostatin®: 100,000 units/g (30 g)
Ointment, topical: 100,000 units/g (15 g, 30 g)
Powder, for prescription compounding: 50 million units (10 g); 150 million units (30 g); 500 million units (100 g); 2 billion units (400 g)
Nystat-Rx®: 50 million units (10 g); 150 million units (30 g); 500 million units (100 g); 1 billion units (190 g); 2 billion units (350 g)
Powder, topical:
Mycostatin®: 100,000 units/g (15 g)
Nyamyc™: 100,000 units/g (15 g, 30 g)
Nystop®: 100,000 units/g (15 g, 30 g, 60 g)
Pedi-Dri®: 100,000 units/g (56.7 g)
Suspension, oral: 100,000 units/mL (5 mL, 60 mL, 480 mL)
Tablet: 500,000 units
Tablet, vaginal: 100,000 units (15s) [packaged with applicator]

## nystatin and triamcinolone (nye STAT in & trye am SIN oh lone)

**Sound-Alike/Look-Alike Issues**
Mycolog®-II may be confused with Halog®

**Synonyms** triamcinolone and nystatin

**Therapeutic Category** Antifungal/Corticosteroid

**Use** Treatment of cutaneous candidiasis

**Usual Dosage** Children and Adults: Topical: Apply sparingly 2-4 times/day. Therapy should be discontinued when control is achieved; if no improvement is seen, reassessment of diagnosis may be necessary.

**Dosage Forms** [DSC] = Discontinued product
Cream (Mycolog®-II [DSC]): Nystatin 100,000 units and triamcinolone acetonide 0.1% (15 g, 30 g, 60 g)
Ointment: Nystatin 100,000 units and triamcinolone acetonide 0.1% (15 g, 30 g, 60 g)
Mycolog®-II: Nystatin 100,000 units and triamcinolone acetonide 0.1% (15 g, 30 g, 60 g) [DSC]

**Nystat-Rx® [US]** *see* nystatin *on this page*

**Nystex®** *(Discontinued)* *see* nystatin *on this page*

Nystop® [US] *see* nystatin *on previous page*

Nytol® [Can] *see* diphenhydramine *on page 254*

Nytol® Extra Strength [Can] *see* diphenhydramine *on page 254*

Nytol® Quick Caps [US-OTC] *see* diphenhydramine *on page 254*

Nytol® Quick Gels [US-OTC] *see* diphenhydramine *on page 254*

Nōstrilla® [US-OTC] *see* oxymetazoline *on page 610*

O-V Staticin® *(Discontinued)* *see* nystatin *on previous page*

OB-20 [US] *see* vitamins (multiple/prenatal) *on page 852*

Obegyn® [US] *see* vitamins (multiple/prenatal) *on page 852*

Obezine® *(Discontinued)* *see* phendimetrazine *on page 637*

OCBZ *see* oxcarbazepine *on page 606*

Occlusal®-HP [US-OTC/Can] *see* salicylic acid *on page 734*

Ocean® [US-OTC] *see* sodium chloride *on page 752*

OCL® *(Discontinued)* *see* polyethylene glycol-electrolyte solution *on page 658*

Octagam® [US] *see* immune globulin (intravenous) *on page 433*

Octamide® *(Discontinued)* *see* metoclopramide *on page 533*

Octicair® Otic *(Discontinued)* *see* neomycin, polymyxin B, and hydrocortisone *on page 568*

Octocaine® *(Discontinued)* *see* lidocaine and epinephrine *on page 480*

Octostim® [Can] *see* desmopressin acetate *on page 230*

## octreotide (ok TREE oh tide)

**Sound-Alike/Look-Alike Issues**
Sandostatin® may be confused with Sandimmune®

**Synonyms** octreotide acetate

**U.S./Canadian Brand Names** Octreotide Acetate Omega [Can]; Sandostatin LAR® [US/Can]; Sandostatin® [US/Can]

**Therapeutic Category** Somatostatin Analog

**Use** Control of symptoms in patients with metastatic carcinoid and vasoactive intestinal peptide-secreting tumors (VIPomas); acromegaly

**Usual Dosage**
Infants and Children: Diarrhea: I.V., SubQ: Doses of 1-10 mcg/kg every 12 hours have been used in children beginning at the low end of the range and increasing by 0.3 mcg/kg/dose at 3-day intervals. Suppression of growth hormone (animal data) is of concern when used as long-term therapy.

Adults: SubQ: Initial: 50 mcg 1-2 times/day and titrate dose based on patient tolerance and response

Carcinoid: 100-600 mcg/day in 2-4 divided doses

VIPomas: 200-300 mcg/day in 2-4 divided doses

Diarrhea: Initial: I.V.: 50-100 mcg every 8 hours; increase by 100 mcg/dose at 48-hour intervals; maximum dose: 500 mcg every 8 hours

Esophageal varices bleeding: I.V. bolus: 25-50 mcg followed by continuous I.V. infusion of 25-50 mcg/hour

Acromegaly: Initial: SubQ: 50 mcg 3 times/day; titrate to achieve growth hormone levels <5 ng/mL or IGF-I (somatomedin C) levels <1.9 U/mL in males and <2.2 U/mL in females; usual effective dose 100 mcg 3 times/day; range 300-1500 mcg/day

**Note:** Should be withdrawn yearly for a 4-week interval in patients who have received irradiation. Resume if levels increase and signs/symptoms recur.

Acromegaly, carcinoid tumors, and VIPomas (depot injection): Patients must be stabilized on subcutaneous octreotide for at least 2 weeks before switching to the long-acting depot: Upon switch: 20 mg I.M. intragluteally every 4 weeks for 2-3 months, then the dose may be modified based upon response

**Dosage adjustment for acromegaly:** After 3 months of depot injections the dosage may be continued or modified as follows:
GH ≤2.5 ng/mL, IGF-1 is normal, symptoms controlled: Maintain octreotide LAR® at 20 mg I.M. every 4 weeks

GH >2.5 ng/mL, IGF-1 is elevated, and/or symptoms uncontrolled: Increase octreotide LAR® to 30 mg I.M. every 4 weeks

GH ≤1 ng/mL, IGF-1 is normal, symptoms controlled: Reduce octreotide LAR® to 10 mg I.M. every 4 weeks

(Continued)

## octreotide *(Continued)*

Dosages >40 mg are not recommended

**Dosage adjustment for carcinoid tumors and VIPomas:** After 2 months of depot injections the dosage may be continued or modified as follows:

Increase to 30 mg I.M. every 4 weeks if symptoms are inadequately controlled

Decrease to 10 mg I.M. every 4 weeks, for a trial period, if initially responsive to 20 mg dose

Dosage >30 mg is not recommended

### Dosage Forms

Injection, microspheres for suspension, as acetate [depot formulation] (Sandostatin LAR®): 10 mg, 20 mg, 30 mg [with diluent and syringe]

Injection, solution, as acetate (Sandostatin®): 0.05 mg/mL (1 mL); 0.1 mg/mL (1 mL); 0.2 mg/mL (5 mL); 0.5 mg/mL (1 mL); 1 mg/mL (5 mL)

**octreotide acetate** *see* octreotide *on previous page*

**Octreotide Acetate Omega [Can]** *see* octreotide *on previous page*

**OcuClear® *(Discontinued)*** *see* oxymetazoline *on page 610*

**OcuCoat® [US-OTC]** *see* artificial tears *on page 71*

**OcuCoat® PF [US-OTC]** *see* artificial tears *on page 71*

**Ocufen® [US/Can]** *see* flurbiprofen *on page 352*

**Ocuflox® [US/Can]** *see* ofloxacin *on this page*

**Ocupress® *(Discontinued)*** *see* carteolol *on page 150*

**Ocupress® Ophthalmic [Can]** *see* carteolol *on page 150*

**Ocusert Pilo-20® *(Discontinued)*** *see* pilocarpine *on page 647*

**Ocusert Pilo-40® *(Discontinued)*** *see* pilocarpine *on page 647*

**Ocu-Sul® *(Discontinued)*** *see* sulfacetamide *on page 771*

**Ocutricin® Topical Ointment *(Discontinued)*** *see* bacitracin, neomycin, and polymyxin B *on page 87*

**Ocuvite® [US-OTC]** *see* vitamins (multiple/oral) *on page 852*

**Ocuvite® Extra® [US-OTC]** *see* vitamins (multiple/oral) *on page 852*

**Ocuvite® Lutein [US-OTC]** *see* vitamins (multiple/oral) *on page 852*

**Oesclim® [Can]** *see* estradiol *on page 299*

## ofloxacin *(oh FLOKS a sin)*

### Sound-Alike/Look-Alike Issues

Floxin® may be confused with Flexeril®

Ocuflox® may be confused with Ocufen®

**U.S./Canadian Brand Names** Apo-Ofloxacin® [Can]; Apo-Oflox® [Can]; Floxin® [US/Can]; Novo-Ofloxacin [Can]; Ocuflox® [US/Can]; PMS-Ofloxacin [Can]

**Therapeutic Category** Antibiotic, Ophthalmic; Antibiotic, Otic; Quinolone

**Use** Quinolone antibiotic for the treatment of acute exacerbations of chronic bronchitis, community-acquired pneumonia, skin and skin structure infections (uncomplicated), urethral and cervical gonorrhea (acute, uncomplicated), urethritis and cervicitis (nongonococcal), mixed infections of the urethra and cervix, pelvic inflammatory disease (acute), cystitis (uncomplicated), urinary tract infections (complicated), prostatitis

Ophthalmic: Treatment of superficial ocular infections involving the conjunctiva or cornea due to strains of susceptible organisms

Otic: Otitis externa, chronic suppurative otitis media, acute otitis media

### Usual Dosage

Oral: Adults:

Chronic bronchitis (acute exacerbation), community-acquired pneumonia, skin and skin structure infections (uncomplicated): 400 mg every 12 hours for 10 days

Urethral and cervical gonorrhea (acute, uncomplicated): 400 mg as a single dose

Cervicitis/urethritis (nongonococcal) due to *C. trachomatis*, mixed infection of urethra and cervix due to *C. trachomatis* and *N. gonorrhoea*: 300 mg every 12 hours for 7 days

Pelvic inflammatory disease (acute): 400 mg every 12 hours for 10-14 days

Cystitis (uncomplicated):
 Due to *E. coli* or *K. pneumoniae*: 200 mg every 12 hours for 3 days
 Due to other organisms: 200 mg every 12 hours for 7 days
 UTI (complicated): 200 mg every 12 hours for 10 days
 Prostatitis: 200 mg every 12 hours for 6 weeks
Ophthalmic: Children >1 year and Adults:
 Conjunctivitis: Instill 1-2 drops in affected eye(s) every 2-4 hours for the first 2 days, then use 4 times/day for an additional 5 days
 Corneal ulcer: Instill 1-2 drops every 30 minutes while awake and every 4-6 hours after retiring for the first 2 days; beginning on day 3, instill 1-2 drops every hour while awake for 4-6 additional days; thereafter, 1-2 drops 4 times/day until clinical cure.
Otic:
 Acute otitis media with tympanostomy tubes: Children 1-12 years: Instill 5 drops (or the contents of 1 single-dose container) into affected ear(s) twice daily for 10 days
 Chronic suppurative otitis media with perforated tympanic membranes: Children >12 years and Adults: Instill 10 drops (or the contents of 2 single-dose containers) into affected ear twice daily for 14 days
 Otitis externa:
  Children 6 months to 13 years: Instill 5 drops (or the contents of 1 single-dose container) into affected ear(s) once daily for 7 days
  Children ≥13 years and Adults: Instill 10 drops (or the contents of 2 single-dose containers) into affected ear(s) once daily for 7 days

**Dosage Forms**
 Solution, ophthalmic (Ocuflox®): 0.3% (5 mL, 10 mL) [contains benzalkonium chloride]
 Solution, otic:
  Floxin®: 0.3% (5 mL, 10 mL) [contains benzalkonium chloride]
  Floxin® Otic Singles™: 0.3% (0.25 mL) [contains benzalkonium chloride; packaged as 2 single-dose containers per pouch, 10 pouches per carton, total net volume 5 mL]
 Tablet (Floxin®): 200 mg, 300 mg, 400 mg

**Ogen® [US/Can]** *see* estropipate *on page 306*

**Ogestrel® [US]** *see* ethinyl estradiol and norgestrel *on page 318*

**OGMT** *see* metyrosine *on page 536*

**OGT-918** *see* miglustat *on page 541*

**OKT3** *see* muromonab-CD3 *on page 554*

# olanzapine (oh LAN za peen)

**Sound-Alike/Look-Alike Issues**
 olanzapine may be confused with olsalazine
 Zyprexa® may be confused with Celexa™, Zyrtec®

**Synonyms** LY170053

**U.S./Canadian Brand Names** Zyprexa® Zydis® [US/Can]; Zyprexa® [US/Can]

**Therapeutic Category** Antipsychotic Agent

**Use** Treatment of the manifestations of schizophrenia; treatment of acute mania episodes associated with bipolar disorder (as monotherapy or in combination with lithium or valproate); maintenance treatment of bipolar disorder; acute agitation (patients with schizophrenia or bipolar mania)

**Usual Dosage**
 Children: Schizophrenia/bipolar disorder: Oral: Initial: 2.5 mg/day; titrate as necessary to 20 mg/day (0.12-0.29 mg/kg/day)
 Adults:
  Schizophrenia: Oral: Usual starting dose: 5-10 mg once daily; increase to 10 mg once daily within 5-7 days, thereafter adjust by 5-10 mg/day at 1-week intervals, up to a maximum of 20 mg/day; doses of 30-50 mg/day have been used; typical dosage range: 10-30 mg/day
  Bipolar mania: Oral:
   Monotherapy: Usual starting dose: 10-15 mg once daily; increase by 5 mg/day at intervals of not less than 24 hours; maintenance: 5-20 mg/day; maximum dose: 20 mg/day
   Combination therapy (olanzapine in combination with lithium or valproate): Initial: 10 mg once daily; dosing range: 5-20 mg/day
  Agitation (acute, associated with bipolar disorder or schizophrenia): I.M.: Initial dose: 5-10 mg (a lower dose of 2.5 mg may be considered when clinical factors warrant); additional doses (2.5-10 mg) may be considered; however, 2-4 hours should be allowed between doses to evaluate response (maximum total daily dose: 30 mg, per manufacturer's recommendation)

(Continued)

## olanzapine *(Continued)*

**Dosage Forms**
Injection, powder for reconstitution (Zyprexa® IntraMuscular): 10 mg [contains lactose 50 mg]
Tablet (Zyprexa®): 2.5 mg, 5 mg, 7.5 mg, 10 mg, 15 mg, 20 mg
Tablet, orally-disintegrating (Zyprexa® Zydis®): 5 mg [contains phenylalanine 0.34 mg/tablet], 10 mg [contains phenylalanine 0.45 mg/tablet], 15 mg [contains phenylalanine 0.67 mg/tablet], 20 mg [contains phenylalanine 0.9 mg/tablet]

## olanzapine and fluoxetine (oh LAN za peen & floo OKS e teen)

**Synonyms** fluoxetine and olanzapine; olanzapine and fluoxetine hydrochloride
**U.S./Canadian Brand Names** Symbyax™ [US]
**Therapeutic Category** Antidepressant, Selective Serotonin Reuptake Inhibitor; Antipsychotic Agent, Thienobenzodiaepine
**Use** Treatment of depressive episodes associated with bipolar disorder
**Usual Dosage** Oral: Adults: Depression associated with bipolar disorder: Initial: Olanzapine 6 mg/fluoxetine 25 mg once daily in the evening. Dosing range: Olanzapine 6-12 mg/fluoxetine 25-50 mg. Use caution adjusting dose in patients predisposed to hypotension, in females, and in nonsmokers (metabolism may be decreased). Safety of daily doses of olanzapine >18 mg/fluoxetine >75 mg have not been evaluated.
**Dosage Forms** Capsule:
6/25: Olanzapine 6 mg and fluoxetine 25 mg
6/50: Olanzapine 6 mg and fluoxetine 50 mg
12/25: Olanzapine 12 mg and fluoxetine 25 mg
12/50: Olanzapine 12 mg and fluoxetine 50 mg

**olanzapine and fluoxetine hydrochloride** *see* olanzapine and fluoxetine *on this page*

**Olay® Vitamins Complete Women's [US-OTC]** *see* vitamins (multiple/oral) *on page 852*

**Olay® Vitamins Complete Women's 50+ [US-OTC]** *see* vitamins (multiple/oral) *on page 852*

**Olay® Vitamins Even Complexion [US-OTC]** *see* vitamins (multiple/oral) *on page 852*

**oleovitamin A** *see* vitamin A *on page 848*

**oleum ricini** *see* castor oil *on page 151*

## olmesartan (ole me SAR tan)

**Synonyms** olmesartan medoxomil
**U.S./Canadian Brand Names** Benicar® [US]
**Therapeutic Category** Angiotensin II Receptor Antagonist
**Use** Treatment of hypertension with or without concurrent use of other antihypertensive agents
**Usual Dosage** Oral: Adults: Initial: Usual starting dose is 20 mg once daily; if initial response is inadequate, may be increased to 40 mg once daily after 2 weeks. May administer with other antihypertensive agents if blood pressure inadequately controlled with olmesartan. Consider lower starting dose in patients with possible depletion of intravascular volume (eg, patients receiving diuretics).
**Dosage Forms** Tablet [film coated], as medoxomil: 5 mg, 20 mg, 40 mg

## olmesartan and hydrochlorothiazide (ole me SAR tan & hye droe klor oh THYE a zide)

**Synonyms** hydrochlorothiazide and olmesartan medoxomil; olmesartan medoxomil and hydrochlorothiazide
**U.S./Canadian Brand Names** Benicar HCT® [US]
**Therapeutic Category** Angiotensin II Receptor Antagonist; Diuretic, Thiazide
**Use** Treatment of hypertension (not recommended for initial treatment)
**Usual Dosage** Oral: Adults: One tablet daily; dosage must be individualized (see below). May be titrated at 2- to 4-week intervals.
Replacement therapy: May be substituted for previously titrated dosages of the individual components. Patients not controlled with single-agent therapy: Initiate by adding the lowest available dose of the alternative component (hydrochlorothiazide 12.5 mg or olmesartan 20 mg). Titrate to effect (maximum daily hydrochlorothiazide dose: 25 mg; maximum daily olmesartan dose: 40 mg).
**Dosage Forms** Tablet:
20/12.5: Olmesartan medoxomil 20 mg and hydrochlorothiazide 12.5 mg
40/12.5: Olmesartan medoxomil 40 mg and hydrochlorothiazide 12.5 mg
40/25: Olmesartan medoxomil 40 mg and hydrochlorothiazide 25 mg

**olmesartan medoxomil** *see* olmesartan *on previous page*

**olmesartan medoxomil and hydrochlorothiazide** *see* olmesartan and hydrochlorothiazide *on previous page*

## olopatadine (oh loe pa TA deen)
**Sound-Alike/Look-Alike Issues**
Patanol® may be confused with Platinol®
**U.S./Canadian Brand Names** Patanol® [US/Can]
**Therapeutic Category** Antihistamine
**Use** Treatment of the signs and symptoms of allergic conjunctivitis
**Usual Dosage** Adults: Ophthalmic: Instill 1 to 2 drops into affected eye(s) twice daily (allowing 6-8 hours between doses); results from an environmental study demonstrated that olopatadine was effective when dosed twice daily for up to 6 weeks
**Dosage Forms** Solution, ophthalmic: 0.1% (5 mL) [contains benzalkonium chloride]

## olsalazine (ole SAL a zeen)
**Sound-Alike/Look-Alike Issues**
olsalazine may be confused with olanzapine
Dipentum® may be confused with Dilantin®
**Synonyms** olsalazine sodium
**U.S./Canadian Brand Names** Dipentum® [US/Can]
**Therapeutic Category** 5-Aminosalicylic Acid Derivative
**Use** Maintenance of remission of ulcerative colitis in patients intolerant to sulfasalazine
**Usual Dosage** Adults: Oral: 1 g/day in 2 divided doses
**Dosage Forms** Capsule, as sodium: 250 mg

**olsalazine sodium** *see* olsalazine *on this page*

**Olux® [US]** *see* clobetasol *on page 194*

**Omacor® [US]** *see* omega-3-acid ethyl esters *on next page*

## omalizumab (oh mah lye ZOO mab)
**Synonyms** rhuMAb-E25
**U.S./Canadian Brand Names** Xolair® [US/Can]
**Therapeutic Category** Monoclonal Antibody
**Use** Treatment of moderate-to-severe, persistent allergic asthma not adequately controlled with inhaled corticosteroids
**Usual Dosage** SubQ: Children ≥12 years and Adults: Asthma: Dose is based on pretreatment IgE serum levels and body weight. Dosing should not be adjusted based on IgE levels taken during treatment or <1 year following therapy; doses should be adjusted during treatment for significant changes in body weight
IgE ≥30-100 int. units/mL:
30-90 kg: 150 mg every 4 weeks
>90-150 kg: 300 mg every 4 weeks
IgE >100-200 int. units/mL:
30-90 kg: 300 mg every 4 weeks
>90-150 kg: 225 mg every 2 weeks
IgE >200-300 int. units/mL:
30-60 kg: 300 mg every 4 weeks
>60-90 kg: 225 mg every 2 weeks
>90-150 kg: 300 mg every 2 weeks
IgE >300-400 int. units/mL:
30-70 kg: 225 mg every 2 weeks
>70-90 kg: 300 mg every 2 weeks
>90 kg: Do not administer dose
IgE >400-500 int. units/mL:
30-70 kg: 300 mg every 2 weeks
>70-90 kg: 375 mg every 2 weeks
>90 kg: Do not administer dose
IgE >500-600 int. units/mL:
30-60 kg: 300 mg every 2 weeks
>60-70 kg: 375 mg every 2 weeks
(Continued)

# omalizumab *(Continued)*

>70 kg: Do not administer dose
IgE >600-700 int. units/mL:
 30-60 kg: 375 mg every 2 weeks
 >60 kg: Do not administer dose
**Dosage Forms** Injection, powder for reconstitution [preservative free]: 150 mg [contains sucrose 145.5 g]

# omega-3-acid ethyl esters (oh MEG a three AS id ETH il ES ters)

**Synonyms** ethyl esters of omega-3 fatty acids; fish oil
**U.S./Canadian Brand Names** Omacor® [US]
**Therapeutic Category** Antilipemic Agent, Miscellaneous
**Use** Omacor®: Treatment of hypertriglyceridemia (≥500 mg/dL)
  **Note:** A number of OTC formulations containing omega-3 fatty acids are marketed as nutritional supplements; these do not have FDA-approved indications.
**Usual Dosage** Oral: Adults: Hypertriglyceridemia: 4 g/day as a single daily dose or in 2 divided doses
**Dosage Forms** Capsule: 1 g [contains EPA ~465 mg and DHA ~375 mg]

# omeprazole (oh ME pray zol)

**Sound-Alike/Look-Alike Issues**
  Prilosec® may be confused with Plendil®, Prevacid®, predniSONE, prilocaine, Prinivil®, Proventil®, Prozac®
**U.S./Canadian Brand Names** Apo-Omeprazole® [Can]; Losec MUPS® [Can]; Losec® [Can]; Prilosec OTC™ [US-OTC]; Prilosec® [US]; Zegerid™ [US]
**Therapeutic Category** Gastric Acid Secretion Inhibitor
**Use** Short-term (4-8 weeks) treatment of active duodenal ulcer disease or active benign gastric ulcer; treatment of heartburn and other symptoms associated with gastroesophageal reflux disease (GERD); short-term (4-8 weeks) treatment of endoscopically-diagnosed erosive esophagitis; maintenance healing of erosive esophagitis; long-term treatment of pathological hypersecretory conditions; as part of a multidrug regimen for *H. pylori* eradication to reduce the risk of duodenal ulcer recurrence; reduction of risk of upper gastrointestinal bleeding in critically-ill patients (Zegerid™)

OTC labeling: Short-term treatment of frequent, uncomplicated heartburn occurring ≥2 days/week
**Usual Dosage** Oral:
Children ≥2 years: GERD or other acid-related disorders:
  <20 kg: 10 mg once daily
  ≥20 kg: 20 mg once daily
Adults:
  Active duodenal ulcer: 20 mg/day for 4-8 weeks
  Gastric ulcers: 40 mg/day for 4-8 weeks
  Symptomatic GERD: 20 mg/day for up to 4 weeks
  Erosive esophagitis: 20 mg/day for 4-8 weeks
  *Helicobacter pylori* eradication: Dose varies with regimen: 20 mg once daily **or** 40 mg/day as single dose or in 2 divided doses; requires combination therapy with antibiotics
  Pathological hypersecretory conditions: Initial: 60 mg once daily; doses up to 120 mg 3 times/day have been administered; administer daily doses >80 mg in divided doses
  Frequent heartburn (OTC labeling): 20 mg/day for 14 days; treatment may be repeated after 4 months if needed
  Risk reduction of upper GI bleeding in critically-ill patients (Zegerid™):
  Loading dose: Day 1: 40 mg every 6-8 hours for two doses
  Maintenance dose: 40 mg/day for up to 14 days; therapy >14 days has not been evaluated
**Dosage Forms**
Capsule, delayed release: 10 mg, 20 mg
  Prilosec®: 10 mg, 20 mg, 40 mg
Powder for oral suspension [packet] (Zegerid™): 20 mg (30s), 40 mg (30s) [both strengths contain sodium bicarbonate 1680 mg, equivalent to sodium 460 mg per packet]
Tablet, delayed release (Prilosec OTC™): 20 mg

**Omnicef® [US/Can]** *see* cefdinir *on page 153*
**Omnicef® [US/Can]** *see* cefdinir *on page 153*
**OmniHIB™ *(Discontinued)***
**Omnipaque® [US]** *see* radiological/contrast media (nonionic) *on page 709*
**Omnipaque® [US]** *see* radiological/contrast media (nonionic) *on page 709*
**Omnipen® *(Discontinued)*** *see* ampicillin *on page 50*
**Omnipen® *(Discontinued)*** *see* ampicillin *on page 50*

Omnipen®-N *(Discontinued)* *see* ampicillin *on page 50*

Oncaspar® [US] *see* pegaspargase *on page 623*

Oncet® *(Discontinued)* *see* hydrocodone and homatropine *on page 413*

Oncotice™ [Can] *see* BCG vaccine *on page 90*

Oncovin® *(Discontinued)* *see* vincristine *on page 846*


# ondansetron (on DAN se tron)

### Sound-Alike/Look-Alike Issues
ondansetron may be confused with dolasetron, granisetron, palonosetron

Zofran® may be confused with Zantac®, Zosyn®

**Synonyms** GR38032R; ondansetron hydrochloride

**U.S./Canadian Brand Names** Zofran® ODT [US/Can]; Zofran® [US/Can]

**Therapeutic Category** Selective 5-HT$_3$ Receptor Antagonist

**Use** Prevention of nausea and vomiting associated with moderately- to highly-emetogenic cancer chemotherapy [not recommended for treatment of **existing** chemotherapy-induced emesis (CIE)]; radiotherapy in patients receiving total body irradiation or fractions to the abdomen; prevention and treatment of postoperative nausea and vomiting

**Usual Dosage Note:** Administration of a single daily dose of 8-12 mg I.V. or 8-24 mg orally is now generally accepted in place of mg/kg dosing.

Children:

I.V.:

Prevention of chemotherapy-induced emesis: 6 months to 18 years: 0.15 mg/kg/dose administered 30 minutes prior to chemotherapy, 4 and 8 hours after the first dose **or** 0.45 mg/kg/day as a single dose

Prevention of postoperative nausea and vomiting: 1 month to 12 years:

≤40 kg: 0.1 mg/kg as a single dose

>40 kg: 4 mg as a single dose

Oral: Prevention of chemotherapy-induced emesis:

4-11 years: 4 mg 30 minutes before chemotherapy; repeat 4 and 8 hours after initial dose, then 4 mg every 8 hours for 1-2 days after chemotherapy completed

≥12 years: Refer to adult dosing.

Adults:

I.V.:

Prevention of chemotherapy-induced emesis:

0.15 mg/kg 3 times/day beginning 30 minutes prior to chemotherapy **or**

0.45 mg/kg once daily **or**

8-10 mg 1-2 times/day **or**

24 mg or 32 mg once daily

I.M., I.V.: Postoperative nausea and vomiting: 4 mg as a single dose approximately 30 minutes before the end of anesthesia, or as treatment if vomiting occurs after surgery

**Note:** Repeat doses given in response to inadequate control of nausea/vomiting from preoperative doses are generally ineffective.

Oral:

Chemotherapy-induced emesis:

Highly-emetogenic agents/single-day therapy: 24 mg given 30 minutes prior to the start of therapy

Moderately-emetogenic agents: 8 mg every 12 hours beginning 30 minutes before chemotherapy, continuously for 1-2 days after chemotherapy completed

Total body irradiation: 8 mg 1-2 hours before daily each fraction of radiotherapy

Single high-dose fraction radiotherapy to abdomen: 8 mg 1-2 hours before irradiation, then 8 mg every 8 hours after first dose for 1-2 days after completion of radiotherapy

Daily fractionated radiotherapy to abdomen: 8 mg 1-2 hours before irradiation, then 8 mg 8 hours after first dose for each day of radiotherapy

Postoperative nausea and vomiting: 16 mg given 1 hour prior to induction of anesthesia

### Dosage Forms

Infusion [premixed in D$_5$W] (Zofran®): 32 mg (50 mL)

Injection, solution (Zofran®): 2 mg/mL (2 mL, 20 mL)

Solution, oral (Zofran®): 4 mg/5 mL (50 mL) [contains sodium benzoate; strawberry flavor]

Tablet (Zofran®): 4 mg, 8 mg, 24 mg

Tablet, orally-disintegrating (Zofran® ODT): 4 mg, 8 mg [each strength contains phenylalanine <0.03 mg/tablet; strawberry flavor]


**ondansetron hydrochloride** *see* ondansetron *on this page*

**One-A-Day® 50 Plus Formula [US-OTC]** *see* vitamins (multiple/oral) *on page 852*

**One-A-Day® Active Formula [US-OTC]** *see* vitamins (multiple/oral) *on page 852*

**One-A-Day® Carb Smart [US-OTC]** *see* vitamins (multiple/oral) *on page 852*

**One-A-Day® Cholesterol Plus™ [US-OTC]** *see* vitamins (multiple/oral) *on page 852*

**One-A-Day® Essential Formula [US-OTC]** *see* vitamins (multiple/oral) *on page 852*

**One-A-Day® Kids Bugs Bunny and Friends Complete [US-OTC]** *see* vitamins (multiple/pediatric) *on page 852*

**One-A-Day® Kids Bugs Bunny and Friends Plus Extra C [US-OTC]** *see* vitamins (multiple/pediatric) *on page 852*

**One-A-Day® Kids Extreme Sports [US-OTC]** *see* vitamins (multiple/pediatric) *on page 852*

**One-A-Day® Kids Scooby-Doo! Complete [US-OTC]** *see* vitamins (multiple/pediatric) *on page 852*

**One-A-Day® Kids Scooby-Doo! Fizzy Vites [US-OTC]** *see* vitamins (multiple/pediatric) *on page 852*

**One-A-Day® Kids Scooby-Doo! Plus Calcium [US-OTC]** *see* vitamins (multiple/pediatric) *on page 852*

**One-A-Day® Maximum Formula [US-OTC]** *see* vitamins (multiple/oral) *on page 852*

**One-A-Day® Men's Formula [US-OTC]** *see* vitamins (multiple/oral) *on page 852*

**One-A-Day® Today [US-OTC]** *see* vitamins (multiple/oral) *on page 852*

**One-A-Day® Weight Smart [US-OTC]** *see* vitamins (multiple/oral) *on page 852*

**One-A-Day® Women's Formula [US-OTC]** *see* vitamins (multiple/oral) *on page 852*

**ONTAK® [US]** *see* denileukin diftitox *on page 228*

**Onxol™ [US]** *see* paclitaxel *on page 612*

**Ony-Clear *(Discontinued)*** *see* benzalkonium chloride *on page 95*

**OPC-13013** *see* cilostazol *on page 183*

**OPC-14597** *see* aripiprazole *on page 70*

**OP-CCK** *see* sincalide *on page 749*

**Opcon-A® [US-OTC]** *see* naphazoline and pheniramine *on page 561*

**Opcon® Ophthalmic *(Discontinued)*** *see* naphazoline *on page 561*

**Operand® [US-OTC]** *see* povidone-iodine *on page 668*

**Operand® Chlorhexidine Gluconate [US-OTC]** *see* chlorhexidine gluconate *on page 168*

**Ophthalgan® Ophthalmic *(Discontinued)*** *see* glycerin *on page 379*

**Ophthetic® [US]** *see* proparacaine *on page 685*

**Ophthifluor® *(Discontinued)*** *see* fluorescein sodium *on page 346*

**Ophthochlor® Ophthalmic *(Discontinued)*** *see* chloramphenicol *on page 167*

**Ophtho-Dipivefrin™ [Can]** *see* dipivefrin *on page 260*

**Ophtho-Tate® [Can]** *see* prednisolone (ophthalmic) *on page 673*

**opium and belladonna** *see* belladonna and opium *on page 92*

## opium tincture (OH pee um TING chur)

**Sound-Alike/Look-Alike Issues**
opium tincture may be confused with camphorated tincture of opium (paregoric)
DTO is an error-prone abbreviation (mistaken as Diluted Tincture of Opium; dose equivalency of paregoric)

**Synonyms** opium tincture, deodorized

**Therapeutic Category** Analgesic, Narcotic

**Controlled Substance** C-II

**Use** Treatment of diarrhea or relief of pain

**Usual Dosage** Oral:

Children:

Diarrhea: 0.005-0.01 mL/kg/dose every 3-4 hours for a maximum of 6 doses/24 hours

Analgesia: 0.01-0.02 mL/kg/dose every 3-4 hours
Adults:
Diarrhea: 0.3-1 mL/dose every 2-6 hours to maximum of 6 mL/24 hours
Analgesia: 0.6-1.5 mL/dose every 3-4 hours
**Dosage Forms** Liquid: 10% (120 mL, 480 mL) [0.6 mL equivalent to morphine 6 mg; contains alcohol 19%]

**opium tincture, deodorized** *see* opium tincture *on previous page*

**oprelvekin** (oh PREL ve kin)
**Sound-Alike/Look-Alike Issues**
oprelvekin may be confused with aldesleukin, Proleukin®
Neumega® may be confused with Neupogen®
**Synonyms** IL-11; interleukin-11; recombinant human interleukin-11; recombinant interleukin-11; rhIL-11; rIL-11
**U.S./Canadian Brand Names** Neumega® [US]
**Therapeutic Category** Platelet Growth Factor
**Use** Prevention of severe thrombocytopenia and the reduction of the need for platelet transfusions following myelosuppressive chemotherapy
**Usual Dosage** SubQ: **Note:** First dose should not be administered until 24-36 hours after the end of chemotherapy. Discontinue the drug at least 48 hours before beginning the next cycle of chemotherapy.
Children: 75-100 mcg/kg once daily for 10-21 days (until postnadir platelet count ≥50,000 cells/μL)
**Note:** The manufacturer states that, until efficacy/toxicity parameters are established, the use of oprelvekin in pediatric patients (particularly those <12 years of age) should be restricted to use in controlled clinical trials.
Adults: 50 mcg/kg once daily for 10-21 days (until postnadir platelet count ≥50,000 cells/μL)
**Dosage Forms** Injection, powder for reconstitution: 5 mg [packaged with diluent]

**Optho-Bunolol®** **[Can]** *see* levobunolol *on page 472*

**Opticrom®** **[US/Can]** *see* cromolyn sodium *on page 211*

**Optigene®** **3 [US-OTC]** *see* tetrahydrozoline *on page 792*

**Optimine®** **[Can]** *see* azatadine *(Canada only) on page 83*

**Optimine®** ***(Discontinued)***

**Optimoist®** **Solution *(Discontinued)*** *see* saliva substitute *on page 737*

**Optimyxin®** **[Can]** *see* bacitracin and polymyxin B *on page 86*

**Optimyxin Plus®** **[Can]** *see* neomycin, polymyxin B, and gramicidin *on page 568*

**OptiPranolol®** **[US/Can]** *see* metipranolol *on page 533*

**Optiray®** **[US]** *see* radiological/contrast media (nonionic) *on page 709*

**Optivar®** **[US]** *see* azelastine *on page 84*

**Optivite®** **P.M.T. [US-OTC]** *see* vitamins (multiple/oral) *on page 852*

**o,p'-DDD** *see* mitotane *on page 544*

**Orabase®-B with Benzocaine [US-OTC]** *see* benzocaine *on page 95*

**Oradex-C®** ***(Discontinued)*** *see* dyclonine *on page 277*

**Oragrafin®** **Calcium [US]** *see* radiological/contrast media (ionic) *on page 707*

**Oragrafin®** **Sodium [US]** *see* radiological/contrast media (ionic) *on page 707*

**Orajel®** **[US-OTC]** *see* benzocaine *on page 95*

**Orajel®** **Baby Teething [US-OTC]** *see* benzocaine *on page 95*

**Orajel®** **Baby Teething Nighttime [US-OTC]** *see* benzocaine *on page 95*

**Orajel®** **Brace-Aid Oral Anesthetic *(Discontinued)*** *see* benzocaine *on page 95*

**Orajel®** **Denture Plus [US-OTC]** *see* benzocaine *on page 95*

**Orajel®** **Maximum Strength [US-OTC]** *see* benzocaine *on page 95*

**Orajel®** **Medicated Toothache [US-OTC]** *see* benzocaine *on page 95*

**Orajel®** **Mouth Sore [US-OTC]** *see* benzocaine *on page 95*

**Orajel®** **Multi-Action Cold Sore [US-OTC]** *see* benzocaine *on page 95*

**Orajel® Perioseptic® Spot Treatment [US-OTC]** *see* carbamide peroxide *on page 141*

**Orajel® PM [US-OTC]** *see* benzocaine *on page 95*

**Orajel® Ultra Mouth Sore [US-OTC]** *see* benzocaine *on page 95*

**Oramorph SR® [US]** *see* morphine sulfate *on page 549*

**Oranyl [US-OTC]** *see* pseudoephedrine *on page 692*

**Orap® [US/Can]** *see* pimozide *on page 648*

**Orapred® [US]** *see* prednisolone (systemic) *on page 674*

**OraRinse™ [US-OTC]** *see* maltodextrin *on page 501*

**Orasone® (Discontinued)** *see* prednisone *on page 674*

**Orazinc® [US-OTC]** *see* zinc sulfate *on page 861*

**orciprenaline sulfate** *see* metaproterenol *on page 518*

**Oreton® Methyl (Discontinued)** *see* methyltestosterone *on page 533*

**Orfadin® [US]** *see* nitisinone *on page 577*

**ORG 946** *see* rocuronium *on page 728*

**Orgalutran® [Can]** *see* ganirelix *on page 367*

**Organ-1 NR [US]** *see* guaifenesin *on page 383*

**Organidin® NR [US]** *see* guaifenesin *on page 383*

**Orgaran® [Can]** *see* danaparoid *on page 222*

**Orgaran® (Discontinued)** *see* danaparoid *on page 222*

**ORG NC 45** *see* vecuronium *on page 842*

**Orinase Diagnostic® (Discontinued)** *see* tolbutamide *on page 808*

**Orinase® Oral (Discontinued)** *see* tolbutamide *on page 808*

**ORLAAM® (Discontinued)**

**orlistat** (OR li stat)
U.S./Canadian Brand Names Xenical® [US/Can]
Therapeutic Category Lipase Inhibitor
Use Management of obesity, including weight loss and weight management when used in conjunction with a reduced-calorie diet; reduce the risk of weight regain after prior weight loss; indicated for obese patients with an initial body mass index (BMI) $\geq$30 kg/m$^2$ or $\geq$27 kg/m$^2$ in the presence of other risk factors
Usual Dosage Oral: Children $\geq$12 years and Adults: 120 mg 3 times/day with each main meal containing fat (during or up to 1 hour after the meal); omit dose if meal is occasionally missed or contains no fat.
Dosage Forms Capsule: 120 mg

**Ormazine® (Discontinued)** *see* chlorpromazine *on page 178*

**Ornex® [US-OTC]** *see* acetaminophen and pseudoephedrine *on page 8*

**Ornex® Maximum Strength [US-OTC]** *see* acetaminophen and pseudoephedrine *on page 8*

**Ornidyl® Injection (Discontinued)** *see* eflornithine *on page 281*

**ORO-Clense [Can]** *see* chlorhexidine gluconate *on page 168*

**Orphenace® [Can]** *see* orphenadrine *on this page*

**orphenadrine** (or FEN a dreen)
Sound-Alike/Look-Alike Issues
Norflex™ may be confused with norfloxacin, Noroxin®
Synonyms orphenadrine citrate
U.S./Canadian Brand Names Norflex™ [US/Can]; Orphenace® [Can]; Rhoxal-orphendrine [Can]
Therapeutic Category Skeletal Muscle Relaxant
Use Treatment of muscle spasm associated with acute painful musculoskeletal conditions; supportive therapy in tetanus
Usual Dosage Adults:
Oral: 100 mg twice daily

I.M., I.V.: 60 mg every 12 hours

**Dosage Forms**

Injection, solution, as citrate: 30 mg/mL (2 mL) [contains sodium bisulfite]

Tablet, extended release, as citrate: 100 mg

## orphenadrine, aspirin, and caffeine (or FEN a dreen, AS pir in, & KAF een)

**Sound-Alike/Look-Alike Issues**

Norgesic™ Forte may be confused with Norgesic 40®

**Synonyms** aspirin, orphenadrine, and caffeine; caffeine, orphenadrine, and aspirin

**U.S./Canadian Brand Names** Norgesic™ Forte [US/Can]; Norgesic™ [US/Can]; Orphengesic Forte [US]; Orphengesic [US]

**Therapeutic Category** Analgesic, Nonnarcotic;  Skeletal Muscle Relaxant

**Use** Relief of discomfort associated with skeletal muscular conditions

**Usual Dosage** Oral: 1-2 tablets 3-4 times/day

**Dosage Forms**

Tablet: Orphenadrine citrate 25 mg, aspirin 385 mg, and caffeine 30 mg; orphenadrine citrate 50 mg, aspirin 770 mg, and caffeine 60 mg

Norgesic™, Orphengesic: Orphenadrine citrate 25 mg, aspirin 385 mg, and caffeine 30 mg

Norgesic™ Forte, Orphengesic Forte: Orphenadrine citrate 50 mg, aspirin 770 mg, and caffeine 60 mg

**orphenadrine citrate** *see* orphenadrine *on previous page*

**Orphengesic [US]** *see* orphenadrine, aspirin, and caffeine *on this page*

**Orphengesic Forte [US]** *see* orphenadrine, aspirin, and caffeine *on this page*

**Ortho® 0.5/35 [Can]** *see* ethinyl estradiol and norethindrone *on page 314*

**Ortho® 1/35 [Can]** *see* ethinyl estradiol and norethindrone *on page 314*

**Ortho® 7/7/7 [Can]** *see* ethinyl estradiol and norethindrone *on page 314*

**ortho cept** *see* ethinyl estradiol and desogestrel *on page 309*

**Orthoclone OKT® 3 [US/Can]** *see* muromonab-CD3 *on page 554*

**Ortho-Cyclen® [US]** *see* ethinyl estradiol and norgestimate *on page 317*

**ortho est** *see* estropipate *on page 306*

**Ortho Evra™ [US]** *see* ethinyl estradiol and norelgestromin *on page 314*

**Ortho-Novum® [US]** *see* ethinyl estradiol and norethindrone *on page 314*

**Ortho-Novum® 1/50 [US/Can]** *see* mestranol and norethindrone *on page 517*

**ortho prefest** *see* estradiol and norgestimate *on page 302*

**Ortho Tri-Cyclen® [US]** *see* ethinyl estradiol and norgestimate *on page 317*

**Ortho Tri-Cyclen® Lo [US]** *see* ethinyl estradiol and norgestimate *on page 317*

**OrthoVisc® [US/Can]** *see* hyaluronate and derivatives *on page 406*

**Or-Tyl® Injection *(Discontinued)*** *see* dicyclomine *on page 245*

**Orudis® KT *(Discontinued)*** *see* ketoprofen *on page 457*

**Oruvail® [Can]** *see* ketoprofen *on page 457*

**Orvaten™ [US]** *see* midodrine *on page 540*

**Os-Cal® [Can]** *see* calcium carbonate *on page 130*

**Os-Cal® 500 [US-OTC]** *see* calcium carbonate *on page 130*

## oseltamivir (oh sel TAM i vir)

**Sound-Alike/Look-Alike Issues**

Tamiflu® may be confused with Thera-Flu®

**U.S./Canadian Brand Names** Tamiflu® [US/Can]

**Therapeutic Category** Antiviral Agent, Oral

**Use** Treatment of uncomplicated acute illness due to influenza (A or B) infection in adults and children >1 year of age who have been symptomatic for no more than 2 days; prophylaxis against influenza (A or B) infection in adults and adolescents ≥13 years of age

(Continued)

## oseltamivir *(Continued)*

**Usual Dosage** Oral:
Treatment: Initiate treatment within 2 days of onset of symptoms; duration of treatment: 5 days:
Children: 1-12 years:
≤15 kg: 30 mg twice daily
>15 kg - ≤23 kg: 45 mg twice daily
>23 kg - ≤40 kg: 60 mg twice daily
>40 kg: 75 mg twice daily
Adolescents ≥13 years and Adults: 75 mg twice daily
Prophylaxis: Adolescents ≥13 years and Adults: 75 mg once daily for at least 7 days; treatment should begin within 2 days of contact with an infected individual. During community outbreaks, dosing is 75 mg once daily. May be used for up to 6 weeks; duration of protection lasts for length of dosing period

**Dosage Forms**
Capsule, as phosphate: 75 mg
Powder for oral suspension: 12 mg/mL (25 mL) [contains sodium benzoate; tutti-frutti flavor]

**OSI-774** *see* erlotinib *on page 294*

**Osmitrol**® **[US/Can]** *see* mannitol *on page 502*

**Osmoglyn**® *(Discontinued) see* glycerin *on page 379*

**Osmolite**® **HN [US-OTC]** *see* nutritional formula, enteral/oral *on page 591*

**Ostac**® **[Can]** *see* clodronate disodium *(Canada only) on page 195*

**Osteocalcin**® *(Discontinued) see* calcitonin *on page 129*

**Osteocit**® **[Can]** *see* calcium citrate *on page 133*

**Ostoforte**® **[Can]** *see* ergocalciferol *on page 292*

**Oticaine [US]** *see* benzocaine *on page 95*

**Otic-Care**® **Otic** *(Discontinued) see* neomycin, polymyxin B, and hydrocortisone *on page 568*

**Otocaine**™ **[US]** *see* benzocaine *on page 95*

**Otocort**® **Otic** *(Discontinued) see* neomycin, polymyxin B, and hydrocortisone *on page 568*

**Otosporin**® **Otic** *(Discontinued) see* neomycin, polymyxin B, and hydrocortisone *on page 568*

**Otrivin**® *(Discontinued)*

**Otrivin**® **Pediatric** *(Discontinued)*

**Outgro**® **[US-OTC]** *see* benzocaine *on page 95*

**Ovace**™ **[US]** *see* sulfacetamide *on page 771*

**Ovcon**® **[US]** *see* ethinyl estradiol and norethindrone *on page 314*

**Ovide**® **[US]** *see* malathion *on page 501*

**Ovidrel**® **[US/Can]** *see* chorionic gonadotropin (recombinant) *on page 181*

**Ovol**® **[Can]** *see* simethicone *on page 748*

**Ovral**® **[Can]** *see* ethinyl estradiol and norgestrel *on page 318*

**Ovral**® *(Discontinued) see* ethinyl estradiol and norgestrel *on page 318*

**Ovrette**® **[Can]** *see* norgestrel *on page 583*

**Ovrette**® *(Discontinued) see* norgestrel *on page 583*

## oxacillin (oks a SIL in)

**Synonyms** methylphenyl isoxazolyl penicillin; oxacillin sodium
**Therapeutic Category** Penicillin
**Use** Treatment of infections such as osteomyelitis, septicemia, endocarditis, and CNS infections caused by susceptible strains of *Staphylococcus*
**Usual Dosage** I.M., I.V.:
Infants and Children:
Mild-to-moderate infections: 100-150 mg/kg/day in divided doses every 6 hours (maximum: 4 g/day)
Severe infections: 150-200 mg/kg/day in divided doses every 6 hours (maximum: 12 g/day)
Adults:
Mild-to-moderate infections: 250-500 mg every 4-6 hours
Severe infections: 1-2 g every 4-6 hours

Dosage Forms
Infusion [premixed iso-osmotic dextrose solution]: 1 g (50 mL); 2 g (50 mL)
Injection, powder for reconstitution, as sodium: 1 g, 2 g, 10 g

**oxacillin sodium** *see* oxacillin *on previous page*

# oxaliplatin (ox AL i pla tin)

**Sound-Alike/Look-Alike Issues**
oxaliplatin may be confused with Aloxi™
**Synonyms** diaminocyclohexane oxalatoplatinum; L-OHP; NSC-266046
**U.S./Canadian Brand Names** Eloxatin™ [US]
**Therapeutic Category** Antineoplastic Agent, Alkylating Agent
**Use** Treatment of advanced colon cancer and advanced rectal carcinoma
**Usual Dosage** I.V.: Colorectal cancer (labeled dosing): Refer to individual protocols.
Adults:
85 mg/m$^2$ every 2 weeks **or**
20-25 mg/m$^2$ days 1-5 every 3 weeks **or**
100-130 mg/m$^2$ every 2-3 weeks
**Dosage Forms**
Injection, powder for reconstitution: 50 mg, 100 mg [contains lactose]
Injection, solution [preservative free]: 5 mg/mL (10 mL, 20 mL)

**Oxandrin® [US]** *see* oxandrolone *on this page*

# oxandrolone (oks AN droe lone)

**U.S./Canadian Brand Names** Oxandrin® [US]
**Therapeutic Category** Androgen
**Controlled Substance** C-III
**Use** Adjunctive therapy to promote weight gain after weight loss following extensive surgery, chronic infections, or severe trauma, and in some patients who, without definite pathophysiologic reasons, fail to gain or to maintain normal weight; to offset protein catabolism with prolonged corticosteroid administration; relief of bone pain associated with osteoporosis
**Usual Dosage**
Children: Total daily dose: ≤0.1 mg/kg **or** ≤0.045 mg/lb
Adults: 2.5-20 mg in divided doses 2-4 times/day based on individual response; a course of therapy of 2-4 weeks is usually adequate. This may be repeated intermittently as needed.
**Dosage Forms** Tablet: 2.5 mg, 10 mg

# oxaprozin (oks a PROE zin)

**Sound-Alike/Look-Alike Issues**
oxaprozin may be confused with oxazepam
Daypro® may be confused with Diupres®
**U.S./Canadian Brand Names** Apo-Oxaprozin® [Can]; Daypro® [US/Can]
**Therapeutic Category** Analgesic, Nonnarcotic; Nonsteroidal Antiinflammatory Drug (NSAID)
**Use** Acute and long-term use in the management of signs and symptoms of osteoarthritis and rheumatoid arthritis; juvenile rheumatoid arthritis
**Usual Dosage** Oral (individualize dosage to lowest effective dose to minimize adverse effects):
Children 6-16 years: Juvenile rheumatoid arthritis:
22-31 kg: 600 mg once daily
32-54 kg: 900 mg once daily
≥55 kg: 1200 mg once daily
Adults:
Osteoarthritis: 600-1200 mg once daily; patients should be titrated to lowest dose possible; patients with low body weight should start with 600 mg daily
Rheumatoid arthritis: 1200 mg once daily; a one-time loading dose of up to 1800 mg/day or 26 mg/kg (whichever is lower) may be given
Maximum daily dose: 1800 mg or 26 mg/kg (whichever is lower) in divided doses
**Dosage Forms** Tablet: 600 mg

# oxazepam (oks A ze pam)

**Sound-Alike/Look-Alike Issues**

oxazepam may be confused with oxaprozin, quazepam

Serax® may be confused with Eurax®, Urex®, Zyrtec®

**U.S./Canadian Brand Names** Apo-Oxazepam® [Can]; Novoxapram® [Can]; Oxpram® [Can]; PMS-Oxazepam [Can]; Serax® [US]

**Therapeutic Category** Anticonvulsant; Benzodiazepine

**Controlled Substance** C-IV

**Use** Treatment of anxiety; management of ethanol withdrawal

**Usual Dosage** Oral:

Children: Anxiety: 1 mg/kg/day has been administered

Adults:

Anxiety: 10-30 mg 3-4 times/day

Ethanol withdrawal: 15-30 mg 3-4 times/day

Hypnotic: 15-30 mg

**Dosage Forms**

Capsule: 10 mg, 15 mg, 30 mg

Tablet: 15 mg [contains tartrazine]

# oxcarbazepine (ox car BAZ e peen)

**Synonyms** GP 47680; OCBZ

**U.S./Canadian Brand Names** Trileptal® [US/Can]

**Therapeutic Category** Anticonvulsant, Miscellaneous

**Use** Monotherapy or adjunctive therapy in the treatment of partial seizures in adults and children (4-16 years of age) with epilepsy

**Usual Dosage** Oral:

Children 4-16 years:

Adjunctive therapy: 8-10 mg/kg/day, not to exceed 600 mg/day, given in 2 divided daily doses. Maintenance dose should be achieved over 2 weeks, and is dependent upon patient weight, according to the following:

20-29 kg: 900 mg/day in 2 divided doses

29.1-39 kg: 1200 mg/day in 2 divided doses

>39 kg: 1800 mg/day in 2 divided doses

Conversion to monotherapy: Oxcarbazepine 8-10 mg/kg/day in twice daily divided doses, while simultaneously initiating the reduction of the dose of the concomitant antiepileptic drug; the concomitant drug should be withdrawn over 3-6 weeks. Oxcarbazepine dose may be increased by a maximum of 10 mg/kg/day at weekly intervals. See below for recommended total daily dose by weight.

Initiation of monotherapy: Oxcarbazepine should be initiated at 8-10 mg/kg/day in twice daily divided doses; doses may be titrated by 5 mg/kg/day every third day. See below for recommended total daily dose by weight.

Range of maintenance doses by weight during monotherapy:

20 kg: 600-900 mg/day

25-30 kg: 900-1200 mg/day

35-40 kg: 900-1500 mg/day

45 kg: 1200-1500 mg/day

50-55 kg: 1200-1800 mg/day

60-65 kg: 1200-2100 mg/day

70 kg: 1500-2100 mg/day

Adults:

Adjunctive therapy: Initial: 300 mg twice daily; dose may be increased by as much as 600 mg/day at weekly intervals; recommended daily dose: 1200 mg/day in 2 divided doses. Although daily doses >1200 mg/day demonstrated greater efficacy, most patients were unable to tolerate 2400 mg/day (due to CNS effects).

Conversion to monotherapy: Oxcarbazepine 600 mg/day in twice daily divided doses while simultaneously initiating the reduction of the dose of the concomitant antiepileptic drug. The concomitant dosage should be withdrawn over 3-6 weeks, while the maximum dose of oxcarbazepine should be reached in about 2-4 weeks. Recommended daily dose: 2400 mg/day.

Initiation of monotherapy: Oxcarbazepine should be initiated at a dose of 600 mg/day in twice daily divided doses; doses may be titrated upward by 300 mg/day every third day to a final dose of 1200 mg/day given in 2 daily divided doses

**Dosage Forms**
  Suspension, oral: 300 mg/5 mL (250 mL) [contains ethanol]
  Tablet [film coated]: 150 mg, 300 mg, 600 mg

**Oxeze® Turbuhaler® [Can]** *see* formoterol *on page 359*

## oxiconazole (oks i KON a zole)

**Synonyms** oxiconazole nitrate
**U.S./Canadian Brand Names** Oxistat® [US/Can]
**Therapeutic Category** Antifungal Agent
**Use** Treatment of tinea pedis (athlete's foot), tinea cruris (jock itch), and tinea corporis (ringworm)
**Usual Dosage** Topical:
  Children and Adults:
    Tinea corporis/tinea cruris: Cream, lotion: Apply to affected areas 1-2 times daily for 2 weeks
    Tinea pedis: Cream, lotion: Apply to affected areas 1-2 times daily for 1 month
    Adults: Tinea versicolor: Cream: Apply to affected areas once daily for 2 weeks
**Dosage Forms**
  Cream: 1% (15 g, 30 g, 60 g) [contains benzoic acid]
  Lotion: 1% (30 mL) [contains benzoic acid]

**oxiconazole nitrate** *see* oxiconazole *on this page*

**oxidized regenerated cellulose** *see* cellulose, oxidized regenerated *on page 160*

**oxilapine succinate** *see* loxapine *on page 494*

**Oxipor® VHC [US-OTC]** *see* coal tar *on page 201*

**Oxistat® [US/Can]** *see* oxiconazole *on this page*

**oxpentifylline** *see* pentoxifylline *on page 632*

**Oxpram® [Can]** *see* oxazepam *on previous page*

## oxprenolol *(Canada only)* (ox PREN oh lole)

**Synonyms** oxprenolol hydrochloride
**U.S./Canadian Brand Names** Slow-Trasicor® [Can]; Trasicor® [Can]
**Therapeutic Category** Beta-Adrenergic Blocker
**Use** Treatment of mild or moderate hypertension
**Usual Dosage** Oral: Adults:
  Initial: 20 mg 3 times/day (regular-release formulation); increase by 60 mg/day (in 3 divided doses) at 1-2 week intervals until adequate control is obtained
  Maintenance: 120-320 mg/day; do not exceed 480 mg; may switch to slow-release formulation once-daily dosing at this time
**Dosage Forms**
  Tablet (Trasicor®): 40 mg, 80 mg
  Tablet, slow release (Slow-Trasicor®): 80 mg, 160 mg

**oxprenolol hydrochloride** *see* oxprenolol *(Canada only)* *on this page*

**Oxsoralen® [US/Can]** *see* methoxsalen *on page 527*

**Oxsoralen-Ultra® [US/Can]** *see* methoxsalen *on page 527*

**Oxy-5® *(Discontinued)*** *see* benzoyl peroxide *on page 98*

**Oxy 10® Balanced Medicated Face Wash [US-OTC]** *see* benzoyl peroxide *on page 98*

**Oxy 10® Balance Spot Treatment [US-OTC]** *see* benzoyl peroxide *on page 98*

**Oxy Balance® [US-OTC]** *see* salicylic acid *on page 734*

**Oxy Balance® Deep Pore [US-OTC]** *see* salicylic acid *on page 734*

## oxybutynin (oks i BYOO ti nin)

**Sound-Alike/Look-Alike Issues**
  oxybutynin may be confused with OxyContin®
  Ditropan® may be confused with Detrol®, diazepam, Diprivan®, dithranol
  (Continued)

# oxybutynin *(Continued)*

**Synonyms** oxybutynin chloride

**U.S./Canadian Brand Names** Ditropan® XL [US/Can]; Ditropan® [US/Can]; Gen-Oxybutynin [Can]; Novo-Oxybutynin [Can]; Nu-Oxybutyn [Can]; Oxytrol™ [US/Can]; PMS-Oxybutynin [Can]

**Therapeutic Category** Antispasmodic Agent, Urinary

**Use** Antispasmodic for neurogenic bladder (urgency, frequency, urge incontinence) and uninhibited bladder

**Usual Dosage**

Oral:

Children:

>5 years: 5 mg twice daily, up to 5 mg 3 times/day maximum

>6 years: Extended release: 5 mg once daily; maximum dose: 20 mg/day

Adults: 5 mg 2-3 times/day up to 5 mg 4 times/day maximum

Extended release: Initial: 5-10 mg once daily, may increase in 5-10 mg increments; maximum: 30 mg daily

Transdermal: Adults: Apply one 3.9 mg/day patch twice weekly (every 3-4 days)

**Note:** Should be discontinued periodically to determine whether the patient can manage without the drug and to minimize resistance to the drug

**Dosage Forms**

Syrup, as chloride (Ditropan®): 5 mg/5 mL (473 mL)

Tablet, as chloride (Ditropan®): 5 mg

Tablet, extended release, as chloride (Ditropan® XL): 5 mg, 10 mg, 15 mg

Transdermal system (Oxytrol™): 3.9 mg/day (8s) [39 cm$^2$; total oxybutynin 36 mg]

**oxybutynin chloride** *see oxybutynin on previous page*

# oxychlorosene *(oks i KLOR oh seen)*

**Synonyms** oxychlorosene sodium

**U.S./Canadian Brand Names** Clorpactin® WCS-90 [US-OTC]

**Therapeutic Category** Antibiotic, Topical

**Use** Treatment of localized infections

**Usual Dosage** Topical (0.1% to 0.5% solutions): Apply by irrigation, instillation, spray, soaks, or wet compresses

**Dosage Forms** Powder for solution, as sodium: 2 g

**oxychlorosene sodium** *see oxychlorosene on this page*

**Oxycocet® [Can]** *see oxycodone and acetaminophen on next page*

**Oxycodan® [Can]** *see oxycodone and aspirin on page 610*

# oxycodone *(oks i KOE done)*

**Sound-Alike/Look-Alike Issues**

oxycodone may be confused with OxyContin®

OxyContin® may be confused with oxybutynin, oxycodone

OxyFast® may be confused with Roxanol™

**Synonyms** dihydrohydroxycodeinone; oxycodone hydrochloride

**U.S./Canadian Brand Names** Oxy.IR® [Can]; OxyContin® [US/Can]; Oxydose™ [US]; OxyFast® [US]; OxyIR® [US]; Roxicodone™ Intensol™ [US]; Roxicodone™ [US]; Supeudol® [Can]

**Therapeutic Category** Analgesic, Narcotic

**Controlled Substance** C-II

**Use** Management of moderate to severe pain, normally used in combination with non-narcotic analgesics

OxyContin® is indicated for around-the-clock management of moderate to severe pain when an analgesic is needed for an extended period of time. **Note:** OxyContin® is not intended for use as an "as needed" analgesic or for immediately-postoperative pain management (should be used postoperatively only if the patient has received it prior to surgery or if severe, persistent pain is anticipated).

**Usual Dosage** Oral:

Immediate release:

Children:

6-12 years: 1.25 mg every 6 hours as needed

>12 years: 2.5 mg every 6 hours as needed

Adults: 5 mg every 6 hours as needed

Controlled release: Adults:
Opioid naive (not currently on opioid): 10 mg every 12 hours
Currently on opioid/ASA or acetaminophen or NSAID combination:
1-5 tablets: 10-20 mg every 12 hours
6-9 tablets: 20-30 mg every 12 hours
10-12 tablets: 30-40 mg every 12 hours
May continue the nonopioid as a separate drug.
Currently on opioids: Use standard conversion chart to convert daily dose to oxycodone equivalent. Divide daily dose in 2 (for every 12-hour dosing) and round down to nearest dosage form.
**Note:** 80 mg or 160 mg tablets are for use **only** in opioid-tolerant patients. Special safety considerations must be addressed when converting to OxyContin® doses ≥160 mg every 12 hours. Dietary caution must be taken when patients are initially titrated to 160 mg tablets.

**Dosage Forms**
Capsule, immediate release, as hydrochloride (OxyIR®): 5 mg
Solution, oral, as hydrochloride: 5 mg/5 mL (500 mL)
Roxicodone™: 5 mg/5 mL (5 mL, 500 mL) [contains alcohol]
Solution, oral concentrate, as hydrochloride: 20 mg/mL (30 mL)
Oxydose™: 20 mg/mL (30 mL) [contains sodium benzoate; berry flavor]
OxyFast®, Roxicodone™ Intensol™: 20 mg/mL (30 mL) [contains sodium benzoate]
Tablet, as hydrochloride: 5 mg, 15 mg, 30 mg
Roxicodone™: 5 mg, 15 mg, 30 mg
Tablet, controlled release, as hydrochloride (OxyContin®): 10 mg, 20 mg, 40 mg, 80 mg, 160 mg
Tablet, extended release, as hydrochloride: 10 mg, 20 mg, 40 mg, 80 mg

# oxycodone and acetaminophen (oks i KOE done & a seet a MIN oh fen)
**Sound-Alike/Look-Alike Issues**
Percocet® may be confused with Percodan®
Roxicet™ may be confused with Roxanol™
Tylox® may be confused with Trimox®, Tylenol®, Wymox®, Xanax®
**Synonyms** acetaminophen and oxycodone
**U.S./Canadian Brand Names** Endocet® [US/Can]; Oxycocet® [Can]; Percocet® [US/Can]; Percocet®-Demi [Can]; PMS-Oxycodone-Acetaminophen [Can]; Roxicet™ 5/500 [US]; Roxicet™ [US]; Tylox® [US]
**Therapeutic Category** Analgesic, Narcotic
**Controlled Substance** C-II
**Use** Management of moderate to severe pain
**Usual Dosage** Oral: Doses should be given every 4-6 hours as needed and titrated to appropriate analgesic effects. **Note:** Initial dose is based on the **oxycodone** content; however, the maximum daily dose is based on the **acetaminophen** content.

Children: Maximum acetaminophen dose: Children <45 kg: 90 mg/kg/day; children >45 kg: 4 g/day
Mild to moderate pain: Initial dose, **based on oxycodone content:** 0.05-0.1 mg/kg/dose
Severe pain: Initial dose, **based on oxycodone content:** 0.3 mg/kg/dose
Adults:
Mild to moderate pain: Initial dose, **based on oxycodone content:** 5 mg
Severe pain: Initial dose, **based on oxycodone content:** 15-30 mg. Do not exceed acetaminophen 4 g/day.

**Dosage Forms**
Caplet (Roxicet™ 5/500): Oxycodone hydrochloride 5 mg and acetaminophen 500 mg
Capsule: Oxycodone hydrochloride 5 mg and acetaminophen 500 mg
Tylox®: Oxycodone hydrochloride 5 mg and acetaminophen 500 mg [contains sodium benzoate and sodium metabisulfite]
Solution, oral (Roxicet™): Oxycodone hydrochloride 5 mg and acetaminophen 325 mg per 5 mL (5 mL, 500 mL) [contains alcohol <0.5%]
Tablet: Oxycodone hydrochloride 5 mg and acetaminophen 325 mg; oxycodone hydrochloride 7.5 mg and acetaminophen 325 mg; oxycodone hydrochloride 7.5 mg and acetaminophen 500 mg; oxycodone hydrochloride 10 mg and acetaminophen 325 mg; oxycodone hydrochloride 10 mg and acetaminophen 650 mg
Endocet® 5/325 [scored]: Oxycodone hydrochloride 5 mg and acetaminophen 325 mg
Endocet® 7.5/325: Oxycodone hydrochloride 7.5 mg and acetaminophen 325 mg
Endocet® 7.5/500: Oxycodone hydrochloride 7.5 mg and acetaminophen 500 mg
Endocet® 10/325: Oxycodone hydrochloride 10 mg and acetaminophen 325 mg
Endocet® 10/650: Oxycodone hydrochloride 10 mg and acetaminophen 650 mg
(Continued)

# oxycodone and acetaminophen *(Continued)*

Percocet® 2.5/325: Oxycodone hydrochloride 2.5 mg and acetaminophen 325 mg
Percocet® 5/325 [scored]: Oxycodone hydrochloride 5 mg and acetaminophen 325 mg
Percocet® 7.5/325: Oxycodone hydrochloride 7.5 mg and acetaminophen 325 mg
Percocet® 7.5/500: Oxycodone hydrochloride 7.5 mg and acetaminophen 500 mg
Percocet® 10/325: Oxycodone hydrochloride 10 mg and acetaminophen 325 mg
Percocet® 10/650: Oxycodone hydrochloride 10 mg and acetaminophen 650 mg
Roxicet™ [scored]: Oxycodone hydrochloride 5 mg and acetaminophen 325 mg

# oxycodone and aspirin (oks i KOE done & AS pir in)
**Sound-Alike/Look-Alike Issues**
Percodan® may be confused with Decadron®, Percocet®, Percogesic®, Periactin®
**Synonyms** aspirin and oxycodone
**U.S./Canadian Brand Names** Endodan® [US/Can]; Oxycodan® [Can]; Percodan® [US/Can]
**Therapeutic Category** Analgesic, Narcotic
**Controlled Substance** C-II
**Use** Management of moderate to severe pain
**Usual Dosage** Oral (based on oxycodone combined salts):
Children: Maximum oxycodone: 5 mg/dose; maximum aspirin dose should not exceed 4 g/day. Doses should be given every 6 hours as needed.
Mild-to-moderate pain: Initial dose, **based on oxycodone content:**: 0.05-0.1 mg/kg/dose
Severe pain: Initial dose, **based on oxycodone content**: 0.3 mg/kg/dose
Adults: Percodan®: 1 tablet every 6 hours as needed for pain; maximum aspirin dose should not exceed 4 g/day.
**Dosage Forms**
Tablet: Oxycodone hydrochloride 4.5 mg, oxycodone terephthalate 0.38 mg, and aspirin 325 mg
Endodan®, Percodan®: Oxycodone hydrochloride 4.5 mg, oxycodone terephthalate 0.38 mg, and aspirin 325 mg

# oxycodone hydrochloride *see* oxycodone *on page 608*

# OxyContin® [US/Can] *see* oxycodone *on page 608*

# Oxyderm™ [Can] *see* benzoyl peroxide *on page 98*

# Oxydose™ [US] *see* oxycodone *on page 608*

# OxyFast® [US] *see* oxycodone *on page 608*

# Oxy.IR® [Can] *see* oxycodone *on page 608*

# oxymetazoline (oks i met AZ oh leen)
**Sound-Alike/Look-Alike Issues**
oxymetazoline may be confused with oxymetholone
Afrin® may be confused with aspirin
Visine® may be confused with Visken®
**Synonyms** oxymetazoline hydrochloride
**U.S./Canadian Brand Names** 4-Way® 12 Hour [US-OTC]; Afrin® Extra Moisturizing [US-OTC]; Afrin® Original [US-OTC]; Afrin® Severe Congestion [US-OTC]; Afrin® Sinus [US-OTC]; Claritin® Allergic Decongestant [Can]; Dristan® Long Lasting Nasal [Can]; Drixoral® Nasal [Can]; Duramist® Plus [US-OTC]; Duration® [US-OTC]; Genasal [US-OTC]; Neo-Synephrine® 12 Hour Extra Moisturizing [US-OTC]; Neo-Synephrine® 12 Hour [US-OTC]; NRS® [US-OTC]; Nōstrilla® [US-OTC]; Vicks Sinex® 12 Hour Ultrafine Mist [US-OTC]; Vicks Sinex® 12 Hour [US-OTC]; Visine® L.R. [US-OTC]
**Therapeutic Category** Adrenergic Agonist Agent
**Use** Adjunctive therapy of middle ear infections, associated with acute or chronic rhinitis, the common cold, sinusitis, hay fever, or other allergies
Ophthalmic: Relief of redness of eye due to minor eye irritations
**Usual Dosage**
Intranasal (therapy should not exceed 3 days): Children ≥6 years and Adults: 0.05% solution: Instill 2-3 sprays into each nostril twice daily
Ophthalmic: Children >6 years and Adults: 0.025% solution: Instill 1-2 drops in affected eye(s) every 6 hours as needed or as directed by healthcare provider
**Dosage Forms**
Solution, intranasal spray, as hydrochloride: 0.05% (15 mL, 30 mL)

Afrin® Extra Moisturizing: 0.05% (15 mL) [contains benzyl alcohol and glycerin; regular or no drip formula]

Afrin® Original: 0.05% (15 mL, 30 mL) [contains benzalkonium chloride]

Afrin® Original: 0.05% (15 mL) [contains benzyl alcohol and benzalkonium chloride; no drip formula]

Afrin® Severe Congestion: 0.05% (15 mL) [contains benzyl alcohol and menthol; regular or no drip formula]

Afrin® Sinus: 0.05% (15 mL) [contains benzyl alcohol, benzalkonium chloride, camphor, phenol; regular or no drip formula]

Duramist® Plus, Neo-Synephrine® 12 Hour, Nōstrilla®, Vicks Sinex® 12 Hour Ultrafine Mist, Vicks Sinex® 12 Hour, 4-Way® 12 Hour: 0.05% (15 mL) [contains benzalkonium chloride]

Duration®: 0.05% (30 mL) [contains benzalkonium chloride]

Genasal, NRS®: 0.05% (15 mL, 30 mL) [contains benzalkonium chloride]

Neo-Synephrine® 12 Hour Extra Moisturizing: 0.05% (15 mL) [contains glycerin]

Solution, ophthalmic, as hydrochloride (Visine® L.R.): 0.025% (15 mL, 30 mL) [contains benzalkonium chloride]

**oxymetazoline hydrochloride** *see* oxymetazoline *on previous page*

## oxymetholone (oks i METH oh lone)

**Sound-Alike/Look-Alike Issues**

oxymetholone may be confused with oxymetazoline, oxymorphone

**U.S./Canadian Brand Names** Anadrol® [US]

**Therapeutic Category** Anabolic Steroid

**Controlled Substance** C-III

**Use** Treatment of anemias caused by deficient red cell production

**Usual Dosage** Children and Adults: Erythropoietic effects: Oral: 1-5 mg/kg/day in one daily dose; usual effective dose: 1-2 mg/kg/day; give for a minimum trial of 3-6 months because response may be delayed

**Dosage Forms** Tablet: 50 mg

## oxymorphone (oks i MOR fone)

**Sound-Alike/Look-Alike Issues**

oxymorphone may be confused with oxymetholone

**Synonyms** oxymorphone hydrochloride

**U.S./Canadian Brand Names** Numorphan® [US]

**Therapeutic Category** Analgesic, Narcotic

**Controlled Substance** C-II

**Use** Management of moderate to severe pain and preoperatively as a sedative and a supplement to anesthesia

**Usual Dosage** Adults: **Note:** More frequent dosing may be required.

I.M., SubQ: 0.5 mg initially, 1-1.5 mg every 4-6 hours as needed

I.V.: 0.5 mg initially

Rectal: 5 mg every 4-6 hours

**Dosage Forms**

Injection, solution, as hydrochloride: 1 mg (1 mL); 1.5 mg/mL (10 mL)

Suppository, rectal, as hydrochloride: 5 mg

**oxymorphone hydrochloride** *see* oxymorphone *on this page*

**oxyphenbutazone** *(Discontinued)*

## oxytetracycline (oks i tet ra SYE kleen)

**Sound-Alike/Look-Alike Issues**

Terramycin® may be confused with Garamycin®

**Synonyms** oxytetracycline hydrochloride

**U.S./Canadian Brand Names** Terramycin® I.M. [US]; Terramycin® [Can]

**Therapeutic Category** Tetracycline Derivative

**Use** Treatment of susceptible bacterial infections; both gram-positive and gram-negative, as well as, *Rickettsia* and *Mycoplasma* organisms

**Usual Dosage** I.M.:

Children >8 years: 15-25 mg/kg/day (maximum: 250 mg/dose) in divided doses every 8-12 hours

Adults: 250 mg every 24 hours or 300 mg/day divided every 8-12 hours

**Dosage Forms** Injection, solution: 5% [50 mg/mL] (10 mL) [contains lidocaine hydrochloride 2%]

## oxytetracycline and polymyxin B (oks i tet ra SYE kleen & pol i MIKS in bee)

**Sound-Alike/Look-Alike Issues**
Terramycin® may be confused with Garamycin®

**Synonyms** polymyxin B and oxytetracycline

**U.S./Canadian Brand Names** Terak™ [US]

**Therapeutic Category** Antibiotic, Ophthalmic

**Use** Treatment of superficial ocular infections involving the conjunctiva and/or cornea

**Usual Dosage** Topical: Apply ½" of ointment onto the lower lid of affected eye 2-4 times/day

**Dosage Forms** Ointment, ophthalmic: Oxytetracycline 5 mg and polymyxin B sulfate 10,000 units per g (3.5 g)

**oxytetracycline hydrochloride** *see* oxytetracycline *on previous page*

## oxytocin (oks i TOE sin)

**Sound-Alike/Look-Alike Issues**
Pitocin® may be confused with Pitressin®

**Synonyms** pit

**U.S./Canadian Brand Names** Pitocin® [US/Can]; Syntocinon® [Can]

**Therapeutic Category** Oxytocic Agent

**Use** Induction of labor at term; control of postpartum bleeding; adjunctive therapy in management of abortion

**Usual Dosage** I.V. administration requires the use of an infusion pump. Adults:
Induction of labor: I.V.: 0.5-1 milliunits/minute; gradually increase dose in increments of 1-2 milliunits/minute until desired contraction pattern is established; dose may be decreased after desired frequency of contractions is reached and labor has progressed to 5-6 cm dilation. Infusion rates of 6 milliunits/minute provide oxytocin levels similar to those at spontaneous labor; rates of >9-10 milliunits/minute are rarely required.
Postpartum bleeding:
I.M.: Total dose of 10 units after delivery
I.V.: 10-40 units by I.V. infusion in 1000 mL of intravenous fluid at a rate sufficient to control uterine atony
Adjunctive treatment of abortion: I.V.: 10-20 milliunits/minute; maximum total dose: 30 units/12 hours

**Dosage Forms**
Injection, solution: 10 units/mL (1 mL, 10 mL)
Pitocin®: 10 units/mL (1 mL)

**Oxytrol™ [US/Can]** *see* oxybutynin *on page 607*

**Oysco 500 [US-OTC]** *see* calcium carbonate *on page 130*

**Oyst-Cal 500 [US-OTC]** *see* calcium carbonate *on page 130*

**P2E1** *(Discontinued)*

**P-V-Tussin® Syrup [US]** *see* pseudoephedrine, hydrocodone, and chlorpheniramine *on page 695*

**P-V Tussin Tablet [US]** *see* hydrocodone and pseudoephedrine *on page 413*

**P-071** *see* cetirizine *on page 162*

**Pacerone® [US]** *see* amiodarone *on page 41*

**Pacis™ [Can]** *see* BCG vaccine *on page 90*

## paclitaxel (PAK li taks el)

**Sound-Alike/Look-Alike Issues**
paclitaxel may be confused with paroxetine, Paxil®
paclitaxel (conventional) may be confused with paclitaxel (protein-bound)
Taxol® may be confused with Abraxane™, Paxil®, Taxotere®

**Synonyms** NSC-125973

**U.S./Canadian Brand Names** Onxol™ [US]; Taxol® [US/Can]

**Therapeutic Category** Antineoplastic Agent

**Use** Treatment of breast, lung (small cell and nonsmall cell), and ovarian cancers

**Usual Dosage** Premedication with dexamethasone (20 mg orally or I.V. at 12 and 6 hours **or** 14 and 7 hours before the dose), diphenhydramine (50 mg I.V. 30-60 minutes prior to the dose), and cimetidine, famotidine or ranitidine (I.V. 30-60 minutes prior to the dose) is recommended

Adults: I.V.: Refer to individual protocols

Ovarian carcinoma: 135-175 mg/m$^2$ over 3 hours every 3 weeks **or**

50-80 mg/m$^2$ over 1-3 hours weekly **or**

1.4-4 mg/m$^2$/day continuous infusion for 14 days every 4 weeks

Metastatic breast cancer: 175-250 mg/m$^2$ over 3 hours every 3 weeks **or**

50-80 mg/m$^2$ weekly **or**

1.4-4 mg/m$^2$/day continuous infusion for 14 days every 4 weeks

Nonsmall cell lung carcinoma: 135 mg/m$^2$ over 24 hours every 3 weeks

AIDS-related Kaposi's sarcoma: 135 mg/m$^2$ over 3 hours every 3 weeks **or**

100 mg/m$^2$ over 3 hours every 2 weeks

**Dosage modification for toxicity (solid tumors, including ovary, breast, and lung carcinoma):** Courses of paclitaxel should not be repeated until the neutrophil count is ≥1500 cells/mm$^3$ and the platelet count is ≥100,000 cells/mm$^3$; reduce dosage by 20% for patients experiencing severe peripheral neuropathy or severe neutropenia (neutrophil <500 cells/mm$^3$ for a week or longer)

**Dosage modification for immunosuppression in advanced HIV disease:** Paclitaxel should not be given to patients with HIV if the baseline or subsequent neutrophil count is <1000 cells/mm$^3$. Additional modifications include: Reduce dosage of dexamethasone in premedication to 10 mg orally; reduce dosage by 20% in patients experiencing severe peripheral neuropathy or severe neutropenia (neutrophil <500 cells/mm$^3$ for a week or longer); initiate concurrent hematopoietic growth factor (G-CSF) as clinically indicated

**Dosage Forms**

Injection, solution: 6 mg/mL (5 mL, 16.7 mL, 50 mL) [contains alcohol and purified Cremophor® EL (polyoxyethylated castor oil)]

Onxol™: 6 mg/mL (5 mL, 25 mL, 50 mL) [contains alcohol] [contains alcohol and purified Cremophor® EL (polyoxyethylated castor oil)]

Taxol®: 6 mg/mL (5 mL, 16.7 mL, 50 mL) [contains alcohol and purified Cremophor® EL (polyoxyethylated castor oil)]

## paclitaxel (protein bound) (PAK li taks el PROE teen bownd)

**Sound-Alike/Look-Alike Issues**

paclitaxel (protein bound) may be confused with paclitaxel (conventional)

Abraxane™ may be confused with Paxil®, Taxol®, Taxotere®

**Synonyms** BI-007; NAB-paclitaxel; protein-bound paclitaxel

**U.S./Canadian Brand Names** Abraxane™ [US]

**Therapeutic Category** Antineoplastic Agent, Antimicrotubular; Antineoplastic Agent, Natural Source (Plant) Derivative

**Use** Treatment of breast cancer (second-line)

**Usual Dosage** I.V.: Adults: Breast cancer: 260 mg/m$^2$ every 3 weeks

**Dosage Forms** Injection, powder for reconstitution: 100 mg [contains human albumin 900 mg]

**Pain-A-Lay® [US-OTC]** see phenol on page 638

**Pain-Off [US-OTC]** see acetaminophen, aspirin, and caffeine on page 9

**Palafer® [Can]** see ferrous fumarate on page 334

**Palgic [US]** see carbinoxamine on page 144

**Palgic®-D [US]** see carbinoxamine and pseudoephedrine on page 144

**Palgic®-DS [US]** see carbinoxamine and pseudoephedrine on page 144

## palifermin (pal ee FER min)

**Synonyms** AMJ 9701; rHu-KGF

**U.S./Canadian Brand Names** Kepivance™ [US]

**Therapeutic Category** Keratinocyte Growth Factor

**Use** Decrease the incidence and severity of severe oral mucositis associated with hematologic malignancies in patients receiving myelotoxic therapy requiring hematopoietic stem cell support

**Usual Dosage** I.V.: Adults: 60 mcg/kg/day for 3 consecutive days before and after myelotoxic therapy; total of 6 doses

**Note:** Administer first 3 doses prior to myelotoxic therapy, with the 3rd dose given 24-48 hours before therapy begins. The last 3 doses should be administered after myelotoxic therapy, with the first of these doses after but on the same day of hematopoietic stem cell infusion and at least 4 days after the most recent dose of palifermin.

(Continued)

## palifermin *(Continued)*

**Dosage Forms** Injection, powder for reconstitution [preservative free]: 6.25 mg [contains mannitol 50 mg, sucrose 25 mg]

## palivizumab *(pah li VIZ u mab)*
**Sound-Alike/Look-Alike Issues**
Synagis® may be confused with Synalgos®-DC, Synvisc®
**U.S./Canadian Brand Names** Synagis® [US/Can]
**Therapeutic Category** Monoclonal Antibody
**Use** Prevention of serious lower respiratory tract disease caused by respiratory syncytial virus (RSV) in infants and children <2 years of age at high risk of RSV disease
**Usual Dosage** I.M.: Infants and Children: 15 mg/kg of body weight, monthly throughout RSV season (First dose administered prior to commencement of RSV season)
**Dosage Forms**
Injection, powder for reconstitution: 50 mg, 100 mg
Injection, solution [preservative free]: 50 mg/0.5 mL (0.5 mL); 100 mg/mL (1 mL)

**Palladone™ [US]** *see* hydromorphone *on page 418*

**Palmer's® Skin Success Acne [US-OTC]** *see* benzoyl peroxide *on page 98*

**Palmer's® Skin Success Acne Cleanser [US-OTC]** *see* salicylic acid *on page 734*

**Palmer's® Skin Success Eventone® Fade Cream [US-OTC]** *see* hydroquinone *on page 420*

**Palmitate-A® [US-OTC]** *see* vitamin A *on page 848*

## palonosetron *(pal oh NOE se tron)*
**Sound-Alike/Look-Alike Issues**
palonosetron may be confused with dolasetron, granisetron, ondansetron
Aloxi™ may be confused with oxaliplatin
**Synonyms** palonosetron hydrochloride; RS-25259-197; RS-25259
**U.S./Canadian Brand Names** Aloxi™ [US]
**Therapeutic Category** Antiemetic; Selective 5-HT$_3$ Receptor Antagonist
**Use** Prevention of acute (within 24 hours) and delayed (2-5 days) chemotherapy-induced nausea and vomiting
**Usual Dosage** I.V.: Adults: Chemotherapy-induced nausea and vomiting: 0.25 mg 30 minutes prior to chemotherapy administration, day 1 of each cycle (doses should not be given more than once weekly)
**Dosage Forms** Injection, solution: 0.05 mg/mL (5 mL)

**palonosetron hydrochloride** *see* palonosetron *on this page*

**2-PAM** *see* pralidoxime *on page 669*

**Pamelor® [US]** *see* nortriptyline *on page 583*

## pamidronate *(pa mi DROE nate)*
**Sound-Alike/Look-Alike Issues**
Aredia® may be confused with Adriamycin
**Synonyms** pamidronate disodium
**U.S./Canadian Brand Names** Aredia® [US/Can]
**Therapeutic Category** Bisphosphonate Derivative
**Use** Treatment of hypercalcemia associated with malignancy; treatment of osteolytic bone lesions associated with multiple myeloma or metastatic breast cancer; moderate to severe Paget disease of bone
**Usual Dosage** Drug must be diluted properly before administration and infused intravenously slowly. Due to risk of nephrotoxicity, doses should not exceed 90 mg. I.V.: Adults:
Hypercalcemia of malignancy:
Moderate cancer-related hypercalcemia (corrected serum calcium: 12-13.5 mg/dL): 60-90 mg, as a single dose
Severe cancer-related hypercalcemia (corrected serum calcium: >13.5 mg/dL): 90 mg, as a single dose
A period of 7 days should elapse before the use of second course; repeat infusions every 2-3 weeks have been suggested, however, could be administered every 2-3 months according to the degree and of severity of hypercalcemia and/or the type of malignancy.
Osteolytic bone lesions with multiple myeloma: 90 mg monthly

Osteolytic bone lesions with metastatic breast cancer: 90 mg repeated every 3-4 weeks

Paget disease: 30 mg for 3 consecutive days

**Dosage Forms**

Injection, powder for reconstitution, as disodium (Aredia®): 30 mg, 90 mg

Injection, solution: 3 mg/mL (10 mL); 6 mg/mL (10 mL); 9 mg/mL (10 mL)

**pamidronate disodium** *see* pamidronate *on previous page*

**Pamine® [US/Can]** *see* methscopolamine *on page 527*

**Pamine® Forte [US]** *see* methscopolamine *on page 527*

**p-aminoclonidine** *see* apraclonidine *on page 67*

**Pamix™ [US-OTC]** *see* pyrantel pamoate *on page 698*

**Pamprin IB® *(Discontinued)*** *see* ibuprofen *on page 427*

**Pamprin® Maximum Strength All Day Relief [US-OTC]** *see* naproxen *on page 562*

**Panadol® *(Discontinued)*** *see* acetaminophen *on page 4*

**Panasal® 5/500 *(Discontinued)*** *see* hydrocodone and aspirin *on page 412*

**pan-B antibody** *see* rituximab *on page 726*

**Pancrease® [US/Can]** *see* pancrelipase *on this page*

**Pancrease® MT [US/Can]** *see* pancrelipase *on this page*

**Pancrecarb MS® [US]** *see* pancrelipase *on this page*

## pancrelipase (pan kre LI pase)

**Synonyms** lipancreatin

**U.S./Canadian Brand Names** Cotazym® [Can]; Creon® 10 [Can]; Creon® 20 [Can]; Creon® 25 [Can]; Creon® 5 [Can]; Creon® [US]; Dygase [US]; Hi-Vegi-Lip [US]; ku-zyme® HP [US]; ku-zyme® [US]; kutrase® [US]; Lapase [US]; Lipram 4500 [US]; Lipram-CR [US]; Lipram-PN [US]; Lipram-UL [US]; Pancrease® MT [US/Can]; Pancrease® [US/Can]; Pancrecarb MS® [US]; Pangestyme™ CN [US]; Pangestyme™ EC [US]; Pangestyme™ MT [US]; Pangestyme™ UL [US]; Panokase® 16 [US]; Panokase® [US]; Plaretase® 8000 [US]; Ultrase® MT [US/Can]; Ultrase® [US/Can]; Viokase® [US/Can]

**Therapeutic Category** Enzyme

**Use** Replacement therapy in symptomatic treatment of malabsorption syndrome caused by pancreatic insufficiency

**Usual Dosage** Oral:

Powder: Actual dose depends on the condition being treated and the digestive requirements of the patient

Children <1 year: Start with ¹/₈ teaspoonful with feedings

Adults: 0.7 g (¹/₄ teaspoonful) with meals

Capsules/tablets: The following dosage recommendations are only an approximation for initial dosages. The actual dosage will depend on the condition being treated and the digestive requirements of the individual patient. Adjust dose based on body weight and stool fat content. Total daily dose reflects ~3 meals/day and 2-3 snacks/day, with half the mealtime dose given with a snack. Older patients may need less units/kg due to increased weight, but decreased ingestion of fat/kg. Maximum dose: 2500 units of lipase/kg/meal (10,000 units of lipase/kg/day)

Children:

<1 year: 2000 units of lipase with meals

1-6 years: 4000-8000 units of lipase with meals and 4000 units with snacks

7-12 years: 4000-12,000 units of lipase with meals and snacks

Adults: 4000-48,000 units of lipase with meals and with snacks

Occluded feeding tubes: One tablet of Viokase® crushed with one 325 mg tablet of sodium bicarbonate (to activate the Viokase®) in 5 mL of water can be instilled into the nasogastric tube and clamped for 5 minutes; then, flushed with 50 mL of tap water

**Dosage Forms**

Capsule:

Dygase: Lipase 2400 units, protease 30,000 units, and amylase 30,000 units

kutrase®: Lipase 2400 units, protease 30,000 units, and amylase 30,000 units

ku-zyme®: Lipase 1200 units, protease 15,000 units, and amylase 15,000 units

ku-zyme® HP: Lipase 8000 units, protease 30,000 units, and amylase 30,000 units

Lapase: Lipase 1200 units, protease 15,000 units, and amylase 15,000 units [contains tartrazine]

(Continued)

## pancrelipase *(Continued)*

Capsule, delayed release, enteric coated granules:

Pangestyme™ CN-10: Lipase 10,000 units, protease 37,500 units, amylase 33,200 units
Pangestyme™ CN-20: Lipase 20,000 units, protease 75,000 units, amylase 66,400 units
Pangestyme™ EC:  Lipase 4500 units, protease 25,000 units, and amylase 20,000 units
Pangestyme™ MT16: Lipase 16,000 units, protease 48,000 units, and amylase 48,000 units
Pangestyme™ UL 12: Lipase 12,000 units, protease 39,000 units, and amylase 39,000 units
Pangestyme™ UL 18: Lipase 18,000 units, protease 58,500 units, and amylase 58,500 units
Pangestyme™ UL 20: Lipase 20,000 units, protease 65,000 units, and amylase 65,000 units

Capsule, delayed release, enteric coated microspheres: Lipase 4,500 units, protease 25,000 units, and amylase 25,000 units

Creon® 5: Lipase 5000 units, protease 18,750 units, and amylase 16,600 units
Creon® 10: Lipase 10,000 units, protease 37,500 units, and amylase 33,200 units
Creon® 20: Lipase 20,000 units, protease 75,000 units, and amylase 66,400 units
Lipram 4500: Lipase 4500 units, protease 25,000 units, and amylase 20,000 units
Lipram-CR5: Lipase 5000 units, protease 18,750 units, and amylase 16,600 units
Lipram-CR10: Lipase 10,000 units, protease 37,500 units, and amylase 33,200 units
Lipram-CR20: Lipase 20,000 units, protease 75,000 units, and amylase 66,400 units
Lipram-PN10: Lipase 10,000 units, protease 30,000 units, and amylase 30,000 units
Lipram-PN16: Lipase 16,000 units, protease 48,000 units, and amylase 48,000 units
Lipram-PN20: Lipase 20,000 units, protease 44,000 units, and amylase 56,000 units
Lipram-UL12: Lipase 12,000 units, protease 39,000 units, and amylase 39,000 units
Lipram-UL18: Lipase 18,000 units, protease 58,500 units, and amylase 58,500 units
Lipram-UL20: Lipase 20,000 units, protease 65,000 units, and amylase 65,000 units
Pancrecarb MS-4®: Lipase 4000 units, protease 25,000 units, and amylase 25,000 units [buffered]
Pancrecarb MS-8®: Lipase 8000 units, protease 45,000 units, and amylase 40,000 units [buffered]

Capsule, enteric coated microspheres (Pancrease®, Ultrase®): Lipase 4500 units, protease 25,000 units, and amylase 20,000 units

Capsule, enteric coated microtablets:

Pancrease® MT 4: Lipase 4000 units, protease 12,000 units, and amylase 12,000 units
Pancrease® MT 10: Lipase 10,000 units, protease 30,000 units, and amylase 30,000 units
Pancrease® MT 16: Lipase 16,000 units, protease 48,000 units, and  amylase 48,000 units
Pancrease® MT 20: Lipase 20,000 units, protease 44,000 units, and amylase 56,000 units

Capsule, enteric coated minitablets:

Ultrase® MT12: Lipase 12,000 units, protease 39,000 units, and amylase 39,000 units
Ultrase® MT18: Lipase 18,000 units, protease 58,500 units, and amylase 58,500 units
Ultrase® MT20: Lipase 20,000 units, protease 65,000 units, and amylase 65,000 units

Powder (Viokase®): Lipase 16,800 units, protease 70,000 units, and amylase 70,000 units per 0.7 g (227 g)

Tablet: Lipase 8000 units, protease 30,000 units, and amylase 30,000 units
Hi-Vegi-Lip: Lipase 4800 units, protease 60,000 units, and amylase 60,000 units
Panokase®: Lipase 8,000 units, protease 30,000 units, and amylase 30,000 units
Panokase® 16: Lipase 16,000 units, protease 60,000 units, and amylase 60,000 units
Plaretase™ 8000: Lipase 8,000 units, protease 30,000 units, and amylase 30,000 units
Viokase® 8: Lipase 8000 units, protease 30,000 units, and amylase 30,000 units
Viokase® 16: Lipase 16,000 units, protease 60,000 units, and amylase 60,000 units

## pancuronium (pan kyoo ROE nee um)

**Sound-Alike/Look-Alike Issues**
pancuronium may be confused with pipecuronium

**Synonyms** pancuronium bromide

**Therapeutic Category** Skeletal Muscle Relaxant

**Use** Adjunct to general anesthesia to facilitate endotracheal intubation and to relax skeletal muscles during surgery; to facilitate mechanical ventilation in ICU patients; does not relieve pain or produce sedation

**Drug of choice** for neuromuscular blockade except in patients with renal failure, hepatic failure, or cardiovascular instability or in situations not suited for pancuronium's long duration of action

**Usual Dosage** Administer I.V.; dose to effect; doses will vary due to interpatient variability; use ideal body weight for obese patients

Surgery:

Neonates <1 month:

Test dose: 0.02 mg/kg to measure responsiveness

Initial: 0.03 mg/kg/dose repeated twice at 5- to 10-minute intervals as needed; maintenance: 0.03-0.09 mg/kg/dose every 30 minutes to 4 hours as needed

Infants >1 month, Children, and Adults: Initial: 0.06-0.1 mg/kg or 0.05 mg/kg after initial dose of succinylcholine for intubation; maintenance dose: 0.01 mg/kg 60-100 minutes after initial dose and then 0.01 mg/kg every 25-60 minutes

Pretreatment/priming: 10% of intubating dose given 3-5 minutes before initial dose

ICU: 0.05-0.1 mg/kg bolus followed by 0.8-1.7 mcg/kg/minute once initial recovery from bolus observed or 0.1-0.2 mg/kg every 1-3 hours

**Dosage Forms** Injection, solution, as bromide: 1 mg/mL (10 mL); 2 mg/mL (2 mL, 5 mL) [may contain benzyl alcohol]

**pancuronium bromide** *see* pancuronium *on previous page*

**Pandel® [US]** *see* hydrocortisone (topical) *on page 417*

**Panectyl® [Can]** *see* trimeprazine *(Canada only) on page 825*

**Pangestyme™ CN [US]** *sec* pancrelipase *on page 615*

**Pangestyme™ EC [US]** *see* pancrelipase *on page 615*

**Pangestyme™ MT [US]** *see* pancrelipase *on page 615*

**Pangestyme™ UL [US]** *see* pancrelipase *on page 615*

**Panglobulin® NF [US]** *see* immune globulin (intravenous) *on page 433*

**Panhematin® [US]** *see* hemin *on page 398*

**Panixine DisperDose™ [US]** *see* cephalexin *on page 161*

**PanMist®-DM [US]** *see* guaifenesin, pseudoephedrine, and dextromethorphan *on page 391*

**PanMist®-JR [US]** *see* guaifenesin and pseudoephedrine *on page 388*

**PanMist®-LA [US]** *see* guaifenesin and pseudoephedrine *on page 388*

**PanMist®-S [US]** *see* guaifenesin and pseudoephedrine *on page 388*

**Panokase® [US]** *see* pancrelipase *on page 615*

**Panokase® 16 [US]** *see* pancrelipase *on page 615*

**PanOxyl® [US/Can]** *see* benzoyl peroxide *on page 98*

**PanOxyl®-AQ [US]** *see* benzoyl peroxide *on page 98*

**PanOxyl® Aqua Gel [US]** *see* benzoyl peroxide *on page 98*

**PanOxyl® Bar [US-OTC]** *see* benzoyl peroxide *on page 98*

**Panretin® [US/Can]** *see* alitretinoin *on page 27*

**Panscol® Lotion *(Discontinued)*** *see* salicylic acid *on page 734*

**Panscol® Ointment *(Discontinued)*** *see* salicylic acid *on page 734*

**Panthoderm® [US-OTC]** *see* dexpanthenol *on page 235*

**Panto™ IV [Can]** *see* pantoprazole *on this page*

**Pantoloc™ [Can]** *see* pantoprazole *on this page*

**Pantopon® *(Discontinued)***

# pantoprazole (pan TOE pra zole)

**Sound-Alike/Look-Alike Issues**

Protonix® may be confused with Lotronex®, Lovenox®, protamine

**U.S./Canadian Brand Names** Pantoloc™ [Can]; Panto™ IV [Can]; Protonix® [US/Can]

**Therapeutic Category** Proton Pump Inhibitor

**Use**

Oral: Treatment and maintenance of healing of erosive esophagitis associated with GERD; reduction in relapse rates of daytime and nighttime heartburn symptoms in GERD; hypersecretory disorders associated with Zollinger-Ellison syndrome or other neoplastic disorders

(Continued)

## pantoprazole *(Continued)*

I.V.: Short-term treatment (7-10 days) of patients with gastroesophageal reflux disease (GERD) and a history of erosive esophagitis; hypersecretory disorders associated with Zollinger-Ellison syndrome or other neoplastic disorders

**Usual Dosage** Adults:

Oral:

Erosive esophagitis associated with GERD:

Treatment: 40 mg once daily for up to 8 weeks; an additional 8 weeks may be used in patients who have not healed after an 8-week course

Maintenance of healing: 40 mg once daily

**Note:** Lower doses (20 mg once daily) have been used successfully in mild GERD treatment and maintenance of healing

Hypersecretory disorders (including Zollinger-Ellison): Initial: 40 mg twice daily; adjust dose based on patient needs; doses up to 240 mg/day have been administered

I.V.:

Erosive esophagitis associated with GERD: 40 mg once daily for 7-10 days

Hypersecretory disorders: 80 mg twice daily; adjust dose based on acid output measurements; 160-240 mg/day in divided doses has been used for a limited period (up to 7 days)

**Dosage Forms** [DSC] = Discontinued product; **Note:** Strength expressed as base

Injection, powder for reconstitution, as sodium: 40 mg [original formulation] [DSC]

Injection, powder for reconstitution, as sodium: 40 mg [contains edetate sodium 1 mg]

Tablet, delayed release, as sodium: 20 mg, 40 mg

## pantothenic acid *(pan toe THEN ik AS id)*

**Synonyms** calcium pantothenate; vitamin $B_5$

**Therapeutic Category** Vitamin, Water Soluble

**Use** Pantothenic acid deficiency

**Usual Dosage** Adults: Oral: Recommended daily dose 4-7 mg/day

**Dosage Forms** Tablet: 100 mg, 200 mg, 250 mg, 500 mg

**pantothenyl alcohol** *see* dexpanthenol *on page 235*

## papain and urea *(pa PAY in & yoor EE a)*

**U.S./Canadian Brand Names** Accuzyme™ [US]

**Therapeutic Category** Enzyme, Topical Debridement; Topical Skin Product

**Use** Enzymatic debriding ointment for treatment of chronic and acute wounds

**Usual Dosage** Cleanse wound with cleanser or saline (not hydrogen peroxide); apply directly to the wound, cover with appropriate dressing, secure into place and reapply 1-2 times/day. Irrigate wound at each dressing.

**Dosage Forms** Ointment, topical: Papain $1.1 \times 10^4$ int. units and urea 10% in hydrophilic ointment (30 g)

## papaverine *(pa PAV er een)*

**Synonyms** papaverine hydrochloride

**U.S./Canadian Brand Names** Para-Time S.R.® [US]

**Therapeutic Category** Vasodilator

**Use** Oral: Relief of peripheral and cerebral ischemia associated with arterial spasm and myocardial ischemia complicated by arrhythmias

**Usual Dosage**

I.M., I.V.:

Children: 6 mg/kg/day in 4 divided doses

Adults: 30-65 mg (rarely up to 120 mg); may repeat every 3 hours

Oral, sustained release: Adults: 150-300 mg every 12 hours; in difficult cases: 150 mg every 8 hours

**Dosage Forms**

Capsule, sustained release, as hydrochloride (Para-Time SR®): 150 mg

Injection, solution, as hydrochloride: 30 mg/mL (2 mL, 10 mL)

**papaverine hydrochloride** *see* papaverine *on this page*

**para-aminosalicylate sodium** *see* aminosalicylic acid *on page 41*

**parabromdylamine** *see* brompheniramine *on page 115*

**paracetamol** *see* acetaminophen *on page 4*

**Paraflex**® *(Discontinued)* *see* chlorzoxazone *on page 179*

**Parafon Forte**® **[Can]** *see* chlorzoxazone *on page 179*

**Parafon Forte**® *(Discontinued)* *see* chlorzoxazone *on page 179*

**Paraplatin**® **[US]** *see* carboplatin *on page 147*

**Paraplatin-AQ [Can]** *see* carboplatin *on page 147*

**parathyroid hormone (1-34)** *see* teriparatide *on page 787*

**Para-Time S.R.**® **[US]** *see* papaverine *on previous page*

**Parcopa**™ **[US]** *see* levodopa and carbidopa *on page 474*

**Paredrine**® *(Discontinued)*

## paregoric (par e GOR ik)

**Sound-Alike/Look-Alike Issues**
   camphorated tincture of opium is an error-prone synonym (mistaken as opium tincture)
   paregoric may be confused with Percogesic®
**Therapeutic Category** Analgesic, Narcotic
**Controlled Substance** C-III
**Use** Treatment of diarrhea or relief of pain; neonatal opiate withdrawal
**Usual Dosage** Oral:
   Neonatal opiate withdrawal: 3-6 drops every 3-6 hours as needed, or initially 0.2 mL every 3 hours;
   increase dosage by approximately 0.05 mL every 3 hours until withdrawal symptoms are controlled; it is
   rare to exceed 0.7 mL/dose. Stabilize withdrawal symptoms for 3-5 days, then gradually decrease
   dosage over a 2- to 4-week period.
   Children: 0.25-0.5 mL/kg 1-4 times/day
   Adults: 5-10 mL 1-4 times/day
**Dosage Forms** Liquid, oral: Morphine equivalent 2 mg/5 mL (473 mL) [equivalent to opium 20 mg
   powder; contains alcohol 45% and benzoic acid]

**Parepectolin**® *(Discontinued)*

## paricalcitol (pah ri KAL si tole)

**U.S./Canadian Brand Names** Zemplar® [US/Can]
**Therapeutic Category** Vitamin D Analog
**Use**
   I.V.: Prevention and treatment of secondary hyperparathyroidism associated with stage 5 chronic kidney
   disease (CKD)
   Oral: Prevention and treatment of secondary hyperparathyroidism associated with stage 3 and 4 CKD
**Usual Dosage Note:** In case hypercalcemia or elevated Ca x P is observed, reduce or interrupt dosing
   until parameters are normalized.
   **Secondary hyperparathyroidism associated with chronic renal failure (stage 5 CKD):** Children >5
   years and Adults: I.V.: 0.04-0.1 mcg/kg (2.8-7 mcg) given as a bolus dose no more frequently than
   every other day at any time during dialysis; doses as high as 0.24 mcg/kg (16.8 mcg) have been
   administered safely; dose may be increased by 2-4 mcg every 2-4 weeks; the dose of paricalcitol
   should be adjusted based on serum PTH levels, as follows:
   Same or increasing serum PTH level: Increase paricalcitol dose
   Serum PTH level decreased by <30%: Increase paricalcitol dose
   Serum PTH level decreased by >30% and <60%: Maintain paricalcitol dose
   Serum PTH level decrease by >60%: Decrease paricalcitol dose
   Serum PTH level 1.5-3 times upper limit of normal: Maintain paricalcitol dose

   **Secondary hyperparathyroidism associated with stage 3 and 4 CKD:** Adults: Oral: Initial dose
   based on baseline iPTH:
   iPTH ≤500 pg/mL: 1 mcg/day or 2 mcg 3 times/week
   iPTH >500 pg/mL: 2 mcg/day or 4 mcg 3 times/week

   *Dosage adjustment based on iPTH level relative to baseline*, adjust dose at 2-4 week intervals:
   iPTH same or increased: Increase paricalcitol dose by 1 mcg/day or 2 mcg 3 times/week
   iPTH decreased by <30%: Increase paricalcitol dose by 1 mcg/day or 2 mcg 3 times//week
   iPTH decreased by ≥30% or ≤60%: Maintain paricalcitol dose
   iPTH decreased by >60%: Decrease paricalcitol dose by 1 mcg/day* or 2 mcg 3 times/week
   iPTH <60 pg/mL: Decrease paricalcitol dose by 1 mcg/day* or 2 mcg 3 times/week
(Continued)

## paricalcitol (Continued)

*If patient is taking the lowest dose on a once-daily regimen, but further dose reduction is needed, decrease dose to 1 mcg 3 times/week. If further dose reduction is required, withhold drug as needed and restart at a lower dose. If applicable, calcium-phosphate binder dosing may also be adjusted or withheld, or switch to noncalcium-based binder

### Dosage Forms

Capsule, gelatin: 1 mcg, 2 mcg, 4 mcg [contains alcohol and coconut or palm kernel oil]

Injection, solution: 2 mcg/mL (1 mL); 5 mcg/mL (1 mL, 2 mL) [contains alcohol 20% v/v and propylene glycol 30% v/v]

**Pariet®** **[Can]** see rabeprazole on page 706

**pariprazole** see rabeprazole on page 706

**Parlodel®** **[US/Can]** see bromocriptine on page 114

**Parnate®** **[US/Can]** see tranylcypromine on page 816

## paromomycin (par oh moe MYE sin)

**Synonyms** paromomycin sulfate

**U.S./Canadian Brand Names** Humatin® [US/Can]

**Therapeutic Category** Amebicide

**Use** Treatment of acute and chronic intestinal amebiasis; hepatic coma

**Usual Dosage** Oral:

Intestinal amebiasis: Children and Adults: 25-35 mg/kg/day in 3 divided doses for 5-10 days

Dientamoeba fragilis: Children and Adults: 25-30 mg/kg/day in 3 divided doses for 7 days

Tapeworm (fish, dog, bovine, porcine):

Children: 11 mg/kg every 15 minutes for 4 doses

Adults: 1 g every 15 minutes for 4 doses

Hepatic coma: Adults: 4 g/day in 2-4 divided doses for 5-6 days

Dwarf tapeworm: Children and Adults: 45 mg/kg/dose every day for 5-7 days

**Dosage Forms** Capsule: 250 mg

**paromomycin sulfate** see paromomycin on this page

## paroxetine (pa ROKS e teen)

**Sound-Alike/Look-Alike Issues**

paroxetine may be confused with paclitaxel, pyridoxine

Paxil® may be confused with Doxil®, paclitaxel, Plavix®, Taxol®

**Synonyms** paroxetine hydrochloride; paroxetine mesylate

**U.S./Canadian Brand Names** Apo-Paroxetine® [Can]; CO Paroxetine [Can]; Gen-Paroxetine [Can]; Novo-Paroxetine [Can]; Paxil CR® [US/Can]; Paxil® [US/Can]; Pexeva® [US]; PMS-Paroxetine [Can]; ratio-Paroxetine [Can]; Rhoxal-paroxetine [Can]

**Therapeutic Category** Antidepressant, Selective Serotonin Reuptake Inhibitor

**Use** Treatment of depression in adults; treatment of panic disorder with or without agoraphobia; obsessive-compulsive disorder (OCD) in adults; social anxiety disorder (social phobia); generalized anxiety disorder (GAD); post-traumatic stress disorder (PTSD)

Paxil CR®: Treatment of depression; panic disorder; premenstrual dysphoric disorder (PMDD); social anxiety disorder (social phobia)

**Usual Dosage** Oral: Adults:

Depression:

Paxil®, Pexeva™: Initial: 20 mg once daily, preferably in the morning; increase if needed by 10 mg/day increments at intervals of at least 1 week; maximum dose: 50 mg/day

Paxil CR™: Initial: 25 mg once daily; increase if needed by 12.5 mg/day increments at intervals of at least 1 week; maximum dose: 62.5 mg/day

GAD (Paxil®): Initial: 20 mg once daily, preferably in the morning; doses of 20-50 mg/day were used in clinical trials, however, no greater benefit was seen with doses >20 mg. If dose is increased, adjust in increments of 10 mg/day at 1-week intervals.

OCD (Paxil®, Pexeva™): Initial: 20 mg once daily, preferably in the morning; increase if needed by 10 mg/day increments at intervals of at least 1 week; recommended dose: 40 mg/day; range: 20-60 mg/day; maximum dose: 60 mg/day

Panic disorder:

Paxil®, Pexeva™: Initial: 10 mg once daily, preferably in the morning; increase if needed by 10 mg/day increments at intervals of at least 1 week; recommended dose: 40 mg/day; range: 10-60 mg/day; maximum dose: 60 mg/day

Paxil CR™: Initial: 12.5 mg once daily; increase if needed by 12.5 mg/day at intervals of at least 1 week; maximum dose: 75 mg/day

PMDD (Paxil CR™): Initial: 12.5 mg once daily in the morning; may be increased to 25 mg/day; dosing changes should occur at intervals of at least 1 week. May be given daily throughout the menstrual cycle or limited to the luteal phase.

PTSD (Paxil®): Initial: 20 mg once daily, preferably in the morning; increase if needed by 10 mg/day increments at intervals of at least 1 week; range: 20-50 mg

Social anxiety disorder:

Paxil®: Initial: 20 mg once daily, preferably in the morning; recommended dose: 20 mg/day; range: 20-60 mg/day; doses >20 mg may not have additional benefit

Paxil CR™: Initial: 12.5 mg once daily, preferably in the morning; may be increased by 12.5 mg/day at intervals of at least 1 week; maximum dose: 37.5 mg/day

**Note:** Upon discontinuation of paroxetine therapy, gradually taper dose:

Paxil®: 10 mg/day at weekly intervals; when 20 mg/day dose is reached, continue for 1 week before treatment is discontinued. Some patients may need to be titrated to 10 mg/day for 1 week before discontinuation.

Paxil CR™: Patients receiving 37.5 mg/day in clinical trials had their dose decreased by 12.5 mg/day to a dose of 25 mg/day and remained at a dose of 25 mg/day for 1 week before treatment was discontinued.

**Dosage Forms Note**: Available as paroxetine hydrochloride or mesylate; mg strength refers to paroxetine

Suspension, oral, as hydrochloride (Paxil®): 10 mg/5 mL (250 mL) [orange flavor]

Tablet, as hydrochloride (Paxil®): 10 mg, 20 mg, 30 mg, 40 mg

Tablet, as mesylate (Pexeva®): 10 mg, 20 mg, 30 mg, 40 mg

Tablet, controlled release, as hydrochloride (Paxil CR®): 12.5 mg, 25 mg, 37.5 mg

**paroxetine hydrochloride** *see* paroxetine *on previous page*

**paroxetine mesylate** *see* paroxetine *on previous page*

**Partuss® LA** *(Discontinued)*

**Parvolex® [Can]** *see* acetylcysteine *on page 15*

**PAS** *see* aminosalicylic acid *on page 41*

**Paser® [US]** *see* aminosalicylic acid *on page 41*

**Patanol® [US/Can]** *see* olopatadine *on page 597*

**Pathilon®** *(Discontinued)*

**Pathocil® [Can]** *see* dicloxacillin *on page 244*

**Pathocil®** *(Discontinued) see* dicloxacillin *on page 244*

**Pavabid®** *(Discontinued) see* papaverine *on page 618*

**Pavatine®** *(Discontinued)*

**Pavulon®** *(Discontinued) see* pancuronium *on page 616*

**Paxene®** *(Discontinued) see* paclitaxel *on page 612*

**Paxil® [US/Can]** *see* paroxetine *on previous page*

**Paxil CR® [US/Can]** *see* paroxetine *on previous page*

**PCE® [US/Can]** *see* erythromycin *on page 295*

**PCEC** *see* rabies virus vaccine *on page 707*

**PCM [US]** *see* chlorpheniramine, phenylephrine, and methscopolamine *on page 175*

**PCM Allergy [US]** *see* chlorpheniramine, phenylephrine, and methscopolamine *on page 175*

**PCV7** *see* pneumococcal conjugate vaccine (7-valent) *on page 654*

**pectin and kaolin** *see* kaolin and pectin *on page 455*

**pectin, gelatin, and methylcellulose** *see* gelatin, pectin, and methylcellulose *on page 369*

**Pedameth® [US]** *see* methionine *on page 523*

**Pediacare® Children's Long Acting Cough Plus Cold [US-OTC]** *see* pseudoephedrine and dextromethorphan *on page 693*

**PediaCare® Children's Medicated Freezer Pops Long Acting Cough [US-OTC]** *see* dextromethorphan *on page 238*

**PediaCare® Cold and Allergy [US-OTC]** *see* chlorpheniramine and pseudoephedrine *on page 172*

**PediaCare® Decongestant Infants [US-OTC]** *see* pseudoephedrine *on page 692*

**Pediacare® Infants' Decongestant & Cough [US-OTC]** *see* pseudoephedrine and dextromethorphan *on page 693*

**PediaCare® Infants' Long-Acting Cough [US-OTC]** *see* dextromethorphan *on page 238*

**PediaCare® Multi-Symptom Cold [US-OTC]** *see* chlorpheniramine, pseudoephedrine, and dextromethorphan *on page 177*

**PediaCare® NightRest Cough and Cold [US-OTC]** *see* chlorpheniramine, pseudoephedrine, and dextromethorphan *on page 177*

**Pediacof® *(Discontinued)*** *see* chlorpheniramine, phenylephrine, codeine, and potassium iodide *on page 176*

**Pediaflor® [US]** *see* fluoride *on page 347*

**PediaHist DM [US]** *see* brompheniramine, pseudoephedrine, and dextromethorphan *on page 116*

**Pedialyte® [US-OTC]** *see* nutritional formula, enteral/oral *on page 591*

**Pediamist® [US-OTC]** *see* sodium chloride *on page 752*

**PediaPatch Transdermal Patch *(Discontinued)*** *see* salicylic acid *on page 734*

**Pediapred® [US/Can]** *see* prednisolone (systemic) *on page 674*

**Pedia-Profen™ *(Discontinued)*** *see* ibuprofen *on page 427*

**Pedia Relief Cough and Cold [US-OTC]** *see* pseudoephedrine and dextromethorphan *on page 693*

**Pedia Relief Infants [US-OTC]** *see* pseudoephedrine and dextromethorphan *on page 693*

**Pediarix™ [US]** *see* diphtheria, tetanus toxoids, acellular pertussis, hepatitis B (recombinant), and poliovirus (inactivated) vaccine *on page 258*

**Pediatex™ [US]** *see* carbinoxamine *on page 144*

**Pediatex™ 12 [US]** *see* carbinoxamine *on page 144*

**Pediatex™-D [US]** *see* carbinoxamine and pseudoephedrine *on page 144*

**Pediatex™-DM [US]** *see* carbinoxamine, pseudoephedrine, and dextromethorphan *on page 145*

**Pediatex™ HC [US]** *see* pseudoephedrine, hydrocodone, and chlorpheniramine *on page 695*

**Pediatric Triban® *(Discontinued)***

**Pediatrix [Can]** *see* acetaminophen *on page 4*

**Pediazole® [US/Can]** *see* erythromycin and sulfisoxazole *on page 296*

**Pedi-Boro® [US-OTC]** *see* aluminum sulfate and calcium acetate *on page 36*

**Pedi-Dri® [US]** *see* nystatin *on page 592*

**PediOtic® [US]** *see* neomycin, polymyxin B, and hydrocortisone *on page 568*

**Pedisilk® [US-OTC]** *see* salicylic acid *on page 734*

**Pedtrace-4® [US]** *see* trace metals *on page 813*

**PedvaxHIB® [US/Can]** *see* Haemophilus B conjugate vaccine *on page 394*

**PEG-L-asparaginase** *see* pegaspargase *on next page*

## pegademase (bovine) (peg A de mase BOE vine)
**U.S./Canadian Brand Names** Adagen® [US/Can]

**Therapeutic Category** Enzyme

**Use Orphan drug:** Enzyme replacement therapy for adenosine deaminase (ADA) deficiency in patients with severe combined immunodeficiency disease (SCID) who can not benefit from bone marrow transplant; not a cure for SCID, unlike bone marrow transplants, injections must be used the rest of the child's life, therefore is not really an alternative

**Usual Dosage** Children: I.M.: Dose given every 7 days, 10 units/kg the first dose, 15 units/kg the second dose, and 20 units/kg the third dose; maintenance dose: 20 units/kg/week is recommended depending on patient's ADA level; maximum single dose: 30 units/kg

**Dosage Forms** Injection, solution: 250 units/mL (1.5 mL)

**Peganone® [US/Can]** *see* ethotoin *on page 320*

## pegaptanib (peg AP ta nib)
**Synonyms** EYE001; pegaptanib sodium

**U.S./Canadian Brand Names** Macugen® [US]

**Therapeutic Category** Ophthalmic Agent; Vaccine, Recombinant

**Use** Treatment of neovascular (wet) age-related macular degeneration (AMD)

**Usual Dosage** Intravitreous injection: Adults: AMD: 0.3 mg into affected eye every 6 weeks

**Dosage Forms** Injection, solution [preservative free]: 0.3 mg/90 µL (90 µL) [prefilled syringe]

**pegaptanib sodium** *see* pegaptanib *on this page*

## pegaspargase (peg AS par jase)
**Sound-Alike/Look-Alike Issues**

pegaspargase may be confused with asparaginase

**Synonyms** NSC-644954; PEG-L-asparaginase

**U.S./Canadian Brand Names** Oncaspar® [US]

**Therapeutic Category** Antineoplastic Agent

**Use** Treatment of acute lymphocytic leukemia, blast crisis of chronic lymphocytic leukemia (CLL), salvage therapy of non-Hodgkin's lymphoma; may be used in some patients who have had hypersensitivity reactions to *E. coli* asparaginase

**Usual Dosage** Refer to individual protocols. I.M. administration is **preferred** over I.V. administration.
Children: I.M., I.V.:
Body surface area <0.6 m$^2$: 82.5 int. units/kg every 14 days
Body surface area ≥0.6 m$^2$: 2500 int. units/m$^2$ every 14 days
Adults: I.M., I.V.: 2500 int. units/m$^2$ every 14 days
Hemodialysis: Significant drug removal is unlikely based on physiochemical characteristics
Peritoneal dialysis: Significant drug removal is unlikely based on physiochemical characteristics

**Dosage Forms** Injection, solution [preservative free]: 750 units/mL (5 mL)

**Pegasys® [US/Can]** *see* peginterferon alfa-2a *on next page*

**Pegasys® RBV [Can]** *see* peginterferon alfa-2b and ribavirin *(Canada only)* *on page 625*

**Pegetron™ [Can]** *see* peginterferon alfa-2b and ribavirin *(Canada only)* *on page 625*

## pegfilgrastim (peg fil GRA stim)
**Synonyms** G-CSF (PEG conjugate); granulocyte colony stimulating factor (PEG conjugate)

**U.S./Canadian Brand Names** Neulasta™ [US/Can]

**Therapeutic Category** Colony-Stimulating Factor

**Use** Decrease the incidence of infection, by stimulation of granulocyte production, in patients with nonmyeloid malignancies receiving myelosuppressive therapy associated with a significant risk of febrile neutropenia

**Usual Dosage** SubQ: Adolescents >45 kg and Adults: 6 mg once per chemotherapy cycle, do not administer in the period between 14 days before and 24 hours after administration of cytotoxic chemotherapy; do not use in patients, infants, children, and smaller adolescents weighing <45 kg

**Dosage Forms** Injection, solution [preservative free]: 10 mg/mL (0.6 mL) [prefilled syringe]

# peginterferon alfa-2a (peg in ter FEER on AL fa too aye)

**Synonyms** interferon alfa-2a (PEG conjugate); pegylated interferon alfa-2a

**U.S./Canadian Brand Names** Pegasys® [US/Can]

**Therapeutic Category** Interferon

**Use** Treatment of chronic hepatitis C (CHC), alone or in combination with ribavirin, in patients with compensated liver disease and histological evidence of cirrhosis (Child-Pugh class A) and patients with clinically-stable HIV disease; treatment of patients with HBeAg positive and HBeAg negative chronic hepatitis B with compensated liver disease and evidence of viral replication and liver inflammation

**Usual Dosage** SubQ: Adults:

**Chronic hepatitis C (monoinfection or coinfection with HIV):**

Monotherapy: 180 mcg once weekly for 48 weeks

Combination therapy with ribavirin: Recommended dosage: 180 mcg once/week with ribavirin (Copegus®)

Duration of therapy: Monoinfection (based on genotype):

Genotype 1,4: 48 weeks

Genotype 2,3: 24 weeks

Duration of therapy: Coinfection with HIV: 48 weeks

**Chronic hepatitis B**: 180 mcg once weekly for 48 weeks

Dose modification:

For moderate-to-severe adverse reactions: Initial: 135 mcg/week; may need decreased to 90 mcg/week in some cases

Based on hematologic parameters:

ANC <750/mm$^3$: 135 mcg/week

ANC <500/mm$^3$: Suspend therapy until >1000/mm$^3$, then restart at 90 mcg/week and monitor

Platelet count <50,000/mm$^3$: 90 mcg/week

Platelet count <25,000/mm$^3$: Discontinue therapy

Depression (severity based on DSM-IV criteria):

Mild depression: No dosage adjustment required; evaluate once weekly by visit/phone call. If depression remains stable, continue weekly visits. If depression improves, resume normal visit schedule

Moderate depression: Decrease interferon dose to 90-135 mcg once/week; evaluate once weekly with an office visit at least every other week. If depression remains stable, consider psychiatric evaluation and continue with reduced dosing. If symptoms improve and remain stable for 4 weeks, resume normal visit schedule; continue reduced dosing or return to normal dose.

Severe depression: Discontinue interferon permanently. Obtain immediate psychiatric consultation. Discontinue ribavirin if using concurrently.

**Dosage Forms** Injection, solution:

180 mcg/0.5 mL (0.5 mL) [prefilled syringe; contains benzyl alcohol; packaged with needles and alcohol swabs]

180 mcg/mL (1 mL) [contains benzyl alcohol]

# peginterferon alfa-2b (peg in ter FEER on AL fa too bee)

**Synonyms** interferon alfa-2b (PEG conjugate); pegylated interferon alfa-2b

**U.S./Canadian Brand Names** PEG-Intron® [US/Can]

**Therapeutic Category** Interferon

**Use** Treatment of chronic hepatitis C (as monotherapy or in combination with ribavirin) in adult patients who have never received interferon alpha and have compensated liver disease

**Usual Dosage** SubQ:

Children: Safety and efficacy have not been established

Adults: Chronic hepatitis C: Administer dose once weekly; **Note:** Usual duration is for 1 year; after 24 weeks of treatment, if serum HCV RNA is not below the limit of detection of the assay, consider discontinuation:

Monotherapy: Initial:

≤45 kg: 40 mcg

46-56 kg: 50 mcg

57-72 kg: 64 mcg

73-88 kg: 80 mcg

89-106 kg: 96 mcg

107-136 kg: 120 mcg

137-160 kg: 150 mcg

Combination therapy with ribavirin (400 mg twice daily): Initial: 1.5 mcg/kg/week

<40 kg: 50 mcg

40-50 kg: 64 mcg
51-60 kg: 80 mcg
61-75 kg: 96 mcg
76-85 kg: 120 mcg
>85 kg: 150 mcg

**Dosage adjustment if serious adverse event occurs:** Depression (severity based upon DSM-IV criteria):

Mild depression: No dosage adjustment required; evaluate once weekly by visit/phone call. If depression remains stable, continue weekly visits. If depression improves, resume normal visit schedule.

Moderate depression: Decrease interferon dose by 50%; evaluate once weekly with an office visit at least every other week. If depression remains stable, consider psychiatric evaluation and continue with reduced dosing. If symptoms improve and remain stable for 4 weeks, resume normal visit schedule; continue reduced dosing or return to normal dose.

Severe depression: Discontinue interferon and ribavirin permanently. Obtain immediate psychiatric consultation.

**Dosage Forms**

Injection, powder for reconstitution [prefilled syringe] (Redipen™): 50 mcg, 80 mcg, 120 mcg, 150 mcg [packaged with alcohol swabs and needle for injection]

Injection, powder for reconstitution [vial]: 50 mcg, 80 mcg, 120 mcg, 150 mcg [packaged with SWFI, alcohol swabs, and syringes]

# peginterferon alfa-2b and ribavirin *(Canada only)*
(peg in ter FEER on AL fa too bee & rye ba VYE rin)

**Synonyms** ribavirin and peginterferon alfa-2b

**U.S./Canadian Brand Names** Pegasys® RBV [Can]; Pegetron™ [Can]

**Therapeutic Category** Antiviral Agent; Interferon

**Use** Combination therapy for the treatment of chronic hepatitis C in patients with compensated liver disease

**Usual Dosage** Chronic hepatitis C:

Recommended dosage of combination therapy:

Intron® A: SubQ: 1.5 mcg/kg/week

**and**

Rebetol®: Oral:

≤64 kg: 800 mg/day (two 200 mg capsules in the morning and two 200 mg capsules in the evening)

64-84 kg: 1000 mg/day (two 200 mg capsules in the morning and three 200 mg capsules in the evening)

≥85 kg: 1200 mg/day (three 200 mg capsules in the morning and three 200 mg capsules in the evening)

Recommended duration of therapy: 1 year. Consider discontinuing therapy in any patient not achieving HCV-RNA below the limit of assay detection by 24 weeks.

**Dosage Forms Combination package:**

Injection, powder for reconstitution (Peginterferon alfa-2b): 50 mcg/0.5 mL
Capsules: Ribavirin (Rebetol®): 200 mg (56s)

Injection, powder for reconstitution (Peginterferon alfa-2b): 80 mcg/0.5 mL
Capsules: Ribavirin (Rebetol®): 200 mg (56s)

Injection, powder for reconstitution (Peginterferon alfa-2b): 100 mcg/0.5 mL
Capsules: Ribavirin (Rebetol®): 200 mg (70s)

Injection, powder for reconstitution (Peginterferon alfa-2b): 120 mcg/0.5 mL
Capsules: Ribavirin (Rebetol®): 200 mg (70s)

Injection, powder for reconstitution (Peginterferon alfa-2b): 150 mcg/0.5 mL
Capsules: Ribavirin (Rebetol®): 200 mg (84s)

**PEG-Intron® [US/Can]** *see* peginterferon alfa-2b *on previous page*

**PegLyte® [Can]** *see* polyethylene glycol-electrolyte solution *on page 658*

# pegvisomant (peg VI soe mant)

**Synonyms** B2036-PEG

**U.S./Canadian Brand Names** Somavert® [US]

**Therapeutic Category** Growth Hormone Receptor Antagonist

**Use** Treatment of acromegaly in patients resistant to or unable to tolerate other therapies

(Continued)

## pegvisomant *(Continued)*

**Usual Dosage** SubQ: Adults: Initial loading dose: 40 mg; maintenance dose: 10 mg once daily; doses may be adjusted by 5 mg in 4- to 6-week intervals based on IGF-I concentrations (maximum dose: 30 mg/day)

**Dosage Forms** Injection, powder for reconstitution [preservative free]: 10 mg, 15 mg, 20 mg [vial stopper contains latex; packaged with SWFI]

**pegylated interferon alfa-2a** *see* peginterferon alfa-2a *on page 624*

**pegylated interferon alfa-2b** *see* peginterferon alfa-2b *on page 624*

**PemADD® CT *(Discontinued)*** *see* pemoline *on this page*

**PemADD® *(Discontinued)*** *see* pemoline *on this page*

## pemetrexed (pem e TREKS ed)

**Synonyms** LY231514; MTA; multitargeted antifolate; NSC-698037; pemetrexed disodium

**U.S./Canadian Brand Names** Alimta® [US/Can]

**Therapeutic Category** Antineoplastic Agent, Antimetabolite; Antineoplastic Agent, Antimetabolite (Antifolate)

**Use** Treatment of malignant pleural mesothelioma in combination with cisplatin; treatment of nonsmall cell lung cancer

**Usual Dosage** I.V.: Adults:

Nonsmall cell lung cancer: 500 mg/m$^2$ on day 1 of each 21-day cycle

Malignant pleural mesothelioma: 500-600 mg/m$^2$ on day 1 of each 21-day cycle

**Note:** Start vitamin supplements 1 week before initial dose of pemetrexed. Folic acid 350-1000 mcg/day orally (continuing for 21 days after last dose of pemetrexed) and vitamin B$_{12}$ 1000 mcg I.M. every 9 weeks. Dexamethasone 4 mg twice daily can be started the day before therapy, and continued the day of and the day after to minimize cutaneous reactions.

**Dosage Forms** Injection, powder for reconstitution: 500 mg

**pemetrexed disodium** *see* pemetrexed *on this page*

## pemirolast (pe MIR oh last)

**U.S./Canadian Brand Names** Alamast® [US/Can]

**Therapeutic Category** Mast Cell Stabilizer; Ophthalmic Agent, Miscellaneous

**Use** Prevention of itching of the eye due to allergic conjunctivitis

**Usual Dosage** Children >3 years and Adults: 1-2 drops instilled in affected eye(s) 4 times/day

**Dosage Forms** Solution, ophthalmic, as potassium: 0.1% (10 mL) [contains lauralkonium chloride]

## pemoline (PEM oh leen)

**Synonyms** phenylisohydantoin; PIO

**Therapeutic Category** Central Nervous System Stimulant, Nonamphetamine

**Controlled Substance** C-IV

**Use** Treatment of attention-deficit/hyperactivity disorder (ADHD) (not first-line)

**Usual Dosage** Children ≥6 years: Oral: Initial: 37.5 mg given once daily in the morning, increase by 18.75 mg/day at weekly intervals; usual effective dose range: 56.25-75 mg/day; maximum: 112.5 mg/day; dosage range: 0.5-3 mg/kg/24 hours; significant benefit may not be evident until third or fourth week of administration

**Dosage Forms** [DSC] = Discontinued product

Tablet (Cylert® [DSC], PemADD® [DSC]): 18.75 mg, 37.5 mg, 75 mg

Tablet, chewable (Cylert® [DSC], PemADD® CT [DSC]): 37.5 mg

## penbutolol (pen BYOO toe lole)

**Sound-Alike/Look-Alike Issues**

Levatol® may be confused with Lipitor®

**Synonyms** penbutolol sulfate

**U.S./Canadian Brand Names** Levatol® [US/Can]

**Therapeutic Category** Beta-Adrenergic Blocker

**Use** Treatment of mild to moderate arterial hypertension

**Usual Dosage** Adults: Oral: Initial: 20 mg once daily, full effect of a 20 or 40 mg dose is seen by the end of a 2-week period, doses of 40-80 mg have been tolerated but have shown little additional antihypertensive effects; usual dose range (JNC 7): 10-40 mg once daily

**Dosage Forms** Tablet, as sulfate: 20 mg

**penbutolol sulfate** *see* penbutolol *on previous page*

# penciclovir (pen SYE kloe veer)

**Sound-Alike/Look-Alike Issues**
Denavir® may be confused with indinavir

**U.S./Canadian Brand Names** Denavir® [US]

**Therapeutic Category** Antiviral Agent

**Use** Topical treatment of herpes simplex labialis (cold sores)

**Usual Dosage** Children ≥12 years and Adults: Topical: Apply cream at the first sign or symptom of cold sore (eg, tingling, swelling); apply every 2 hours during waking hours for 4 days

**Dosage Forms** Cream: 1% (1.5 g)

**Penetrex® *(Discontinued)***

# penicillamine (pen i SIL a meen)

**Sound-Alike/Look-Alike Issues**
penicillamine may be confused with penicillin
Depen® may be confused with Endal®

**Synonyms** D-3-mercaptovaline; D-penicillamine; B,B-dimethylcysteine

**U.S./Canadian Brand Names** Cuprimine® [US/Can]; Depen® [US/Can]

**Therapeutic Category** Chelating Agent

**Use** Treatment of Wilson disease, cystinuria; adjunctive treatment of rheumatoid arthritis

**Usual Dosage** Oral:
Rheumatoid arthritis:
Adults: 125-250 mg/day, may increase dose at 1- to 3-month intervals up to 1-1.5 g/day; maximum in older adults: 750 mg/day

Wilson disease (doses titrated to maintain urinary copper excretion >2 mg/day); decrease dose for surgery and during last trimester of pregnancy
Children <12 years: 20 mg/kg/day in 2-3 divided doses, round off to the nearest 250 mg dose; maximum 1 g/day
Adults: 250 mg 4 times/day (maximum in older adults: 750 mg/day)

Cystinuria: **Note:** Adjust dose to limit cystine excretion to 100-200 mg/day (<100 mg/day with history of stone formation)
Children: 30 mg/kg/day in 4 divided doses
Adults: 1-4 g/day in divided doses every 6 hours; usual dose: 2 g/day

**Dosage Forms**
Capsule (Cuprimine®): 125 mg [DSC], 250 mg
Tablet (Depen®): 250 mg

# penicillin V potassium (pen i SIL in vee poe TASS ee um)

**Sound-Alike/Look-Alike Issues**
penicillin V procaine may be confused with penicillin G potassium

**Synonyms** pen VK; phenoxymethyl penicillin

**U.S./Canadian Brand Names** Apo-Pen VK® [Can]; Novo-Pen-VK [Can]; Nu-Pen-VK [Can]; Veetids® [US]

**Therapeutic Category** Penicillin

**Use** Treatment of infections caused by susceptible organisms involving the respiratory tract, otitis media, sinusitis, skin, and urinary tract; prophylaxis in rheumatic fever

**Usual Dosage** Oral:
Systemic infections:
Children <12 years: 25-50 mg/kg/day in divided doses every 6-8 hours; maximum dose: 3 g/day
Children ≥12 years and Adults: 125-500 mg every 6-8 hours
Prophylaxis of pneumococcal infections:
Children <5 years: 125 mg twice daily
Children ≥5 years and Adults: 250 mg twice daily
(Continued)

## penicillin V potassium *(Continued)*

Prophylaxis of recurrent rheumatic fever:
Children <5 years: 125 mg twice daily
Children ≥5 years and Adults: 250 mg twice daily
**Dosage Forms Note**: 250 mg = 400,000 units
Powder for oral solution: 125 mg/5 mL (100 mL, 200 mL); 250 mg/5 mL (100 mL, 200 mL)
Tablet: 250 mg, 500 mg

## penicillin G benzathine (pen i SIL in jee BENZ a theen)

**Sound-Alike/Look-Alike Issues**
penicillin may be confused with penicillamine
Bicillin® may be confused with Wycillin®
Bicillin® C-R (penicillin G benzathine and penicillin G procaine) may be confused with Bicillin® L-A (penicillin G benzathine). Penicillin G benzathine is the only product currently approved for the treatment of syphilis. Administration of penicillin G benzathine and penicillin G procaine combination instead of Bicillin® L-A may result in inadequate treatment response.
**Synonyms** benzathine benzylpenicillin; benzathine penicillin G; benzylpenicillin benzathine
**U.S./Canadian Brand Names** Bicillin® L-A [US]
**Therapeutic Category** Penicillin
**Use** Active against some gram-positive organisms, few gram-negative organisms such as *Neisseria gonorrhoeae*, and some anaerobes and spirochetes; used in the treatment of syphilis; used only for the treatment of mild to moderately severe infections caused by organisms susceptible to low concentrations of penicillin G or for prophylaxis of infections caused by these organisms
**Usual Dosage** I.M.: Administer undiluted injection; higher doses result in more sustained rather than higher levels. Use a penicillin G benzathine-penicillin G procaine combination to achieve early peak levels in acute infections.

Infants and Children:
Group A streptococcal upper respiratory infection: 25,000-50,000 units/kg as a single dose; maximum: 1.2 million units
Prophylaxis of recurrent rheumatic fever: 25,000-50,000 units/kg every 3-4 weeks; maximum: 1.2 million units/dose
Early syphilis: 50,000 units/kg as a single injection; maximum: 2.4 million units
Syphilis of more than 1-year duration: 50,000 units/kg every week for 3 doses; maximum: 2.4 million units/dose
Adults:
Group A streptococcal upper respiratory infection: 1.2 million units as a single dose
Prophylaxis of recurrent rheumatic fever: 1.2 million units every 3-4 weeks or 600,000 units twice monthly
Early syphilis: 2.4 million units as a single dose in 2 injection sites
Syphilis of more than 1-year duration: 2.4 million units in 2 injection sites once weekly for 3 doses
Not indicated as single drug therapy for neurosyphilis, but may be given 1 time/week for 3 weeks following I.V. treatment; refer to Penicillin G Parenteral/Aqueous monograph for dosing
**Dosage Forms** Injection, suspension [prefilled syringe]: 600,000 units/mL (1 mL, 2 mL, 4 mL)

## penicillin G benzathine and penicillin G procaine

(pen i SIL in jee BENZ a theen & pen i SIL in jee PROE kane)
**Sound-Alike/Look-Alike Issues**
penicillin may be confused with penicillamine
Bicillin® may be confused with Wycillin®
Bicillin® C-R (penicillin G benzathine and penicillin G procaine) may be confused with Bicillin® L-A (penicillin G benzathine). Penicillin G benzathine is the only product currently approved for the treatment of syphilis. Administration of penicillin G benzathine and penicillin G procaine combination instead of Bicillin® L-A may result in inadequate treatment response.
**Synonyms** penicillin G procaine and benzathine combined
**U.S./Canadian Brand Names** Bicillin® C-R 900/300 [US]; Bicillin® C-R [US]
**Therapeutic Category** Penicillin
**Use** May be used in specific situations in the treatment of streptococcal infections
**Usual Dosage** I.M.:
Children:
<30 lb: 600,000 units in a single dose

30-60 lb: 900,000 units to 1.2 million units in a single dose

Children >60 lb and Adults: 2.4 million units in a single dose

**Dosage Forms** Injection, suspension [prefilled syringe]:

Bicillin® C-R:

600,000 units: Penicillin G benzathine 300,000 units and penicillin G procaine 300,000 units per 1 mL (1 mL)

1,200,000 units: Penicillin G benzathine 600,000 units and penicillin G procaine 600,000 units per 2 mL (2 mL)

2,400,000 units: Penicillin G benzathine 1,200,000 units and penicillin G procaine 1,200,000 units per 4 mL (4 mL)

Bicillin® C-R 900/300: 1,200,000 units: Penicillin G benzathine 900,000 units and penicillin G procaine 300,000 units per 2 mL (2 mL)

# penicillin G (parenteral/aqueous) (pen i SIL in jee, pa REN ter al, AYE kwee us)

**Sound-Alike/Look-Alike Issues**

penicillin may be confused with penicillamine

**Synonyms** benzylpenicillin potassium; benzylpenicillin sodium; crystalline penicillin; penicillin G potassium; penicillin G sodium

**U.S./Canadian Brand Names** Pfizerpen® [US/Can]

**Therapeutic Category** Penicillin

**Use** Active against some gram-positive organisms, generally not *Staphylococcus aureus*; some gram-negative organisms such as *Neisseria gonorrhoeae*, and some anaerobes and spirochetes

**Usual Dosage** I.M., I.V.:

Neonates:

<7 days, <2000 g: 25,000-50,000 units/kg every 12 hours

<7 days, >2000 g: 25,000-50,000 units/kg every 8 hours

>7 days, <2000 g: 25,000-50,000 units/kg every 8 hours

>7 days, >2000 g: 25,000-50,000 units/kg every 6 hours

Infants and Children:

Mild-to-moderate infections: 25,000-50,000 units/kg/day in 4 divided doses

Severe infections: 250,000 to 400,000 units/kg/day in divided doses every 4-6 hours; maximum dose: 24 million units/day

Congenital syphilis:

Neonates:

≤7 days: 50,000 units/kg I.V. every 12 hours for a total of 10 days

>7 days: 50,000 units/kg I.V. every 8 hours for a total of 10 days

Infants: 50,000 units/kg every 4-6 hours for 10 days

Adults: 2-24 million units/day in divided doses every 4 hours depending on sensitivity of the organism and severity of the infection

Neurosyphilis: 18-24 million units/day in divided doses every 4 hours (or by continuous infusion) for 10-14 days

**Dosage Forms**

Infusion, as potassium [premixed iso-osmotic dextrose solution, frozen]: 1 million units (50 mL), 2 million units (50 mL), 3 million units (50 mL) [contains sodium 1.02 mEq and potassium 1.7 mEq per 1 million units]

Injection, powder for reconstitution, as potassium (Pfizerpen®): 5 million units, 20 million units [contains sodium 6.8 mg (0.3 mEq) and potassium 65.6 mg (1.68 mEq) per 1 million units]

Injection, powder for reconstitution, as sodium: 5 million units [contains sodium 1.68 mEq per 1 million units]

**penicillin G potassium** *see* penicillin G (parenteral/aqueous) *on this page*

# penicillin G procaine (pen i SIL in jee PROE kane)

**Sound-Alike/Look-Alike Issues**

penicillin G procaine may be confused with penicillin V potassium

Wycillin® may be confused with Bicillin®

**Synonyms** APPG; aqueous procaine penicillin G; procaine benzylpenicillin; procaine penicillin G

**U.S./Canadian Brand Names** Pfizerpen-AS® [Can]; Wycillin® [Can]

**Therapeutic Category** Penicillin

**Use** Moderately severe infections due to *Treponema pallidum* and other penicillin G-sensitive microorganisms that are susceptible to low, but prolonged serum penicillin concentrations; anthrax due to (Continued)

## penicillin G procaine *(Continued)*

*Bacillus anthracis* (postexposure) to reduce the incidence or progression of disease following exposure to aerolized *Bacillus anthracis*

**Usual Dosage** I.M.:

Children: 25,000-50,000 units/kg/day in divided doses 1-2 times/day; not to exceed 4.8 million units/24 hours

Anthrax, inhalational (postexposure prophylaxis): 25,000 units/kg every 12 hours (maximum: 1,200,000 units every 12 hours); see "Note" in Adults dosing

Congenital syphilis: 50,000 units/kg/day for 10-14 days

Adults: 0.6-4.8 million units/day in divided doses every 12-24 hours

Anthrax:

Inhalational (postexposure prophylaxis): 1,200,000 units every 12 hours

**Note:** Overall treatment duration should be 60 days. Available safety data suggest continued administration of penicillin G procaine for longer than 2 weeks may incur additional risk for adverse reactions. Clinicians may consider switching to effective alternative treatment for completion of therapy beyond 2 weeks.

Cutaneous (treatment): 600,000-1,200,000 units/day; alternative therapy is recommended in severe cutaneous or other forms of anthrax infection

Endocarditis caused by susceptible viridans *Streptococcus* (when used in conjunction with an aminoglycoside): 1.2 million units every 6 hours for 2-4 weeks

Neurosyphilis: I.M.: 2-4 million units/day with 500 mg probenecid by mouth 4 times/day for 10-14 days; **penicillin G aqueous I.V. is the preferred agent**

**Dosage Forms** Injection, suspension: 600,000 units/mL (1 mL, 2 mL)

**penicillin G procaine and benzathine combined** *see* penicillin G benzathine and penicillin G procaine *on page 628*

**penicillin G sodium** *see* penicillin G (parenteral/aqueous) *on previous page*

**penicilloyl-polylysine** *see* benzylpenicilloyl-polylysine *on page 100*

**Penlac® [US/Can]** *see* ciclopirox *on page 182*

**Pennsaid® [Can]** *see* diclofenac *on page 243*

**Penta/3B®+C [Can]** *see* vitamin B complex with vitamin C *on page 850*

**Pentacarinat® Injection *(Discontinued)*** *see* pentamidine *on this page*

**pentahydrate** *see* sodium thiosulfate *on page 758*

**Pentam-300® [US]** *see* pentamidine *on this page*

## pentamidine *(pen TAM i deen)*

**Synonyms** pentamidine isethionate

**U.S./Canadian Brand Names** NebuPent® [US]; Pentam-300® [US]

**Therapeutic Category** Antiprotozoal

**Use** Treatment and prevention of pneumonia caused by *Pneumocystis carinii* (PCP)

**Usual Dosage**

Children:

Treatment of PCP pneumonia: I.M., I.V. (I.V. preferred): 4 mg/kg/day once daily for 10-14 days

Prevention of PCP pneumonia:

I.M., I.V.: 4 mg/kg monthly or every 2 weeks

Inhalation (aerosolized pentamidine in children ≥5 years): 300 mg/dose given every 3-4 weeks via Respirgard® II inhaler (8 mg/kg dose has also been used in children <5 years)

Adults:

Treatment: I.M., I.V. (I.V. preferred): 4 mg/kg/day once daily for 14-21 days

Prevention: Inhalation: 300 mg every 4 weeks via Respirgard® II nebulizer

**Dosage Forms**

Injection, powder for reconstitution, as isethionate (Pentam-300®): 300 mg

Powder for nebulization, as isethionate (NebuPent®): 300 mg

**pentamidine isethionate** *see* pentamidine *on this page*

**Pentamycetin® [Can]** *see* chloramphenicol *on page 167*

**Pentasa® [US/Can]** *see* mesalamine *on page 516*

**Pentaspan® [US/Can]** *see* pentastarch *on next page*

# pentastarch (PEN ta starch)

**U.S./Canadian Brand Names** Pentaspan® [US/Can]

**Therapeutic Category** Blood Modifiers

**Use Orphan drug:** Adjunct in leukapheresis to improve harvesting and increase yield of leukocytes by centrifugal means

**Usual Dosage** 250-700 mL to which citrate anticoagulant has been added is administered by adding to the input line of the centrifugation apparatus at a ratio of 1:8-1:13 to venous whole blood

**Dosage Forms** Infusion [premixed in NS]: 10% (500 mL)

**Penta-Triamterene HCTZ [Can]** *see* hydrochlorothiazide and triamterene *on page 410*

# pentazocine (pen TAZ oh seen)

**Synonyms** naloxone hydrochloride and pentazocine hydrochloride; pentazocine hydrochloride and naloxone hydrochloride; pentazocine hydrochloride; pentazocine lactate

**U.S./Canadian Brand Names** Talwin® NX [US]; Talwin® [US/Can]

**Therapeutic Category** Analgesic, Narcotic

**Controlled Substance** C-IV

**Use** Relief of moderate to severe pain; has also been used as a sedative prior to surgery and as a supplement to surgical anesthesia

**Usual Dosage**

Preoperative/preanesthetic: Children 1-16 years: I.M.: 0.5 mg/kg

Analgesia:

Children: I.M.:

5-8 years: 15 mg

8-14 years: 30 mg

Children >12 years and Adults: Oral: 50 mg every 3-4 hours; may increase to 100 mg/dose if needed, but should not exceed 600 mg/day

Adults:

I.M., SubQ: 30-60 mg every 3-4 hours, not to exceed total daily dose of 360 mg

I.V.: 30 mg every 3-4 hours (maximum: 360 mg/day)

**Dosage Forms**

Injection, solution (Talwin®): 30 mg/mL (1 mL, 10 mL) [10 mL size contains sodium bisulfite]

Tablet (Talwin® NX): Pentazocine 50 mg and naloxone 0.5 mg

**pentazocine hydrochloride** *see* pentazocine *on this page*

**pentazocine hydrochloride and naloxone hydrochloride** *see* pentazocine *on this page*

**pentazocine lactate** *see* pentazocine *on this page*

**pentetate calcium trisodium** *see* diethylene triamine penta-acetic acid *on page 246*

**pentetate zinc trisodium** *see* diethylene triamine penta-acetic acid *on page 246*

**Penthrane® *(Discontinued)***

# pentobarbital (pen toe BAR bi tal)

**Sound-Alike/Look-Alike Issues**

pentobarbital may be confused with phenobarbital

Nembutal® may be confused with Myambutol®

**Synonyms** pentobarbital sodium

**U.S./Canadian Brand Names** Nembutal® Sodium [Can]; Nembutal® [US]

**Therapeutic Category** Barbiturate

**Controlled Substance** C-II

**Use** Sedative/hypnotic; preanesthetic; high-dose barbiturate coma for treatment of increased intracranial pressure or status epilepticus unresponsive to other therapy

**Usual Dosage**

Children:

Hypnotic: I.M.: 2-6 mg/kg; maximum: 100 mg/dose

Preoperative/preprocedure sedation: ≥6 months:

**Note:** Limited information is available for infants <6 months of age.

I.M.: 2-6 mg/kg; maximum: 100 mg/dose

I.V.: 1-3 mg/kg to a maximum of 100 mg until asleep

(Continued)

## pentobarbital *(Continued)*

Conscious sedation prior to a procedure: Children 5-12 years: I.V.: 2 mg/kg 5-10 minutes before procedures, may repeat one time

Adolescents: Conscious sedation: I.V.: 100 mg prior to a procedure

Children and Adults: Barbiturate coma in head injury patients: I.V.: Loading dose: 5-10 mg/kg given slowly over 1-2 hours; monitor blood pressure and respiratory rate; Maintenance infusion: Initial: 1 mg/kg/hour; may increase to 2-3 mg/kg/hour; maintain burst suppression on EEG

Status epilepticus: I.V.: **Note:** Intubation required; monitor hemodynamics

Children: Loading dose: 5-15 mg/kg given slowly over 1-2 hours; maintenance infusion: 0.5-5 mg/kg/hour

Adults: Loading dose: 2-15 mg/kg given slowly over 1-2 hours; maintenance infusion: 0.5-3 mg/kg/hour

Adults:

Hypnotic:

I.M.: 150-200 mg

I.V.: Initial: 100 mg, may repeat every 1-3 minutes up to 200-500 mg total dose

Preoperative sedation: I.M.: 150-200 mg

**Dosage Forms** Injection, solution, as sodium: 50 mg/mL (20 mL, 50 mL) [contains alcohol 10% and propylene glycol 40%]

**pentobarbital sodium** *see* pentobarbital *on previous page*

## pentosan polysulfate sodium (PEN toe san pol i SUL fate SOW dee um)

**Sound-Alike/Look-Alike Issues**

pentosan may be confused with pentostatin

Elmiron® may be confused with Imuran®

**Synonyms** PPS

**U.S./Canadian Brand Names** Elmiron® [US/Can]

**Therapeutic Category** Analgesic, Urinary

**Use Orphan drug:** Relief of bladder pain or discomfort due to interstitial cystitis

**Usual Dosage** Adults: Oral: 100 mg 3 times/day taken with water 1 hour before or 2 hours after meals

Patients should be evaluated at 3 months and may be continued an additional 3 months if there has been no improvement and if there are no therapy-limiting side effects. **The risks and benefits of continued use beyond 6 months in patients who have not responded is not yet known.**

**Dosage Forms** Capsule: 100 mg

## pentostatin (PEN toe stat in)

**Sound-Alike/Look-Alike Issues**

pentostatin may be confused with pentosan

**Synonyms** 2'-deoxycoformycin; CL-825; co-vidarabine; dCF; deoxycoformycin; NSC-218321

**U.S./Canadian Brand Names** Nipent® [US/Can]

**Therapeutic Category** Antineoplastic Agent

**Use** Treatment of hairy cell leukemia; non-Hodgkin lymphoma, cutaneous T-cell lymphoma

**Usual Dosage** Refractory hairy cell leukemia: Adults (refer to individual protocols):

4 mg/m² every other week **or**

4 mg/m² weekly for 3 weeks, then every 2 weeks **or**

5 mg/m² daily for 3 days every 3 weeks

**Dosage Forms** Injection, powder for reconstitution: 10 mg

**Pentothal® [US/Can]** *see* thiopental *on page 797*

**Pentothal® Sodium Rectal Suspension *(Discontinued)*** *see* thiopental *on page 797*

## pentoxifylline (pen toks I fi leen)

**Sound-Alike/Look-Alike Issues**

pentoxifylline may be confused with tamoxifen

Trental® may be confused with Bentyl®, Tegretol®, Trandate®

**Synonyms** oxpentifylline

**U.S./Canadian Brand Names** Albert® Pentoxifylline [Can]; Apo-Pentoxifylline SR® [Can]; Nu-Pentoxifylline SR [Can]; Pentoxil® [US]; ratio-Pentoxifylline [Can]; Trental® [US/Can]

**Therapeutic Category** Blood Viscosity Reducer Agent

**Use** Treatment of intermittent claudication on the basis of chronic occlusive arterial disease of the limbs; may improve function and symptoms, but not intended to replace more definitive therapy

**Usual Dosage** Adults: Oral: 400 mg 3 times/day with meals; maximal therapeutic benefit may take 2-4 weeks to develop; recommended to maintain therapy for at least 8 weeks. May reduce to 400 mg twice daily if GI or CNS side effects occur.

**Dosage Forms** Tablet, extended release (Pentoxil®, Trental®): 400 mg

**Pentoxil® [US]** *see* pentoxifylline *on previous page*

**Pentrax® [US-OTC]** *see* coal tar *on page 201*

**Pen.Vee® K *(Discontinued)*** *see* penicillin V potassium *on page 627*

**pen VK** *see* penicillin V potassium *on page 627*

**Pepcid® [US/Can]** *see* famotidine *on page 327*

**Pepcid® AC [US-OTC/Can]** *see* famotidine *on page 327*

**Pepcid® Complete [US-OTC/Can]** *see* famotidine, calcium carbonate, and magnesium hydroxide *on page 328*

**Pepcid® I.V. [Can]** *see* famotidine *on page 327*

**Pepcid RPD® *(Discontinued)*** *see* famotidine *on page 327*

**Pepto-Bismol® [OTC]** *see* bismuth subsalicylate *on page 108*

**Pepto-Bismol® Maximum Strength [OTC]** *see* bismuth subsalicylate *on page 108*

**Pepto® Diarrhea Control *(Discontinued)*** *see* loperamide *on page 489*

**Perchloracap® [US]** *see* radiological/contrast media (ionic) *on page 707*

**Percocet® [US/Can]** *see* oxycodone and acetaminophen *on page 609*

**Percocet®-Demi [Can]** *see* oxycodone and acetaminophen *on page 609*

**Percodan® [US/Can]** *see* oxycodone and aspirin *on page 610*

**Percodan®-Demi *(Discontinued)*** *see* oxycodone and aspirin *on page 610*

**Percogesic® [US-OTC]** *see* acetaminophen and phenyltoloxamine *on page 8*

**Percogesic® Extra Strength [US-OTC]** *see* acetaminophen and diphenhydramine *on page 7*

**Percolone® *(Discontinued)*** *see* oxycodone *on page 608*

**Perdiem® Overnight Relief [US-OTC]** *see* senna *on page 743*

**Perfectoderm® Gel *(Discontinued)*** *see* benzoyl peroxide *on page 98*

## perflutren lipid microspheres (per FLOO tren LIP id MIKE roe sfeers)

**U.S./Canadian Brand Names** Definity® [US/Can]

**Therapeutic Category** Diagnostic Agent

**Use** Opacification of left ventricular chamber and improvement of delineation of the left ventricular endocardial border in patients with suboptimal echocardiograms

**Usual Dosage** Adults: Dose should be given following baseline noncontrast echocardiography. Imaging should begin immediately following dose and compared to noncontrast image. Mechanical index for the ultrasound device should be set at ≤0.8.

I.V. bolus: 10 μL/kg of activated product, followed by 10 mL saline flush. May repeat in 30 minutes if needed (maximum dose: 2 bolus infusions).

I.V. infusion: Initial: 4 mL/minute of prepared infusion; titrate to achieve optimal image; maximum rate: 10 mL/minute (maximum dose: 1 intravenous infusion).

**Dosage Forms** Injection, solution [preservative free]: OFP 6.52 mg/mL and lipid blend 0.75 mg/mL (2 mL) [following activation, forms a suspension containing perflutren lipid microspheres 1.2 x $10^{10}$/mL and OFP 1.1 mg/mL]

## pergolide (PER go lide)

**Sound-Alike/Look-Alike Issues**

Permax® may be confused with Bumex®, Pentrax®, Pernox®

(Continued)

## pergolide *(Continued)*

**Synonyms** pergolide mesylate

**U.S./Canadian Brand Names** Permax® [US/Can]

**Therapeutic Category** Anti-Parkinson Agent; Dopaminergic Agent (Anti-Parkinson); Ergot Alkaloid and Derivative

**Use** Adjunctive treatment to levodopa/carbidopa in the management of Parkinson disease

**Usual Dosage** When adding pergolide to levodopa/carbidopa, the dose of the latter can usually and should be decreased. Patients no longer responsive to bromocriptine may benefit by being switched to pergolide.

Oral: Adults: Parkinson disease: Start with 0.05 mg/day for 2 days, then increase dosage by 0.1 or 0.15 mg/day every 3 days over next 12 days, increase dose by 0.25 mg/day every 3 days until optimal therapeutic dose is achieved, up to 5 mg/day maximum; usual dosage range: 2-3 mg/day in 3 divided doses

**Dosage Forms** Tablet: 0.05 mg, 0.25 mg, 1 mg

**pergolide mesylate** *see* pergolide *on previous page*

**Pergonal® *(Discontinued)*** *see* menotropins *on page 511*

**Periactin® *(Discontinued)*** *see* cyproheptadine *on page 217*

**Peri-Colace® *(reformulation)* [US-OTC]** *see* docusate and senna *on page 264*

## pericyazine *(Canada only)* (per ee CYE ah zeen)

**U.S./Canadian Brand Names** Neuleptil® [Can]

**Therapeutic Category** Phenothiazine Derivative

**Use** As adjunctive medication in some psychotic patients, for the control of residual prevailing hostility, impulsiveness and aggressiveness

**Usual Dosage** Oral:

Children and adolescents (5 years of age and over): 2.5-10 mg in the morning and 5-30 mg in the evening. These dosages approximate a daily dosage range of 1-3 mg/year of age.

Adults: 5-20 mg in the morning and 10-40 mg in the evening. For maintenance therapy, the dosage should be reduced to the minimum effective dose. Lower doses of 2.5-15 mg in the morning, and 5-30 mg in the evening have been suggested. Children and adolescents (5 years of age and over): 2.5-10 mg in the morning and 5-30 mg in the evening. These dosages approximate a daily dosage range of 1-3 mg/year of age.

**Dosage Forms**

Capsule: 5 mg, 10 mg, 20 mg

Drops, oral: 10 mg/mL (100 mL)

**Peridex® [US]** *see* chlorhexidine gluconate *on page 168*

**Peridol [Can]** *see* haloperidol *on page 396*

## perindopril and indapamide *(Canada only)* (per IN doe pril & in DAP a mide)

**U.S./Canadian Brand Names** Coversyl® Plus [Can]; Preterax® [Can]

**Therapeutic Category** Miscellaneous Product

**Use** Hypertension

**Usual Dosage** Oral: Adults: One tablet daily

**Dosage Forms** Tablet: Perindopril 2 mg and indapamide 0.625 mg

## perindopril erbumine (per IN doe pril er BYOO meen)

**U.S./Canadian Brand Names** Aceon® [US]; Coversyl® [Can]

**Therapeutic Category** Miscellaneous Product

**Use** Treatment of essential hypertension; reduction of cardiovascular mortality or nonfatal myocardial infarction in patients with stable coronary artery disease

**Usual Dosage** Oral: Adults:

Essential hypertension: Initial: 4 mg/day but may be titrated to response; usual range: 4-8 mg/day (may be given in 2 divided doses); increase at 1- to 2-week intervals (maximum: 16 mg/day)

Concomitant therapy with diuretics: To reduce the risk of hypotension, discontinue diuretic, if possible, 2-3 days prior to initiating perindopril. If unable to stop diuretic, initiate perindopril at 2-4 mg/day and monitor blood pressure closely for the first 2 weeks of therapy, and after any dose adjustment of perindopril or diuretic.

Stable coronary artery disease: Initial: 4 mg once daily for 2 weeks; increase as tolerated to 8 mg once daily.

Dosage Forms Tablet: 2 mg, 4 mg, 8 mg

**PerioChip**® **[US]** *see* chlorhexidine gluconate *on page 168*

**PerioGard**® **[US]** *see* chlorhexidine gluconate *on page 168*

**Periostat**® **[US/Can]** *see* doxycycline *on page 271*

**Permax**® **[US/Can]** *see* pergolide *on page 633*

## permethrin (per METH rin)

**U.S./Canadian Brand Names** A200® Lice [US-OTC]; Acticin® [US]; Elimite® [US]; Kwellada-P™ [Can]; Nix® [US-OTC/Can]; Rid® Spray [US-OTC]

**Therapeutic Category** Scabicides/Pediculicides

**Use** Single-application treatment of infestation with *Pediculus humanus capitis* (head louse) and its nits or *Sarcoptes scabiei* (scabies); indicated for prophylactic use during epidemics of lice

**Usual Dosage** Topical:

Head lice: Children >2 months and Adults: After hair has been washed with shampoo, rinsed with water, and towel dried, apply a sufficient volume of topical liquid (lotion or cream rinse) to saturate the hair and scalp. Leave on hair for 10 minutes before rinsing off with water; remove remaining nits; may repeat in 1 week if lice or nits still present.

Scabies: Apply cream from head to toe; leave on for 8-14 hours before washing off with water; for infants, also apply on the hairline, neck, scalp, temple, and forehead; may reapply in 1 week if live mites appear

Permethrin 5% cream was shown to be safe and effective when applied to an infant <1 month of age with neonatal scabies; time of application was limited to 6 hours before rinsing with soap and water

**Dosage Forms**

Cream, topical (Acticin®, Elimite®): 5% (60 g) [contains coconut oil]

Lotion, topical: 1% (59 mL)

Liquid, topical [creme rinse formulation] (Nix®): 1% (60 mL) [contains isopropyl alcohol 20%]

Solution, spray [for bedding and furniture]:

A200® Lice: 0.5% (180 mL)

Nix®: 0.25% (148 mL)

Rid®: 0.5% (150 mL)

**Permitil**® **Oral** *(Discontinued)* *see* fluphenazine *on page 351*

**Peroxin A5**® *(Discontinued)* *see* benzoyl peroxide *on page 98*

**Peroxin A10**® *(Discontinued)* *see* benzoyl peroxide *on page 98*

## perphenazine (per FEN a zeen)

**Sound-Alike/Look-Alike Issues**

Trilafon® may be confused with Tri-Levlen®

**U.S./Canadian Brand Names** Apo-Perphenazine® [Can]

**Therapeutic Category** Phenothiazine Derivative

**Use** Treatment of schizophrenia; nausea and vomiting

**Usual Dosage** Oral:

Children:

Schizophrenia/psychoses:

1-6 years: 4-6 mg/day in divided doses

6-12 years: 6 mg/day in divided doses

>12 years: 4-16 mg 2-4 times/day

Adults:

Schizophrenia/psychoses: 4-16 mg 2-4 times/day not to exceed 64 mg/day

Nausea/vomiting: 8-16 mg/day in divided doses up to 24 mg/day

**Dosage Forms** Tablet: 2 mg, 4 mg, 8 mg, 16 mg

**perphenazine and amitriptyline** *see* amitriptyline and perphenazine *on page 43*

**Persa-Gel**® *(Discontinued)* *see* benzoyl peroxide *on page 98*

**Persantine**® **[US/Can]** *see* dipyridamole *on page 260*

**Pertussin**® **CS** *(Discontinued)* *see* dextromethorphan *on page 238*

**Pertussin**® **ES** *(Discontinued)* *see* dextromethorphan *on page 238*

**pethidine hydrochloride** *see* meperidine *on page 512*

**Pexeva**® **[US]** *see* paroxetine *on page 620*

**Pexicam**® **[Can]** *see* piroxicam *on page 650*

**PFA** *see* foscarnet *on page 360*

**Pfizerpen**® **[US/Can]** *see* penicillin G (parenteral/aqueous) *on page 629*

**Pfizerpen-AS**® **[Can]** *see* penicillin G procaine *on page 629*

**PGE₁** *see* alprostadil *on page 31*

**PGE₂** *see* dinoprostone *on page 253*

**PGI₂** *see* epoprostenol *on page 291*

**PGX** *see* epoprostenol *on page 291*

**Phanasin [US-OTC]** *see* guaifenesin *on page 383*

**Phanasin**® **Diabetic Choice [US-OTC]** *see* guaifenesin *on page 383*

**Phanatuss**® **DM [US-OTC]** *see* guaifenesin and dextromethorphan *on page 385*

**Pharmaflur**® **[US]** *see* fluoride *on page 347*

**Pharmaflur**® **1.1 [US]** *see* fluoride *on page 347*

**Pharmorubicin**® **[Can]** *see* epirubicin *on page 289*

**Phazyme**™ **[Can]** *see* simethicone *on page 748*

**Phazyme**® *(Discontinued)* *see* simethicone *on page 748*

**Phazyme**® **Quick Dissolve [US-OTC]** *see* simethicone *on page 748*

**Phazyme**® **Ultra Strength [US-OTC]** *see* simethicone *on page 748*

**Phenadex**® **Senior** *(Discontinued)* *see* guaifenesin and dextromethorphan *on page 385*

**Phenadoz**™ **[US]** *see* promethazine *on page 682*

**Phenameth**® **DM** *(Discontinued)* *see* promethazine and dextromethorphan *on page 683*

**Phenaphen**® *(Discontinued)* *see* acetaminophen *on page 4*

**PhenaVent**™ **[US]** *see* guaifenesin and phenylephrine *on page 387*

**PhenaVent**™ **D [US]** *see* guaifenesin and phenylephrine *on page 387*

**PhenaVent**™ **Ped [US]** *see* guaifenesin and phenylephrine *on page 387*

**Phenazine**® **Injection** *(Discontinued)* *see* promethazine *on page 682*

**Phenazo**™ **[Can]** *see* phenazopyridine *on this page*

## phenazopyridine (fen az oh PEER i deen)

**Sound-Alike/Look-Alike Issues**
Pyridium® may be confused with Dyrenium®, Perdiem®, pyridoxine, pyrithione

**Synonyms** phenazopyridine hydrochloride; phenylazo diamino pyridine hydrochloride

**U.S./Canadian Brand Names** AZO-Gesic® [US-OTC]; AZO-Standard® [US-OTC]; Baridium® [US-OTC]; Phenazo™ [Can]; Pyridium® [US]; ReAzo [US-OTC]; Uristat® [US-OTC]; UTI Relief® [US-OTC]

**Therapeutic Category** Analgesic, Urinary

**Use** Symptomatic relief of urinary burning, itching, frequency and urgency in association with urinary tract infection or following urologic procedures

**Usual Dosage** Oral:
Children: 12 mg/kg/day in 3 divided doses administered after meals for 2 days
Adults: 100-200 mg 3 times/day after meals for 2 days when used concomitantly with an antibacterial agent

**Dosage Forms**
Tablet, as hydrochloride: 100 mg, 200 mg
AZO-Gesic®, AZO-Standard®, Uristat®: 95 mg
Baridium®: 97.2 mg
ReAzo: 95 mg
Pyridium®: 100 mg, 200 mg
UTI Relief®: 97.2 mg

**phenazopyridine hydrochloride** *see* phenazopyridine *on previous page*

# phendimetrazine (fen dye ME tra zeen)
**Sound-Alike/Look-Alike Issues**
   Bontril PDM® may be confused with Bentyl®
**Synonyms** phendimetrazine tartrate
**U.S./Canadian Brand Names** Bontril® PDM [US]; Bontril® Slow-Release [US]; Bontril® [Can]; Melfiat® [US]; Plegine® [Can]; Statobex® [Can]
**Therapeutic Category** Anorexiant
**Controlled Substance** C-III
**Use** Appetite suppressant during the first few weeks of dieting to help establish new eating habits; its effectiveness lasts only for short periods (3-12 weeks)
**Usual Dosage** Adults: Oral:
   Tablet: 35 mg 2 or 3 times daily, 1 hour before meals
   Capsule, timed release: 105 mg once daily in the morning before breakfast
**Dosage Forms** [DSC] = Discontinued product
   Capsule, slow release, as tartrate (Bontril® Slow Release, Prelu-2® [DSC]): 105 mg
   Capsule, sustained release, as tartrate (Melfiat®): 105 mg
   Tablet, as tartrate (Bontril PDM®, Obezine® [DSC]): 35 mg

**phendimetrazine tartrate** *see* phendimetrazine *on this page*

**Phendry® Oral *(Discontinued)*** *see* diphenhydramine *on page 254*

# phenelzine (FEN el zeen)
**Sound-Alike/Look-Alike Issues**
   phenelzine may be confused with phenytoin
   Nardil® may be confused with Norinyl®
**Synonyms** phenelzine sulfate
**U.S./Canadian Brand Names** Nardil® [US/Can]
**Therapeutic Category** Antidepressant, Monoamine Oxidase Inhibitor
**Use** Symptomatic treatment of atypical, nonendogenous, or neurotic depression
**Usual Dosage** Oral: Adults: Depression: 15 mg 3 times/day; may increase to 60-90 mg/day during early phase of treatment, then reduce dose for maintenance therapy slowly after maximum benefit is obtained; takes 2-4 weeks for a significant response to occur
**Dosage Forms** Tablet: 15 mg

**phenelzine sulfate** *see* phenelzine *on this page*

**Phenerbel-S® *(Discontinued)***

**Phenergan® [US/Can]** *see* promethazine *on page 682*

**Phenergan® VC With Codeine *(Discontinued)*** *see* promethazine, phenylephrine, and codeine *on page 684*

**Phenergan® With Dextromethorphan *(Discontinued)*** *see* promethazine and dextromethorphan *on page 683*

# phenindamine (fen IN dah meen)
**Synonyms** phenindamine tartrate
**U.S./Canadian Brand Names** Nolahist® [US-OTC/Can]
**Therapeutic Category** Antihistamine
**Use** Treatment of perennial and seasonal allergic rhinitis and chronic urticaria
**Usual Dosage** Oral:
   Children <6 years: As directed by physician
   Children 6 to <12 years: 12.5 mg every 4-6 hours, up to 75 mg/24 hours
   Adults: 25 mg every 4-6 hours, up to 150 mg/24 hours
**Dosage Forms** Tablet, as tartrate: 25 mg [DSC]

**phenindamine tartrate** *see* phenindamine *on this page*

**pheniramine and naphazoline** *see* naphazoline and pheniramine *on page 561*

# phenobarbital (fee noe BAR bi tal)

**Sound-Alike/Look-Alike Issues**
phenobarbital may be confused with pentobarbital
Luminal® may be confused with Tuinal®

**Synonyms** phenobarbital sodium; phenobarbitone; phenylethylmalonylurea

**U.S./Canadian Brand Names** Luminal® Sodium [US]; PMS-Phenobarbital [Can]

**Therapeutic Category** Anticonvulsant; Barbiturate

**Controlled Substance** C-IV

**Use** Management of generalized tonic-clonic (grand mal) and partial seizures; sedative

**Usual Dosage**
Children:
Sedation: Oral: 2 mg/kg 3 times/day
Hypnotic: I.M., I.V., SubQ: 3-5 mg/kg at bedtime
Preoperative sedation: Oral, I.M., I.V.: 1-3 mg/kg 1-1.5 hours before procedure
Adults:
Sedation: Oral, I.M.: 30-120 mg/day in 2-3 divided doses
Hypnotic: Oral, I.M., I.V., SubQ: 100-320 mg at bedtime
Preoperative sedation: I.M.: 100-200 mg 1-1.5 hours before procedure

Anticonvulsant: Status epilepticus: **Loading dose:** I.V.:
Infants and Children: 10-20 mg/kg in a single or divided dose; in select patients may administer additional 5 mg/kg/dose every 15-30 minutes until seizure is controlled or a total dose of 40 mg/kg is reached
Adults: 300-800 mg initially followed by 120-240 mg/dose at 20-minute intervals until seizures are controlled or a total dose of 1-2 g
Anticonvulsant maintenance dose: Oral, I.V.:
Infants: 5-8 mg/kg/day in 1-2 divided doses
Children:
1-5 years: 6-8 mg/kg/day in 1-2 divided doses
5-12 years: 4-6 mg/kg/day in 1-2 divided doses
Children >12 years and Adults: 1-3 mg/kg/day in divided doses or 50-100 mg 2-3 times/day

**Dosage Forms**
Elixir: 20 mg/5 mL (473 mL) [contains alcohol]
Injection, solution, as sodium: 65 mg/mL (1 mL); 130 mg/mL (1 mL) [contains alcohol and propylene glycol]
Luminal® Sodium: 60 mg/mL (1 mL); 130 mg/mL (1 mL) [contains alcohol 10% and propylene glycol]
Tablet: 15 mg, 30 mg, 32 mg, 60 mg, 65 mg, 100 mg

**phenobarbital, belladonna, and ergotamine tartrate** *see* belladonna, phenobarbital, and ergotamine tartrate *on page 92*

**phenobarbital, hyoscyamine, atropine, and scopolamine** *see* hyoscyamine, atropine, scopolamine, and phenobarbital *on page 425*

**phenobarbital sodium** *see* phenobarbital *on this page*

**phenobarbitone** *see* phenobarbital *on this page*

# phenol (FEE nol)

**Sound-Alike/Look-Alike Issues**
Cēpastat® may be confused with Capastat®

**Synonyms** carbolic acid

**U.S./Canadian Brand Names** Castellani Paint Modified [US]; Cepastat® Extra Strength [US-OTC]; Cepastat® [US-OTC]; Chloraseptic® Gargle [US-OTC]; Chloraseptic® Mouth Pain Spray [US-OTC]; Chloraseptic® Rinse [US-OTC]; Chloraseptic® Spray for Kids [US-OTC]; Chloraseptic® Spray [US-OTC]; P & S™ Liquid Phenol [Can]; Pain-A-Lay® [US-OTC]; Ulcerease® [US-OTC]

**Therapeutic Category** Pharmaceutical Aid

**Use** Relief of sore throat pain, mouth, gum, and throat irritations; neurologic pain, rectal prolapse, hemorrhoids, hydrocele

**Usual Dosage**
Allow to dissolve slowly in mouth; may be repeated every 2 hours as needed
For each neurolysis procedure: 0.5-2 mL (up to 7.5 mL may be needed)

**Dosage Forms**
Liquid, oral (Ulcerease®): 0.6% (180 mL) [contains glycerin; sugar free]

Lozenge:

Cēpastat®: 14.5 mg (18s) [ contains eucalyptus oil and menthol; sugar free; cherry flavor]

Cēpastat® Extra Strength: 29 mg (18s) [contains eucalyptus oil and menthol; sugar free; eucalyptus flavor]

Solution, oral:

Chloraseptic® [gargle]: 1.4% (296 mL) [cool mint flavor]

Chloraseptic® [rinse]: 1.4% (240 mL) [cinnamon flavor]

Pain-A-Lay®: 1.4% (240 mL) [gargle; contains tartrazine]

Solution, oral spray: 1.4% (180 mL)

Chloraseptic®: 1.4% (180 mL) [cherry flavor]

Chloraseptic® for Kids: 0.5% (177 mL) [grape flavor]

Chloraseptic® Mouth Pain Spray: 1.4% (30 mL) [cherry blast or cool mint flavor]

Pain-A-Lay®: 1.4% (180 mL) [contains tartrazine]

Solution, topical: Phenol 1.5%, alcohol 13%, basic fuchsin, resorcinol, acetone (30 mL, 480 mL)

**phenol and camphor** *see* camphor and phenol *on page 136*

**Phenoptic® [US]** *see* phenylephrine *on next page*

**Phenoxine® *(Discontinued)***

# phenoxybenzamine (fen oks ee BEN za meen)

**Synonyms** phenoxybenzamine hydrochloride

**U.S./Canadian Brand Names** Dibenzyline® [US/Can]

**Therapeutic Category** Alpha-Adrenergic Blocking Agent

**Use** Symptomatic management of pheochromocytoma; treatment of hypertensive crisis caused by sympathomimetic amines

**Usual Dosage** Oral:

Children: Initial: 0.2 mg/kg (maximum: 10 mg) once daily, increase by 0.2 mg/kg increments; usual maintenance dose: 0.4-1.2 mg/kg/day every 6-8 hours, higher doses may be necessary

Adults: Initial: 10 mg twice daily, increase by 10 mg every other day until optimum dose is achieved; usual range: 20-40 mg 2-3 times/day

**Dosage Forms** Capsule, as hydrochloride: 10 mg [contains benzyl alcohol]

**phenoxybenzamine hydrochloride** *see* phenoxybenzamine *on this page*

**phenoxymethyl penicillin** *see* penicillin V potassium *on page 627*

# phentermine (FEN ter meen)

**Sound-Alike/Look-Alike Issues**

phentermine may be confused with phentolamine, phenytoin

Ionamin® may be confused with Imodium®

**Synonyms** phentermine hydrochloride

**U.S./Canadian Brand Names** Adipex-P® [US]; Ionamin® [US/Can]

**Therapeutic Category** Anorexiant

**Controlled Substance** C-IV

**Use** Short-term adjunct in a regimen of weight reduction based on exercise, behavioral modification, and caloric reduction in the management of exogenous obesity for patients with an initial body mass index $\geq$30 kg/m$^2$ or $\geq$27 kg/m$^2$ in the presence of other risk factors (diabetes, hypertension)

**Usual Dosage** Oral: Adults: Obesity: 8 mg 3 times/day 30 minutes before meals or food or 15-37.5 mg/day before breakfast or 10-14 hours before retiring

**Dosage Forms**

Capsule, as hydrochloride: 15 mg, 30 mg

Adipex-P®: 37.5 mg

Capsule, resin complex (Ionamin®): 15 mg, 30 mg

Tablet, as hydrochloride (Adipex-P®): 37.5 mg

**phentermine hydrochloride** *see* phentermine *on this page*

# phentolamine (fen TOLE a meen)

**Sound-Alike/Look-Alike Issues**

phentolamine may be confused with phentermine, Ventolin®

(Continued)

# phentolamine *(Continued)*

**Synonyms** phentolamine mesylate

**U.S./Canadian Brand Names** Regitine® [Can]; Rogitine® [Can]

**Therapeutic Category** Alpha-Adrenergic Blocking Agent; Diagnostic Agent

**Use** Diagnosis of pheochromocytoma and treatment of hypertension associated with pheochromocytoma or other forms of hypertension caused by excess sympathomimetic amines; as treatment of dermal necrosis after extravasation of drugs with alpha-adrenergic effects (norepinephrine, dopamine, epinephrine)

**Usual Dosage**

Treatment of alpha-adrenergic drug extravasation: SubQ:

Children: 0.1-0.2 mg/kg diluted in 10 mL 0.9% sodium chloride infiltrated into area of extravasation within 12 hours

Adults: Infiltrate area with small amount of solution made by diluting 5-10 mg in 10 mL 0.9% sodium chloride within 12 hours of extravasation; do not exceed 0.1-0.2 mg/kg or 5 mg total

If dose is effective, normal skin color should return to the blanched area within 1 hour

Diagnosis of pheochromocytoma: I.M., I.V.:

Children: 0.05-0.1 mg/kg/dose, maximum single dose: 5 mg

Adults: 5 mg

Surgery for pheochromocytoma: Hypertension: I.M., I.V.:

Children: 0.05-0.1 mg/kg/dose given 1-2 hours before procedure; repeat as needed every 2-4 hours until hypertension is controlled; maximum single dose: 5 mg

Adults: 5 mg given 1-2 hours before procedure and repeated as needed every 2-4 hours

Hypertensive crisis: Adults: 5-20 mg

**Dosage Forms** Injection, powder for reconstitution, as mesylate: 5 mg

**phentolamine mesylate** *see* phentolamine *on previous page*

**phenylalanine mustard** *see* melphalan *on page 509*

**phenylazo diamino pyridine hydrochloride** *see* phenazopyridine *on page 636*

**Phenyldrine® *(Discontinued)***

# phenylephrine *(fen il EF rin)*

**Sound-Alike/Look-Alike Issues**

Mydfrin® may be confused with Midrin®

**Synonyms** phenylephrine hydrochloride

**U.S./Canadian Brand Names** AK-Dilate® [US]; AK-Nefrin® [US]; Dionephrine® [Can]; Formulation R™ [US-OTC]; Medicone® [US-OTC]; Mydfrin® [US/Can]; Neo-Synephrine® Extra Strength [US-OTC]; Neo-Synephrine® Mild [US-OTC]; Neo-Synephrine® Ophthalmic [US]; Neo-Synephrine® Regular Strength [US-OTC]; Neo-Synephrine® [Can]; Nostril® [US-OTC]; Phenoptic® [US]; Relief® [US-OTC]; Vicks® Sinex® Nasal Spray [US-OTC]; Vicks® Sinex® UltraFine Mist [US-OTC]

**Therapeutic Category** Adrenergic Agonist Agent

**Use** Treatment of hypotension, vascular failure in shock; as a vasoconstrictor in regional analgesia; as a mydriatic in ophthalmic procedures and treatment of wide-angle glaucoma; supraventricular tachycardia

For OTC use as symptomatic relief of nasal and nasopharyngeal mucosal congestion, treatment of hemorrhoids, relief of redness of the eye due to irritation

**Usual Dosage**

Ocular procedures:

Infants <1 year: Instill 1 drop of 2.5% 15-30 minutes before procedures

Children and Adults: Instill 1 drop of 2.5% or 10% solution, may repeat in 10-60 minutes as needed

Ophthalmic irritation (OTC formulation for relief of eye redness): Adults: Instill 1-2 drops 0.12% solution into affected eye, up to 4 times/day; do not use for >72 hours

Nasal decongestant (therapy should not exceed 3 continuous days):

Children:

2-6 years: Instill 1 drop every 2-4 hours of 0.125% solution as needed

6-12 years: Instill 1-2 sprays or instill 1-2 drops every 4 hours of 0.25% solution as needed

Children >12 years and Adults: Instill 1-2 sprays or instill 1-2 drops every 4 hours of 0.25% to 0.5% solution as needed; 1% solution may be used in adult in cases of extreme nasal congestion; do not use nasal solutions more than 3 days

Hypotension/shock:

Children:

I.V. bolus: 5-20 mcg/kg/dose every 10-15 minutes as needed

I.V. infusion: 0.1-0.5 mcg/kg/minute

Adults:

I.V. bolus: 0.1-0.5 mg/dose every 10-15 minutes as needed (initial dose should not exceed 0.5 mg)

I.V. infusion: 10 mg in 250 mL D$_5$W or NS (1:25,000 dilution) (40 mcg/mL); start at 100-180 mcg/minute (2-5 mL/minute; 50-90 drops/minute) initially; when blood pressure is stabilized, maintenance rate: 40-60 mcg/minute (20-30 drops/minute); rates up to 360 mcg/minute have been reported; dosing range: 0.4-9.1 mcg/kg/minute

**Note:** Concentrations up to 100-500 mg in 250 mL have been used.

Paroxysmal supraventricular tachycardia: I.V.:

Children: 5-10 mcg/kg/dose over 20-30 seconds

Adults: 0.25-0.5 mg/dose over 20-30 seconds

Hemorrhoids: Children ≥12 years and Adults: Rectal:

Cream/ointment: Apply to clean dry area, up to 4 times/day; may be used externally or inserted rectally using applicator.

Suppository: Insert 1 suppository rectally, up to 4 times/day

**Dosage Forms** [DSC] = Discontinued product

Cream, rectal, as hydrochloride (Formulation R™): 0.25% (54 g) [contains sodium benzoate]

Injection, solution, as hydrochloride: 1% [10 mg/mL] (1 mL, 5 mL) [may contain sodium metabisulfite]

Neo Synephrine®: 1% (1 mL) [contains sodium metabisulfite]

Ointment, rectal, as hydrochloride:

Formulation R™: 0.25% (30 g, 60 g) [contains benzoic acid]

Rectacaine: 0.25% (30 g) [contains shark liver oil]

Solution, intranasal drops, as hydrochloride:

Neo-Synephrine® Extra Strength: 1% (15 mL) [contains benzalkonium chloride]

Neo-Synephrine® Regular Strength: 0.5% (15 mL) [contains benzalkonium chloride]

Rhinall: 0.25% (30 mL) [contains benzalkonium chloride and sodium bisulfite]

Solution, intranasal spray, as hydrochloride:

Neo-Synephrine® Extra Strength: 1% (15 mL) [contains benzalkonium chloride]

Neo-Synephrine® Mild: 0.25% (15 mL) [contains benzalkonium chloride]

Neo-Synephrine® Regular Strength: 0.5% (15 mL) [contains benzalkonium chloride]

Rhinall: 0.25% (40 mL) [contains benzalkonium chloride and sodium bisulfite]

Vicks® Sinex®, Vicks® Sinex® UltraFine Mist: 0.5% (15 mL) [contains benzalkonium chloride]

Solution, ophthalmic, as hydrochloride: 2.5% (1 mL, 2 mL, 3 mL, 5 mL, 15 mL) [may contain sodium bisulfite]

AK-Dilate®: 2.5% (2 mL, 15 mL); 10% (5 mL)

Altrafrin: 0.12% (15 mL) [OTC]; 2.5% (5 mL, 15 mL) [RX; contains benzalkonium chloride]; 10% (5 mL) [RX; contains benzalkonium chloride]

Mydfrin®: 2.5% (3 mL, 5 mL) [contains sodium bisulfite]

Neo-Synephrine®: 2.5% (15 mL); 10% (5 mL) [contains benzalkonium chloride] [DSC]

Neo-Synephrine® Viscous: 10% (5 mL) [contains benzalkonium chloride] [DSC]

Suppository, rectal, as hydrochloride: 0.25% (12s)

Anu-Med, Tronolane®: 0.25% (12s)

Medicone®: 0.25% (18s, 24s)

Rectacaine: 0.25% (12s) [contains shark liver oil]

Suspension, oral, as tannate (NāSop™): 7.5 mg/5 mL (120 mL) [orange flavor]

Tablet, as hydrochloride (Sudafed PE™): 10 mg

Tablet, chewable, as hydrochloride (AH-chew® D): 10 mg

Tablet, orally dissolving, as hydrochloride (NāSop™): 10 mg [contains phenylalanine 4 mg/tablet; bubble gum flavor]

**phenylephrine and chlorpheniramine** *see* chlorpheniramine and phenylephrine *on page 171*

**phenylephrine and cyclopentolate** *see* cyclopentolate and phenylephrine *on page 214*

**phenylephrine and promethazine** *see* promethazine and phenylephrine *on page 684*

# phenylephrine and pyrilamine (fen il EF rin & peer IL a meen)

**Synonyms** pyrilamine tannate and phenylephrine tannate

**U.S./Canadian Brand Names** Pyrilafen Tannate-12™ [US]; Ry-T 12 [US]; Ryna-12 S™ [US]; Ryna-12™ [US]; V-Tann [US]; Viravan® [US]

**Therapeutic Category** Antihistamine; Antihistamine/Decongestant Combination; Sympathomimetic

**Use** Symptomatic relief of nasal congestion and discharge associated with the common cold, sinusitis, allergic rhinitis, and other respiratory tract conditions

(Continued)

## phenylephrine and pyrilamine (Continued)

**Usual Dosage** Oral: Relief of cough, congestion (Viravan®):
Children 2-6 years: 2.5 mL of the suspension or ½ tablet every 12 hours
Children 6-12 years: 5 mL of the suspension or ½ to 1 tablet every 12 hours
Children >12 years and Adults: 5-10 mL of the suspension or 1-2 tablets every 12 hours

**Dosage Forms**
Suspension:
Pyrilafen Tannate-12™: Phenylephrine tannate 5 mg and pyrilamine tannate 30 mg per 5 mL (120 mL, 480 mL) [strawberry-black currant flavor]
Ryna-12 S™: Phenylephrine tannate 5 mg and pyrilamine tannate 30 mg per 5 mL (120 mL) [contains benzoic acid; strawberry-currant flavor]
Ry-T 12: Phenylephrine tannate 5 mg and pyrilamine tannate 30 mg per 5 mL (120 mL, 480 mL)
Viravan®, V-Tann: Phenylephrine tannate 12.5 mg and pyrilamine tannate 30 mg per 5 mL (120 mL, 480 mL) [contains sodium benzoate; grape flavor]
Tablet (Ryna-12™): Phenylephrine tannate 25 mg and pyrilamine tannate 60 mg
Tablet, chewable (Viravan®): Phenylephrine tannate 25 mg and pyrilamine tannate 30 mg [dye free; grape flavor]

## phenylephrine and scopolamine (fen il EF rin & skoe POL a meen)

**Sound-Alike/Look-Alike Issues**
Murocoll-2® may be confused with Murocel®
**Synonyms** scopolamine and phenylephrine
**U.S./Canadian Brand Names** Murocoll-2® [US]
**Therapeutic Category** Anticholinergic/Adrenergic Agonist
**Use** Mydriasis, cycloplegia, and to break posterior synechiae in iritis
**Usual Dosage** Ophthalmic: Instill 1-2 drops into eye(s); repeat in 5 minutes
**Dosage Forms** Solution, ophthalmic: Phenylephrine hydrochloride 10% and scopolamine hydrobromide 0.3% (5 mL) [contains benzalkonium chloride and sodium metabisulfite]

## phenylephrine and zinc sulfate (fen il EF rin & zingk SUL fate)

**Synonyms** zinc sulfate and phenylephrine
**U.S./Canadian Brand Names** Zincfrin® [US-OTC/Can]
**Therapeutic Category** Adrenergic Agonist Agent
**Use** Soothe, moisturize, and remove redness due to minor eye irritation
**Usual Dosage** Ophthalmic: Instill 1-2 drops in eye(s) 2-4 times/day as needed
**Dosage Forms** Solution, ophthalmic: Phenylephrine hydrochloride 0.12% and zinc sulfate 0.25% (15 mL)

**phenylephrine, chlorpheniramine, and carbetapentane** *see carbetapentane, phenylephrine, and chlorpheniramine on page 142*

**phenylephrine, chlorpheniramine, and dextromethorphan** *see chlorpheniramine, phenylephrine, and dextromethorphan on page 174*

**phenylephrine, chlorpheniramine, and methscopolamine** *see chlorpheniramine, phenylephrine, and methscopolamine on page 175*

**phenylephrine, chlorpheniramine, and phenyltoloxamine** *see chlorpheniramine, phenylephrine, and phenyltoloxamine on page 176*

**phenylephrine, chlorpheniramine, codeine, and potassium iodide** *see chlorpheniramine, phenylephrine, codeine, and potassium iodide on page 176*

**phenylephrine, diphenhydramine, and hydrocodone** *see hydrocodone, phenylephrine, and diphenhydramine on page 414*

**phenylephrine, ephedrine, chlorpheniramine, and carbetapentane** *see chlorpheniramine, ephedrine, phenylephrine, and carbetapentane on page 173*

**phenylephrine hydrochloride** *see phenylephrine on page 640*

**phenylephrine hydrochloride and guaifenesin** *see guaifenesin and phenylephrine on page 387*

**phenylephrine hydrochloride, hydrocodone bitartrate, and chlorpheniramine maleate** *see phenylephrine, hydrocodone, and chlorpheniramine on next page*

# phenylephrine, hydrocodone, and chlorpheniramine

(fen il EF rin, hye droe KOE done, & klor fen IR a meen)

**Synonyms** chlorpheniramine, phenylephrine, and hydrocodone; dihydrocodeine bitartrate, phenylephrine hydrochloride, and chlorpheniramine maleate; hydrocodone, phenylephrine, and chlorpheniramine; phenylephrine hydrochloride, hydrocodone bitartrate, and chlorpheniramine maleate

**U.S./Canadian Brand Names** Coughtuss [US]; Cytuss HC [US]; De-Chlor HC [US]; De-Chlor HD [US]; Endagen™-HD [US]; Endal® HD Plus [US]; H-C Tussive [US]; Histinex® HC [US]; Histussin® HC [US]; Hydro PC II Plus [US]; Hydro-PC II [US]; Hydron CP [US]; Maxi-Tuss HCX [US]; Maxi-Tuss HC® [US]; Mintuss HC [US]; Mintuss HD [US]; Mintuss MS [US]; Relacon-HC [US]; Rindal HD Plus [US]; Uni-Tricof HC [US]; Uni-Tuss HC [US]; Vanex-HD® [US]; Z-Cof HC [US]

**Therapeutic Category** Antihistamine; Antihistamine/Decongestant/Antitussive; Antitussive; Decongestant

**Controlled Substance** C-III

**Use** Symptomatic relief of cough and congestion associated with the common cold, sinusitis, or acute upper respiratory tract infections

**Usual Dosage** Oral:

Children 2-6 years: Z-Cof HC: 1.25-2.5 mL every 4-6 hours (maximum: 10 mL/24 hours)

Children 6-12 years:

Endagen™-HD, Vanex-HD®: 5 mL 3-4 times/day (maximum: 20 mL/24 hours)

Histinex® HC, Cytuss HC, Endal® HD Plus: 5 mL every 4 hours (maximum: 20 mL/24 hours)

Maxi-Tuss HC®, Maxi-Tuss HCX: 2.5 mL every 4 hours (maximum: 15 mL/24 hours)

Z-Cof HC: 2.5-5 mL every 4-6 hours as needed (maximum: 20 mL/24 hours)

Adults:

Endagen™-HD, Vanex-HD®: 10 mL 3-4 times/day (maximum: 40 mL/24 hours)

Histinex® HC, Cytuss HC, Endal® HD Plus: 10 mL every 4 hours (maximum: 40 mL/24 hours)

Maxi-Tuss HC®, Maxi-Tuss HCX: 5 mL every 4 hours (maximum: 30 mL/24 hours)

Z-Cof HC: 5-10 mL every 4-6 hours (maximum: 40 mL/24 hours)

**Dosage Forms**

Liquid: Phenylephrine hydrochloride 5 mg, hydrocodone bitartrate 5 mg, and chlorpheniramine maleate 2 mg per 5 mL (480 mL); phenylephrine hydrochloride 10 mg, hydrocodone bitartrate 2.5 mg, and chlorpheniramine maleate 4 mg per 5 mL (480 mL); phenylephrine hydrochloride 10 mg, hydrocodone bitartrate 5 mg, and chlorpheniramine maleate 2 mg per 5 mL (480 mL)

Coughtuss: Phenylephrine hydrochloride 5 mg, hydrocodone bitartrate 5 mg, and chlorpheniramine maleate 2 mg per 5 mL (480 mL) [alcohol free, sugar free]

De-Chlor HC: Phenylephrine hydrochloride 10 mg, hydrocodone bitartrate 2.5 mg, and chlorpheniramine maleate 2 mg per 5 mL (480 mL) [cherry flavor]

De-Chlor HD: Phenylephrine hydrochloride 10 mg, hydrocodone bitartrate 2.5 mg, and chlorpheniramine maleate 4 mg per 5 mL (480 mL) [cherry flavor]

Endal® HD Plus: Phenylephrine hydrochloride 7.5 mg, hydrocodone bitartrate 3.5 mg, and chlorpheniramine maleate 2 mg per 5 mL (480 mL) [alcohol free, sugar free; black raspberry flavor]

Hydron CP: Phenylephrine hydrochloride 10 mg, hydrocodone bitartrate 5 mg, and chlorpheniramine maleate 2 mg per 5 mL (480 mL) [pineapple-orange flavor]

Hydro PC II Plus: Phenylephrine hydrochloride 7.5 mg, hydrocodone bitartrate 3.5 mg, and chlorpheniramine maleate 2 mg per 5 mL (480 mL) [strawberry flavor]

Maxi-Tuss HCX: Phenylephrine hydrochloride 12 mg, hydrocodone bitartrate 6 mg and chlorpheniramine maleate 2 mg per 5 mL (480 mL) [alcohol free, sugar free; contains aspartame; vanilla bean flavor]

Relacon-HC: Phenylephrine hydrochloride 10 mg, hydrocodone bitartrate 3.5 mg, and chlorpheniramine maleate 2.5 mg per 5 mL (480 mL) [raspberry flavor]

Uni-Tricof HC: Phenylephrine hydrochloride 5 mg, hydrocodone bitartrate 1.67 mg, and chlorpheniramine maleate 2 mg per 5 mL (480 mL) [strawberry flavor]

Vanex-HD®: Phenylephrine hydrochloride 5 mg, hydrocodone bitartrate 1.7 mg, and chlorpheniramine maleate 2 mg per 5mL (480 mL) [dye free; cherry flavor]

Z-Cof HC: Phenylephrine hydrochloride 10 mg, hydrocodone bitartrate 3.5 mg, and chlorpheniramine maleate 2.5 mg per 5 mL (480 mL) [alcohol free, sugar free; raspberry flavor]

Syrup:

Cytuss HC: Phenylephrine hydrochloride 5 mg, hydrocodone bitartrate 2.5 mg, and chlorpheniramine maleate 2 mg per 5 mL (480 mL) [peach flavor]

Endagen™-HD: Phenylephrine hydrochloride 5 mg, hydrocodone bitartrate 1.7 mg, and chlorpheniramine maleate 2 mg per 5 mL (480 mL) [cherry flavor]

H-C Tussive: Phenylephrine hydrochloride 5 mg, hydrocodone bitartrate 2.5 mg, and chlorpheniramine maleate 2 mg per 5 mL (120 mL, 480 mL, 4000 mL) [orange-pineapple flavor]

(Continued)

## phenylephrine, hydrocodone, and chlorpheniramine *(Continued)*

Histinex® HC: Phenylephrine hydrochloride 5 mg, hydrocodone bitartrate 2.5 mg, and chlorpheniramine maleate 2 mg per 5 mL (480 mL, 960 mL) [alcohol free, sugar free; contains sodium benzoate]

Histussin® HC: Phenylephrine hydrochloride 5 mg, hydrocodone bitartrate 2.5 mg, and chlorpheniramine maleate 2 mg per 5 mL (480 mL) [alcohol free, sugar free; orange-pineapple flavor]

Hydro-PC II: Phenylephrine hydrochloride 7.5 mg, hydrocodone bitartrate 2 mg, and chlorpheniramine maleate 2 mg per 5 mL (480 mL) [strawberry flavor]

Maxi-Tuss HC®: Phenylephrine hydrochloride 10 mg, hydrocodone bitartrate 2.5 mg, and chlorpheniramine maleate 4 mg per 5 mL (480 mL) [orange flavor]

Mintuss HC: Phenylephrine hydrochloride 10 mg, hydrocodone bitartrate 2.5 mg, and chlorpheniramine maleate 2 mg per 5 mL (480 mL) [alcohol free; contains sodium benzoate; black cherry flavor]

Mintuss HD: Phenylephrine hydrochloride 10 mg, hydrocodone bitartrate 2.5 mg, and chlorpheniramine maleate 4 mg per 5 mL (480 mL) [alcohol free; contains sodium benzoate; cherry flavor]

Mintuss MS: Phenylephrine hydrochloride 10 mg, hydrocodone bitartrate 5 mg, and chlorpheniramine maleate 2 mg per 5 mL (480 mL) [alcohol free; contains sodium benzoate; orange flavor]

Rindal HD Plus: Phenylephrine hydrochloride 7.5 mg, hydrocodone bitartrate 3.5 mg, and chlorpheniramine maleate 2 mg per 5 mL (480 mL) [alcohol free, sugar free; contains sodium benzoate; black raspberry flavor]

Uni-Tuss HC: Phenylephrine hydrochloride 5 mg, hydrocodone bitartrate 1.67 mg, and chlorpheniramine maleate 2 mg per 5 mL (480 mL) [sugar free; orange flavor]

**phenylephrine, hydrocodone, chlorpheniramine, acetaminophen, and caffeine** *see* hydrocodone, chlorpheniramine, phenylephrine, acetaminophen, and caffeine *on page 414*

**phenylephrine, promethazine, and codeine** *see* promethazine, phenylephrine, and codeine *on page 684*

## phenylephrine, pyrilamine, and dextromethorphan

(fen il EF rin, peer IL a meen, & deks troe meth OR fan)

**Synonyms** dextromethorphan tannate, pyrilamine tannate, and phenylephrine tannate; pyrilamine maleate, dextromethorphan hydrobromide, and phenylephrine hydrochloride

**U.S./Canadian Brand Names** Codal-DM [US-OTC]; Codimal® DM [US-OTC]; Codituss DM [US-OTC]; Viravan®-DM [US]

**Therapeutic Category** Antihistamine; Antihistamine/Decongestant/Antitussive; Antitussive; Sympathomimetic

**Use** Symptomatic relief of cough, nasal congestion, and discharge associated with the common cold, sinusitis, allergic rhinitis, and other respiratory tract conditions

**Usual Dosage** Oral: Relief of cough, congestion:

Children 2-6 years (Viravan®-DM): 2.5 mL of the suspension or ½ tablet every 12 hours

Children 6-12 years:
Codimal® DM: 5 mL every 4 hours; maximum: 30 mL/24 hours
Viravan®-DM: 5 mL of the suspension or ½ to 1 tablet every 12 hours

Children >12 years and Adults:
Codimal® DM: 10 mL every 4 hours; maximum: 60 mL/24 hours
Viravan®-DM: 5-10 mL of the suspension or 1-2 tablets every 12 hours

**Dosage Forms**

Suspension (Viravan®-DM): Phenylephrine tannate 12.5 mg, pyrilamine tannate 30 mg, and dextromethorphan tannate 25 mg per 5 mL (480 mL) [contains sodium benzoate; grape flavor]

Syrup:
Codal-DM: Phenylephrine hydrochloride 5 mg, pyrilamine maleate 8.33 mg, and dextromethorphan hydrobromide 10 mg (480 mL) [cherry flavor]

Codimal® DM: Phenylephrine hydrochloride 5 mg, pyrilamine maleate 8.33 mg, and dextromethorphan hydrobromide 10 mg (120 mL, 480 mL) [alcohol free, dye free, sugar free; contains benzoic acid]

Codituss DM: Phenylephrine hydrochloride 5 mg, pyrilamine maleate 8.33 mg, and dextromethorphan hydrobromide 10 mg (120 mL, 480 mL) [alcohol free, dye free, sugar free; cherry punch flavor]

Tablet, chewable (Viravan®-DM): Phenylephrine tannate 25 mg, pyrilamine tannate 30 mg, and dextromethorphan tannate 25 mg [dye free; grape flavor]

**phenylethylmalonylurea** *see* phenobarbital *on page 638*

**Phenylfenesin® L.A.** *(Discontinued)*

**Phenylgesic® [US-OTC]** *see* acetaminophen and phenyltoloxamine *on page 8*

**phenylisohydantoin** *see* pemoline *on page 626*

**phenyltoloxamine and acetaminophen** *see* acetaminophen and phenyltoloxamine *on page 8*

**phenyltoloxamine, chlorpheniramine, and phenylephrine** *see* chlorpheniramine, phenylephrine, and phenyltoloxamine *on page 176*

**Phenytek™ [US]** *see* phenytoin *on this page*

## phenytoin (FEN i toyn)

**Sound-Alike/Look-Alike Issues**
    phenytoin may be confused with phenelzine, phentermine
    Dilantin® may be confused with Dilaudid®, diltiazem, Dipentum®

**Synonyms** diphenylhydantoin; DPH; phenytoin sodium, extended; phenytoin sodium, prompt; phenytoin sodium

**U.S./Canadian Brand Names** Dilantin® [US/Can]; Phenytek™ [US]

**Therapeutic Category** Antiarrhythmic Agent, Class I-B; Hydantoin

**Use** Management of generalized tonic-clonic (grand mal), complex partial seizures; prevention of seizures following head trauma/neurosurgery

**Usual Dosage**
  Status epilepticus: I.V.:
    Infants and Children: Loading dose: 15-20 mg/kg in a single or divided dose; maintenance dose: Initial: 5 mg/kg/day in 2 divided doses; usual doses:
      6 months to 3 years: 8-10 mg/kg/day
      4-6 years: 7.5-9 mg/kg/day
      7-9 years: 7-8 mg/kg/day
      10-16 years: 6-7 mg/kg/day, some patients may require every 8 hours dosing
    Adults: Loading dose: Manufacturer recommends 10-15 mg/kg, however, 15-25 mg/kg has been used clinically; maintenance dose: 300 mg/day or 5-6 mg/kg/day in 3 divided doses or 1-2 divided doses using extended release
  Anticonvulsant: Children and Adults: Oral:
    Loading dose: 15-20 mg/kg; based on phenytoin serum concentrations and recent dosing history; administer oral loading dose in 3 divided doses given every 2-4 hours to decrease GI adverse effects and to ensure complete oral absorption; maintenance dose: same as I.V.
    Neurosurgery (prophylactic): 100-200 mg at approximately 4-hour intervals during surgery and during the immediate postoperative period

**Dosage Forms**
  Capsule, extended release, as sodium:
    Dilantin®: 30 mg [contains sodium benzoate], 100 mg
    Phenytek™: 200 mg, 300 mg
  Capsule, prompt release, as sodium: 100 mg
  Injection, solution, as sodium: 50 mg/mL (2 mL, 5 mL) [contains alcohol and propylene glycol]
  Suspension, oral (Dilantin®): 125 mg/5 mL (240 mL) [contains alcohol <0.6%, sodium benzoate; banana flavor]
  Tablet, chewable (Dilantin®): 50 mg

**phenytoin sodium** *see* phenytoin *on this page*

**phenytoin sodium, extended** *see* phenytoin *on this page*

**phenytoin sodium, prompt** *see* phenytoin *on this page*

**Pherazine® VC With Codeine *(Discontinued)*** *see* promethazine, phenylephrine, and codeine *on page 684*

**Pherazine® With Codeine *(Discontinued)*** *see* promethazine and codeine *on page 683*

**Pherazine® With DM *(Discontinued)*** *see* promethazine and dextromethorphan *on page 683*

**Phillips'® M-O [US-OTC]** *see* magnesium hydroxide and mineral oil emulsion *on page 499*

**Phillips'® Fibercaps [US-OTC]** *see* polycarbophil *on page 657*

**Phillips'® Milk of Magnesia [US-OTC]** *see* magnesium hydroxide *on page 498*

**Phillips'® Stool Softener Laxative [US-OTC]** *see* docusate *on page 263*

**pHisoHex® [US/Can]** *see* hexachlorophene *on page 403*

**Phos-Flur® [US]** *see* fluoride *on page 347*

**Phos-Flur® Rinse [US-OTC]** *see* fluoride *on page 347*

**PhosLo**® **[US]** *see* calcium acetate *on page 130*

**phosphate, potassium** *see* potassium phosphate *on page 666*

**Phospholine Iodide**® **[US]** *see* echothiophate iodide *on page 278*

**phosphonoformate** *see* foscarnet *on page 360*

**phosphonoformic acid** *see* foscarnet *on page 360*

**phosphorated carbohydrate solution** *see* fructose, dextrose, and phosphoric acid *on page 362*

**phosphoric acid, levulose and dextrose** *see* fructose, dextrose, and phosphoric acid *on page 362*

**Photofrin**® **[US/Can]** *see* porfimer *on page 661*

**Phoxal-timolol [Can]** *see* timolol *on page 803*

**Phrenilin**® **With Caffeine and Codeine [US]** *see* butalbital, aspirin, caffeine, and codeine *on page 125*

***p*-hydroxyampicillin** *see* amoxicillin *on page 46*

**Phyllocontin**® **[Can]** *see* aminophylline *on page 41*

**Phyllocontin**®**-350 [Can]** *see* aminophylline *on page 41*

**phylloquinone** *see* phytonadione *on this page*

## physostigmine (fye zoe STIG meen)
**Sound-Alike/Look-Alike Issues**
physostigmine may be confused with Prostigmin®, pyridostigmine
**Synonyms** eserine salicylate; physostigmine salicylate; physostigmine sulfate
**U.S./Canadian Brand Names** Eserine® [Can]; Isopto® Eserine [Can]
**Therapeutic Category** Cholinesterase Inhibitor
**Use** Reverse toxic CNS effects caused by anticholinergic drugs
**Usual Dosage**
Children: Anticholinergic drug overdose: Reserve for life-threatening situations only: I.V.: 0.01-0.03 mg/kg/dose (maximum: 0.5 mg/minute); may repeat after 5-10 minutes to a maximum total dose of 2 mg or until response occurs or adverse cholinergic effects occur
Adults: Anticholinergic drug overdose:
I.M., I.V., SubQ: 0.5-2 mg to start, repeat every 20 minutes until response occurs or adverse effect occurs
Repeat 1-4 mg every 30-60 minutes as life-threatening signs (arrhythmias, seizures, deep coma) recur; maximum I.V. rate: 1 mg/minute
**Dosage Forms** Injection, solution, as salicylate: 1 mg/mL (2 mL) [contains benzyl alcohol and sodium metabisulfite]

**physostigmine salicylate** *see* physostigmine *on this page*

**physostigmine sulfate** *see* physostigmine *on this page*

**phytomenadione** *see* phytonadione *on this page*

## phytonadione (fye toe na DYE one)
**Sound-Alike/Look-Alike Issues**
Mephyton® may be confused with melphalan, methadone
**Synonyms** methylphytyl napthoquinone; phylloquinone; phytomenadione; vitamin $K_1$
**U.S./Canadian Brand Names** AquaMEPHYTON® [Can]; Konakion [Can]; Mephyton® [US/Can]
**Therapeutic Category** Vitamin, Fat Soluble
**Use** Prevention and treatment of hypoprothrombinemia caused by drug-induced or anticoagulant-induced vitamin K deficiency, hemorrhagic disease of the newborn; phytonadione is more effective and is preferred to other vitamin K preparations in the presence of impending hemorrhage; oral absorption depends on the presence of bile salts
**Usual Dosage** SubQ is the preferred (per manufacturer) parenteral route; I.V. route should be restricted for emergency use only
Minimum daily requirement: Not well established
Infants: 1-5 mcg/kg/day
Adults: 0.03 mcg/kg/day

Hemorrhagic disease of the newborn:
 Prophylaxis: I.M.: 0.5-1 mg within 1 hour of birth
 Treatment: I.M., SubQ: 1-2 mg/dose/day
Oral anticoagulant overdose:
Infants and Children:
 No bleeding, rapid reversal needed, patient **will require** further oral anticoagulant therapy: SubQ, I.V.:
  0.5-2 mg
 No bleeding, rapid reversal needed, patient **will not require** further oral anticoagulant therapy: SubQ,
  I.V.: 2-5 mg
 Significant bleeding, not life-threatening: SubQ, I.V.: 0.5-2 mg
 Significant bleeding, life-threatening: I.V.: 5 mg over 10-20 minutes
 Adults: Oral, I.V., SubQ: 1-10 mg/dose depending on degree of INR elevation
 Serious bleeding or major overdose: 10 mg I.V. (slow infusion); may repeat every 12 hours (have
  required doses up to 25 mg)
Vitamin K deficiency: Due to drugs, malabsorption, or decreased synthesis of vitamin K
Infants and Children:
 Oral: 2.5-5 mg/24 hours
 I.M., I.V., SubQ: 1-2 mg/dose as a single dose
Adults:
 Oral: 5-25 mg/24 hours
 I.M., I.V., SubQ: 10 mg
 **Dosage Forms**
Injection, aqueous colloidal: 2 mg/mL (0.5 mL); 10 mg/mL (1 mL) [contains benzyl alcohol]
Tablet: 5 mg

$\alpha_1$**-PI** *see* alpha$_1$-proteinase inhibitor *on page 30*

**pidorubicin** *see* epirubicin *on page 289*

**pidorubicin hydrochloride** *see* epirubicin *on page 289*

**Pilagan**® **Ophthalmic *(Discontinued)*** *see* pilocarpine *on this page*

# pilocarpine (pye loe KAR peen)
 **Sound-Alike/Look-Alike Issues**
Isopto® Carpine may be confused with Isopto® Carbachol
Salagen® may be confused with Salacid®
 **Synonyms** pilocarpine hydrochloride
 **U.S./Canadian Brand Names** Diocarpine [Can]; Isopto® Carpine [US/Can]; Pilopine HS® [US/Can];
Salagen® [US/Can]
 **Therapeutic Category** Cholinergic Agent
 **Use**
Ophthalmic: Management of chronic simple glaucoma, chronic and acute angle-closure glaucoma
Oral: Symptomatic treatment of xerostomia caused by salivary gland hypofunction resulting from radio-
therapy for cancer of the head and neck or Sjögren syndrome
 **Usual Dosage** Adults:
Ophthalmic: Glaucoma:
 Solution: Instill 1-2 drops up to 6 times/day; adjust the concentration and frequency as required to
 control elevated intraocular pressure
 Gel: Instill 0.5" ribbon into lower conjunctival sac once daily at bedtime
Oral: Xerostomia:
 Following head and neck cancer: 5 mg 3 times/day, titration up to 10 mg 3 times/day may be
 considered for patients who have not responded adequately; do not exceed 2 tablets/dose
 Sjögren's syndrome: 5 mg 4 times/day
 **Dosage Forms**
Gel, ophthalmic, as hydrochloride (Pilopine HS®): 4% (4 g) [contains benzalkonium chloride]
Solution, ophthalmic, as hydrochloride: 0.5% (15 mL); 1% (2 mL, 15 mL); 2% (2 mL, 15 mL); 3% (15
mL); 4% (2 mL, 15 mL); 6% (15 mL) [may contain benzalkonium chloride]
Isopto® Carpine: 1% (15 mL); 2% (15 mL); 4% (15 mL) [contains benzalkonium chloride]
Tablet, as hydrochloride: 5 mg
Salagen®: 5 mg, 7.5 mg

**pilocarpine hydrochloride** *see* pilocarpine *on this page*

**Pilopine HS**® **[US/Can]** *see* pilocarpine *on this page*

**Pilostat**® **Ophthalmic** *(Discontinued)* *see* pilocarpine *on previous page*

**Pima**® **[US]** *see* potassium iodide *on page 665*

**pimaricin** *see* natamycin *on page 564*

# pimecrolimus (pim e KROE li mus)

**U.S./Canadian Brand Names** Elidel® [US/Can]

**Therapeutic Category** Immunosuppressant Agent; Topical Skin Product

**Use** Short-term and intermittent long-term treatment of mild to moderate atopic dermatitis in patients not responsive to conventional therapy or when conventional therapy is not appropriate

**Usual Dosage** Children ≥2 years and Adults: Topical: Apply thin layer to affected area twice daily; rub in gently and completely. **Note:** Continue as long as signs and symptoms persist; discontinue if resolution occurs; re-evaluate if symptoms persist >6 weeks.

**Dosage Forms** Cream, topical: 1% (30 g, 60 g, 100 g)

# pimozide (PI moe zide)

**U.S./Canadian Brand Names** Apo-Pimozide® [Can]; Orap® [US/Can]

**Therapeutic Category** Neuroleptic Agent

**Use** Suppression of severe motor and phonic tics in patients with Tourette disorder who have failed to respond satisfactorily to standard treatment

**Usual Dosage** Oral: **Note:** An ECG should be performed baseline and periodically thereafter, especially during dosage adjustment:

Children ≤12 years: Tourette disorder: Initial: 0.05 mg/kg preferably once at bedtime; may be increased every third day; usual range: 2-4 mg/day; do not exceed 10 mg/day (0.2 mg/kg/day)

Children >12 years and Adults: Tourette disorder: Initial: 1-2 mg/day in divided doses, then increase dosage as needed every other day; range is usually 7-16 mg/day, maximum dose: 10 mg/day or 0.2 mg/kg/day are not generally recommended

**Note:** Sudden unexpected deaths have occurred in patients taking doses >10 mg. Therefore, dosages exceeding 10 mg/day are generally not recommended.

**Dosage Forms** Tablet: 1 mg, 2 mg

**Pin-X**® **[US-OTC]** *see* pyrantel pamoate *on page 698*

**pinaverium bromide** *see* pinaverium *(Canada only)* *on this page*

# pinaverium *(Canada only)* (pin ah VEER ee um)

**Synonyms** pinaverium bromide

**U.S./Canadian Brand Names** Dicetel® [Can]

**Therapeutic Category** Calcium Antagonist; Gastrointestinal Agent, Miscellaneous

**Use** Treatment and relief of symptoms associated with irritable bowel syndrome (IBS); treatment of symptoms related to functional disorders of the biliary tract

**Usual Dosage** Oral: Adults: 50 mg 3 times/day; in exceptional cases, the dosage may be increased up to 100 mg 3 times/day (maximum dose: 300 mg/day). Tablets should be taken with a full glass of water during a meal/snack.

**Dosage Forms** Tablet, as bromide: 50 mg, 100 mg

# pindolol (PIN doe lole)

**Sound-Alike/Look-Alike Issues**

pindolol may be confused with Parlodel®, Plendil®

Visken® may be confused with Visine®

**U.S./Canadian Brand Names** Apo-Pindol® [Can]; Gen-Pindolol [Can]; Novo-Pindol [Can]; Nu-Pindol [Can]; PMS-Pindolol [Can]; Visken® [Can]

**Therapeutic Category** Beta-Adrenergic Blocker

**Use** Management of hypertension

**Usual Dosage** Oral: Adults:

Hypertension: Initial: 5 mg twice daily, increase as necessary by 10 mg/day every 3-4 weeks (maximum daily dose: 60 mg); usual dose range (JNC 7): 10-40 mg twice daily

Antidepressant augmentation: 2.5 mg 3 times/day

**Dosage Forms** Tablet: 5 mg, 10 mg

**pink bismuth** *see* bismuth subsalicylate *on page 108*

**Pin-Rid**® *(Discontinued)* see pyrantel pamoate on page 698

**PIO** see pemoline on page 626

## pioglitazone (pye oh GLI ta zone)

**Sound-Alike/Look-Alike Issues**
Actos® may be confused with Actidose®, Actonel®

**U.S./Canadian Brand Names** Actos® [US/Can]

**Therapeutic Category** Antidiabetic Agent; Thiazolidinedione Derivative

**Use**
Type 2 diabetes mellitus (noninsulin dependent, NIDDM), monotherapy: Adjunct to diet and exercise, to improve glycemic control

Type 2 diabetes mellitus (noninsulin dependent, NIDDM), combination therapy with sulfonylurea, metformin, or insulin: When diet, exercise, and a single agent alone does not result in adequate glycemic control

**Usual Dosage** Oral: Adults:
Monotherapy: Initial: 15-30 mg once daily; if response is inadequate, the dosage may be increased in increments up to 45 mg once daily; maximum recommended dose: 45 mg once daily

Combination therapy: Maximum recommended dose: 45 mg/day
With sulfonylureas: Initial: 15-30 mg once daily; dose of sulfonylurea should be reduced if the patient reports hypoglycemia

With metformin: Initial: 15-30 mg once daily; it is unlikely that the dose of metformin will need to be reduced due to hypoglycemia

With insulin: Initial: 15-30 mg once daily; dose of insulin should be reduced by 10% to 25% if the patient reports hypoglycemia or if the plasma glucose falls to <100 mg/dL.

Dosage adjustment in patients with CHF (NYHA Class II) in mono- or combination therapy: Initial: 15 mg once daily; may be increased after several months of treatment, with close attention to heart failure symptoms

**Dosage Forms** Tablet: 15 mg, 30 mg, 45 mg

## piperacillin (pi PER a sil in)

**Synonyms** piperacillin sodium

**Therapeutic Category** Penicillin

**Use** Treatment of susceptible infections such as septicemia, acute and chronic respiratory tract infections, skin and soft tissue infections, and urinary tract infections due to susceptible strains of *Pseudomonas*, *Proteus*, and *Escherichia coli* and *Enterobacter*; active against some streptococci and some anaerobic bacteria; febrile neutropenia (as part of combination regimen)

**Usual Dosage**
Neonates: 100 mg/kg every 12 hours
Infants and Children: I.M., I.V.: 200-300 mg/kg/day in divided doses every 4-6 hours
Higher doses have been used in cystic fibrosis: 350-500 mg/kg/day in divided doses every 4-6 hours
Adults: I.M., I.V.:
Moderate infections (urinary tract infections): 2-3 g/dose every 6-12 hours; maximum: 2 g I.M./site
Serious infections: 3-4 g/dose every 4-6 hours; maximum: 24 g/24 hours
Uncomplicated gonorrhea: 2 g I.M. in a single dose accompanied by 1 g probenecid 30 minutes prior to injection

**Dosage Forms** Injection, powder for reconstitution: 2 g, 3 g, 4 g, 40 g

## piperacillin and tazobactam sodium (pi PER a sil in & ta zoe BAK tam SOW dee um)

**Sound-Alike/Look-Alike Issues**
Zosyn® may be confused with Zofran®, Zyvox™

**Synonyms** piperacillin sodium and tazobactam sodium

**U.S./Canadian Brand Names** Tazocin® [Can]; Zosyn® [US]

**Therapeutic Category** Penicillin

**Use** Treatment of infections caused by susceptible organisms, including infections of the lower respiratory tract (community-acquired pneumonia, nosocomial pneumonia); urinary tract; skin and skin structures; gynecologic (endometritis, pelvic inflammatory disease); bone and joint infections; intra-abdominal infections (appendicitis with rupture/abscess, peritonitis); and septicemia. Tazobactam expands activity of piperacillin to include beta-lactamase producing strains of *S. aureus*, *H. influenzae*, *Bacteroides*, and other gram-negative bacteria.
(Continued)

## piperacillin and tazobactam sodium *(Continued)*

### Usual Dosage

Infants and Children ≥6 months: **Note:** Not FDA-approved for use in children <12 years of age:

I.V.: 240 mg of piperacillin component/kg/day in divided doses every 8 hours; higher doses have been used for serious pseudomonal infections: 300-400 mg of piperacillin component/kg/day in divided doses every 6 hours.

Children >12 years and Adults:

Nosocomial pneumonia: I.V.: Piperacillin/tazobactam 4/0.5 g every 6 hours for 7-14 days (when used empirically, combination with an aminoglycoside is recommended; consider discontinuation of aminoglycoside if *P. aeruginosa* is not isolated)

Severe infections: I.V.: Piperacillin/tazobactam 4/0.5 g every 8 hours or 3/0.375 g every 6 hours for 7-10 days

Moderate infections: I.M.: Piperacillin/tazobactam 2/0.25 g every 6-8 hours; treatment should be continued for ≥7-10 days depending on severity of disease (**Note:** I.M. route not FDA-approved)

**Dosage Forms Note**: 8:1 ratio of piperacillin sodium/tazobactam sodium

Infusion [premixed iso-osmotic solution, frozen]:

2.25 g: Piperacillin 2 g and tazobactam 0.25 g (50 mL) [contains sodium 5.7 mEq (131 mg)]

3.375 g: Piperacillin 3 g and tazobactam 0.375 g (50 mL) [contains sodium 8.6 mEq (197 mg)]

4.5 g: Piperacillin 4 g and tazobactam 0.5 g (50 mL) [contains sodium 11.4 mEq (263 mg)]

Injection, powder for reconstitution:

2.25 g: Piperacillin 2 g and tazobactam 0.25 g [contains sodium 4.69 mEq (108 mg)]

3.375 g: Piperacillin 3 g and tazobactam 0.375 g [contains sodium 7.04 mEq (162 mg)]

4.5 g: Piperacillin 4 g and tazobactam 0.5 g [contains sodium 9.39 mEq (216 mg)]

40.5 g: Piperacillin 36 g and tazobactam 4.5 g [contains sodium 84.5 mEq (1944 mg); bulk pharmacy vial]

**piperacillin sodium** *see* piperacillin *on previous page*

**piperacillin sodium and tazobactam sodium** *see* piperacillin and tazobactam sodium *on previous page*

**piperazine estrone sulfate** *see* estropipate *on page 306*

**piperonyl butoxide and pyrethrins** *see* pyrethrins and piperonyl butoxide *on page 699*

**Pipracil®** *(Discontinued)* *see* piperacillin *on previous page*

## pirbuterol *(peer BYOO ter ole)*

**Synonyms** pirbuterol acetate

**U.S./Canadian Brand Names** Maxair™ Autohaler™ [US]

**Therapeutic Category** Adrenergic Agonist Agent

**Use** Prevention and treatment of reversible bronchospasm including asthma

**Usual Dosage** Children ≥12 years and Adults: 2 inhalations every 4-6 hours for prevention; two inhalations at an interval of at least 1-3 minutes, followed by a third inhalation in treatment of bronchospasm, not to exceed 12 inhalations/day

**Dosage Forms** Aerosol for oral inhalation, as acetate:

Maxair™ Autohaler™: 14 g [400 inhalations; contains chlorofluorocarbons]

**pirbuterol acetate** *see* pirbuterol *on this page*

## piroxicam *(peer OKS i kam)*

**U.S./Canadian Brand Names** Apo-Piroxicam® [Can]; Feldene® [US]; Gen-Piroxicam [Can]; Novo-Pirocam [Can]; Nu-Pirox [Can]; Pexicam® [Can]

**Therapeutic Category** Analgesic, Nonnarcotic; Nonsteroidal Antiinflammatory Drug (NSAID)

**Use** Symptomatic treatment of acute and chronic rheumatoid arthritis and osteoarthritis

**Usual Dosage** Oral: Adults: 10-20 mg/day once daily; although associated with increase in GI adverse effects, doses >20 mg/day have been used (ie, 30-40 mg/day)

**Dosage Forms** Capsule: 10 mg, 20 mg

**p-isobutylhydratropic acid** *see* ibuprofen *on page 427*

**pit** *see* oxytocin *on page 612*

**Pitocin®** **[US/Can]** *see* oxytocin *on page 612*

**Pitressin®** **[US]** *see* vasopressin *on page 842*

**Pitrex [Can]** *see* tolnaftate *on page 809*

**pit viper antivenin** *see* antivenin *(Crotalidae)* polyvalent *on page 60*

## pivampicillin *(Canada only)* (piv am pi SIL in)
U.S./Canadian Brand Names Pondocillin® [Can]
Therapeutic Category Antibiotic, Penicillin
Use For the treatment of respiratory tract infections (including acute bronchitis, acute exacerbations of chronic bronchitis and pneumonia); ear, nose and throat infections; gynecological infections; urinary tract infections (including acute uncomplicated gonococcal urethritis) when caused by nonpenicillinase-producing susceptible strains of the following organisms: gram-positive organisms, ie, streptococci, pneumococci and staphylococci; gram-negative organisms, ie, *H. influenzae, N. gonorrhoeae, E. coli, P. mirabilis.*
Usual Dosage Oral:
Suspension:
Infants 3 to 12 months: 40-60 mg/kg body weight daily divided into 2 equal doses
Children:
1 to 3 years: 5 mL (175 mg) twice daily
4 to 6 years: 7.5 mL (262.5 mg) twice daily
7 to 10 years: 10 mL (350 mg) twice daily
Children ≤10 years: Dosage range: 25-35 mg/kg/day ; should not exceed the recommended adult dose of 500 mg twice daily
Children ≥10 years and Adults: 15 mL (525 mg) twice daily; for severe infections: Dosage may be doubled
Tablet: Children ≥10 years and Adults: 500 mg twice daily; for severe infections: Dosage may be doubled
In gonococcal urethritis: 1.5 g as a single dose with 1 g probenecid concurrently
Dosage Forms
Suspension, oral: 35 mg/5 mL (100 mL, 150 mL, 200 mL)
Tablet: 500 mg (equivalent to ampicillin 377 mg)

**pix carbonis** *see* coal tar *on page 201*

## pizotifen *(Canada only)* (pi ZOE ti fen)
Synonyms pizotifen malate
U.S./Canadian Brand Names Sandomigran DS® [Can]; Sandomigran® [Can]
Therapeutic Category Antimigraine Agent
Use Migraine prophylaxis
Usual Dosage Oral: Children ≥12 years and Adults: Migraine prophylaxis: Initial: 0.5 mg at bedtime; increase gradually to 0.5 mg 3 times/day; usual dosage range: 1-6 mg/day
Note: Therapeutic response may require several weeks of therapy. Do not discontinue abruptly (reduce gradually over 2-week period).
Dosage Forms
Tablet (Sandomigran®): 0.5 mg [pizotifen malate 0.73 mg]
Tablet, double strength (Sandomigran® DS): 1 mg [pizotifen malate 1.46 mg]

**pizotifen malate** *see* pizotifen *(Canada only)* on this page

## plague vaccine (plaig vak SEEN)
Therapeutic Category Vaccine, Inactivated Bacteria
Use Selected travelers to countries reporting cases for whom avoidance of rodents and fleas is impossible; all laboratory and field personnel working with *Yersinia pestis* organisms possibly resistant to antimicrobials; those engaged in *Yersinia pestis* aerosol experiments or in field operations in areas with enzootic plague where regular exposure to potentially infected wild rodents, rabbits, or their fleas cannot be prevented. Prophylactic antibiotics may be indicated following definite exposure, whether or not the exposed persons have been vaccinated.
Usual Dosage Three I.M. doses: First dose 1 mL, second dose (0.2 mL) 1 month later, third dose (0.2 mL) 5 months after the second dose; booster doses (0.2 mL) at 1- to 2-year intervals if exposure continues
Dosage Forms Injection: 2 mL, 20 mL

**Plan B**® **[US/Can]** *see* levonorgestrel *on page 476*

**plantago seed** *see* psyllium *on page 697*

**plantain seed** *see* psyllium *on page 697*

**Plaquase®** *(Discontinued) see* collagenase *on page 206*

**Plaquenil®** **[US/Can]** *see* hydroxychloroquine *on page 421*

**Plaretase®** **8000 [US]** *see* pancrelipase *on page 615*

**Plasbumin®** **[US]** *see* albumin *on page 22*

**Plasbumin®-5 [Can]** *see* albumin *on page 22*

**Plasbumin®-25 [Can]** *see* albumin *on page 22*

**Plasmanate®** **[US]** *see* plasma protein fraction *on this page*

**Plasma-Plex®** *(Discontinued) see* plasma protein fraction *on this page*

**plasma protein fraction** (PLAS mah PROE teen FRAK shun)
U.S./Canadian Brand Names Plasmanate® [US]
Therapeutic Category Blood Product Derivative
Use Plasma volume expansion and maintenance of cardiac output in the treatment of certain types of shock or impending shock
Usual Dosage I.V.: 250-1500 mL/day
Dosage Forms Injection, solution [human]: 5% (50 mL, 250 mL) [contains sodium 145 mEq/L]

**Plasmatein®** *(Discontinued) see* plasma protein fraction *on this page*

**Platinol®-AQ** *(Discontinued) see* cisplatin *on page 187*

**Plavix®** **[US/Can]** *see* clopidogrel *on page 198*

**Plegine®** **[Can]** *see* phendimetrazine *on page 637*

**Plegine®** *(Discontinued) see* phendimetrazine *on page 637*

**Plenaxis™** *(Discontinued) see* abarelix *on page 2*

**Plendil®** **[US/Can]** *see* felodipine *on page 330*

**Pletal®** **[US/Can]** *see* cilostazol *on page 183*

**Plexion®** **[US]** *see* sulfur and sulfacetamide *on page 776*

**Plexion SCT™ [US]** *see* sulfur and sulfacetamide *on page 776*

**Plexion TS®** **[US]** *see* sulfur and sulfacetamide *on page 776*

**PMPA** *see* tenofovir *on page 786*

**PMS-Amantadine [Can]** *see* amantadine *on page 37*

**PMS-Amitriptyline [Can]** *see* amitriptyline *on page 42*

**PMS-Amoxicillin [Can]** *see* amoxicillin *on page 46*

**PMS-Atenolol [Can]** *see* atenolol *on page 76*

**PMS-Baclofen [Can]** *see* baclofen *on page 88*

**PMS-Benzydamine [Can]** *see* benzydamine *(Canada only) on page 100*

**PMS-Bethanechol [Can]** *see* bethanechol *on page 104*

**PMS-Bezafibrate [Can]** *see* bezafibrate *(Canada only) on page 106*

**PMS-Brimonidine Tartrate [Can]** *see* brimonidine *on page 113*

**PMS-Bromocriptine [Can]** *see* bromocriptine *on page 114*

**PMS-Buspirone [Can]** *see* buspirone *on page 123*

**PMS-Butorphanol [Can]** *see* butorphanol *on page 126*

**PMS-Captopril [Can]** *see* captopril *on page 139*

**PMS-Carbamazepine [Can]** *see* carbamazepine *on page 140*

**PMS-Carvedilol [Can]** *see* carvedilol *on page 150*

**PMS-Cefaclor [Can]** *see* cefaclor *on page 152*

**PMS-Chloral Hydrate [Can]** *see* chloral hydrate *on page 166*

**PMS-Cholestyramine [Can]** *see* cholestyramine resin *on page 180*

**PMS-Minocycline [Can]** *see* minocycline *on page 542*

**PMS-Mirtazapine [Can]** *see* mirtazapine *on page 543*

**PMS-Moclobemide [Can]** *see* moclobemide *(Canada only) on page 546*

**PMS-Morphine Sulfate SR [Can]** *see* morphine sulfate *on page 549*

**PMS-Nizatidine [Can]** *see* nizatidine *on page 580*

**PMS-Norfloxacin [Can]** *see* norfloxacin *on page 582*

**PMS-Nortriptyline [Can]** *see* nortriptyline *on page 583*

**PMS-Nystatin [Can]** *see* nystatin *on page 592*

**PMS-Ofloxacin [Can]** *see* ofloxacin *on page 594*

**PMS-Oxazepam [Can]** *see* oxazepam *on page 606*

**PMS-Oxybutynin [Can]** *see* oxybutynin *on page 607*

**PMS-Oxycodone-Acetaminophen [Can]** *see* oxycodone and acetaminophen *on page 609*

**PMS-Paroxetine [Can]** *see* paroxetine *on page 620*

**PMS-Phenobarbital [Can]** *see* phenobarbital *on page 638*

**PMS-Pindolol [Can]** *see* pindolol *on page 648*

**PMS-Polytrimethoprim [Can]** *see* trimethoprim and polymyxin B *on page 826*

**PMS-Pravastatin [Can]** *see* pravastatin *on page 671*

**PMS-Procyclidine [Can]** *see* procyclidine *on page 681*

**PMS-Pseudoephedrine [Can]** *see* pseudoephedrine *on page 692*

**PMS-Ranitidine [Can]** *see* ranitidine hydrochloride *on page 710*

**PMS-Salbutamol [Can]** *see* albuterol *on page 22*

**PMS-Sertraline [Can]** *see* sertraline *on page 744*

**PMS-Simvastatin [Can]** *see* simvastatin *on page 748*

**PMS-Sodium Polystyrene Sulfonate [Can]** *see* sodium polystyrene sulfonate *on page 758*

**PMS-Sotalol [Can]** *see* sotalol *on page 762*

**PMS-Sucralate [Can]** *see* sucralfate *on page 769*

**PMS-Temazepam [Can]** *see* temazepam *on page 784*

**PMS-Terazosin [Can]** *see* terazosin *on page 786*

**PMS-Theophylline [Can]** *see* theophylline *on page 793*

**PMS-Tiaprofenic [Can]** *see* tiaprofenic acid *(Canada only) on page 801*

**PMS-Timolol [Can]** *see* timolol *on page 803*

**PMS-Tobramycin [Can]** *see* tobramycin *on page 807*

**PMS-Trazodone [Can]** *see* trazodone *on page 817*

**PMS-Trifluoperazine [Can]** *see* trifluoperazine *on page 823*

**PMS-Valproic Acid [Can]** *see* valproic acid and derivatives *on page 837*

**PMS-Valproic Acid E.C. [Can]** *see* valproic acid and derivatives *on page 837*

**PMS-Yohimbine [Can]** *see* yohimbine *on page 857*

**PMS-Zopiclone [Can]** *see* zopiclone *(Canada only) on page 864*

**Pneumo 23™ [Can]** *see* pneumococcal polysaccharide vaccine (polyvalent) *on next page*

**pneumococcal 7-valent conjugate vaccine** *see* pneumococcal conjugate vaccine (7-valent) *on this page*

# pneumococcal conjugate vaccine (7-valent)
(noo moe KOK al KON ju gate vak SEEN, seven vay lent)
### Sound-Alike/Look-Alike Issues
Prevnar® may be confused with PREVEN®

**Synonyms** diphtheria CRM$_{197}$ protein; PCV7; pneumococcal 7-valent conjugate vaccine

**U.S./Canadian Brand Names** Prevnar® [US/Can]

**Therapeutic Category** Vaccine

**Use** Immunization of infants and toddlers against *Streptococcus pneumoniae* infection caused by serotypes included in the vaccine

Advisory Committee on Immunization Practices (ACIP) guidelines also recommend PCV7 for use in:
All children 2-23 months
Children ≥2-59 months with cochlear implants
Children ages 24-59 months with: Sickle cell disease (including other sickle cell hemoglobinopathies, asplenia, splenic dysfunction), HIV infection, immunocompromising conditions (congenital immunodeficiencies, renal failure, nephrotic syndrome, diseases associated with immunosuppressive or radiation therapy, solid organ transplant), chronic illnesses (cardiac disease, cerebrospinal fluid leaks, diabetes mellitus, pulmonary disease excluding asthma unless on high dose corticosteroids)
Consider use in all children 24-59 months with priority given to:
Children 24-35 months
Children 24-59 months who are of Alaska native, American Indian, or African-American descent
Children 24-59 months who attend group day care centers

**Usual Dosage** I.M.:
Infants: 2-6 months: 0.5 mL at approximately 2-month intervals for 3 consecutive doses, followed by a fourth dose of 0.5 mL at 12-15 months of age; first dose may be given as young as 6 weeks of age, but is typically given at 2 months of age. In case of a moderate shortage of vaccine, defer the fourth dose until shortage is resolved; in case of a severe shortage of vaccine, defer third and fourth doses until shortage is resolved.

**Previously Unvaccinated Older Infants and Children:**
7-11 months: 0.5 mL for a total of 3 doses; 2 doses at least 4 weeks apart, followed by a third dose after the 1-year birthday (12-15 months), separated from the second dose by at least 2 months. In case of a severe shortage of vaccine, defer the third dose until shortage is resolved.
12-23 months: 0.5 mL for a total of 2 doses, separated by at least 2 months. In case of a severe shortage of vaccine, defer the second dose until shortage is resolved.
24-59 months:
Healthy Children: 0.5 mL as a single dose. In case of a severe shortage of vaccine, defer dosing until shortage is resolved.
Children with sickle cell disease, asplenia, HIV infection, chronic illness or immunocompromising conditions (not including bone marrow transplants - results pending; use PPV23 [pneumococcal polysaccharide vaccine, polyvalent] at 12- and 24-months until studies are complete): 0.5 mL for a total of 2 doses, separated by 2 months

**Previously Vaccinated Children with a lapse in vaccine administration:**
7-11 months: Previously received 1 or 2 doses PCV7: 0.5 mL dose at 7-11 months of age, followed by a second dose ≥2 months later at 12-15 months of age
12-23 months:
Previously received 1 dose before 12 months of age: 0.5 mL dose, followed by a second dose ≥2 months later
Previously received 2 doses before age 12 months: 0.5 mL dose ≥2 months after the most recent dose
24-59 months: Any incomplete schedule: 0.5 mL as a single dose; **Note:** Patients with chronic diseases or immunosuppressing conditions should receive 2 doses ≥2 months apart

**Dosage Forms** Injection, suspension: 2 mcg of each saccharide for serotypes 4, 9V, 14, 18C, 19F, and 23F, and 4 mcg of serotype 6B per 0.5 mL (0.5 mL) [contains 16 mcg total saccharide; also contains diphtheria CRM197 carrier protein ~20 mcg/0.5 mL and aluminum 0.125 mg/0.5 mL (as aluminum phosphate adjuvant); serotypes grown in soy peptone broth; vial stopper contains latex]

# pneumococcal polysaccharide vaccine (polyvalent)
(noo moe KOK al pol i SAK a ride vak SEEN, pol i VAY lent)

**Synonyms** 23-valent pneumococcal polysaccharide vaccine; 23PS; PPV23

**U.S./Canadian Brand Names** Pneumo 23™ [Can]; Pneumovax® 23 [US/Can]

**Therapeutic Category** Vaccine, Inactivated Bacteria

**Use** Children ≥2 years of age and adults who are at increased risk of pneumococcal disease and its complications because of underlying health conditions (including patients with cochlear implants); routine use in older adults >50 years of age, including all those ≥65 years

Current Advisory Committee on Immunization Practices (ACIP) guidelines recommend **pneumococcal 7-valent conjugate vaccine (PCV7)** be used for children 2-23 months of age and, in certain situations, children up to 59 months of age

(Continued)

## pneumococcal polysaccharide vaccine (polyvalent) *(Continued)*

Usual Dosage I.M., SubQ:

Children >2 years and Adults: 0.5 mL

**Previously vaccinated with PCV7 vaccine**: Children ≥2 years and Adults:

With sickle cell disease, asplenia, immunocompromised or HIV infection: 0.5 mL at ≥2 years of age and ≥2 months after last dose of PCV7; revaccination with PPV23 should be given ≥5 years for children >10 years of age and every 3-5 years for children ≤10 years of age; revaccination should not be administered <3 years after the previous PPV23 dose

With chronic illness: 0.5 mL at ≥2 years of age and ≥2 months after last dose of PCV7; revaccination with PPV23 is not recommended

Following bone marrow transplant (use of PCV7 under study): Administer one dose PPV23 at 12- and 24-months following BMT

**Revaccination should be considered:**

1. If ≥6 years since initial vaccination has elapsed, or
2. In patients who received 14-valent pneumococcal vaccine and are at highest risk (asplenic) for fatal infection or
3. At ≥6 years in patients with nephrotic syndrome, renal failure, or transplant recipients, or
4. 3-5 years in children with nephrotic syndrome, asplenia, or sickle cell disease

Dosage Forms Injection, solution: 25 mcg each of 23 polysaccharide isolates/0.5 mL (0.5 mL, 2.5 mL)

**Pneumomist**® *(Discontinued)* *see guaifenesin on page 383*

**Pneumotussin**® **[US]** *see hydrocodone and guaifenesin on page 412*

**Pneumovax**® **23 [US/Can]** *see pneumococcal polysaccharide vaccine (polyvalent) on previous page*

**PNU-140690E** *see tipranavir on page 806*

**Pnu-Imune**® **23** *(Discontinued)*

**Podactin Cream [US-OTC]** *see miconazole on page 537*

**Podactin Powder [US-OTC]** *see tolnaftate on page 809*

**Pod-Ben-25**® *(Discontinued)* *see podophyllum resin on this page*

**Podocon-25**® **[US]** *see podophyllum resin on this page*

**Podofilm**® **[Can]** *see podophyllum resin on this page*

## podofilox *(po do FIL oks)*

U.S./Canadian Brand Names Condyline™ [Can]; Condylox® [US]; Wartec® [Can]

Therapeutic Category Keratolytic Agent

Use Treatment of external genital warts

Usual Dosage Topical: Adults: Apply twice daily (morning and evening) for 3 consecutive days, then withhold use for 4 consecutive days; this cycle may be repeated up to 4 times until there is no visible wart tissue

Dosage Forms

Gel: 0.5% (3.5 g) [contains alcohol]

Solution, topical: 0.5% (3.5 mL) [contains alcohol]

**Podofin**® *(Discontinued)* *see podophyllum resin on this page*

**podophyllin** *see podophyllum resin on this page*

## podophyllum resin *(po DOF fil um REZ in)*

Synonyms mandrake; may apple; podophyllin

U.S./Canadian Brand Names Podocon-25® [US]; Podofilm® [Can]

Therapeutic Category Keratolytic Agent

Use Topical treatment of benign growths including external genital and perianal warts, papillomas, fibroids; compound benzoin tincture generally is used as the medium for topical application

Usual Dosage Topical:

Children and Adults: 10% to 25% solution in compound benzoin tincture; apply drug to dry surface, use 1 drop at a time allowing drying between drops until area is covered; total volume should be limited to <0.5 mL per treatment session

Condylomata acuminatum: 25% solution is applied daily; use a 10% solution when applied to or near mucous membranes

Verrucae: 25% solution is applied 3-5 times/day directly to the wart

Dosage Forms Liquid, topical: 25% (15 mL) [in benzoin tincture]

**Point-Two**® *(Discontinued)* see fluoride *on page 347*

**Poladex**® *(Discontinued)* see dexchlorpheniramine *on page 234*

**Polaramine**® *(Discontinued)* see dexchlorpheniramine *on page 234*

## poliovirus vaccine (inactivated) (POE lee oh VYE rus vak SEEN, in ak ti VAY ted)
**Synonyms** enhanced-potency inactivated poliovirus vaccine; IPV; salk vaccine
**U.S./Canadian Brand Names** IPOL® [US/Can]
**Therapeutic Category** Vaccine, Live Virus and Inactivated Virus
**Use**

As the global eradication of poliomyelitis continues, the risk for importation of wild-type poliovirus into the United States decreases dramatically. To eliminate the risk for vaccine-associated paralytic poliomyelitis (VAPP), an all-IPV schedule is recommended for routine childhood vaccination in the United States. All children should receive four doses of IPV (at age 2 months, age 4 months, between ages 6-18 months, and between ages 4-6 years). Oral poliovirus vaccine (OPV), if available, may be used only for the following special circumstances:

Mass vaccination campaigns to control outbreaks of paralytic polio

Unvaccinated children who will be traveling within 4 weeks to areas where polio is endemic or epidemic

Children of parents who do not accept the recommended number of vaccine injections; these children may receive OPV only for the third or fourth dose or both. In this situation, healthcare providers should administer OPV only after discussing the risk for VAPP with parents or caregivers.

OPV supplies are expected to be very limited in the United States after inventories are depleted. ACIP reaffirms its support for the global eradication initiative and use of OPV as the vaccine of choice to eradicate polio where it is endemic.

**Usual Dosage** SubQ: **Enhanced-potency inactivated poliovirus vaccine (E-IPV) is preferred for primary vaccination of adults**, two doses SubQ 4-8 weeks apart, a third dose 6-12 months after the second. For adults with a completed primary series and for whom a booster is indicated, either OPV or E-IPV can be given (E-IPV preferred). If immediate protection is needed, either OPV or E-IPV is recommended.

**Dosage Forms** Injection, suspension: Type 1 poliovirus 40 D antigen units/0.5 mL, Type 2 poliovirus 8 D antigen units/0.5 mL, and Type 3 poliovirus 32 D antigen units/0.5 mL (5 mL) [contains calf serum protein, neomycin, streptomycin, and polymyxin B]

**Polocaine**® **[US/Can]** see mepivacaine *on page 514*

**Polocaine**® **MPF [US]** see mepivacaine *on page 514*

## polycarbophil (pol i KAR boe fil)
**U.S./Canadian Brand Names** Equalactin® [US-OTC]; Fiber-Lax® [US-OTC]; FiberCon® [US-OTC]; Konsyl® Fiber Tablets [US-OTC]; Phillips'® Fibercaps [US-OTC]
**Therapeutic Category** Gastrointestinal Agent, Miscellaneous; Laxative
**Use** Treatment of constipation or diarrhea
**Usual Dosage** Oral: General dosing guidelines (OTC labeling):
Children 6-12 years: 625 mg calcium polycarbophil 1-4 times/day
Children ≥12 years and Adults: 1250 mg calcium polycarbophil 1-4 times/day
**Dosage Forms**
Caplet:
FiberCon®: Calcium polycarbophil 625 mg [equivalent to polycarbophil 500 mg; contains calcium 122 mg/caplet]
Phillips'® Fibercaps: Calcium polycarbophil 625 mg [equivalent to polycarbophil 500 mg]
Captab (Fiber-Lax®): Calcium polycarbophil 625 mg [equivalent to polycarbophil 500 mg; contains calcium 170 mg/captab]
Tablet (Konsyl® Fiber): Calcium polycarbophil 625 mg [equivalent to polycarbophil 500 mg; contains calcium 125 mg/tablet]
Tablet, chewable (Equalactin®): Calcium polycarbophil 625 mg [equivalent to polycarbophil 500 mg; citrus flavor]

**Polycitra**® **[US]** see citric acid, sodium citrate, and potassium citrate *on page 189*

**Polycitra**®**-K [Can]** see potassium citrate *on page 664*

**Polycitra®-LC [US]** *see* citric acid, sodium citrate, and potassium citrate *on page 189*

**Polycose® [US-OTC]** *see* glucose polymers *on page 377*

# polyethylene glycol-electrolyte solution
(pol i ETH i leen GLY kol ee LEK troe lite soe LOO shun)

## Sound-Alike/Look-Alike Issues
GoLYTELY® may be confused with NuLYTELY®

MiraLax™ may be confused with Mirapex®

NuLYTELY® may be confused with GoLYTELY®

**Synonyms** electrolyte lavage solution

**U.S./Canadian Brand Names** Colyte® [US/Can]; GlycoLax™ [US]; GoLYTELY® [US]; Klean-Prep® [Can]; MiraLax™ [US]; NuLYTELY® [US]; PegLyte® [Can]; TriLyte™ [US]

**Therapeutic Category** Laxative

**Use** Bowel cleansing prior to GI examination or following toxic ingestion (electrolyte containing solutions only); treatment of occasional constipation (MiraLax™)

## Usual Dosage
Oral:

Children ≥6 months: Bowel cleansing prior to GI exam (solutions with electrolytes only): 25-40 mL/kg/hour for 4-10 hours (until rectal effluent is clear). Ideally, patients should fast for ~3-4 hours prior to administration; absolutely no solid food for at least 2 hours before the solution is given. The solution may be given via nasogastric tube to patients who are unwilling or unable to drink the solution. Patients <2 years should be monitored closely.

Adults:

Bowel cleansing prior to GI exam (solutions with electrolytes only): 240 mL (8 oz) every 10 minutes, until 4 L are consumed or the rectal effluent is clear; rapid drinking of each portion is preferred to drinking small amounts continuously. Ideally, patients should fast for ~3-4 hours prior to administration; absolutely no solid food for at least 2 hours before the solution is given. The solution may be given via nasogastric tube to patients who are unwilling or unable to drink the solution.

Occasional constipation (MiraLax™): 17 g of powder (~1 heaping tablespoon) dissolved in 8 oz of water; once daily; do not use for >2 weeks.

Nasogastric tube:

Children ≥6 months: Bowel cleansing prior to GI exam (solutions with electrolytes only): 25 mL/kg/hour until rectal effluent is clear. Ideally, patients should fast for ~3-4 hours prior to administration; absolutely no solid food for at least 2 hours before the solution is given.

Adults: Bowel cleansing prior to GI exam (solutions with electrolytes only): 20-30 mL/minute (1.2-1.8 L/hour); the first bowel movement should occur ~1 hour after the start of administration. Ideally, patients should fast for ~3-4 hours prior to administration; absolutely no solid food for at least 2 hours before the solution is given.

## Dosage Forms
Powder, for oral solution: PEG 3350 240 g, sodium sulfate 22.72 g, sodium bicarbonate 6.72 g, sodium chloride 5.84 g, and potassium chloride 2.98 g (4000 mL)

Colyte®:

PEG 3350 240 g, sodium sulfate 22.72 g, sodium bicarbonate 6.72 g, sodium chloride 5.84 g, and potassium chloride 2.98 g (4000 mL) [available with citrus berry, lemon lime, cherry, and pineapple flavor packets]

PEG 3350 227.1 g, sodium sulfate 21.5 g, sodium bicarbonate 6.36 g, sodium chloride 5.53 g, and potassium chloride 2.82 g (4000 mL) [regular and pineapple flavor]

GlycoLax™: PEG 3350 17 g/packet (14s); PEG 3350 255 g (16 oz); PEG 3350 527 g (24 oz)

GoLYTELY®:

Disposable jug: PEG 3350 236 g, sodium sulfate 22.74 g, sodium bicarbonate 6.74 g, sodium chloride 5.86 g, and potassium chloride 2.97 g (4000 mL) [regular and pineapple flavor]

Packets: PEG 3350 227.1 g, sodium sulfate 21.5 g, sodium bicarbonate 6.36 g, sodium chloride 5.53 g, and potassium chloride 2.82 g (4000 mL) [regular flavor]

MiraLax™: PEG 3350 17 g/packet (12s); PEG 3350 255 g (14 oz); PEG 3350 527 g (26 oz)

NuLYTELY®: PEG 3350 420 g, sodium bicarbonate 5.72 g, sodium chloride 11.2 g, and potassium chloride 1.48 (4000 mL) [cherry, lemon-lime, and orange flavors]

TriLyte™: PEG 3350 420 g, sodium bicarbonate 5.72 g, sodium chloride 11.2 g, and potassium chloride 1.48 (4000 mL) [supplied with flavor packets]

# polyethylene glycol-electrolyte solution and bisacodyl
(pol i ETH i leen GLY kol ee LEK troe lite soe LOO shun & bis a KOE dil)

**U.S./Canadian Brand Names** HalfLytely® and Bisacodyl [US]

**Therapeutic Category** Laxative, Bowel Evacuant; Laxative, Stimulant

**Use** Bowel cleansing prior to GI examination

**Usual Dosage** Oral: Adults: Bowel cleansing:
Bisacodyl: 4 tablets as a single dose. After bowel movement or 6 hours (whichever occurs first), initiate polyethylene glycol-electrolyte solution
Polyethylene glycol-electrolyte solution: 8 ounces every 10 minutes until 2 L are consumed

**Dosage Forms** Kit (HalfLytely® and Bisacodyl) [each kit contains]:
Powder for oral solution (HalfLytely®):PEG 3350 210 g, sodium bicarbonate 2.86 g, sodium chloride 5.6 g, potassium chloride 0.74 g (2000 mL) [sulfate-free, regular, cherry, lemon-lime, orange flavor]
Tablet, delayed release: Bisacodyl: 5 mg (4s)

**Polygam® S/D [US]** *see* immune globulin (intravenous) *on page 433*

**Poly-Histine-D® Capsule *(Discontinued)***

# polymyxin B (pol i MIKS in bee)

**Synonyms** polymyxin B sulfate

**U.S./Canadian Brand Names** Poly-Rx [US]

**Therapeutic Category** Antibiotic, Irrigation; Antibiotic, Miscellaneous

**Use** Treatment of acute infections caused by susceptible strains of *Pseudomonas aeruginosa*; used occasionally for gut decontamination; parenteral use of polymyxin B has mainly been replaced by less toxic antibiotics, reserved for life-threatening infections caused by organisms resistant to the preferred drugs (eg, pseudomonal meningitis - intrathecal administration)

**Usual Dosage**
Otic (in combination with other drugs): 1-2 drops, 3-4 times/day; should be used sparingly to avoid accumulation of excess debris
Infants <2 years:
I.M.: Up to 40,000 units/kg/day divided every 6 hours (not routinely recommended due to pain at injection sites)
I.V.: Up to 40,000 units/kg/day divided every 12 hours
Intrathecal: 20,000 units/day for 3-4 days, then 25,000 units every other day for at least 2 weeks after CSF cultures are negative and CSF (glucose) has returned to within normal limits
Children ≥2 years and Adults:
I.M.: 25,000-30,000 units/kg/day divided every 4-6 hours (not routinely recommended due to pain at injection sites)
I.V.: 15,000-25,000 units/kg/day divided every 12 hours
Intrathecal: 50,000 units/day for 3-4 days, then every other day for at least 2 weeks after CSF cultures are negative and CSF (glucose) has returned to within normal limits
Total daily dose should not exceed 2,000,000 units/day
Bladder irrigation: Continuous irrigant or rinse in the urinary bladder for up to 10 days using 20 mg (equal to 200,000 units) added to 1 L of normal saline; usually no more than 1 L of irrigant is used per day unless urine flow rate is high; administration rate is adjusted to patient's urine output
Topical irrigation or topical solution: 500,000 units/L of normal saline; topical irrigation should not exceed 2 million units/day in adults
Gut sterilization: Oral: 15,000-25,000 units/kg/day in divided doses every 6 hours
*Clostridium difficile* enteritis: Oral: 25,000 units every 6 hours for 10 days
Ophthalmic: A concentration of 0.1% to 0.25% is administered as 1-3 drops every hour, then increasing the interval as response indicates to 1-2 drops 4-6 times/day

**Dosage Forms**
Injection, powder for reconstitution: 500,000 units
Powder [for prescription compounding] (Poly-Rx): 100 million units (13 g)

**polymyxin B and bacitracin** *see* bacitracin and polymyxin B *on page 86*

**polymyxin B and neomycin** *see* neomycin and polymyxin B *on page 567*

**polymyxin B and oxytetracycline** *see* oxytetracycline and polymyxin B *on page 612*

**polymyxin B and trimethoprim** *see* trimethoprim and polymyxin B *on page 826*

**polymyxin B, bacitracin, and neomycin** *see* bacitracin, neomycin, and polymyxin B *on page 87*

**polymyxin B, bacitracin, neomycin, and hydrocortisone** *see* bacitracin, neomycin, polymyxin B, and hydrocortisone *on page 87*

**polymyxin B, neomycin, and dexamethasone** *see* neomycin, polymyxin B, and dexamethasone *on page 567*

**polymyxin B, neomycin, and gramicidin** *see* neomycin, polymyxin B, and gramicidin *on page 568*

**polymyxin B, neomycin, and hydrocortisone** *see* neomycin, polymyxin B, and hydrocortisone *on page 568*

**polymyxin B, neomycin, and prednisolone** *see* neomycin, polymyxin B, and prednisolone *on page 568*

**polymyxin B sulfate** *see* polymyxin B *on previous page*

**Poly-Pred® [US]** *see* neomycin, polymyxin B, and prednisolone *on page 568*

**Poly-Rx [US]** *see* polymyxin B *on previous page*

## polysaccharide-iron complex (pol i SAK a ride-EYE ern KOM pleks)
**Sound-Alike/Look-Alike Issues**
Niferex® may be confused with Nephrox®
**Synonyms** iron-polysaccharide complex
**U.S./Canadian Brand Names** Ferrex 150 [US-OTC]; Hytinic® [US-OTC]; Niferex® 150 [US-OTC]; Niferex® [US-OTC]; Nu-Iron® 150 [US-OTC]
**Therapeutic Category** Electrolyte Supplement, Oral
**Use** Prevention and treatment of iron-deficiency anemias
**Usual Dosage**
Children ≥6 years: Tablets/elixir: 50-100 mg/day; may be given in divided doses
Adults:
 Tablets/elixir: 50-100 mg twice daily
 Capsules: 150-300 mg/day
**Dosage Forms** [DSC] = Discontinued product
Capsule (Ferrex 150, Fe-Tinic™ 150 [DSC], Hytinic®, Niferex® 150, Nu-Iron® 150): Elemental iron 150 mg
Elixir (Niferex®): Elemental iron 100 mg/5 mL (240 mL) [contains alcohol 10%]
Tablet (Niferex®): Elemental iron 50 mg

**Polysporin® Ophthalmic [US]** *see* bacitracin and polymyxin B *on page 86*

**Polysporin® Topical [US-OTC]** *see* bacitracin and polymyxin B *on page 86*

**Polytapp® Allergy Dye-Free Medication [US-OTC]** *see* brompheniramine *on page 115*

**Polytar® [US-OTC]** *see* coal tar *on page 201*

## polythiazide (pol i THYE a zide)
**U.S./Canadian Brand Names** Renese® [US]
**Therapeutic Category** Diuretic, Thiazide
**Use** Adjunctive therapy in treatment of edema and hypertension
**Usual Dosage** Adults: Oral:
 Edema: 1-4 mg/day
 Hypertension: 2-4 mg/day
**Dosage Forms** Tablet: 2 mg

**polythiazide and prazosin** *see* prazosin and polythiazide *on page 672*

**Polytrim® [US/Can]** *see* trimethoprim and polymyxin B *on page 826*

**Poly-Vi-Flor® [US]** *see* vitamins (multiple/pediatric) *on page 852*

**Poly-Vi-Flor® With Iron [US]** *see* vitamins (multiple/pediatric) *on page 852*

**polyvinyl alcohol** *see* artificial tears *on page 71*

**Poly-Vi-Sol® [US-OTC]** *see* vitamins (multiple/pediatric) *on page 852*

**Poly-Vi-Sol® with Iron [US-OTC]** *see* vitamins (multiple/pediatric) *on page 852*

**Pondocillin® [Can]** *see* pivampicillin *(Canada only)* *on page 651*

**Ponstel® [US/Can]** *see* mefenamic acid *on page 508*

**Pontocaine**® **[US/Can]** *see* tetracaine *on page 791*

**Pontocaine**® **Niphanoid**® **[US]** *see* tetracaine *on page 791*

**Pontocaine**® **With Dextrose [US]** *see* tetracaine and dextrose *on page 791*

## poractant alfa (por AKT ant AL fa)
**U.S./Canadian Brand Names** Curosurf® [US/Can]
**Therapeutic Category** Lung Surfactant
**Use Orphan drug:** Treatment and prevention of respiratory distress syndrome (RDS) in premature infants
**Usual Dosage** Intratracheal use **only**: Premature infant with RDS: Initial dose is 2.5 mL/kg of birth weight. Up to 2 subsequent doses of 1.25 mL/kg birth weight can be administered at 12-hour intervals if needed in infants who continue to require mechanical ventilation and supplemental oxygen.
**Dosage Forms** Suspension for intratracheal instillation [preservative free; porcine derived]: 80 mg/mL (1.5 mL, 3 mL)

**Porcelana**® **Sunscreen** *(Discontinued)* *see* hydroquinone *on page 420*

## porfimer (POR fi mer)
**Synonyms** CL-184116; dihematoporphyrin ether; porfimer sodium
**U.S./Canadian Brand Names** Photofrin® [US/Can]
**Therapeutic Category** Antineoplastic Agent
**Use** Adjunct to laser light therapy for obstructing esophageal cancer, obstructing endobronchial nonsmall cell lung cancer (NSCLC), ablation of high-grade dysplasia in Barrett esophagus
**Usual Dosage** I.V. (refer to individual protocols):
Children: Safety and efficacy have not been established
Adults: 2 mg/kg, followed by exposure to the appropriate laser light
**Dosage Forms** Injection, powder for reconstitution, as sodium: 75 mg

**porfimer sodium** *see* porfimer *on this page*

**Portagen**® **[US-OTC]** *see* nutritional formula, enteral/oral *on page 591*

**Portia**™ **[US]** *see* ethinyl estradiol and levonorgestrel *on page 312*

**Post Peel Healing Balm [US-OTC]** *see* hydrocortisone (topical) *on page 417*

**Posture**® **[US-OTC]** *see* calcium phosphate (tribasic) *on page 135*

**Potasalan**® *(Discontinued)* *see* potassium chloride *on page 663*

## potassium acetate (poe TASS ee um AS e tate)
**Therapeutic Category** Electrolyte Supplement, Oral
**Use** Potassium deficiency; to avoid chloride when high concentration of potassium is needed, source of bicarbonate
**Usual Dosage** I.V. doses should be incorporated into the patient's maintenance I.V. fluids, intermittent I.V. potassium administration should be reserved for severe depletion situations and requires ECG monitoring; doses listed as mEq of potassium

Children:
Treatment of hypokalemia: I.V.: 2-5 mEq/kg/day
I.V. intermittent infusion (must be diluted prior to administration): 0.5-1 mEq/kg/dose (maximum: 30 mEq/dose) to infuse at 0.3-0.5 mEq/kg/hour (maximum: 1 mEq/kg/hour)
**Note:** Use caution in premature neonates; potassium acetate for injection contains aluminum.
Adults:
Treatment of hypokalemia: I.V.: 40-100 mEq/day
I.V. intermittent infusion (must be diluted prior to administration): 5-10 mEq/dose (maximum: 40 mEq/dose) to infuse over 2-3 hours (maximum: 40 mEq over 1 hour)

**Note:** Continuous cardiac monitor recommended for rates >0.5 mEq/hour
Potassium dosage/rate of infusion guidelines:
Serum potassium >2.5 mEq/L: Maximum infusion rate: 10 mEq/hour; maximum concentration: 40 mEq/L; maximum 24-hour dose: 200 mEq
Serum potassium <2.5 mEq/L: Maximum infusion rate: 40 mEq/hour; maximum concentration: 80 mEq/L; maximum 24-hour dose: 400 mEq
(Continued)

## potassium acetate *(Continued)*

**Dosage Forms** Injection, solution: 2 mEq/mL (20 mL, 50 mL, 100 mL); 4 mEq/mL (50 mL) [contains aluminum ≤200 mcg/mL]

## potassium acetate, potassium bicarbonate, and potassium citrate

(poe TASS ee um AS e tate, poe TASS ee um bye KAR bun ate, & poe TASS ee um SIT rate)

**Synonyms** potassium acetate, potassium citrate, and potassium bicarbonate; potassium bicarbonate, potassium acetate, and potassium citrate; potassium bicarbonate, potassium citrate, and potassium acetate; potassium citrate, potassium acetate, and potassium bicarbonate; potassium citrate, potassium bicarbonate, and potassium acetate

**U.S./Canadian Brand Names** Tri-K® [US]

**Therapeutic Category** Electrolyte Supplement, Oral

**Use** Treatment or prevention of hypokalemia

**Usual Dosage** Oral:

Children: 1-4 mEq/kg/24 hours in divided doses as required to maintain normal serum potassium

Adults:

Prevention: 16-24 mEq/day in 2-4 divided doses

Treatment: 40-100 mEq/day in 2-4 divided doses

**Dosage Forms** Solution, oral: Potassium 45 mEq/15 mL (480 mL) [from potassium acetate 1500 mg, potassium bicarbonate 1500 mg, and potassium citrate 1500 mg per 15 mL]

**potassium acetate, potassium citrate, and potassium bicarbonate** *see* potassium acetate, potassium bicarbonate, and potassium citrate *on this page*

## potassium acid phosphate (poe TASS ee um AS id FOS fate)

**U.S./Canadian Brand Names** K-Phos® Original [US]

**Therapeutic Category** Urinary Acidifying Agent

**Use** Acidifies urine and lowers urinary calcium concentration; reduces odor and rash caused by ammoniacal urine; increases the antibacterial activity of methenamine

**Usual Dosage** Adults: Oral: 1000 mg dissolved in 6-8 oz of water 4 times/day with meals and at bedtime; for best results, soak tablets in water for 2-5 minutes, then stir and swallow

**Dosage Forms** Tablet [scored]: 500 mg [phosphorus 114 mg and potassium 144 mg (3.7 mEq) per tablet; sodium free]

## potassium bicarbonate (poe TASS ee um bye KAR bun ate)

**Therapeutic Category** Electrolyte Supplement, Oral

**Use** Potassium deficiency, hypokalemia

**Usual Dosage** Oral:

Children: 1-4 mEq/kg/day

Adults: 25 mEq 2-4 times/day

**Dosage Forms** Tablet for oral solution, effervescent: Potassium 25 mEq

## potassium bicarbonate and potassium chloride, effervescent

(poe TASS ee um bye KAR bun ate & poe TASS ee um KLOR ide, ef er VES ent)

**U.S./Canadian Brand Names** K-Lyte/Cl® 50 [US]; K-Lyte/Cl® [US]

**Therapeutic Category** Electrolyte Supplement, Oral

**Use** Treatment or prevention of hypokalemia

**Usual Dosage** Oral:

Children: 1-4 mEq/kg/24 hours in divided doses as required to maintain normal serum potassium

Adults:

Prevention: 16-24 mEq/day in 2-4 divided doses

Treatment: 40-100 mEq/day in 2-4 divided doses

**Dosage Forms** Tablet for oral solution, effervescent:

K-Lyte/Cl®: Potassium chloride 25 mEq [potassium chloride 1.5 g and potassium bicarbonate 0.5 g; citrus or fruit punch flavor]

K-Lyte/Cl® 50: Potassium chloride 50 mEq [potassium chloride 2.24 g and potassium bicarbonate 2 g; citrus flavor]

## potassium bicarbonate and potassium citrate, effervescent
(poe TASS ee um bye KAR bun ate & poe TASS ee um SIT rate, ef er VES ent)

**Sound-Alike/Look-Alike Issues**
Klor-Con® may be confused with Klaron®, K-Lor®

**U.S./Canadian Brand Names** Effer-K™ [US]; K-Lyte® DS [US]; K-Lyte® [US]; Klor-Con®/EF [US]

**Therapeutic Category** Electrolyte Supplement, Oral

**Use** Treatment or prevention of hypokalemia

**Usual Dosage** Oral:
Children: 1-4 mEq/kg/24 hours in divided doses as required to maintain normal serum potassium
Adults:
Prevention: 16-24 mEq/day in 2-4 divided doses
Treatment: 40-100 mEq/day in 2-4 divided doses

**Dosage Forms**
Tablet, effervescent: Potassium 25 mEq
Effer-K™: Potassium 25 mEq
Klor-Con®/EF: Potassium 25 mEq [orange flavor]
K-Lyte®: Potassium 25 mEq [lime or orange flavor]
K-Lyte® DS: Potassium 50 mEq [lime or orange flavor]

**potassium bicarbonate, potassium acetate, and potassium citrate** *see* potassium acetate, potassium bicarbonate, and potassium citrate *on previous page*

**potassium bicarbonate, potassium citrate, and potassium acetate** *see* potassium acetate, potassium bicarbonate, and potassium citrate *on previous page*

## potassium chloride (poe TASS ee um KLOR ide)

**Sound-Alike/Look-Alike Issues**
Kaon-Cl-10® may be confused with kaolin
KCl may be confused with HCl
K-Dur® may be confused with Cardura®, Imdur®
K-Lor® may be confused with Kaochlor®, Klor-Con®
Klor-Con® may be confused with Klaron®, K-Lor®
Klotrix® may be confused with liotrix
microK® may be confused with Micronase®

**Synonyms** KCl

**U.S./Canadian Brand Names** Apo-K® [Can]; K+ Potassium [US]; K-10® [Can]; K-Dur® 10 [US]; K-Dur® 20 [US]; K-Dur® [Can]; K-Lor® [US/Can]; K-Lyte®/Cl [Can]; K-Tab® [US]; Kaon-Cl-10® [US]; Kaon-Cl® 20 [US]; Kay Ciel® [US]; Klor-Con® 10 [US]; Klor-Con® 8 [US]; Klor-Con® M [US]; Klor-Con® [US]; Klor-Con®/25 [US]; Micro-K Extencaps® [Can]; microK® 10 [US]; microK® [US]; Roychlor® [Can]; Rum-K® [US]; Slow-K® [Can]

**Therapeutic Category** Electrolyte Supplement, Oral

**Use** Treatment or prevention of hypokalemia

**Usual Dosage** I.V. doses should be incorporated into the patient's maintenance I.V. fluids; intermittent I.V. potassium administration should be reserved for severe depletion situations in patients undergoing ECG monitoring.

Normal daily requirements: Oral, I.V.:
Premature infants: 2-6 mEq/kg/24 hours
Term infants 0-24 hours: 0-2 mEq/kg/24 hours
Infants >24 hours: 1-2 mEq/kg/24 hours
Children: 2-3 mEq/kg/day
Adults: 40-80 mEq/day
Prevention during diuretic therapy: Oral:
Children: 1-2 mEq/kg/day in 1-2 divided doses
Adults: 20-40 mEq/day in 1-2 divided doses
Treatment of hypokalemia: Children:
Oral: 1-2 mEq/kg initially, then as needed based on frequently obtained lab values. If deficits are severe or ongoing losses are great, I.V. route should be considered.
I.V.: 1 mEq/kg over 1-2 hours initially, then repeated as needed based on frequently obtained lab values; severe depletion or ongoing losses may require >200% of normal limit needs
I.V. intermittent infusion: Dose should not exceed 1 mEq/kg/hour, or 40 mEq/hour; if it exceeds 0.5 mEq/kg/hour, physician should be at bedside and patient should have continuous ECG monitoring; usual pediatric maximum: 3 mEq/kg/day or 40 mEq/m$^2$/day

(Continued)

# potassium chloride (Continued)

Treatment of hypokalemia: Adults:

I.V. intermittent infusion: 5-10 mEq/hour (continuous cardiac monitor recommended for rates >5 mEq/hour), not to exceed 40 mEq/hour; usual adult maximum per 24 hours: 400 mEq/day.

Potassium dosage/rate of infusion guidelines:

Serum potassium >2.5 mEq/L: Maximum infusion rate: 10 mEq/hour; maximum concentration: 40 mEq/L; maximum 24-hour dose: 200 mEq

Serum potassium <2.5 mEq/L: Maximum infusion rate: 40 mEq/hour; maximum concentration: 80 mEq/L; maximum 24-hour dose: 400 mEq

Potassium >2.5 mEq/L:

Oral: 60-80 mEq/day plus additional amounts if needed

I.V.: 10 mEq over 1 hour with additional doses if needed

Potassium <2.5 mEq/L:

Oral: Up to 40-60 mEq initial dose, followed by further doses based on lab values

I.V.: Up to 40 mEq over 1 hour, with doses based on frequent lab monitoring; deficits at a plasma level of 2 mEq/L may be as high as 400-800 mEq of potassium

Dosage Forms [DSC] = Discontinued product

Capsule, extended release: 10 mEq [750 mg]

microK® [microencapsulated]: 8 mEq [600 mg]

microK® 10 [microencapsulated]: 10 mEq [750 mg]

Infusion [premixed in $D_5W$]: 20 mEq (1000 mL); 30 mEq (1000 mL); 40 mEq (1000 mL)

Infusion [premixed in $D_5W$ and LR]: 20 mEq (1000 mL); 30 mEq (1000 mL); 40 mEq (1000 mL)

Infusion [premixed in $D_5W$ and $\frac{1}{4}NS$]: 10 mEq (500 mL, 1000 mL); 20 mEq (250 mL, 500 mL, 1000 mL); 30 mEq (1000 mL); 40 mEq (1000 mL)

Infusion [premixed in $D_5W$ and $\frac{1}{2}NS$]: 10 mEq (500 mL, 1000 mL); 20 mEq (500 mL, 1000 mL); 30 mEq (1000 mL); 40 mEq (1000 mL)

Infusion [premixed in $D_5$ and NS]: 20 mEq (1000 mL); 40 mEq (1000 mL)

Infusion [premixed in $D_5W$ and sodium chloride 0.3%]: 10 mEq (500 mL); 20 mEq (1000 mL); 30 mEq (1000 mL); 40 mEq (1000 mL)

Infusion [premixed in $D_{10}W$ and sodium chloride 0.2%]: 20 mEq (250 mL)

Infusion [premixed in NS]: 20 mEq (1000 mL); 40 mEq (1000 mL)

Infusion [premixed in SWFI; concentrate]: 10 mEq (50 mL, 100 mL); 20 mEq (50 mL, 100 mL); 30 mEq (100 mL); 40 mEq (100 mL)

Injection, solution [concentrate]: 2 mEq/mL (5 mL, 10 mL, 15 mL, 20 mL, 30 mL, 250 mL, 500 mL)

Powder, for oral solution: 20 mEq/packet (30s, 100s, 1000s)

K-Lor™: 20 mEq/packet (30s, 100s) [fruit flavor]

K+ Potassium: 20 mEq/packet (30s) [orange flavor]

Kay Ciel® 10%: 20 mEq/packet (30s, 100s) [sugar free]

Klor-Con®: 20 mEq/packet (30s, 100s) [sugar free; fruit flavor]

Klor-Con®/25: 25 mEq/packet (30s, 100s) [sugar free; fruit flavor]

Solution, oral: 20 mEq/15 mL (480 mL, 3840 mL); 40 mEq/15 mL (480 mL)

Kaon-Cl® 20: 40 mEq/15 mL (480 mL) [sugar free; contains alcohol; cherry flavor]

Kay Ciel® 10%: 20 mEq/15 mL (480 mL) [sugar free; contains alcohol] [DSC]

Rum-K®: 20 mEq/10 mL (480 mL) [alcohol free, sugar free; butter/rum flavor]

Tablet, extended release: 8 mEq [600 mg]; 10 mEq [750 mg]; 20 mEq [1500 mg]

K-Dur® 10 [microencapsulated]: 10 mEq [750 mg]

K-Dur® 20 [microencapsulated]: 20 mEq [1500 mg; scored]

K-Tab®: 10 mEq [750 mg]

Kaon-Cl® 10 [film coated]: 10 mEq [750 mg]

Klor-Con® 8: 8 mEq [600 mg; wax matrix]

Klor-Con® 10: 10 mEq [750 mg; wax matrix]

Klor-Con® M10 [microencapsulated]: 10 mEq [750 mg]

Klor-Con® M15 [microencapsulated]: 15 mEq [1125 mg; scored]

Klor-Con® M20 [microencapsulated]: 20 mEq [1500 mg; scored]

# potassium citrate (poe TASS ee um SIT rate)

## Sound-Alike/Look-Alike Issues

Urocit®-K may be confused with Urised®

U.S./Canadian Brand Names K-Citra® [Can]; K-Lyte® [Can]; Polycitra®-K [Can]; Urocit®-K [US]

Therapeutic Category Alkalinizing Agent

Use Prevention of uric acid nephrolithiasis; prevention of calcium renal stones in patients with hypocitraturia; urinary alkalinizer when sodium citrate is contraindicated

Usual Dosage Adults: Oral: 10-20 mEq 3 times/day with meals up to 100 mEq/day

Dosage Forms Tablet: 540 mg [5 mEq]; 1080 mg [10 mEq]

## potassium citrate and citric acid (poe TASS ee um SIT rate & SI trik AS id)

Synonyms citric acid and potassium citrate

U.S./Canadian Brand Names Cytra-K [US]; Polycitra®-K [US]

Therapeutic Category Alkalinizing Agent

Use Treatment of metabolic acidosis; alkalinizing agent in conditions where long-term maintenance of an alkaline urine is desirable

Usual Dosage Urine alkalizing agent:
Children: Solution: 5-15 mL after meals and at bedtime; adjust dose based on urinary pH
Adults:
Powder: One packet dissolved in water after meals and at bedtime; adjust dose to urinary pH
Solution: 15-30 mL after meals and at bedtime; adjust dose based on urinary pH

Dosage Forms Note: Equivalent to potassium 2 mEq/mL and bicarbonate 2 mEq/mL
Powder:
Cytra-K: Potassium citrate 3300 mg and citric acid 1002 mg per packet (100s) [sugar free; fruit flavor]
Polycitra®-K: Potassium citrate 3300 mg and citric acid 1002 mg per packet (100s) [sugar free]
Solution:
Cytra-K: Potassium citrate 1100 mg and citric acid monohydrate 334 mg per 5 mL (480 mL) [alcohol free, sugar free; contains sodium benzoate; cherry flavor]
Polycitra®-K: Potassium citrate 1100 mg and citric acid monohydrate 334 mg per 5 mL (480 mL) [alcohol free, sugar free]

## potassium citrate, citric acid, and sodium citrate see citric acid, sodium citrate, and potassium citrate on page 189

## potassium citrate, potassium acetate, and potassium bicarbonate see potassium acetate, potassium bicarbonate, and potassium citrate on page 662

## potassium citrate, potassium bicarbonate, and potassium acetate see potassium acetate, potassium bicarbonate, and potassium citrate on page 662

## potassium gluconate (poe TASS ee um GLOO coe nate)

U.S./Canadian Brand Names Glu-K® [US-OTC]

Therapeutic Category Electrolyte Supplement, Oral

Use Treatment or prevention of hypokalemia

Usual Dosage Oral (doses listed as mEq of potassium):
Normal daily requirement:
Children: 2-3 mEq/kg/day
Adults: 40-80 mEq/day
Prevention of hypokalemia during diuretic therapy:
Children: 1-2 mEq/kg/day in 1-2 divided doses
Adults: 16-24 mEq/day in 1-2 divided doses
Treatment of hypokalemia:
Children: 2-5 mEq/kg/day in 2-4 divided doses
Adults: 40-100 mEq/day in 2-4 divided doses

Dosage Forms
Tablet: 500 mg, 610 mg
Glu-K®: 486 mg
Tablet, timed release: 595 mg

## potassium iodide (poe TASS ee um EYE oh dide)

Sound-Alike/Look-Alike Issues
Potassium iodide products, including saturated solution of potassium iodide (SSKI®) may be confused with potassium iodide and iodine (Strong Iodide Solution or Lugol's solution)

(Continued)

## potassium iodide *(Continued)*

**Synonyms** KI

**U.S./Canadian Brand Names** Iosat™ [US-OTC]; Pima® [US]; SSKI® [US]; ThyroSafe™ [US-OTC]; ThyroShield™ [US-OTC]

**Therapeutic Category** Antithyroid Agent; Expectorant

**Use** Expectorant for the symptomatic treatment of chronic pulmonary diseases complicated by mucous; reduce thyroid vascularity prior to thyroidectomy and management of thyrotoxic crisis; block thyroidal uptake of radioactive isotopes of iodine in a radiation emergency or other exposure to radioactive iodine

**Usual Dosage** Oral:

Adults: RDA: 150 mcg (iodine)

Expectorant:

Children (Pima®):

<3 years: 162 mg 3 times day

>3 years: 325 mg 3 times/day

Adults:

Pima®: 325-650 mg 3 times/day

SSKI®: 300-600 mg 3-4 times/day

Preoperative thyroidectomy: Children and Adults: 50-250 mg (1-5 drops SSKI®) 3 times/day; administer for 10 days before surgery

Radiation protectant to radioactive isotopes of iodine (Pima®):

Children:

Infants up to 1 year: 65 mg once daily for 10 days; start 24 hours prior to exposure

>1 year: 130 mg once daily for 10 days; start 24 hours prior to exposure

Adults: 195 mg once daily for 10 days; start 24 hours prior to exposure 7

To reduce risk of thyroid cancer following nuclear accident (Iosat™, ThyroSafe™, ThyroShield™): Dosing should continue until risk of exposure has passed or other measures are implemented:

Children (see adult dose for children >68 kg):

Infants <1 month: 16.25 mg once daily

1 month to 3 years: 32.5 mg once daily

3-18 years: 65 mg once daily

Children >68 kg and Adults (including pregnant/lactating women): 130 mg once daily

Thyrotoxic crisis:

Infants <1 year: 150-250 mg (3-5 drops SSKI®) 3 times/day

Children and Adults: 300-500 mg (6-10 drops SSKI®) 3 times/day

**Dosage Forms**

Solution, oral:

SSKI®: 1 g/mL (30 mL, 240 mL) [contains sodium thiosulfate]

ThyroShield™: 65 mg/mL (30 mL) [black raspberry flavor]

Syrup (Pima®): 325 mg/5 mL (473 mL) [equivalent to iodide 249 mg/5 mL; black raspberry flavor]

Tablet:

Iosat™: 130 mg

ThyroSafe™: 65 mg [equivalent to iodine 50 mg]

**potassium iodide, chlorpheniramine, phenylephrine, and codeine** *see* chlorpheniramine, phenylephrine, codeine, and potassium iodide *on page 176*

**potassium perchlorate** *see* radiological/contrast media (ionic) *on page 707*

## potassium phosphate *(poe TASS ee um FOS fate)*

**Sound-Alike/Look-Alike Issues**

Neutra-Phos®-K may be confused with K-Phos Neutral®

**Synonyms** phosphate, potassium

**U.S./Canadian Brand Names** Neutra-Phos®-K [US-OTC]

**Therapeutic Category** Electrolyte Supplement, Oral

**Use** Treatment and prevention of hypophosphatemia or hypokalemia

**Usual Dosage** I.V. doses should be incorporated into the patient's maintenance I.V. fluids; intermittent I.V. infusion should be reserved for severe depletion situations in patients undergoing continuous ECG monitoring. It is difficult to determine total body phosphorus deficit; the following dosages are empiric guidelines:

Normal requirements elemental phosphorus: Oral:

0-6 months: 240 mg

6-12 months: 360 mg

1-10 years: 800 mg

>10 years: 1200 mg

Pregnancy lactation: Additional 400 mg/day

Adults: 800 mg

Treatment: It is difficult to provide concrete guidelines for the treatment of severe hypophosphatemia because the extent of total body deficits and response to therapy are difficult to predict. Aggressive doses of phosphate may result in a transient serum elevation followed by redistribution into intracellular compartments or bone tissue. It is recommended that repletion of severe hypophosphatemia (<1 mg/dL in adults) be done I.V. because large doses of oral phosphate may cause diarrhea and intestinal absorption may be unreliable

**Pediatric I.V. phosphate repletion:**

Children: 0.25-0.5 mmol/kg **administer over 4-6 hours and repeat if symptomatic hypophosphatemia persists**; to assess the need for further phosphate administration, obtain serum inorganic phosphate after administration of the first dose and base further doses on serum levels and clinical status

**Adult I.V. phosphate repletion:**

Initial dose: 0.08 mmol/kg if recent uncomplicated hypophosphatemia

Initial dose: 0.16 mmol/kg if prolonged hypophosphatemia with presumed total body deficits; increase dose by 25% to 50% if patient symptomatic with severe hypophosphatemia

**Do not exceed 0.24 mmol/kg/dose; administer over 6-12 hours by I.V. infusion.** Some investigators have used more rapid infusions.

**With orders for I.V. phosphate, there is considerable confusion associated with the use of millimoles (mmol) versus milliequivalents (mEq) to express the phosphate requirement.** Because inorganic phosphate exists as monobasic and dibasic anions, with the mixture of valences dependent on pH, ordering by mEq amounts is unreliable and may lead to large dosing errors. In addition, I.V. phosphate is available in the sodium and potassium salt; therefore, the content of these cations must be considered when ordering phosphate. The most reliable method of ordering I.V. phosphate is by millimoles, then specifying the potassium or sodium salt. For example, an order for 15 mmol of phosphate as potassium phosphate in one liter of normal saline. The dosing of phosphate should be 0.2-0.3 mmol/kg with a usual daily requirement of 30-60 mmol/day or 15 mmol of phosphate per liter of TPN or 15 mmol phosphate per 1000 calories of dextrose. Would also provide 22 mEq of potassium.

Maintenance:

I.V. solutions:

Children: 0.5-1.5 mmol/kg/24 hours I.V. or 2-3 mmol/kg/24 hours orally in divided doses

Adults: 15-30 mmol/24 hours I.V. or 50-150 mmol/24 hours orally in divided doses

Oral:

Children <4 years: 1 capsule (250 mg phosphorus/8 mmol) 4 times/day; dilute as instructed

Children >4 years and Adults: 1-2 capsules (250-500 mg phosphorus/8-16 mmol) 4 times/day; dilute as instructed

**Dosage Forms**

Injection, solution: Phosphate 3 mmol and potassium 4.4 mEq per mL (5 mL, 15 mL, 50 mL) [equivalent to phosphate 285 mg and potassium 170 mg per mL]

Powder for oral solution [packet] (Neutra-Phos®-K): Monobasic potassium phosphate and dibasic potassium phosphate/packet (100s) [equivalent to elemental phosphorus 250 mg and potassium 556 mg (14.2 mEq) per packet; sodium free]

# potassium phosphate and sodium phosphate

(poe TASS ee um FOS fate & SOW dee um FOS fate)

**Sound-Alike/Look-Alike Issues**

K-Phos® Neutral may be confused with Neutra-Phos-K®

**Synonyms** sodium phosphate and potassium phosphate

**U.S./Canadian Brand Names** K-Phos® MF [US]; K-Phos® Neutral [US]; K-Phos® No. 2 [US]; Neutra-Phos® [US-OTC]; Uro-KP-Neutral® [US]

**Therapeutic Category** Electrolyte Supplement, Oral

**Use** Treatment of conditions associated with excessive renal phosphate loss or inadequate GI absorption of phosphate; to acidify the urine to lower calcium concentrations; to increase the antibacterial activity of methenamine; reduce odor and rash caused by ammonia in urine

**Usual Dosage** All dosage forms to be mixed in 6-8 oz of water prior to administration

Children ≥4 years: Elemental phosphorus 250 mg 4 times/day after meals and at bedtime

Adults: Elemental phosphorus 250-500 mg 4 times/day after meals and at bedtime

(Continued)

# potassium phosphate and sodium phosphate *(Continued)*

## Dosage Forms

Powder, for oral solution (Neutra-Phos®, Phos-NaK): Monobasic sodium, dibasic sodium, and potassium phosphate/packet (100s) [equivalent to elemental phosphorus 250 mg, sodium 164 mg (7.1 mEq), and potassium 278 mg (7.1 mEq) per packet]

Tablet:

K-Phos® MF: Potassium acid phosphate 155 mg and sodium acid phosphate 350 mg [equivalent to elemental phosphorus 125.6 mg, sodium 67 mg (2.9 mEq), and potassium 44.5 mg (1.1 mEq)]

K-Phos® Neutral: Dibasic sodium phosphate 852 mg, monobasic potassium phosphate 155 mg, and monobasic sodium phosphate 130 mg [equivalent to elemental phosphorus 250 mg, sodium 298 mg (13 mEq), and potassium 45 mg (1.1 mEq)]

K-Phos® No. 2: Potassium acid phosphate 305 mg and sodium acid phosphate 700 mg [equivalent to elemental phosphorus 250 mg, sodium 134 mg (5.8 mEq), and potassium 88 mg (2.3 mEq)]

Phospha 250™ Neutral: Dibasic sodium phosphate 852 mg, monobasic potassium phosphate 155 mg, and monobasic sodium phosphate 130 mg [equivalent to elemental phosphorus 250 mg, sodium 298 mg (13 mEq), and potassium 45 mg (1.1 mEq)]

Uro-KP-Neutral®: Sodium phosphate monobasic, dipotassium phosphate, and disodium phosphate [equivalent to elemental phosphorus 258 mg, sodium 262.4 mg (10.8 mEq), and potassium 49.4 mg (1.3 mEq)]

# povidone-iodine (POE vi done EYE oh dyne)

## Sound-Alike/Look-Alike Issues

Betadine® may be confused with Betagan®, betaine

**U.S./Canadian Brand Names** ACU-dyne® [US-OTC]; Betadine® Ophthalmic [US]; Betadine® [US-OTC/Can]; Minidyne® [US-OTC]; Operand® [US-OTC]; Proviodine [Can]; Summer's Eve® Medicated Douche [US-OTC]; Vagi-Gard® [US-OTC]

**Therapeutic Category** Antibacterial, Topical

**Use** External antiseptic with broad microbicidal spectrum against bacteria, fungi, viruses, protozoa, and yeasts

## Usual Dosage

Shampoo: Apply 2 teaspoons to hair and scalp, lather and rinse; repeat application 2 times/week until improvement is noted, then shampoo weekly

Topical: Apply as needed for treatment and prevention of susceptible microbial infections

## Dosage Forms

Gel, topical (Operand®): 10% (120 g)

Liquid, topical: 7.5% (120 mL)

ACU-dyne®: 7.5% (60 mL, 240 mL, 480 mL, 960 mL, 3840 mL)

Betadine®: 7.5% (120 mL)

Liquid, topical scrub: 7.5% (120 mL)

Betadine®: 7.5% (120 mL, 480 mL, 960 mL, 3840 mL)

Operand®: 7.5% (960 mL)

Ointment, topical: 10% (1 g, 3.5 g, 30 g)

Betadine®: 10% (0.9 g, 3.7 g, 30 g)

Pad [prep pads]: 10% (200s)

Solution, ophthalmic (Betadine®): 5% (50 mL)

Solution, perineal (Betadine®, Operand®): 10% (240 mL)

Solution, topical: 10% (30 mL, 120 mL, 240 mL, 480 mL, 3840 mL)

Betadine®: 10% (15 mL, 120 mL, 240 mL, 480 mL, 960 mL, 3840 mL)

Minidyne®: 10% (15 mL)

Operand®: 10% (60 mL, 120 mL, 240 mL, 480 mL, 960 mL, 3840 mL)

Solution, topical scrub: 7.5% (120 mL, 240 mL, 480 mL, 3840 mL)

Operand®: 7.5% (60 mL, 120 mL, 240 mL, 480 mL, 960 mL, 3840 mL)

Solution, topical spray (Betadine®): 5% (90 mL)

Solution, vaginal douche: 10% (240 mL) [concentrate]

Betadine®: 10% (180 mL, 240 mL) [concentrate]

Operand®: 10% (240 mL) [concentrate]

Summer's Eve® Medicated Douche: 0.3% (135 mL)

Vagi-Gard®: 10% (240 mL) [concentrate]

Solution, whirlpool: 10% (3840 mL) [concentrate]

Operand®: 1% (3840 mL)

Swabsticks: 7.5% (25s, 50s); 10% (25s, 50s)

Betadine®: 10% (50s, 150s, 200s, 1000s)

**PPD** *see* tuberculin tests *on page 830*

**PPI-149** *see* abarelix *on page 2*

**PPL** *see* benzylpenicilloyl-polylysine *on page 100*

**PPS** *see* pentosan polysulfate sodium *on page 632*

**PPV23** *see* pneumococcal polysaccharide vaccine (polyvalent) *on page 655*

## pralidoxime (pra li DOKS eem)

**Sound-Alike/Look-Alike Issues**

pralidoxime may be confused with pramoxine, pyridoxine

Protopam® may be confused with Proloprim®, protamine, Protropin®

**Synonyms** 2-PAM; 2-pyridine aldoxime methochloride; pralidoxime chloride

**U.S./Canadian Brand Names** Protopam® [US/Can]

**Therapeutic Category** Antidote

**Use** Reverse muscle paralysis caused by toxic exposure to organophosphate anticholinesterase pesticides and chemicals; control of overdose of anticholinesterase medications used to treat myasthenia gravis (ambenonium, neostigmine, pyridostigmine)

**Usual Dosage**

Organic phosphorus poisoning (use in conjunction with atropine; atropine effects should be established before pralidoxime is administered): I.V. (may be given I.M. or SubQ if I.V. is not feasible):

Children: 20-50 mg/kg/dose; repeat in 1-2 hours if muscle weakness has not been relieved, then at 8- to 12-hour intervals if cholinergic signs recur

Adults: 1-2 g; repeat in 1 hour if muscle weakness has not been relieved, then at 8- to 12-hour intervals if cholinergic signs recur. When the poison has been ingested, continued absorption from the lower bowel may require additional doses; patients should be titrated as long as signs of poisoning recur; dosing may need repeated every 3-8 hours.

Treatment of acetylcholinesterase inhibitor toxicity: Adults: I.V.: Initial: 1-2 g followed by increments of 250 mg every 5 minutes until response is observed

Infants and Children:

Prehospital ("in the field"): Mild-to-moderate symptoms: I.M.: 15 mg/kg; severe symptoms: 25 mg/kg

Hospital/emergency department: Mild-to-severe symptoms: I.V.: 15 mg/kg (up to 1 g)

Adults:

Prehospital ("in the field"): Mild-to-moderate symptoms: I.M.: 600 mg; severe symptoms: 1800 mg

Hospital/emergency department: Mild-to-severe symptoms: I.V.: 15 mg/kg (up to 1 g)

Frail patients:

Prehospital ("in the field"): Mild-to-moderate symptoms: I.M.: 10 mg/kg; severe symptoms: 25 mg/kg

Hospital/emergency department: Mild-to-severe symptoms: I.V.: 5-10 mg/kg

**Dosage Forms** Injection, powder for reconstitution, as chloride: 1 g

## pralidoxime chloride *see* pralidoxime *on this page*

## Pramet® FA *(Discontinued)*

## Pramilet® FA *(Discontinued)*

## pramipexole (pra mi PEKS ole)

**Sound-Alike/Look-Alike Issues**

Mirapex® may be confused with Mifeprex®, MiraLax™

**U.S./Canadian Brand Names** Mirapex® [US/Can]

**Therapeutic Category** Dopaminergic Agent (Anti-Parkinson)

**Use** Treatment of the signs and symptoms of idiopathic Parkinson disease

**Usual Dosage** Adults: Oral: Initial: 0.375 mg/day given in 3 divided doses, increase gradually by 0.125 mg/dose every 5-7 days; range: 1.5-4.5 mg/day

**Dosage Forms** Tablet, as dihydrochloride monohydrate: 0.125 mg, 0.25 mg, 0.5 mg, 1 mg, 1.5 mg

# pramlintide (PRAM lin tide)

**Synonyms** pramlintide acetate

**U.S./Canadian Brand Names** Symlin® [US]

**Therapeutic Category** Antidiabetic Agent

**Use**

Adjunctive treatment with mealtime insulin in type 1 diabetes mellitus (insulin dependent, IDDM) patients who have failed to achieve desired glucose control despite optimal insulin therapy

Adjunctive treatment with mealtime insulin in type 2 diabetes mellitus (noninsulin dependent, NIDDM) patients who have failed to achieve desired glucose control despite optimal insulin therapy, with or without concurrent sulfonylurea and/or metformin

**Usual Dosage** SubQ: Adults: **Note:** When initiating pramlintide, reduce current insulin dose (including rapidly- and mixed-acting preparations) by 50% to avoid hypoglycemia.

Type 1 diabetes mellitus (insulin dependent, IDDM): Initial: 15 mcg immediately prior to meals; titrate in 15 mcg increments every 3 days (if no significant nausea occurs) to target dose of 30-60 mcg (consider discontinuation if intolerant of 30 mcg dose)

Type 2 diabetes mellitus (noninsulin dependent, NIDDM): Initial: 60 mcg immediately prior to meals; after 3-7 days, increase to 120 mcg prior to meals if no significant nausea occurs (if nausea occurs at 120 mcg dose, reduce to 60 mcg)

If pramlintide is discontinued for any reason, restart therapy with same initial titration protocol.

**Dosage Forms** Injection, solution: Pramlintide acetate 0.6 mg/mL (5 mL) [contains phenol-derivative metacresol]

**pramlintide acetate** see pramlintide on this page

**Pramosone® [US]** see pramoxine and hydrocortisone on next page

**Pramox® HC [Can]** see pramoxine and hydrocortisone on next page

# pramoxine (pra MOKS een)

**Sound-Alike/Look-Alike Issues**

pramoxine may be confused with pralidoxime

Anusol® may be confused with Anusol-HC®, Aplisol®, Aquasol®

Tronolane® may be confused with Tronothane®

**Synonyms** pramoxine hydrochloride

**U.S./Canadian Brand Names** Anusol® Ointment [US-OTC]; Caladryl® Clear [US-OTC]; CalaMycin® Cool and Clear [US-OTC]; Callergy Clear [US-OTC]; Curasore [US-OTC]; Itch-X® [US-OTC]; Prax® [US-OTC]; ProctoFoam® NS [US-OTC]; Sarna® Sensitive [US]; Tronolane® [US-OTC]; Tucks® Hemorrhoidal [US-OTC]

**Therapeutic Category** Local Anesthetic

**Use** Temporary relief of pain and itching associated with anogenital pruritus or irritation; dermatosis, minor burns, or hemorrhoids

**Usual Dosage** Adults: Topical: Apply as directed, usually every 3-4 hours to affected area (maximum adult dose: 200 mg)

**Dosage Forms**

Aerosol, foam, topical, as hydrochloride (ProctoFoam® NS): 1% (15 g)

Cream, topical, as hydrochloride (Tronolane®): 1% (30 g, 60 g) [contains zinc oxide 5%]

Gel, topical, as hydrochloride (Itch-X®): 1% (35.4 g) [contains benzyl alcohol]

Liquid, topical, as hydrochloride (Curasore): 1% (15 mL) [contains ethyl alcohol; packaged with cotton applicators]

Lotion, topical, as hydrochloride:

Caladryl® Clear: 1% (177 mL) [contains zinc acetate 0.1%]

Callergy Clear: 1% (180 mL) [contains zinc acetate 0.1%]

Prax®: 1% (15 mL, 120 mL, 240 mL)

Sarna® Sensitive: 1% (222 mL)

Ointment, rectal, as hydrochloride (Anusol®, Tucks® Hemorrhoidal): 1% (30 g) [contains zinc oxide 12.5% and mineral oil; Anusol® ointment renamed Tucks® Hemorrhoidal]

Solution, topical spray, as hydrochloride:

CalaMycin® Cool and Clear: 1% (60 mL) [contains zinc acetate 0.1%]

Itch-X®: 1% (60 mL) [contains zinc oxide 1% and benzyl alcohol]

## pramoxine and hydrocortisone (pra MOKS een & hye droe KOR ti sone)
**Sound-Alike/Look-Alike Issues**
pramosone® may be confused with predniSONE
Zone-A Forte® may be confused with Zonalon®
**Synonyms** hydrocortisone and pramoxine
**U.S./Canadian Brand Names** Analpram-HC® [US]; Enzone® [US]; Epifoam® [US]; Pramosone® [US]; Pramox® HC [Can]; ProctoFoam®-HC [US/Can]; Zone-A Forte® [US]; Zone-A® [US]
**Therapeutic Category** Anesthetic/Corticosteroid
**Use** Relief of inflammatory and pruritic manifestations of corticosteroid-responsive dermatoses
**Usual Dosage** Topical/rectal: Apply to affected areas 3-4 times/day
**Dosage Forms**
Cream, topical:
Analpram-HC®: Pramoxine hydrochloride 1% and hydrocortisone acetate 1% (30 g); pramoxine hydrochloride 1% and hydrocortisone acetate 2.5% (30 g)
Enzone®: Pramoxine hydrochloride 1% and hydrocortisone acetate 1% (30 g)
Pramosone®: Pramoxine hydrochloride 1% and hydrocortisone acetate 1% (30 g, 60 g); pramoxine hydrochloride 1% and hydrocortisone acetate 2.5% (30 g, 60 g)
Foam, rectal (ProctoFoam®-HC): Pramoxine hydrochloride 1% and hydrocortisone acetate 1% (10 g)
Foam, topical (Epifoam®): Pramoxine hydrochloride 1% and hydrocortisone acetate 1% (10 g)
Lotion, topical:
Analpram-HC®: Pramoxine hydrochloride 1% and hydrocortisone 2.5% (60 mL)
Pramosone®: Pramoxine hydrochloride 1% and hydrocortisone 1% (60 mL, 120 mL, 240 mL); pramoxine hydrochloride 1% and hydrocortisone 2.5% (60 mL, 120 mL)
Zone-A®: Pramoxine hydrochloride 1% and hydrocortisone 1% (60 mL)
Zone-A Forte®: Pramoxine hydrochloride 1% and hydrocortisone 2.5% (60 mL)
Ointment, topical (Pramosone®): Pramoxine hydrochloride 1% and hydrocortisone 1% (30 g); pramoxine hydrochloride 1% and hydrocortisone 2.5% (30 g)

## pramoxine hydrochloride see pramoxine on previous page

## Prandase® [Can] see acarbose on page 3

## Prandin® [US/Can] see repaglinide on page 715

## Pravachol® [US/Can] see pravastatin on this page

## pravastatin (PRA va stat in)
**Sound-Alike/Look-Alike Issues**
Pravachol® may be confused with Prevacid®, Prinivil®, propranolol
**Synonyms** pravastatin sodium
**U.S./Canadian Brand Names** Apo-Pravastatin® [Can]; CO Pravastatin [Can]; Novo-Pravastatin [Can]; PMS-Pravastatin [Can]; Pravachol® [US/Can]; ratio-Pravastatin [Can]
**Therapeutic Category** HMG-CoA Reductase Inhibitor
**Use** Use with dietary therapy for the following:
Primary prevention of coronary events: In hypercholesterolemic patients without established coronary heart disease to reduce cardiovascular morbidity (myocardial infarction, coronary revascularization procedures) and mortality.
Secondary prevention of cardiovascular events in patients with established coronary heart disease: To slow the progression of coronary atherosclerosis; to reduce cardiovascular morbidity (myocardial infarction, coronary vascular procedures) and to reduce mortality; to reduce the risk of stroke and transient ischemic attacks
Hyperlipidemias: Reduce elevations in total cholesterol, LDL-C, apolipoprotein B, and triglycerides (elevations of 1 or more components are present in Fredrickson type IIa, IIb, III, and IV hyperlipidemias)
Heterozygous familial hypercholesterolemia (HeFH): In pediatric patients, 8-18 years of age, with HeFH having LDL-C ≥190 mg/dL **or** LDL ≥160 mg/dL with positive family history of premature cardiovascular disease (CVD) or 2 or more CVD risk factors in the pediatric patient
**Usual Dosage** Oral: **Note:** Doses should be individualized according to the baseline LDL-cholesterol levels, the recommended goal of therapy, and patient response; adjustments should be made at intervals of 4 weeks or more; doses may need adjusted based on concomitant medications
Children: HeFH:
8-13 years: 20 mg/day
14-18 years: 40 mg/day
(Continued)

# pravastatin *(Continued)*

**Dosage adjustment for pravastatin based on concomitant immunosuppressants (ie, cyclosporine):** Refer to Adults dosing section

Adults: Hyperlipidemias, primary prevention of coronary events, secondary prevention of cardiovascular events: Initial: 40 mg once daily; titrate dosage to response; usual range: 10-80 mg; (maximum dose: 80 mg once daily)

**Dosage adjustment for pravastatin based on concomitant immunosuppressants (ie, cyclosporine):** Initial: 10 mg/day, titrate with caution (maximum dose: 20 mg/day)

Dosage Forms Tablet, as sodium: 10 mg, 20 mg, 40 mg, 80 mg

**pravastatin and aspirin** *see* aspirin and pravastatin *on page 75*

**pravastatin sodium** *see* pravastatin *on previous page*

**Pravigard™ PAC *(Discontinued)*** *see* aspirin and pravastatin *on page 75*

**Prax® [US-OTC]** *see* pramoxine *on page 670*

# praziquantel *(pray zi KWON tel)*

U.S./Canadian Brand Names Biltricide® [US/Can]

Therapeutic Category Anthelmintic

Use All stages of schistosomiasis caused by all *Schistosoma* species pathogenic to humans; clonorchiasis and opisthorchiasis

Usual Dosage Children >4 years and Adults: Oral:

Schistosomiasis: 20 mg/kg/dose 2-3 times/day for 1 day at 4- to 6-hour intervals

Clonorchiasis/opisthorchiasis: 3 doses of 25 mg/kg as a 1-day treatment

Dosage Forms Tablet [tri-scored]: 600 mg

# prazosin *(PRA zoe sin)*

Sound-Alike/Look-Alike Issues

prazosin may be confused with prazepam, predniSONE

Synonyms furazosin; prazosin hydrochloride

U.S./Canadian Brand Names Apo-Prazo® [Can]; Minipress® [US/Can]; Novo-Prazin [Can]; Nu-Prazo [Can]

Therapeutic Category Alpha-Adrenergic Blocking Agent

Use Treatment of hypertension

Usual Dosage Oral:

Children: Initial: 5 mcg/kg/dose (to assess hypotensive effects); usual dosing interval: every 6 hours; increase dosage gradually up to maximum of 25 mcg/kg/dose every 6 hours

Adults:

Hypertension: Initial: 1 mg/dose 2-3 times/day; usual maintenance dose: 3-15 mg/day in divided doses 2-4 times/day; maximum daily dose: 20 mg

Hypertensive urgency: 10-20 mg once, may repeat in 30 minutes

Dosage Forms Capsule, as hydrochloride: 1 mg, 2 mg, 5 mg

# prazosin and polythiazide *(PRA zoe sin & pol i THYE a zide)*

Sound-Alike/Look-Alike Issues

Minizide® may be confused with Minocin®

Synonyms polythiazide and prazosin

U.S./Canadian Brand Names Minizide® [US]

Therapeutic Category Antihypertensive Agent, Combination

Use Management of mild to moderate hypertension

Usual Dosage Adults: Oral: 1 capsule 2-3 times/day

Dosage Forms Capsule:

Minizide® 1: Prazosin 1 mg and polythiazide 0.5 mg

Minizide® 2: Prazosin 2 mg and polythiazide 0.5 mg

Minizide® 5: Prazosin 5 mg and polythiazide 0.5 mg

**prazosin hydrochloride** *see* prazosin *on this page*

**PreCare® [US]** *see* vitamins (multiple/prenatal) *on page 852*

**PreCare® Conceive™ [US]** *see* vitamins (multiple/prenatal) *on page 852*

**PreCare® Prenatal [US]** *see* vitamins (multiple/prenatal) *on page 852*

**Precedex™ [US/Can]** *see* dexmedetomidine *on page 235*

**Precose® [US]** *see* acarbose *on page 3*

**Pred Forte® [US/Can]** *see* prednisolone (ophthalmic) *on this page*

**Pred-G® [US]** *see* prednisolone and gentamicin *on this page*

**Pred Mild® [US/Can]** *see* prednisolone (ophthalmic) *on this page*

## prednicarbate (PRED ni kar bate)

**Sound-Alike/Look-Alike Issues**
Dermatop® may be confused with Dimetapp®

**U.S./Canadian Brand Names** Dermatop® [US/Can]

**Therapeutic Category** Corticosteroid, Topical

**Use** Relief of the inflammatory and pruritic manifestations of corticosteroid-responsive dermatoses (medium potency topical corticosteroid)

**Usual Dosage** Adults: Topical: Apply a thin film to affected area twice daily. Therapy should be discontinued when control is achieved; if no improvement is seen, reassessment of diagnosis may be necessary.

**Dosage Forms**
Cream: 0.1% (15 g, 60 g)
Ointment: 0.1% (15 g, 60 g)

**Prednicen-M® *(Discontinued)*** *see* prednisone *on next page*

**prednisolone acetate** *see* prednisolone (systemic) *on next page*

**prednisolone acetate, ophthalmic** *see* prednisolone (ophthalmic) *on this page*

## prednisolone and gentamicin (pred NIS oh lone & jen ta MYE sin)

**Synonyms** gentamicin and prednisolone

**U.S./Canadian Brand Names** Pred-G® [US]

**Therapeutic Category** Antibiotic/Corticosteroid, Ophthalmic

**Use** Treatment of steroid responsive inflammatory conditions and superficial ocular infections due to microorganisms susceptible to gentamicin

**Usual Dosage** Ophthalmic: Children and Adults:
Ointment: Apply ½ inch ribbon in the conjunctival sac 1-3 times/day
Suspension: 1 drop 2-4 times/day; during the initial 24-48 hours, the dosing frequency may be increased if necessary up to 1 drop every hour

**Dosage Forms**
Ointment, ophthalmic: Prednisolone acetate 0.6% and gentamicin sulfate 0.3% (3.5 g)
Suspension, ophthalmic: Prednisolone acetate 1% and gentamicin sulfate 0.3% (2 mL, 5 mL, 10 mL) [contains benzalkonium chloride]

**prednisolone and sulfacetamide** *see* sulfacetamide and prednisolone *on page 771*

**prednisolone, neomycin, and polymyxin B** *see* neomycin, polymyxin B, and prednisolone *on page 568*

## prednisolone (ophthalmic) (pred NISS oh lone op THAL mik)

**Sound-Alike/Look-Alike Issues**
prednisoLONE may be confused with predniSONE

**Synonyms** prednisolone acetate, ophthalmic; prednisolone sodium phosphate, ophthalmic

**Tall-Man** prednisoLONE (ophthalmic)

**U.S./Canadian Brand Names** AK-Pred® [US]; Econopred® Plus [US]; Inflamase® Mild [Can]; Ophtho-Tate® [Can]; Pred Forte® [US/Can]; Pred Mild® [US/Can]

**Therapeutic Category** Adrenal Corticosteroid

**Use** Treatment of palpebral and bulbar conjunctivitis; corneal injury from chemical, radiation, thermal burns, or foreign body penetration

**Usual Dosage** Ophthalmic suspension/solution: Conjunctivitis, corneal injury: Children and Adults: Instill 1-2 drops into conjunctival sac every hour during day, every 2 hours at night until favorable response is obtained, then use 1 drop every 4 hours.

**Dosage Forms**
Solution, ophthalmic, as sodium phosphate: 1% (5 mL, 10 mL, 15 mL) [contains benzalkonium chloride]
AK-Pred®: 1% (5 mL, 15 mL) [contains benzalkonium chloride]
(Continued)

## prednisolone (ophthalmic) *(Continued)*

Suspension, ophthalmic, as acetate: 1% (5 mL, 10 mL, 15 mL) [contains benzalkonium chloride]
Econopred® Plus: 1% (5 mL, 10 mL) [contains benzalkonium chloride]
Pred Forte®: 1% (1 mL, 5 mL, 10 mL, 15 mL) [contains benzalkonium chloride and sodium bisulfite]
Pred Mild®: 0.12% (5 mL, 10 mL) [contains benzalkonium chloride and sodium bisulfite]

**prednisolone sodium phosphate** *see* prednisolone (systemic) *on this page*

**prednisolone sodium phosphate, ophthalmic** *see* prednisolone (ophthalmic) *on previous page*

## prednisolone (systemic) (pred NISS oh lone sis TEM ik)

**Sound-Alike/Look-Alike Issues**
prednisoLONE may be confused with predniSONE
Pediapred® may be confused with Pediazole®
**Synonyms** deltahydrocortisone; metacortandralone; prednisolone acetate; prednisolone sodium phosphate
**Tall-Man** predniso**LONE** (systemic)
**U.S./Canadian Brand Names** Bubbli-Pred™ [US]; Diopred® [Can]; Hydeltra T.B.A.® [Can]; Novo-Prednisolone [Can]; Orapred® [US]; Pediapred® [US/Can]; Prelone® [US]
**Therapeutic Category** Adrenal Corticosteroid
**Use** Treatment of endocrine disorders, rheumatic disorders, collagen diseases, dermatologic diseases, allergic states, ophthalmic diseases, respiratory diseases, hematologic disorders, neoplastic diseases, edematous states, and gastrointestinal diseases; resolution of acute exacerbations of multiple sclerosis
**Usual Dosage** Dose depends upon condition being treated and response of patient; dosage for infants and children should be based on severity of the disease and response of the patient rather than on strict adherence to dosage indicated by age, weight, or body surface area. Consider alternate day therapy for long-term therapy. Discontinuation of long-term therapy requires gradual withdrawal by tapering the dose. Patients undergoing unusual stress while receiving corticosteroids, should receive increased doses prior to, during, and after the stressful situation.

Children: Oral:
Acute asthma: 1-2 mg/kg/day in divided doses 1-2 times/day for 3-5 days
Anti-inflammatory or immunosuppressive dose: 0.1-2 mg/kg/day in divided doses 1-4 times/day
Nephrotic syndrome:
Initial (first 3 episodes): 2 mg/kg/day **or** 60 mg/m²/day (maximum: 80 mg/day) in divided doses 3-4 times/day until urine is protein free for 3 consecutive days (maximum: 28 days); followed by 1-1.5 mg/kg/dose **or** 40 mg/m²/dose given every other day for 4 weeks
Maintenance (long-term maintenance dose for frequent relapses): 0.5-1 mg/kg/dose given every other day for 3-6 months
Adults: Oral:
Usual range: 5-60 mg/day
Multiple sclerosis: 200 mg/day for 1 week followed by 80 mg every other day for 1 month
Rheumatoid arthritis: Initial: 5-7.5 mg/day; adjust dose as necessary
**Dosage Forms**
Solution, oral, as sodium phosphate: Prednisolone base 5 mg/5 mL (120 mL)
Bubbli-Pred™: Prednisolone base 5 mg/5 mL (120 mL) [bubble gum flavor]
Orapred®: 20 mg/5 mL (240 mL) [equivalent to prednisolone base 15 mg/5 mL; dye free; contains alcohol 2%, sodium benzoate; grape flavor]
Pediapred®: 6.7 mg/5 mL (120 mL) [equivalent to prednisolone base 5 mg/5 mL; dye free; raspberry flavor]
Syrup, as base: 5 mg/5 mL (120 mL); 15 mg/5 mL (240 mL, 480 mL)
Prelone®: 15 mg/5 mL (240 mL, 480 mL) [contains alcohol 5%, benzoic acid; cherry flavor]
Tablet, as base: 5 mg

## prednisone (PRED ni sone)

**Sound-Alike/Look-Alike Issues**
predniSONE may be confused with methylPREDNISolone, Pramosone®, prazosin, prednisoLONE, Prilosec®, primidone, promethazine
**Synonyms** deltacortisone; deltadehydrocortisone
**Tall-Man** predni**SONE**
**U.S./Canadian Brand Names** Apo-Prednisone® [Can]; Novo-Prednisone [Can]; Prednisone Intensol™ [US]; Sterapred® DS [US]; Sterapred® [US]; Winpred™ [Can]

**Therapeutic Category** Adrenal Corticosteroid

**Use** Treatment of a variety of diseases including adrenocortical insufficiency, hypercalcemia, rheumatic, and collagen disorders; dermatologic, ocular, respiratory, gastrointestinal, and neoplastic diseases; organ transplantation and a variety of diseases including those of hematologic, allergic, inflammatory, and autoimmune in origin; not available in injectable form, prednisolone must be used

**Usual Dosage** Oral: Dose depends upon condition being treated and response of patient; dosage for infants and children should be based on severity of the disease and response of the patient rather than on strict adherence to dosage indicated by age, weight, or body surface area. Consider alternate day therapy for long-term therapy. Discontinuation of long-term therapy requires gradual withdrawal by tapering the dose.

Children:
Anti-inflammatory or immunosuppressive dose: 0.05-2 mg/kg/day divided 1-4 times/day
Acute asthma: 1-2 mg/kg/day in divided doses 1-2 times/day for 3-5 days
Alternatively (for 3- to 5-day "burst"):
<1 year: 10 mg every 12 hours
1-4 years: 20 mg every 12 hours
5-13 years: 30 mg every 12 hours
>13 years: 40 mg every 12 hours
Asthma long-term therapy (alternative dosing by age):
<1 year: 10 mg every other day
1-4 years: 20 mg every other day
5-13 years: 30 mg every other day
>13 years: 40 mg every other day
Nephrotic syndrome:
Initial (first 3 episodes): 2 mg/kg/day **or** 60 mg/m$^2$/day (maximum: 80 mg/day) in divided doses 3-4 times/day until urine is protein free for 3 consecutive days (maximum: 28 days); followed by 1-1.5 mg/kg/dose **or** 40 mg/m$^2$/dose given every other day for 4 weeks
Maintenance dose (long-term maintenance dose for frequent relapses): 0.5-1 mg/kg/dose given every other day for 3-6 months
Children and Adults: Physiologic replacement: 4-5 mg/m$^2$/day
Children ≥5 years and Adults: Asthma:
Moderate persistent: Inhaled corticosteroid (medium dose) or inhaled corticosteroid (low-medium dose) with a long-acting bronchodilator
Severe persistent: Inhaled corticosteroid (high dose) and corticosteroid tablets or syrup long term: 2 mg/kg/day, generally not to exceed 60 mg/day
Adults:
Immunosuppression/chemotherapy adjunct: Range: 5-60 mg/day in divided doses 1-4 times/day
Allergic reaction (contact dermatitis):
Day 1: 30 mg divided as 10 mg before breakfast, 5 mg at lunch, 5 mg at dinner, 10 mg at bedtime
Day 2: 5 mg at breakfast, 5 mg at lunch, 5 mg at dinner, 10 mg at bedtime
Day 3: 5 mg 4 times/day (with meals and at bedtime)
Day 4: 5 mg 3 times/day (breakfast, lunch, bedtime)
Day 5: 5 mg 2 times/day (breakfast, bedtime)
Day 6: 5 mg before breakfast
*Pneumocystis carinii* pneumonia (PCP):
40 mg twice daily for 5 days **followed by**
40 mg once daily for 5 days **followed by**
20 mg once daily for 11 days or until antimicrobial regimen is completed
Thyrotoxicosis: Oral: 60 mg/day
Chemotherapy (refer to individual protocols): Oral: Range: 20 mg/day to 100 mg/m$^2$/day
Rheumatoid arthritis: Oral: Use lowest possible daily dose (often ≤7.5 mg/day)
Idiopathic thrombocytopenia purpura (ITP): Oral: 60 mg daily for 4-6 weeks, gradually tapered over several weeks
Systemic lupus erythematosus (SLE): Oral:
Acute: 1-2 mg/kg/day in 2-3 divided doses
Maintenance: Reduce to lowest possible dose, usually <1 mg/kg/day as single dose (morning)

**Dosage Forms**
Solution, oral: 1 mg/mL (5 mL, 120 mL, 500 mL) [contains alcohol 5%, sodium benzoate; vanilla flavor]
Solution, oral concentrate (Prednisone Intensol™): 5 mg/mL (30 mL) [contains alcohol 30%]
Tablet: 1 mg, 2.5 mg, 5 mg, 10 mg, 20 mg, 50 mg
Sterapred®: 5 mg [supplied as 21 tablet 6-day unit-dose package or 48 tablet 12-day unit-dose package]
(Continued)

## prednisone *(Continued)*

Sterapred® DS: 10 mg [supplied as 21 tablet 6-day unit-dose package or 48 tablet 12-day unit-dose package]

**Prednisone Intensol**™ **[US]** *see* prednisone *on page 674*

**Prefest**™ **[US]** *see* estradiol and norgestimate *on page 302*

**Prefrin**™ *(Discontinued) see* phenylephrine *on page 640*

**Pregestimil**® **[US-OTC]** *see* nutritional formula, enteral/oral *on page 591*

**pregnenedione** *see* progesterone *on page 682*

**Pregnyl**® **[US/Can]** *see* chorionic gonadotropin (human) *on page 181*

**Prelone**® **[US]** *see* prednisolone (systemic) *on page 674*

**Prelu-2**® *(Discontinued) see* phendimetrazine *on page 637*

**Premarin**® **[US/Can]** *see* estrogens (conjugated/equine) *on page 304*

**Premarin**® **With Methyltestosterone** *(Discontinued)*

**Premjact**® **[US-OTC]** *see* lidocaine *on page 479*

**Premphase**® **[US/Can]** *see* estrogens (conjugated/equine) and medroxyprogesterone *on page 304*

**Premplus**® **[Can]** *see* estrogens (conjugated/equine) and medroxyprogesterone *on page 304*

**Prempro**™ **[US/Can]** *see* estrogens (conjugated/equine) and medroxyprogesterone *on page 304*

**Prenatal 1-A-Day [US]** *see* vitamins (multiple/prenatal) *on page 852*

**Prenatal AD [US]** *see* vitamins (multiple/prenatal) *on page 852*

**Prenatal H [US]** *see* vitamins (multiple/prenatal) *on page 852*

**Prenatal MR 90 Fe**™ **[US]** *see* vitamins (multiple/prenatal) *on page 852*

**Prenatal MTR with Selenium [US]** *see* vitamins (multiple/prenatal) *on page 852*

**Prenatal Plus [US]** *see* vitamins (multiple/prenatal) *on page 852*

**Prenatal Rx 1 [US]** *see* vitamins (multiple/prenatal) *on page 852*

**Prenatal U [US]** *see* vitamins (multiple/prenatal) *on page 852*

**prenatal vitamins** *see* vitamins (multiple/prenatal) *on page 852*

**Prenatal Z [US]** *see* vitamins (multiple/prenatal) *on page 852*

**Prenate Elite**™ **[US]** *see* vitamins (multiple/prenatal) *on page 852*

**Prenate GT**™ **[US]** *see* vitamins (multiple/prenatal) *on page 852*

**Preparation H**® **Cleansing Pads [Can]** *see* witch hazel *on page 855*

**Preparation H**® **Hydrocortisone [US-OTC]** *see* hydrocortisone (rectal) *on page 416*

**Preparation H**® **Medicated Wipes [US-OTC]** *see* witch hazel *on page 855*

**Prepcat**® **[US]** *see* radiological/contrast media (ionic) *on page 707*

**Pre-Pen**® *(Discontinued) see* benzylpenicilloyl-polylysine *on page 100*

**Prepidil**® **[US/Can]** *see* dinoprostone *on page 253*

**Prescription Strength Desenex**® *(Discontinued) see* miconazole *on page 537*

**PreserVision**® **AREDS [US-OTC]** *see* vitamins (multiple/oral) *on page 852*

**PreserVision**® **Lutein [US-OTC]** *see* vitamins (multiple/oral) *on page 852*

**Pressyn**® **[Can]** *see* vasopressin *on page 842*

**Pressyn**® **AR [Can]** *see* vasopressin *on page 842*

**PreSun**® **29 [US-OTC]** *see* methoxycinnamate and oxybenzone *on page 527*

**Preterax**® **[Can]** *see* perindopril and indapamide *(Canada only) on page 634*

**Pretz-D**® **[US-OTC]** *see* ephedrine *on page 287*

**Pretz**® **Irrigation [US-OTC]** *see* sodium chloride *on page 752*

**Prevacid**® **[US/Can]** *see* lansoprazole *on page 467*

**Prevacid**® **NapraPAC**™ **[US]** *see* lansoprazole and naproxen *on page 468*

**Prevacid**® **SoluTab**™ **[US]** *see* lansoprazole *on page 467*

**Prevalite**® **[US]** *see* cholestyramine resin *on page 180*

**PREVEN**® **[US]** *see* ethinyl estradiol and levonorgestrel *on page 312*

**Prevex**® **B [Can]** *see* betamethasone (topical) *on page 103*

**Prevex**® **HC [Can]** *see* hydrocortisone (topical) *on page 417*

**PreviDent**® **[US]** *see* fluoride *on page 347*

**PreviDent**® **5000 Plus**™ **[US]** *see* fluoride *on page 347*

**Previfem**™ **[US]** *see* ethinyl estradiol and norgestimate *on page 317*

**Prevnar**® **[US/Can]** *see* pneumococcal conjugate vaccine (7-valent) *on page 654*

**Prevpac**® **[US/Can]** *see* lansoprazole, amoxicillin, and clarithromycin *on page 468*

**Prialt**® **[US]** *see* ziconotide *on page 859*

**Priftin**® **[US/Can]** *see* rifapentine *on page 723*

## prilocaine (PRIL oh kane)

**Sound-Alike/Look-Alike Issues**
prilocaine may be confused with Polocaine®, Prilosec®
**U.S./Canadian Brand Names** Citanest® Plain [US/Can]
**Therapeutic Category** Local Anesthetic
**Usual Dosage**
Children <10 years: Doses >40 mg (1 mL) as a 4% solution per procedure rarely needed
Children >10 years and Adults: Dental anesthesia, infiltration, or conduction block: Initial: 40-80 mg (1-2 mL) as a 4% solution; up to a maximum of 400 mg (10 mL) as a 4% solution within a 2-hour period. Manufacturer's maximum recommended dose is not more than 600 mg to normal healthy adults. The effective anesthetic dose varies with procedure, intensity of anesthesia needed, duration of anesthesia required and physical condition of the patient. Always use the lowest effective dose along with careful aspiration.
**Dosage Forms** Injection, solution: Prilocaine hydrochloride 4% (1.8 mL) [prefilled cartridge]

**prilocaine and lidocaine** *see* lidocaine and prilocaine *on page 482*

**Prilosec**® **[US]** *see* omeprazole *on page 598*

**Prilosec OTC**™ **[US-OTC]** *see* omeprazole *on page 598*

**primaclone** *see* primidone *on next page*

**Primacor**® **[US/Can]** *see* milrinone *on page 541*

## primaquine (PRIM a kween)

**Synonyms** primaquine phosphate; prymaccone
**Therapeutic Category** Aminoquinoline (Antimalarial)
**Use** Treatment of malaria
**Usual Dosage** Oral: Dosage expressed as mg of base (15 mg base = 26.3 mg primaquine phosphate):
Treatment of malaria (decrease risk of delayed primary attacks and prevent relapse):
Children: 0.3 mg base/kg/day once daily for 14 days (not to exceed 15 mg/day) or 0.9 mg base/kg once weekly for 8 weeks not to exceed 45 mg base/week
Adults: 15 mg/day (base) once daily for 14 days or 45 mg base once weekly for 8 weeks
CDC treatment recommendations: Begin therapy during last 2 weeks of, or following a course of, suppression with chloroquine or a comparable drug
**Note:** A second course (30 mg/day) for 14 days may be required in patients with relapse. Higher initial doses (30 mg/day) have also been used following exposure in S.E. Asia or Somalia.
**Dosage Forms** Tablet, as phosphate: 26.3 mg [15 mg base]

**primaquine phosphate** *see* primaquine *on this page*

**Primatene**® **Mist [US-OTC]** *see* epinephrine *on page 287*

**Primaxin**® **[US/Can]** *see* imipenem and cilastatin *on page 431*

## primidone (PRI mi done)

**Sound-Alike/Look-Alike Issues**
primidone may be confused with predniSONE
**Synonyms** desoxyphenobarbital; primaclone
**U.S./Canadian Brand Names** Apo-Primidone® [Can]; Mysoline® [US]
**Therapeutic Category** Anticonvulsant; Barbiturate
**Use** Management of grand mal, psychomotor, and focal seizures
**Usual Dosage** Oral:

Children <8 years: Initial: 50-125 mg/day given at bedtime; increase by 50-125 mg/day increments every 3-7 days; usual dose: 10-25 mg/kg/day in divided doses 3-4 times/day

Children ≥8 years and Adults: Initial: 125-250 mg/day at bedtime; increase by 125-250 mg/day every 3-7 days; usual dose: 750-1500 mg/day in divided doses 3-4 times/day with maximum dosage of 2 g/day

**Dosage Forms** Tablet: 50 mg, 250 mg [generic tablet may contain sodium benzoate]

**Primsol® [US]** *see* trimethoprim *on page 825*

**Principen® [US]** *see* ampicillin *on page 50*

**Prinivil® [US/Can]** *see* lisinopril *on page 485*

**Prinzide® [US/Can]** *see* lisinopril and hydrochlorothiazide *on page 486*

**Priorix™ [Can]** *see* measles, mumps, and rubella vaccines, combined *on page 504*

**pristinamycin** *see* quinupristin and dalfopristin *on page 706*

**Privine® [US-OTC]** *see* naphazoline *on page 561*

**ProAmatine® [US]** *see* midodrine *on page 540*

**Pro-Banthine® *(Discontinued)*** *see* propantheline *on page 685*

## probenecid (proe BEN e sid)

**Sound-Alike/Look-Alike Issues**
probenecid may be confused with Procanbid®
**U.S./Canadian Brand Names** Benuryl™ [Can]
**Therapeutic Category** Uricosuric Agent
**Use** Prevention of gouty arthritis; hyperuricemia; prolongation of beta-lactam effect (ie, serum levels)
**Usual Dosage** Oral:

Children:

<2 years: Not recommended

2-14 years: Prolong penicillin serum levels: 25 mg/kg starting dose, then 40 mg/kg/day given 4 times/day

Gonorrhea: <45 kg: 25 mg/kg x 1 (maximum: 1 g/dose) 30 minutes before penicillin, ampicillin or amoxicillin

Adults:

Hyperuricemia with gout: 250 mg twice daily for one week; increase to 250-500 mg/day; may increase by 500 mg/month, if needed, to maximum of 2-3 g/day (dosages may be increased by 500 mg every 6 months if serum urate concentrations are controlled)

Prolong penicillin serum levels: 500 mg 4 times/day

Gonorrhea: 1 g 30 minutes before penicillin, ampicillin, procaine, or amoxicillin

Pelvic inflammatory disease: Cefoxitin 2 g I.M. plus probenecid 1 g orally as a single dose

Neurosyphilis: Aqueous procaine penicillin 2.4 million units/day I.M. plus probenecid 500 mg 4 times/day for 10-14 days

**Dosage Forms** Tablet: 500 mg

**probenecid and colchicine** *see* colchicine and probenecid *on page 204*

**Pro-Bionate® *(Discontinued)***

## procainamide (proe kane A mide)

**Sound-Alike/Look-Alike Issues**
Procanbid® may be confused with probenecid
Pronestyl® may be confused with Ponstel®
PCA is an error-prone abbreviation (mistaken as patient controlled analgesia)

**Synonyms** procainamide hydrochloride; procaine amide hydrochloride

**U.S./Canadian Brand Names** Apo-Procainamide® [Can]; Procanbid® [US]; Procan® SR [Can]; Pronestyl®-SR [Can]

**Therapeutic Category** Antiarrhythmic Agent, Class I-A

**Use** Treatment of ventricular tachycardia (VT), premature ventricular contractions, paroxysmal atrial tachycardia (PSVT), and atrial fibrillation (AF); prevent recurrence of ventricular tachycardia, paroxysmal supraventricular tachycardia, atrial fibrillation or flutter

**Usual Dosage** Must be titrated to patient's response

Children:

Oral: 15-50 mg/kg/24 hours divided every 3-6 hours

I.M.: 50 mg/kg/24 hours divided into doses of $1/8$ to $1/4$ every 3-6 hours in divided doses until oral therapy is possible

I.V. (infusion requires use of an infusion pump):

Load: 3-6 mg/kg/dose over 5 minutes not to exceed 100 mg/dose; may repeat every 5-10 minutes to maximum of 15 mg/kg/load

Maintenance as continuous I.V. infusion: 20-80 mcg/kg/minute; maximum: 2 g/24 hours

Adults:

Oral: 250-500 mg/dose every 3-6 hours or 500 mg to 1 g every 6 hours extended release; usual dose: 50 mg/kg/24 hours; maximum: 4 g/24 hours (**Note:** Twice daily dosing approved for Procanbid®)

I.M.: 0.5-1 g every 4-8 hours until oral therapy is possible

I.V. (infusion requires use of an infusion pump): Loading dose: 15-18 mg/kg administered as slow infusion over 25-30 minutes or 100-200 mg/dose repeated every 5 minutes as needed to a total dose of 1 g; maintenance dose: 1-4 mg/minute by continuous infusion

Infusion rate: **2 g/250 mL** (I.V. infusion requires use of an infusion pump):

1 mg/minute: 7.5 mL/hour

2 mg/minute: 15 mL/hour

3 mg/minute: 22.5 mL/hour

4 mg/minute: 30 mL/hour

5 mg/minute: 37.5 mL/hour

6 mg/minute: 45 mL/hour

Intermittent/recurrent VF or pulseless VT:

Initial: 20-30 mg/minute (maximum: 50 mg/minute if necessary), up to a total of 17 mg/kg. ACLS guidelines: I.V.: Infuse 20 mg/minute until arrhythmia is controlled, hypotension occurs, QRS complex widens by 50% of its original width, or total of 17 mg/kg is given.

**Note:** Reduce to 12 mg/kg in setting of cardiac or renal dysfunction

I.V. maintenance infusion: 1-4 mg/minute; monitor levels and do not exceed 3 mg/minute for >24 hours in adults with renal failure.

**Dosage Forms**

Capsule, as hydrochloride: 250 mg, 500 mg

Injection, solution, as hydrochloride: 100 mg/mL (10 mL); 500 mg/mL (2 mL) [contains sodium metabisulfite]

Tablet, extended release, as hydrochloride: 500 mg, 750 mg, 1000 mg

Procanbid®: 500 mg, 1000 mg

**procainamide hydrochloride** *see* procainamide *on previous page*

# procaine (PROE kane)

**Synonyms** procaine hydrochloride

**U.S./Canadian Brand Names** Novocain® [US]

**Therapeutic Category** Local Anesthetic

**Use** Produces spinal anesthesia and epidural and peripheral nerve block by injection and infiltration methods

**Usual Dosage** Dose varies with procedure, desired depth, and duration of anesthesia, desired muscle relaxation, vascularity of tissues, physical condition, and age of patient

**Dosage Forms** Injection, solution, as hydrochloride: 1% [10 mg/mL] (2 mL) [contains sodium bisulfite]; 10% (2 mL) [contains sodium bisulfite]

**procaine amide hydrochloride** *see* procainamide *on previous page*

**procaine benzylpenicillin** *see* penicillin G procaine *on page 629*

**procaine hydrochloride** *see* procaine *on this page*

**procaine penicillin G** *see* penicillin G procaine *on page 629*

**Pro-Cal-Sof**® *(Discontinued)* see docusate *on page 263*

**Procanbid**® **[US]** see procainamide *on page 678*

**Procan**® **SR [Can]** see procainamide *on page 678*

**Procan**™ **SR** *(Discontinued)* see procainamide *on page 678*

## procarbazine (proe KAR ba zeen)
**Sound-Alike/Look-Alike Issues**
   procarbazine may be confused with dacarbazine
   Matulane® may be confused with Modane®
**Synonyms** benzmethyzin; N-methylhydrazine; NSC-77213; procarbazine hydrochloride
**U.S./Canadian Brand Names** Matulane® [US/Can]; Natulan® [Can]
**Therapeutic Category** Antineoplastic Agent
**Use** Treatment of Hodgkin disease
**Usual Dosage** Refer to individual protocols. Dose based on patient's ideal weight if the patient is obese or has abnormal fluid retention. Oral (may be given as a single daily dose or in 2-3 divided doses):

  Children:
    BMT aplastic anemia conditioning regimen: 12.5 mg/kg/dose every other day for 4 doses
    Hodgkin's disease: MOPP/IC-MOPP regimens: 100 mg/m$^2$/day for 14 days and repeated every 4 weeks
    Neuroblastoma and medulloblastoma: Doses as high as 100-200 mg/m$^2$/day once daily have been used
    Adults: Initial: 2-4 mg/kg/day in single or divided doses for 7 days then increase dose to 4-6 mg/kg/day until response is obtained or leukocyte count decreased <4000/mm$^3$ or the platelet count decreased <100,000/mm$^3$; maintenance: 1-2 mg/kg/day
**Dosage Forms** Capsule, as hydrochloride: 50 mg

**procarbazine hydrochloride** see procarbazine *on this page*

**Procardia**® **[US/Can]** see nifedipine *on page 575*

**Procardia XL**® **[US]** see nifedipine *on page 575*

**procetofene** see fenofibrate *on page 330*

**Prochieve**™ **[US]** see progesterone *on page 682*

## prochlorperazine (proe klor PER a zeen)
**Sound-Alike/Look-Alike Issues**
   prochlorperazine may be confused with chlorproMAZINE
   Compazine® may be confused with Copaxone®, Coumadin®
   CPZ (occasional abbreviation for Compazine®) is an error-prone abbreviation (mistaken as chlorpromazine)
**Synonyms** chlormeprazine; prochlorperazine edisylate; prochlorperazine maleate
**U.S./Canadian Brand Names** Apo-Prochlorperazine® [Can]; Compazine® [Can]; Compro™ [US]; Nu-Prochlor [Can]; Stemetil® [Can]
**Therapeutic Category** Phenothiazine Derivative
**Use** Management of nausea and vomiting; psychotic disorders including schizophrenia; anxiety
**Usual Dosage**
  Antiemetic: Children (therapy >1 day usually not required): **Note:** Not recommended for use in children <9 kg or <2 years:
    Oral, rectal: >9 kg: 0.4 mg/kg/24 hours in 3-4 divided doses; **or**
    9-13 kg: 2.5 mg every 12-24 hours as needed; maximum: 7.5 mg/day
    13.1-17 kg: 2.5 mg every 8-12 hours as needed; maximum: 10 mg/day
    17.1-37 kg: 2.5 mg every 8 hours or 5 mg every 12 hours as needed; maximum: 15 mg/day
    I.M.: 0.13 mg/kg/dose; change to oral as soon as possible
  Antiemetic: Adults:
    Oral (tablet): 5-10 mg 3-4 times/day; usual maximum: 40 mg/day; larger doses may rarely be required
    I.M. (deep): 5-10 mg every 3-4 hours; usual maximum: 40 mg/day
    I.V.: 2.5-10 mg; maximum 10 mg/dose or 40 mg/day; may repeat dose every 3-4 hours as needed
    Rectal: 25 mg twice daily
  Surgical nausea/vomiting: Adults: **Note:** Should not exceed 40 mg/day
    I.M.: 5-10 mg 1-2 hours before induction or to control symptoms during or after surgery; may repeat once if necessary

I.V. (administer slow IVP <5 mg/minute): 5-10 mg 15-30 minutes before induction or to control symptoms during or after surgery; may repeat once if necessary

Antipsychotic:

Children 2-12 years (not recommended in children <9 kg or <2 years):

Oral, rectal: 2.5 mg 2-3 times/day; do not give more than 10 mg the first day; increase dosage as needed to maximum daily dose of 20 mg for 2-5 years and 25 mg for 6-12 years

I.M.: 0.13 mg/kg/dose; change to oral as soon as possible

Adults:

Oral: 5-10 mg 3-4 times/day; titrate dose slowly every 2-3 days; doses up to 150 mg/day may be required in some patients for treatment of severe disturbances

I.M.: Initial: 10-20 mg; if necessary repeat initial dose every 1-4 hours to gain control; more than 3-4 doses are rarely needed. If parenteral administration is still required; give 10-20 mg every 4-6 hours; change to oral as soon as possible.

Nonpsychotic anxiety: Oral (tablet): Adults: Usual dose: 15-20 mg/day in divided doses; do not give doses >20 mg/day or for longer than 12 weeks

**Dosage Forms**

Injection, solution, as edisylate: 5 mg/mL (2 mL, 10 mL) [contains benzyl alcohol]

Suppository, rectal: 2.5 mg (12s), 5 mg (12s), 25 mg (12s) [may contain coconut and palm oil]

Compro™: 25 mg (12s) [contains coconut and palm oils]

Tablet, as maleate: 5 mg, 10 mg

**prochlorperazine edisylate** *see* prochlorperazine *on previous page*

**prochlorperazine maleate** *see* prochlorperazine *on previous page*

**Procrit**® **[US]** *see* epoetin alfa *on page 290*

**Proctocort**® **[US]** *see* hydrocortisone (rectal) *on page 416*

**ProctoCream**® **HC [US]** *see* hydrocortisone (rectal) *on page 416*

**proctofene** *see* fenofibrate *on page 330*

**ProctoFoam**®**-HC [US/Can]** *see* pramoxine and hydrocortisone *on page 671*

**ProctoFoam**® **NS [US-OTC]** *see* pramoxine *on page 670*

**Procto-Kit**™ **[US]** *see* hydrocortisone (rectal) *on page 416*

**Procto-Pak**™ **[US]** *see* hydrocortisone (rectal) *on page 416*

**Proctosert [US]** *see* hydrocortisone (rectal) *on page 416*

**Proctosol-HC**® **[US]** *see* hydrocortisone (rectal) *on page 416*

**Proctozone-HC**™ **[US]** *see* hydrocortisone (rectal) *on page 416*

**procyclidine** (proe SYE kli deen)

**Sound-Alike/Look-Alike Issues**

Kemadrin® may be confused with Coumadin®

**Synonyms** procyclidine hydrochloride

**U.S./Canadian Brand Names** Kemadrin® [US]; PMS-Procyclidine [Can]

**Therapeutic Category** Anti-Parkinson Agent; Anticholinergic Agent

**Use** Relieves symptoms of parkinsonian syndrome and drug-induced extrapyramidal symptoms

**Usual Dosage** Adults: Oral: 2.5 mg 3 times/day after meals; if tolerated, gradually increase dose, maximum of 20 mg/day if necessary

**Dosage Forms** Tablet, as hydrochloride [scored]: 5 mg

**procyclidine hydrochloride** *see* procyclidine *on this page*

**Procytox**® **[Can]** *see* cyclophosphamide *on page 214*

**Prodrox**® **[US]** *see* hydroxyprogesterone caproate *on page 422*

**Profasi**® **HP [Can]** *see* chorionic gonadotropin (human) *on page 181*

**Profen II**® **[US]** *see* guaifenesin and pseudoephedrine *on page 388*

**Profen II DM**® **[US]** *see* guaifenesin, pseudoephedrine, and dextromethorphan *on page 391*

**Profen Forte**® **[US]** *see* guaifenesin and pseudoephedrine *on page 388*

**Profen Forte**™ **DM [US]** *see* guaifenesin, pseudoephedrine, and dextromethorphan *on page 391*

**Profen LA**® *(Discontinued)*

**Profilnine**® **SD [US]** *see* factor IX complex (human) *on page 326*

**Proflavanol C**™ **[Can]** *see* ascorbic acid *on page 71*

## progesterone (proe JES ter one)

**Synonyms** pregnenedione; progestin

**U.S./Canadian Brand Names** Crinone® [US/Can]; Prochieve™ [US]; Prometrium® [US/Can]

**Therapeutic Category** Progestin

**Use**

Oral: Prevention of endometrial hyperplasia in nonhysterectomized, postmenopausal women who are receiving conjugated estrogen tablets; secondary amenorrhea

I.M.: Amenorrhea; abnormal uterine bleeding due to hormonal imbalance

Intravaginal gel: Part of assisted reproductive technology (ART) for infertile women with progesterone deficiency; secondary amenorrhea

**Usual Dosage** Adults:

I.M.: Female:

Amenorrhea: 5-10 mg/day for 6-8 consecutive days

Functional uterine bleeding: 5-10 mg/day for 6 doses

Oral: Female:

Prevention of endometrial hyperplasia (in postmenopausal women with a uterus who are receiving daily conjugated estrogen tablets): 200 mg as a single daily dose every evening for 12 days sequentially per 28-day cycle

Amenorrhea: 400 mg every evening for 10 days

Intravaginal gel: Female:

ART in women who require progesterone supplementation: 90 mg (8% gel) once daily; if pregnancy occurs, may continue treatment for up to 10-12 weeks

ART in women with partial or complete ovarian failure: 90 mg (8% gel) intravaginally twice daily; if pregnancy occurs, may continue up to 10-12 weeks

Secondary amenorrhea: 45 mg (4% gel) intravaginally every other day for up to 6 doses; women who fail to respond may be increased to 90 mg (8% gel) every other day for up to 6 doses

**Dosage Forms**

Capsule (Prometrium®): 100 mg, 200 mg [contains peanut oil]

Gel, vaginal (Crinone®, Prochieve™): 4% (45 mg); 8% (90 mg) [contains palm oil; prefilled applicators]

Injection, oil: 50 mg/mL (10 mL) [contains benzyl alcohol 10%, sesame oil]

**progestin** *see* progesterone *on this page*

**Proglycem**® **[US/Can]** *see* diazoxide *on page 242*

**Prograf**® **[US/Can]** *see* tacrolimus *on page 778*

**proguanil and atovaquone** *see* atovaquone and proguanil *on page 78*

**ProHance**® **[US]** *see* radiological/contrast media (nonionic) *on page 709*

**ProHIBiT**® *(Discontinued)*

**Prolastin**® **[US/Can]** *see* alpha₁-proteinase inhibitor *on page 30*

**Proleukin**® **[US/Can]** *see* aldesleukin *on page 25*

**Prolex**™**-D [US]** *see* guaifenesin and phenylephrine *on page 387*

**Prolixin Decanoate**® **[US]** *see* fluphenazine *on page 351*

**Prolixin**® *(Discontinued)* *see* fluphenazine *on page 351*

**Prolixin Enanthate**® *(Discontinued)* *see* fluphenazine *on page 351*

**Prolopa**® **[Can]** *see* benserazide and levodopa *(Canada only)* *on page 94*

**Proloprim**® **[US]** *see* trimethoprim *on page 825*

**Prometa**® *(Discontinued)*

## promethazine (proe METH a zeen)

**Sound-Alike/Look-Alike Issues**

promethazine may be confused with chlorproMAZINE, predniSONE, promazine

Phenergan® may be confused with Phenaphen®, Phrenilin®, Theragran®

**Synonyms** promethazine hydrochloride

**U.S./Canadian Brand Names** Phenadoz™ [US]; Phenergan® [US/Can]; Promethegan™ [US]

**Therapeutic Category** Antiemetic; Phenothiazine Derivative

**Use** Symptomatic treatment of various allergic conditions; antiemetic; motion sickness; sedative; postoperative pain (adjunctive therapy); anesthetic (adjunctive therapy); anaphylactic reactions (adjunctive therapy)

**Usual Dosage**

Children ≥2 years:

Allergic conditions: Oral, rectal: 0.1 mg/kg/dose (maximum: 12.5 mg) every 6 hours during the day and 0.5 mg/kg/dose (maximum: 25 mg) at bedtime as needed

Antiemetic: Oral, I.M., I.V., rectal: 0.25-1 mg/kg 4-6 times/day as needed (maximum: 25 mg/dose)

Motion sickness: Oral, rectal: 0.5 mg/kg/dose 30 minutes to 1 hour before departure, then every 12 hours as needed (maximum dose: 25 mg twice daily)

Sedation: Oral, I.M., I.V., rectal: 0.5-1 mg/kg/dose every 6 hours as needed (maximum: 50 mg/dose)

Adults:

Allergic conditions (including allergic reactions to blood or plasma):

Oral, rectal: 25 mg at bedtime **or** 12.5 mg before meals and at bedtime (range: 6.25-12.5 mg 3 times/day)

I.M., I.V.: 25 mg, may repeat in 2 hours when necessary; switch to oral route as soon as feasible

Antiemetic: Oral, I.M., I.V., rectal: 12.5-25 mg every 4-6 hours as needed

Motion sickness: Oral, rectal: 25 mg 30-60 minutes before departure, then every 12 hours as needed

Sedation: Oral, I.M., I.V., rectal: 12.5-50 mg/dose

**Dosage Forms** [DSC] = Discontinued product

Injection, solution, as hydrochloride: 25 mg/mL (1 mL); 50 mg/mL (1 mL)

Phenergan®: 25 mg/mL (1 mL); 50 mg/mL (1 mL) [contains sodium metabisulfite]

Suppository, rectal, as hydrochloride: 12.5 mg, 25 mg, 50 mg

Phenadoz™: 12.5 mg, 25 mg

Phenergan®: 12.5 mg, 25 mg; 50 mg [DSC]

Promethegan™: 12.5 mg, 25 mg, 50 mg

Syrup, as hydrochloride: 6.25 mg/5 mL (120 mL, 480 mL) [contains alcohol]

Tablet, as hydrochloride: 12.5 mg, 25 mg, 50 mg

Phenergan®: 12.5 mg [DSC], 25 mg, 50 mg [DSC]

## promethazine and codeine (proe METH a zeen & KOE deen)

**Sound-Alike/Look-Alike Issues**

Phenergan® may be confused with Phenaphen®, Phrenilin®, Theragran®

**Synonyms** codeine and promethazine

**Therapeutic Category** Antihistamine/Antitussive

**Controlled Substance** C-V

**Use** Temporary relief of coughs and upper respiratory symptoms associated with allergy or the common cold

**Usual Dosage** Oral (in terms of codeine):

Children: 1-1.5 mg/kg/day every 4 hours as needed; maximum: 30 mg/day **or**

2-6 years: 1.25-2.5 mL every 4-6 hours or 2.5-5 mg/dose every 4-6 hours as needed; maximum: 30 mg codeine/day

6-12 years: 2.5-5 mL every 4-6 hours as needed or 5-10 mg/dose every 4-6 hours as needed; maximum: 60 mg codeine/day

Adults: 10-20 mg/dose every 4-6 hours as needed; maximum: 120 mg codeine/day; or 5-10 mL every 4-6 hours as needed

**Dosage Forms** Syrup: Promethazine hydrochloride 6.25 mg and codeine phosphate 10 mg per 5 mL (120 mL, 473 mL, 3840 mL) [contains alcohol]

## promethazine and dextromethorphan (proe METH a zeen & deks troe meth OR fan)

**Synonyms** dextromethorphan and promethazine

**Therapeutic Category** Antihistamine/Antitussive

**Use** Temporary relief of coughs and upper respiratory symptoms associated with allergy or the common cold

**Usual Dosage** Oral:

Children:

2-6 years: 1.25-2.5 mL every 4-6 hours up to 10 mL in 24 hours

6-12 years: 2.5-5 mL every 4-6 hours up to 20 mL in 24 hours

(Continued)

## promethazine and dextromethorphan (Continued)

Adults: 5 mL every 4-6 hours up to 30 mL in 24 hours

Dosage Forms Syrup: Promethazine hydrochloride 6.25 mg and dextromethorphan hydrobromide 15 mg per 5 mL (120 mL, 480 mL, 4000 mL) [contains alcohol 7%]

**promethazine and meperidine** see meperidine and promethazine on page 513

## promethazine and phenylephrine (proe METH a zeen & fen il EF rin)

Synonyms phenylephrine and promethazine

Therapeutic Category Antihistamine/Decongestant Combination

Use Temporary relief of upper respiratory symptoms associated with allergy or the common cold

Usual Dosage Oral:

Children:

2-6 years: 1.25 mL every 4-6 hours, not to exceed 7.5 mL in 24 hours

6-12 years: 2.5 mL every 4-6 hours, not to exceed 15 mL in 24 hours

Children >12 years and Adults: 5 mL every 4-6 hours, not to exceed 30 mL in 24 hours

Dosage Forms Syrup: Promethazine hydrochloride 6.25 mg and phenylephrine hydrochloride 5 mg per 5 mL (120 mL, 473 mL) [contains alcohol]

**promethazine hydrochloride** see promethazine on page 682

## promethazine, phenylephrine, and codeine

(proe METH a zeen, fen il EF rin, & KOE deen)

Synonyms codeine, promethazine, and phenylephrine; phenylephrine, promethazine, and codeine

Therapeutic Category Antihistamine/Decongestant/Antitussive

Controlled Substance C-V

Use Temporary relief of coughs and upper respiratory symptoms including nasal congestion

Usual Dosage Oral:

Children (expressed in terms of codeine dosage): 1-1.5 mg/kg/day every 4 hours, maximum: 30 mg/day

**or**

<2 years: Not recommended

2-6 years:

Weight 25 lb: 1.25-2.5 mL every 4-6 hours, not to exceed 6 mL/24 hours

Weight 30 lb: 1.25-2.5 mL every 4-6 hours, not to exceed 7 mL/24 hours

Weight 35 lb: 1.25-2.5 mL every 4-6 hours, not to exceed 8 mL/24 hours

Weight 40 lb: 1.25-2.5 mL every 4-6 hours, not to exceed 9 mL/24 hours

6 to <12 years: 2.5-5 mL every 4-6 hours, not to exceed 15 mL/24 hours

Adults: 5 mL every 4-6 hours, not to exceed 30 mL/24 hours

Dosage Forms Syrup: Promethazine hydrochloride 6.25 mg, phenylephrine hydrochloride 5 mg, and codeine phosphate 10 mg per 5 mL with alcohol 7% (120 mL, 480 mL) [contains alcohol]

**Promethegan™ [US]** see promethazine on page 682

**Promethist® With Codeine (Discontinued)** see promethazine, phenylephrine, and codeine on this page

**Prometh® VC Plain Liquid (Discontinued)** see promethazine and phenylephrine on this page

**Prometh® VC With Codeine (Discontinued)** see promethazine, phenylephrine, and codeine on this page

**Prometrium® [US/Can]** see progesterone on page 682

**Promit® [US]** see dextran 1 on page 236

**Pronap-100® [US]** see propoxyphene and acetaminophen on page 687

**Pronestyl® (Discontinued)** see procainamide on page 678

**Pronestyl®-SR [Can]** see procainamide on page 678

**Pronestyl-SR® (Discontinued)** see procainamide on page 678

**Pronto® Complete Lice Killing Kit [US-OTC]** see pyrethrins and piperonyl butoxide on page 699

**Pronto® Lice Control [Can]** see pyrethrins and piperonyl butoxide on page 699

**Pronto® Plus Hair and Scalp Masque [US-OTC]** *see* pyrethrins and piperonyl butoxide *on page 699*

**Pronto® Plus Mousse [US-OTC]** *see* pyrethrins and piperonyl butoxide *on page 699*

**Pronto® Plus Warm Oil Treatment and Conditioner [US-OTC]** *see* pyrethrins and piperonyl butoxide *on page 699*

**Pronto® Plus with Natural Extracts and Oils [US-OTC]** *see* pyrethrins and piperonyl butoxide *on page 699*

**Propac™ [US-OTC]** *see* nutritional formula, enteral/oral *on page 591*

**Propacet® (Discontinued)** *see* propoxyphene and acetaminophen *on page 687*

**Propaderm® [Can]** *see* beclomethasone *on page 91*

## propafenone (proe pa FEEN one)

**Synonyms** propafenone hydrochloride
**U.S./Canadian Brand Names** Apo-Propafenone® [Can]; Rythmol® Gen-Propafenone [Can]; Rythmol® SR [US]; Rythmol® [US]
**Therapeutic Category** Antiarrhythmic Agent, Class I-C
**Use** Treatment of life-threatening ventricular arrhythmias
Rythmol® SR: Maintenance of normal sinus rhythm in patients with symptomatic atrial fibrillation
**Usual Dosage** Oral: Adults: **Note:** Patients who exhibit significant widening of QRS complex or second- or third-degree AV block may need dose reduction.
Immediate release tablet: Initial: 150 mg every 8 hours, increase at 3- to 4-day intervals up to 300 mg every 8 hours.
Extended release capsule: Initial: 225 mg every 12 hours; dosage increase may be made at a minimum of 5-day intervals; may increase to 325 mg every 12 hours; if further increase is necessary, may increase to 425 mg every 12 hours
**Dosage Forms**
Capsule, extended release, as hydrochloride (Rythmol® SR): 225 mg, 325 mg, 425 mg  [contains soy lecithin]
Tablet, as hydrochloride (Rythmol®): 150 mg, 225 mg, 300 mg

**propafenone hydrochloride** *see* propafenone *on this page*

**Propagest® (Discontinued)**

## propantheline (proe PAN the leen)

**Synonyms** propantheline bromide
**Therapeutic Category** Anticholinergic Agent
**Use** Adjunctive treatment of peptic ulcer, irritable bowel syndrome, pancreatitis, ureteral and urinary bladder spasm; reduce duodenal motility during diagnostic radiologic procedures
**Usual Dosage** Oral:
Antisecretory:
Children: 1-2 mg/kg/day in 3-4 divided doses
Adults: 15 mg 3 times/day before meals or food and 30 mg at bedtime
Antispasmodic:
Children: 2-3 mg/kg/day in divided doses every 4-6 hours and at bedtime
Adults: 15 mg 3 times/day before meals or food and 30 mg at bedtime
**Dosage Forms** Tablet, as bromide: 15 mg [contains lactose 23.2 mg]

**propantheline bromide** *see* propantheline *on this page*

**Propa pH [US-OTC]** *see* salicylic acid *on page 734*

## proparacaine (proe PAR a kane)

**Sound-Alike/Look-Alike Issues**
proparacaine may be confused with propoxyphene
**Synonyms** proparacaine hydrochloride; proxymetacaine
**U.S./Canadian Brand Names** Alcaine® [US/Can]; Diocaine® [Can]; Ophthetic® [US]
**Therapeutic Category** Local Anesthetic
**Use** Anesthesia for tonometry, gonioscopy; suture removal from cornea; removal of corneal foreign body; cataract extraction, glaucoma surgery; short operative procedure involving the cornea and conjunctiva
(Continued)

# proparacaine *(Continued)*

Usual Dosage Children and Adults:
Ophthalmic surgery: Instill 1 drop of 0.5% solution in eye every 5-10 minutes for 5-7 doses
Tonometry, gonioscopy, suture removal: Instill 1-2 drops of 0.5% solution in eye just prior to procedure
Dosage Forms Solution, ophthalmic, as hydrochloride: 0.5% (15 mL) [contains benzalkonium chloride]

# proparacaine and fluorescein (proe PAR a kane & FLURE e seen)

Synonyms fluorescein and proparacaine
U.S./Canadian Brand Names Flucaine® [US]; Fluoracaine® [US]
Therapeutic Category Diagnostic Agent; Local Anesthetic
Use Anesthesia for tonometry, gonioscopy; suture removal from cornea; removal of corneal foreign body; cataract extraction, glaucoma surgery
Usual Dosage
Ophthalmic surgery: Children and Adults: Instill 1 drop in each eye every 5-10 minutes for 5-7 doses
Tonometry, gonioscopy, suture removal: Adults: Instill 1-2 drops in each eye just prior to procedure
Dosage Forms Solution, ophthalmic: Proparacaine hydrochloride 0.5% and fluorescein sodium 0.25% (5 mL)

**proparacaine hydrochloride** *see* proparacaine *on previous page*

**Propecia**® **[US/Can]** *see* finasteride *on page 339*

**Propine**® **[US/Can]** *see* dipivefrin *on page 260*

**Proplex**® **T [US]** *see* factor IX complex (human) *on page 326*

# propofol (PROE po fole)

Sound-Alike/Look-Alike Issues
Diprivan® may be confused with Diflucan®, Ditropan®
U.S./Canadian Brand Names Diprivan® [US/Can]
Therapeutic Category General Anesthetic
Use Induction of anesthesia for inpatient or outpatient surgery in patients ≥3 years of age; maintenance of anesthesia for inpatient or outpatient surgery in patients >2 months of age; in adults, for the induction and maintenance of monitored anesthesia care sedation during diagnostic procedures; treatment of agitation in intubated, mechanically-ventilated ICU patients
Usual Dosage Dosage must be individualized based on total body weight and titrated to the desired clinical effect; wait at least 3-5 minutes between dosage adjustments to clinically assess drug effects; smaller doses are required when used with narcotics; the following are general dosing guidelines:

**General anesthesia:**
Induction: I.V.:
Children 3-16 years, ASA I or II: 2.5-3.5 mg/kg over 20-30 seconds; use a lower dose for children ASA III or IV
Adults, ASA I or II, <55 years: 2-2.5 mg/kg (~40 mg every 10 seconds until onset of induction)
Cardiac anesthesia: 0.5-1.5 mg/kg (~20 mg every 10 seconds until onset of induction)
Neurosurgical patients: 1-2 mg/kg (~20 mg every 10 seconds until onset of induction)
Maintenance: I.V. infusion:
Children 2 months to 16 years, ASA I or II: Initial: 200-300 mcg/kg/minute; decrease dose after 30 minutes if clinical signs of light anesthesia are absent; usual infusion rate: 125-150 mcg/kg/minute (range: 125-300 mcg/kg/minute; 7.5-18 mg/kg/hour); children ≤5 years may require larger infusion rates compared to older children
Adults, ASA I or II, <55 years: Initial: 150-200 mcg/kg/minute for 10-15 minutes; decrease by 30% to 50% during first 30 minutes of maintenance; usual infusion rate: 100-200 mcg/kg/minute (6-12 mg/kg/hour)
Cardiac anesthesia:
Low-dose propofol with primary opioid: 50-100 mcg/kg/minute (see manufacturer's labeling)
Primary propofol with secondary opioid: 100-150 mcg/kg/minute
Neurosurgical patients: 100-200 mcg/kg/minute (6-12 mg/kg/hour)
Maintenance: I.V. intermittent bolus: Adults, ASA I or II, <55 years: 20-50 mg increments as needed

**Monitored anesthesia care sedation:**
Initiation: Adults, ASA I or II, <55 years: Slow I.V. infusion: 100-150 mcg/kg/minute for 3-5 minutes **or** slow injection: 0.5 mg/kg over 3-5 minutes

Maintenance: Adults, ASA I or II, <55 years: I.V. infusion using variable rates (preferred over intermittent boluses): 25-75 mcg/kg/minute **or** incremental bolus doses: 10 mg or 20 mg

**ICU sedation in intubated mechanically-ventilated patients:** Avoid rapid bolus injection; individualize dose and titrate to response Continuous infusion: Initial: 0.3 mg/kg/hour (5 mcg/kg/min); increase by 0.3-0.6 mg/kg/hour (5-10 mcg/kg/min) every 5-10 minutes until desired sedation level is achieved; usual maintenance: 0.3-4.8 mg/kg/hour (5-80 mcg/kg/min) or higher; reduce dose by 80% in elderly, debilitated, and ASA III or IV patients; reduce dose after adequate sedation established and adjust to response (ie, evaluate frequently to use minimum dose for sedation). Some clinicians recommend daily interruption of infusion to perform clinical evaluation.

**Dosage Forms**

Injection, emulsion: 10 mg/mL (20 mL, 50 mL, 100 mL) [contains egg lecithin, and soybean oil; may contain either benzyl alcohol or sodium metabisulfite]

Diprivan®: 10 mg/mL (20 mL, 50 mL, 100 mL) [contains egg lecithin, soybean oil, and disodium edetate]

**Propoxacet-N® (Discontinued)** see propoxyphene and acetaminophen *on this page*

# propoxyphene (proe POKS i feen)

**Sound-Alike/Look-Alike Issues**

propoxyphene may be confused with proparacaine

Darvon® may be confused with Devrom®, Diovan®

Darvon-N® may be confused with Darvocet-N®

**Synonyms** dextropropoxyphene; propoxyphene hydrochloride; propoxyphene napsylate

**U.S./Canadian Brand Names** 642® Tablet [Can]; Darvon-N® [US/Can]; Darvon® [US]

**Therapeutic Category** Analgesic, Narcotic

**Controlled Substance** C-IV

**Use** Management of mild to moderate pain

**Usual Dosage** Oral:

Children: Doses for children are not well established; doses of the hydrochloride of 2-3 mg/kg/d divided every 6 hours have been used

Adults:

Hydrochloride: 65 mg every 3-4 hours as needed for pain; maximum: 390 mg/day

Napsylate: 100 mg every 4 hours as needed for pain; maximum: 600 mg/day

**Dosage Forms**

Capsule, as hydrochloride (Darvon®): 65 mg

Tablet, as napsylate (Darvon-N®): 100 mg

# propoxyphene and acetaminophen (proe POKS i feen & a seet a MIN oh fen)

**Sound-Alike/Look-Alike Issues**

Darvocet-N® may be confused with Darvon-N®

**Synonyms** propoxyphene hydrochloride and acetaminophen; propoxyphene napsylate and acetaminophen

**U.S./Canadian Brand Names** Balacet 325™ [US]; Darvocet A500™ [US]; Darvocet-N® 100 [US/Can]; Darvocet-N® 50 [US/Can]; Pronap-100® [US]

**Therapeutic Category** Analgesic, Narcotic

**Controlled Substance** C-IV

**Use** Management of mild to moderate pain

**Usual Dosage** Oral: Adults:

Darvocet A500™, Darvocet-N® 100: 1 tablet every 4 hours as needed; maximum: 600 mg propoxyphene napsylate/day

Darvocet-N® 50: 1-2 tablets every 4 hours as needed; maximum: 600 mg propoxyphene napsylate/day

**Note:** Dosage of acetaminophen should not exceed 4 g/day (6 tablets of Darvocet-N® 100); possibly less in patients with ethanol

**Dosage Forms**

Tablet: Propoxyphene hydrochloride 65 mg and acetaminophen 650 mg, propoxyphene napsylate 100 mg, and acetaminophen 650 mg

Balacet 325™: Propoxyphene napsylate 100 mg and acetaminophen 325 mg

Darvocet A500™: Propoxyphene napsylate 100 mg and acetaminophen 500 mg [contains lactose]

Darvocet-N® 50: Propoxyphene napsylate 50 mg and acetaminophen 325 mg

Darvocet-N® 100, Pronap-100®: Propoxyphene napsylate 100 mg and acetaminophen 650 mg

## propoxyphene, aspirin, and caffeine (proe POKS i feen, AS pir in, & KAF een)

**Sound-Alike/Look-Alike Issues**
Darvon® may be confused with Devrom®, Diovan®

**Synonyms** aspirin, caffeine, and propoxyphene; caffeine, propoxyphene, and aspirin; propoxyphene hydrochloride, aspirin, and caffeine

**U.S./Canadian Brand Names** Darvon® Compound [US]

**Therapeutic Category** Analgesic Combination (Narcotic)

**Controlled Substance** C-IV

**Use** Treatment of mild-to-moderate pain

**Usual Dosage** Oral: Adults: Pain: One capsule (providing propoxyphene 65 mg) every 4 hours as needed; maximum propoxyphene 390 mg/day. This will also provide aspirin 389 mg and caffeine 32.4 mg per capsule.

**Dosage Forms** Capsule (Darvon® Compound 65): Propoxyphene hydrochloride 65 mg, aspirin 389 mg, and caffeine 32.4 mg

**propoxyphene hydrochloride** *see propoxyphene on previous page*

**propoxyphene hydrochloride and acetaminophen** *see propoxyphene and acetaminophen on previous page*

**propoxyphene hydrochloride, aspirin, and caffeine** *see propoxyphene, aspirin, and caffeine on this page*

**propoxyphene napsylate** *see propoxyphene on previous page*

**propoxyphene napsylate and acetaminophen** *see propoxyphene and acetaminophen on previous page*

## propranolol (proe PRAN oh lole)

**Sound-Alike/Look-Alike Issues**
propranolol may be confused with Pravachol®, Propulsid®
Inderal® may be confused with Adderall®, Enduron®, Enduronyl®, Imdur®, Imuran®, Inderide®, Isordil®, Toradol®
Inderal® 40 may be confused with Enduronyl® Forte

**Synonyms** propranolol hydrochloride

**U.S./Canadian Brand Names** Apo-Propranolol® [Can]; Inderal® LA [US/Can]; Inderal® [US/Can]; InnoPran XL™ [US]; Novo-Pranol [Can]; Nu-Propranolol [Can]

**Therapeutic Category** Antiarrhythmic Agent, Class II; Beta-Adrenergic Blocker

**Use** Management of hypertension; angina pectoris; pheochromocytoma; essential tremor; tetralogy of Fallot cyanotic spells; arrhythmias (such as atrial fibrillation and flutter, AV nodal re-entrant tachycardias, and catecholamine-induced arrhythmias); prevention of myocardial infarction; migraine headache; symptomatic treatment of hypertrophic subaortic stenosis

**Usual Dosage**
Akathisia: Oral: Adults: 30-120 mg/day in 2-3 divided doses
Angina: Oral: Adults: 80-320 mg/day in doses divided 2-4 times/day
Long-acting formulation: Initial: 80 mg once daily; maximum dose: 320 mg once daily
Essential tremor: Oral: Adults: 20-40 mg twice daily initially; maintenance doses: usually 120-320 mg/day
Hypertension:
Oral:
Children: Initial: 0.5-1 mg/kg/day in divided doses every 6-12 hours; increase gradually every 5-7 days; maximum: 16 mg/kg/24 hours
Adults: Initial: 40 mg twice daily; increase dosage every 3-7 days; usual dose: ≤320 mg divided in 2-3 doses/day; maximum daily dose: 640 mg; usual dosage range (JNC 7): 40-160 mg/day in 2 divided doses
Long-acting formulation: Initial: 80 mg once daily; usual maintenance: 120-160 mg once daily; maximum daily dose: 640 mg; usual dosage range (JNC 7): 60-180 mg/day once daily
I.V.: Children: 0.01-0.05 mg/kg over 1 hour; maximum dose: 10 mg
Hypertrophic subaortic stenosis: Oral: Adults: 20-40 mg 3-4 times/day
Long-acting formulation: 80-160 mg once daily
Migraine headache prophylaxis: Oral:
Children: Initial: 2-4 mg/kg/day **or**
≤35 kg: 10-20 mg 3 times/day
>35 kg: 20-40 mg 3 times/day

Adults: Initial: 80 mg/day divided every 6-8 hours; increase by 20-40 mg/dose every 3-4 weeks to a maximum of 160-240 mg/day given in divided doses every 6-8 hours; if satisfactory response not achieved within 6 weeks of starting therapy, drug should be withdrawn gradually over several weeks

Long-acting formulation: Initial: 80 mg once daily; effective dose range: 160-240 mg once daily

Myocardial infarction prophylaxis: Oral: Adults: 180-240 mg/day in 3-4 divided doses

Pheochromocytoma: Oral: Adults: 30-60 mg/day in divided doses

Tachyarrhythmias:

Oral:

Children: Initial: 0.5-1 mg/kg/day in divided doses every 6-8 hours; titrate dosage upward every 3-7 days; usual dose: 2-6 mg/kg/day; higher doses may be needed; do not exceed 16 mg/kg/day or 60 mg/day

Adults: 10-30 mg/dose every 6-8 hours

I.V.:

Children: 0.01-0.1 mg/kg/dose slow IVP over 10 minutes; maximum dose: 1 mg for infants; 3 mg for children

Adults (in patients having nonfunctional GI tract): 1 mg/dose slow IVP; repeat every 5 minutes up to a total of 5 mg; titrate initial dose to desired response

Tetralogy spells: Children:

Oral: Palliation: Initial: 1 mg/kg/day every 6 hours; if ineffective, may increase dose after 1 week by 1 mg/kg/day to a maximum of 5 mg/kg/day; if patient becomes refractory, may increase slowly to a maximum of 10-15 mg/kg/day. Allow 24 hours between dosing changes.

I.V.: 0.01-0.2 mg/kg/dose infused over 10 minutes; maximum initial dose: 1 mg

Thyrotoxicosis:

Oral:

Children: 2 mg/kg/day, divided every 6-8 hours, titrate to effective dose

Adolescents and Adults: Oral: 10-40 mg/dose every 6 hours

I.V.: Adults: 1-3 mg/dose slow IVP as a single dose

**Dosage Forms**

Capsule, extended release, as hydrochloride (InnoPran XL™): 80 mg, 120 mg

Capsule, sustained release, as hydrochloride (Inderal® LA): 60 mg, 80 mg, 120 mg, 160 mg

Injection, solution, as hydrochloride (Inderal®): 1 mg/mL (1 mL)

Solution, oral, as hydrochloride: 4 mg/mL (5 mL, 500 mL); 8 mg/mL (500 mL) [strawberry-mint flavor; contains alcohol 0.6%]

Tablet, as hydrochloride (Inderal®): 10 mg, 20 mg, 40 mg, 60 mg, 80 mg

# propranolol and hydrochlorothiazide

(proe PRAN oh lole & hye droe klor oh THYE a zide)

**Sound-Alike/Look-Alike Issues**

Inderide® may be confused with Inderal®

**Synonyms** hydrochlorothiazide and propranolol

**U.S./Canadian Brand Names** Inderide® [US]

**Therapeutic Category** Antihypertensive Agent, Combination

**Use** Management of hypertension

**Usual Dosage** Oral: Adults: Hypertension: Dose is individualized; typical dosages of **hydrochlorothiazide**: 12.5-50 mg/day; initial dose of **propranolol**: 80 mg/day

Daily dose of tablet form should be divided into 2 daily doses; may be used to maximum dosage of up to 160 mg of propranolol; higher dosages would result in higher than optimal thiazide dosages.

**Dosage Forms** [DSC] = Discontinued product

Tablet: Propranolol hydrochloride 40 mg and hydrochlorothiazide 25 mg; propranolol hydrochloride 80 mg and hydrochlorothiazide 25 mg

Inderide®:

40/25: Propranolol hydrochloride 40 mg and hydrochlorothiazide 25 mg

80/25: Propranolol hydrochloride 80 mg and hydrochlorothiazide 25 mg [DSC]

**propranolol hydrochloride** *see* propranolol *on previous page*

**Proprinal [US-OTC]** *see* ibuprofen *on page 427*

**Proprinal® Cold and Sinus [US-OTC]** *see* pseudoephedrine and ibuprofen *on page 694*

**Propulsid® [US]** *see* cisapride *on page 186*

**propylene glycol and salicylic acid** *see* salicylic acid and propylene glycol *on page 736*

**propylene glycol diacetate, acetic acid, and hydrocortisone** *see* acetic acid, propylene glycol diacetate, and hydrocortisone *on page 14*

**propylene glycol diacetate, hydrocortisone, and acetic acid** *see* acetic acid, propylene glycol diacetate, and hydrocortisone *on page 14*

**propylhexedrine** (proe pil HEKS e dreen)
**U.S./Canadian Brand Names** Benzedrex® [US-OTC]
**Therapeutic Category** Adrenergic Agonist Agent
**Use** Topical nasal decongestant
**Usual Dosage** Nasal: Children 6-12 years and Adults: Two inhalations in each nostril, not more frequently than every 2 hours
**Dosage Forms** Inhaler, nasal: 0.4-0.5 mg/inhalation (1s) [total content 250 mg]

**propyliodone** *see* radiological/contrast media (ionic) *on page 707*

**2-propylpentanoic acid** *see* valproic acid and derivatives *on page 837*

**propylthiouracil** (proe pil thye oh YOOR a sil)
**Sound-Alike/Look-Alike Issues**
propylthiouracil may be confused with Purinethol®
PTU is an error-prone abbreviation (mistaken as mercaptopurine [Purinethol®; 6-MP])
**U.S./Canadian Brand Names** Propyl-Thyracil® [Can]
**Therapeutic Category** Antithyroid Agent
**Use** Palliative treatment of hyperthyroidism as an adjunct to ameliorate hyperthyroidism in preparation for surgical treatment or radioactive iodine therapy; management of thyrotoxic crisis
**Usual Dosage** Oral: Administer in 3 equally divided doses at approximately 8-hour intervals. Adjust dosage to maintain $T_3$, $T_4$, and TSH levels in normal range; elevated $T_3$ may be sole indicator of inadequate treatment. Elevated TSH indicates excessive antithyroid treatment.

Children: Initial: 5-7 mg/kg/day **or** 150-200 mg/m$^2$/day in divided doses every 8 hours
**or**
6-10 years: 50-150 mg/day
>10 years: 150-300 mg/day
Maintenance: Determined by patient response **or** $1/3$ to $2/3$ of the initial dose in divided doses every 8-12 hours. This usually begins after 2 months on an effective initial dose.
Adults: Initial: 300 mg/day in divided doses every 8 hours. In patients with severe hyperthyroidism, very large goiters, or both, the initial dosage is usually 450 mg/day; an occasional patient will require 600-900 mg/day; maintenance: 100-150 mg/day in divided doses every 8-12 hours
Withdrawal of therapy: Therapy should be withdrawn gradually with evaluation of the patient every 4-6 weeks for the first 3 months then every 3 months for the first year after discontinuation of therapy to detect any reoccurrence of a hyperthyroid state.
**Dosage Forms** Tablet: 50 mg

**Propyl-Thyracil® [Can]** *see* propylthiouracil *on this page*

**2-propylvaleric acid** *see* valproic acid and derivatives *on page 837*

**Proquin® XR [US]** *see* ciprofloxacin *on page 184*

**Proscar® [US/Can]** *see* finasteride *on page 339*

**ProSom® [US]** *see* estazolam *on page 299*

**prostacyclin** *see* epoprostenol *on page 291*

**prostaglandin E₁** *see* alprostadil *on page 31*

**prostaglandin E₂** *see* dinoprostone *on page 253*

**ProStep® Patch *(Discontinued)*** *see* nicotine *on page 574*

**Prostigmin® [US/Can]** *see* neostigmine *on page 569*

**Prostin E₂® [US/Can]** *see* dinoprostone *on page 253*

**Prostin F₂ Alpha® *(Discontinued)***

**Prostin® VR [Can]** *see* alprostadil *on page 31*

**Prostin VR Pediatric® [US]** *see* alprostadil *on page 31*

# protamine sulfate (PROE ta meen SUL fate)
**Sound-Alike/Look-Alike Issues**
protamine may be confused with ProAmatine®, protamine, Protopam®, Protropin®
**Therapeutic Category** Antidote
**Use** Treatment of heparin overdosage; neutralize heparin during surgery or dialysis procedures
**Usual Dosage**
Heparin neutralization: I.V.: Protamine dosage is determined by the dosage of heparin; 1 mg of protamine neutralizes 90 USP units of heparin (lung) and 115 USP units of heparin (intestinal); maximum dose: 50 mg
Heparin overdosage, following intravenous administration: I.V.: Since blood heparin concentrations decrease rapidly **after** administration, adjust the protamine dosage depending upon the duration of time since heparin administration.
**Note:** Excessive protamine doses may worsen bleeding potential.
**Dosage Forms** Injection, solution, as sulfate [preservative free]: 10 mg/mL (5 mL, 25 mL)

**protein C (activated), human, recombinant** see drotrecogin alfa on page 274

**protein-bound paclitaxel** see paclitaxel (protein bound) on page 613

**Protenate® (Discontinued)** see plasma protein fraction on page 652

**Prothazine-DC® (Discontinued)** see promethazine and codeine on page 683

**prothrombin complex concentrate** see factor IX complex (human) on page 326

**Protilase® (Discontinued)** see pancrelipase on page 615

**Protonix® [US/Can]** see pantoprazole on page 617

**Protopam® [US/Can]** see pralidoxime on page 669

**Protopic® [US/Can]** see tacrolimus on page 778

**Protostat® Oral (Discontinued)** see metronidazole on page 535

# protriptyline (proe TRIP ti leen)
**Synonyms** protriptyline hydrochloride
**U.S./Canadian Brand Names** Vivactil® [US]
**Therapeutic Category** Antidepressant, Tricyclic (Secondary Amine)
**Use** Treatment of depression
**Usual Dosage** Oral:
Adolescents: 15-20 mg/day
Adults: 15-60 mg in 3-4 divided doses
**Dosage Forms** Tablet, as hydrochloride [film coated]: 5 mg, 10 mg

**protriptyline hydrochloride** see protriptyline on this page

**Protuss®-DM (Discontinued)** see guaifenesin, pseudoephedrine, and dextromethorphan on page 391

**Proventil® [US]** see albuterol on page 22

**Proventil® HFA [US]** see albuterol on page 22

**Proventil® Inhaler (Discontinued)** see albuterol on page 22

**Proventil® Repetabs® [US]** see albuterol on page 22

**Proventil® Solution (Discontinued)** see albuterol on page 22

**Proventil® Tablet (Discontinued)** see albuterol on page 22

**Provera® [US/Can]** see medroxyprogesterone acetate on page 507

**Provigil® [US/Can]** see modafinil on page 546

**Proviodine [Can]** see povidone-iodine on page 668

**Provisc® [US]** see hyaluronate and derivatives on page 406

**Provocholine® [US/Can]** see methacholine on page 520

**proxymetacaine** see proparacaine on page 685

**Prozac® [US/Can]** see fluoxetine on page 349

**Prozac® Weekly™ [US]** see fluoxetine on page 349

**PRP-OMP** see Haemophilus B conjugate vaccine on page 394

**PRP-T** *see Haemophilus* B conjugate vaccine *on page 394*

**Prudoxin**™ **[US]** *see* doxepin *on page 269*

**prussian blue** *see* ferric hexacyanoferrate *on page 334*

**prymaccone** *see* primaquine *on page 677*

**23PS** *see* pneumococcal polysaccharide vaccine (polyvalent) *on page 655*

**PS-341** *see* bortezomib *on page 110*

## pseudoephedrine (soo doe e FED rin)

**Sound-Alike/Look-Alike Issues**
Dimetapp® may be confused with Dermatop®, Dimetabs®, Dimetane®
Sudafed® may be confused with Sufenta®

**Synonyms** d-isoephedrine hydrochloride; pseudoephedrine hydrochloride; pseudoephedrine sulfate

**U.S./Canadian Brand Names** Balminil Decongestant [Can]; Benylin® D for Infants [Can]; Biofed [US-OTC]; Contact® Cold [US-OTC]; Contac® Cold 12 Hour Relief Non Drowsy [Can]; Dimetapp® 12-Hour Non-Drowsy Extentabs® [US-OTC]; Dimetapp® Decongestant Infant [US-OTC]; Drixoral® ND [Can]; ElixSure™ Congestion [US-OTC]; Eltor® [Can]; Genaphed® [US-OTC]; Kidkare Decongestant [US-OTC]; Kodet SE [US-OTC]; Oranyl [US-OTC]; PediaCare® Decongestant Infants [US-OTC]; PMS-Pseudoephedrine [Can]; Pseudofrin [Can]; Robidrine® [Can]; Silfedrine Children's [US-OTC]; Simply Stuffy™ [US-OTC]; Sudafed® 12 Hour [US-OTC]; Sudafed® 24 Hour [US-OTC]; Sudafed® Children's [US-OTC]; Sudafed® Decongestant [Can]; Sudafed® [US-OTC]; Sudo-Tab® [US-OTC]; Sudodrin [US-OTC]; SudoGest [US-OTC]

**Therapeutic Category** Adrenergic Agonist Agent

**Use** Temporary symptomatic relief of nasal congestion due to common cold, upper respiratory allergies, and sinusitis; also promotes nasal or sinus drainage

**Usual Dosage** Oral: General dosing guidelines:
Children:
<2 years: 4 mg/kg/day in divided doses every 6 hours
2-5 years: 15 mg every 4-6 hours; maximum: 60 mg/24 hours
6-12 years: 30 mg every 4-6 hours; maximum: 120 mg/24 hours
Adults: 30-60 mg every 4-6 hours, sustained release: 120 mg every 12 hours; maximum: 240 mg/24 hours

**Dosage Forms**
Caplet, extended release, as hydrochloride (Contact® Cold, Sudafed® 12 Hour): 120 mg
Liquid, as hydrochloride: 30 mg/5 mL (120 mL, 480 mL)
Silfedrine Children's: 15 mg/5 mL (120 mL, 480 mL) [alcohol and sugar free; grape flavor]
Simply Stuffy™: 15 mg/5 mL (120 mL) [alcohol free; contains sodium benzoate; cherry berry flavor]
Sudafed® Children's: 15 mg/5 mL (120 mL) [alcohol and sugar free; contains sodium benzoate; grape flavor]
Liquid, oral drops, as hydrochloride:
Dimetapp® Decongestant Infant Drops: 7.5 mg/0.8 mL (15 mL) [alcohol free; contains sodium benzoate; grape flavor]
Kidkare Decongestant: 7.5 mg/0.8 mL (30 mL) [alcohol free; contains benzoic acid and sodium benzoate; cherry flavor]
PediaCare® Decongestant: 7.5 mg/0.8 mL (15 mL) [alcohol free, dye free; contains benzoic acid, sodium benzoate; fruit flavor]
Syrup, as hydrochloride:
Biofed: 30 mg/5 mL (120 mL, 240 mL, 480 mL, 3840 mL) [alcohol free; contains sodium benzoate]
ElixSure™ Congestion: 15 mg/5 mL (120 mL) [grape bubble gum flavor]
Tablet, as hydrochloride: 30 mg, 60 mg
Genaphed®, Kodet SE, Oranyl, Sudafed®, Sudodrin, Sudo-Tab®: 30 mg
SudoGest: 30 mg, 60 mg
Tablet, chewable, as hydrochloride (Sudafed® Children's): 15 mg [sugar free; contains phenylalanine 0.78 mg/tablet; orange flavor]
Tablet, extended release, as hydrochloride:
Dimetapp® 12-Hour Non-Drowsy Extentabs®: 120 mg
Sudafed® 24 Hour: 240 mg

## pseudoephedrine, acetaminophen, and chlorpheniramine *see* acetaminophen, chlorpheniramine, and pseudoephedrine *on page 10*

**pseudoephedrine, acetaminophen, and dextromethorphan** *see* acetaminophen, dextromethorphan, and pseudoephedrine *on page 11*

**pseudoephedrine and acetaminophen** *see* acetaminophen and pseudoephedrine *on page 8*

**pseudoephedrine and acrivastine** *see* acrivastine and pseudoephedrine *on page 16*

**pseudoephedrine and azatadine** *see* azatadine and pseudoephedrine *on page 83*

**pseudoephedrine and brompheniramine** *see* brompheniramine and pseudoephedrine *on page 115*

**pseudoephedrine and carbetapentane** *see* carbetapentane and pseudoephedrine *on page 142*

**pseudoephedrine and carbinoxamine** *see* carbinoxamine and pseudoephedrine *on page 144*

**pseudoephedrine and chlorpheniramine** *see* chlorpheniramine and pseudoephedrine *on page 172*

**pseudoephedrine and dexbrompheniramine** *see* dexbrompheniramine and pseudoephedrine *on page 234*

## pseudoephedrine and dextromethorphan (soo doe e FED rin & deks troe meth OR fan)

**Synonyms** dextromethorphan and pseudoephedrine

**U.S./Canadian Brand Names** Balminil DM D [Can]; Benylin® DM-D [Can]; Dimetapp® Infant Decongestant Plus Cough [US-OTC]; Koffex DM-D [Can]; Novahistex® DM Decongestant [Can]; Novahistine® DM Decongestant [Can]; Pedia Relief Cough and Cold [US-OTC]; Pedia Relief Infants [US-OTC]; Pediacare® Children's Long Acting Cough Plus Cold [US-OTC]; Pediacare® Infants' Decongestant & Cough [US-OTC]; Robitussin® Childrens Cough & Cold [Can]; Robitussin® Maximum Strength Cough & Cold [US-OTC]; Robitussin® Pediatric Cough & Cold [US-OTC]; Sudafed® Children's Cold & Cough [US-OTC]; SudoGest Children's [US-OTC]; Triaminic® Cough & Nasal Congestion [US-OTC]; Triaminic® Cough [US-OTC]; Vicks® 44D Cough & Head Congestion [US-OTC]

**Therapeutic Category** Antitussive/Decongestant

**Use** Temporary symptomatic relief of nasal congestion and cough due to common cold, hay fever, upper respiratory allergies

**Usual Dosage** Relief of nasal congestion and cough: Oral:
General dosing guidelines base on pseudoephedrine component:
Children 2-6 years: 15 mg every 4-6 hours (maximum: 60 mg/24 hours)
Children 6-12 years: 30 mg every 4-6 hours (maximum: 120 mg/24 hours)
Children ≥12 years and Adults: 60 mg every 4-6 hours (maximum: 240 mg/24 hours)

Product-specific dosing:
Children 2-3 years (PediaCare® Infants Decongestant & Cough): 1.6 mL every 4-6 hours (maximum: 6.4 mL/24 hours)
Children 2-6 years:
Pediacare® Children's Long Acting Cough Plus Cold: One chewable tablet or 5 mL every 6-8 hours (maximum: 4 doses/24 hours)
Robitussin® Pediatric Cough & Cold, Triaminic® Cough and Nasal Congestion: 5 mL every 6 hours (maximum: 20 mL/24 hours)
Sudafed® Children's Cold & Cough: 5 mL every 4 hours (maximum: 20 mL/24 hours)
Triaminic® Cough: 5 mL every 4-6 hours (maximum: 20 mL/24 hours)
Children 6-12 years:
Pediacare® Children's Long Acting Cough Plus Cold: Two chewable tablets or 10 mL every 6-8 hours (maximum: 4 doses/24 hours)
Robitussin® Pediatric Cough & Cold, Triaminic® Cough and Nasal Congestion: 10 mL every 6 hours (maximum: 40 mL/24 hours)
Sudafed® Children's Cold & Cough: 10 mL every 4 hours (maximum: 40 mL/24 hours)
Triaminic® Cough: 10 mL every 4-6 hours (maximum: 40 mL/24 hours)
Vicks® 44D Cough & Head Congestion: 7.5 mL every 6 hours (maximum: 30 mL/24 hours)
Children ≥12 years and Adults:
Robitussin® Maximum Strength Cough & Cold: 10 mL every 6 hours as needed (maximum: 40 mL/24 hours)
Sudafed® Children's Cold & Cough: 20 mL every 4 hours (maximum: 80 mL/24 hours)
Vicks® 44D Cough & Head Congestion: 15 mL every 6 hours (maximum: 60 mL/24 hours)

**Dosage Forms**
Liquid: Pseudoephedrine hydrochloride 15 mg and dextromethorphan hydrobromide 7.5 mg per 5 mL (120 mL)
(Continued)

## pseudoephedrine and dextromethorphan *(Continued)*

PediaCare® Children's Long Acting Cough Plus Cold: Pseudoephedrine hydrochloride 15 mg and dextromethorphan hydrobromide 7.5 mg per 5 mL (120 mL) [alcohol free; contains sodium benzoate; grape flavor]

Sudafed® Children's Cold & Cough: Pseudoephedrine hydrochloride 15 mg and dextromethorphan hydrobromide 5 mg per 5 mL (120 mL) [alcohol free, sugar free; contains sodium benzoate; cherry berry flavor]

Triaminic® Cough: Pseudoephedrine hydrochloride 15 mg and dextromethorphan hydrobromide 5 mg per 5 mL (120 mL, 150 mL) [alcohol free; contains benzoic acid, sodium 20 mg/5 mL; berry flavor]

Triaminic® Cough & Nasal Congestion: Pseudoephedrine hydrochloride 15 mg and dextromethorphan hydrobromide 7.5 mg per 5 mL (120 mL) [alcohol free; contains benzoic acid, sodium 7 mg/5 mL; orange strawberry flavor]

Vicks® 44D Cough & Head Congestion: Pseudoephedrine hydrochloride 20 mg and dextromethorphan hydrobromide 10 mg per 5 mL (120 mL, 240 mL) [contains alcohol 5%, sodium 10.3 mg/5 mL and sodium benzoate; cherry flavor]

Liquid, oral drops:

Dimetapp® Infant Decongestant Plus Cough: Pseudoephedrine hydrochloride 7.5 mg and dextromethorphan hydrobromide 2.5 mg per 0.8 mL (15 mL) [alcohol free, sugar free; grape flavor]

PediaCare® Infants' Decongestant & Cough: Pseudoephedrine hydrochloride 7.5 mg and dextromethorphan hydrobromide 2.5 mg per 0.8 mL (15 mL) [alcohol free; contains sodium benzoate; cherry flavor]

Pedia Relief Infants: Pseudoephedrine hydrochloride 7.5 mg and dextromethorphan hydrobromide 2.5 mg per 0.8 mL (15 mL) [cherry flavor]

Syrup:

Pedia Relief Cough and Cold: Pseudoephedrine hydrochloride 15 mg and dextromethorphan hydrobromide 7.5 mg per 5 mL (120 mL) [cherry flavor]

Robitussin® Maximum Strength Cough & Cold: Pseudoephedrine hydrochloride 30 mg and dextromethorphan hydrobromide 15 mg per 5 mL (120 mL, 240 mL) [contains alcohol 1.4% and sodium benzoate]

Robitussin® Pediatric Cough & Cold: Pseudoephedrine hydrochloride 15 mg and dextromethorphan hydrobromide 7.5 mg per 5 mL (120 mL, 240 mL) [alcohol free; contains sodium benzoate; fruit punch flavor]

SudoGest Children's: Pseudoephedrine hydrochloride 15 mg and dextromethorphan hydrobromide 5 mg per 5 mL (120 mL)

Tablets, chewable (PediaCare® Children's Long Acting Cough Plus Cold): Pseudoephedrine hydrochloride 15 mg and dextromethorphan hydrobromide 7.5 mg [contains phenylalanine 5 mg per tablet; grape flavor]

## pseudoephedrine and diphenhydramine *see* diphenhydramine and pseudoephedrine *on* *page 256*

## pseudoephedrine and fexofenadine *see* fexofenadine and pseudoephedrine *on page 337*

## pseudoephedrine and guaifenesin *see* guaifenesin and pseudoephedrine *on page 388*

## pseudoephedrine and hydrocodone *see* hydrocodone and pseudoephedrine *on page 413*

## pseudoephedrine and ibuprofen (soo doe e FED rin & eye byoo PROE fen)

**Synonyms** ibuprofen and pseudoephedrine

**U.S./Canadian Brand Names** Advil® Cold & Sinus [US-OTC/Can]; Advil® Cold, Children's [US-OTC]; Children's Advil® Cold [Can]; Dristan® Sinus [US-OTC]; Motrin® Cold and Sinus [US-OTC]; Motrin® Cold, Children's [US-OTC]; Proprinal® Cold and Sinus [US-OTC]; Sudafed® Sinus Advance [Can]

**Therapeutic Category** Decongestant/Analgesic

**Use** For temporary relief of cold, sinus and flu symptoms (including nasal congestion, headache, sore throat, minor body aches and pains, and fever)

**Usual Dosage** OTC labeling: Oral:

Children: Ibuprofen 100 mg and pseudoephedrine 15 mg per 5 mL: May repeat dose every 6 hours (maximum: 4 doses/24 hours); dose should be based on weight when possible. Contact healthcare provider if symptoms have not improved within 3 days (2 days if treating sore throat accompanied by fever).

2-5 years or 11 to <22 kg (24-47 pounds): 5 mL

6-11 years or 22-43 kg (48-95 pounds): 10 mL

Children ≥12 years and Adults: Ibuprofen 200 mg and pseudoephedrine 30 mg per dose: One dose every 4-6 hours as needed; may increase to 2 doses if necessary (maximum: 6 doses/24 hours).

Contact healthcare provider if symptoms have not improved within 7 days when treating cold symptoms or within 3 days when treating fever.

**Dosage Forms**

Caplet (Advil® Cold and Sinus, Dristan® Sinus, Motrin® Cold and Sinus, Proprinal® Cold and Sinus): Pseudoephedrine hydrochloride 30 mg and ibuprofen 200 mg

Capsule, liquid filled (Advil® Cold and Sinus): Pseudoephedrine hydrochloride 30 mg and ibuprofen 200 mg [solubilized ibuprofen as free acid and potassium salt; contains coconut oil]

Suspension:

Advil® Cold, Children's: Pseudoephedrine hydrochloride 15 mg and ibuprofen 100 mg per 5 mL (120 mL) [alcohol free; contains sodium benzoate; grape flavor]

Motrin® Cold, Children's: Pseudoephedrine hydrochloride 15 mg and ibuprofen 100 mg per 5 mL (120 mL) [contains sodium benzoate; berry, dye free berry, and grape flavors]

Tablet (Advil® Cold and Sinus): Pseudoephedrine hydrochloride 30 mg and ibuprofen 200 mg

**pseudoephedrine and loratadine** *see* loratadine and pseudoephedrine *on page 491*

**pseudoephedrine and triprolidine** *see* triprolidine and pseudoephedrine *on page 827*

**pseudoephedrine, carbinoxamine, and dextromethorphan** *see* carbinoxamine, pseudoephedrine, and dextromethorphan *on page 145*

**pseudoephedrine, chlorpheniramine, and acetaminophen** *see* acetaminophen, chlorpheniramine, and pseudoephedrine *on page 10*

**pseudoephedrine, chlorpheniramine, and codeine** *see* chlorpheniramine, pseudoephedrine, and codeine *on page 176*

**pseudoephedrine, chlorpheniramine, and dextromethorphan** *see* chlorpheniramine, pseudoephedrine, and dextromethorphan *on page 177*

**pseudoephedrine, codeine, and triprolidine** *see* triprolidine, pseudoephedrine, and codeine *(Canada only) on page 827*

**pseudoephedrine, dextromethorphan, and acetaminophen** *see* acetaminophen, dextromethorphan, and pseudoephedrine *on page 11*

**pseudoephedrine, dextromethorphan, and brompheniramine** *see* brompheniramine, pseudoephedrine, and dextromethorphan *on page 116*

**pseudoephedrine, dextromethorphan, and carbinoxamine** *see* carbinoxamine, pseudoephedrine, and dextromethorphan *on page 145*

**pseudoephedrine, dextromethorphan, and guaifenesin** *see* guaifenesin, pseudoephedrine, and dextromethorphan *on page 391*

**pseudoephedrine, guaifenesin, and codeine** *see* guaifenesin, pseudoephedrine, and codeine *on page 391*

**pseudoephedrine hydrochloride** *see* pseudoephedrine *on page 692*

**pseudoephedrine hydrochloride and cetirizine hydrochloride** *see* cetirizine and pseudoephedrine *on page 163*

**pseudoephedrine hydrochloride, hydrocodone bitartrate, and chlorpheniramine maleate** *see* pseudoephedrine, hydrocodone, and chlorpheniramine *on this page*

**pseudoephedrine, hydrocodone, and carbinoxamine** *see* hydrocodone, carbinoxamine, and pseudoephedrine *on page 414*

# pseudoephedrine, hydrocodone, and chlorpheniramine

(soo doe e FED rin, hye droe KOE done, & klor fen IR a meen)

**Synonyms** chlorpheniramine, pseudoephedrine, and hydrocodone; hydrocodone, chlorpheniramine, and pseudoephedrine; pseudoephedrine hydrochloride, hydrocodone bitartrate, and chlorpheniramine maleate

**U.S./Canadian Brand Names** Coldcough HC [US]; Cordron-HC [US]; Detuss [US]; Histinex® PV [US]; Hydro-Tussin™ HC [US]; Hydron PSC [US]; Hyphed [US]; P-V-Tussin® Syrup [US]; Pediatex™ HC [US]; Q-V Tussin [US]; Tussend® Syrup [US]; Tussend® Tablet [US]; Vasophrinic DH [Can]

**Therapeutic Category** Antihistamine; Antihistamine/Decongestant/Antitussive; Antitussive; Decongestant

**Controlled Substance** C-III

**Use** Temporary relief of cough, congestion, and sneezing due to colds, respiratory infections, or hay fever

(Continued)

## pseudoephedrine, hydrocodone, and chlorpheniramine *(Continued)*

**Usual Dosage** Oral:
Children:
2-6 years:
Hydro-Tussin™ HC: 1.25-2.5 mL every 4-6 hours; do not exceed 4 doses in 24 hours
Histinex® PV, Pediatex™ HC, P-V-Tussin®: 2.5 mL every 4-6 hours; do not exceed 4 doses in 24 hours
6-12 years:
Histinex® PV, Pediatex™ HC, P-V-Tussin®, Tussend®: 5 mL or ½ tablet every 4-6 hours; do not exceed 4 doses in 24 hours
Hydro-Tussin™ HC: 2.5-5 mL or ½ tablet every 4-6 hours; do not exceed 4 doses in 24 hours
Children >12 years and Adults:
Histinex® PV, Pediatex™ HC, P-V-Tussin®, Tussend®: 10 mL or 1 tablet every 4-6 hours; do not exceed 4 doses in 24 hours
Hydro-Tussin™ HC: 5-10 mL or 1 tablet every 4-6 hours; do not exceed 4 doses in 24 hours

**Dosage Forms**
Liquid:
Cordron-HC: Pseudoephedrine hydrochloride 20 mg, hydrocodone bitartrate 1.67 mg, and chlorpheniramine maleate 2.5 mg per 5 mL (480 mL) [vanilla mint flavor]
Detuss: Pseudoephedrine hydrochloride 30 mg, hydrocodone bitartrate 5 mg, and chlorpheniramine maleate 2 mg per 5 mL (480 mL) [alcohol free; vanilla flavor]
Hydron PSC: Pseudoephedrine hydrochloride 30 mg, hydrocodone bitartrate 5 mg, and chlorpheniramine maleate 2 mg per 5 mL (480 mL) [vanilla flavor]
Pediatex™ HC: Pseudoephedrine hydrochloride 20 mg, hydrocodone bitartrate 1.67 mg, and chlorpheniramine maleate 2.5 mg per 5 mL (480 mL) [alcohol free, sugar free; vanilla mint flavor]
Syrup:
Coldcough HC: Pseudoephedrine hydrochloride 15 mg, hydrocodone bitartrate 3 mg, and chlorpheniramine maleate 2 mg per 5 mL (480 mL) [alcohol free, dye free, sugar free; grape flavor]
Histinex® PV: Pseudoephedrine hydrochloride 30 mg, hydrocodone bitartrate 2.5 mg, and chlorpheniramine maleate 2 mg per 5 mL (480 mL) [alcohol free, sugar free; apricot flavor]
Hydro-Tussin™ HC: Pseudoephedrine hydrochloride 15 mg, hydrocodone bitartrate 3 mg, and chlorpheniramine maleate 2 mg per 5 mL (480 mL) [alcohol free, dye free, sugar free]
Hyphed: Pseudoephedrine hydrochloride 30 mg, hydrocodone bitartrate 2.5 mg, and chlorpheniramine maleate 2 mg per 5 mL (480 mL) [contains alcohol 5%; raspberry flavor]
P-V-Tussin®, Q-V Tussin, Tussend®: Pseudoephedrine hydrochloride 30 mg, hydrocodone bitartrate 2.5 mg, and chlorpheniramine maleate 2 mg per 5 mL (480 mL) [contains alcohol 5%; banana flavor]
Tablet [scored] (Tussend®): Pseudoephedrine hydrochloride 60 mg, hydrocodone bitartrate 5 mg, and chlorpheniramine maleate 4 mg

**pseudoephedrine, hydrocodone, and guaifenesin** *see* hydrocodone, pseudoephedrine, and guaifenesin *on page 415*

**pseudoephedrine sulfate** *see* pseudoephedrine *on page 692*

**pseudoephedrine, triprolidine, and codeine** *see* triprolidine, pseudoephedrine, and codeine *(Canada only) on page 827*

**Pseudofrin [Can]** *see* pseudoephedrine *on page 692*

**Pseudo-Gest Plus® Tablet *(Discontinued)*** *see* chlorpheniramine and pseudoephedrine *on page 172*

**Pseudo GG TR [US]** *see* guaifenesin and pseudoephedrine *on page 388*

**pseudomonic acid A** *see* mupirocin *on page 553*

**Pseudovent™ [US]** *see* guaifenesin and pseudoephedrine *on page 388*

**Pseudovent™ 400 [US]** *see* guaifenesin and pseudoephedrine *on page 388*

**Pseudovent™ DM [US]** *see* guaifenesin, pseudoephedrine, and dextromethorphan *on page 391*

**Pseudovent™-Ped [US]** *see* guaifenesin and pseudoephedrine *on page 388*

**P & S™ Liquid Phenol [Can]** *see* phenol *on page 638*

**Psorcon® [Can]** *see* diflorasone *on page 247*

**Psorcon® *(Discontinued)*** *see* diflorasone *on page 247*

**Psorcon® e™ [US]** *see* diflorasone *on page 247*

**Psoriatec**™ **[US]** *see* anthralin *on page 54*

**PsoriGel**® **[US-OTC]** *see* coal tar *on page 201*

**Psorion**® **Topical** *(Discontinued)*

# psyllium (SIL i yum)

**Sound-Alike/Look-Alike Issues**

Fiberall® may be confused with Feverall®

Hydrocil® may be confused with Hydrocet®

Modane® may be confused with Matulane®, Moban®

Perdiem® may be confused with Pyridium®

**Synonyms** plantago seed; plantain seed; psyllium hydrophilic mucilloid

**U.S./Canadian Brand Names** Fiberall® [US]; Fibro-Lax [US-OTC]; Fibro-XL [US-OTC]; Genfiber® [US-OTC]; Hydrocil® Instant [US-OTC]; Konsyl-D® [US-OTC]; Konsyl® Easy Mix [US-OTC]; Konsyl® Orange [US-OTC]; Konsyl® [US-OTC]; Metamucil® Plus Calcium [US-OTC]; Metamucil® Smooth Texture [US-OTC]; Metamucil® [US-OTC/Can]; Modane® Bulk [US-OTC]; Natural Fiber Therapy [US-OTC]; Reguloid® [US-OTC]; Serutan® [US-OTC]

**Therapeutic Category** Laxative

**Use** Treatment of chronic atonic or spastic constipation and in constipation associated with rectal disorders; management of irritable bowel syndrome; labeled for OTC use as fiber supplement, treatment of constipation

**Usual Dosage** Oral (administer at least 2 hours before or after other drugs):

Children 6-11 years: Approximately $1/2$ adult dosage

Children ≥12 years and Adults: Take 1 dose up to 3 times/day; all doses should be followed with 8 oz of water or liquid

Capsule: 4 capsules/dose (range: 2-6); swallow capsules one at a time

Powder: 1 rounded tablespoonful/dose (1 teaspoonful/dose for many sugar free or select concentrated products) mixed in 8 oz liquid

Tablet: 1 tablet/dose

Wafer: 2 wafers/dose

**Dosage Forms**

Capsule:

Fibro XL: 675 mg

Metamucil®: 0.52 g [contains potassium 5 mg/capsule; provides 3 g dietary fiber 2.4 g per 6 capsules]

Metamucil® Plus Calcium: 0.42 g [contains potassium 6 mg/capsule; provides dietary fiber 2.1 g and calcium 300 mg per 5 capsules]

Granules (Serutan®): 2.5 g/teaspoon (510 g) [contains sodium benzoate]

Powder: 3.4 g/dose (390 g, 570 g)

Bulk-K: 4.725 g/dose (392 g)

Fiberall®: 3.5 g/dose (454 g) [sugar free; contains phenylalanine; orange flavor]

Fibro-Lax: 4.725 g /dose (140 g, 392g)

Genfiber®: 3.4 g/dose (397 g, 595 g) [regular flavor]

Genfiber®: 3.5 g/dose (283 g) [sugar free; orange flavor]

Hydrocil® Instant: 3.5 g/dose (3.7 g unit-dose packets, 300 g) [sugar free]

Konsyl®: 6 g/dose (6 g unit-dose packets, 300 g, 450 g) [sugar free; contains sodium 4.1 mg/dose; regular flavor]

Konsyl-D®: 3.4 g/dose (6.5 g unit-dose packets, 325 g, 397 g,  500 g) [contains sodium 2.3 mg/dose and dextrose]

Konsyl® Easy Mix: 6 g/dose (6 g unit-dose packets, 250 g) [sugar free; contains sodium 4.4 mg/dose]

Konsyl® Orange: 3.4 g/dose (12 g unit-dose packets, 538 g) [contains sodium 2.3 mg/dose and sucrose; orange flavor]

Konsyl® Orange: 3.4 g/dose (425 g) [sugar free; contains sodium 2.3 mg/dose; orange flavor]

Metamucil®: 3.4 g/dose:

(390 g, 570 g, 870 g) [contains sodium 3 mg and potassium 30 mg per dose; regular flavor]

(570 g, 870 g, 1254 g) [contains sodium 5 mg and potassium 30 mg per dose; orange flavor]

Metamucil® Smooth Texture: 3.4 g/dose:

(unit-dose packets, 609 g, 912 g, 1446 g) [contains sodium 5 mg and potassium 30 mg per dose; orange flavor]

(300 g, 450 g, 690 g) [contains sodium 4 mg and potassium 30 mg per dose; regular flavor]

(unit-dose packets, 183 g, 300 g, 450 g, 699 g, 1104 g) [sugar free; contains phenylalanine 25 mg, sodium 5 mg, and potassium 30 mg per dose; orange flavor]

Modane® Bulk: 3.4 g/dose (390 g) [contains dextrose; flavor free]

(Continued)

## psyllium *(Continued)*

Natural Fiber Therapy: 3.4 g/dose (369 g, 539 g) [natural and orange flavors]

Reguloid®: 3.4 g/dose (300 g, 450 g) [sugar free; regular or orange flavors]; (390 g, 570g) [regular or orange flavors]

Wafers (Metamucil®): 3.4 g/dose (24s) [one dose= 2 wafers; contains sodium 20 mg and potassium 60 mg per dose; apple crisp and cinnamon spice flavors]

**psyllium hydrophilic mucilloid** *see* psyllium *on previous page*

**P.T.E.-4® [US]** *see* trace metals *on page 813*

**P.T.E.-5® [US]** *see* trace metals *on page 813*

**pteroylglutamic acid** *see* folic acid *on page 356*

**Pulmicort® [Can]** *see* budesonide *on page 118*

**Pulmicort Respules® [US]** *see* budesonide *on page 118*

**Pulmicort Turbuhaler® [US]** *see* budesonide *on page 118*

**Pulmophylline [Can]** *see* theophylline *on page 793*

**Pulmozyme® [US/Can]** *see* dornase alfa *on page 267*

**Puralube® Tears [US-OTC]** *see* artificial tears *on page 71*

**Purge® [US-OTC]** *see* castor oil *on page 151*

**Puri-Clens™ [US-OTC]** *see* methylbenzethonium chloride *on page 528*

**purified chick embryo cell** *see* rabies virus vaccine *on page 707*

**Purinethol® [US/Can]** *see* mercaptopurine *on page 515*

## pyrantel pamoate *(pi RAN tel PAM oh ate)*

**U.S./Canadian Brand Names** Combantrin™ [Can]; Pamix™ [US-OTC]; Pin-X® [US-OTC]; Reese's® Pinworm Medicine [US-OTC]

**Therapeutic Category** Anthelmintic

**Use** Treatment of pinworms (*Enterobius vermicularis*) and roundworms (*Ascaris lumbricoides*)

**Usual Dosage** Children and Adults (purgation is not required prior to use): Oral: Roundworm, pinworm, or trichostrongyliasis: 11 mg/kg administered as a single dose; maximum dose: 1 g. (**Note:** For pinworm infection, dosage should be repeated in 2 weeks and all family members should be treated).

**Dosage Forms**

Suspension, oral as pamoate:

Pamix™: 144 mg/mL (30 mL, 60 mL, 240 mL) [equivalent to pyrantel base 50 mg/mL; contains sodium benzoate]

Pin-X®: 144 mg/mL (30 mL, 60 mL) [equivalent to pyrantel base 50 mg/mL; contains sodium benzoate; caramel flavor]

Reese's® Pinworm Medicine: 144 mg/mL (30 mL) [equivalent to pyrantel base 50 mg/mL]

Tablet, as pamoate (Reese's® Pinworm Medicine): 180 mg [equivalent to pyrantel base 62.5 mg/tablet]

## pyrazinamide *(peer a ZIN a mide)*

**Synonyms** pyrazinoic acid amide

**U.S./Canadian Brand Names** Tebrazid™ [Can]

**Therapeutic Category** Antitubercular Agent

**Use** Adjunctive treatment of tuberculosis in combination with other antituberculosis agents

**Usual Dosage** Oral: Treatment of tuberculosis:

**Note:** Used as part of a multidrug regimen. Treatment regimens consist of an initial 2-month phase, followed by a continuation phase of 4 or 7 additional months; frequency of dosing may differ depending on phase of therapy.

**Children:**

Daily therapy: 15-30 mg/kg/day (maximum: 2 g/day)

Twice weekly directly observed therapy (DOT): 50 mg/kg/dose (maximum: 4 g/dose)

**Adults (dosing is based on lean body weight):**

Daily therapy: 15-30 mg/kg/day

40-55 kg: 1000 mg

56-75 kg: 1500 mg

76-90 kg: 2000 mg (maximum dose regardless of weight)

Twice weekly directly observed therapy (DOT): 50 mg/kg

40-55 kg: 2000 mg
56-75 kg: 3000 mg
76-90 kg: 4000 mg (maximum dose regardless of weight)
Three times/week DOT: 25-30 mg/kg (maximum: 2.5 g)
40-55 kg: 1500 mg
56-75 kg: 2500 mg
76-90 kg: 3000 mg (maximum dose regardless of weight)
**Dosage Forms** Tablet: 500 mg

**pyrazinamide, rifampin, and isoniazid** *see* rifampin, isoniazid, and pyrazinamide *on page 723*

**pyrazinoic acid amide** *see* pyrazinamide *on previous page*

# pyrethrins and piperonyl butoxide (pye RE thrins & pi PER oh nil byo TOKS ide)

**Synonyms** piperonyl butoxide and pyrethrins

**U.S./Canadian Brand Names** A-200® Maximum Strength [US-OTC]; Lice-Aid [US-OTC]; Licide® [US-OTC]; Pronto® Complete Lice Killing Kit [US-OTC]; Pronto® Lice Control [Can]; Pronto® Plus Hair and Scalp Masque [US-OTC]; Pronto® Plus Mousse [US-OTC]; Pronto® Plus Warm Oil Treatment and Conditioner [US-OTC]; Pronto® Plus with Natural Extracts and Oils [US-OTC]; Pyrinyl Plus® [US-OTC]; R & C™ II [Can]; R & C™ Shampoo/Conditioner [Can]; RID® Maximum Strength [US-OTC]; RID® Mousse [Can]; Tisit® Blue Gel [US-OTC]; Tisit® [US-OTC]

**Therapeutic Category** Scabicides/Pediculicides

**Use** Treatment of *Pediculus humanus* infestations (head lice, body lice, pubic lice and their eggs)

**Usual Dosage** Application of pyrethrins:
Topical products:
Apply enough solution to completely wet infested area, including hair
Allow to remain on area for 10 minutes
Wash and rinse with large amounts of warm water.
Use fine-toothed comb to remove lice and eggs from hair
Shampoo hair to restore body and luster
Treatment may be repeated if necessary once in a 24-hour period
Repeat treatment in 7-10 days to kill newly hatched lice
**Note:** Keep out of eyes when rinsing hair; protect eyes with a wash cloth or towel
Solution for furniture, bedding: Spray on entire area to be treated; allow to dry before use. Intended for use on items which cannot be laundered or dry cleaned. **Not for use on humans or animals.**

**Dosage Forms**
Cream, topical (Pronto® Plus Hair and Scalp Masque): Pyrethrins 0.33% and piperonyl butoxide 4% (60 g) [green cream shampoo; contains coconut and sesame oil; apple herb scent; packaged with nit removal comb]
Foam, topical [mousse] (RID® Maximum Strength): Pyrethrins 0.33% and piperonyl butoxide 4% (156 g) [packaged with nit removal comb]
Gel (Tisit® Blue Gel): Pyrethrins 0.33% and piperonyl butoxide 3% (30 g)
Liquid, topical (Tisit®): Pyrethrins 0.33% and piperonyl butoxide 2% (60 mL, 120 mL) [packaged with nit removal comb]
Oil, topical (Pronto® Plus Warm Oil Treatment and Conditioner): Pyrethrins 0.33% and piperonyl butoxide 4% (36 mL) [fruity herbal scent; packaged with nit removal comb]
Shampoo: Pyrethrins 0.33% and piperonyl butoxide 4% (60 mL, 120 mL)
A-200® Maximum Strength: Pyrethrins 0.33% and piperonyl butoxide 4% (60 mL, 120 mL) [contains benzyl alcohol; packaged with nit removal comb]
Lice-Aid: Pyrethrins 0.33% and piperonyl butoxide 4% (120 mL)
Licide®: Pyrethrins 0.33% and piperonyl butoxide 4% (120 mL) [packaged with nit removal comb; also available in a kit containing shampoo, household spray and nit removal comb]
Pronto® Complete Lice Killing kit: Pyrethrins 0.33% and piperonyl butoxide 4% (120 mL) [contains benzyl alcohol; packaged in a kit containing shampoo, creme rinse, hair separators, nit removal comb, magnifying glass, and furniture spray]
Pronto® Plus Mousse: Pyrethrins 0.33% and piperonyl butoxide 4% (120 mL) [blue mousse shampoo; contains vitamin E; packaged with nit removal comb]
Pronto® Plus with Natural Extracts and Oils: Pyrethrins 0.33% and piperonyl butoxide 4% (60 mL) [orange scent; packaged with metal nit removal comb; also available in a kit packaged with lice/egg remover and household spray]
Pyrinyl Plus®: Pyrethrins 0.33% and piperonyl butoxide 4% (60 mL) [contains benzyl alcohol; packaged with nit removal comb]

(Continued)

## pyrethrins and piperonyl butoxide *(Continued)*

RID® Maximum Strength: Pyrethrins 0.33% and piperonyl butoxide 4% (60 mL, 120 mL, 180 mL, 240 mL) [packaged with nit removal comb; also available in a kit containing shampoo, gel, and furniture spray]

Tisit®: Pyrethrins 0.33% and piperonyl butoxide 3% (60 mL, 120 mL) [also available in a kit containing shampoo, nit removal comb, and furniture spray]

Solution, spray [for furniture, garments, bedding; not for human or animal use] (Tisit®): Pyrethrins 0.4% and piperonyl butoxide 2% (150 mL)

## 2-pyridine aldoxime methochloride *see* pralidoxime *on page 669*

## Pyridium® [US] *see* phenazopyridine *on page 636*

## pyridostigmine (peer id oh STIG meen)

### Sound-Alike/Look-Alike Issues
pyridostigmine may be confused with physostigmine
Mestinon® may be confused with Metatensin®
Regonol® may be confused with Reglan®, Renagel®

**Synonyms** pyridostigmine bromide

**U.S./Canadian Brand Names** Mestinon® Timespan® [US]; Mestinon® [US/Can]; Mestinon®-SR [Can]; Regonol® [US]

**Therapeutic Category** Cholinergic Agent

**Use** Symptomatic treatment of myasthenia gravis; antidote for nondepolarizing neuromuscular blockers
Military use: Pretreatment for Soman nerve gas exposure

### Usual Dosage
Myasthenia gravis:
Oral:
Children: 7 mg/kg/24 hours divided into 5-6 doses
Adults: Highly individualized dosing ranges: 60-1500 mg/day, usually 600 mg/day divided into 5-6 doses, spaced to provide maximum relief
Sustained release formulation: Highly individualized dosing ranges: 180-540 mg once or twice daily (doses separated by at least 6 hours); **Note:** Most clinicians reserve sustained release dosage form for bedtime dose only.
I.M., slow I.V. push:
Children: 0.05-0.15 mg/kg/dose
Adults: To supplement oral dosage pre- and postoperatively during labor and postpartum, during myasthenic crisis, or when oral therapy is impractical: ~1/30th of oral dose; observe patient closely for cholinergic reactions
**or**
I.V. infusion: Initial: 2 mg/hour with gradual titration in increments of 0.5-1 mg/hour, up to a maximum rate of 4 mg/hour
Pretreatment for Soman nerve gas exposure (military use): Oral: Adults: 30 mg every 8 hours beginning several hours prior to exposure; discontinue at first sign of nerve agent exposure, then begin atropine and pralidoxime
Reversal of nondepolarizing muscle relaxants: **Note:** Atropine sulfate (0.6-1.2 mg) I.V. immediately prior to pyridostigmine to minimize side effects: I.V.:
Children: Dosing range: 0.1-0.25 mg/kg/dose*
Adults: 0.1-0.25 mg/kg/dose; 10-20 mg is usually sufficient*
*Full recovery usually occurs ≤15 minutes, but ≥30 minutes may be required

### Dosage Forms
Injection, solution, as bromide:
Mestinon®: 5 mg/mL (2 mL)
Regonol®: 5 mg/mL (2 mL) [contains benzyl alcohol]
Syrup, as bromide (Mestinon®): 60 mg/5 mL (480 mL) [raspberry flavor; contains alcohol 5%, sodium benzoate]
Tablet, as bromide (Mestinon®): 60 mg
Tablet, sustained release, as bromide (Mestinon® Timespan®): 180 mg

## pyridostigmine bromide *see* pyridostigmine *on this page*

## pyridoxine (peer i DOKS een)

**Sound-Alike/Look-Alike Issues**
pyridoxine may be confused with paroxetine, pralidoxime, Pyridium®
**Synonyms** pyridoxine hydrochloride; vitamin B₆
**U.S./Canadian Brand Names** Aminoxin® [US-OTC]
**Therapeutic Category** Vitamin, Water Soluble
**Use** Prevention and treatment of vitamin B₆ deficiency, pyridoxine-dependent seizures in infants; adjunct to treatment of acute toxicity from isoniazid, cycloserine, or hydrazine overdose

**Usual Dosage**
Recommended daily allowance (RDA):
Children:
1-3 years: 0.9 mg
4-6 years: 1.3 mg
7-10 years: 1.6 mg
Adults:
Male: 1.7-2.0 mg
Female: 1.4-1.6 mg
Pyridoxine-dependent Infants:
Oral: 2-100 mg/day
I.M., I.V., SubQ: 10-100 mg
Dietary deficiency: Oral:
Children: 5-25 mg/24 hours for 3 weeks, then 1.5-2.5 mg/day in multiple vitamin product
Adults: 10-20 mg/day for 3 weeks
Drug-induced neuritis (eg, isoniazid, hydralazine, penicillamine, cycloserine): Oral:
Children:
Treatment: 10-50 mg/24 hours
Prophylaxis: 1-2 mg/kg/24 hours
Adults:
Treatment: 100-200 mg/24 hours
Prophylaxis: 25-100 mg/24 hours
Treatment of seizures and/or coma from acute isoniazid toxicity, a dose of pyridoxine hydrochloride equal to the amount of INH ingested can be given I.M./I.V. in divided doses together with other anticonvulsants; if the amount INH ingested is not known, administer 5 g I.V. pyridoxine
Treatment of acute hydrazine toxicity, a pyridoxine dose of 25 mg/kg in divided doses I.M./I.V. has been used

**Dosage Forms**
Capsule, as hydrochloride: 250 mg
Injection, solution, as hydrochloride: 100 mg/mL (1 mL)
Tablet, as hydrochloride: 25 mg, 50 mg, 100 mg, 200 mg, 250 mg, 500 mg
Tablet, enteric coated, as hydrochloride (Aminoxin®): 20 mg

**pyridoxine and doxylamine** *see* doxylamine and pyridoxine *(Canada only) on page 273*

**pyridoxine, folic acid, and cyanocobalamin** *see* folic acid, cyanocobalamin, and pyridoxine *on page 357*

**pyridoxine hydrochloride** *see* pyridoxine *on this page*

**Pyrilafen Tannate-12™ [US]** *see* phenylephrine and pyrilamine *on page 641*

**pyrilamine maleate, dextromethorphan hydrobromide, and phenylephrine hydrochloride** *see* phenylephrine, pyrilamine, and dextromethorphan *on page 644*

**pyrilamine tannate and phenylephrine tannate** *see* phenylephrine and pyrilamine *on page 641*

## pyrimethamine (peer i METH a meen)

**Sound-Alike/Look-Alike Issues**
Daraprim® may be confused with Dantrium®, Daranide®
**U.S./Canadian Brand Names** Daraprim® [US/Can]
**Therapeutic Category** Folic Acid Antagonist (Antimalarial)
**Use** Prophylaxis of malaria due to susceptible strains of plasmodia; used in conjunction with quinine and sulfadiazine for the treatment of uncomplicated attacks of chloroquine-resistant *P. falciparum* malaria; used in conjunction with fast-acting schizonticide to initiate transmission control and suppression cure; synergistic combination with sulfonamide in treatment of toxoplasmosis
(Continued)

## pyrimethamine *(Continued)*

**Usual Dosage**

Malaria chemoprophylaxis (for areas where chloroquine-resistant *P. falciparum* exists): Begin prophylaxis 2 weeks before entering endemic area:

Children: 0.5 mg/kg once weekly; not to exceed 25 mg/dose

**or**

Children:

<4 years: 6.25 mg once weekly

4-10 years: 12.5 mg once weekly

Children >10 years and Adults: 25 mg once weekly

Dosage should be continued for all age groups for at least 6-10 weeks after leaving endemic areas

Chloroquine-resistant *P. falciparum* malaria (when used in conjunction with quinine and sulfadiazine):

Children:

<10 kg: 6.25 mg/day once daily for 3 days

10-20 kg: 12.5 mg/day once daily for 3 days

20-40 kg: 25 mg/day once daily for 3 days

Adults: 25 mg twice daily for 3 days

Toxoplasmosis:

Infants (congenital toxoplasmosis): Oral: 1 mg/kg once daily for 6 months with sulfadiazine then every other month with sulfa, alternating with spiramycin.

Children: Loading dose: 2 mg/kg/day divided into 2 equal daily doses for 1-3 days (maximum: 100 mg/day) followed by 1 mg/kg/day divided into 2 doses for 4 weeks; maximum: 25 mg/day

With sulfadiazine or trisulfapyrimidines: 2 mg/kg/day divided every 12 hours for 3 days, followed by 1 mg/kg/day once daily or divided twice daily for 4 weeks given with trisulfapyrimidines or sulfadiazine

Adults: 50-75 mg/day together with 1-4 g of a sulfonamide for 1-3 weeks depending on patient's tolerance and response, then reduce dose by 50% and continue for 4-5 weeks **or** 25-50 mg/day for 3-4 weeks

Prophylaxis for first episode of *Toxoplasma gondii*:

Children ≥1 month of age: 1 mg/kg/day once daily with dapsone, plus oral folinic acid 5 mg every 3 days

Adolescents and Adults: 50 mg once weekly with dapsone, plus oral folinic acid 25 mg once weekly

Prophylaxis to prevent recurrence of *Toxoplasma gondii*:

Children ≥1 month of age: 1 mg/kg/day once daily given with sulfadiazine or clindamycin, plus oral folinic acid 5 mg every 3 days

Adolescents and Adults: 25-50 mg once daily in combination with sulfadiazine or clindamycin, plus oral folinic acid 10-25 mg daily; atovaquone plus oral folinic acid has also been used in combination with pyrimethamine.

**Dosage Forms** Tablet: 25 mg

**pyrimethamine and sulfadoxine** *see* sulfadoxine and pyrimethamine *on page 773*

**Pyrinyl Plus® [US-OTC]** *see* pyrethrins and piperonyl butoxide *on page 699*

## pyrithione zinc *(peer i THYE one zingk)*

**Sound-Alike/Look-Alike Issues**

pyrithione may be confused with Pyridium®

**U.S./Canadian Brand Names** DHS™ Zinc [US-OTC]; Head & Shoulders® Classic Clean 2-In-1 [US-OTC]; Head & Shoulders® Classic Clean [US-OTC]; Head & Shoulders® Dry Scalp Care [US-OTC]; Head & Shoulders® Extra Fullness [US-OTC]; Head & Shoulders® Refresh [US-OTC]; Head & Shoulders® Smooth & Silky 2-In-1 [US-OTC]; Zincon® [US-OTC]; ZNP® Bar [US-OTC]

**Therapeutic Category** Antiseborrheic Agent, Topical

**Use** Relieves the itching, irritation and scalp flaking associated with dandruff and/or seborrheal dermatitis

**Usual Dosage** Adults: Products should be used at least twice weekly for best results, but may be used with each washing.

Bar: May be used on body and or scalp; wet area, massage in, and rinse.

Shampoo: Should be applied to wet hair and massaged into scalp; rinse. May be followed with conditioner

**Dosage Forms**

Conditioner, topical:

Head & Shoulders® Dry Scalp Care: 0.5% (400 mL)

Head & Shoulders® Extra Volume: 0.5% (200 mL, 400 mL)

Conditioner, topical (DermaZinc™): 0.25% (120 g)

Lotion, topical:
 Head & Shoulders® Leave-in Treatment: 0.1% (200 mL)
 Skin Care™: 0.25% (120 mL) [pump spray]
Shampoo, topical:
 BetaMed: 2% (480 mL) [dye free]
 DermaZinc™: 2% (240 mL)
 DHS™ Zinc: 2% (240 mL, 360 mL)
 Head & Shoulders® Citrus Breeze: 1% (400 mL, 700 mL)
 Head & Shoulders® Classic Clean: 1% (50 mL, 200 mL, 400 mL, 700 mL, 1000 mL, 1200 mL)
 Head & Shoulders® Dry Scalp Care: 1% (400 mL, 700 mL, 1200 mL)
 Head & Shoulders® Extra Volume: 1% (400 mL, 700 mL)
 Head & Shoulders® Refresh: 1% (400 mL, 700 mL, 1200 mL)
 Head & Shoulders® Sensitive Care: 1% (400 mL, 700 mL, 1200 mL)
 Zincon®: 1% (120 mL, 240 mL)
Shampoo, topical [with conditioner]:
 Head & Shoulders® Classic Clean 2-in-1: 1% (200 mL, 400 mL, 700 mL)
 Head & Shoulders® Dry Scalp Care: 0.5% (400 mL, 700 mL)
 Head & Shoulders® Smooth and Silky 2-in-1: 1% (400 mL)
Soap, topical (ZNP®): 2% (119 g) [bar]
Solution, topical (DermaZinc™): 0.25% (120 mL) [spray/drops]

**Q-V Tussin [US]** *see* pseudoephedrine, hydrocodone, and chlorpheniramine *on page 695*

**Q-Bid DM [US]** *see* guaifenesin and dextromethorphan *on page 385*

**Q-Dryl [US-OTC]** *see* diphenhydramine *on page 254*

**Q-Naftate [US-OTC]** *see* tolnaftate *on page 809*

**Q-Tussin [US-OTC]** *see* guaifenesin *on page 383*

**Q-Tussin DM [US-OTC]** *see* guaifenesin and dextromethorphan *on page 385*

**quaternium-18 bentonite** *see* bentoquatam *on page 94*

**quazepam** (KWAY ze pam)
 **Sound-Alike/Look-Alike Issues**
  quazepam may be confused with oxazepam
 **U.S./Canadian Brand Names** Doral® [US/Can]
 **Therapeutic Category** Benzodiazepine
 **Controlled Substance** C-IV
 **Use** Treatment of insomnia
 **Usual Dosage** Adults: Oral: Initial: 15 mg at bedtime, in some patients the dose may be reduced to 7.5 mg after a few nights
 **Dosage Forms** Tablet: 7.5 mg, 15 mg

**Quelicin® [US/Can]** *see* succinylcholine *on page 768*

**Queltuss® *(Discontinued)*** *see* guaifenesin and dextromethorphan *on page 385*

**Quenalin [US-OTC]** *see* diphenhydramine *on page 254*

**Questran® [US/Can]** *see* cholestyramine resin *on page 180*

**Questran® Light [US]** *see* cholestyramine resin *on page 180*

**Questran® Light Sugar Free [Can]** *see* cholestyramine resin *on page 180*

**quetiapine** (kwe TYE a peen)
 **Sound-Alike/Look-Alike Issues**
  Seroquel® may be confused with Serentil®, Serzone®, Sinequan®
 **Synonyms** quetiapine fumarate
 **U.S./Canadian Brand Names** Seroquel® [US/Can]
 **Therapeutic Category** Antipsychotic Agent
 **Use** Treatment of schizophrenia; treatment of acute manic episodes associated with bipolar disorder (as monotherapy or in combination with lithium or valproate)
 **Usual Dosage** Oral: Adults:
  Schizophrenia/psychoses: Initial: 25 mg twice daily; increase in increments of 25-50 mg 2-3 times/day on the second and third day, if tolerated, to a target dose of 300-400 mg in 2-3 divided doses by day 4.
  (Continued)

## quetiapine *(Continued)*

Make further adjustments as needed at intervals of at least 2 days in adjustments of 25-50 mg twice daily. Usual maintenance range: 300-800 mg/day

Mania: Initial: 50 mg twice daily on day 1, increase dose in increments of 100 mg/day to 200 mg twice daily on day 4; may increase to a target dose of 800 mg/day by day 6 at increments of ≤200 mg/day. Usual dosage range: 400-800 mg/day

**Note:** Dose reductions should be attempted periodically to establish lowest effective dose in patients with psychosis or to establish need to continue treating agitated symptoms in demented older adults. Patients being restarted after 1 week of no drug need to be titrated as above.

Dosage Forms Tablet, as fumarate: 25 mg, 100 mg, 200 mg, 300 mg [contains lactose]

**quetiapine fumarate** *see* quetiapine *on previous page*

**Quibron®  [US]** *see* theophylline and guaifenesin *on page 795*

**Quibron®-T [US]** *see* theophylline *on page 793*

**Quibron®-T/SR [US]** *see* theophylline *on page 793*

**Quiess® Injection *(Discontinued)*** *see* hydroxyzine *on page 423*

**Quinaglute® Dura-Tabs® *(Discontinued)*** *see* quinidine *on next page*

**quinagolide *(Discontinued)***

**Quinalan® *(Discontinued)*** *see* quinidine *on next page*

**quinalbarbitone sodium** *see* secobarbital *on page 741*

## quinapril (KWIN a pril)

Sound-Alike/Look-Alike Issues

Accupril® may be confused with Accolate®, Accutane®, AcipHex®, Monopril®

Synonyms quinapril hydrochloride

U.S./Canadian Brand Names Accupril® [US/Can]

Therapeutic Category Angiotensin-Converting Enzyme (ACE) Inhibitor

Use Management of hypertension; treatment of congestive heart failure

Usual Dosage Adults: Oral:

Hypertension: Initial: 10-20 mg once daily, adjust according to blood pressure response at peak and trough blood levels; initial dose may be reduced to 5 mg in patients receiving diuretic therapy if the diuretic is continued; usual dose range (JNC 7): 10-40 mg once daily

Congestive heart failure or post-MI: Initial: 5 mg once daily, titrated at weekly intervals to 20-40 mg daily in 2 divided doses

Dosage Forms Tablet, as hydrochloride: 5 mg, 10 mg, 20 mg, 40 mg

## quinapril and hydrochlorothiazide (KWIN a pril & hye droe klor oh THYE a zide)

Synonyms hydrochlorothiazide and quinapril

U.S./Canadian Brand Names Accuretic® [US/Can]; Quinarectic [US]

Therapeutic Category Antihypertensive Agent, Combination

Use Treatment of hypertension (not for initial therapy)

Usual Dosage Oral:

Children: Safety and efficacy have not been established.

Adults: Initial:

Patients who have failed quinapril monotherapy:

Quinapril 10 mg/hydrochlorothiazide 12.5 mg **or**

Quinapril 20 mg/hydrochlorothiazide 12.5 mg once daily

Patients with adequate blood pressure control on hydrochlorothiazide 25 mg/day, but significant potassium loss:

Quinapril 10 mg/hydrochlorothiazide 12.5 mg **or**

Quinapril 20 mg/hydrochlorothiazide 12.5 mg once daily

**Note:** Clinical trials of quinapril/hydrochlorothiazide combinations used quinapril doses of 2.5-40 mg/day and hydrochlorothiazide doses of 6.25-25 mg/day.

Dosage Forms Tablet:

10/12.5: Quinapril 10 mg and hydrochlorothiazide 12.5 mg

20/12.5: Quinapril 20 mg and hydrochlorothiazide 12.5 mg

20/25: Quinapril 20 mg and hydrochlorothiazide 25 mg

**quinapril hydrochloride** *see* quinapril *on previous page*

**Quinarectic [US]** *see* quinapril and hydrochlorothiazide *on previous page*

**Quinate® [Can]** *see* quinidine *on this page*

## quinidine (KWIN i deen)

**Sound-Alike/Look-Alike Issues**
  quinidine may be confused with clonidine, quinine, Quinora®

**Synonyms** quinidine gluconate; quinidine polygalacturonate; quinidine sulfate

**U.S./Canadian Brand Names** Apo-Quin-G® [Can]; Apo-Quinidine® [Can]; BioQuin® Durules™ [Can]; Novo-Quinidin [Can]; Quinate® [Can]

**Therapeutic Category** Antiarrhythmic Agent, Class I-A

**Use** Prophylaxis after cardioversion of atrial fibrillation and/or flutter to maintain normal sinus rhythm; prevent recurrence of paroxysmal supraventricular tachycardia, paroxysmal AV junctional rhythm, paroxysmal ventricular tachycardia, paroxysmal atrial fibrillation, and atrial or ventricular premature contractions; has activity against *Plasmodium falciparum* malaria

**Usual Dosage Dosage expressed in terms of the salt: 267 mg of quinidine gluconate = 200 mg of quinidine sulfate.**

  Children: Test dose for idiosyncratic reaction (sulfate, oral or gluconate, I.M.): 2 mg/kg or 60 mg/m$^2$
    Oral (quinidine sulfate): 15-60 mg/kg/day in 4-5 divided doses or 6 mg/kg every 4-6 hours; usual 30 mg/kg/day or 900 mg/m$^2$/day given in 5 daily doses
    I.V. **not** recommended (quinidine gluconate): 2-10 mg/kg/dose given at a rate ≤10 mg/minute every 3-6 hours as needed
  Adults: Test dose: Oral, I.M.: 200 mg administered several hours before full dosage (to determine possibility of idiosyncratic reaction)
    Oral (for malaria):
    Sulfate: 100-600 mg/dose every 4-6 hours; begin at 200 mg/dose and titrate to desired effect (maximum daily dose: 3-4 g)
    Gluconate: 324-972 mg every 8-12 hours
    I.M.: 400 mg/dose every 2-6 hours; initial dose: 600 mg (gluconate)
    I.V.: 200-400 mg/dose diluted and given at a rate ≤10 mg/minute; may require as much as 500-750 mg

**Dosage Forms**
  Injection, solution, as gluconate: 80 mg/mL (10 mL) [equivalent to quinidine base 50 mg]
  Tablet, as sulfate: 200 mg, 300 mg
  Tablet, extended release, as gluconate: 324 mg [equivalent to quinidine base 202 mg]
  Tablet, extended release, as sulfate: 300 mg [equivalent to quinidine base 249 mg]

**quinidine gluconate** *see* quinidine *on this page*

**quinidine polygalacturonate** *see* quinidine *on this page*

**quinidine sulfate** *see* quinidine *on this page*

## quinine (KWYE nine)

**Sound-Alike/Look-Alike Issues**
  quinine may be confused with quinidine

**Synonyms** quinine sulfate

**U.S./Canadian Brand Names** Apo-Quinine® [Can]; Novo-Quinine [Can]; Quinine-Odan™ [Can]

**Therapeutic Category** Antimalarial Agent

**Use** In conjunction with other antimalarial agents, suppression or treatment of chloroquine-resistant *P. falciparum* malaria; treatment of *Babesia microti* infection in conjunction with clindamycin

**Usual Dosage** Oral:
  Children:
    Treatment of chloroquine-resistant malaria: 25-30 mg/kg/day in divided doses every 8 hours for 3-7 days with tetracycline (consider risk versus benefit in children <8 years of age)
    Babesiosis: 25 mg/kg/day divided every 8 hours for 7 days
  Adults:
    Treatment of chloroquine-resistant malaria: 650 mg every 8 hours for 3-7 days with tetracycline
    Suppression of malaria: 325 mg twice daily and continued for 6 weeks after exposure
    Babesiosis: 650 mg every 6-8 hours for 7 days
    Leg cramps: 200-300 mg at bedtime

**Dosage Forms**
  Capsule, as sulfate: 200 mg, 325 mg
  Tablet, as sulfate: 260 mg

**Quinine-Odan**™ **[Can]** *see* quinine *on previous page*

**quinine sulfate** *see* quinine *on previous page*

**quinol** *see* hydroquinone *on page 420*

**Quinora**® *(Discontinued) see* quinidine *on previous page*

**Quintabs [US-OTC]** *see* vitamins (multiple/oral) *on page 852*

**Quintabs-M [US-OTC]** *see* vitamins (multiple/oral) *on page 852*

**Quintasa**® **[Can]** *see* mesalamine *on page 516*

## quinupristin and dalfopristin (kwi NYOO pris tin & dal FOE pris tin)

**Synonyms** pristinamycin; RP-59500
**U.S./Canadian Brand Names** Synercid® [US/Can]
**Therapeutic Category** Antibiotic, Streptogramin
**Use** Treatment of serious or life-threatening infections associated with vancomycin-resistant *Enterococcus faecium* bacteremia; treatment of complicated skin and skin structure infections caused by methcillin-susceptible *Staphylococcus aureus* or *Streptococcus pyogenes*

Has been studied in the treatment of a variety of infections caused by *Enterococcus faecium* (not *E. fecalis*) including vancomycin-resistant strains. May also be effective in the treatment of serious infections caused by *Staphylococcus* species including those resistant to methicillin.

**Usual Dosage** I.V.:
Children (limited information): Dosages similar to adult dosing have been used in the treatment of complicated skin/soft tissue infections and infections caused by vancomycin-resistant *Enterococcus faecium*
CNS shunt infection due to vancomycin-resistant *Enterococcus faecium*: 7.5 mg/kg/dose every 8 hours; concurrent intrathecal doses of 1-2 mg/day have been administered for up to 68 days
Adults:
Vancomycin-resistant *Enterococcus faecium*: 7.5 mg/kg every 8 hours
Complicated skin and skin structure infection: 7.5 mg/kg every 12 hours
**Dosage Forms** Injection, powder for reconstitution:
500 mg: Quinupristin 150 mg and dalfopristin 350 mg
600 mg: Quinupristin 180 mg and dalfopristin 420 mg

**Quixin**™ **[US]** *see* levofloxacin *on page 475*

**QVAR**® **[US/Can]** *see* beclomethasone *on page 91*

**R 14-15** *see* erlotinib *on page 294*

**R & C**™ **II [Can]** *see* pyrethrins and piperonyl butoxide *on page 699*

**R & C**® **Lice** *(Discontinued) see* permethrin *on page 635*

**R & C**™ **Shampoo/Conditioner [Can]** *see* pyrethrins and piperonyl butoxide *on page 699*

**R-3827** *see* abarelix *on page 2*

**RabAvert**® **[US/Can]** *see* rabies virus vaccine *on next page*

## rabeprazole (ra BE pray zole)

**Sound-Alike/Look-Alike Issues**
rabeprazole may be confused with aripiprazole
AcipHex® may be confused with Acephen®, Accupril®, Aricept®
**Synonyms** pariprazole
**U.S./Canadian Brand Names** AcipHex® [US/Can]; Pariet® [Can]
**Therapeutic Category** Gastric Acid Secretion Inhibitor
**Use** Short-term (4-8 weeks) treatment and maintenance of erosive or ulcerative gastroesophageal reflux disease (GERD); symptomatic GERD; short-term (up to 4 weeks) treatment of duodenal ulcers; long-term treatment of pathological hypersecretory conditions, including Zollinger-Ellison syndrome; *H. pylori* eradication (in combination with amoxicillin and clarithromycin)
**Usual Dosage** Oral: Adults >18 years:
GERD: 20 mg once daily for 4-8 weeks; maintenance: 20 mg once daily
Duodenal ulcer: 20 mg/day before breakfast for 4 weeks

*H. pylori* eradication: 20 mg twice daily for 7 days; to be administered with amoxicillin 1000 mg and clarithromycin 500 mg, also given twice daily for 7 days.

Hypersecretory conditions: 60 mg once daily; dose may need to be adjusted as necessary. Doses as high as 100 mg once daily and 60 mg twice daily have been used.

**Dosage Forms** Tablet, delayed release, enteric coated, as sodium: 20 mg

## rabies immune globulin (human) (RAY beez i MYUN GLOB yoo lin, HYU man)

**Synonyms** RIG

**U.S./Canadian Brand Names** BayRab® [US/Can]; Imogam® Rabies Pasteurized [Can]; Imogam® Rabies-HT [US]

**Therapeutic Category** Immune Globulin

**Use** Part of postexposure prophylaxis of persons with rabies exposure who lack a history of pre-exposure or postexposure prophylaxis with rabies vaccine or a recently documented neutralizing antibody response to previous rabies vaccination; although it is preferable to administer RIG with the first dose of vaccine, it can be given up to 8 days after vaccination

**Usual Dosage** Children and Adults: I.M.: 20 units/kg in a single dose (RIG should always be administered as part of rabies vaccine (HDCV)) regimen (as soon as possible after the first dose of vaccine, up to 8 days); infiltrate 1/2 of the dose locally around the wound; administer the remainder I.M.

**Note:** Persons known to have an adequate titer or who have been completely immunized with rabies vaccine should not receive RIG, only booster doses of HDCV

**Dosage Forms** Injection, solution:

BayRab®: 150 int. units/mL (2 mL, 10 mL) [solvent/detergent treated]

Imogam® Rabies-HT: 150 int. units/mL (2 mL, 10 mL) [heat treated]

## rabies virus vaccine (RAY beez VYE rus vak SEEN)

**Synonyms** HDCV; human diploid cell cultures rabies vaccine; PCEC; purified chick embryo cell

**U.S./Canadian Brand Names** Imovax® Rabies [US/Can]; RabAvert® [US/Can]

**Therapeutic Category** Vaccine, Inactivated Virus

**Use** Pre-exposure immunization: Vaccinate persons with greater than usual risk due to occupation or avocation including veterinarians, rangers, animal handlers, certain laboratory workers, and persons living in or visiting countries for longer than 1 month where rabies is a constant threat.

Postexposure prophylaxis: If a bite from a carrier animal is unprovoked, if it is not captured and rabies is present in that species and area, administer rabies immune globulin (RIG) and the vaccine as indicated

**Usual Dosage**

**Pre-exposure prophylaxis:** 1 mL I.M. on days 0, 7, and 21 to 28. **Note:** Prolonging the interval between doses does not interfere with immunity achieved after the concluding dose of the basic series.

**Postexposure prophylaxis:** All postexposure treatment should begin with immediate cleansing of the wound with soap and water

Persons not previously immunized as above: I.M.: 5 doses (1 mL each) on days 0, 3, 7, 14, 28. In addition, patients should receive rabies immune globulin 20 units/kg body weight, half infiltrated at bite site if possible, remainder I.M.)

Persons who have previously received postexposure prophylaxis with rabies vaccine, received a recommended I.M. pre-exposure series of rabies vaccine or have a previously documented rabies antibody titer considered adequate: 1 mL of either vaccine I.M. only on days 0 and 3; do not administer RIG

Booster (for occupational or other continuing risk): 1 mL I.M. every 2-5 years or based on antibody titers

**Dosage Forms** Injection, powder for reconstitution:

Imovax® Rabies: 2.5 int. units [HDCV; grown in human diploid cell culture; contains albumin <100 mg, neomycin <150 mcg]

RabAvert®: 2.5 int. units [PCEC; grown in chicken fibroblasts; contains amphotericin <2 ng, chlortetracycline <20 ng, and neomycin <1 mcg]

**Radiogardase™ [US]** *see* ferric hexacyanoferrate *on page 334*

## radiological/contrast media (ionic) (ray deo LOG ik al/KON trast MEE dia eye ON ik)

**Synonyms** barium sulfate; diatrizoate meglumine and diatrizoate sodium; diatrizoate meglumine and iodipamide meglumine; diatrizoate meglumine; diatrizoate sodium; ethiodized oil; gadopentetate dimeglumine; iocetamic acid; iodamide meglumine; iodipamide meglumine; iopanoic acid; iothalamate meglumine and iothalamate sodium; iothalamate sodium; ipodate calcium; ipodate sodium; isosulfan blue; potassium perchlorate; propyliodone; tyropanoate sodium

(Continued)

# radiological/contrast media (ionic) *(Continued)*

**U.S./Canadian Brand Names** Anatrast® [US]; Angio Conray® [US]; Angiovist® [US]; Bar-Test® [US]; Baricon® [US]; Baro-CAT® [US]; Barobag® [US]; Baroflave® [US]; Barosperse® [US]; Cholebrine® [US]; Cholografin® Meglumine [US]; Conray® [US]; Cystografin® [US]; Dionosil Oily® [US]; Enecat® [US]; Entrobar® [US]; Epi-C® [US]; Ethiodol® [US]; Flo-Coat® [US]; Gastrografin® [US]; HD 200 Plus® [US]; HD 85® [US]; Hexabrix™ [US]; Hypaque-Cysto® [US]; Hypaque® Meglumine [US]; Hypaque® Sodium [US]; Liquid Barosperse® [US]; Liquipake® [US]; Lymphazurin® [US/Can]; Magnevist® [US/Can]; MD-Gastroview® [US]; Oragrafin® Calcium [US]; Oragrafin® Sodium [US]; Perchloracap® [US]; Prepcat® [US]; Reno-M-30® [US]; Reno-M-60® [US]; Reno-M-DIP® [US]; Renovue®-65 [US]; Renovue®-DIP [US]; Sinografin® [US]; Telepaque® [US]; Tomocat® [US]; Tonopaque® [US]; Urovist Cysto® [US]; Urovist® Meglumine [US]; Urovist® Sodium 300 [US]; Vascoray® [US]

**Therapeutic Category** Radiopaque Agents

**Use** Enhance visualization of structures during radiologic procedures

**Usual Dosage** Varies with procedure

**Dosage Forms** [DSC] = Discontinued product

**Oral cholecystographic agents:**
Iocetamic acid: Tablet (Cholebrine®): 750 mg
Iopanoic acid: Tablet (Telepaque®): 500 mg
Ipodate calcium: Granules for oral suspension (Oragrafin® Calcium): 3 g
Ipodate sodium: Capsule (Bilivist®, Oragrafin® Sodium): 500 mg
Tyropanoate sodium: Capsule (Bilopaque®): 750 mg [DSC]

**GI contrast agents: Barium sulfate:**
Paste (Anatrast®): 100% (500 g)
Powder:
  Baroflave®: 100%
  Baricon®, HD 200 Plus®: 98%
  Barosperse®, Tonopaque®: 95%
Suspension:
  Baro-CAT®, Prepcat®: 1.5%
  Enecat®, Tomocat®: 5%
  Entrobar®: 50%
  Liquid Barasperse®: 60%
  HD 85®: 85%
  Barobag®: 97%
  Flo-Coat®, Liquipake®: 100%
  Epi-C®: 150%
Tablet (Bar-Test®): 650 mg

**Parenteral agents: Injection:**
**Diatrizoate meglumine:**
  Hypaque® Meglumine
  Reno-M-DIP®
  Urovist® Meglumine
  Angiovist® 282
  Hypaque® Meglumine
  Reno-M-60®
**Diatrizoate sodium:**
  Hypaque® Sodium
  Urovist® Sodium 300
**Gadopentetate dimeglumine:** Magnevist®
**Iodamide meglumine:**
  Renovue®-DIP
  Renovue®-65
**Iodipamide meglumine:** Cholografin® meglumine
**Iothalamate meglumine:**
  Conray® 30
  Conray® 43
  Conray®
**Iothalamate sodium:**
  Angio Conray®
  Conray® 325
  Conray® 400

**Diatrizoate meglumine and diatrizoate sodium**:
Angiovist® 292
Angiovist® 370
Hypaque-76®
Hypaque-M®, 75%
Hypaque-M®, 90%
MD-60®
MD-76®
Renografin-60®
Renografin-76®
Renovist® II
Renovist®
**Iothalamate meglumine and iothalamate sodium**:
Vascoray®
Hexabrix™

**Miscellaneous agents** (**NOT** for intravascular use, for instillation into various cavities):
**Diatrizoate meglumine**: Urogenital solution, sterile:
Crystografin®
Crystografin® Dilute
Hypaque-Cysto®
Reno-M-30®
Urovist Cysto®
**Diatrizoate meglumine and diatrizoate sodium**: Solution, oral or rectal:
Gastrografin®
MD-Gastroview®
**Diatrizoate sodium**:
Solution, oral or rectal (Hypaque® sodium oral)
Solution, urogenital (Hypaque® sodium 20%)
**Iothalamate meglumine**: Solution, urogenital:
Cysto-Conray®
Cysto-Conray® II

**Diatrizoate meglumine and iodipamide meglumine**:
Injection, urogenital for intrauterine instillation (Sinografin®)
**Ethiodized oil**: Injection (Ethiodol®)
**Propyliodone**: Suspension (Dionosil Oily®)
**Isosulfan blue**: Injection (Lymphazurin® 1%)
**Potassium perchlorate**: Capsule (Perchloracap®): 200 mg

# radiological/contrast media (nonionic)
(ray deo LOG ik al/KON trast MEE dia non eye ON ik)
**Sound-Alike/Look-Alike Issues**
Optiray® may be confused with Optivar™
**Synonyms** gadoteridol; iohexol; iopamidol; ioversol; metrizamide
**U.S./Canadian Brand Names** Isovue® [US]; Omnipaque® [US]; Optiray® [US]; ProHance® [US]
**Therapeutic Category** Radiopaque Agents
**Use** Enhance visualization of structures during radiologic procedures
**Usual Dosage** Dose varies with procedure
**Dosage Forms** [DSC] = Discontinued product
Injection, solution:
Gadoteridol (ProHance®): 279.3 mg/mL (15 mL, 30 mL, 50 mL) [single use vial]; 279.3 mg/mL (20 mL) [prefilled syringe]
Iohexol (Omnipaque®): 140 mg/mL, 180 mg/mL, 210 mg/mL, 240 mg/mL, 300 mg/mL, 350 mg/mL
Iopamidol:
Isovue-128®
Isovue-200®
Isovue-300®
Isovue-370®
Isovue-M 200®
Isovue-M 300®
Ioversol:
Optiray® 160
(Continued)

# radiological/contrast media (nonionic) *(Continued)*

Optiray® 240
Optiray® 320
Metrizamide: Amipaque® [DSC]

**rAHF** *see* antihemophilic factor (recombinant) *on page 57*

**R-albuterol** *see* levalbuterol *on page 472*

## raloxifene (ral OKS i feen)

**Sound-Alike/Look-Alike Issues**
Evista® may be confused with Avinza™
**Synonyms** keoxifene hydrochloride; raloxifene hydrochloride
**U.S./Canadian Brand Names** Evista® [US/Can]
**Therapeutic Category** Selective Estrogen Receptor Modulator (SERM)
**Use** Prevention and treatment of osteoporosis in postmenopausal women
**Usual Dosage** Adults: Female: Oral: 60 mg/day which may be administered any time of the day without regard to meals
**Dosage Forms** Tablet, as hydrochloride: 60 mg

**raloxifene hydrochloride** *see* raloxifene *on this page*

## raltitrexed *(Canada only)* (ral ti TREX ed)

**Synonyms** ICI-D1694; NSC-639186; raltitrexed disodium; ZD1694
**U.S./Canadian Brand Names** Tomudex® [Can]
**Therapeutic Category** Antineoplastic Agent
**Use** Treatment of advanced colorectal neoplasms
**Usual Dosage** Refer to individual protocols.
I.V.: 3 mg/m$^2$ every 3 weeks
**Dosage Forms** Injection, powder for reconstitution, as disodium: 2 mg

**raltitrexed disodium** *see* raltitrexed *(Canada only)* *on this page*

## ramipril (ra MI pril)

**Sound-Alike/Look-Alike Issues**
ramipril may be confused with enalapril, Monopril®
Altace® may be confused with alteplase, Amaryl®, Amerge®, Artane®
**U.S./Canadian Brand Names** Altace® [US/Can]
**Therapeutic Category** Angiotensin-Converting Enzyme (ACE) Inhibitor
**Use** Treatment of hypertension, alone or in combination with thiazide diuretics; treatment of left ventricular dysfunction after myocardial infarction; to reduce risk of heart attack, stroke, and death in patients at increased risk for these problems
**Usual Dosage** Adults: Oral:
Hypertension: 2.5-5 mg once daily, maximum: 20 mg/day
Reduction in risk of MI, stroke, and death from cardiovascular causes: Initial: 2.5 mg once daily for 1 week, then 5 mg once daily for the next 3 weeks, then increase as tolerated to 10 mg once daily (may be given as divided dose)
Heart failure postmyocardial infarction: Initial: 2.5 mg twice daily titrated upward, if possible, to 5 mg twice daily.
**Note:** The dose of any concomitant diuretic should be reduced. If the diuretic cannot be discontinued, initiate therapy with 1.25 mg. After the initial dose, the patient should be monitored carefully until blood pressure has stabilized.
**Dosage Forms** Capsule: 1.25 mg, 2.5 mg, 5 mg, 10 mg

**Raniclor™ [US]** *see* cefaclor *on page 152*

## ranitidine hydrochloride (ra NI ti deen hye droe KLOR ide)

**Sound-Alike/Look-Alike Issues**
ranitidine may be confused with amantadine, rimantadine
Zantac® may be confused with Xanax®, Zarontin®, Zofran®, Zyrtec®

**U.S./Canadian Brand Names** Alti-Ranitidine [Can]; Apo-Ranitidine® [Can]; CO Ranitidine [Can]; Gen-Ranidine [Can]; Novo-Ranidine [Can]; Nu-Ranit [Can]; PMS-Ranitidine [Can]; Rhoxal-ranitidine [Can]; Zantac 150™ [US-OTC]; Zantac 75® [US-OTC/Can]; Zantac® EFFERdose® [US]; Zantac® [US/Can]

**Therapeutic Category** Histamine $H_2$ Antagonist

**Use**

Zantac®: Short-term and maintenance therapy of duodenal ulcer, gastric ulcer, gastroesophageal reflux, active benign ulcer, erosive esophagitis, and pathological hypersecretory conditions; as part of a multidrug regimen for *H. pylori* eradication to reduce the risk of duodenal ulcer recurrence

Zantac® 75 [OTC]: Relief of heartburn, acid indigestion, and sour stomach

**Usual Dosage**

Children 1 month to 16 years:

Duodenal and gastric ulcer:

Oral:

Treatment: 2-4 mg/kg/day divided twice daily; maximum treatment dose: 300 mg/day

Maintenance: 2-4 mg/kg once daily; maximum maintenance dose: 150 mg/day

I.V.: 2-4 mg/kg/day divided every 6-8 hours; maximum: 150 mg/day

GERD and erosive esophagitis:

Oral: 5-10 mg/kg/day divided twice daily; maximum: GERD: 300 mg/day, erosive esophagitis: 600 mg/day

I.V.: 2-4 mg/kg/day divided every 6-8 hours; maximum: 150 mg/day **or as an alternative**

Continuous infusion: Initial: 1 mg/kg/dose for one dose followed by infusion of 0.08-0.17 mg/kg/hour or 2-4 mg/kg/day

Children ≥12 years: Prevention of heartburn: Oral: Zantac® 75 [OTC]: 75 mg 30-60 minutes before eating food or drinking beverages which cause heartburn; maximum: 150 mg/24 hours; do not use for more than 14 days

Adults:

Duodenal ulcer: Oral: Treatment: 150 mg twice daily, or 300 mg once daily after the evening meal or at bedtime; maintenance: 150 mg once daily at bedtime

*Helicobacter pylori* eradication: 150 mg twice daily; requires combination therapy

Pathological hypersecretory conditions:

Oral: 150 mg twice daily; adjust dose or frequency as clinically indicated; doses of up to 6 g/day have been used

I.V.: Continuous infusion for Zollinger-Ellison: 1 mg/kg/hour; measure gastric acid output at 4 hours, if >10 mEq or if patient is symptomatic, increase dose in increments of 0.5 mg/kg/hour; doses of up to 2.5 mg/kg/hour have been used

Gastric ulcer, benign: Oral: 150 mg twice daily; maintenance: 150 mg once daily at bedtime

Erosive esophagitis: Oral: Treatment: 150 mg 4 times/day; maintenance: 150 mg twice daily

Prevention of heartburn: Oral: Zantac® 75 [OTC]: 75 mg 30-60 minutes before eating food or drinking beverages which cause heartburn; maximum: 150 mg in 24 hours; do not use for more than 14 days

Patients not able to take oral medication:

I.M.: 50 mg every 6-8 hours

I.V.: Intermittent bolus or infusion: 50 mg every 6-8 hours

Continuous I.V. infusion: 6.25 mg/hour

**Dosage Forms**

Capsule, as hydrochloride: 150 mg, 300 mg

Infusion, as hydrochloride [premixed in NaCl 0.45%; preservative free] (Zantac®): 50 mg (50 mL)

Injection, solution, as hydrochloride: 25 mg/mL (2 mL, 6 mL)

Zantac®: 25 mg/mL (2 mL, 6 mL, 40 mL) [contains phenol 0.5% as preservative]

Syrup, as hydrochloride: 15 mg/mL (10 mL) [contains alcohol 7.5%; peppermint flavor]

Zantac®: 15 mg/mL (473 mL) [contains alcohol 7.5%; peppermint flavor]

Tablet, as hydrochloride: 75 mg [OTC], 150 mg, 300 mg

Zantac®: 150 mg, 300 mg

Zantac 75® : 75 mg

Zantac 150™: 150 mg

Tablet, effervescent, as hydrochloride (Zantac® EFFERdose®): 25 mg [contains sodium 1.33 mEq/tablet, phenylalanine 2.81 mg/tablet, and sodium benzoate]; 150 mg [contains sodium 7.96 mEq/tablet, phenylalanine 16.84 mg/tablet, and sodium benzoate]

**Rapamune® [US/Can]** *see* sirolimus *on page 750*

**Raplon® *(Discontinued)***

**Raptiva® [US]** *see* efalizumab *on page 280*

# rasburicase (ras BYOOR i kayse)

**U.S./Canadian Brand Names** Elitek™ [US]; Fasturtec® [Can]

**Therapeutic Category** Enzyme

**Use** Initial management of uric acid levels in pediatric patients with leukemia, lymphoma, and solid tumor malignancies receiving anticancer therapy expected to result in tumor lysis and elevation of plasma uric acid

**Usual Dosage** I.V.:

Children: Management of uric acid levels: 0.15 mg/kg or 0.2 mg/kg once daily for 5 days (manufacturer-recommended duration); begin chemotherapy 4-24 hours after the first dose

Limited data suggest that a single prechemotherapy dose (versus multiple-day administration) may be sufficiently efficacious. Monitoring electrolytes, hydration status, and uric acid concentrations are necessary to identify the need for additional doses. Other clinical manifestations of tumor lysis syndrome (eg, hyperphosphatemia, hypocalcemia, and hyperkalemia) may occur.

Adults: Refer to pediatric dosing; insufficient data collected in adult/geriatric patients to determine response to treatment

**Dosage Forms** Injection, powder for reconstitution: 1.5 mg [packaged with three 1 mL ampuls of diluent]

Raudixin® *(Discontinued)*

Rauverid® *(Discontinued)*

Raxar® *(Discontinued)*

Razadyne™ **[US]** *see* galantamine *on page 365*

Razadyne™ **ER [US]** *see* galantamine *on page 365*

Reactine™ **[Can]** *see* cetirizine *on page 162*

Reactine® **Allergy and Sinus [Can]** *see* cetirizine and pseudoephedrine *on page 163*

Rea-Lo® **[US-OTC]** *see* urea *on page 834*

ReAzo **[US-OTC]** *see* phenazopyridine *on page 636*

Rebetol® **[US]** *see* ribavirin *on page 720*

Rebetron® **[US]** *see* interferon alfa-2b and ribavirin *on page 441*

Rebif® **[US/Can]** *see* interferon beta-1a *on page 443*

recombinant α-L-iduronidase (glycosaminoglycan α-L-iduronohydrolase) *see* laronidase *on page 468*

recombinant hirudin *see* lepirudin *on page 469*

recombinant human deoxyribonuclease *see* dornase alfa *on page 267*

recombinant human interleukin-11 *see* oprelvekin *on page 601*

recombinant human parathyroid hormone (1-34) *see* teriparatide *on page 787*

recombinant human platelet-derived growth factor B *see* becaplermin *on page 91*

recombinant interleukin-11 *see* oprelvekin *on page 601*

recombinant N-acetylgalactosamine 4-sulfatase *see* galsulfase *on page 366*

recombinant plasminogen activator *see* reteplase *on page 717*

Recombinate™ **[US/Can]** *see* antihemophilic factor (recombinant) *on page 57*

Recombivax HB® **[US/Can]** *see* hepatitis B vaccine *on page 401*

Red Cross™ **Canker Sore [US-OTC]** *see* benzocaine *on page 95*

Redisol® *(Discontinued) see* cyanocobalamin *on page 212*

Redutemp® **[US-OTC]** *see* acetaminophen *on page 4*

Reese's® **Pinworm Medicine [US-OTC]** *see* pyrantel pamoate *on page 698*

ReFacto® **[US/Can]** *see* antihemophilic factor (recombinant) *on page 57*

Refenesen Plus **[US-OTC]** *see* guaifenesin and pseudoephedrine *on page 388*

Refludan® **[US/Can]** *see* lepirudin *on page 469*

Refresh® **[US-OTC]** *see* artificial tears *on page 71*

Refresh Liquigel™ **[US-OTC]** *see* carboxymethylcellulose *on page 148*

Refresh Plus® **[US-OTC]** *see* artificial tears *on page 71*

Refresh Tears® **[US-OTC]** *see* artificial tears *on page 71*

Regitine® **[Can]** *see* phentolamine *on page 639*

Regitine® *(Discontinued) see* phentolamine *on page 639*

Reglan® **[US]** *see* metoclopramide *on page 533*

Reglan® **Syrup** *(Discontinued) see* metoclopramide *on page 533*

Regonol® **[US]** *see* pyridostigmine *on page 700*

Regranex® **[US/Can]** *see* becaplermin *on page 91*

Regular Iletin® **I Insulin** *(Discontinued)*

Regular Iletin® **II** *(Discontinued) see* insulin preparations *on page 438*

regular, insulin *see* insulin preparations *on page 438*

Regulax SS® *(Discontinued) see* docusate *on page 263*

Regulex® **[Can]** *see* docusate *on page 263*

Reguloid® **[US-OTC]** *see* psyllium *on page 697*

**Rejuva-A**® **[Can]** *see* tretinoin (topical) *on page 818*

**Relacon-DM [US]** *see* guaifenesin, pseudoephedrine, and dextromethorphan *on page 391*

**Relacon-HC [US]** *see* phenylephrine, hydrocodone, and chlorpheniramine *on page 643*

**Relafen**® **[US/Can]** *see* nabumetone *on page 556*

**Relenza**® **[US/Can]** *see* zanamivir *on page 858*

**Relief**® **[US-OTC]** *see* phenylephrine *on page 640*

**Relief**® **Ophthalmic Solution** *(Discontinued) see* phenylephrine *on page 640*

**Relpax**® **[US/Can]** *see* eletriptan *on page 281*

**Remeron**® **[US/Can]** *see* mirtazapine *on page 543*

**Remeron**® **RD [Can]** *see* mirtazapine *on page 543*

**Remeron SolTab**® **[US]** *see* mirtazapine *on page 543*

**Reme-t**™ **[US-OTC]** *see* coal tar *on page 201*

**Remicade**® **[US/Can]** *see* infliximab *on page 436*

## remifentanil (rem i FEN ta nil)

**Sound-Alike/Look-Alike Issues**
  remifentanil may be confused with alfentanil
**Synonyms** GI87084B
**U.S./Canadian Brand Names** Ultiva® [US/Can]
**Therapeutic Category** Analgesic, Narcotic
**Controlled Substance** C-II
**Use** Analgesic for use during the induction and maintenance of general anesthesia; for continued analgesia into the immediate postoperative period; analgesic component of monitored anesthesia
**Usual Dosage** I.V. continuous infusion: Dose should be based on ideal body weight (IBW) in obese patients (>30% over IBW).

Children birth to 2 months: Maintenance of anesthesia with nitrous oxide (70%): 0.4 mcg/kg/minute (range: 0.4-1 mcg/kg/minute); supplemental bolus dose of 1 mcg/kg may be administered, smaller bolus dose may be required with potent inhalation agents, potent neuraxial anesthesia, significant comorbidities, significant fluid shifts, or without atropine pretreatment. Clearance in neonates is highly variable; dose should be carefully titrated.

Children 1-12 years: Maintenance of anesthesia with halothane, sevoflurane or isoflurane: 0.25 mcg/kg/minute (range 0.05-1.3 mcg/kg/minute); supplemental bolus dose of 1 mcg/kg may be administered every 2-5 minutes. Consider increasing concomitant anesthetics with infusion rate >1 mcg/kg/minute. Infusion rate can be titrated upward in increments up to 50% or titrated downward in decrements of 25% to 50%. May titrate every 2-5 minutes.

Adults:
  Induction of anesthesia: 0.5-1 mcg/kg/minute; if endotracheal intubation is to occur in <8 minutes, an initial dose of 1 mcg/kg may be given over 30-60 seconds
  Coronary bypass surgery: 1 mcg/kg/minute
  Maintenance of anesthesia: **Note:** Supplemental bolus dose of 1 mcg/kg may be administered every 2-5 minutes. Consider increasing concomitant anesthetics with infusion rate >1 mcg/kg/minute. Infusion rate can be titrated upward in increments of 25% to 100% or downward in decrements of 25% to 50%. May titrate every 2-5 minutes.
    With nitrous oxide (66%): 0.4 mcg/kg/minute (range: 0.1-2 mcg/kg/minute)
    With isoflurane: 0.25 mcg/kg/minute (range: 0.05-2 mcg/kg/minute)
    With propofol: 0.25 mcg/kg/minute (range: 0.05-2 mcg/kg/minute)
    Coronary bypass surgery: 1 mcg/kg/minute (range: 0.125-4 mcg/kg/minute); supplemental dose: 0.5-1 mcg/kg
  Continuation as an analgesic in immediate postoperative period: 0.1 mcg/kg/minute (range: 0.025-0.2 mcg/kg/minute). Infusion rate may be adjusted every 5 minutes in increments of 0.025 mcg/kg/minute. Bolus doses are not recommended. Infusion rates >0.2 mcg/kg/minute are associated with respiratory depression.
    Coronary bypass surgery, continuation as an analgesic into the ICU: 1 mcg/kg/minute (range: 0.05-1 mcg/kg/minute)
  Analgesic component of monitored anesthesia care: **Note:** Supplemental oxygen is recommended:
    Single I.V. dose given 90 seconds prior to local anesthetic:
      Remifentanil alone: 1 mcg/kg over 30-60 seconds
      With midazolam: 0.5 mcg/kg over 30-60 seconds

Continuous infusion beginning 5 minutes prior to local anesthetic:
Remifentanil alone: 0.1 mcg/kg minute
With midazolam: 0.05 mcg/kg/minute
Continuous infusion given after local anesthetic:
Remifentanil alone: 0.05 mcg/kg/minute (range: 0.025-0.2 mcg/kg/minute)
With midazolam: 0.025 mcg/kg/minute (range: 0.025-0.2 mcg/kg/minute)
**Note:** Following local or anesthetic block, infusion rate should be decreased to 0.05 mcg/kg/minute; rate adjustments of 0.025 mcg/kg/minute may be done at 5-minute intervals
Dosage Forms Injection, powder for reconstitution: 1 mg, 2 mg, 5 mg [contains glycine 15 mg]

**Reminyl**® **[US/Can]** see galantamine on page 365

**Remodulin**® **[US]** see treprostinil on page 817

**Renacidin**® **[US]** see citric acid, magnesium carbonate, and glucono-delta-lactone on page 188

**Renagel**® **[US/Can]** see sevelamer on page 745

**Renedil**® **[Can]** see felodipine on page 330

**Renese**® **[US]** see polythiazide on page 660

**Reno-M-30**® **[US]** see radiological/contrast media (ionic) on page 707

**Reno-M-60**® **[US]** see radiological/contrast media (ionic) on page 707

**Reno-M-DIP**® **[US]** see radiological/contrast media (ionic) on page 707

**Renografin-60**® **(Discontinued)** see radiological/contrast media (ionic) on page 707

**Renografin-76**® **(Discontinued)** see radiological/contrast media (ionic) on page 707

**Renoquid**® **(Discontinued)**

**Renova**® **[US]** see tretinoin (topical) on page 818

**Renovist**® **II (Discontinued)** see radiological/contrast media (ionic) on page 707

**Renovist**® **(Discontinued)** see radiological/contrast media (ionic) on page 707

**Renovue**®**-65 [US]** see radiological/contrast media (ionic) on page 707

**Renovue**®**-DIP [US]** see radiological/contrast media (ionic) on page 707

**ReoPro**® **[US/Can]** see abciximab on page 3

# repaglinide (re pa GLI nide)

Sound-Alike/Look-Alike Issues
Prandin® may be confused with Avandia®
U.S./Canadian Brand Names GlucoNorm® [Can]; Prandin® [US/Can]
Therapeutic Category Hypoglycemic Agent, Oral
Use Management of type 2 diabetes mellitus (noninsulin-dependent, NIDDM); may be used in combination with metformin or thiazolidinediones
Usual Dosage Adults: Oral: Should be taken within 15 minutes of the meal, but time may vary from immediately preceding the meal to as long as 30 minutes before the meal

Initial: For patients not previously treated or whose Hb $A_{1c}$ is <8%, the starting dose is 0.5 mg. For patients previously treated with blood glucose-lowering agents whose Hb $A_{1c}$ is ≥8%, the initial dose is 1 or 2 mg before each meal.
Dose adjustment: Determine dosing adjustments by blood glucose response, usually fasting blood glucose. Double the preprandial dose up to 4 mg until satisfactory blood glucose response is achieved. At least 1 week should elapse to assess response after each dose adjustment.
Dose range: 0.5-4 mg taken with meals. Repaglinide may be dosed preprandial 2, 3 or 4 times/day in response to changes in the patient's meal pattern. Maximum recommended daily dose: 16 mg.
**Patients receiving other oral hypoglycemic agents:** When repaglinide is used to replace therapy with other oral hypoglycemic agents, it may be started the day after the final dose is given. Observe patients carefully for hypoglycemia because of potential overlapping of drug effects. When transferred from longer half-life sulfonylureas (eg, chlorpropamide), close monitoring may be indicated for up to ≥1 week.
**Combination therapy:** If repaglinide monotherapy does not result in adequate glycemic control, metformin or a thiazolidinedione may be added. Or, if metformin or thiazolidinedione therapy does not provide adequate control, repaglinide may be added. The starting dose and dose adjustments for combination therapy are the same as repaglinide monotherapy. Carefully adjust the dose of each drug to determine the minimal dose required to achieve the desired pharmacologic effect. Failure to do so
(Continued)

## repaglinide *(Continued)*

could result in an increase in the incidence of hypoglycemic episodes. Use appropriate monitoring of FPG and Hb $A_{1c}$ measurements to ensure that the patient is not subjected to excessive drug exposure or increased probability of secondary drug failure. If glucose is not achieved after a suitable trial of combination therapy, consider discontinuing these drugs and using insulin.

Dosage Forms Tablet: 0.5 mg, 1 mg, 2 mg

**Repan**® **[US]** *see* butalbital, acetaminophen, and caffeine *on page 124*

**Replace [US-OTC]** *see* vitamins (multiple/oral) *on page 852*

**Replace with Iron [US-OTC]** *see* vitamins (multiple/oral) *on page 852*

**Reposans-10**® **Oral *(Discontinued)*** *see* chlordiazepoxide *on page 167*

**Reprexain**™ **[US]** *see* hydrocodone and ibuprofen *on page 413*

**Repronex**® **[US/Can]** *see* menotropins *on page 511*

**Requip**® **[US/Can]** *see* ropinirole *on page 730*

**Resa**® ***(Discontinued)*** *see* reserpine *on this page*

**Rescon DM [US-OTC]** *see* chlorpheniramine, pseudoephedrine, and dextromethorphan *on page 177*

**Rescon GG [US]** *see* guaifenesin and phenylephrine *on page 387*

**Rescon-Jr. [US]** *see* chlorpheniramine and pseudoephedrine *on page 172*

**Rescriptor**® **[US/Can]** *see* delavirdine *on page 227*

**Rescula**® ***(Discontinued)***

**Resectisol**® **[US]** *see* mannitol *on page 502*

## reserpine *(re SER peen)*

**Sound-Alike/Look-Alike Issues**
reserpine may be confused with Risperdal®, risperidone

**Therapeutic Category** Rauwolfia Alkaloid

**Use** Management of mild-to-moderate hypertension; treatment of agitated psychotic states (schizophrenia)

**Usual Dosage Note:** When used for management of hypertension, full antihypertensive effects may take as long as 3 weeks.
Oral:
Children: Hypertension: 0.01-0.02 mg/kg/24 hours divided every 12 hours; maximum dose: 0.25 mg/day (not recommended in children)
Adults: Hypertension:
Manufacturer's labeling: Initial: 0.5 mg/day for 1-2 weeks; maintenance: 0.1-0.25 mg/day
**Note:** Clinically, the need for a "loading" period (as recommended by the manufacturer) is not well supported, and alternative dosing is preferred.
Usual dose range (JNC 7): 0.05-0.25 mg once daily; 0.1 mg every other day may be given to achieve 0.05 mg once daily

**Dosage Forms** Tablet: 0.1 mg, 0.25 mg

**reserpine, hydralazine, and hydrochlorothiazide** *see* hydralazine, hydrochlorothiazide, and reserpine *on page 409*

**Respa-DM**® **[US]** *see* guaifenesin and dextromethorphan *on page 385*

**Respa-GF**® ***(Discontinued)*** *see* guaifenesin *on page 383*

**Respaire**®**-60 SR [US]** *see* guaifenesin and pseudoephedrine *on page 388*

**Respaire**®**-120 SR [US]** *see* guaifenesin and pseudoephedrine *on page 388*

**Respbid**® ***(Discontinued)*** *see* theophylline *on page 793*

**Respi-Tann**™ **[US]** *see* carbetapentane and pseudoephedrine *on page 142*

**Resporal**® ***(Discontinued)*** *see* dexbrompheniramine and pseudoephedrine *on page 234*

**Restall**® ***(Discontinued)*** *see* hydroxyzine *on page 423*

**Restasis**™ **[US]** *see* cyclosporine *on page 215*

**Restoril**® **[US/Can]** *see* temazepam *on page 784*

**Restylane**® **[US]** *see* hyaluronate and derivatives *on page 406*

**Retavase**® **[US/Can]** *see* reteplase *on this page*

**reteplase** (RE ta plase)
Synonyms r-PA; recombinant plasminogen activator
U.S./Canadian Brand Names Retavase® [US/Can]
Therapeutic Category Fibrinolytic Agent
Use Management of acute myocardial infarction (AMI); improvement of ventricular function; reduction of the incidence of CHF and the reduction of mortality following AMI
Usual Dosage
Children: Not recommended
Adults: 10 units I.V. over 2 minutes, followed by a second dose 30 minutes later of 10 units I.V. over 2 minutes
Withhold second dose if serious bleeding or anaphylaxis occurs
Dosage Forms Injection, powder for reconstitution [preservative free]: 10.4 units [equivalent to reteplase 18.1 mg; contains sucrose and polysorbate 80; packaged with sterile water for injection]

**Retin-A**® **[US/Can]** *see* tretinoin (topical) *on page 818*

**Retin-A**® **Micro [US/Can]** *see* tretinoin (topical) *on page 818*

**retinoic acid** *see* tretinoin (topical) *on page 818*

**Retinova**® **[Can]** *see* tretinoin (topical) *on page 818*

**Retisert**™ **[US]** *see* fluocinolone *on page 344*

**Retrovir**® **[US/Can]** *see* zidovudine *on page 859*

**Revatio**™ **[US]** *see* sildenafil *on page 746*

**Reversol**® **[US]** *see* edrophonium *on page 279*

**Revex**® **[US]** *see* nalmefene *on page 559*

**ReVia**® **[US/Can]** *see* naltrexone *on page 560*

**Revitalose C-1000**® **[Can]** *see* ascorbic acid *on page 71*

**Rexigen Forte**® ***(Discontinued)*** *see* phendimetrazine *on page 637*

**Reyataz**® **[US/Can]** *see* atazanavir *on page 76*

**Rezulin**® ***(Discontinued)***

**rFVIIa** *see* factor VIIa (recombinant) *on page 325*

**R-Gel**® ***(Discontinued)*** *see* capsaicin *on page 138*

**R-Gene**® **[US]** *see* arginine *on page 69*

**rGM-CSF** *see* sargramostim *on page 739*

**rhASB** *see* galsulfase *on page 366*

**r-hCG** *see* chorionic gonadotropin (recombinant) *on page 181*

**Rheaban**® ***(Discontinued)*** *see* attapulgite *on page 81*

**Rheomacrodex**® ***(Discontinued)*** *see* dextran *on page 236*

**Rheumatrex**® **[US]** *see* methotrexate *on page 524*

**r-h α-GAL** *see* agalsidase beta *on page 20*

**RhIG** *see* Rh$_o$(D) immune globulin *on this page*

**rhIL-11** *see* oprelvekin *on page 601*

**Rhinalar**® **[Can]** *see* flunisolide *on page 344*

**Rhinocort**® **Aqua**® **[US]** *see* budesonide *on page 118*

**Rhinocort**® **Nasal Inhaler** ***(Discontinued)*** *see* budesonide *on page 118*

**Rhinocort**® **Turbuhaler**® **[Can]** *see* budesonide *on page 118*

**Rh$_o$(D) immune globulin** (ar aych oh (dee) i MYUN GLOB yoo lin)
Synonyms RhIG; Rho(D) immune globulin (human); RhoIGIV; RhoIVIM
U.S./Canadian Brand Names BayRho-D® Full-Dose [US/Can]; BayRho-D® Mini-Dose [US]; MICRhoGAM® [US]; RhoGAM® [US]; Rhophylac® [US]; WinRho SDF® [US]
(Continued)

# Rh$_o$(D) immune globulin *(Continued)*

**Therapeutic Category** Immune Globulin

**Use**

Suppression of Rh isoimmunization: Use in the following situations when an Rh$_o$(D)-negative individual is exposed to Rh$_o$(D)-positive blood: During delivery of an Rh$_o$(D)-positive infant; abortion; amniocentesis; chorionic villus sampling; ruptured tubal pregnancy; abdominal trauma; transplacental hemorrhage. Used when the mother is Rh$_o$(D) negative, the father of the child is either Rh$_o$(D) positive or Rh$_o$(D) unknown, the baby is either Rh$_o$(D) positive or Rh$_o$(D) unknown.

Transfusion: Suppression of Rh isoimmunization in Rh$_o$(D)-negative female children and female adults in their childbearing years transfused with Rh$_o$(D) antigen-positive RBCs or blood components containing Rh$_o$(D) antigen-positive RBCs

Treatment of idiopathic thrombocytopenic purpura (ITP): Used in the following nonsplenectomized Rh$_o$(D) positive individuals: Children with acute or chronic ITP, adults with chronic ITP, children and adults with ITP secondary to HIV infection

**Usual Dosage**

**ITP:** Children and Adults: WinRho SDF®: I.V.:

Initial: 50 mcg/kg as a single injection, or can be given as a divided dose on separate days. If hemoglobin is <10 g/dL: Dose should be reduced to 25-40 mcg/kg.

Subsequent dosing: 25-60 mcg/kg can be used if required to elevate platelet count

Maintenance dosing if patient **did respond** to initial dosing: 25-60 mcg/kg based on platelet and hemoglobin levels:

Maintenance dosing if patient **did not respond** to initial dosing:

Hemoglobin 8-10 g/dL: Redose between 25-40 mcg/kg

Hemoglobin >10 g/dL: Redose between 50-60 mcg/kg

Hemoglobin <8 g/dL: Use with caution

**Rh$_o$(D) suppression:** Adults: **Note:** One "full dose" (300 mcg) provides enough antibody to prevent Rh sensitization if the volume of RBC entering the circulation is ≤15 mL. When >15 mL is suspected, a fetal red cell count should be performed to determine the appropriate dose.

Pregnancy:

Antepartum prophylaxis: In general, dose is given at 28 weeks. If given early in pregnancy, administer every 12 weeks to ensure adequate levels of passively acquired anti-Rh

BayRho-D® Full Dose, RhoGAM®: I.M.: 300 mcg

Rhophylac®, WinRho SDF®: I.M., I.V.: 300 mcg

Postpartum prophylaxis: In general, dose is administered as soon as possible after delivery, preferably within 72 hours. Can be given up to 28 days following delivery

BayRho-D® Full Dose, RhoGAM®: I.M.: 300 mcg

Rhophylac®: I.M., I.V.: 300 mcg

WinRho SDF®: I.M., I.V.: 120 mcg

Threatened abortion, any time during pregnancy (with continuation of pregnancy):

BayRho-D® Full Dose, RhoGAM®: I.M.: 300 mcg; administer as soon as possible

Rhophylac®, WinRho SDF®: I.M., I.V.: 300 mcg; administer as soon as possible

Abortion, miscarriage, termination of ectopic pregnancy:

BayRho-D®, RhoGAM®: I.M.: ≥13 weeks gestation: 300 mcg.

BayRho-D® Mini Dose, MICRhoGAM®: <13 weeks gestation: I.M.: 50 mcg

Rhophylac®: I.M., I.V.: 300 mcg

WinRho SDF®: I.M., I.V.: After 34 weeks gestation: 120 mcg; administer immediately or within 72 hours

Amniocentesis, chorionic villus sampling:

BayRho-D®, RhoGAM®: I.M.: At 15-18 weeks gestation or during the 3rd trimester: 300 mcg. If dose is given between 13-18 weeks, repeat at 26-28 weeks and within 72 hours of delivery.

Rhophylac®: I.M., I.V.: 300 mcg

WinRho SDF®: I.M., I.V.: Before 34 weeks gestation: 300 mcg; administer immediately, repeat dose every 12 weeks during pregnancy; After 34 weeks gestation: 120 mcg, administered immediately or within 72 hours

Abdominal trauma, manipulation:

BayRho-D®, RhoGAM®: I.M.: 2nd or 3rd trimester: 300 mcg. If dose is given between 13-18 weeks, repeat at 26-28 weeks and within 72 hours of delivery

WinRho SDF®: I.M./I.V.: After 34 weeks gestation: 120 mcg; administer immediately or within 72 hours

**Transfusion:**

Children and Adults: WinRho SDF®: Administer within 72 hours after exposure of incompatible blood transfusions or massive fetal hemorrhage.

I.V.: Calculate dose as follows; administer 600 mcg every 8 hours until the total dose is administered:
Exposure to Rh$_o$(D) positive whole blood: 9 mcg/mL blood
Exposure to Rh$_o$(D) positive red blood cells: 18 mcg/mL cells
I.M.: Calculate dose as follows; administer 1200 mcg every 12 hours until the total dose is administered:
Exposure to Rh$_o$(D) positive whole blood: 12 mcg/mL blood
Exposure to Rh$_o$(D) positive red blood cells: 24 mcg/mL cells
Adults:
BayRho-D®, RhoGAM®: I.M.: Multiply the volume of Rh positive whole blood administered by the hematocrit of the donor unit to equal the volume of RBCs transfused. The volume of RBCs is then divided by 15 mL, providing the number of 300 mcg doses (vials/syringes) to administer. If the dose calculated results in a fraction, round up to the next higher whole 300 mcg dose (vial/syringe).
Rhophylac®: I.M., I.V.: 20 mcg/2 mL transfused blood or 20 mcg/mL erythrocyte concentrate

**Dosage Forms**
Injection, solution [preservative free]:
BayRho-D® Full-Dose, RhoGAM®: 300 mcg [for I.M. use only]
BayRho-D® Mini-Dose, MICRhoGAM®: 50 mcg [for I.M. use only]
Rhophylac®: 300 mcg/2 mL (2 mL) [1500 int. units; for I.M. or I.V. use]
Injection, powder for reconstitution [preservative free] (WinRho SDF®): 120 mcg [600 int. units], 300 mcg [1500 int. units], 1000 mcg [5000 int. units] [for I.M. or I.V. use]

**Rho(D) immune globulin (human)** *see* Rh$_o$(D) immune globulin *on page 717*

**Rho-Clonazepam [Can]** *see* clonazepam *on page 197*

**Rhodacine® [Can]** *see* indomethacin *on page 436*

**Rhodis™ [Can]** *see* ketoprofen *on page 457*

**Rhodis-EC™ [Can]** *see* ketoprofen *on page 457*

**Rhodis SR™ [Can]** *see* ketoprofen *on page 457*

**RhoGAM® [US]** *see* Rh$_o$(D) immune globulin *on page 717*

**RhoIGIV** *see* Rh$_o$(D) immune globulin *on page 717*

**RhoIVIM** *see* Rh$_o$(D) immune globulin *on page 717*

**Rho®-Loperamine [Can]** *see* loperamide *on page 489*

**Rho®-Metformin [Can]** *see* metformin *on page 519*

**Rho-Nitro [Can]** *see* nitroglycerin *on page 578*

**Rhophylac® [US]** *see* Rh$_o$(D) immune globulin *on page 717*

**Rho®-Sotalol [Can]** *see* sotalol *on page 762*

**Rhotral [Can]** *see* acebutolol *on page 4*

**Rhotrimine® [Can]** *see* trimipramine *on page 826*

**Rhovane® [Can]** *see* zopiclone *(Canada only) on page 864*

**Rhoxal-Acebutolol [Can]** *see* acebutolol *on page 4*

**Rhoxal-amiodarone [Can]** *see* amiodarone *on page 41*

**Rhoxal-Anagrelide [Can]** *see* anagrelide *on page 52*

**Rhoxal-atenolol [Can]** *see* atenolol *on page 76*

**Rhoxal-ciprofloxacin [Can]** *see* ciprofloxacin *on page 184*

**Rhoxal-citalopram [Can]** *see* citalopram *on page 188*

**Rhoxal-cyclosporine [Can]** *see* cyclosporine *on page 215*

**Rhoxal-diltiazem CD [Can]** *see* diltiazem *on page 251*

**Rhoxal-diltiazem SR [Can]** *see* diltiazem *on page 251*

**Rhoxal-fluoxetine [Can]** *see* fluoxetine *on page 349*

**Rhoxal-fluvoxamine [Can]** *see* fluvoxamine *on page 356*

**Rhoxal-gliclazide [Can]** *see* gliclazide *(Canada only) on page 375*

**Rhoxal-minocycline [Can]** *see* minocycline *on page 542*

**Rhoxal-mirtazapine [Can]** *see* mirtazapine *on page 543*

**Rhoxal-nabumetone [Can]** *see* nabumetone *on page 556*

**Rhoxal-orphendrine [Can]** *see* orphenadrine *on page 602*

**Rhoxal-paroxetine [Can]** *see* paroxetine *on page 620*

**Rhoxal-ranitidine [Can]** *see* ranitidine hydrochloride *on page 710*

**Rhoxal-salbutamol [Can]** *see* albuterol *on page 22*

**Rhoxal-Sertraline [Can]** *see* sertraline *on page 744*

**Rhoxal-ticlopidine [Can]** *see* ticlopidine *on page 802*

**Rhoxal-valproic [Can]** *see* valproic acid and derivatives *on page 837*

**Rhoxal-zopiclone [Can]** *see* zopiclone *(Canada only) on page 864*

**rhPTH(1-34)** *see* teriparatide *on page 787*

***r*HuEPO-α** *see* epoetin alfa *on page 290*

**rHu-KGF** *see* palifermin *on page 613*

**Rhulicaine®** ***(Discontinued)*** *see* benzocaine *on page 95*

**rhuMAb-E25** *see* omalizumab *on page 597*

**rhuMAb-VEGF** *see* bevacizumab *on page 105*

**Ribasphere™ [US]** *see* ribavirin *on this page*

## ribavirin (rye ba VYE rin)

**Sound-Alike/Look-Alike Issues**
ribavirin may be confused with riboflavin

**Synonyms** RTCA; tribavirin

**U.S./Canadian Brand Names** Copegus® [US]; Rebetol® [US]; Ribasphere™ [US]; Virazole® [US/Can]

**Therapeutic Category** Antiviral Agent

**Use**
Inhalation: Treatment of patients with respiratory syncytial virus (RSV) infections; specially indicated for treatment of severe lower respiratory tract RSV infections in patients with an underlying compromising condition (prematurity, bronchopulmonary dysplasia and other chronic lung conditions, congenital heart disease, immunodeficiency, immunosuppression), and recent transplant recipients

Oral capsule:
In combination with interferon alfa-2b (Intron® A) injection for the treatment of chronic hepatitis C in patients with compensated liver disease who have relapsed after alpha interferon therapy or were previously untreated with alpha interferons

In combination with peginterferon alfa-2b (PEG-Intron®) injection for the treatment of chronic hepatitis C in patients with compensated liver disease who were previously untreated with alpha interferons

Oral solution: In combination with interferon alfa 2b (Intron® A) injection for the treatment of chronic hepatitis C in patients ≥3 years of age with compensated liver disease who were previously untreated with alpha interferons or patients ≥18 years of age who have relapsed after alpha interferon therapy

Oral tablet: In combination with peginterferon alfa-2a (Pegasys®) injection for the treatment of chronic hepatitis C in patients with compensated liver disease who were previously untreated with alpha interferons (includes patients with histological evidence of cirrhosis [Child-Pugh class A] and patients with clinically-stable HIV disease)

**Usual Dosage**
Aerosol inhalation: Infants and children: Use with Viratek® small particle aerosol generator (SPAG-2) at a concentration of 20 mg/mL (6 g reconstituted with 300 mL of sterile water without preservatives). Continuous aerosol administration: 12-18 hours/day for 3 days, up to 7 days in length

Oral capsule or solution: Children ≥3 years: Chronic hepatitis C (in combination with interferon alfa-2b):
Rebetol®: Oral: **Note:** Oral solution should be used in children 3-5 years of age, children ≤25 kg, or those unable to swallow capsules.

Capsule/solution: 15 mg/kg/day in 2 divided doses (morning and evening)

Capsule dosing recommendations:
25-36 kg: 400 mg/day (200 mg morning and evening)
37-49 kg: 600 mg/day (200 mg in the morning and two 200 mg capsules in the evening)
50-61 kg: 800 mg/day (two 200 mg capsules morning and evening)
>61 kg: Refer to Adults dosing

**Note:** Duration of therapy is 48 weeks in pediatric patients with genotype 1 and 24 weeks in patients with genotype 2,3. Discontinue treatment in any patient if HCV-RNA is not below the limit of detection of the assay after 24 weeks of therapy.

**Note:** Also refer to Interferon Alfa-2b/Ribavirin combination pack monograph.

Oral capsule (Rebetol®, Ribasphere™): Adults:

Chronic hepatitis C (in combination with interferon alfa-2b):

≤75 kg: 400 mg in the morning, then 600 mg in the evening

>75 kg: 600 mg in the morning, then 600 mg in the evening

**Note:** If HCV-RNA is undetectable at 24 weeks, duration of therapy is 48 weeks. In patients who relapse following interferon therapy, duration of dual therapy is 24 weeks.

**Note:** Also refer to Interferon Alfa-2b/Ribavirin combination pack monograph.

Chronic hepatitis C (in combination with peginterferon alfa-2b): 400 mg twice daily; duration of therapy is 1 year; after 24 weeks of treatment, if serum HCV-RNA is not below the limit of detection of the assay, consider discontinuation.

Oral tablet (Copegus®, in combination with peginterferon alfa-2b): Adults: Chronic hepatitis C:

Monoinfection, genotype 1,4:

<75kg: 1000 mg/day in 2 divided doses for 48 weeks

≥75kg: 1200 mg/day in 2 divided doses for 48 weeks

Monoinfection, genotype 2,3: 800 mg/day in 2 divided doses for 24 weeks

Coinfection with HIV: 800 mg/day in 2 divided doses for 48 weeks

**Note:** Also refer to Peginterferon Alfa-2a monograph.

**Dosage Forms**

Capsule (Rebetol®, Ribasphere™): 200 mg

Powder for aerosol (Virazole®): 6 g

Powder for solution, inhalation [for aerosol administration] (Virazole®): 6 g [reconstituted product provides 20 mg/mL]

Tablet (Copegus®): 200 mg

**ribavirin and interferon alfa-2b combination pack** *see* interferon alfa-2b and ribavirin *on* *page 441*

**ribavirin and peginterferon alfa-2b** *see* peginterferon alfa-2b and ribavirin *(Canada only) on* *page 625*

**Ribo-100 [US]** *see* riboflavin *on this page*

# riboflavin (RYE boe flay vin)

**Sound-Alike/Look-Alike Issues**

riboflavin may be confused with ribavirin

**Synonyms** lactoflavin; vitamin B$_2$; vitamin G

**U.S./Canadian Brand Names** Ribo-100 [US]

**Therapeutic Category** Vitamin, Water Soluble

**Use** Prevention of riboflavin deficiency and treatment of ariboflavinosis

**Usual Dosage** Oral:

Riboflavin deficiency:

Children: 2.5-10 mg/day in divided doses

Adults: 5-30 mg/day in divided doses

Recommended daily allowance:

Children: 0.4-1.8 mg

Adults: 1.2-1.7 mg

**Dosage Forms**

Tablet: 25 mg, 50 mg, 100 mg

Ribo-100: 100 mg

**Rid-A-Pain Dental Drops [US-OTC]** *see* benzocaine *on page 95*

**Ridaura® [US/Can]** *see* auranofin *on page 81*

**RID® *(Discontinued)*** *see* pyrethrins and piperonyl butoxide *on page 699*

**RID® Maximum Strength [US-OTC]** *see* pyrethrins and piperonyl butoxide *on page 699*

**RID® Mousse [Can]** *see* pyrethrins and piperonyl butoxide *on page 699*

**Rid® Spray [US-OTC]** *see* permethrin *on page 635*

# rifabutin (rif a BYOO tin)

**Sound-Alike/Look-Alike Issues**

rifabutin may be confused with rifampin

(Continued)

# rifabutin *(Continued)*

**Synonyms** ansamycin

**U.S./Canadian Brand Names** Mycobutin® [US/Can]

**Therapeutic Category** Antibiotic, Miscellaneous

**Use** Prevention of disseminated *Mycobacterium avium* complex (MAC) in patients with advanced HIV infection

**Usual Dosage** Oral:

Children >1 year: Prophylaxis: 5 mg/kg daily; higher dosages have been used in limited trials

Adults: Prophylaxis: 300 mg once daily (alone or in combination with azithromycin)

Patients receiving nelfinavir, amprenavir, indinavir: Reduce dose to 150 mg/day; no change in dose if administered twice weekly

**Dosage Forms** Capsule: 150 mg

**Rifadin® [US/Can]** *see* rifampin *on this page*

**Rifamate® [US/Can]** *see* rifampin and isoniazid *on this page*

**rifampicin** *see* rifampin *on this page*

# rifampin *(RIF am pin)*

**Sound-Alike/Look-Alike Issues**

rifampin may be confused with rifabutin, Rifamate®, rifapentine, rifaximin

Rifadin® may be confused with Ritalin®

Rimactane® may be confused with rimantadine

**Synonyms** rifampicin

**U.S./Canadian Brand Names** Rifadin® [US/Can]; Rofact™ [Can]

**Therapeutic Category** Antibiotic, Miscellaneous

**Use** Management of active tuberculosis in combination with other agents; elimination of meningococci from the nasopharynx in asymptomatic carriers

**Usual Dosage** Oral (I.V. infusion dose is the same as for the oral route):

**Tuberculosis therapy (drug susceptible): Note:** A four-drug regimen (isoniazid, rifampin, pyrazinamide, and ethambutol) is preferred for the initial, empiric treatment of TB. When the drug susceptibility results are available, the regimen should be altered as appropriate.

Infants and Children <12 years:

Daily therapy: 10-20 mg/kg/day usually as a single dose (maximum: 600 mg/day)

Twice weekly directly observed therapy (DOT): 10-20 mg/kg (maximum: 600 mg)

Adults:

Daily therapy: 10 mg/kg/day (maximum: 600 mg/day)

Twice weekly directly observed therapy (DOT): 10 mg/kg (maximum: 600 mg); 3 times/week: 10 mg/kg (maximum: 600 mg)

**Latent tuberculosis infection (LTBI):** As an alternative to isoniazid:

Children: 10-20 mg/kg/day (maximum: 600 mg/day) for 6 months

Adults: 10 mg/kg/day (maximum: 600 mg/day) for 4 months. **Note:** Combination with pyrazinamide should not generally be offered (*MMWR*, Aug 8, 2003).

**Meningococcal meningitis prophylaxis:**

Infants <1 month: 10 mg/kg/day in divided doses every 12 hours for 2 days

Infants ≥1 month and Children: 20 mg/kg/day in divided doses every 12 hours for 2 days (maximum: 600 mg/dose)

Adults: 600 mg every 12 hours for 2 days

**Dosage Forms**

Capsule: 150 mg, 300 mg

Injection, powder for reconstitution: 600 mg

# rifampin and isoniazid *(RIF am pin & eye soe NYE a zid)*

**Sound-Alike/Look-Alike Issues**

Rifamate® may be confused with rifampin

**Synonyms** isoniazid and rifampin

**U.S./Canadian Brand Names** Rifamate® [US/Can]

**Therapeutic Category** Antibiotic, Miscellaneous

**Use** Management of active tuberculosis; see individual agents for additional information

**Usual Dosage** Oral: 2 capsules/day

**Dosage Forms** Capsule: Rifampin 300 mg and isoniazid 150 mg

## rifampin, isoniazid, and pyrazinamide
(RIF am pin, eye soe NYE a zid, & peer a ZIN a mide)
**Synonyms** isoniazid, rifampin, and pyrazinamide; pyrazinamide, rifampin, and isoniazid
**U.S./Canadian Brand Names** Rifater® [US/Can]
**Therapeutic Category** Antibiotic, Miscellaneous
**Use** Initial phase, short-course treatment of pulmonary tuberculosis; see individual agents for additional information
**Usual Dosage** Adults: Oral: Patients weighing:
≤44 kg: 4 tablets
45-54 kg: 5 tablets
≥55 kg: 6 tablets
Doses should be administered in a single daily dose
**Dosage Forms** Tablet: Rifampin 120 mg, isoniazid 50 mg, and pyrazinamide 300 mg

## rifapentine (RIF a pen teen)
**Sound-Alike/Look-Alike Issues**
rifapentine may be confused with rifampin
**U.S./Canadian Brand Names** Priftin® [US/Can]
**Therapeutic Category** Antitubercular Agent
**Use** Treatment of pulmonary tuberculosis; rifapentine must always be used in conjunction with at least one other antituberculosis drug to which the isolate is susceptible; it may also be necessary to add a third agent (either streptomycin or ethambutol) until susceptibility is known.
**Usual Dosage**
Children: No dosing information available
Adults: **Rifapentine should not be used alone**; initial phase should include a 3- to 4-drug regimen
Intensive phase (initial 2 months) of short-term therapy: 600 mg (four 150 mg tablets) given twice weekly (with an interval of not less than 72 hours between doses); following the intensive phase, treatment should continue with rifapentine 600 mg once weekly for 4 months in combination with INH or appropriate agent for susceptible organisms
**Dosage Forms** Tablet [film coated]: 150 mg

**Rifater® [US/Can]** see rifampin, isoniazid, and pyrazinamide *on this page*

## rifaximin (rif AX i min)
**Sound-Alike/Look-Alike Issues**
rifaximin may be confused with rifampin
**U.S./Canadian Brand Names** Xifaxan™ [US]
**Therapeutic Category** Antibiotic, Miscellaneous
**Use** Treatment of travelers' diarrhea caused by noninvasive strains of *E. coli*
**Usual Dosage** Oral: Children ≥12 years and Adults: Travelers' diarrhea: 200 mg 3 times/day for 3 days
**Dosage Forms** Tablet: 200 mg

**rIFN-A** *see* interferon alfa-2a *on page 440*

**rIFN beta-1a** *see* interferon beta-1a *on page 443*

**rIFN beta-1b** *see* interferon beta-1b *on page 443*

**RIG** *see* rabies immune globulin (human) *on page 707*

**rIL-11** *see* oprelvekin *on page 601*

**Rilutek® [US/Can]** *see* riluzole *on this page*

## riluzole (RIL yoo zole)
**Synonyms** 2-amino-6-trifluoromethoxy-benzothiazole; RP-54274
**U.S./Canadian Brand Names** Rilutek® [US/Can]
**Therapeutic Category** Miscellaneous Product
**Use** Treatment of amyotrophic lateral sclerosis (ALS); riluzole can extend survival or time to tracheostomy
**Usual Dosage** Adults: Oral: 50 mg every 12 hours; no increased benefit can be expected from higher daily doses, but adverse events are increased
**Dosage adjustment in smoking:** Cigarette smoking is known to induce CYP1A2; patients who smoke cigarettes would be expected to eliminate riluzole faster. There is no information, however, on the effect of, or need for, dosage adjustment in these patients.
(Continued)

## riluzole *(Continued)*

**Dosage adjustment in special populations:** Females and Japanese patients may possess a lower metabolic capacity to eliminate riluzole compared with male and Caucasian subjects, respectively

**Dosage Forms** Tablet: 50 mg [film coated]

## rimantadine (ri MAN ta deen)

**Sound-Alike/Look-Alike Issues**
rimantadine may be confused with amantadine, ranitidine, Rimactane®
Flumadine® may be confused with fludarabine, flunisolide, flutamide

**Synonyms** rimantadine hydrochloride

**U.S./Canadian Brand Names** Flumadine® [US/Can]

**Therapeutic Category** Antiviral Agent

**Use** Prophylaxis (adults and children >1 year of age) and treatment (adults) of influenza A viral infection

**Usual Dosage** Oral:
Prophylaxis:
Children 1-10 years or <40 kg: 5 mg/kg/day in 2 divided doses; maximum: 150 mg/day
Children >10 years and Adults: 100 mg twice daily
Treatment: Adults: 100 mg twice daily

**Dosage Forms**
Syrup, as hydrochloride: 50 mg/5 mL (240 mL) [raspberry flavor]
Tablet, as hydrochloride: 100 mg

**rimantadine hydrochloride** *see* rimantadine *on this page*

## rimexolone (ri MEKS oh lone)

**Sound-Alike/Look-Alike Issues**
Vexol® may be confused with VoSol®

**U.S./Canadian Brand Names** Vexol® [US/Can]

**Therapeutic Category** Adrenal Corticosteroid

**Use** Treatment of inflammation after ocular surgery and the treatment of anterior uveitis

**Usual Dosage** Adults: Ophthalmic: Instill 1 drop in conjunctival sac 2-4 times/day up to every 4 hours; may use every 1-2 hours during first 1-2 days

**Dosage Forms** Suspension, ophthalmic: 1% (5 mL, 10 mL) [contains benzalkonium chloride]

**Rimso®-50 [US/Can]** *see* dimethyl sulfoxide *on page 253*

**Rindal HD Plus [US]** *see* phenylephrine, hydrocodone, and chlorpheniramine *on page 643*

**Riobin® *(Discontinued)*** *see* riboflavin *on page 721*

**Riomet™ [US]** *see* metformin *on page 519*

**Riopan® Plus *(Discontinued)*** *see* magaldrate and simethicone *on page 496*

**Riopan® Plus Double Strength *(Discontinued)*** *see* magaldrate and simethicone *on page 496*

**Riphenidate [Can]** *see* methylphenidate *on page 530*

## risedronate (ris ED roe nate)

**Synonyms** risedronate sodium

**U.S./Canadian Brand Names** Actonel® [US/Can]

**Therapeutic Category** Bisphosphonate Derivative

**Use** Paget disease of the bone; treatment and prevention of glucocorticoid-induced osteoporosis; treatment and prevention of osteoporosis in postmenopausal women

**Usual Dosage** Risedronate should be taken at least 30 minutes before the first food or drink of the day other than water. Oral:
Adults (patients should receive supplemental calcium and vitamin D if dietary intake is inadequate):
Paget disease of bone: 30 mg once daily for 2 months
Retreatment may be considered (following post-treatment observation of at least 2 months) if relapse occurs, or if treatment fails to normalize serum alkaline phosphatase. For retreatment, the dose and duration of therapy are the same as for initial treatment. No data are available on more than one course of retreatment.

Osteoporosis (postmenopausal) prevention and treatment: 5 mg once daily; efficacy for use longer than 1 year has not been established; **alternatively,** a dose of 35 mg once weekly has been demonstrated effective for treatment and may be considered for prevention

Osteoporosis (glucocorticoid-induced) prevention and treatment: 5 mg once daily

**Dosage Forms** Tablet, as sodium: 5 mg, 30 mg, 35 mg

**risedronate sodium** *see* risedronate *on previous page*

**Risperdal**® **[US/Can]** *see* risperidone *on this page*

**Risperdal**® **Consta**™ **[US/Can]** *see* risperidone *on this page*

## risperidone (ris PER i done)

**Sound-Alike/Look-Alike Issues**

risperidone may be confused with reserpine

Risperdal® may be confused with lisinopril, reserpine

**U.S./Canadian Brand Names** Risperdal® Consta™ [US/Can]; Risperdal® M-Tab™ [US/Can]; Risperdal® [US/Can]

**Therapeutic Category** Antipsychotic Agent, Benzisoxazole

**Use** Treatment of schizophrenia; treatment of acute mania or mixed episodes associated with bipolar I disorder (as monotherapy or in combination with lithium or valproate)

**Usual Dosage**

Oral: Adults:

Schizophrenia:

Initial: 1 mg twice daily; may be increased to 2 mg/day to a target dose of 6 mg/day; usual range: 4-8 g/day; may be given as a single daily dose once maintenance dose is achieved; daily dosages >6 mg do not appear to confer any additional benefit, and the incidence of extrapyramidal symptoms is higher than with lower doses. Further dose adjustments should be made in increments/decrements of 1-2 mg/day on a weekly basis. Dose range studied in clinical trials: 4-16 mg/day.

Maintenance: Target dose: 4 mg once daily (range 2-8 mg/day)

Bipolar mania:

Initial: 2-3 mg once daily; if needed, adjust dose by 1 mg/day in intervals ≥24 hours; dosing range: 1-6 mg/day

Maintenance: No dosing recommendation available for treatment >3 weeks duration.

I.M.: Adults: Schizophrenia (Risperdal® Consta™): 25 mg every 2 weeks; some patients may benefit from larger doses; maximum dose not to exceed 50 mg every 2 weeks. Dosage adjustments should not be made more frequently than every 4 weeks.

**Note:** Oral risperidone (or other antipsychotic) should be administered with the initial injection of Risperdal® Consta™ and continued for 3 weeks (then discontinued) to maintain adequate therapeutic plasma concentrations prior to main release phase of risperidone from injection site. When switching from depot administration to a short-acting formulation, administer short-acting agent in place of the next regularly-scheduled depot injection.

**Dosage Forms**

Injection, microspheres for reconstitution, extended release (Risperdal® Consta™): 25 mg, 37.5 mg, 50 mg [supplied in a dose-pack containing vial with active ingredient in microsphere formulation, prefilled syringe with diluent, needle-free vial access device, and safety needle]

Solution, oral: 1 mg/mL (30 mL) [contains benzoic acid]

Tablet: 0.25 mg, 0.5 mg, 1 mg, 2 mg, 3 mg, 4 mg

Tablet, orally disintegrating (Risperdal® M-Tabs™): 0.5 mg [contains phenylalanine 0.14 mg]; 1 mg [contains phenylalanine 0.28 mg]; 2 mg [contains phenylalanine 0.56 mg]

**Ritalin**® **[US/Can]** *see* methylphenidate *on page 530*

**Ritalin**® **LA [US]** *see* methylphenidate *on page 530*

**Ritalin-SR**® **[US/Can]** *see* methylphenidate *on page 530*

## ritonavir (ri TOE na veer)

**Sound-Alike/Look-Alike Issues**

ritonavir may be confused with Retrovir®

Norvir® may be confused with Norvasc®

**U.S./Canadian Brand Names** Norvir® SEC [Can]; Norvir® [US/Can]

**Therapeutic Category** Antiviral Agent

**Use** Treatment of HIV infection; should always be used as part of a multidrug regimen (at least three antiretroviral agents); may be used as a pharmacokinetic 'booster' for other protease inhibitors

(Continued)

## ritonavir *(Continued)*

**Usual Dosage Treatment of HIV infection: Oral:**
Children ≥2 years: 250 mg/m$^2$ twice daily; titrate dose upward to 400 mg/m$^2$ twice daily (maximum: 600 mg twice daily)

Adults: 600 mg twice daily; dose escalation tends to avoid nausea that many patients experience upon initiation of full dosing. Escalate the dose as follows: 300 mg twice daily for 1 day, 400 mg twice daily for 2 days, 500 mg twice daily for 1 day, then 600 mg twice daily. Ritonavir may be better tolerated when used in combination with other antiretrovirals by initiating the drug alone and subsequently adding the second agent within 2 weeks.

**Pharmacokinetic "booster" in combination with other protease inhibitors:** 100-400 mg/day
Refer to individual monographs; specific dosage recommendations often require adjustment of both agents.

**Note:** Dosage adjustments for ritonavir when administered in combination therapy:
Amprenavir: Adjustments necessary for each agent:
Amprenavir 1200 mg with ritonavir 200 mg once daily **or**
Amprenavir 600 mg with ritonavir 100 mg twice daily
Amprenavir plus efavirenz (3-drug regimen): Amprenavir 1200 mg twice daily plus ritonavir 200 mg twice daily plus efavirenz at standard dose
Indinavir: Adjustments necessary for both agents:
Indinavir 800 mg twice daily plus ritonavir 100-200 mg twice daily **or**
Indinavir 400 mg twice daily plus ritonavir 400 mg twice daily
Nelfinavir or saquinavir: Ritonavir 400 mg twice daily
Rifabutin: Decrease rifabutin dose to 150 mg every other day

**Dosage Forms**
Capsule: 100 mg [contains ethanol and polyoxyl 35 castor oil]
Solution: 80 mg/mL (240 mL) [contains ethanol and polyoxyl 35 castor oil; peppermint and caramel flavor]

**ritonavir and lopinavir** *see* lopinavir and ritonavir *on page 490*

**Rituxan® [US/Can]** *see* rituximab *on this page*

## rituximab (ri TUK si mab)

**Sound-Alike/Look-Alike Issues**
Rituxan® may be confused with Remicade®

**Synonyms** anti-CD20 monoclonal antibody; C2B8 monoclonal antibody; C2B8; IDEC-C2B8; pan-B antibody

**U.S./Canadian Brand Names** Rituxan® [US/Can]

**Therapeutic Category** Antineoplastic Agent

**Use** Treatment of relapsed or refractory CD20 positive, B-cell non-Hodgkin lymphoma

**Usual Dosage** Adults: I.V. infusion (refer to individual protocols):
Manufacturer's labeling: 375 mg/m$^2$ once weekly for 4-8 weeks
**or**
100 mg/m$^2$ I.V. day 1, then 375 mg/m$^2$ 3 times/week for 11 doses has also been reported (cycles may be repeated in patients with refractory or relapsed disease)
Retreatment following disease progression: 375 mg/m$^2$ once weekly for 4 doses
Combination therapy with ibritumomab: 250 mg/m$^2$ I.V. day 1; repeat in 7-9 days with ibritumomab (also see Ibritumomab monograph *on page 427*):

**Dosage Forms** Injection, solution [preservative free]: 10 mg/mL (10 mL, 50 mL)

**Riva-Cloxacillin [Can]** *see* cloxacillin *on page 200*

**Riva-Diclofenac [Can]** *see* diclofenac *on page 243*

**Riva-Diclofenac-K [Can]** *see* diclofenac *on page 243*

**Riva-Dicyclomine [Can]** *see* dicyclomine *on page 245*

**Riva-Famotidine [Can]** *see* famotidine *on page 327*

**Riva-Loperamine [Can]** *see* loperamide *on page 489*

**Riva-Lorazepam [Can]** *see* lorazepam *on page 491*

**Riva-Naproxen [Can]** *see* naproxen *on page 562*

**Rivanase AQ [Can]** *see* beclomethasone *on page 91*

**Riva-Norfloxacin [Can]** *see* norfloxacin *on page 582*

**Riva-Simvastatin [Can]** *see* simvastatin *on page 748*

**Rivasol [Can]** *see* zinc sulfate *on page 861*

## rivastigmine (ri va STIG meen)

**Synonyms** ENA 713; rivastigmine tartrate; SDZ ENA 713
**U.S./Canadian Brand Names** Exelon® [US/Can]
**Therapeutic Category** Acetylcholinesterase Inhibitor; Cholinergic Agent
**Use** Mild to moderate dementia from Alzheimer disease
**Usual Dosage** Adults: Mild to moderate Alzheimer dementia: Oral: Initial: 1.5 mg twice daily to start; if dose is tolerated for at least 2 weeks then it may be increased to 3 mg twice daily; increases to 4.5 mg twice daily and 6 mg twice daily should only be attempted after at least 2 weeks at the previous dose; maximum dose: 6 mg twice daily. If adverse events such as nausea, vomiting, abdominal pain, or loss of appetite occur, the patient should be instructed to discontinue treatment for several doses then restart at the same or next lower dosage level; antiemetics have been used to control GI symptoms. If treatment is interrupted for longer than several days, restart the treatment at the lowest dose and titrate as previously described.
**Dosage Forms**
Capsule: 1.5 mg, 3 mg, 4.5 mg, 6 mg
Solution, oral: 2 mg/mL (120 mL) [contains sodium benzoate]

**rivastigmine tartrate** *see* rivastigmine *on this page*

**Riva-Zide [Can]** *see* hydrochlorothiazide and triamterene *on page 410*

**Rivotril® [Can]** *see* clonazepam *on page 197*

## rizatriptan (rye za TRIP tan)

**Synonyms** MK462
**U.S./Canadian Brand Names** Maxalt RPD™ [Can]; Maxalt-MLT® [US]; Maxalt® [US/Can]
**Therapeutic Category** Antimigraine Agent; Serotonin Agonist
**Use** Acute treatment of migraine with or without aura
**Usual Dosage Note:** In patients with risk factors for coronary artery disease, following adequate evaluation to establish the absence of coronary artery disease, the initial dose should be administered in a setting where response may be evaluated (physician's office or similarly staffed setting). ECG monitoring may be considered.
Oral: 5-10 mg, repeat after 2 hours if significant relief is not attained; maximum: 30 mg in a 24-hour period (use 5 mg dose in patients receiving propranolol with a maximum of 15 mg in 24 hours)
**Note:** For orally-disintegrating tablets (Maxalt-MLT®): Patient should be instructed to place tablet on tongue and allow to dissolve. Dissolved tablet will be swallowed with saliva.
**Dosage Forms**
Tablet, as benzoate (Maxalt®): 5 mg, 10 mg
Tablet, orally-disintegrating, as benzoate (Maxalt-MLT®): 5 mg [contains phenylalanine 1.05 mg/tablet; peppermint flavor]; 10 mg [contains phenylalanine 2.1 mg/tablet; peppermint flavor]

**rLFN-α2** *see* interferon alfa-2b *on page 440*

**RMS® [US]** *see* morphine sulfate *on page 549*

**Ro 5488** *see* tretinoin (oral) *on page 817*

**Robafen® AC [US]** *see* guaifenesin and codeine *on page 384*

**Robafen® CF *(Discontinued)***

**Robafen DM [US-OTC]** *see* guaifenesin and dextromethorphan *on page 385*

**Robaxin® [US/Can]** *see* methocarbamol *on page 524*

**Robidrine® [Can]** *see* pseudoephedrine *on page 692*

**Robinul® [US]** *see* glycopyrrolate *on page 379*

**Robinul® Forte [US]** *see* glycopyrrolate *on page 379*

**Robitussin® [US-OTC/Can]** *see* guaifenesin *on page 383*

**Robitussin® A-C *(Discontinued)*** *see* guaifenesin and codeine *on page 384*

**Robitussin® CF [US-OTC]** *see* guaifenesin, pseudoephedrine, and dextromethorphan *on page 391*

**Robitussin® Childrens Cough & Cold [Can]** *see* pseudoephedrine and dextromethorphan *on page 693*

**Robitussin® Cold and Congestion [US-OTC]** *see* guaifenesin, pseudoephedrine, and dextromethorphan *on page 391*

**Robitussin® Cough and Cold Infant [US-OTC]** *see* guaifenesin, pseudoephedrine, and dextromethorphan *on page 391*

**Robitussin® Cough and Congestion [US-OTC]** *see* guaifenesin and dextromethorphan *on page 385*

**Robitussin® Cough & Cold® [Can]** *see* guaifenesin, pseudoephedrine, and dextromethorphan *on page 391*

**Robitussin® CoughGels™ [US-OTC]** *see* dextromethorphan *on page 238*

**Robitussin®-DAC *(Discontinued)*** *see* guaifenesin, pseudoephedrine, and codeine *on page 391*

**Robitussin® DM [US-OTC/Can]** *see* guaifenesin and dextromethorphan *on page 385*

**Robitussin® DM Infant [US-OTC]** *see* guaifenesin and dextromethorphan *on page 385*

**Robitussin® Honey Cough [US-OTC]** *see* dextromethorphan *on page 238*

**Robitussin® Maximum Strength Cough [US-OTC]** *see* dextromethorphan *on page 238*

**Robitussin® Maximum Strength Cough & Cold [US-OTC]** *see* pseudoephedrine and dextromethorphan *on page 693*

**Robitussin-PE® [US-OTC]** *see* guaifenesin and pseudoephedrine *on page 388*

**Robitussin® Pediatric Cough [US-OTC]** *see* dextromethorphan *on page 238*

**Robitussin® Pediatric Cough & Cold [US-OTC]** *see* pseudoephedrine and dextromethorphan *on page 693*

**Robitussin® Pediatric Night Relief [US-OTC]** *see* chlorpheniramine, pseudoephedrine, and dextromethorphan *on page 177*

**Robitussin® Severe Congestion [US-OTC]** *see* guaifenesin and pseudoephedrine *on page 388*

**Robitussin® Sugar Free Cough [US-OTC]** *see* guaifenesin and dextromethorphan *on page 385*

**Rocaltrol® [US/Can]** *see* calcitriol *on page 129*

**Rocephin® [US/Can]** *see* ceftriaxone *on page 158*

**rocuronium** (roe kyoor OH nee um)

**Sound-Alike/Look-Alike Issues**
Zemuron® may be confused with Remeron®

**Synonyms** ORG 946; rocuronium bromide

**U.S./Canadian Brand Names** Zemuron® [US/Can]

**Therapeutic Category** Skeletal Muscle Relaxant

**Use** Adjunct to general anesthesia to facilitate both rapid sequence and routine endotracheal intubation and to relax skeletal muscles during surgery; to facilitate mechanical ventilation in ICU patients; does not relieve pain or produce sedation

**Usual Dosage** Administer I.V.; dose to effect; doses will vary due to interpatient variability; use ideal body weight for obese patients

Children:

Initial: 0.6 mg/kg under halothane anesthesia produce excellent to good intubating conditions within 1 minute and will provide a median time of 41 minutes of clinical relaxation in children 3 months to 1 year of age, and 27 minutes in children 1-12 years

Maintenance: 0.075-0.125 mg/kg administered upon return of $T_1$ to 25% of control provides clinical relaxation for 7-10 minutes

Adults:

Tracheal intubation: I.V.:

Initial: 0.6 mg/kg is expected to provide approximately 31 minutes of clinical relaxation under opioid/nitrous oxide/oxygen anesthesia with neuromuscular block sufficient for intubation attained in 1-2 minutes; lower doses (0.45 mg/kg) may be used to provide 22 minutes of clinical relaxation with median time to neuromuscular block of 1-3 minutes; maximum blockade is achieved in <4 minutes

Maximum: 0.9-1.2 mg/kg may be given during surgery under opioid/nitrous oxide/oxygen anesthesia without adverse cardiovascular effects and is expected to provide 58-67 minutes of clinical relaxation; neuromuscular blockade sufficient for intubation is achieved in <2 minutes with maximum blockade in <3 minutes

Maintenance: 0.1, 0.15, and 0.2 mg/kg administered at 25% recovery of control $T_1$ (defined as 3 twitches of train-of-four) provides a median of 12, 17, and 24 minutes of clinical duration under anesthesia

Rapid sequence intubation: 0.6-1.2 mg/kg in appropriately premedicated and anesthetized patients with excellent or good intubating conditions within 2 minutes

Continuous infusion: Initial: 0.01-0.012 mg/kg/minute only after early evidence of spontaneous recovery of neuromuscular function is evident; infusion rates have ranged from 4-16 mcg/kg/minute

ICU: 10 mcg/kg/minute; adjust dose to maintain appropriate degree of neuromuscular blockade (eg, 1 or 2 twitches on train-of-four)

**Dosage Forms** Injection, solution, as bromide: 10 mg/mL (5 mL, 10 mL)

**rocuronium bromide** *see* rocuronium *on previous page*

**Rofact™ [Can]** *see* rifampin *on page 722*

## rofecoxib (roe fe COX ib)

**Sound-Alike/Look-Alike Issues**
Vioxx® may be confused with Zyvox™

**Therapeutic Category** Nonsteroidal Antiinflammatory Drug (NSAID), COX-2 Selective

**Use** Relief of the signs and symptoms of osteoarthritis, rheumatoid arthritis, and juvenile rheumatoid arthritis (JRA); management of acute pain; treatment of primary dysmenorrhea; treatment of migraine attacks

**Usual Dosage** Oral:
Children 2-17 years and ≥10 kg: JRA: 0.6 mg/kg/day (maximum: 25 mg/day)
Adults:
Osteoarthritis: 12.5 mg once daily; may be increased to a maximum of 25 mg once daily
Acute pain and management of dysmenorrhea: 50 mg once daily as needed (use for longer than 5 days has not been studied)
Migraine attack: 25 mg once daily, as needed; may be increased to a maximum of 50 mg once daily
Rheumatoid arthritis: 25 mg once daily

**Dosage Forms** [DSC] = Discontinued product
Suspension, oral [DSC]: 12.5 mg/5 mL (150 mL); 25 mg/5 mL (150 mL) [strawberry flavor]
Tablet [DSC]: 12.5 mg, 25 mg, 50 mg

**Roferon-A® [US/Can]** *see* interferon alfa-2a *on page 440*

**Rogaine® [Can]** *see* minoxidil *on page 543*

**Rogaine® Extra Strength for Men [US-OTC]** *see* minoxidil *on page 543*

**Rogaine® for Men [US-OTC]** *see* minoxidil *on page 543*

**Rogaine® for Women [US-OTC]** *see* minoxidil *on page 543*

**Rogitine® [Can]** *see* phentolamine *on page 639*

**Rolaids® [US-OTC]** *see* calcium carbonate and magnesium hydroxide *on page 132*

**Rolaids® Extra Strength [US-OTC]** *see* calcium carbonate and magnesium hydroxide *on page 132*

**Rolatuss® Plain Liquid (Discontinued)** *see* chlorpheniramine and phenylephrine *on page 171*

**Romazicon® [US/Can]** *see* flumazenil *on page 343*

**Romilar® AC [US]** *see* guaifenesin and codeine *on page 384*

**Romycin® [US]** *see* erythromycin *on page 295*

**Rondec®-DM Drops [US]** *see* carbinoxamine, pseudoephedrine, and dextromethorphan *on page 145*

**Rondec®-DM Syrup [US]** *see* brompheniramine, pseudoephedrine, and dextromethorphan *on page 116*

**Rondec® Drops [US]** *see* carbinoxamine and pseudoephedrine *on page 144*

**Rondec® Syrup [US]** *see* brompheniramine and pseudoephedrine *on page 115*

**Rondec® Tablets [US]** *see* carbinoxamine and pseudoephedrine *on page 144*

**Rondec-TR® [US]** *see* carbinoxamine and pseudoephedrine *on page 144*

**Rondomycin® Capsule** *(Discontinued)*

## ropinirole (roe PIN i role)

**Sound-Alike/Look-Alike Issues**
ropinirole may be confused with ropivacaine

**Synonyms** ropinirole hydrochloride

**U.S./Canadian Brand Names** Requip® [US/Can]

**Therapeutic Category** Anti-Parkinson Agent

**Use** Treatment of idiopathic Parkinson disease; in patients with early Parkinson disease who were not receiving concomitant levodopa therapy as well as in patients with advanced disease on concomitant levodopa; treatment of moderate-to-severe primary Restless Legs Syndrome (RLS)

**Usual Dosage** Oral: Adults:

**Parkinson's disease:** The dosage should be increased to achieve a maximum therapeutic effect, balanced against the principal side effects of nausea, dizziness, somnolence and dyskinesia. Recommended starting dose is 0.25 mg 3 times/day; based on individual patient response, the dosage should be titrated with weekly increments as described below:

- Week 1: 0.25 mg 3 times/day; total daily dose: 0.75 mg
- Week 2: 0.5 mg 3 times/day; total daily dose: 1.5 mg
- Week 3: 0.75 mg 3 times/day; total daily dose: 2.25 mg
- Week 4: 1 mg 3 times/day; total daily dose: 3 mg

**Note:** After week 4, if necessary, daily dosage may be increased by 1.5 mg per day on a weekly basis up to a dose of 9 mg/day, and then by up to 3 mg/day weekly to a total of 24 mg/day

*Parkinson's disease discontinuation taper:* Ropinirole should be gradually tapered over 7 days as follows: reduce frequency of administration from 3 times daily to twice daily for 4 days, then reduce to once daily for remaining 3 days.

**Restless Legs Syndrome:** Initial: 0.25 mg once daily 1-3 hours before bedtime. Dose may be increased after 2 days to 0.5 mg daily, and after 7 days to 1 mg daily. Dose may be further titrated upward in 0.5 mg increments every week until reaching a daily dose of 3 mg during week 6. If symptoms persist or reappear, the daily dose may be increased to a maximum of 4 mg beginning week 7.

**Note:** Doses up to 4 mg per day may be discontinued without tapering.

**Dosage Forms** Tablet: 0.25 mg, 0.5 mg, 1 mg, 2 mg, 3 mg, 4 mg, 5 mg

**ropinirole hydrochloride** *see* ropinirole *on this page*

## ropivacaine (roe PIV a kane)

**Sound-Alike/Look-Alike Issues**
ropivacaine may be confused with bupivacaine, ropinirole

**Synonyms** ropivacaine hydrochloride

**U.S./Canadian Brand Names** Naropin® [US/Can]

**Therapeutic Category** Local Anesthetic

**Use** Local anesthetic for use in surgery, postoperative pain management, and obstetrical procedures when local or regional anesthesia is needed

**Usual Dosage** Dose varies with procedure, onset and depth of anesthesia desired, vascularity of tissues, duration of anesthesia, and condition of patient: Adults:

Surgical anesthesia:
Lumbar epidural: 15-30 mL of 0.5% to 1% solution
Lumbar epidural block for cesarean section:
20-30 mL dose of 0.5% solution
15-20 mL dose of 0.75% solution
Thoracic epidural block: 5-15 mL dose of 0.5% to 0.75% solution
Major nerve block:
35-50 mL dose of 0.5% solution (175-250 mg)
10-40 mL dose of 0.75% solution (75-300 mg)
Field block: 1-40 mL dose of 0.5% solution (5-200 mg)
Labor pain management: Lumbar epidural: Initial: 10-20 mL 0.2% solution; continuous infusion dose: 6-14 mL/hour of 0.2% solution with incremental injections of 10-15 mL/hour of 0.2% solution

Postoperative pain management:
Lumbar or thoracic epidural: Continuous infusion dose: 6-14 mL/hour of 0.2% solution
Infiltration/minor nerve block:
1-100 mL dose of 0.2% solution
1-40 mL dose of 0.5% solution
**Dosage Forms**
Infusion, as hydrochloride: 2 mg/mL (100 mL, 200 mL)
Injection, solution, as hydrochloride [preservative free]: 2 mg/mL (10 mL, 20 mL); 5 mg/mL (20 mL, 30 mL); 7.5 mg/mL (20 mL); 10 mg/mL (10 mL, 20 mL)

**ropivacaine hydrochloride** *see* ropivacaine *on previous page*

**Rosanil® [US]** *see* sulfur and sulfacetamide *on page 776*

# rosiglitazone (roh si GLI ta zone)
**Sound-Alike/Look-Alike Issues**
Avandia® may be confused with Avalide®, Coumadin®, Prandin®
**U.S./Canadian Brand Names** Avandia® [US/Can]
**Therapeutic Category** Hypoglycemic Agent, Oral; Thiazolidinedione Derivative
**Use** Type 2 diabetes mellitus (noninsulin-dependent, NIDDM):
Monotherapy: Improve glycemic control as an adjunct to diet and exercise
Combination therapy: In combination with a sulfonylurea, metformin, or insulin, or sulfonylurea plus metformin when diet, exercise, and a single agent do not result in adequate glycemic control
**Usual Dosage** Oral: Adults:
Monotherapy: Initial: 4 mg daily as a single daily dose or in divided doses twice daily. If response is inadequate after 8-12 weeks of treatment, the dosage may be increased to 8 mg daily as a single daily dose or in divided doses twice daily. In clinical trials, the 4 mg twice-daily regimen resulted in the greatest reduction in fasting plasma glucose and Hb $A_{1c}$.
Combination therapy: When adding rosiglitazone to existing therapy, continue current dose(s) of previous agents:
With sulfonylureas or metformin (or sulfonylurea plus metformin): Initial: 4 mg daily as a single daily dose or in divided doses twice daily. If response is inadequate after 8-12 weeks of treatment, the dosage may be increased to 8 mg daily as a single daily dose or in divided doses twice daily. Reduce dose of sulfonylurea if hypoglycemia occurs. It is unlikely that the dose of metformin will need to be reduced to hypoglycemia.
With insulin: Initial: 4 mg daily as a single daily dose or in divided doses twice daily. Dose of insulin should be reduced by 10% to 25% if the patient reports hypoglycemia or if the plasma glucose falls to <100 mg/dL. Doses of rosiglitazone >4 mg/day are not indicated in combination with insulin.
**Dosage Forms** Tablet: 2 mg, 4 mg, 8 mg

# rosiglitazone and metformin (roh si GLI ta zone & met FOR min)
**Synonyms** metformin and rosiglitazone; metformin hydrochloride and rosiglitazone maleate; rosiglitazone maleate and metformin hydrochloride
**U.S./Canadian Brand Names** Avandamet™ [US/Can]
**Therapeutic Category** Antidiabetic Agent (Biguanide); Antidiabetic Agent (Thiazolidinedione)
**Use** Management of type 2 diabetes mellitus (noninsulin-dependent, NIDDM) in patients who are already treated with the combination of rosiglitazone and metformin, or who are not adequately controlled on metformin alone. Used as an adjunct to diet and exercise to lower the blood glucose when hyperglycemia cannot be controlled satisfactorily by diet and exercise alone
**Usual Dosage** Oral: Adults: Type 2 diabetes mellitus: Initial dose should be based on current dose of rosiglitazone and/or metformin; daily dose should be divided and given with meals
Patients inadequately controlled on **metformin alone**: Initial dose: Rosiglitazone 4 mg/day plus current dose of metformin
Patients inadequately controlled on **rosiglitazone alone**: Initial dose: Metformin 1000 mg/day plus current dose of rosiglitazone
**Note:** When switching from combination rosiglitazone and metformin as separate tablets: Use current dose
Dose adjustment: Doses may be increased as increments of rosiglitazone 4 mg and/or metformin 500 mg, up to the maximum dose; doses should be titrated gradually.
After a change in the metformin dosage, titration can be done after 1-2 weeks
After a change in the rosiglitazone dosage, titration can be done after 8-12 weeks
Maximum dose: Rosiglitazone 8 mg/metformin 2000 mg daily
(Continued)

## rosiglitazone and metformin *(Continued)*

Dosage Forms Tablet [film coated]:
1/500: Rosiglitazone 1 mg and metformin hydrochloride 500 mg
2/500: Rosiglitazone 2 mg and metformin hydrochloride 500 mg
4/500: Rosiglitazone 4 mg and metformin hydrochloride 500 mg
2/1000: Rosiglitazone 2 mg and metformin hydrochloride 1000 mg
4/1000: Rosiglitazone 4 mg and metformin hydrochloride 1000 mg

**rosiglitazone maleate and metformin hydrochloride** *see* rosiglitazone and metformin *on previous page*

**Rosula**® **[US]** *see* sulfur and sulfacetamide *on page 776*

## rosuvastatin (roe SOO va sta tin)

Synonyms rosuvastatin calcium
U.S./Canadian Brand Names Crestor® [US/Can]
Therapeutic Category Antilipemic Agent, HMG-CoA Reductase Inhibitor
Use Used with dietary therapy for hyperlipidemias to reduce elevations in total cholesterol (TC), LDL-C, apolipoprotein B, and triglycerides (TG) in patients with primary hypercholesterolemia (elevations of 1 or more components are present in Fredrickson type IIa, IIb, and IV hyperlipidemias); treatment of homozygous familial hypercholesterolemia (FH)
Usual Dosage Adults: Oral:
Heterozygous familial and nonfamilial hypercholesterolemia; mixed dyslipidemia:
Initial dose:
General dosing: 10 mg once daily (20 mg in patients with severe hypercholesterolemia)
Conservative dosing: Patients requiring less aggressive treatment or predisposed to myopathy (including patients of Asian descent): 5 mg once daily
Titration: After 2 weeks, may be increased by 5-10 mg once daily; dosing range: 5-40 mg/day (maximum dose: 40 mg once daily)
**Note:** The 40 mg dose should be reserved for patients who have not achieved goal cholesterol levels on a dose of 20 mg/day, including patients switched from another HMG-CoA reductase inhibitor.
Homozygous FH: Initial: 20 mg once daily (maximum dose: 40 mg/day)
**Dosage adjustment with concomitant medications:**
Cyclosporine: Rosuvastatin dose should not exceed 5 mg/day
Gemfibrozil: Rosuvastatin dose should not exceed 10 mg/day
**Dosage adjustment for persistent, unexplained proteinuria while on 40 mg/day:** Reduce dose and evaluate causes
Dosage Forms Tablet, as calcium: 5 mg, 10 mg, 20 mg, 40 mg

**rosuvastatin calcium** *see* rosuvastatin *on this page*

**RotaShield**® *(Discontinued)*

**Rovamycine**® **[Can]** *see* spiramycin *(Canada only) on page 764*

**Rowasa**® **[US/Can]** *see* mesalamine *on page 516*

**Roxanol**™ **[US]** *see* morphine sulfate *on page 549*

**Roxanol 100**™ **[US]** *see* morphine sulfate *on page 549*

**Roxanol SR**™ **Oral** *(Discontinued) see* morphine sulfate *on page 549*

**Roxanol**™**-T [US]** *see* morphine sulfate *on page 549*

**Roxicet**™ **[US]** *see* oxycodone and acetaminophen *on page 609*

**Roxicet**™ **5/500 [US]** *see* oxycodone and acetaminophen *on page 609*

**Roxicodone**™ **[US]** *see* oxycodone *on page 608*

**Roxicodone**™ **Intensol**™ **[US]** *see* oxycodone *on page 608*

**Roxiprin**® *(Discontinued) see* oxycodone and aspirin *on page 610*

**Roychlor**® **[Can]** *see* potassium chloride *on page 663*

**RP-54274** *see* riluzole *on page 723*

**RP-59500** *see* quinupristin and dalfopristin *on page 706*

**RP-6976** *see* docetaxel *on page 263*

**r-PA** *see* reteplase *on page 717*

**rPDGF-BB** *see* becaplermin *on page 91*

**RS-25259** *see* palonosetron *on page 614*

**RS-25259-197** *see* palonosetron *on page 614*

**RTCA** *see* ribavirin *on page 720*

**RU-486** *see* mifepristone *on page 540*

**RU-23908** *see* nilutamide *on page 576*

**RU-38486** *see* mifepristone *on page 540*

**rubella, measles and mumps vaccines, combined** *see* measles, mumps, and rubella vaccines, combined *on page 504*

## rubella virus vaccine (live) (rue BEL a VYE rus vak SEEN, live)

**Sound-Alike/Look-Alike Issues**
Meruvax® II may be confused with Attenuvax®
**Synonyms** German measles vaccine
**U.S./Canadian Brand Names** Meruvax® II [US]
**Therapeutic Category** Vaccine, Live Virus
**Use** Selective active immunization against rubella; vaccination is routinely recommended for persons from 12 months of age to puberty. All adults, both male and female, lacking documentation of live vaccine on or after first birthday, or laboratory evidence of immunity (particularly women of childbearing age and young adults who work in or congregate in hospitals, colleges, and on military bases) should be vaccinated. Susceptible travelers should be vaccinated.
**Note:** Trivalent measles - mumps - rubella (MMR) vaccine is the preferred immunizing agent for most children and many adults.
**Usual Dosage** Children ≥12 months and Adults: SubQ: 0.5 mL in outer aspect of upper arm; children vaccinated before 12 months of age should be revaccinated. Recommended age for primary immunization is 12-15 months; revaccination with MMR-II is recommended prior to elementary school.
**Dosage Forms** Injection, powder for reconstitution [single dose]: 1000 $TCID_{50}$ (Wistar RA 27/3 Strain) [contains gelatin, human albumin, and neomycin]

**rubeola vaccine** *see* measles virus vaccine (live) *on page 504*

**Rubex® [US]** *see* doxorubicin *on page 270*

**rubidomycin hydrochloride** *see* daunorubicin hydrochloride *on page 225*

**Rubramin-PC® (Discontinued)** *see* cyanocobalamin *on page 212*

**Rulox [US]** *see* aluminum hydroxide and magnesium hydroxide *on page 35*

**Rulox No. 1 [US]** *see* aluminum hydroxide and magnesium hydroxide *on page 35*

**Rum-K® [US]** *see* potassium chloride *on page 663*

**Ru-Tuss® Liquid (Discontinued)** *see* chlorpheniramine and phenylephrine *on page 171*

**Ru-Vert-M® (Discontinued)** *see* meclizine *on page 506*

**Rymed® (Discontinued)** *see* guaifenesin and pseudoephedrine *on page 388*

**Rymed-TR® (Discontinued)**

**Ryna-12™ [US]** *see* phenylephrine and pyrilamine *on page 641*

**Ryna-12 S™ [US]** *see* phenylephrine and pyrilamine *on page 641*

**Ryna-C® (Discontinued)** *see* chlorpheniramine, pseudoephedrine, and codeine *on page 176*

**Ryna® (Discontinued)** *see* chlorpheniramine, pseudoephedrine, and codeine *on page 176*

**Rynatan® [US]** *see* chlorpheniramine and phenylephrine *on page 171*

**Rynatan® Pediatric Suspension [US]** *see* chlorpheniramine and phenylephrine *on page 171*

**Rynatuss® [US]** *see* chlorpheniramine, ephedrine, phenylephrine, and carbetapentane *on page 173*

**Rynatuss® Pediatric [US]** *see* chlorpheniramine, ephedrine, phenylephrine, and carbetapentane *on page 173*

**Ry-T 12 [US]** *see* phenylephrine and pyrilamine *on page 641*

**Rythmodan® [Can]** *see* disopyramide *on page 261*

**Rythmodan®-LA [Can]** *see* disopyramide *on page 261*

**Rythmol**® **[US]** *see* propafenone *on page 685*

**Rythmol**® **Gen-Propafenone [Can]** *see* propafenone *on page 685*

**Rythmol**® **SR [US]** *see* propafenone *on page 685*

**Rēv-Eyes**™ **[US]** *see* dapiprazole *on page 223*

**SAB-Gentamicin [Can]** *see* gentamicin *on page 372*

**Sabril**® **[Can]** *see* vigabatrin *(Canada only) on page 846*

**SAB-Trifluridine [Can]** *see* trifluridine *on page 823*

**sacrosidase** (sak ROE si dase)
    U.S./Canadian Brand Names Sucraid® [US/Can]
    Therapeutic Category Enzyme
    Use Orphan drug: Oral replacement therapy in sucrase deficiency, as seen in congenital sucrase-isomaltase deficiency (CSID)
    Usual Dosage Oral:
        Infants ≥5 months and Children <15 kg: 8500 int. units (1 mL) per meal or snack
        Children >15 kg and Adults: 17,000 int. units (2 mL) per meal or snack
        Doses should be diluted with 2-4 oz of water, milk, or formula with each meal or snack. Approximately one-half of the dose may be taken before, and the remainder of a dose taken at the completion of each meal or snack.
    Dosage Forms Solution, oral: 8500 int. units per mL (118 mL)

**Safe Tussin**® **30 [US-OTC]** *see* guaifenesin and dextromethorphan *on page 385*

**Saizen**® **[US/Can]** *see* somatropin *on page 760*

**SalAc**® **[US-OTC]** *see* salicylic acid *on this page*

**Sal-Acid**® **[US-OTC]** *see* salicylic acid *on this page*

**Salacid**® **Ointment** *(Discontinued)* *see* salicylic acid *on this page*

**Salactic**® **[US-OTC]** *see* salicylic acid *on this page*

**Salagen**® **[US/Can]** *see* pilocarpine *on page 647*

**Salazopyrin**® **[Can]** *see* sulfasalazine *on page 774*

**Salazopyrin En-Tabs**® **[Can]** *see* sulfasalazine *on page 774*

**Salbu-2 [Can]** *see* albuterol *on page 22*

**Salbu-4 [Can]** *see* albuterol *on page 22*

**salbutamol** *see* albuterol *on page 22*

**Saleto-200**® *(Discontinued)* *see* ibuprofen *on page 427*

**Saleto-400**® *(Discontinued)* *see* ibuprofen *on page 427*

**Salflex**® **[Can]** *see* salsalate *on page 738*

**Salgesic**® *(Discontinued)* *see* salsalate *on page 738*

**salicylazosulfapyridine** *see* sulfasalazine *on page 774*

**salicylic acid** (sal i SIL ik AS id)
    U.S./Canadian Brand Names Compound W® One Step Wart Remover [US-OTC]; Compound W® [US-OTC]; DHS™ Sal [US-OTC]; Dr. Scholl's® Callus Remover [US-OTC]; Dr. Scholl's® Clear Away [US-OTC]; DuoFilm® [US-OTC/Can]; Duoforte® 27 [Can]; Freezone® [US-OTC]; Fung-O® [US-OTC]; Gordofilm® [US-OTC]; Hydrisalic™ [US-OTC]; Ionil® Plus [US-OTC]; Ionil® [US-OTC]; Keralyt® [US-OTC]; LupiCare™ Dandruff [US-OTC]; LupiCare™ II Psoriasis [US-OTC]; LupiCare™ Psoriasis [US-OTC]; Mediplast® [US-OTC]; MG217 Sal-Acid® [US-OTC]; Mosco® Corn and Callus Remover [US-OTC]; NeoCeuticals™ Acne Spot Treatment [US-OTC]; Neutrogena® Acne Wash [US-OTC]; Neutrogena® Body Clear™ [US-OTC]; Neutrogena® Clear Pore Shine Control [US-OTC]; Neutrogena® Clear Pore [US-OTC]; Neutrogena® Healthy Scalp [US-OTC]; Neutrogena® Maximum Strength T/Sal® [US-OTC]; Neutrogena® On The Spot® Acne Patch [US-OTC]; Occlusal®-HP [US-OTC/Can]; Oxy Balance® Deep Pore [US-OTC]; Oxy Balance® [US-OTC]; Palmer's® Skin Success Acne Cleanser [US-OTC]; Pedisilk® [US-OTC]; Propa pH [US-OTC]; Sal-Acid® [US-OTC]; Sal-Plant® [US-OTC]; Salactic® [US-OTC]; SalAc® [US-OTC]; Sebcur® [Can]; Soluver® Plus [Can]; Soluver® [Can]; Stri-dex® Body Focus [US-OTC]; Stri-dex® Facewipes To Go™ [US-OTC]; Stri-dex® Maximum Strength [US-OTC]; Stri-

dex® [US-OTC]; Tinamed® [US-OTC]; Tiseb® [US-OTC]; Trans-Plantar® [Can]; Trans-Ver-Sal® [US-OTC/Can]; Wart-Off® Maximum Strength [US-OTC]; Zapzyt® Acne Wash [US-OTC]; Zapzyt® Pore Treatment [US-OTC]

**Therapeutic Category** Keratolytic Agent

**Use** Topically for its keratolytic effect in controlling seborrheic dermatitis or psoriasis of body and scalp, dandruff, and other scaling dermatoses; also used to remove warts, corns, and calluses; acne

**Usual Dosage** Children and Adults (consult specific product labeling for use in children <12 years):

**Acne:**
Cream, cloth, foam, or liquid cleansers (2%): Use to cleanse skin once or twice daily. Massage gently into skin, work into lather and rinse thoroughly. Cloths should be wet with water prior to using and disposed of (not flushed) after use.

Gel (0.5% or 2%): Apply small amount to face in the morning or evening; if peeling occurs, may be used every other day. Some products may be labeled for OTC use up to 3 or 4 times per day. Apply to clean, dry skin

Pads (0.5% or 2%): Use pad to cover affected area with thin layer of salicylic acid one to three times a day. Apply to clean, dry skin. Do not leave pad on skin.

Patch (2%): At bedtime, after washing face, allow skin to dry at least 5 minutes. Apply patch directly over pimple being treated. Remove in the morning.

Shower/bath gels or soap (2%): Use once daily in shower or bath to massage over skin prone to acne. Rinse well.

**Callus, corns, or warts:**
Gel or liquid (17%): Apply to each wart and allow to dry. May repeat once or twice daily, up to 12 weeks. Apply to clean dry area.

Gel (6%): Apply to affected area once daily, generally used at night and rinsed off in the morning.

Plaster or transdermal patch (40%): Apply directly over affected area, leave in place for 48 hours. Some products may be cut to fit area or secured with adhesive strips. May repeat procedure for up to 12 weeks. Apply to clean, dry skin

Transdermal patch (15%): Apply directly over affected area at bedtime, leave in place overnight and remove in the morning. Patch should be trimmed to cover affected area. May repeat daily for up to 12 weeks.

**Dandruff, psoriasis, or seborrheic dermatitis:**
Cream (2.5%): Apply to affected area 3-4 times daily. Apply to clean, dry skin. Some products may be left in place overnight.

Ointment (3%): Apply to scales or plaques on skin up to 4 times per day (not for scalp or face)

Shampoo (1.8% to 3%): Massage into wet hair or affected area; leave in place for several minutes; rinse thoroughly. Labeled for OTC use 2-3 times a week, or as directed by healthcare provider. Some products may be left in place overnight.

**Dosage Forms** [DSC] = Discontinued product
Cream:
LupiCare™ Dandruff, LupiCare™ Psoriasis: 2.5% (120 g, 240 g) [contains alcohol]
LupiCare™ II Psoriasis: 2.5% (60 g, 240 g) [contains alcohol]
Neutrogena® Acne Wash: 2% (200 mL) [contains alcohol]
Cloths: Neutrogena® Acne Wash: 2% (30s) [disposable cloths]
Foam:
Neutrogena® Acne Wash: 2% (150 mL) [foaming cleanser]
SalAc®: 2% (100 g)
Gel: 17% (15 g)
Compound W®: 17% (7 g) [contains alcohol]
DuoPlant® [DSC]: 17% (15 g)
Hydrisalic™: 6% (28 g) [contains alcohol and propylene glycol]
Keralyt®: 6% (30 g) [contains alcohol and propylene glycol]
NeoCeuticals™ Acne Spot Treatment: 2% (15 g) [contains alcohol]
Neutrogena® Clear Pore: 2% (60 g) [contains alcohol]
Neutrogena® Clear Pore Shine Control: 0.5% (10 g)
Oxy Balance®: 2% (240 mL) [shower gel]
Sal-Plant®: 17% (14 g) [contains alcohol]
Stri-dex® Body Focus™: 2% (300 mL)
Zapzyt® Acne Wash: 2% (190 g) [alcohol free]
Zapzyt® Pore Treatment: 2% (23 g) [alcohol free]
Liquid, topical:
Compound W®: 17% (9 mL) [contains alcohol]
DuoFilm®: 17% (15 mL) [contains alcohol]
(Continued)

# salicylic acid (Continued)

Freezone®: 17.6% (9.3 mL) [contains alcohol]
Fung-O®: 17% (15 mL)
Gordofilm®: 16.7% (15 mL)
Mosco® Corn and Callus Remover: 17.6% (10 mL)
NeoCeuticals™ Acne Spot Treatment: 2% (60 mL) [contains alcohol]
Neutrogena® Acne Wash: 2% (180 mL) [contains tartrazine]
Neutrogena® Body Clear™ [body scrub with microbeads]: 2% (250 mL) [contains tartrazine]
Neutrogena® Body Clear™ [body wash]: 2% (250 mL) [contains tartrazine]
Occlusal®-HP: 17% (10 mL)
Palmer's® Skin Success Acne Cleanser: 0.5% (240 mL)
Pedisilk®: 17% (15 mL)
Propa pH: 2% (80 mL) [alcohol free; contains aloe vera]
SalAc®: 2% (180 mL)
Salactic®: 17% (15 mL) [contains alcohol]
Tinamed®: 17% (15 mL)
Wart-Off®: 17% (13 mL) [contains alcohol]
Ointment (MG217 Sal-Acid®): 3% (56 g) [contains vitamin E]
Pads:
Oxy Balance®, Oxy Balance® Deep Pore: 0.5% (55s, 90s) [contains alcohol]
Stri-dex®: 0.5% (55s)
Stri-dex® Facewipes To Go™ : 0.5% (32s) [contains alcohol]
Stri-dex® Maximum Strength: 2% (32s, 55s, 90s)
Patch, transdermal:
Compound W® One Step Wart Remover: 40% (12s, 14s)
Dr. Scholl's® Callus Remover: 40% (4s)
Dr. Scholl's® Clear Away: 40% (14s, 16s, 18s, 24s)
DuoFilm®: 40% (18s)
Neutrogena® On The Spot® Acne Patch: 2% (27s)
Trans-Ver-Sal®: 15% [6 mm PediaPatch, 12 mm AdultPatch, 20 mm PlantarPatch] (10s, 12s, 15s, 25s, 40s)
Plaster:
Mediplast®: 40% (25s)
Sal-Acid®: 40% (14s)
Tinamed®: 40% (24s)
Shampoo:
DHS™ Sal: 3% (120 mL)
Ionil®: 2% (240 mL, 480 mL, 960 mL)
Ionil® Plus: 2% (240 mL) [conditioning shampoo]
LupiCare™ Dandruff, LupiCare™ Psoriasis: 2% (120 mL, 240 mL)
Neutrogena® Healthy Scalp: 1.8% (90 mL, 180 mL)
Neutrogena® Maximum Strength T/Sal®: 3% (135 mL)
Tiseb®: 2% (240 mL)
Soap: 2% (114 g)

**salicylic acid and coal tar** *see* coal tar and salicylic acid *on page 202*

# salicylic acid and propylene glycol (sal i SIL ik AS id & PROE pi leen GLYE cole)

**Synonyms** propylene glycol and salicylic acid
**U.S./Canadian Brand Names** Keralyt® [Can]
**Therapeutic Category** Keratolytic Agent
**Use** Removal of excessive keratin in hyperkeratotic skin disorders, including various ichthyosis, keratosis palmaris and plantaris and psoriasis; may be used to remove excessive keratin in dorsal and plantar hyperkeratotic lesions
**Usual Dosage** Topical: Apply to area at night after soaking region for at least 5 minutes to hydrate area, and place under occlusion; medication is washed off in morning
**Dosage Forms** Gel, topical: Salicylic acid 6% and propylene glycol 60% in ethyl alcohol 19.4% with hydroxypropyl methylcellulose and water (30 g)

**salicylic acid and sulfur** *see* sulfur and salicylic acid *on page 775*

**salicylsalicylic acid** *see* salsalate *on page 738*

**SalineX**® **[US-OTC]** *see* sodium chloride *on page 752*

**Salivart**® **[US-OTC]** *see* saliva substitute *on this page*

## saliva substitute (sa LYE va SUB stee tute)

**U.S./Canadian Brand Names** Entertainer's Secret® [US-OTC]; Moi-Stir® [US-OTC]; Mouthkote® [US-OTC]; Saliva Substitute™ [US-OTC]; Salivart® [US-OTC]; Salix® [US-OTC]

**Therapeutic Category** Gastrointestinal Agent, Miscellaneous

**Use** Relief of dry mouth and throat in xerostomia

**Usual Dosage** Use as needed

**Dosage Forms**

Lozenge (Salix®): Sorbitol, malic acid, sodium citrate, citric acid, dibasic calcium phosphate, sodium carboxymethylcellulose, propylene glycol, hydrogenated cottonseed oil, silicon dioxide, magnesium stearate [fruit flavor]

Solution, oral:

Entertainer's Secret®: Sodium carboxymethylcellulose, aloe vera gel, glycerin (60 mL) [honey-apple flavor]

Saliva Substitute®: Sorbitol, sodium carboxymethylcellulose, methylparaben (5 mL, 120 mL)

Spray, oral:

Moi-Stir®: Water, sorbitol, sodium carboxymethylcellulose, methylparaben, propylparaben, potassium chloride, dibasic sodium phosphate, calcium chloride, magnesium chloride, sodium chloride (120 mL)

Mouthkote®: Water, xylitol, sorbitol, yerba santa, citric acid, ascorbic acid, sodium saccharin, sodium benzoate (60 mL, 240 mL) [lemon-lime flavor]

Salivart®: Water, sodium carboxymethylcellulose, sorbitol, sodium chloride, potassium chloride, calcium chloride, magnesium chloride, potassium phosphate (70 mL)

Swabsticks, oral (Moi-Stir®): Water, sorbitol, sodium carboxymethylcellulose, methylparaben, propylparaben, potassium chloride, dibasic sodium phosphate, calcium chloride, magnesium chloride, sodium chloride (300s)

**Salix**® **[US-OTC]** *see* saliva substitute *on this page*

**salk vaccine** *see* poliovirus vaccine (inactivated) *on page 657*

## salmeterol (sal ME te role)

**Sound-Alike/Look-Alike Issues**

salmeterol may be confused with Salbutamol

Serevent® may be confused with Serentil®

**Synonyms** salmeterol xinafoate

**U.S./Canadian Brand Names** Serevent® Diskus® [US]; Serevent® [Can]

**Therapeutic Category** Adrenergic Agonist Agent

**Use** Maintenance treatment of asthma and in prevention of bronchospasm with reversible obstructive airway disease, including patients with symptoms of nocturnal asthma, who require regular treatment with inhaled, short-acting beta$_2$ agonists; prevention of exercise-induced bronchospasm; maintenance treatment of bronchospasm associated with COPD

**Usual Dosage** Inhalation, powder (Serevent® Diskus®):

Asthma, maintenance and prevention: Children ≥4 years and Adults: One inhalation (50 mcg) twice daily (~12 hours apart)

Exercise-induced asthma, prevention: Children ≥4 years and Adults: One inhalation (50 mcg) at least 30 minutes prior to exercise; additional doses should not be used for 12 hours; should not be used in individuals already receiving salmeterol twice daily

COPD (maintenance treatment of associated bronchospasm): Adults: One inhalation (50 mcg) twice daily (~12 hours apart)

**Dosage Forms** Powder for oral inhalation: 50 mcg (28s, 60s) [delivers 47 mcg/inhalation; contains lactose]

**salmeterol and fluticasone** *see* fluticasone and salmeterol *on page 353*

**salmeterol xinafoate** *see* salmeterol *on this page*

## *Salmonella typhi* Vi capsular polysaccharide vaccine *(Canada only)*
(sal mo NEL la TI fi vi CAP su lar po le SAK ar ide VAK seen)
**U.S./Canadian Brand Names** Typherix™ [Can]
**Therapeutic Category** Vaccine
**Use** For active immunization against typhoid fever in persons 2 years of age and older.
**Usual Dosage** One dose administered I.M. ensures protection for at least 3 years. The vaccine must be given at least 2 weeks prior to travel to endemic areas.
**Dosage Forms** Injection: Vi polysaccharide vaccine of *S. typhi* 25 mcg (0.5 mL)

**Salmonine®** *(Discontinued)* see calcitonin *on page 129*

**Salofalk®** [Can] *see* mesalamine *on page 516*

**Sal-Plant®** [US-OTC] *see* salicylic acid *on page 734*

## salsalate (SAL sa late)
**Sound-Alike/Look-Alike Issues**
salsalate may be confused with sucralfate, sulfasalazine
**Synonyms** disalicylic acid; salicylsalicylic acid
**U.S./Canadian Brand Names** Amigesic® [US/Can]; Salflex® [Can]
**Therapeutic Category** Analgesic, Nonnarcotic; Antipyretic; Nonsteroidal Antiinflammatory Drug (NSAID)
**Use** Treatment of minor pain or fever; arthritis
**Usual Dosage** Adults: Oral: 3 g/day in 2-3 divided doses
**Dosage Forms**
Tablet: 500 mg, 750 mg
Amigesic®: 500 mg, 750 mg

**Salsitab®** *(Discontinued)* see salsalate *on this page*

**salt** *see* sodium chloride *on page 752*

**salt poor albumin** *see* albumin *on page 22*

**Sal-Tropine™** [US] *see* atropine *on page 79*

**Sanctura™** [US] *see* trospium *on page 830*

**Sandimmune®** [US] *see* cyclosporine *on page 215*

**Sandimmune®** I.V. [Can] *see* cyclosporine *on page 215*

**Sandomigran®** [Can] *see* pizotifen *(Canada only) on page 651*

**Sandomigran DS®** [Can] *see* pizotifen *(Canada only) on page 651*

**Sandostatin®** [US/Can] *see* octreotide *on page 593*

**Sandostatin LAR®** [US/Can] *see* octreotide *on page 593*

**SangCya™** *(Discontinued)* see cyclosporine *on page 215*

**Sani-Supp®** [US-OTC] *see* glycerin *on page 379*

**Sans Acne®** [Can] *see* erythromycin *on page 295*

**Santyl®** [US] *see* collagenase *on page 206*

## saquinavir (sa KWIN a veer)
**Sound-Alike/Look-Alike Issues**
saquinavir may be confused with Sinequan®
Fortovase® may be confused with Invirase®
Invirase® may be confused with Fortovase®
**Synonyms** saquinavir mesylate
**U.S./Canadian Brand Names** Fortovase® [Can]; Invirase® [US/Can]
**Therapeutic Category** Antiviral Agent
**Use** Treatment of HIV infection; used in combination with at least two other antiretroviral agents
**Usual Dosage** Oral: Children ≥16 years and Adults: **Note:** Fortovase® and Invirase® are not bioequivalent and should not be used interchangeably; only Fortovase® should be used to initiate therapy:
Unboosted regimen: Fortovase®: 1200 mg (six 200 mg capsules) 3 times/day or 1600 mg twice daily within 2 hours after a meal in combination with a nucleoside analog
**Note:** Saquinavir hard-gel capsules (Invirase®) should not be used in "unboosted regimens."

Ritonavir-boosted regimens:

*Fortovase®:* 1000 mg (five 200 mg capsules) twice daily in combination with ritonavir 100 mg twice daily

*Invirase®:* 1000 mg (five 200 mg capsules or two 500 mg tablets) twice daily given in combination with ritonavir 100 mg twice daily. This combination should be given together and within 2 hours after a full meal in combination with a nucleoside analog.

**Dosage Forms Note:** Strength expressed as base; [DSC] = Discontinued product

Capsule, as mesylate (Invirase®): 200 mg [contains lactose 63.3 mg/capsule]

Capsule, soft gelatin, as base (Fortovase®): 200 mg [DSC]

Tablet, as base (Invirase®): 500 mg

## saquinavir mesylate *see* saquinavir *on previous page*

## Sarafem™ [US] *see* fluoxetine *on page 349*

# sargramostim (sar GRAM oh stim)

**Sound-Alike/Look-Alike Issues**

Leukine® may be confused with Leukeran®

**Synonyms** GM-CSF; granulocyte-macrophage colony stimulating factor; rGM-CSF

**U.S./Canadian Brand Names** Leukine® [US/Can]

**Therapeutic Category** Colony-Stimulating Factor

**Use**

**Myeloid reconstitution after autologous bone marrow transplantation:** Non-Hodgkin's lymphoma (NHL), acute lymphoblastic leukemia (ALL), Hodgkin's lymphoma, metastatic breast cancer

**Myeloid reconstitution after allogeneic bone marrow transplantation**

**Peripheral stem cell transplantation:** Metastatic breast cancer, non-Hodgkin's lymphoma, Hodgkin's lymphoma, multiple myeloma

**Orphan drug:**

**Acute myelogenous leukemia (AML)** following induction chemotherapy in older adults to shorten time to neutrophil recovery and to reduce the incidence of severe and life-threatening infections and infections resulting in death

**Bone marrow transplant (allogeneic or autologous) failure or engraftment delay**

Safety and efficacy of GM-CSF given simultaneously with cytotoxic chemotherapy have not been established. Concurrent treatment may increase myelosuppression.

**Usual Dosage**

Children and Adults: I.V. infusion over ≥2 hours or SubQ: **Rounding the dose to the nearest vial size enhances patient convenience and reduces costs without clinical detriment**

**Myeloid reconstitution after peripheral stem cell, allogeneic or autologous bone marrow transplant:** I.V.: 250 mcg/m$^2$/day for 21 days to begin 2-4 hours after the marrow infusion or ≥24 hours after chemotherapy or 12 hours after last dose of radiotherapy

If a severe adverse reaction occurs, reduce or temporarily discontinue the dose until the reaction abates

If blast cells appear or progression of the underlying disease occurs, disrupt treatment

Interrupt or reduce the dose by half if ANC is >20,000 cells/mm$^3$

Patients should not receive sargramostim until the postmarrow infusion ANC is <500 cells/mm$^3$

**Neutrophil recovery following chemotherapy in AML:** I.V.: 250 mcg/m$^2$/day over a 4-hour period starting approximately day 11 or 4 days following the completion of induction chemotherapy, if day 10 bone marrow is hypoblastic with <5% blasts

If a second cycle of chemotherapy is necessary, administer ~4 days after the completion of chemotherapy if the bone marrow is hypoblastic with <5% blasts

Continue sargramostim until ANC is >1500 cells/mm$^3$ for consecutive days or a maximum of 42 days

Discontinue sargramostim immediately if leukemic regrowth occurs

If a severe adverse reaction occurs, reduce the dose by 50% or temporarily discontinue the dose until the reaction abates

**Mobilization of peripheral blood progenitor cells:** I.V.: 250 mcg/m$^2$/day over 24 hours or SubQ once daily

Continue the same dose through the period of PBPC collection

The optimal schedule for PBPC collection has not been established (usually begun by day 5 and performed daily until protocol specified targets are achieved)

If WBC >50,000 cells/mm$^3$, reduce the dose by 50%

If adequate numbers of progenitor cells are not collected, consider other mobilization therapy

**Postperipheral blood progenitor cell transplantation:** I.V.: 250 mcg/m$^2$/day or SubQ once daily beginning immediately following infusion of progenitor cells and continuing until ANC is >1500 for 3 consecutive days is attained

(Continued)

## sargramostim *(Continued)*

**BMT failure or engraftment delay:** I.V.: 250 mcg/m$^2$/day for 14 days

The dose can be repeated after 7 days off therapy if engraftment has not occurred

If engraftment still has not occurred, a third course of 500 mcg/m$^2$/day for 14 days may be tried after another 7 days off therapy; if there is still no improvement, it is unlikely that further dose escalation will be beneficial

If a severe adverse reaction occurs, reduce or temporarily discontinue the dose until the reaction abates

If blast cells appear or disease progression occurs, discontinue treatment

**Dosage Forms**

Injection, powder for reconstitution: 250 mcg [contains sucrose 10 mg/mL]

Injection, solution: 500 mcg/mL (1 mL) [contains benzyl alcohol and sucrose 10 mg/mL]

**Sarna® HC [Can]** *see* hydrocortisone *(topical) on page 417*

**Sarna® Sensitive [US]** *see* pramoxine *on page 670*

**Sarnol®-HC [US-OTC]** *see* hydrocortisone *(topical) on page 417*

**SB-265805** *see* gemifloxacin *on page 370*

**SC 33428** *see* idarubicin *on page 429*

**SCH 13521** *see* flutamide *on page 353*

**S-citalopram** *see* escitalopram *on page 297*

**Scleromate® [US]** *see* morrhuate sodium *on page 551*

**Scopace™ [US]** *see* scopolamine derivatives *on this page*

**scopolamine and phenylephrine** *see* phenylephrine and scopolamine *on page 642*

**scopolamine butylbromide** *see* scopolamine derivatives *on this page*

## scopolamine derivatives *(skoe POL a meen dah RIV ah tives)*

**Synonyms** hyoscine butylbromide; hyoscine hydrobromide; scopolamine butylbromide; scopolamine hydrobromide

**U.S./Canadian Brand Names** Buscopan® [Can]; Isopto® Hyoscine [US]; Scopace™ [US]; Transderm Scōp® [US]; Transderm-V® [Can]

**Therapeutic Category** Anticholinergic Agent

**Use**

**Scopolamine hydrobromide:**

**Injection:** Preoperative medication to produce amnesia, sedation, and decrease salivary and respiratory secretions

**Ophthalmic:** Produce cycloplegia and mydriasis; treatment of iridocyclitis

**Oral:** Symptomatic treatment of postencephalitic parkinsonism and paralysis agitans; inhibits excessive motility and hypertonus of the genitourinary or gastrointestinal tract in such conditions as the irritable colon syndrome, mild dysentery, diverticulitis, pylorospasm, and cardiospasm

**Transdermal:** Prevention of nausea/vomiting associated with anesthesia or opiate analgesia; prevention of motion sickness

**Scopolamine butylbromide:**

**Oral/injection:** Treatment of smooth muscle spasm of the genitourinary or gastrointestinal tract; injection may also be used to prior to radiological/diagnostic procedures to prevent spasm

**Usual Dosage**

**Scopolamine hydrobromide:**

Preoperative:

Children: I.M., SubQ: 6 mcg/kg/dose (maximum: 0.3 mg/dose) every 6-8 hours

Adults:

I.M., I.V., SubQ: 0.3-0.65 mg; may be repeated every 4-6 hours

Transdermal patch: Apply 2.5 cm$^2$ patch to hairless area behind ear the night before surgery or 1 hour prior to cesarean section (the patch should be applied no sooner than 1 hour before surgery for best results and removed 24 hours after surgery)

Motion sickness: Transdermal: Adults: Apply 1 disc behind the ear at least 4 hours prior to exposure and every 3 days as needed; effective if applied as soon as 2-3 hours before anticipated need, best if 12 hours before

Refraction: Ophthalmic:

Children: Instill 1 drop of 0.25% to eye(s) twice daily for 2 days before procedure

Adults: Instill 1-2 drops of 0.25% to eye(s) 1 hour before procedure

Iridocyclitis: Ophthalmic:

Children: Instill 1 drop of 0.25% to eye(s) up to 3 times/day

Adults: Instill 1-2 drops of 0.25% to eye(s) up to 4 times/day

Parkinsonism, spasticity, motion sickness: Oral: 0.4-0.8 mg as a range; the dosage may be cautiously increased in parkinsonism and spastic states.

**Scopolamine butylbromide:**

Gastrointestinal/genitourinary spasm (Buscopan® [CAN]; not available in the U.S.): Adults:

Oral: 10-20 mg daily (1-2 tablets); maximum: 6 tablets/day

I.M., I.V., SubQ: 10-20 mg; maximum: 100 mg/day. Intramuscular injections should be administered 10-15 minutes prior to radiological/diagnostic procedures

**Dosage Forms** [CAN] = Canadian brand name

Injection, solution, as hydrobromide: 0.4 mg/mL (1 mL)

Injection, solution, as hyoscine-N-butylbromide (Buscopan® [CAN]): 20 mg/mL [not available in U.S.]

Solution, ophthalmic, as hydrobromide (Isopto® Hyoscine): 0.25% (5 mL, 15 mL) [contains benzalkonium chloride]

Tablet, as hyoscine-N-butylbromide (Buscopan® [CAN]): 10 mg [not available in U.S.]

Tablet, soluble, as hydrobromide (Scopace™): 0.4 mg

Transdermal system (Transderm Scōp®): 1.5 mg (4s, 10s, 24s) [releases ~1 mg over 72 hours]

**scopolamine hydrobromide** see scopolamine derivatives on previous page

**scopolamine, hyoscyamine, atropine, and phenobarbital** see hyoscyamine, atropine, scopolamine, and phenobarbital on page 425

**Scot-Tussin DM® Cough Chasers [US-OTC]** see dextromethorphan on page 238

**Scot-Tussin® Expectorant [US-OTC]** see guaifenesin on page 383

**Scot-Tussin® Senior [US-OTC]** see guaifenesin and dextromethorphan on page 385

**SDZ ENA 713** see rivastigmine on page 727

**SeaMist® [US-OTC]** see sodium chloride on page 752

**Seasonale® [US]** see ethinyl estradiol and levonorgestrel on page 312

**Seba-Gel™ [US]** see benzoyl peroxide on page 98

**Sebcur® [Can]** see salicylic acid on page 734

**Sebcur/T® [Can]** see coal tar and salicylic acid on page 202

**Sebizon® (Discontinued)** see sulfacetamide on page 771

# secobarbital (see koe BAR bi tal)

**Sound-Alike/Look-Alike Issues**

Seconal® may be confused with Sectral®

**Synonyms** quinalbarbitone sodium; secobarbital sodium

**U.S./Canadian Brand Names** Seconal® [US]

**Therapeutic Category** Barbiturate

**Controlled Substance** C-II

**Use** Preanesthetic agent; short-term treatment of insomnia

**Usual Dosage** Oral:

Children:

Preoperative sedation: 2-6 mg/kg (maximum dose: 100 mg/dose) 1-2 hours before procedure

Sedation: 6 mg/kg/day divided every 8 hours

Adults:

Hypnotic: Usual: 100 mg/dose at bedtime; range 100-200 mg/dose

Preoperative sedation: 100-300 mg 1-2 hours before procedure

**Dosage Forms** Capsule, as sodium: 100 mg

**secobarbital and amobarbital** see amobarbital and secobarbital on page 45

**secobarbital sodium** see secobarbital on this page

**Seconal® [US]** see secobarbital on this page

**Secran® (Discontinued)**

**SecreFlo™ [US]** see secretin on next page

# secretin (SEE kre tin)

**Synonyms** secretin, human; secretin, porcine

**U.S./Canadian Brand Names** SecreFlo™ [US]

**Therapeutic Category** Diagnostic Agent

**Use** Secretin-stimulation testing to aid in diagnosis of pancreatic exocrine dysfunction; diagnosis of gastrinoma (Zollinger-Ellison syndrome); facilitation of ERCP visualization

**Usual Dosage** I.V.: Adults: **Note:** A test dose of 0.2 mcg (0.1 mL) is injected to test for possible allergy. Dosing may be completed if no reaction occurs after 1 minute.

Diagnosis of pancreatic dysfunction, facilitation of ERCP: 0.2 mcg/kg over 1 minute

Diagnosis of gastrinoma: 0.4 mcg/kg over 1 minute

**Dosage Forms**

Injection, powder for reconstitution [human]: 16 mcg

Injection, powder for reconstitution [porcine] (SecreFlo™): 16 mcg

**secretin, human** *see* secretin *on this page*

**secretin, porcine** *see* secretin *on this page*

**Sectral® [US/Can]** *see* acebutolol *on page 4*

**Secura® Antifungal [US-OTC]** *see* miconazole *on page 537*

**Selax® [Can]** *see* docusate *on page 263*

**Select™ 1/35 [Can]** *see* ethinyl estradiol and norethindrone *on page 314*

# selegiline (se LE ji leen)

**Sound-Alike/Look-Alike Issues**

selegiline may be confused with Serentil®, sertraline, Serzone®, Stelazine®

Eldepryl® may be confused with Elavil®, enalapril

**Synonyms** deprenyl; L-deprenyl; selegiline hydrochloride

**U.S./Canadian Brand Names** Apo-Selegiline® [Can]; Eldepryl® [US]; Gen-Selegiline [Can]; Novo-Selegiline [Can]; Nu-Selegiline [Can]

**Therapeutic Category** Anti-Parkinson Agent; Dopaminergic Agent (Anti-Parkinson)

**Use** Adjunct in the management of parkinsonian patients in which levodopa/carbidopa therapy is deteriorating

**Usual Dosage** Oral: Adults: Parkinson's disease: 5 mg twice daily with breakfast and lunch or 10 mg in the morning

**Dosage Forms**

Capsule, as hydrochloride (Eldepryl®): 5 mg

Tablet, as hydrochloride: 5 mg

**selegiline hydrochloride** *see* selegiline *on this page*

**selenium** *see* trace metals *on page 813*

# selenium sulfide (se LEE nee um SUL fide)

**U.S./Canadian Brand Names** Head & Shoulders® Intensive Treatment [US-OTC]; Selsun Blue® 2-in-1 Treatment [US-OTC]; Selsun Blue® Balanced Treatment [US-OTC]; Selsun Blue® Medicated Treatment [US-OTC]; Selsun Blue® Moisturizing Treatment [US-OTC]; Selsun® [US]; Versel® [Can]

**Therapeutic Category** Antiseborrheic Agent, Topical

**Use** Treatment of itching and flaking of the scalp associated with dandruff, to control scalp seborrheic dermatitis; treatment of tinea versicolor

**Usual Dosage** Topical:

Dandruff, seborrhea: Massage 5-10 mL into wet scalp, leave on scalp 2-3 minutes, rinse thoroughly

Tinea versicolor: Apply the 2.5% lotion to affected area and lather with small amounts of water; leave on skin for 10 minutes, then rinse thoroughly; apply every day for 7 days

**Dosage Forms** [DSC] = Discontinued product

Lotion, topical: 2.5% (120 mL)

Shampoo, topical: 1% (210 mL)

Exsel® [DSC], Selsun®: 2.5% (120 mL)

Head & Shoulders® Intensive Treatment: 1% (400 mL)

Selsun Blue® Balanced Treatment, Selsun Blue® Medicated Treatment, Selsun Blue® Moisturizing Treatment, Selsun Blue® 2-in-1 Treatment: 1% (120 mL, 210 mL, 330 mL)

**Selepen® [US]** *see* trace metals *on page 813*

**Selpak® *(Discontinued)*** *see* selegiline *on previous page*

**Selsun® [US]** *see* selenium sulfide *on previous page*

**Selsun Blue® 2-in-1 Treatment [US-OTC]** *see* selenium sulfide *on previous page*

**Selsun Blue® Balanced Treatment [US-OTC]** *see* selenium sulfide *on previous page*

**Selsun Blue® Medicated Treatment [US-OTC]** *see* selenium sulfide *on previous page*

**Selsun Blue® Moisturizing Treatment [US-OTC]** *see* selenium sulfide *on previous page*

**Selsun Gold® for Women *(Discontinued)*** *see* selenium sulfide *on previous page*

**Semprex®-D [US]** *see* acrivastine and pseudoephedrine *on page 16*

**Senexon® [US-OTC]** *see* senna *on this page*

**senna** (SEN na)
  **Sound-Alike/Look-Alike Issues**
    Senexon® may be confused with Cenestin®
    Senokot® may be confused with Depakote®
  **U.S./Canadian Brand Names** Black Draught Tablets [US-OTC]; Evac-U-Gen [US-OTC]; Ex-lax® Maximum Strength [US-OTC]; Ex-lax® [US-OTC]; Fletcher's® Castoria® [US-OTC]; Perdiem® Overnight Relief [US-OTC]; Senexon® [US-OTC]; Senna-Gen® [US-OTC]; Sennatural™ [US-OTC]; Senokot® [US-OTC]; Uni-Senna [US-OTC]; X-Prep® [US-OTC]
  **Therapeutic Category** Laxative
  **Use** Short-term treatment of constipation; evacuate the colon for bowel or rectal examinations
  **Usual Dosage** Oral:
    Bowel evacuation: OTC labeling: Children ≥12 years and Adults: Usual dose: Sennosides 130 mg (X-Prep® 75 mL) between 2-4 PM the afternoon of the day prior to procedure
    Constipation : OTC ranges:
    Children :
     2-6 years:
      Sennosides: Initial: 3.75 mg once daily (maximum: 15 mg/day, divided twice daily)
      Senna concentrate: 33.3 mg/mL: 5-10 mL up to twice daily
     6-12 years:
      Sennosides: Initial: 8.6 mg once daily  (maximum: 50 mg/day, divided twice daily)
      Senna concentrate: 33.3 mg/mL: 10-30 mL up to twice daily
    Children ≥12 years and Adults: Sennosides 15 mg once daily (maximum: 70-100 mg/day, divided twice daily)
  **Dosage Forms**
    Granules (Senokot®): Sennosides 15 mg/teaspoon (60 g, 180 g, 360 g) [cocoa flavor] [DSC]
    Liquid:
     Senexon: Sennosides 8.8 mg/5 mL (240 mL)
     X-Prep®: Sennosides 8.8 mg/5 mL (75 mL) [alcohol free; contains sugar 50 g/75 mL; available individually or in a kit]
    Liquid concentrate (Fletcher's® Castoria®): Senna concentrate 33.3 mg/mL (75 mL) [alcohol free; contains sodium benzoate; root beer flavor]
    Syrup (Uni-Senna): Sennosides 8.8 mg/5 mL (240 mL)[contains alcohol; butterscotch flavor]
    Tablet: Sennosides 8.6 mg, 15 mg, 25 mg
     ex-lax®: Sennosides USP 15 mg
     ex-lax® Maximum Strength: Sennosides USP 25 mg
     Perdiem® Overnight Relief: Sennosides USP 15 mg
     Sennatural™, Senokot®, Senexon®, Senna-Gen®, Uni-Senna: Sennosides 8.6 mg
    Tablet, chewable:
     ex-lax®: Sennosides USP 15 mg [chocolate flavor]
     Evac-U-Gen: Sennosides 10 mg

**senna and docusate** *see* docusate and senna *on page 264*

**Senna-Gen® [US-OTC]** *see* senna *on this page*

**senna-S** *see* docusate and senna *on page 264*

**Sennatural™ [US-OTC]** *see* senna *on this page*

**Senokot® [US-OTC]** *see* senna *on this page*

**Senokot-S**® **[US-OTC]** *see* docusate and senna *on page 264*

**Sensipar**™ **[US]** *see* cinacalcet *on page 183*

**Sensorcaine**® **[US/Can]** *see* bupivacaine *on page 120*

**Sensorcaine**®**-MPF [US]** *see* bupivacaine *on page 120*

**Septa**® **Topical Ointment** *(Discontinued) see* bacitracin, neomycin, and polymyxin B *on page 87*

**Septisol**® *(Discontinued) see* hexachlorophene *on page 403*

**Septra**® **[US]** *see* sulfamethoxazole and trimethoprim *on page 773*

**Septra**® **DS [US]** *see* sulfamethoxazole and trimethoprim *on page 773*

**Septra**® **Injection [Can]** *see* sulfamethoxazole and trimethoprim *on page 773*

**Ser-A-Gen**® *(Discontinued) see* hydralazine, hydrochlorothiazide, and reserpine *on page 409*

**Ser-Ap-Es**® *(Discontinued) see* hydralazine, hydrochlorothiazide, and reserpine *on page 409*

**Serax**® **[US]** *see* oxazepam *on page 606*

**Serc**® **[Can]** *see* betahistine *(Canada only) on page 102*

**Serentil**® **[Can]** *see* mesoridazine *on page 517*

**Serentil**® *(Discontinued) see* mesoridazine *on page 517*

**Serevent**® **[Can]** *see* salmeterol *on page 737*

**Serevent**® *(Discontinued) see* salmeterol *on page 737*

**Serevent**® **Diskus**® **[US]** *see* salmeterol *on page 737*

## sermorelin acetate (ser moe REL in AS e tate )
**U.S./Canadian Brand Names** Geref® Diagnostic [US]
**Therapeutic Category**  Diagnostic Agent
**Use**  Geref® Diagnostic: For evaluation of the ability of the pituitary gland to secrete growth hormone (GH)
**Usual Dosage** Children and Adults: Diagnostic: I.V.: 1 mcg/kg as a single dose in the morning following an overnight fast
**Note:** Response to diagnostic test may be decreased in patients >40 years
**Dosage Forms** Injection, powder for reconstitution, as acetate: 50 mcg [packaged with diluent]

**Seromycin**® **[US]** *see* cycloserine *on page 215*

**Serophene**® **[US/Can]** *see* clomiphene *on page 196*

**Seroquel**® **[US/Can]** *see* quetiapine *on page 703*

**Serostim**® **[US/Can]** *see* somatropin *on page 760*

**Serpalan**® *(Discontinued) see* reserpine *on page 716*

**Serpatabs**® *(Discontinued) see* reserpine *on page 716*

## sertaconazole (ser ta KOE na zole)
**Synonyms** sertaconazole nitrate
**U.S./Canadian Brand Names** Ertaczo™ [US]
**Therapeutic Category**  Antifungal Agent, Topical
**Use** Topical treatment of tinea pedis (athlete's foot)
**Usual Dosage** Topical: Children ≥12 years and Adults: Apply between toes and to surrounding healthy skin twice daily for 4 weeks
**Dosage Forms** Cream, topical, as nitrate: 2% (30 g)

**sertaconazole nitrate** *see* sertaconazole *on this page*

## sertraline (SER tra leen)
**Sound-Alike/Look-Alike Issues**
sertraline may be confused with selegiline, Serentil®
Zoloft® may be confused with Zocor®

**Synonyms** sertraline hydrochloride

**U.S./Canadian Brand Names** Apo-Sertraline® [Can]; Gen-Sertraline [Can]; Novo-Sertraline [Can]; Nu-Sertraline [Can]; PMS-Sertraline [Can]; ratio-Sertraline [Can]; Rhoxal-Sertraline [Can]; Zoloft® [US/Can]

**Therapeutic Category** Antidepressant, Selective Serotonin Reuptake Inhibitor

**Use** Treatment of major depression; obsessive-compulsive disorder (OCD); panic disorder; post-traumatic stress disorder (PTSD); premenstrual dysphoric disorder (PMDD); social anxiety disorder

**Usual Dosage** Oral:

Children and Adolescents: OCD:

6-12 years: Initial: 25 mg once daily

13-17 years: Initial: 50 mg once daily

**Note:** May increase daily dose, at intervals of not less than 1 week, to a maximum of 200 mg/day. If somnolence is noted, give at bedtime.

Adults:

Depression/OCD: Oral: Initial: 50 mg/day (see "Note" above)

Panic disorder, PTSD, social anxiety disorder: Initial: 25 mg once daily; increase to 50 mg once daily after 1 week (see "Note" above)

PMDD: 50 mg/day either daily throughout menstrual cycle **or** limited to the luteal phase of menstrual cycle, depending on physician assessment. Patients not responding to 50 mg/day may benefit from dose increases (50 mg increments per menstrual cycle) up to 150 mg/day when dosing throughout menstrual cycle **or** up to 100 mg day when dosing during luteal phase only. If a 100 mg/day dose has been established with luteal phase dosing, a 50 mg/day titration step for 3 days should be utilized at the beginning of each luteal phase dosing period.

**Dosage Forms Note:** Available as sertraline hydrochloride; mg strength refers to sertraline

Solution, oral concentrate: 20 mg/mL (60 mL) [contains alcohol 12%]

Tablet: 25 mg, 50 mg, 100 mg

**sertraline hydrochloride** *see* sertraline *on previous page*

**Serutan® [US-OTC]** *see* psyllium *on page 697*

**Serzone® (Discontinued)** *see* nefazodone *on page 565*

**sevelamer** (se VEL a mer)

**Sound-Alike/Look-Alike Issues**

Renagel® may be confused with Reglan®, Regonol®

**Synonyms** sevelamer hydrochloride

**U.S./Canadian Brand Names** Renagel® [US/Can]

**Therapeutic Category** Phosphate Binder

**Use** Reduction of serum phosphorous in patients with chronic kidney disease on hemodialysis

**Usual Dosage**

Adults: Oral: Patients not taking a phosphate binder: 800-1600 mg 3 times/day with meals; the initial dose may be based on serum phosphorous levels:

>5.5 mg/dL to <7.5 mg/dL: 800 mg 3 times/day

≥7.5 mg/dL to <9.0 mg/dL: 1200-1600 mg 3 times/day

≥9.0 mg/dL: 1600 mg 3 times/day

Maintenance dose adjustment based on serum phosphorous concentration (goal of lowering to <5.5 mg/dL; maximum daily dose studied was equivalent to 13 g/day):

>5.5 mg/dL: Increase by 1 tablet per meal every 2 weeks

3.5-5.5 mg/dL: Maintain current dose

<3.5 mg/dL: Decrease by 1 tablet per meal

Dosage adjustment when switching between phosphate binder products: 667 mg of calcium acetate is equivalent to 800 mg sevelamer

**Dosage Forms** Tablet, as hydrochloride: 400 mg, 800 mg

**sevelamer hydrochloride** *see* sevelamer *on this page*

**sevoflurane** (see voe FLOO rane)

**Sound-Alike/Look-Alike Issues**

Ultane® may be confused with Ultram®

**U.S./Canadian Brand Names** Sevorane™ [Can]; Ultane® [US]

**Therapeutic Category** General Anesthetic

**Use** Induction and maintenance of general anesthesia

(Continued)

## sevoflurane *(Continued)*

**Usual Dosage** Minimum alveolar concentration (MAC), the concentration that abolishes movement in response to a noxious stimulus (surgical incision) in 50% of patients, is 2.6% (25 years of age) for sevoflurane. Surgical levels of anesthesia are generally achieved with concentrations from 0.5% to 3%; the concentration at which amnesia and loss of awareness occur is 0.6%.

Minimum alveolar concentrations (MAC) values for surgical levels of anesthesia:
0 to 1 month old full-term neonates: Sevoflurane in oxygen: 3.3%
1 to <6 months: Sevoflurane in oxygen: 3%
6 months to <3 years:
  Sevoflurane in oxygen: 2.8%
  Sevoflurane in 60% $N_2O$/40% oxygen: 2%
3-12 years: Sevoflurane in oxygen: 2.5%
25 years:
  Sevoflurane in oxygen: 2.6%
  Sevoflurane in 65% $N_2O$/35% oxygen: 1.4%
40 years:
  Sevoflurane in oxygen: 2.1%
  Sevoflurane in 65% $N_2O$/35% oxygen: 1.1%
60 years:
  Sevoflurane in oxygen: 1.7%
  Sevoflurane in 65% $N_2O$/35% oxygen: 0.9%
80 years:
  Sevoflurane in oxygen: 1.4%
  Sevoflurane in 65% $N_2O$/35% oxygen: 0.7%

**Dosage Forms** Liquid for inhalation: 100% (250 mL)

**Sevorane™ [Can]** *see* sevoflurane *on previous page*

**Shur-Seal® *(Discontinued)*** *see* nonoxynol 9 *on page 580*

**Sibelium® [Can]** *see* flunarizine *(Canada only) on page 344*

## sibutramine (si BYOO tra meen)

**Synonyms** sibutramine hydrochloride monohydrate
**U.S./Canadian Brand Names** Meridia® [US/Can]
**Therapeutic Category** Anorexiant
**Controlled Substance** C-IV
**Use** Management of obesity, including weight loss and maintenance of weight loss; should be used in conjunction with a reduced-calorie diet
**Usual Dosage** Adults ≥16 years: Initial: 10 mg once daily; after 4 weeks may titrate up to 15 mg once daily as needed and tolerated (may be used for up to 2 years, per manufacturer labeling)
**Dosage Forms** Capsule, as hydrochloride: 5 mg, 10 mg, 15 mg

**sibutramine hydrochloride monohydrate** *see* sibutramine *on this page*

**Silace [US-OTC]** *see* docusate *on page 263*

**Siladryl® Allergy [US-OTC]** *see* diphenhydramine *on page 254*

**Siladryl® DAS [US-OTC]** *see* diphenhydramine *on page 254*

**Silafed® [US-OTC]** *see* triprolidine and pseudoephedrine *on page 827*

**Silain® *(Discontinued)*** *see* simethicone *on page 748*

**Silaminic® Expectorant *(Discontinued)***

**Silapap® Children's [US-OTC]** *see* acetaminophen *on page 4*

**Silapap® Infants [US-OTC]** *see* acetaminophen *on page 4*

**Sildec [US]** *see* carbinoxamine and pseudoephedrine *on page 144*

**Sildec-DM [US]** *see* carbinoxamine, pseudoephedrine, and dextromethorphan *on page 145*

## sildenafil (sil DEN a fil)

**Sound-Alike/Look-Alike Issues**
Viagra® may be confused with Allegra®, Vaniqa™

Synonyms UK92480
**U.S./Canadian Brand Names** Revatio™ [US]; Viagra® [US/Can]
**Therapeutic Category** Phosphodiesterase (Type 5) Enzyme Inhibitor
**Use** Treatment of erectile dysfunction; treatment of pulmonary arterial hypertension
**Usual Dosage** Adults: Oral:
  Erectile dysfunction (Viagra®): For most patients, the recommended dose is 50 mg taken as needed, approximately 1 hour before sexual activity. However, sildenafil may be taken anywhere from 30 minutes to 4 hours before sexual activity. Based on effectiveness and tolerance, the dose may be increased to a maximum recommended dose of 100 mg or decreased to 25 mg. The maximum recommended dosing frequency is once daily.
  Pulmonary arterial hypertension (Revatio™): 20 mg 3 times/day, taken 4-6 hours apart
  **Dosage considerations for patients taking alpha blockers:** Viagra®: Doses of 50 or 100 mg, should not be taken within 4 hours of an alpha blocker; doses of 25 mg may be given at any time
  **Dosage adjustment for concomitant use of potent CYP304A inhibitors:**
    Revatio™:
    Erythromycin, saquinavir: No dosage adjustment
    Itraconazole, ketoconazole, ritonavir: Not recommended
    Viagra®:
    Erythromycin, itraconazole, ketoconazole, saquinavir: Starting dose of 25 mg should be considered
    Ritonavir: Maximum: 25 mg every 48 hours
**Dosage Forms** Tablet:
  Revatio™: 20 mg
  Viagra®: 25 mg, 50 mg, 100 mg

**Sildicon-E® *(Discontinued)***

**Silexin® [US-OTC]** *see* guaifenesin and dextromethorphan *on page 385*

**Silfedrine Children's [US-OTC]** *see* pseudoephedrine *on page 692*

**Silphen® [US-OTC]** *see* diphenhydramine *on page 254*

**Silphen DM® [US-OTC]** *see* dextromethorphan *on page 238*

**Sil-Tex [US]** *see* guaifenesin and phenylephrine *on page 387*

**Siltussin-CF® *(Discontinued)***

**Siltussin DAS [US-OTC]** *see* guaifenesin *on page 383*

**Siltussin DM [US-OTC]** *see* guaifenesin and dextromethorphan *on page 385*

**Siltussin DM DAS [US-OTC]** *see* guaifenesin and dextromethorphan *on page 385*

**Siltussin SA [US-OTC]** *see* guaifenesin *on page 383*

**Silvadene® [US]** *see* silver sulfadiazine *on this page*

## silver nitrate (SIL ver NYE trate)

Synonyms AgNO₃
**Therapeutic Category** Topical Skin Product
**Use** Cauterization of wounds and sluggish ulcers, removal of granulation tissue and warts; aseptic prophylaxis of burns
**Usual Dosage** Children and Adults:
  Sticks: Apply to mucous membranes and other moist skin surfaces only on area to be treated 2-3 times/week for 2-3 weeks
  Topical solution: Apply a cotton applicator dipped in solution on the affected area 2-3 times/week for 2-3 weeks
**Dosage Forms**
  Applicator sticks, topical: Silver nitrate 75% and potassium nitrate 25% (6", 12", 18")
  Solution, topical: 10% (30 mL); 25% (30 mL); 50% (30 mL)

## silver sulfadiazine (SIL ver sul fa DYE a zeen)

**U.S./Canadian Brand Names** Flamazine® [Can]; Silvadene® [US]; SSD® AF [US]; SSD® [US]; Thermazene® [US]
**Therapeutic Category** Antibacterial, Topical
**Use** Prevention and treatment of infection in second and third degree burns
**Usual Dosage** Children and Adults: Topical: Apply once or twice daily with a sterile-gloved hand; apply to a thickness of ¹/₁₆"; burned area should be covered with cream at all times
(Continued)

## silver sulfadiazine *(Continued)*
**Dosage Forms**
Cream, topical: 1% (25 g, 50  mg, 85 g, 400 g)
Silvadene®, Thermazene®: 1% (20 g, 50 g, 85 g, 400 g, 1000 g)
SSD®: 1% (25 g, 50 g, 85 g, 400 g)
SSD® AF: 1% (50 g, 400 g)

## simethicone (sye METH i kone)
**Sound-Alike/Look-Alike Issues**
simethicone may be confused with cimetidine
Mylanta® may be confused with Mynatal®
Mylicon® may be confused with Modicon®, Myleran®
Phazyme® may be confused with Pherazine®
**Synonyms** activated dimethicone; activated methylpolysiloxane
**U.S./Canadian Brand Names** Equalizer Gas Relief [US-OTC]; Gas-X® Extra Strength [US-OTC]; Gas-X® Maximum Strength [US-OTC]; Gas-X® [US-OTC]; Genasyme® [US-OTC]; Infantaire Gas Drops [US-OTC]; Mylanta® Gas Maximum Strength [US-OTC]; Mylanta® Gas [US-OTC]; Mylicon® Infants [US-OTC]; Ovol® [Can]; Phazyme® Quick Dissolve [US-OTC]; Phazyme® Ultra Strength [US-OTC]; Phazyme™ [Can]
**Therapeutic Category** Antiflatulent
**Use** Relieves flatulence and functional gastric bloating, and postoperative gas pains
**Usual Dosage** Oral:
Infants: 20 mg 4 times/day
Children <12 years: 40 mg 4 times/day
Children >12 years and Adults: 40-120 mg after meals and at bedtime as needed, not to exceed 500 mg/day
**Dosage Forms**
Softgels: 125 mg
GasAid, Gas-X® Extra Strength, Mylanta® Gas Maximum Strength: 125 mg
Gas-X® Maximum Strength: 166 mg
Phazyme® Ultra Strength: 180 mg
Suspension, oral drops:  40 mg/0.6 mL (30 mL)
Equalizer Gas Relief, Genasyme®, Infantaire Gas: 40 mg/0.6 mL (30 mL)
Mylicon® Infants: 40 mg/0.6 mL (15 mL, 30 mL) [alcohol free; contains sodium benzoate; available in a nonstaining formula]
Tablet, chewable: 80 mg, 125 mg
Gas-X®: 80 mg [sodium free; peppermint crème or cherry crème flavor]
Gas-X® Extra Strength: 125 mg [peppermint crème or cherry crème flavor]
Genasyme®: 80 mg
Mylanta® Gas: 80 mg [mint flavor]
Mylanta® Gas Maximum Strength: 125 mg [cherry and mint flavors]
Phazyme® Quick Dissolve: 125 mg [contains phenylalanine 0.4 mg per tablet; mint flavor]

**simethicone, aluminum hydroxide, and magnesium hydroxide** *see* aluminum hydroxide, magnesium hydroxide, and simethicone *on page 35*

**simethicone and calcium carbonate** *see* calcium carbonate and simethicone *on page 132*

**simethicone and magaldrate** *see* magaldrate and simethicone *on page 496*

**Simply Cough® [US-OTC]** *see* dextromethorphan *on page 238*

**Simply Saline™ [US-OTC]** *see* sodium chloride *on page 752*

**Simply Sleep® [US-OTC/Can]** *see* diphenhydramine *on page 254*

**Simply Stuffy™ [US-OTC]** *see* pseudoephedrine *on page 692*

**Simulect® [US/Can]** *see* basiliximab *on page 89*

## simvastatin (SIM va stat in)
**Sound-Alike/Look-Alike Issues**
Zocor® may be confused with Cozaar®, Yocon®, Zoloft®
**U.S./Canadian Brand Names** Apo-Simvastatin® [Can]; CO Simvastatin [Can]; Gen-Simvastatin [Can]; Novo-Simvastatin [Can]; PMS-Simvastatin [Can]; ratio-Simvastatin [Can]; Riva-Simvastatin [Can]; Zocor® [US/Can]

**Therapeutic Category** HMG-CoA Reductase Inhibitor

**Use** Used with dietary therapy for the following:

Secondary prevention of cardiovascular events in hypercholesterolemic patients with established coronary heart disease (CHD) or at high risk for CHD: To reduce cardiovascular morbidity (myocardial infarction, coronary revascularization procedures) and mortality; to reduce the risk of stroke and transient ischemic attacks

Hyperlipidemias: To reduce elevations in total cholesterol, LDL-C, apolipoprotein B, and triglycerides in patients with primary hypercholesterolemia (elevations of 1 or more components are present in Fredrickson type IIa, IIb, III, and IV hyperlipidemias); treatment of homozygous familial hypercholesterolemia

Heterozygous familial hypercholesterolemia (HeFH): In adolescent patients (10-17 years of age, females >1 year postmenarche) with HeFH having LDL-C ≥190 mg/dL **or** LDL ≥160 mg/dL with positive family history of premature cardiovascular disease (CVD), or 2 or more CVD risk factors in the adolescent patient

**Usual Dosage** Oral: **Note:** Doses should be individualized according to the baseline LDL-cholesterol levels, the recommended goal of therapy, and the patient's response; adjustments should be made at intervals of 4 weeks or more; doses may need adjusted based on concomitant medications

Children 10-17 years (females >1 year postmenarche): HeFH: 10 mg once daily in the evening; range: 10-40 mg/day (maximum: 40 mg/day)

**Dosage adjustment for simvastatin with concomitant cyclosporine, danazol, fibrates, niacin, amiodarone, or verapamil:** Refer to drug-specific dosing in Adults dosing section

Adults:

Homozygous familial hypercholesterolemia: 40 mg once daily in the evening **or** 80 mg/day (given as 20 mg, 20 mg, and 40 mg evening dose)

Prevention of cardiovascular events, hyperlipidemias: 20-40 mg once daily in the evening; range: 5-80 mg/day

Patients requiring only moderate reduction of LDL-cholesterol may be started at 10 mg once daily

Patients requiring reduction of >45% in low-density lipoprotein (LDL) cholesterol may be started at 40 mg once daily in the evening

Patients with CHD or at high risk for CHD: Dosing should be started at 40 mg once daily in the evening; simvastatin may be started simultaneously with diet

**Dosage Forms** Tablet: 5 mg, 10 mg, 20 mg, 40 mg, 80 mg

**Sina-12X [US]** *see* guaifenesin and phenylephrine *on page 387*

## sincalide (SIN ka lide)

**Synonyms** C8-CCK; OP-CCK

**U.S./Canadian Brand Names** Kinevac® [US]

**Therapeutic Category** Diagnostic Agent

**Use** Postevacuation cholecystography; gallbladder bile sampling; stimulate pancreatic secretion for analysis

**Usual Dosage** Adults: I.V.:

Contraction of gallbladder: 0.02 mcg/kg over 30 seconds to 1 minute, may repeat in 15 minutes a 0.04 mcg/kg dose

Pancreatic function: 0.02 mcg/kg over 30 minutes administered after secretin

**Dosage Forms** Injection, powder for reconstitution: 5 mcg [contains sodium chloride 45 mg/vial]

**Sine-Aid® IB (Discontinued)** *see* pseudoephedrine and ibuprofen *on page 694*

**Sinemet® [US/Can]** *see* levodopa and carbidopa *on page 474*

**Sinemet® CR [US/Can]** *see* levodopa and carbidopa *on page 474*

**Sinequan® [US/Can]** *see* doxepin *on page 269*

**Singulair® [US/Can]** *see* montelukast *on page 549*

**Sinografin® [US]** *see* radiological/contrast media (ionic) *on page 707*

**Sinubid® (Discontinued)**

**Sinufed® Timecelles® (Discontinued)** *see* guaifenesin and pseudoephedrine *on page 388*

**Sinumed® (Discontinued)** *see* acetaminophen, chlorpheniramine, and pseudoephedrine *on page 10*

**Sinumist®-SR Capsulets® (Discontinued)** *see* guaifenesin *on page 383*

**Sinus-Relief® [US-OTC]** *see* acetaminophen and pseudoephedrine *on page 8*

**Sinutab® Non Drowsy [Can]** *see* acetaminophen and pseudoephedrine *on page 8*

**Sinutab® Sinus [US-OTC]** *see* acetaminophen and pseudoephedrine *on page 8*

**Sinutab® Sinus & Allergy [Can]** *see* acetaminophen, chlorpheniramine, and pseudoephedrine *on page 10*

**Sinutab® Sinus Allergy Maximum Strength [US-OTC]** *see* acetaminophen, chlorpheniramine, and pseudoephedrine *on page 10*

**SINUvent® PE [US]** *see* guaifenesin and phenylephrine *on page 387*

**Sirdalud® *(Discontinued)*** *see* tizanidine *on page 806*

**sirolimus** (sir OH li mus)
  U.S./Canadian Brand Names Rapamune® [US/Can]
  Therapeutic Category Immunosuppressant Agent
  Use Prophylaxis of organ rejection in patients receiving renal transplants, in combination with corticosteroids and cyclosporine (cyclosporine may be withdrawn in low-to-moderate immunological risk patients after 2-4 months, in conjunction with an increase in sirolimus dosage)
  Usual Dosage Oral:
    Combination therapy with cyclosporine: For *de novo* transplant recipients, a loading dose of 3 times the daily maintenance dose should be administered on day 1 of dosing. Doses should be taken 4 hours after cyclosporine, and should be taken consistently either with or without food.
    Children ≥13 years and Adults: Dosing by body weight:
      <40 kg: Loading dose: Loading dose: 3 mg/m$^2$ on day 1, followed by a maintenance dosing of 1 mg/m$^2$
      ≥40 kg: Loading dose: 6 mg on day 1; maintenance: 2 mg/day
  **Maintenance therapy after withdrawal of cyclosporine:**
    Following 2-4 months of combined therapy, withdrawal of cyclosporine may be considered in low-to-moderate risk patients. Cyclosporine withdrawal in not recommended in high immunological risk patients. Cyclosporine should be discontinued over 4-8 weeks, and a necessary increase in the dosage of sirolimus (up to fourfold) should be anticipated due to removal of metabolic inhibition by cyclosporine and to maintain adequate immunosuppressive effects.
    Sirolimus dosages should be adjusted to maintain trough concentrations of 12-24 ng/mL. Dosage should be adjusted at intervals of 7-14 days to account for the long half-life of sirolimus. Considerable increases in dosage may require an additional loading dose, calculated as the difference between the target concentration and the current concentration, multiplied by a factor of 3. Loading doses >40 mg may be administered over two days. Serum concentrations should not be used as the sole basis for dosage adjustment (monitor clinical signs/symptoms, tissue biopsy, and laboratory parameters).
  Dosage Forms
    Solution, oral [bottle]: 1 mg/mL (60 mL) [contains ethanol 1.5% to 2.5%; packaged with oral syringes and a carrying case]
    Tablet: 1 mg, 2 mg

**SK** *see* streptokinase *on page 766*

**SK and F 104864** *see* topotecan *on page 811*

**Skeeter Stik [US-OTC]** *see* benzocaine *on page 95*

**Skelaxin® [US/Can]** *see* metaxalone *on page 519*

**Skelid® [US]** *see* tiludronate *on page 803*

**SKF 104864** *see* topotecan *on page 811*

**SKF 104864-A** *see* topotecan *on page 811*

**Sleep-Aid® [US-OTC]** *see* doxylamine *on page 273*

**Sleep-ettes D [US-OTC]** *see* diphenhydramine *on page 254*

**Sleep-eze 3® Oral *(Discontinued)*** *see* diphenhydramine *on page 254*

**Sleepinal® [US-OTC]** *see* diphenhydramine *on page 254*

**Sleepwell 2-nite® *(Discontinued)*** *see* diphenhydramine *on page 254*

**Slim-Mint® *(Discontinued)*** *see* benzocaine *on page 95*

**Slo-bid™ *(Discontinued)*** *see* theophylline *on page 793*

**Slo-Niacin® [US-OTC]** *see* niacin *on page 571*

**Slo-Phyllin® (all products) *(Discontinued)*** *see* theophylline *on page 793*

**Slo-Phyllin**® **GG** *(Discontinued)* *see* theophylline and guaifenesin *on page 795*

**Slow FE**® **[US-OTC]** *see* ferrous sulfate *on page 335*

**Slow-K**® **[Can]** *see* potassium chloride *on page 663*

**Slow-K**® *(Discontinued)* *see* potassium chloride *on page 663*

**Slow-Mag**® **[US-OTC]** *see* magnesium chloride *on page 497*

**Slow-Trasicor**® **[Can]** *see* oxprenolol *(Canada only)* *on page 607*

## smallpox vaccine (SMAL poks vak SEEN)
**Synonyms** dried smallpox vaccine; vaccinia vaccine
**U.S./Canadian Brand Names** Dryvax® [US]
**Therapeutic Category** Vaccine
**Use** Active immunization against vaccinia virus, the causative agent of smallpox in persons determined to be at risk for smallpox infection. The ACIP recommends vaccination of laboratory workers at risk of exposure from cultures or contaminated animals which may be a source of vaccinia or related Orthopoxviruses capable of causing infections in humans (monkeypox, cowpox, or variola). The ACIP also recommends that consideration be given for vaccination in healthcare workers having contact with clinical specimens, contaminated material, or patients receiving vaccinia or recombinant vaccinia viruses. Revaccination is recommended every 10 years. The Armed Forces recommend vaccination of certain personnel categories. Recommendations for use in response to bioterrorism are regularly updated by the CDC, and may be found at www.cdc.gov.
**Usual Dosage** Not for I.M., I.V., or SubQ injection: Vaccination by scarification (multiple-puncture technique) only: **Note:** A trace of blood should appear at vaccination site after 15-20 seconds; if no trace of blood is visible, an additional 3 insertions should be made using the same needle, without reinserting the needle into the vaccine bottle.
Adults (children ≥12 months in emergency conditions only):
  Primary vaccination: Use a single drop of vaccine suspension and 2 or 3 needle punctures (using the same needle) into the superficial skin
  Revaccination: Use a single drop of vaccine suspension and 15 needle punctures (using the same needle) into the superficial skin
**Dosage Forms** Injection, powder for reconstitution [calf liver source]: ~100 million vaccinia virions per mL following reconstitution [contains polymyxin B, neomycin, dihydrostreptomycin sulfate, and chlortetracycline (trace amounts); packed with diluent, venting needle, and 100 bifurcated needles; vial stopper contains latex]

**smelling salts** *see* ammonia spirit (aromatic) *on page 45*

**SMZ-TMP** *see* sulfamethoxazole and trimethoprim *on page 773*

**snake (pit vipers) antivenin** *see* antivenin *(Crotalidae)* polyvalent *on page 60*

**Snaplets-EX**® *(Discontinued)*

**(+)-(S)-N-methyl-γ-(1-naphthyloxy)-2-thiophenepropylamine hydrochloride** *see* duloxetine *on page 275*

**sodium 2-mercaptoethane sulfonate** *see* mesna *on page 516*

**sodium 4-hydroxybutyrate** *see* sodium oxybate *on page 755*

**sodium L-triiodothyronine** *see* liothyronine *on page 484*

## sodium acetate (SOW dee um AS e tate)
**Therapeutic Category** Alkalinizing Agent; Electrolyte Supplement, Oral
**Use** Sodium source in large volume I.V. fluids to prevent or correct hyponatremia in patients with restricted intake; used to counter acidosis through conversion to bicarbonate
**Usual Dosage** Sodium acetate is metabolized to bicarbonate on an equimolar basis outside the liver; administer in large volume I.V. fluids as a sodium source. Refer to Sodium Bicarbonate monograph.
Maintenance electrolyte requirements of sodium in parenteral nutrition solutions:
  Daily requirements: 3-4 mEq/kg/24 hours or 25-40 mEq/1000 kcal/24 hours
  Maximum: 100-150 mEq/24 hours
**Dosage Forms** Injection, solution: 2 mEq/mL (20 mL, 50 mL, 100 mL); 4 mEq/mL (50 mL, 100 mL)

**sodium acid carbonate** *see* sodium bicarbonate *on next page*

**sodium benzoate and caffeine** *see* caffeine and sodium benzoate *on page 127*

**sodium benzoate and sodium phenylacetate** *see* sodium phenylacetate and sodium benzoate *on page 755*

**sodium bicarbonate** (SOW dee um bye KAR bun ate)

**Synonyms** baking soda; $NaHCO_3$; sodium acid carbonate; sodium hydrogen carbonate

**U.S./Canadian Brand Names** Brioschi® [US-OTC]; Neut® [US]

**Therapeutic Category** Alkalinizing Agent; Antacid; Electrolyte Supplement, Oral

**Use** Management of metabolic acidosis; gastric hyperacidity; as an alkalinization agent for the urine; treatment of hyperkalemia; management of overdose of certain drugs, including tricyclic antidepressants and aspirin

**Usual Dosage**

Cardiac arrest: **Routine use of $NaHCO_3$ is not recommended and should be given only after adequate alveolar ventilation has been established and effective cardiac compressions are provided**

Infants and Children: I.V.: 0.5-1 mEq/kg/dose repeated every 10 minutes or as indicated by arterial blood gases; rate of infusion should not exceed 10 mEq/minute; neonates and children <2 years of age should receive 4.2% (0.5 mEq/mL) solution

Adults: I.V.: Initial: 1 mEq/kg/dose one time; maintenance: 0.5 mEq/kg/dose every 10 minutes or as indicated by arterial blood gases

Metabolic acidosis: Infants, Children, and Adults: Dosage should be based on the following formula if blood gases and pH measurements are available:

$HCO_3^-$(mEq) = 0.3 x weight (kg) x base deficit (mEq/L)

Administer $^1/_2$ dose initially, then remaining $^1/_2$ dose over the next 24 hours; monitor pH, serum $HCO_3^-$, and clinical status

**Note:** If acid-base status is not available: Dose for older Children and Adults: 2-5 mEq/kg I.V. infusion over 4-8 hours; subsequent doses should be based on patient's acid-base status

Chronic renal failure: Oral: Initiate when plasma $HCO_3^-$ <15 mEq/L

Children: 1-3 mEq/kg/day

Adults: Start with 20-36 mEq/day in divided doses, titrate to bicarbonate level of 18-20 mEq/L

Hyperkalemia: Adults: I.V.: 1 mEq/kg over 5 minutes

Renal tubular acidosis: Oral:

Distal:

Children: 2-3 mEq/kg/day

Adults: 0.5-2 mEq/kg/day in 4-5 divided doses

Proximal: Children and Adults: Initial: 5-10 mEq/kg/day; maintenance: Increase as required to maintain serum bicarbonate in the normal range

Urine alkalinization: Oral:

Children: 1-10 mEq (84-840 mg)/kg/day in divided doses every 4-6 hours; dose should be titrated to desired urinary pH

Adults: Initial: 48 mEq (4 g), then 12-24 mEq (1-2 g) every 4 hours; dose should be titrated to desired urinary pH; doses up to 16 g/day (200 mEq) in patients <60 years and 8 g (100 mEq) in patients >60 years

Antacid: Adults: Oral: 325 mg to 2 g 1-4 times/day

**Dosage Forms**

Granules, effervescent (Brioschi®): 2.69 g/packet (6 g) [unit-dose packets; contains sodium 770 mg/packet; lemon flavor]; 2.69 g/capful (120 g, 240 g) [contains sodium 770 mg/capful; lemon flavor]

Infusion [premixed in sterile water]: 5% (500 mL)

Injection, solution:

4.2% [42 mg/mL = 5 mEq/10 mL] (10 mL)

7.5% [75 mg/mL = 8.92 mEq/10 mL] (50 mL)

8.4% [84 mg/mL = 10 mEq/10 mL] (10 mL, 50 mL)

Neut®: 4% [40 mg/mL = 2.4 mEq/5 mL] (5 mL)

Powder: Sodium bicarbonate USP (120 g, 480 g) [contains sodium 30 mEq per $^1/_2$ teaspoon]

Tablet: 325 mg [3.8 mEq]; 650 mg [7.6 mEq]

**sodium cellulose phosphate** *see* cellulose sodium phosphate *on page 160*

**sodium chloride** (SOW dee um KLOR ide)

**Synonyms** NaCl; normal saline; salt

**U.S./Canadian Brand Names** Altamist [US-OTC]; Ayr® Baby Saline [US-OTC]; Ayr® Saline Mist [US-OTC]; Ayr® Saline [US-OTC]; Breathe Right® Saline [US-OTC]; Broncho Saline® [US-OTC]; Entsol® [US-OTC]; Muro 128® [US-OTC]; Na-Zone® [US-OTC]; Nasal Moist® [US-OTC]; NaSal™ [US-OTC];

Ocean® [US-OTC]; Pediamist® [US-OTC]; Pretz® Irrigation [US-OTC]; SalineX® [US-OTC]; SeaMist® [US-OTC]; Simply Saline™ [US-OTC]; Wound Wash Saline™ [US-OTC]

**Therapeutic Category** Electrolyte Supplement, Oral; Lubricant, Ocular

**Use**

Parenteral: Restores sodium ion in patients with restricted oral intake (especially hyponatremia states or low salt syndrome). In general, parenteral saline uses:

Bacteriostatic sodium chloride: Dilution or dissolving drugs for I.M., I.V., or SubQ injections

Concentrated sodium chloride: Additive for parenteral fluid therapy

Hypertonic sodium chloride: For severe hyponatremia and hypochloremia

Hypotonic sodium chloride: Hydrating solution

Normal saline: Restores water/sodium losses

Pharmaceutical aid/diluent for infusion of compatible drug additives

Ophthalmic: Reduces corneal edema

Oral: Restores sodium losses

Inhalation: Restores moisture to pulmonary system; loosens and thins congestion caused by colds or allergies; diluent for bronchodilator solutions that require dilution before inhalation

Intranasal: Restores moisture to nasal membranes

Irrigation: Wound cleansing, irrigation, and flushing

**Usual Dosage**

Children: I.V.: Hypertonic solutions (>0.9%) should only be used for the initial treatment of acute serious symptomatic hyponatremia; maintenance: 3-4 mEq/kg/day; maximum: 100-150 mEq/day; dosage varies widely depending on clinical condition

Replacement: Determined by laboratory determinations mEq

Sodium deficiency (mEq/kg) = [% dehydration (L/kg)/100 x 70 (mEq/L)] + [0.6 (L/kg) x (140 - serum sodium) (mEq/L)]

Children ≥2 years and Adults:

Intranasal: 2-3 sprays in each nostril as needed

Irrigation: Spray affected area

Children and Adults: Inhalation: Bronchodilator diluent: 1-3 sprays (1-3 mL) to dilute bronchodilator solution in nebulizer prior to administration

Adults:

GU irrigant: 1-3 L/day by intermittent irrigation

Heat cramps: Oral: 0.5-1 g with full glass of water, up to 4.8 g/day

Replacement I.V.: Determined by laboratory determinations mEq

Sodium deficiency (mEq/kg) = [% dehydration (L/kg)/100 x 70 (mEq/L)] + [0.6 (L/kg) x (140 - serum sodium) (mEq/L)]

To correct acute, serious hyponatremia: mEq sodium = [desired sodium (mEq/L) - actual sodium (mEq/L)] x [0.6 x wt (kg)]; for acute correction use 125 mEq/L as the desired serum sodium; acutely correct serum sodium in 5 mEq/L/dose increments; more gradual correction in increments of 10 mEq/L/day is indicated in the asymptomatic patient

Chloride maintenance electrolyte requirement in parenteral nutrition: 2-4 mEq/kg/24 hours or 25-40 mEq/1000 kcals/24 hours; maximum: 100-150 mEq/24 hours

Sodium maintenance electrolyte requirement in parenteral nutrition: 3-4 mEq/kg/24 hours or 25-40 mEq/1000 kcals/24 hours; maximum: 100-150 mEq/24 hours.

Ophthalmic:

Ointment: Apply once daily or more often

Solution: Instill 1-2 drops into affected eye(s) every 3-4 hours

**Dosage Forms**

Gel, intranasal (Nasal Moist®): 0.65% (30 g)

Injection, solution: 0.45% (25 mL, 50 mL, 100 mL, 250 mL, 500 mL, 1000 mL, 1500 mL, 2000 mL); 0.9% (1 mL, 2 mL, 3 mL, 5 mL, 10 mL, 20 mL, 25 mL, 30 mL, 50 mL, 100 mL, 150 mL, 250 mL, 500 mL, 1000 mL); 2.5 % (250 mL); 3% (500 mL); 5% (500 mL)

Injection, solution [preservative free]: 0.9% (2 mL, 3 mL, 5 mL, 10 mL, 20 mL, 50 mL, 100 mL)

Injection, solution, bacteriostatic: 0.9% (10 mL, 20 mL, 30 mL)

Injection, solution, concentrate: 14.6% [2.5 mEq/mL] (20 mL, 40 mL, 250 mL); 23.4% [4 mEq/mL] (30 mL, 50 mL, 100 mL, 200 mL, 250 mL)

Ointment, ophthalmic (Muro 128®): 5% (3.5 g)

Powder, for nasal solution:

Broncho Saline®: 0.9% (90 mL, 240 mL)

Entsol®: 3% (10.5 g)

Solution, for inhalation: 0.45% (3 mL, 5 mL); 0.9% (3 mL, 5 mL, 15 mL); 3% (15 mL); 10% (15 mL)

Solution, intranasal: 0.65% (45 mL)

(Continued)

# sodium chloride *(Continued)*

Altamist: 0.65% (60 mL) [spray]
Ayr® Baby Saline: 0.65% (30 mL) [spray/drops]
Ayr® Saline: 0.65% (50 mL) [drops]
Ayr® Saline Mist: 0.65% (50 mL) [spray]
Breathe Right® Saline: 0.65% (44 mL) [spray]
Entsol® [preservative free]: 3% (100 mL) [spray]
Entsol® Mist: 3% (30 mL) [spray]
Enstol® Single Use [preservative free]: 3% (240 mL) [nasal wash]
Na-Zone®: 0.75% (60 mL) [spray]
NāSal™: 0.65% (15 mL) [drops]; (30 mL) [spray]
Nasal Moist®: 0.65% (15 mL, 45 mL) [spray]
Ocean®: 0.65% (45 mL) [spray/drops]
Pediamist®: 0.5% (15 mL) [spray]
Pretz® Irrigation: 0.75% (240 mL)
SalineX®: 0.4% (15 mL) [drops]; (50 mL) [spray]
SeaMist®: 0.65% (15 mL) [spray]
Simply Saline™: 0.9% (44 mL) [mist]
Solution for irrigation: 0.45% (2000 mL); 0.9% (250 mL, 500 mL, 1000 mL, 1500 mL, 2000 mL, 3000 mL, 4000 mL, 5000 mL)
Wound Wash Saline™: 0.9% (90 mL, 210 mL)
Solution, ophthalmic: 5% (15 mL)
Muro 128®: 2% (15 mL), 5% (15 mL, 30 mL)
Tablet: 1 g

**sodium citrate, citric acid, and potassium citrate** *see* citric acid, sodium citrate, and potassium citrate *on page 189*

**sodium edetate** *see* edetate disodium *on page 279*

**sodium etidronate** *see* etidronate disodium *on page 321*

**sodium ferric gluconate** *see* ferric gluconate *on page 333*

**sodium fluoride** *see* fluoride *on page 347*

**sodium fusidate** *see* fusidic acid *(Canada only) on page 364*

**sodium hyaluronate** *see* hyaluronate and derivatives *on page 406*

**sodium hyaluronate-chrondroitin sulfate** *see* chondroitin sulfate and sodium hyaluronate *on page 180*

**sodium hydrogen carbonate** *see* sodium bicarbonate *on page 752*

# sodium hypochlorite solution (SOW dee um hye poe KLOR ite soe LOO shun)

**Synonyms** modified Dakin's solution
**U.S./Canadian Brand Names** Dakin's Solution [US]; Di-Dak-Sol [US]
**Therapeutic Category** Disinfectant
**Use** Treatment of athlete's foot (0.5%); wound irrigation (0.5%); disinfection of utensils and equipment (5%)
**Usual Dosage** Topical irrigation
**Dosage Forms** Solution, topical:
Dakin's: 0.25% (480 mL); 0.5% (480 mL, 3840 mL)
Di-Dak-Sol: 0.0125% (480 mL)

**sodium hyposulfate** *see* sodium thiosulfate *on page 758*

# sodium lactate (SOW dee um LAK tate)

**Therapeutic Category** Alkalinizing Agent
**Use** Source of bicarbonate for prevention and treatment of mild to moderate metabolic acidosis
**Usual Dosage** Dosage depends on degree of acidosis
**Dosage Forms** Injection, solution: 560 mg/mL [sodium 5 mEq and lactate 5 mEq per mL] (10 mL)

**sodium nafcillin** *see* nafcillin *on page 557*

## sodium nitrite, sodium thiosulfate, and amyl nitrite
(SOW dee um NYE trite, SOW dee um thye oh SUL fate, & AM il NYE trite)

**Synonyms** amyl nitrite, sodium thiosulfate, and sodium nitrite; cyanide antidote kit; sodium thiosulfate, sodium nitrite, and amyl nitrite

**U.S./Canadian Brand Names** Cyanide Antidote Package [US]

**Therapeutic Category** Antidote

**Use** Treatment of cyanide poisoning

**Usual Dosage** Cyanide poisoning:

Children: 0.3 mL ampul of amyl nitrite is crushed every minute and vapor is inhaled for 15-30 seconds until an I.V. sodium nitrite infusion is available. Following administration of sodium nitrite I.V. 6-8 mL/m$^2$ ($\sim$0.2 mL/kg, maximum: 10 mL), inject sodium thiosulfate I.V. 7 g/m$^2$ (maximum 12.5 g) over $\sim$10 minutes, if needed; injection of both may be repeated at $^1/_2$ the original dose.

Adults: 0.3 mL ampul of amyl nitrite is crushed every minute and vapor is inhaled for 15-30 seconds until an I.V. sodium nitrite infusion is available. Following administration of 300 mg I.V. sodium nitrite, inject 12.5 g sodium thiosulfate I.V. (over $\sim$10 minutes), if needed; injection of both may be repeated at $^1/_2$ the original dose.

**Dosage Forms** Kit [each kit contains] (Cyanide Antidote Package):

Injection, solution:

Sodium nitrite 300 mg/10 mL (2)

Sodium thiosulfate 12.5 g/50 mL (2)

Inhalant: Amyl nitrite 0.3 mL (12)

[kit also includes disposable syringes, stomach tube, tourniquet, and instructions]

**sodium nitroferricyanide** *see* nitroprusside *on page 579*

**sodium nitroprusside** *see* nitroprusside *on page 579*

## sodium oxybate (SOW dee um ox i BATE)
**Synonyms** 4-hydroxybutyrate; gamma hydroxybutyric acid; GHB; sodium 4-hydroxybutyrate

**U.S./Canadian Brand Names** Xyrem® [US]

**Therapeutic Category** Central Nervous System Depressant

**Controlled Substance** C-I (illicit use); C-III (medical use)

**Use Orphan drug:** Treatment of cataplexy in patients with narcolepsy

**Usual Dosage** Oral: Children ≥16 years and Adults: Treatment of cataplexy in patients with narcolepsy: Initial: 4.5 g/day, in 2 equal doses; first dose to be given at bedtime after the patient is in bed, and second dose to be given 2.5-4 hours later. Dose may be increased or adjusted in 2-week intervals; average dose: 6-9 g/day (maximum: 9 g/day)

**Dosage Forms** Solution, oral: 500 mg/mL (180 mL) [supplied in a kit containing two dosing cups and measuring device]

**sodium PAS** *see* aminosalicylic acid *on page 41*

**sodium-PCA and lactic acid** *see* lactic acid *on page 462*

## sodium phenylacetate and sodium benzoate
(SOW dee um fen il AS e tate & SOW dee um BENZ oh ate)

**Synonyms** NAPA and NABZ; sodium benzoate and sodium phenylacetate

**U.S./Canadian Brand Names** Ammonul® [US]

**Therapeutic Category** Ammonium Detoxicant

**Use** Adjunct to treatment of acute hyperammonemia and encephalopathy in patients with urea cycle disorders involving partial or complete deficiencies of carbamyl-phosphate synthetase (CPS), ornithine transcarbamoylase (OTC), argininosuccinate lysase (ASL), or argininosuccinate synthetase (ASS); for use with hemodialysis in acute neonatal hyperammonemic coma, moderate-to-severe hyperammonemic encephalopathy and hyperammonemia which fails to respond to initial therapy

**Usual Dosage** Administer as a loading dose over 90-120 minutes, followed by an equivalent maintenance infusion given over 24 hours. Dosage based on weight and specific enzyme deficiency; therapy should continue until ammonia levels are in normal range.

≤20 kg:

CPS and OTC deficiency: Ammonul® 2.5 mL/kg and arginine 10% 2 mL/kg (provides sodium phenylacetate 250 mg/kg, sodium benzoate 250 mg/kg, and arginine hydrochloride 200 mg/kg).

ASS and ASL deficiency: Ammonul® 2.5 mL/kg and arginine 10% 6 mL/kg (provides sodium phenylacetate 250 mg/kg, sodium benzoate 250 mg/kg, and arginine hydrochloride 600 mg/kg)

(Continued)

## sodium phenylacetate and sodium benzoate *(Continued)*

**Note:** Pending a specific diagnosis in infants, the bolus and maintenance dose of arginine should be 6 mL/kg. If ASS or ASL are excluded as diagnostic possibilities, reduce dose of arginine to 2 mL/kg/day.
>20 kg:
CPS and OTC deficiency: Ammonul® 55 mL/m$^2$ and arginine 10% 2 mL/kg (provides sodium phenylacetate 5.5 g/m$^2$, sodium benzoate 5.5 g/m$^2$, and arginine hydrochloride 200 mg/kg)
ASS and ASL deficiency: Ammonul® 55 mL/m$^2$ and arginine 10% 6 mL/kg (provides sodium phenylacetate 5.5 g/m$^2$, sodium benzoate 5.5 g/m$^2$, and arginine hydrochloride 600 mg/kg)

**Dosage Forms** Injection, solution: Sodium phenylacetate 100 mg and sodium benzoate 100 mg per mL (50 mL)

## sodium phenylbutyrate (SOW dee um fen il BYOO ti rate)

**Synonyms** ammonapse
**U.S./Canadian Brand Names** Buphenyl® [US]
**Therapeutic Category** Miscellaneous Product
**Use Orphan drug:** Adjunctive therapy in the chronic management of patients with urea cycle disorder involving deficiencies of carbamoylphosphate synthetase, ornithine transcarbamylase, or argininosuccinic acid synthetase
**Usual Dosage** Oral:
Powder: Patients weighing <20 kg: 450-600 mg/kg/day or 9.9-13 g/m$^2$/day, administered in equally divided amounts with each meal or feeding, four to six times daily; safety and efficacy of doses >20 g/day has not been established
Tablet: Children >20 kg and Adults: 450-600 mg/kg/day or 9.9-13 g/m$^2$/day, administered in equally divided amounts with each meal; safety and efficacy of doses >20 g/day have not been established
**Dosage Forms**
Powder, for oral solution: 3 g/level teaspoon (250 g) [contains sodium 125 mg/g; packaged with measuring device]
Tablet: 500 mg [contains sodium 124 mg/g]

## sodium phosphate and potassium phosphate *see* potassium phosphate and sodium phosphate *on page 667*

## sodium phosphates (SOW dee um FOS fates)

**U.S./Canadian Brand Names** Fleet Enema® [Can]; Fleet® Accu-Prep® [US-OTC]; Fleet® Enema [US-OTC]; Fleet® Phospho-Soda® Oral Laxative [Can]; Fleet® Phospho-Soda® [US-OTC]; Visicol® [US]
**Therapeutic Category** Electrolyte Supplement, Oral; Laxative
**Use**
Oral, rectal: Short-term treatment of constipation and to evacuate the colon for rectal and bowel exams
I.V.: Source of phosphate in large volume I.V. fluids and parenteral nutrition; treatment and prevention of hypophosphatemia
**Usual Dosage**
Normal requirements elemental phosphorus: Oral:
0-6 months: Adequate intake: 100 mg/day
6-12 months: Adequate intake: 275 mg/day
1-3 years: RDA: 460 mg
4-8 years: RDA: 500 mg
9-18 years: RDA: 1250 mg
≥19 years: RDA: 700 mg

**Hypophosphatemia:** It is difficult to provide concrete guidelines for the treatment of severe hypophosphatemia because the extent of total body deficits and response to therapy are difficult to predict. Aggressive doses of phosphate may result in a transient serum elevation followed by redistribution into intracellular compartments or bone tissue. Intermittent I.V. infusion should be reserved for severe depletion situations (<1 mg/dL in adults); large doses of oral phosphate may cause diarrhea and intestinal absorption may be unreliable. I.V. solutions should be infused slowly. Use caution when mixing with calcium and magnesium, precipitate may form. The following dosages are empiric guidelines. **Note:** 1 mmol phosphate = 31 mg phosphorus; 1 mg phosphorus = 0.032 mmol phosphate

Hypophosphatemia treatment: Doses listed as mmol of phosphate:
Intermittent I.V. infusion: Acute repletion or replacement:
Children:
Low dose: 0.08 mmol/kg over 6 hours; use if losses are recent and uncomplicated

Intermediate dose: 0.16-0.24 mmol/kg over 4-6 hours; use if serum phosphorus level 0.5-1 mg/dL
High dose: 0.36 mmol/kg over 6 hours; use if serum phosphorus <0.5 mg/dL
Adults: Varying dosages: 0.15-0.3 mmol/kg/dose over 12 hours; may repeat as needed to achieve desired serum level **or**
15 mmol/dose over 2 hours; use if serum phosphorus <2 mg/dL **or**
Low dose: 0.16 mmol/kg over 4-6 hours; use if serum phosphorus level 2.3-3 mg/dL
Intermediate dose: 0.32 mmol/kg over 4-6 hours; use if serum phosphorus level 1.6-2.2 mg/dL
High dose: 0.64 mmol/kg over 8-12 hours; use if serum phosphorus <1.5 mg/dL
Oral: Adults: 0.5-1 g elemental phosphorus 2-3 times/day may be used when serum phosphorus level is 1-2.5 mg/dL
Maintenance: Doses listed as mmol of phosphate:
Children:
Oral: 2-3 mmol/kg/day in divided doses
I.V.: 0.5-1.5 mmol/kg/day
Adults:
Oral: 50-150 mmol/day in divided doses
I.V.: 50-70 mmol/day

**Laxative (Fleet®):** Rectal:
Children 2-<5 years: One-half contents of one 2.25 oz pediatric enema
Children 5-12 years: Contents of one 2.25 oz pediatric enema, may repeat
Children ≥12 years and Adults: Contents of one 4.5 oz enema as a single dose, may repeat

**Laxative (Fleet® Phospho-Soda®):** Oral: Take on an empty stomach; dilute dose with 4 ounces cool water, then follow dose with 8 ounces water; **do not repeat dose within 24 hours**
Children 5-9 years: 5-10 mL as a single dose
Children 10-12 years: 10-20 mL as a single dose
Children ≥12 years and Adults: 20-45 mL as a single dose

**Bowel cleansing prior to colonoscopy:** Adults:
Fleet® Phospho-Soda® Accu-Prep™: Oral: Prior to procedure (timing of doses determined by prescriber): One dose is equal to 45 mL (2 doses are recommended): Each dose is diluted as follows:
Mix 45 mL with 120 mL clear liquid; drink, then follow with at least 240 mL of clear liquid; **or**
Mix 15 mL with 240 mL clear liquid; drink, then follow with 240 mL clear liquid; repeat every 10 minutes for a total of 45 mL
Visicol™: Oral: Adults: A total of 40 tablets divided as follows:
Evening before colonoscopy: 3 tablets every 15 minutes for 6 doses, then 2 additional tablets in 15 minutes (total of 20 tablets)
3-5 hours prior to colonoscopy: 3 tablets every 15 minutes for 6 doses, then 2 additional tablets in 15 minutes (total of 20 tablets)
**Note:** Each dose should be taken with a minimum of 8 ounces of clear liquids. Do not repeat treatment within 7 days. Do not use additional agents, especially sodium phosphate products.

## Dosage Forms
Kit (Fleet® Accu-Prep®):
Solution, oral (Fleet® Phosph-Soda®): Monobasic sodium phosphate monohydrate 2.4 g and dibasic sodium phosphate heptahydrate 0.9 g per 5 mL (15 mL) [contains sodium benzoate; kit contains six 15 mL unit-dose containers (equal to two 45 mL doses)]
Pads, anorectal (Fleet® Relief™): Pramoxine hydrochloride 1% and glycerin 12% (4s)
Injection, solution [preservative free]: Phosphorus 3 mmol and sodium 4 mEq per mL (5 mL, 15 mL, 50 mL)
Solution, oral (Fleet® Phospho-Soda®): Monobasic sodium phosphate monohydrate 2.4 g and dibasic sodium phosphate heptahydrate 0.9 g per 5 mL (45 mL, 90 mL) [contains sodium benzoate; unflavored or ginger-lemon flavor]
Solution, rectal [enema]: Monobasic sodium phosphate 19 g and dibasic sodium phosphate 7 g per 118 mL delivered dose (135 mL)
Fleet® Enema: Monobasic sodium phosphate 19 g and dibasic sodium phosphate 7 g per 118 mL delivered dose (135 mL)
Fleet® Enema for Children: Monobasic sodium phosphate 9.5 g and dibasic sodium phosphate 3.5 g per 59 mL delivered dose (68 mL)
Tablet, oral (Visicol®): Sodium phosphate monobasic monohydrate 1.102 g and sodium phosphate dibasic anhydrous 0.398 g [1.5 g total sodium phosphate per tablet]

# sodium polystyrene sulfonate (SOW dee um pol ee STYE reen SUL fon ate)

**Sound-Alike/Look-Alike Issues**
Kayexalate® may be confused with Kaopectate®

**U.S./Canadian Brand Names** Kayexalate® [US/Can]; Kionex™ [US]; PMS-Sodium Polystyrene Sulfonate [Can]; SPS® [US]

**Therapeutic Category** Antidote

**Use** Treatment of hyperkalemia

**Usual Dosage**
Children:
Oral: 1 g/kg/dose every 6 hours
Rectal: 1 g/kg/dose every 2-6 hours (In small children and infants, employ lower doses by using the practical exchange ratio of 1 mEq K⁺/g of resin as the basis for calculation)
Adults: Hyperkalemia:
Oral: 15 g (60 mL) 1-4 times/day
Rectal: 30-50 g every 6 hours

**Dosage Forms**
Powder for suspension, oral/rectal:
Kayexalate®: 15 g/4 level teaspoons (480 g) [contains sodium 100 mg (4.1 mEq)/g]
Kionex™: 15 g/4 level teaspoons (454 g) [contains sodium 100 mg (4.1 mEq)/g]
Suspension, oral/rectal: 15 g/60 mL (60 mL, 120 mL, 200 mL, 500 mL) [contains sodium 1500 mg (65 mEq)/60 mL, sorbitol, and alcohol 0.1%; cherry/caramel flavor]
SPS®: 15 g/60 mL (60 mL, 120 mL, 480 mL) [contains alcohol 0.3%, sodium 1500 mg (65 mEq)/60 mL, and sorbitol; cherry flavor]

# sodium salicylate (SOW dee um sa LIS i late)

**Therapeutic Category** Analgesic, Nonnarcotic; Antipyretic

**Use** Treatment of minor pain or fever; arthritis

**Usual Dosage** Adults: Oral: 325-650 mg every 4 hours

**Dosage Forms** Tablet, enteric coated: 325 mg, 650 mg

**sodium sulfacetamide** *see* sulfacetamide *on page 771*

**sodium sulfacetamide and sulfur** *see* sulfur and sulfacetamide *on page 776*

# sodium tetradecyl

**Synonyms** sodium tetradecyl sulfate

**U.S./Canadian Brand Names** Sotradecol® [US]; Trombovar® [Can]

**Therapeutic Category** Sclerosing Agent

**Use** Treatment of small, uncomplicated varicose veins of the lower extremities

**Usual Dosage** I.V.: Test dose: 0.5 mL given several hours prior to administration of larger dose; 0.5-2 mL (preferred maximum: 1 mL) in each vein, maximum: 10 mL per treatment session; 3% solution reserved for large varices

**Dosage Forms** Injection, as sulfate: 1% [10 mg/mL] (2 mL) [contains benzyl alcohol]; 3% [30 mg/mL] (2 mL) [contains benzyl alcohol]

**sodium tetradecyl sulfate** *see* sodium tetradecyl *on this page*

# sodium thiosulfate (SOW dee um thye oh SUL fate)

**Synonyms** disodium thiosulfate pentahydrate; pentahydrate; sodium hyposulfate; sodium thiosulphate; thiosulfuric acid disodium salt

**U.S./Canadian Brand Names** Versiclear™ [US]

**Therapeutic Category** Antidote; Antifungal Agent

**Use**
Parenteral: Used alone or with sodium nitrite or amyl nitrite in cyanide poisoning; reduce the risk of nephrotoxicity associated with cisplatin therapy
Topical: Treatment of tinea versicolor

**Usual Dosage**
Cyanide and nitroprusside antidote: I.V.:
Children <25 kg: 50 mg/kg after receiving 4.5-10 mg/kg sodium nitrite; a half dose of each may be repeated if necessary

Children >25 kg and Adults: 12.5 g after 300 mg of sodium nitrite; a half dose of each may be repeated if necessary

Cyanide poisoning: I.V.: Dose should be based on determination as with nitrite, at rate of 2.5-5 mL/minute to maximum of 50 mL.

Cisplatin rescue should be given before or during cisplatin administration: I.V. infusion (in sterile water): 12 g/m$^2$ over 6 hours or 9 g/m$^2$ I.V. push followed by 1.2 g/m$^2$ continuous infusion for 6 hours

Arsenic poisoning: I.V.: 1 mL first day, 2 mL second day, 3 mL third day, 4 mL fourth day, 5 mL on alternate days thereafter

Children and Adults: Topical: 20% to 25% solution: Apply a thin layer to affected areas twice daily

**Dosage Forms**

Injection, solution [preservative free]: 100 mg/mL (10 mL); 250 mg/mL (50 mL)

Lotion: Sodium thiosulfate 25% and salicylic acid 1% (120 mL) [contains isopropyl alcohol 10%]

**sodium thiosulfate, sodium nitrite, and amyl nitrite** *see* sodium nitrite, sodium thiosulfate, and amyl nitrite *on page 755*

**sodium thiosulphate** *see* sodium thiosulfate *on previous page*

**Soflax**ᴵᴹ **[Can]** *see* docusate *on page 263*

**Sofra-Tulle**® **[Can]** *see* framycetin *(Canada only) on page 362*

**Soft Plug**® **[US]** *see* collagen implants *on page 206*

**Solagé**ᵀᴹ **[US/Can]** *see* mequinol and tretinoin *on page 514*

**Solaquin**® **[US-OTC/Can]** *see* hydroquinone *on page 420*

**Solaquin Forte**® **[US/Can]** *see* hydroquinone *on page 420*

**Solaraze**ᵀᴹ **[US]** *see* diclofenac *on page 243*

**Solarcaine**® **[US-OTC]** *see* benzocaine *on page 95*

**Solarcaine**® **Aloe Extra Burn Relief [US-OTC]** *see* lidocaine *on page 479*

**Solfoton**® *(Discontinued) see* phenobarbital *on page 638*

**Solia**ᵀᴹ **[US]** *see* ethinyl estradiol and desogestrel *on page 309*

## solifenacin (sol i FEN a sin)

**Synonyms** solifenacin succinate

**U.S./Canadian Brand Names** VESIcare® [US]

**Therapeutic Category** Anticholinergic Agent

**Use** Treatment of overactive bladder with symptoms of urinary frequency, urgency, or urge incontinence

**Usual Dosage** Oral:

Children: Use is not recommended.

Adults: 5 mg/day; if tolerated, may increase to 10 mg/day

**Dosage Forms** Tablet: 5 mg, 10 mg

**solifenacin succinate** *see* solifenacin *on this page*

**soluble fluorescein** *see* fluorescein sodium *on page 346*

**Solu-Cortef**® **[US/Can]** *see* hydrocortisone (systemic) *on page 416*

**Solugel**® **[Can]** *see* benzoyl peroxide *on page 98*

**Solu-Medrol**® **[US/Can]** *see* methylprednisolone *on page 531*

**Soluver**® **[Can]** *see* salicylic acid *on page 734*

**Soluver**® **Plus [Can]** *see* salicylic acid *on page 734*

**Soluvite-F [US]** *see* vitamins (multiple/pediatric) *on page 852*

**Soma**® **[US/Can]** *see* carisoprodol *on page 148*

**Soma**® **Compound [US]** *see* carisoprodol and aspirin *on page 148*

**Soma**® **Compound w/Codeine [US]** *see* carisoprodol, aspirin, and codeine *on page 149*

# somatostatin *(Canada only)* (soe mat oh STA tin)

**U.S./Canadian Brand Names** Stilamin® [Can]

**Therapeutic Category** Variceal Bleeding (Acute) Agent

**Use** For the symptomatic treatment of acute bleeding from esophageal varices. Other treatment options for long-term management of the condition may be considered if necessary, once initial control has been established.

**Usual Dosage** Slow 250 mcg I.V. bolus injection over 3 to 5 minutes, followed by a continuous infusion at a rate of 250 mcg/hour until bleeding from the varices has stopped (usually within 12 to 24 hours). Once bleeding has been controlled, it is recommended that the infusion be continued for at least another 48 to 72 hours, or out to a maximum of 120 hours to prevent recurrent bleeding.

**Dosage Forms** Injection: 250 mcg, 3 mg

**somatrem** *see* somatropin *on this page*

# somatropin (soe ma TROE pin)

**Sound-Alike/Look-Alike Issues**

somatropin may be confused with somatrem, sumatriptan

somatrem may be confused with somatropin

**Synonyms** human growth hormone; somatrem

**U.S./Canadian Brand Names** Genotropin Miniquick® [US]; Genotropin® [US]; Humatrope® [US/Can]; Norditropin® NordiFlex® [US]; Norditropin® [US]; Nutropin AQ® [US]; Nutropine® [Can]; Nutropin® AQ [Can]; Nutropin® [US]; Saizen® [US/Can]; Serostim® [US/Can]; Tev-Tropin™ [US]; Zorbtive™ [US]

**Therapeutic Category** Growth Hormone

**Use**

Children:

Long-term treatment of growth failure due to inadequate endogenous growth hormone secretion (Genotropin®, Humatrope®, Norditropin®, Nutropin®, Nutropin AQ®, Saizen®, Tev-Tropin™)

Long-term treatment of short stature associated with Turner syndrome (Humatrope®, Nutropin®, Nutropin AQ®)

Treatment of Prader-Willi syndrome (Genotropin®)

Treatment of growth failure associated with chronic renal insufficiency (CRI) up until the time of renal transplantation (Nutropin®, Nutropin AQ®)

Long-term treatment of growth failure in children born small for gestational age who fail to manifest catch-up growth by 2 years of age (Genotropin®)

Long-term treatment of idiopathic short stature (nongrowth hormone-deficient short stature) defined by height standard deviation score (SDS) less than or equal to -2.25 and growth rate not likely to attain normal adult height (Humatrope®, Nutropin®, Nutropin AQ®)

Adults:

AIDS-wasting or cachexia with concomitant antiviral therapy (Serostim®)

Replacement of endogenous growth hormone in patients with adult growth hormone deficiency who meet both of the following criteria (Genotropin®, Humatrope®, Norditropin®, Nutropin®, Nutropin AQ®, Saizen®):

Biochemical diagnosis of adult growth hormone deficiency by means of a subnormal response to a standard growth hormone stimulation test (peak growth hormone ≤5 mcg/L)

**and**

Adult-onset: Patients who have adult growth hormone deficiency whether alone or with multiple hormone deficiencies (hypopituitarism) as a result of pituitary disease, hypothalamic disease, surgery, radiation therapy, or trauma

**or**

Childhood-onset: Patients who were growth hormone deficient during childhood, confirmed as an adult before replacement therapy is initiated

Treatment of short-bowel syndrome (Zorbtive™)

**Usual Dosage**

**Children (individualize dose):**

**Growth hormone deficiency:**

Genotropin®: SubQ: Weekly dosage: 0.16-0.24 mg/kg divided into 6-7 doses

Humatrope®: I.M., SubQ: Weekly dosage: 0.18 mg/kg; maximum replacement dose: 0.3 mg/kg/week; dosing should be divided into equal doses given 3 times/week on alternating days, 6 times/week, or daily

Norditropin®: SubQ: 0.024-0.034 mg/kg/day, 6-7 times/week

Nutropin®, Nutropin® AQ: SubQ: Weekly dosage: 0.3 mg/kg divided into daily doses; pubertal patients: ≤0.7 mg/kg/week divided daily

Tev-Tropin™: SubQ: Up to 0.1 mg/kg administered 3 times/week

Saizen®: I.M., SubQ: 0.06 mg/kg/dose administered 3 times/week

**Note:** Therapy should be discontinued when patient has reached satisfactory adult height, when epiphyses have fused, or when the patient ceases to respond. Growth of 5 cm/year or more is expected, if growth rate does not exceed 2.5 cm in a 6-month period, double the dose for the next 6 months; if there is still no satisfactory response, discontinue therapy

**Chronic renal insufficiency (CRI):** Nutropin®, Nutropin® AQ: SubQ: Weekly dosage: 0.35 mg/kg divided into daily injections; continue until the time of renal transplantation

Dosage recommendations in patients treated for CRI who require dialysis:

Hemodialysis: Administer dose at night prior to bedtime or at least 3-4 hours after hemodialysis to prevent hematoma formation from heparin

CCPD: Administer dose in the morning following dialysis

CAPD: Administer dose in the evening at the time of overnight exchange

**Turner syndrome:** Humatrope®, Nutropin®, Nutropin® AQ: SubQ: Weekly dosage: ≤0.375 mg/kg divided into equal doses 3-7 times per week

**Prader-Willi syndrome:** Genotropin®: SubQ: Weekly dosage: 0.24 mg/kg divided into 6-7 doses

**Small for gestational age:** Genotropin®: SubQ: Weekly dosage: 0.48 mg/kg divided into 6-7 doses

**Idiopathic short stature:**

Humatrope®: SubQ: Weekly dosage: 0.37 mg/kg divided into equal doses 6-7 times per week

Nutropin®, Nutropin AQ®: SubQ: Weekly dosage: Up to 0.3 mg/kg divided into daily doses

## Adults:

**Growth hormone deficiency:** To minimize adverse events in older or overweight patients, reduced dosages may be necessary. During therapy, dosage should be decreased if required by the occurrence of side effects or excessive IGF-I levels.

Norditropin®: SubQ: Initial dose ≤0.004 mg/kg/day; after 6 weeks of therapy, may increase dose to 0.016 mg/kg/day

Nutropin®, Nutropin® AQ: SubQ: ≤0.006 mg/kg/day; dose may be increased according to individual requirements, up to a maximum of 0.025 mg/kg/day in patients <35 years of age, or up to a maximum of 0.0125 mg/kg/day in patients ≥35 years of age

Humatrope®: SubQ: ≤0.006 mg/kg/day; dose may be increased according to individual requirements, up to a maximum of 0.0125 mg/kg/day

Genotropin®: SubQ: Weekly dosage: ≤0.04 mg/kg divided into 6-7 doses; dose may be increased at 4- to 8-week intervals according to individual requirements, to a maximum of 0.08 mg/kg/week

Saizen®: SubQ: ≤0.005 mg/kg/day; dose may be increased to not more than 0.01 mg/kg/day after 4 weeks, based on individual requirements.

**AIDS-wasting or cachexia:**

Serostim®: SubQ: Dose should be given once daily at bedtime; patients who continue to lose weight after 2 weeks should be re-evaluated for opportunistic infections or other clinical events; rotate injection sites to avoid lipodystrophy

Daily dose based on body weight:

<35 kg: 0.1 mg/kg

35-45 kg: 4 mg

45-55 kg: 5 mg

>55 kg: 6 mg

**Short-bowel syndrome** (Zorbtive™): SubQ: 0.1 mg/kg once daily for 4 weeks (maximum: 8 mg/day)

Fluid retention (moderate) or arthralgias: Treat symptomatically or reduce dose by 50%

Severe toxicity: Discontinue therapy for up to 5 days; when symptoms resolve, restart at 50% of dose. If severe toxicity recurs or does not disappear within 5 days after discontinuation, permanently discontinue treatment.

Dosage Forms [DSC] = Discontinued product

Injection, powder for reconstitution [rDNA origin]:

Genotropin® [preservative free]: 1.5 mg [4 int. units/mL] [delivers 1.3 mg/mL] [DSC]

Genotropin® [with preservative]:

5.8 mg [15 int. units/mL] [delivers 5 mg/mL]

13.8 mg [36 int. units/mL] [delivers 12 mg/mL]

Genotropin Miniquick® [preservative free]: 0.2 mg, 0.4 mg, 0.6 mg, 0.8 mg, 1 mg, 1.2 mg, 1.4 mg, 1.6 mg, 1.8 mg, 2 mg [each strength delivers 0.25 mL]

Humatrope®: 5 mg [~15 int. units], 6 mg [18 int. units], 12 mg [36 int. units], 24 mg [72 int. units]

Nutropin® [diluent contains benzyl alcohol]: 5 mg [~15 int. units]; 10 mg [~30 int. units]

Tev-Tropin™: 5 mg [15 int. units/mL] [diluent contains benzyl alcohol]

(Continued)

# somatropin *(Continued)*

Saizen® [diluent contains benzyl alcohol]: 5 mg [~15 int. units; contains sucrose 34.2 mg]; 8.8 mg [~26.4 int. units; contains sucrose 60.2 mg]

Serostim®: 4 mg [12 int. units; contains sucrose 27.3 mg]; 5 mg [15 int. units; contains sucrose 34.2 mg]; 6 mg [18 int. units; contains sucrose 41 mg]

Zorbtive™: 8.8 mg [~26.4 int. units; contains sucrose 60.19 mg; packaged with diluent containing benzyl alcohol]

Injection, solution [rDNA origin]:

Norditropin®: 5 mg/1.5 mL (1.5 mL); 15 mg/1.5 mL (1.5 mL) [cartridge]

Norditropin® NordiFlex®: 5 mg/1.5 mL (1.5 mL); 15 mg/1.5 mL (1.5 mL) [prefilled pen]

Nutropin AQ®: 5 mg/mL [~15 int. units/mL] (2 mL) [vial or cartridge]

**Somavert® [US]** *see* pegvisomant *on page 625*

**Sominex® [US-OTC]** *see* diphenhydramine *on page 254*

**Sominex® Maximum Strength [US-OTC]** *see* diphenhydramine *on page 254*

**Somnote™ [US]** *see* chloral hydrate *on page 166*

**Sonata® [US/Can]** *see* zaleplon *on page 857*

# sorbitol *(SOR bi tole)*

**Therapeutic Category** Genitourinary Irrigant; Laxative

**Use** Genitourinary irrigant in transurethral prostatic resection or other transurethral resection or other transurethral surgical procedures; diuretic; humectant; sweetening agent; hyperosmotic laxative; facilitate the passage of sodium polystyrene sulfonate through the intestinal tract

**Usual Dosage** Hyperosmotic laxative (as single dose, at infrequent intervals):

Children 2-11 years:

Oral: 2 mL/kg (as 70% solution)

Rectal enema: 30-60 mL as 25% to 30% solution

Children >12 years and Adults:

Oral: 30-150 mL (as 70% solution)

Rectal enema: 120 mL as 25% to 30% solution

Adjunct to sodium polystyrene sulfonate: 15 mL as 70% solution orally until diarrhea occurs (10-20 mL/2 hours) or 20-100 mL as an oral vehicle for the sodium polystyrene sulfonate resin

When administered with charcoal:

Oral:

Children: 4.3 mL/kg of 35% sorbitol with 1 g/kg of activated charcoal

Adults: 4.3 mL/kg of 70% sorbitol with 1 g/kg of activated charcoal every 4 hours until first stool containing charcoal is passed

Topical: 3% to 3.3% as transurethral surgical procedure irrigation

**Dosage Forms**

Solution, genitourinary irrigation: 3% (3000 mL, 5000 mL); 3.3% (2000 mL, 4000 mL)

Solution, oral: 70% (30 mL, 480 mL, 3840 mL)

**Sorbitrate® *(Discontinued)*** *see* isosorbide dinitrate *on page 451*

**Soriatane® [US/Can]** *see* acitretin *on page 15*

**Sorine® [US]** *see* sotalol *on this page*

**Sotacor® [Can]** *see* sotalol *on this page*

# sotalol *(SOE ta lole)*

**Sound-Alike/Look-Alike Issues**

sotalol may be confused with Stadol®

Betapace® may be confused with Betapace AF®

Betapace AF® may be confused with Betapace®

**Synonyms** sotalol hydrochloride

**U.S./Canadian Brand Names** Alti-Sotalol [Can]; Apo-Sotalol® [Can]; Betapace AF® [US/Can]; Betapace® [US]; Gen-Sotalol [Can]; Lin-Sotalol [Can]; Novo-Sotalol [Can]; Nu-Sotalol [Can]; PMS-Sotalol [Can]; Rho®-Sotalol [Can]; Sorine® [US]; Sotacor® [Can]

**Therapeutic Category** Antiarrhythmic Agent, Class II; Antiarrhythmic Agent, Class III; Beta-Adrenergic Blocker, Nonselective

**Use** Treatment of documented ventricular arrhythmias (ie, sustained ventricular tachycardia), that in the judgment of the physician are life-threatening; maintenance of normal sinus rhythm in patients with symptomatic atrial fibrillation and atrial flutter who are currently in sinus rhythm. Manufacturer states substitutions should not be made for Betapace AF® since Betapace AF® is distributed with a patient package insert specific for atrial fibrillation/flutter.

**Usual Dosage** Sotalol should be initiated and doses increased in a hospital with facilities for cardiac rhythm monitoring and assessment. Proarrhythmic events can occur after initiation of therapy and with each upward dosage adjustment.

Children: Oral: The safety and efficacy of sotalol in children have not been established
**Note:** Dosing per manufacturer, based on pediatric pharmacokinetic data; wait at least 36 hours between dosage adjustments to allow monitoring of QT intervals
≤2 years: Dosage should be adjusted (decreased) by plotting of the child's age on a logarithmic scale; refer to manufacturer's package labeling.
>2 years: Initial: 90 mg/m$^2$/day in 3 divided doses; may be incrementally increased to a maximum of 180 mg/m$^2$/day
Adults: Oral:
Ventricular arrhythmias (Betapace®, Sorine®):
Initial: 80 mg twice daily
Dose may be increased gradually to 240-320 mg/day; allow 3 days between dosing increments in order to attain steady-state plasma concentrations and to allow monitoring of QT intervals
Most patients respond to a total daily dose of 160-320 mg/day in 2-3 divided doses.
Some patients, with life-threatening refractory ventricular arrhythmias, may require doses as high as 480-640 mg/day; however, these doses should only be prescribed when the potential benefit outweighs the increased of adverse events.
Atrial fibrillation or atrial flutter (Betapace AF®): Initial: 80 mg twice daily
If the initial dose does not reduce the frequency of relapses of atrial fibrillation/flutter and is tolerated without excessive QT prolongation (not >520 msec) after 3 days, the dose may be increased to 120 mg twice daily. This may be further increased to 160 mg twice daily if response is inadequate and QT prolongation is not excessive.

**Dosage Forms**
Tablet, as hydrochloride: 80 mg, 80 mg [AF], 120 mg, 120 mg [AF], 160 mg, 160 mg [AF], 240 mg
Betapace® [light blue]: 80 mg, 120 mg, 160 mg, 240 mg
Betapace AF® [white]: 80 mg, 120 mg, 160 mg
Sorine® [white]: 80 mg, 120 mg, 160 mg, 240 mg

**sotalol hydrochloride** *see* sotalol *on previous page*

**Sotradecol® [US]** *see* sodium tetradecyl *on page 758*

**Sotret® [US]** *see* isotretinoin *on page 452*

**Soyacal® *(Discontinued)*** *see* fat emulsion *on page 328*

**Soyalac® [US-OTC]** *see* nutritional formula, enteral/oral *on page 591*

**SPA** *see* albumin *on page 22*

**Spacol *(Discontinued)*** *see* hyoscyamine *on page 424*

**Spacol T/S *(Discontinued)*** *see* hyoscyamine *on page 424*

**Span-FF® *(Discontinued)*** *see* ferrous fumarate *on page 334*

## sparfloxacin (spar FLOKS a sin)
**Sound-Alike/Look-Alike Issues**
Zagam® may be confused with Zyban®
**Therapeutic Category** Quinolone
**Use** Treatment of adults with community-acquired pneumonia caused by *C. pneumoniae*, *H. influenzae*, *H. parainfluenzae*, *M. catarrhalis*, *M. pneumoniae* or *S. pneumoniae*; treatment of acute bacterial exacerbations of chronic bronchitis caused by *C. pneumoniae*, *E. cloacae*, *H. influenzae*, *H. parainfluenzae*, *K. pneumoniae*, *M. catarrhalis*, *S. aureus* or *S. pneumoniae*
**Usual Dosage** Adults: Oral:
Loading dose: 400 mg on day 1
Maintenance: 200 mg/day for 10 days total therapy
**Dosage Forms** [DSC] = Discontinued product
Tablet [film coated]: 200 mg [DSC]

**Spasmolin**® *(Discontinued)* *see* hyoscyamine, atropine, scopolamine, and phenobarbital *on page 425*

**SPD417** *see* carbamazepine *on page 140*

**Spectazole**® **[US/Can]** *see* econazole *on page 278*

**Spec-T**® *(Discontinued)* *see* benzocaine *on page 95*

## spectinomycin (spek ti noe MYE sin)
**Sound-Alike/Look-Alike Issues**
Trobicin® may be confused with tobramycin
**Synonyms** spectinomycin hydrochloride
**U.S./Canadian Brand Names** Trobicin® [US]
**Therapeutic Category** Antibiotic, Miscellaneous
**Use** Treatment of uncomplicated gonorrhea
**Usual Dosage** I.M.:
Children:
<45 kg: 40 mg/kg/dose 1 time (ceftriaxone preferred)
≥45 kg: Refer to adult dosing.
Children >8 years who are allergic to PCNS/cephalosporins may be treated with oral tetracycline
Adults:
Uncomplicated urethral, cervical, pharyngeal, or rectal gonorrhea: 2 g deep I.M. or 4 g where antibiotic resistance is prevalent 1 time; 4 g (10 mL) dose should be given as two 5 mL injections, followed by adequate chlamydial treatment (doxycycline 100 mg twice daily for 7 days)
Disseminated gonococcal infection: 2 g every 12 hours
**Dosage Forms** Injection, powder for reconstitution, as hydrochloride: 2 g [diluent contains benzyl alcohol]

**spectinomycin hydrochloride** *see* spectinomycin *on this page*

**Spectracef**™ **[US]** *see* cefditoren *on page 153*

## spiramycin *(Canada only)* (speer a MYE sin)
**U.S./Canadian Brand Names** Rovamycine® [Can]
**Therapeutic Category** Antibiotic, Macrolide
**Use** Treatment of infections of the respiratory tract, buccal cavity, skin and soft tissues due to susceptible organisms. *N. gonorrhoeae*: as an alternate choice of treatment for gonorrhea in patients allergic to the penicillins. Before treatment of gonorrhea, the possibility of concomitant infection due to *T. pallidum* should be excluded.
**Usual Dosage** Oral:
Children: Dosage by body weight; usual dosage 150,000 int. units/kg; expressed as the number of 750,000 int. unit (Rovamycine® "250") capsules per day. Daily dose should be administered in 2-3 divided doses.
15 kg = 3 capsules per day
20 kg = 4 capsules per day
30 kg = 6 capsules per day
**Note:** In severe infections, dosage may be increased by 50%.
Adults:
Mild to moderate infections: 6,000,000 to 9,000,000 int. units (4-6 capsules of Rovamycine® "500" per day) in 2 divided doses
Severe infections: 12,000,000 to 15,000,000 int. units (8-10 capsules of Rovamycine® "500" per day) in 2 divided doses
Gonorrhea: 12,000,000 to 13,500,000 int. units (8-9 capsules of Rovamycine® "500") as a single dose
**Dosage Forms** Capsule:
Rovamycine® "250": 750,000 int. units
Rovamycine® "500": 1,500,000 int. units

**Spiriva**® **[US/Can]** *see* tiotropium *on page 805*

**Spironazide**® *(Discontinued)* *see* hydrochlorothiazide and spironolactone *on page 410*

## spironolactone (speer on oh LAK tone)
**Sound-Alike/Look-Alike Issues**
Aldactone® may be confused with Aldactazide®

**U.S./Canadian Brand Names** Aldactone® [US/Can]; Novo-Spiroton [Can]

**Therapeutic Category** Diuretic, Potassium Sparing

**Use** Management of edema associated with excessive aldosterone excretion; hypertension; congestive heart failure; primary hyperaldosteronism; hypokalemia; treatment of hirsutism; cirrhosis of liver accompanied by edema or ascites

**Usual Dosage** To reduce delay in onset of effect, a loading dose of 2 or 3 times the daily dose may be administered on the first day of therapy. Oral: Adults:

Edema, hypokalemia: 25-200 mg/day in 1-2 divided doses

Hypertension (JNC 7): 25-50 mg/day in 1-2 divided doses

Diagnosis of primary aldosteronism: 100-400 mg/day in 1-2 divided doses

CHF, severe (with ACE inhibitor and a loop diuretic ± digoxin): 25 mg/day, increased or reduced depending on individual response and evidence of hyperkalemia

**Dosage Forms** Tablet: 25 mg, 50 mg, 100 mg

**spironolactone and hydrochlorothiazide** *see* hydrochlorothiazide and spironolactone *on page 410*

**Spirozide®** *(Discontinued)* *see* hydrochlorothiazide and spironolactone *on page 410*

**Sporanox®** **[US/Can]** *see* itraconazole *on page 453*

**Sportscreme®** **[US-OTC]** *see* triethanolamine salicylate *on page 823*

**Sprintec™** **[US]** *see* ethinyl estradiol and norgestimate *on page 317*

**SPS®** **[US]** *see* sodium polystyrene sulfonate *on page 758*

**SRC® Expectorant** *(Discontinued)* *see* hydrocodone, pseudoephedrine, and guaifenesin *on page 415*

**SSD®** **[US]** *see* silver sulfadiazine *on page 747*

**SSD® AF** **[US]** *see* silver sulfadiazine *on page 747*

**SSKI®** **[US]** *see* potassium iodide *on page 665*

**S.T. 37®** **[US-OTC]** *see* hexylresorcinol *on page 404*

**Stadol®** **[US]** *see* butorphanol *on page 126*

**Stadol® NS** *(Discontinued)* *see* butorphanol *on page 126*

**Stagesic®** **[US]** *see* hydrocodone and acetaminophen *on page 411*

**Stalevo™** **[US]** *see* levodopa, carbidopa, and entacapone *on page 475*

**Stan-gard®** **[US]** *see* fluoride *on page 347*

**stannous fluoride** *see* fluoride *on page 347*

**stanozolol** (stan OH zoe lole)

**U.S./Canadian Brand Names** Winstrol® [US]

**Therapeutic Category** Anabolic Steroid

**Controlled Substance** C-III

**Use** Prophylactic use against hereditary angioedema

**Usual Dosage**

Children: Acute attacks:

<6 years: 1 mg/day

6-12 years: 2 mg/day

Adults: Oral: Initial: 2 mg 3 times/day, may then reduce to a maintenance dose of 2 mg/day or 2 mg every other day after 1-3 months

**Dosage Forms** Tablet: 2 mg

**Starlix®** **[US/Can]** *see* nateglinide *on page 564*

**Starnoc®** **[Can]** *see* zaleplon *on page 857*

**Statex®** **[Can]** *see* morphine sulfate *on page 549*

**Staticin®** *(Discontinued)*

**Statobex®** **[Can]** *sec* phendimetrazine *on page 637*

**stavudine** (STAV yoo deen)

**Sound-Alike/Look-Alike Issues**

Zerit® may be confused with Ziac®

(Continued)

## stavudine *(Continued)*

**Synonyms** d4T
**U.S./Canadian Brand Names** Zerit® [US/Can]
**Therapeutic Category** Antiviral Agent
**Use** Treatment of HIV infection in combination with other antiretroviral agents
**Usual Dosage** Oral:
  Newborns (Birth to 13 days): 0.5 mg/kg every 12 hours
  Children:
   >14 days and <30 kg: 1 mg/kg every 12 hours
   ≥30 kg: Refer to Adults dosing
  Adults:
   ≥60 kg: 40 mg every 12 hours
   <60 kg: 30 mg every 12 hours
**Dosage Forms**
  Capsule: 15 mg, 20 mg, 30 mg, 40 mg
  Powder, for oral solution: 1 mg/mL (200 mL) [dye-free; fruit flavor]

**Stelazine®** *(Discontinued)* *see* trifluoperazine *on page 823*

**Stemetil®** **[Can]** *see* prochlorperazine *on page 680*

**Sterapred®** **[US]** *see* prednisone *on page 674*

**Sterapred®** **DS [US]** *see* prednisone *on page 674*

**STI571** *see* imatinib *on page 430*

**Stilamin®** **[Can]** *see* somatostatin *(Canada only) on page 760*

**Stimate™** **[US]** *see* desmopressin acetate *on page 230*

**Sting-Kill [US-OTC]** *see* benzocaine *on page 95*

**St. Joseph®** **Adult Aspirin [US-OTC]** *see* aspirin *on page 73*

**St. Joseph®** **Cough Suppressant** *(Discontinued)* *see* dextromethorphan *on page 238*

**St. Joseph®** **Measured Dose Nasal Solution** *(Discontinued)* *see* phenylephrine *on page 640*

**Stop®** **[US]** *see* fluoride *on page 347*

**Strattera®** **[US/Can]** *see* atomoxetine *on page 77*

**Streptase®** **[US/Can]** *see* streptokinase *on this page*

## streptokinase (strep toe KYE nase)

**Synonyms** SK
**U.S./Canadian Brand Names** Streptase® [US/Can]
**Therapeutic Category** Fibrinolytic Agent
**Use** Thrombolytic agent used in treatment of recent severe or massive deep vein thrombosis, pulmonary emboli, myocardial infarction, and occluded arteriovenous cannulas
**Usual Dosage** I.V.:
  Children: Safety and efficacy have not been not established. Limited studies have used 3500-4000 units/kg over 30 minutes followed by 1000-1500 units/kg/hour.
  Clotted catheter: I.V.: **Note:** Not recommended due to possibility of allergic reactions with repeated doses: 10,000-25,000 units diluted in NS to a final volume equivalent to catheter volume; instill into catheter and leave in place for 1 hour, then aspirate contents out of catheter and flush catheter with normal saline.
  Adults: Antibodies to streptokinase remain for at least 3-6 months after initial dose: Administration requires the use of an infusion pump.
  An intradermal skin test of 100 units has been suggested to predict allergic response to streptokinase. If a positive reaction is not seen after 15-20 minutes, a therapeutic dose may be administered.
  **Guidelines for acute myocardial infarction** (AMI): 1.5 million units over 60 minutes
  Administration:
   Dilute two 750,000 unit vials of streptokinase with 5 mL dextrose 5% in water ($D_5W$) each, gently swirl to dissolve.
   Add this dose of the 1.5 million units to 150 mL $D_5W$.
   This should be infused over 60 minutes; an in-line filter ≥0.45 micron should be used.

Monitor for the first few hours for signs of anaphylaxis or allergic reaction. **Infusion should be slowed if blood pressure falls by 25 mm Hg or terminated if asthmatic symptoms appear**.

Following completion of streptokinase, initiate heparin, if directed, when aPTT returns to less than 2 times the upper limit of control; do not use a bolus, but initiate infusion adjusted to a target aPTT of 1.5-2 times the upper limit of control. If prolonged (>48 hours) heparin is required, infusion may be switched to subcutaneous therapy.

**Guidelines for acute pulmonary embolism** (APE): 3 million unit dose over 24 hours

Administration:

Dilute four 750,000 unit vials of streptokinase with 5 mL dextrose 5% in water ($D_5W$) each, gently swirl to dissolve.

Add this dose of 3 million units to 250 mL $D_5W$, an in-line filter ≥0.45 micron should be used.

Administer 250,000 units (23 mL) over 30 minutes followed by 100,000 units/hour (9 mL/hour) for 24 hours.

Monitor for the first few hours for signs of anaphylaxis or allergic reaction. **Infusion should be slowed if blood pressure is lowered by 25 mm Hg or if asthmatic symptoms appear**.

Begin heparin 1000 units/hour about 3-4 hours after completion of streptokinase infusion or when PTT is <100 seconds.

Monitor PT, PTT, and fibrinogen levels during therapy.

Thromboses: 250,000 units to start, then 100,000 units/hour for 24-72 hours depending on location.

**Cannula occlusion:** 250,000 units into cannula, clamp for 2 hours, then aspirate contents and flush with normal saline

Dosage Forms [DSC] = Discontinued product

Injection, powder for reconstitution: 250,000 int. units; 750,000 int. units; 1,500,000 int. units [DSC]

# streptomycin (strep toe MYE sin)

**Sound-Alike/Look-Alike Issues**

streptomycin may be confused with streptozocin

**Synonyms** streptomycin sulfate

**Therapeutic Category** Antibiotic, Aminoglycoside; Antitubercular Agent

**Use** Part of combination therapy of active tuberculosis; used in combination with other agents for treatment of streptococcal or enterococcal endocarditis, mycobacterial infections, plague, tularemia, and brucellosis

**Usual Dosage**

Children:

Tuberculosis:

Daily therapy: 20-40 mg/kg/day (maximum: 1 g/day)

Directly observed therapy (DOT): Twice weekly: 20-40 mg/kg (maximum: 1 g)

DOT: 3 times/week: 25-30 mg/kg (maximum: 1 g)

Adults:

Tuberculosis:

Daily therapy: 15 mg/kg/day (maximum: 1 g)

Directly observed therapy (DOT): Twice weekly: 25-30 mg/kg (maximum: 1.5 g)

DOT: 3 times/week: 25-30 mg/kg (maximum: 1 g)

Enterococcal endocarditis: 1 g every 12 hours for 2 weeks, 500 mg every 12 hours for 4 weeks in combination with penicillin

Streptococcal endocarditis: 1 g every 12 hours for 1 week, 500 mg every 12 hours for 1 week

Tularemia: 1-2 g/day in divided doses for 7-10 days or until patient is afebrile for 5-7 days

Plague: 2-4 g/day in divided doses until the patient is afebrile for at least 3 days

**Dosage Forms** Injection, powder for reconstitution: 1 g

# streptomycin sulfate *see* streptomycin *on this page*

# streptozocin (strep toe ZOE sin)

**Sound-Alike/Look-Alike Issues**

streptozocin may be confused with streptomycin

**Synonyms** NSC-85998

**U.S./Canadian Brand Names** Zanosar® [US/Can]

**Therapeutic Category** Antineoplastic Agent

**Use** Treatment of metastatic islet cell carcinoma of the pancreas, carcinoid tumor and syndrome, Hodgkin's disease, palliative treatment of colorectal cancer

**Usual Dosage** I.V. (refer to individual protocols): Children and Adults:

Single agent therapy: 1-1.5 g/m$^2$ weekly for 6 weeks followed by a 4-week rest period

(Continued)

## streptozocin *(Continued)*

Combination therapy: 0.5-1 g/m$^2$ for 5 consecutive days followed by a 4- to 6-week rest period
**Dosage Forms** Injection, powder for reconstitution: 1 g

**Stresstabs® B-Complex [US-OTC]** *see* vitamin B complex combinations *on page 849*
**Stresstabs® B-Complex + Iron [US-OTC]** *see* vitamin B complex combinations *on page 849*
**Stresstabs® B-Complex + Zinc [US-OTC]** *see* vitamin B complex combinations *on page 849*
**Striant® [US]** *see* testosterone *on page 788*
**Stri-dex® [US-OTC]** *see* salicylic acid *on page 734*
**Stri-dex® Body Focus [US-OTC]** *see* salicylic acid *on page 734*
**Stri-dex® Facewipes To Go™ [US-OTC]** *see* salicylic acid *on page 734*
**Stri-dex® Maximum Strength [US-OTC]** *see* salicylic acid *on page 734*
**Strifon Forte® [Can]** *see* chlorzoxazone *on page 179*
**Stromectol® [US]** *see* ivermectin *on page 454*
**StrongStart™ [US]** *see* vitamins (multiple/prenatal) *on page 852*

## strontium-89 (STRON shee um atey nine)

**Synonyms** strontium-89 chloride
**U.S./Canadian Brand Names** Metastron® [US/Can]
**Therapeutic Category** Radiopharmaceutical
**Use** Relief of bone pain in patients with skeletal metastases
**Usual Dosage** Adults: I.V.: 148 megabecquerel (4 millicurie) administered by slow I.V. injection over 1-2 minutes or 1.5-2.2 megabecquerel (40-60 microcurie)/kg; repeated doses are generally not recommended at intervals <90 days; measure the patient dose by a suitable radioactivity calibration system immediately prior to administration
**Dosage Forms** Injection, solution, as chloride [preservative free]: 10.9-22.6 mg/mL [148 megabecquerel, 4 millicurie] (10 mL)

**strontium-89 chloride** *see* strontium-89 *on this page*
**Strovite® Forte [US]** *see* vitamins (multiple/oral) *on page 852*
**Stuartnatal® Plus 3™ [US-OTC]** *see* vitamins (multiple/prenatal) *on page 852*
**Stuart Prenatal® [US-OTC]** *see* vitamins (multiple/prenatal) *on page 852*
**Sublimaze® [US]** *see* fentanyl *on page 332*
**Suboxone® [US]** *see* buprenorphine and naloxone *on page 122*
**Subutex® [US/Can]** *see* buprenorphine *on page 121*

## succimer (SUKS si mer)

**Synonyms** DMSA
**U.S./Canadian Brand Names** Chemet® [US/Can]
**Therapeutic Category** Chelating Agent
**Use** Orphan drug: Treatment of lead poisoning in children with blood levels >45 mcg/dL. It is not indicated for prophylaxis of lead poisoning in a lead-containing environment. Following oral administration, succimer is generally well tolerated and produces a linear dose-dependent reduction in serum lead concentrations. This agent appears to offer advantages over existing lead chelating agents.
**Usual Dosage** Children and Adults: Oral: 10 mg/kg/dose every 8 hours for 5 days followed by 10 mg/kg/dose every 12 hours for 14 days
**Dosage Forms** Capsule: 100 mg

## succinylcholine (suks in il KOE leen)

**Synonyms** succinylcholine chloride; suxamethonium chloride
**U.S./Canadian Brand Names** Quelicin® [US/Can]
**Therapeutic Category** Skeletal Muscle Relaxant
**Use** Adjunct to general anesthesia to facilitate both rapid sequence and routine endotracheal intubation and to relax skeletal muscles during surgery; to reduce the intensity of muscle contractions of pharmacologically- or electrically-induced convulsions; does not relieve pain or produce sedation

**Usual Dosage** I.M., I.V.: Dose to effect; doses will vary due to interpatient variability; use ideal body weight for obese patients

I.M.: 2.5-4 mg/kg, total dose should not exceed 150 mg

I.V.:

Children: Initial: 1-2 mg/kg; maintenance: 0.3-0.6 mg/kg every 5-10 minutes as needed; because of the risk of malignant hyperthermia, use of continuous infusions is not recommended in infants and children

Adults: 1-1.5 mg/kg, up to 150 mg total dose

Maintenance: 0.04-0.07 mg/kg every 5-10 minutes as needed

Continuous infusion: 10-100 mcg/kg/minute (or 0.5-10 mg/minute); dilute to concentration of 1-2 mg/mL in $D_5W$ or NS

**Note:** Initial dose of succinylcholine must be increased when nondepolarizing agent pretreatment used because of the antagonism between succinylcholine and nondepolarizing neuromuscular blocking agents

**Dosage Forms** Injection, solution, as chloride: 20 mg/mL (5 mL, 10 mL); 50 mg/mL (10 mL); 100 mg/mL (10 mL)

**succinylcholine chloride** *see* succinylcholine *on previous page*

**Sucraid**® **[US/Can]** *see* sacrosidase *on page 734*

## sucralfate (soo KRAL fate)

**Sound-Alike/Look-Alike Issues**

sucralfate may be confused with salsalate

Carafate® may be confused with Cafergot®

**Synonyms** Aluminum Sucrose Sulfate, Basic

**U.S./Canadian Brand Names** Apo-Sucralate® [Can]; Carafate® [US]; Novo-Sucralate [Can]; Nu-Sucra-late [Can]; PMS-Sucralate [Can]; Sulcrate® Suspension Plus [Can]; Sulcrate® [Can]

**Therapeutic Category** Gastrointestinal Agent, Gastric or Duodenal Ulcer Treatment

**Use** Short-term management of duodenal ulcers; maintenance of duodenal ulcers

**Usual Dosage** Oral:

Children: Dose not established, doses of 40-80 mg/kg/day divided every 6 hours have been used

Adults:

Stress ulcer prophylaxis: 1 g 4 times/day

Stress ulcer treatment: 1 g every 4 hours

Duodenal ulcer:

Treatment: 1 g 4 times/day on an empty stomach and at bedtime for 4-8 weeks, or alternatively 2 g twice daily; treatment is recommended for 4-8 weeks in adults

Maintenance: Prophylaxis: 1 g twice daily

**Dosage Forms**

Suspension, oral: 1 g/10 mL (10 mL) [DSC]

Carafate®: 1 g/10 mL (420 mL)

Tablet (Carafate®): 1 g

**Sucrets**® **[US-OTC]** *see* dyclonine *on page 277*

**Sucrets**® **Cough Calmers** *(Discontinued)* *see* dextromethorphan *on page 238*

**Sucrets**® **Original [US-OTC]** *see* hexylresorcinol *on page 404*

**Sudafed**® **[US-OTC]** *see* pseudoephedrine *on page 692*

**Sudafed**® **12 Hour [US-OTC]** *see* pseudoephedrine *on page 692*

**Sudafed**® **24 Hour [US-OTC]** *see* pseudoephedrine *on page 692*

**Sudafed**® **Children's [US-OTC]** *see* pseudoephedrine *on page 692*

**Sudafed**® **Children's Cold & Cough [US-OTC]** *see* pseudoephedrine and dextromethorphan *on page 693*

**Sudafed**® **Cold & Cough Extra Strength [Can]** *see* acetaminophen, dextromethorphan, and pseudoephedrine *on page 11*

**Sudafed**® **Decongestant [Can]** *see* pseudoephedrine *on page 692*

**Sudafed**® **Head Cold and Sinus Extra Strength [Can]** *see* acetaminophen and pseudoephedrine *on page 8*

**Sudafed**® **Non-Drying Sinus [US-OTC]** *see* guaifenesin and pseudoephedrine *on page 388*

**Sudafed® Severe Cold [US-OTC]** *see* acetaminophen, dextromethorphan, and pseudoephedrine *on page 11*

**Sudafed® Sinus Advance [Can]** *see* pseudoephedrine and ibuprofen *on page 694*

**Sudafed® Sinus & Allergy [US-OTC]** *see* chlorpheniramine and pseudoephedrine *on page 172*

**Sudafed® Sinus and Cold [US-OTC]** *see* acetaminophen and pseudoephedrine *on page 8*

**Sudafed® Sinus Headache [US-OTC]** *see* acetaminophen and pseudoephedrine *on page 8*

**Sudafed® Sinus Nighttime [US-OTC]** *see* triprolidine and pseudoephedrine *on page 827*

**Sudal® 12 [US]** *see* chlorpheniramine and pseudoephedrine *on page 172*

**Sudex® *(Discontinued)*** *see* guaifenesin and pseudoephedrine *on page 388*

**Sudodrin [US-OTC]** *see* pseudoephedrine *on page 692*

**SudoGest [US-OTC]** *see* pseudoephedrine *on page 692*

**SudoGest Children's [US-OTC]** *see* pseudoephedrine and dextromethorphan *on page 693*

**SudoGest Sinus [US-OTC]** *see* acetaminophen and pseudoephedrine *on page 8*

**Sudo-Tab® [US-OTC]** *see* pseudoephedrine *on page 692*

**Sufedrin® *(Discontinued)*** *see* pseudoephedrine *on page 692*

**Sufenta® [US/Can]** *see* sufentanil *on this page*

## sufentanil (soo FEN ta nil)
**Sound-Alike/Look-Alike Issues**
sufentanil may be confused with alfentanil, fentanyl
Sufenta® may be confused with Alfenta®, Sudafed®, Survanta®
**Synonyms** sufentanil citrate
**U.S./Canadian Brand Names** Sufenta® [US/Can]
**Therapeutic Category** Analgesic, Narcotic; General Anesthetic
**Controlled Substance** C-II
**Use** Analgesic supplement in maintenance of balanced general anesthesia
**Usual Dosage**
Children 2-12 years: 10-25 mcg/kg (10-15 mcg/kg most common dose) with 100% $O_2$, maintenance: up to 1-2 mcg/kg total dose

Adults: Dose should be based on body weight. **Note:** In obese patients (ie, >20% above ideal body weight), use lean body weight to determine dosage.
1-2 mcg/kg with $N_2O/O_2$ for endotracheal intubation; maintenance: 10-25 mcg as needed
2-8 mcg/kg with $N_2O/O_2$ more complicated major surgical procedures; maintenance: 10-50 mcg as needed
8-30 mcg/kg with 100% $O_2$ and muscle relaxant produces sleep; at doses ≥8 mcg/kg maintains a deep level of anesthesia; maintenance: 10-50 mcg as needed
**Dosage Forms** Injection, solution [preservative free]: 50 mcg/mL (1 mL, 2 mL, 5 mL)

**sufentanil citrate** *see* sufentanil *on this page*

**Sular® [US]** *see* nisoldipine *on page 576*

**sulbactam and ampicillin** *see* ampicillin and sulbactam *on page 51*

## sulconazole (sul KON a zole)
**Synonyms** sulconazole nitrate
**U.S./Canadian Brand Names** Exelderm® [US/Can]
**Therapeutic Category** Antifungal Agent
**Use** Treatment of superficial fungal infections of the skin, including tinea cruris (jock itch), tinea corporis (ringworm), tinea versicolor, and possibly tinea pedis (athlete's foot, cream only)
**Usual Dosage** Adults: Topical: Apply a small amount to the affected area and gently massage once or twice daily for 3 weeks (tinea cruris, tinea corporis, tinea versicolor) to 4 weeks (tinea pedis).
**Dosage Forms**
Cream, as nitrate: 1% (15 g, 30 g, 60 g)
Solution, topical, as nitrate: 1% (30 mL)

**sulconazole nitrate** *see* sulconazole *on this page*

Sulcrate® [Can] *see* sucralfate *on page 769*

Sulcrate® Suspension Plus [Can] *see* sucralfate *on page 769*

# sulfabenzamide, sulfacetamide, and sulfathiazole
(sul fa BENZ a mide, sul fa SEE ta mide, & sul fa THYE a zole)

**Synonyms** triple sulfa

**U.S./Canadian Brand Names** V.V.S.® [US]

**Therapeutic Category** Antibiotic, Vaginal

**Use** Treatment of *Haemophilus vaginalis* vaginitis

**Usual Dosage** Intravaginal: Adults: Female: Cream: Insert one applicatorful into vagina twice daily for 4-6 days; dosage may then be decreased to $1/2$ to $1/4$ of an applicatorful twice daily

**Dosage Forms** Cream, vaginal: Sulfabenzamide 3.7%, sulfacetamide 2.86%, and sulfathiazole 3.42% (78 g with applicator)

## sulfacetamide (sul fa SEE ta mide)

**Sound-Alike/Look-Alike Issues**

Bleph®-10 may be confused with Blephamide®

Klaron® may be confused with Klor-Con®

**Synonyms** sodium sulfacetamide; sulfacetamide sodium

**U.S./Canadian Brand Names** Bleph®-10 [US]; Carmol® Scalp [US]; Cetamide™ [Can]; Diosulf™ [Can]; Klaron® [US]; Ovace™ [US]

**Therapeutic Category** Antibiotic, Ophthalmic

**Use**

Ophthalmic: Treatment and prophylaxis of conjunctivitis due to susceptible organisms; corneal ulcers; adjunctive treatment with systemic sulfonamides for therapy of trachoma

Dermatologic: Scaling dermatosis (seborrheic); bacterial infections of the skin; acne vulgaris

**Usual Dosage**

Children >2 months and Adults: Ophthalmic:

Ointment: Apply to lower conjunctival sac 1-4 times/day and at bedtime

Solution: Instill 1-2 drops several times daily up to every 2-3 hours in lower conjunctival sac during waking hours and less frequently at night; increase dosing interval as condition responds. Usual duration of treatment: 7-10 days

Trachoma: Instill 2 drops into the conjunctival sac every 2 hours; must be used in conjunction with systemic therapy

Children >12 years and Adults: Topical:

Acne: Apply thin film to affected area twice daily

Seborrheic dermatitis: Apply at bedtime and allow to remain overnight; in severe cases, may apply twice daily. Duration of therapy is usually 8-10 applications; dosing interval may be increased as eruption subsides. Applications once or twice weekly, or every other week may be used to prevent eruptions.

Secondary cutaneous bacterial infections: Apply 2-4 times/day until infection clears

**Dosage Forms** [DSC] = Discontinued product

Cream, topical, as sodium (Ovace™): 10% (30 g, 60 g)

Foam, topical, as sodium (Ovace™): 10% (50 g, 100 g)

Gel, topical, as sodium (Ovace™): 10% (30 g, 60 g)

Lotion, as sodium:

Carmol® Scalp: 10% (85 g) [contains urea 10%]

Klaron®: 10% (120 mL) [contains sodium metabisulfite]

Ovace™: 10% (180 mL, 360 mL)

Ointment, ophthalmic, as sodium: 10% (3.5 g)

Solution, ophthalmic, as sodium: 10% (15 mL)

Bleph®-10: 10% (5 mL; 15 mL [DSC]) [contains benzalkonium chloride]

## sulfacetamide and prednisolone (sul fa SEE ta mide & pred NIS oh lone)

**Sound-Alike/Look-Alike Issues**

Blephamide® may be confused with Bleph®-10

Vasocidin® may be confused with Vasodilan®

(Continued)

771

## sulfacetamide and prednisolone *(Continued)*

**Synonyms** prednisolone and sulfacetamide

**U.S./Canadian Brand Names** Blephamide® [US/Can]; Dioptimyd® [Can]

**Therapeutic Category** Antibiotic/Corticosteroid, Ophthalmic

**Use** Steroid-responsive inflammatory ocular conditions where infection is present or there is a risk of infection; ophthalmic suspension may be used as an otic preparation

**Usual Dosage** Children >2 months and Adults: Ophthalmic:
Ointment: Apply to lower conjunctival sac 1-4 times/day
Solution, suspension: Instill 1-3 drops every 2-3 hours while awake

**Dosage Forms**
Ointment, ophthalmic (Blephamide®): Sulfacetamide sodium 10% and prednisolone acetate 0.2% (3.5 g)
Solution, ophthalmic: Sulfacetamide sodium 10% and prednisolone sodium phosphate 0.25% (5 mL, 10 mL)
Suspension, ophthalmic (Blephamide®): Sulfacetamide sodium 10% and prednisolone acetate 0.2% (5 mL, 10 mL) [contains benzalkonium chloride]

**sulfacetamide and sulfur** *see* sulfur and sulfacetamide *on page 776*

**sulfacetamide sodium** *see* sulfacetamide *on previous page*

## sulfacetamide sodium and fluorometholone

(sul fa SEE ta mide SOW dee um & flure oh METH oh lone)

**Synonyms** fluorometholone and sulfacetamide

**U.S./Canadian Brand Names** FML-S® [US]

**Therapeutic Category** Antibiotic/Corticosteroid, Ophthalmic

**Use** Steroid-responsive inflammatory ocular conditions where infection is present or there is a risk of infection

**Usual Dosage** Ophthalmic: Children >2 years and Adults: Instill 1 drop into affected eye(s) 4 times/day
**Note:** Dose may be decreased but should not be discontinued prematurely; re-evaluation should occur if improvement is not seen within 2 days; in chronic conditions, dosing frequency should be gradually decreased prior to discontinuing treatment

**Dosage Forms** Suspension, ophthalmic: Sulfacetamide sodium 10% and fluorometholone 0.1% (5 mL, 10 mL) [contains benzalkonium chloride]

**Sulfacet-R® [US/Can]** *see* sulfur and sulfacetamide *on page 776*

## sulfadiazine (sul fa DYE a zeen)

**Sound-Alike/Look-Alike Issues**
sulfaDIAZINE may be confused with sulfasalazine, sulfiSOXAZOLE

**Tall-Man** sulfaDIAZINE

**Therapeutic Category** Sulfonamide

**Use** Treatment of urinary tract infections and nocardiosis; adjunctive treatment in toxoplasmosis; uncomplicated attack of malaria

**Usual Dosage** Oral:
Asymptomatic meningococcal carriers:
Infants 1-12 months: 500 mg once daily for 2 days
Children 1-12 years: 500 mg twice daily for 2 days
Adults: 1 g twice daily for 2 days
Congenital toxoplasmosis:
Newborns and Children <2 months: 100 mg/kg/day divided every 6 hours in conjunction with pyrimethamine 1 mg/kg/day once daily and supplemental folinic acid 5 mg every 3 days for 6 months
Children >2 months: 25-50 mg/kg/dose 4 times/day
Nocardiosis: 4-8 g/day for a minimum of 6 weeks
Toxoplasmosis:
Children >2 months: Loading dose: 75 mg/kg; maintenance dose: 120-150 mg/kg/day, maximum dose: 6 g/day; divided every 4-6 hours in conjunction with pyrimethamine 2 mg/kg/day divided every 12 hours for 3 days followed by 1 mg/kg/day once daily with supplemental folinic acid
Adults: 2-6 g/day in divided doses every 6 hours in conjunction with pyrimethamine 50-75 mg/day and with supplemental folinic acid

**Dosage Forms** Tablet: 500 mg

## sulfadoxine and pyrimethamine (sul fa DOKS een & peer i METH a meen)

**Synonyms** pyrimethamine and sulfadoxine

**U.S./Canadian Brand Names** Fansidar® [US]

**Therapeutic Category** Antimalarial Agent

**Use** Treatment of *Plasmodium falciparum* malaria in patients in whom chloroquine resistance is suspected; malaria prophylaxis for travelers to areas where chloroquine-resistant malaria is endemic

**Usual Dosage** Children and Adults: Oral:

Treatment of acute attack of malaria: A single dose of the following number of Fansidar® tablets is used in sequence with quinine or alone:

2-11 months: $^1/_4$ tablet

1-3 years: $^1/_2$ tablet

4-8 years: 1 tablet

9-14 years: 2 tablets

>14 years: 3 tablets

Malaria prophylaxis: A single dose should be carried for self-treatment in the event of febrile illness when medical attention is not immediately available:

2-11 months: $^1/_4$ tablet

1-3 years: $^1/_2$ tablet

4-8 years: 1 tablet

9-14 years: 2 tablets

>14 years and Adults: 3 tablets

**Dosage Forms** Tablet: Sulfadoxine 500 mg and pyrimethamine 25 mg

**Sulfa-Gyn®** *(Discontinued)* *see* sulfabenzamide, sulfacetamide, and sulfathiazole *on page 771*

**Sulfamethoprim®** *(Discontinued)*

## sulfamethoxazole and trimethoprim (sul fa meth OKS a zole & trye METH oh prim)

**Sound-Alike/Look-Alike Issues**

Bactrim™ may be confused with bacitracin, Bactine®

co-trimoxazole may be confused with clotrimazole

Septra® may be confused with Ceptaz®, Sectral®, Septa®

**Synonyms** co-trimoxazole; SMZ-TMP; sulfatrim; TMP-SMZ; trimethoprim and sulfamethoxazole

**U.S./Canadian Brand Names** Apo-Sulfatrim® [Can]; Bactrim™ DS [US]; Bactrim™ [US]; Novo-Trimel D.S. [Can]; Novo-Trimel [Can]; Nu-Cotrimox [Can]; Septra® DS [US]; Septra® Injection [Can]; Septra® [US]

**Therapeutic Category** Sulfonamide

**Use**

Oral treatment of urinary tract infections due to *E. coli*, *Klebsiella* and *Enterobacter* sp, *M. morganii*, *P. mirabilis* and *P. vulgaris*; acute otitis media in children; acute exacerbations of chronic bronchitis in adults due to susceptible strains of *H. influenzae* or *S. pneumoniae*; treatment and prophylaxis of *Pneumocystis carinii* pneumonitis (PCP); traveler's diarrhea due to enterotoxigenic *E. coli*; treatment of enteritis caused by *Shigella flexneri* or *Shigella sonnei*

I.V. treatment or severe or complicated infections when oral therapy is not feasible, for documented PCP, empiric treatment of PCP in immune compromised patients; treatment of documented or suspected shigellosis, typhoid fever, *Nocardia asteroides* infection, or other infections caused by susceptible bacteria

**Usual Dosage** Dosage recommendations are based on the trimethoprim component. Double-strength tablets are equivalent to sulfamethoxazole 800 mg and trimethoprim 160 mg.

Children >2 months:

**General dosing guidelines:**

Mild-to-moderate infections: Oral: 8-12 mg TMP/kg/day in divided doses every 12 hours

Serious infection:

Oral: 20 mg TMP/kg/day in divided doses every 6 hours

I.V.: 8-12 mg TMP/kg/day in divided doses every 6 hours

Acute otitis media: Oral: 8 mg TMP/kg/day in divided doses every 12 hours for 10 days

Urinary tract infection:

Treatment:

Oral: 6-12 mg TMP/kg/day in divided doses every 12 hours

I.V.: 8-10 mg TMP/kg/day in divided doses every 6, 8, or 12 hours for up to 4 days with serious infections

Prophylaxis: Oral: 2 mg TMP/kg/dose daily or 5 mg TMP/kg/dose twice weekly

(Continued)

## sulfamethoxazole and trimethoprim *(Continued)*

*Pneumocystis*:
Treatment: Oral, I.V.: 15-20 mg TMP/kg/day in divided doses every 6-8 hours
Prophylaxis: Oral, 150 mg TMP/m$^2$/day in divided doses every 12 hours for 3 days/week; dose should not exceed trimethoprim 320 mg and sulfamethoxazole 1600 mg daily
Alternative prophylaxis dosing schedules include:
150 mg TMP/m$^2$/day as a single daily dose 3 times/week on consecutive days
**or**
150 mg TMP/m$^2$/day in divided doses every 12 hours administered 7 days/week
**or**
150 mg TMP/m$^2$/day in divided doses every 12 hours administered 3 times/week on alternate days
Shigellosis:
Oral: 8 mg TMP/kg/day in divided doses every 12 hours for 5 days
I.V.: 8-10 mg TMP/kg/day in divided doses every 6, 8, or 12 hours for up to 5 days
Adults:
Urinary tract infection:
Oral: One double-strength tablet every 12 hours
Duration of therapy: Uncomplicated: 3-5 days; Complicated: 7-10 days
Pyelonephritis: 14 days
Prostatitis: Acute: 2 weeks; Chronic: 2-3 months
I.V.: 8-10 mg TMP/kg/day in divided doses every 6, 8, or 12 hours for up to 14 days with severe infections
Chronic bronchitis: Oral: One double-strength tablet every 12 hours for 10-14 days
Shigellosis:
Oral: One double strength tablet every 12 hours for 5 days
I.V.: 8-10 mg TMP/kg/day in divided doses every 6, 8, or 12 hours for up to 5 days
Travelers' diarrhea: Oral: One double strength tablet every 12 hours for 5 days
Sepsis: I.V.: 20 TMP/kg/day divided every 6 hours
*Pneumocystis carinii*:
Prophylaxis: Oral: 1 double strength tablet daily or 3 times/week
Treatment: Oral, I.V.: 15-20 mg TMP/kg/day in 3-4 divided doses
**Dosage Forms Note:** The 5:1 ratio (SMX:TMP) remains constant in all dosage forms.
Injection, solution: Sulfamethoxazole 80 mg and trimethoprim 16 mg per mL (5 mL, 10 mL, 30 mL) [contains propylene glycol ~400 mg/mL, alcohol, benzyl alcohol, and sodium metabisulfite]
Suspension, oral: Sulfamethoxazole 200 mg and trimethoprim 40 mg per 5 mL (480 mL) [contains alcohol]
Septra®: Sulfamethoxazole 200 mg and trimethoprim 40 mg per 5 mL (480 mL) [contains alcohol 0.26% and sodium benzoate; cherry and grape flavors]
Tablet: Sulfamethoxazole 400 mg and trimethoprim 80 mg
Bactrim™: Sulfamethoxazole 400 mg and trimethoprim 80 mg [contains sodium benzoate]
Septra®: Sulfamethoxazole 400 mg and trimethoprim 80 mg
Tablet, double strength: Sulfamethoxazole 800 mg and trimethoprim 160 mg
Bactrim™ DS: Sulfamethoxazole 800 mg and trimethoprim 160 mg [contains sodium benzoate]
Septra® DS: Sulfamethoxazole 800 mg and trimethoprim 160 mg

**Sulfamylon®  [US]** *see* mafenide *on page 496*

## sulfasalazine (sul fa SAL a zeen)

**Sound-Alike/Look-Alike Issues**
sulfasalazine may be confused with salsalate, sulfaDIAZINE, sulfiSOXAZOLE
Azulfidine® may be confused with Augmentin®, azathioprine
**Synonyms** salicylazosulfapyridine
**U.S./Canadian Brand Names** Alti-Sulfasalazine [Can]; Azulfidine® EN-tabs® [US]; Azulfidine® [US]; Salazopyrin En-Tabs® [Can]; Salazopyrin® [Can]; Sulfazine EC [US]; Sulfazine [US]
**Therapeutic Category** 5-Aminosalicylic Acid Derivative
**Use** Management of ulcerative colitis; enteric coated tablets are also used for rheumatoid arthritis (including juvenile rheumatoid arthritis) in patients who inadequately respond to analgesics and NSAIDs
**Usual Dosage** Oral:
Children ≥2 years: Ulcerative colitis: Initial: 40-60 mg/kg/day in 3-6 divided doses; maintenance dose: 20-30 mg/kg/day in 4 divided doses

Children ≥6 years: Juvenile rheumatoid arthritis: Enteric coated tablet: 30-50 mg/kg/day in 2 divided doses; Initial: Begin with ¼ to ⅓ of expected maintenance dose; increase weekly; maximum: 2 g/day typically

Adults:

Ulcerative colitis: Initial: 1 g 3-4 times/day, 2 g/day maintenance in divided doses; may initiate therapy with 0.5-1 g/day

Rheumatoid arthritis: Enteric coated tablet: Initial: 0.5-1 g/day; increase weekly to maintenance dose of 2 g/day in 2 divided doses; maximum: 3 g/day (if response to 2 g/day is inadequate after 12 weeks of treatment)

**Dosage Forms**
Tablet (Azulfidine®, Sulfazine): 500 mg
Tablet, delayed release, enteric coated (Azulfidine® EN-tabs®, Sulfazine EC): 500 mg

**sulfatrim** *see sulfamethoxazole and trimethoprim* *on page 773*

**Sulfa-Trip®** *(Discontinued)* *see sulfabenzamide, sulfacetamide, and sulfathiazole* *on page 771*

**Sulfazine [US]** *see sulfasalazine* *on previous page*

**Sulfazine EC [US]** *see sulfasalazine* *on previous page*

## sulfinpyrazone (sul fin PEER a zone)
**U.S./Canadian Brand Names** Apo-Sulfinpyrazone® [Can]; Nu-Sulfinpyrazone [Can]
**Therapeutic Category** Uricosuric Agent
**Use** Treatment of chronic gouty arthritis and intermittent gouty arthritis
**Usual Dosage** Adults: Oral: 100-200 mg twice daily; maximum daily dose: 800 mg
**Dosage Forms** Tablet: 100 mg

## sulfisoxazole (sul fi SOKS a zole)
**Sound-Alike/Look-Alike Issues**
sulfiSOXAZOLE may be confused with sulfaDIAZINE, sulfamethoxazole, sulfasalazine
Gantrisin® may be confused with Gastrosed™
**Synonyms** sulfisoxazole acetyl; sulphafurazole
**Tall-Man** sulfiSOXAZOLE
**U.S./Canadian Brand Names** Gantrisin® [US]; Novo-Soxazole [Can]; Sulfizole® [Can]
**Therapeutic Category** Sulfonamide
**Use** Treatment of urinary tract infections, otitis media, *Chlamydia*; nocardiosis
**Usual Dosage** Oral: Not for use in patients <2 months of age:
Children >2 months: Initial: 75 mg/kg, followed by 120-150 mg/kg/day in divided doses every 4-6 hours; not to exceed 6 g/day
Adults: Initial: 2-4 g, then 4-8 g/day in divided doses every 4-6 hours
**Dosage Forms**
Suspension, oral, pediatric, as acetyl (Gantrisin®): 500 mg/5 mL (480 mL) [contains alcohol 0.3%; raspberry flavor]
Tablet: 500 mg

**sulfisoxazole acetyl** *see sulfisoxazole* *on this page*

**sulfisoxazole and erythromycin** *see erythromycin and sulfisoxazole* *on page 296*

**Sulfizole® [Can]** *see sulfisoxazole* *on this page*

## sulfur and salicylic acid (SUL fur & sal i SIL ik AS id)
**Synonyms** salicylic acid and sulfur
**Therapeutic Category** Antiseborrheic Agent, Topical
**Use** Therapeutic shampoo for dandruff and seborrheal dermatitis; acne skin cleanser
**Usual Dosage** Children and Adults: Topical:
Shampoo: Initial: Use daily or every other day; 1-2 treatments/week will usually maintain control
Soap: Use daily or every other day
**Dosage Forms**
Cake: Sulfur 2% and salicylic acid 2% (123 g)
Cleanser: Sulfur 2% and salicylic acid 1.5% (60 mL, 120 mL)
Shampoo: Micropulverized sulfur 2% and salicylic acid 2% (120 mL, 240 mL)
Soap: Micropulverized sulfur 2% and salicylic acid 2% (113 g)
Wash: Sulfur 1.6% and salicylic acid 1.6% (75 mL)

## sulfur and sulfacetamide (SUL fur & sul fa SEE ta mide)

**Synonyms** sodium sulfacetamide and sulfur; sulfacetamide and sulfur; sulfur and sulfacetamide sodium

**U.S./Canadian Brand Names** AVAR™ Cleanser [US]; AVAR™ Green [US]; AVAR™ [US]; Clenia™ [US]; Nocosyn™ [US]; Plexion SCT™ [US]; Plexion TS® [US]; Plexion® [US]; Rosanil® [US]; Rosula® [US]; Sulfacet-R® [US/Can]; Zetacet® [US]

**Therapeutic Category** Antiseborrheic Agent, Topical

**Use** Aid in the treatment of acne vulgaris, acne rosacea, and seborrheic dermatitis

**Usual Dosage** Topical: Children ≥12 years and Adults: Apply in a thin film 1-3 times/day. Cleansing products should be used 1-2 times/day.

**Dosage Forms**
Cream, topical:
Clenia™: Sulfur 5% and sulfacetamide sodium 10% (28 g)
Plexion SCT™: Sulfur 5% and sulfacetamide sodium 10% (120 g) [contains benzyl alcohol]
Rosanil®: Sulfur 5% and sulfacetamide sodium 10% (170 g) [cleanser]
Gel, topical:
AVAR™: Sulfur 5% and sulfacetamide sodium 10% (45 g) [contains benzyl alcohol]
AVAR™ Green: Sulfur 5% and sulfacetamide sodium 10% (45 g) [contains benzyl alcohol; color corrective gel]
Rosula®: Sulfur 5% and sulfacetamide sodium 10% (45 g) [contains urea 10% and benzyl alcohol]
Liquid soap (Clenia™): Sulfur 5% and sulfacetamide sodium 10% (170 g, 340 g)
Lotion, topical: Sulfur 5% and sulfacetamide sodium 10% (25 g)
AVAR™ Cleanser: Sulfur 5% and sulfacetamide sodium 10% (228 g)
Nicosyn™: Sulfur 5% and sulfacetamide sodium 10% (45 g) [contains benzyl alcohol]
Plexion®: Sulfur 5% and sulfacetamide sodium 10% (170 g, 340 g) [cleanser]
Rosula®: Sulfur 5% and sulfacetamide sodium 10% (45 g) [contains urea 10% and benzyl alcohol]
Sulfacet-R®: Sulfur 5% and sulfacetamide sodium 10% (25 g) [contains sodium metabisulfate; available with tint or tint-free formulations]
Suspension, topical (Plexion TS®, Zetacet®): Sulfur 5% and sulfacetamide sodium 10% (30 g) [contains benzyl alcohol]

## sulfur and sulfacetamide sodium *see* sulfur and sulfacetamide *on this page*

## sulindac (sul IN dak)

**Sound-Alike/Look-Alike Issues**
Clinoril® may be confused with Cleocin®, Clozaril®, Oruvail®

**U.S./Canadian Brand Names** Apo-Sulin® [Can]; Clinoril® [US]; Novo-Sundac [Can]; Nu-Sundac [Can]

**Therapeutic Category** Analgesic, Nonnarcotic; Nonsteroidal Antiinflammatory Drug (NSAID)

**Use** Management of inflammatory disease, osteoarthritis, rheumatoid disorders, acute gouty arthritis, ankylosing spondylitis, bursitis/tendonitis of shoulder

**Usual Dosage** Maximum therapeutic response may not be realized for up to 3 weeks
Oral:
Children: Dose not established
Adults: 150-200 mg twice daily or 300-400 mg once daily; not to exceed 400 mg/day

**Dosage Forms**
Tablet: 150 mg, 200 mg
Clinoril®: 200 mg

## sulphafurazole *see* sulfisoxazole *on previous page*

## Sultrin™ *(Discontinued)* *see* sulfabenzamide, sulfacetamide, and sulfathiazole *on page 771*

## sumatriptan succinate (soo ma TRIP tan SUKS i nate)

**Sound-Alike/Look-Alike Issues**
sumatriptan may be confused with somatropin, zolmitriptan

**Synonyms** sumatriptan succinate

**U.S./Canadian Brand Names** Imitrex® DF [Can]; Imitrex® [US]

**Therapeutic Category** Antimigraine Agent

**Use**
Oral, SubQ: Acute treatment of migraine with or without aura
SubQ: Acute treatment of cluster headache episodes

**Usual Dosage** Adults:

Oral: A single dose of 25 mg, 50 mg, or 100 mg (taken with fluids). If a satisfactory response has not been obtained at 2 hours, a second dose may be administered. Results from clinical trials show that initial doses of 50 mg and 100 mg are more effective than doses of 25 mg, and that 100 mg doses do not provide a greater effect than 50 mg and may have increased incidence of side effects. Although doses of up to 300 mg/day have been studied, the total daily dose should not exceed 200 mg. The safety of treating an average of >4 headaches in a 30-day period have not been established.

Intranasal: A single dose of 5 mg, 10 mg, or 20 mg administered in one nostril. A 10 mg dose may be achieved by administering a single 5 mg dose in each nostril. If headache returns, the dose may be repeated once after 2 hours, not to exceed a total daily dose of 40 mg. The safety of treating an average of >4 headaches in a 30-day period has not been established.

SubQ: 6 mg; a second injection may be administered at least 1 hour after the initial dose, but not more than 2 injections in a 24-hour period. If side effects are dose-limiting, lower doses may be used.

**Dosage Forms Note:** Strength expressed as sumatriptan base

Injection, solution, as succinate: 12 mg/mL (0.5 mL)

Solution, intranasal spray: 5 mg (100 µL unit dose spray device); 20 mg (100 µL unit dose spray device)

Tablet, as succinate: 25 mg, 50 mg, 100 mg

**Summer's Eve® Medicated Douche [US-OTC]** *see* povidone-iodine *on page 668*

**Summer's Eve® SpecialCare™ Medicated Anti-Itch Cream [US-OTC]** *see* hydrocortisone (topical) *on page 417*

**Sumycin® [US]** *see* tetracycline *on page 791*

**Sun-Benz® [Can]** *see* benzydamine *(Canada only) on page 100*

**sunscreen (paba-free)** *see* methoxycinnamate and oxybenzone *on page 527*

**Supartz™ [US]** *see* hyaluronate and derivatives *on page 406*

**Superdophilus® [US-OTC]** *see* Lactobacillus *on page 462*

**Supeudol® [Can]** *see* oxycodone *on page 608*

**Suplasyn® [Can]** *see* hyaluronate and derivatives *on page 406*

**Suppress® *(Discontinued)*** *see* dextromethorphan *on page 238*

**Suprane® [US/Can]** *see* desflurane *on page 229*

**Suprax® [US/Can]** *see* cefixime *on page 154*

**Surbex-T® [US-OTC]** *see* vitamin B complex combinations *on page 849*

**Surbex-T® Filmtabs® [US-OTC]** *see* vitamin B complex with vitamin C *on page 850*

**Surbex® With C Filmtabs® [US-OTC]** *see* vitamin B complex with vitamin C *on page 850*

**Sureprin 81™ [US-OTC]** *see* aspirin *on page 73*

**Surfak® [US-OTC]** *see* docusate *on page 263*

**Surgam® [Can]** *see* tiaprofenic acid *(Canada only) on page 801*

**Surgam® SR [Can]** *see* tiaprofenic acid *(Canada only) on page 801*

**Surmontil® [US/Can]** *see* trimipramine *on page 826*

**Survanta® [US/Can]** *see* beractant *on page 101*

**Sus-Phrine® *(Discontinued)*** *see* epinephrine *on page 287*

**Sustaire® *(Discontinued)*** *see* theophylline *on page 793*

**Sustiva® [US/Can]** *see* efavirenz *on page 280*

**Su-Tuss DM [US]** *see* guaifenesin and dextromethorphan *on page 385*

**Su-Tuss®-HD [US]** *see* hydrocodone, pseudoephedrine, and guaifenesin *on page 415*

**suxamethonium chloride** *see* succinylcholine *on page 768*

**Sween Cream® [US-OTC]** *see* vitamin A and vitamin D *on page 849*

**Symadine® *(Discontinued)***

**Symax SL [US]** *see* hyoscyamine *on page 424*

**Symax SR [US]** *see* hyoscyamine *on page 424*

**Symbicort® [Can]** *see* budesonide and formoterol *(Canada only) on page 119*

**Symbyax™ [US]** *see* olanzapine and fluoxetine *on page 596*

**Symlin**® **[US]** *see* pramlintide *on page 670*

**Symmetrel**® **[US/Can]** *see* amantadine *on page 37*

**synacthen** *see* cosyntropin *on page 210*

**Synagis**® **[US/Can]** *see* palivizumab *on page 614*

**Synalar**® **[US/Can]** *see* fluocinolone *on page 344*

**Synalar-HP**® **Topical** *(Discontinued)* *see* fluocinolone *on page 344*

**Synalgos**®**-DC [US]** *see* dihydrocodeine, aspirin, and caffeine *on page 249*

**Synarel**® **[US/Can]** *see* nafarelin *on page 557*

**Syn-Diltiazem**® **[Can]** *see* diltiazem *on page 251*

**Synemol**® **Topical** *(Discontinued)* *see* fluocinolone *on page 344*

**Synercid**® **[US/Can]** *see* quinupristin and dalfopristin *on page 706*

**Synphasic**® **[Can]** *see* ethinyl estradiol and norethindrone *on page 314*

**Syntest D.S. [US]** *see* estrogens (esterified) and methyltestosterone *on page 306*

**Syntest H.S. [US]** *see* estrogens (esterified) and methyltestosterone *on page 306*

**Synthroid**® **[US/Can]** *see* levothyroxine *on page 477*

**Syntocinon**® **[Can]** *see* oxytocin *on page 612*

**Synvisc**® **[US]** *see* hyaluronate and derivatives *on page 406*

**Syprine**® **[US/Can]** *see* trientine *on page 822*

**SyringeAvitene**™ **[US]** *see* collagen hemostat *on page 206*

**syrup of ipecac** *see* ipecac syrup *on page 445*

**Sytobex**® *(Discontinued)* *see* cyanocobalamin *on page 212*

**T₃/T₄ liotrix** *see* liotrix *on page 484*

**T₄** *see* levothyroxine *on page 477*

**T-20** *see* enfuvirtide *on page 285*

**642**® **Tablet [Can]** *see* propoxyphene *on page 687*

**Tabloid**® **[US]** *see* thioguanine *on page 797*

**Tac**™**-40 Injection** *(Discontinued)*

## tacrine (TAK reen)
**Sound-Alike/Look-Alike Issues**
   Cognex® may be confused with Corgard®
**Synonyms** tacrine hydrochloride; tetrahydroaminoacrine; THA
**U.S./Canadian Brand Names** Cognex® [US]
**Therapeutic Category** Acetylcholinesterase Inhibitor; Cholinergic Agent
**Use** Treatment of mild to moderate dementia of the Alzheimer type
**Usual Dosage** Adults: Initial: 10 mg 4 times/day; may increase by 40 mg/day adjusted every 6 weeks; maximum: 160 mg/day; best administered separate from meal times.
   Dose adjustment based upon transaminase elevations:
   ALT ≤3 times ULN*: Continue titration
   ALT >3 to ≤5 times ULN*: Decrease dose by 40 mg/day, resume when ALT returns to normal
   ALT >5 times ULN*: Stop treatment, may rechallenge upon return of ALT to normal
   *ULN = upper limit of normal
   Patients with clinical jaundice confirmed by elevated total bilirubin (>3 mg/dL) should not be rechallenged with tacrine
**Dosage Forms** Capsule, as hydrochloride: 10 mg, 20 mg, 30 mg, 40 mg

**tacrine hydrochloride** *see* tacrine *on this page*

## tacrolimus (ta KROE li mus)
**Sound-Alike/Look-Alike Issues**
   Prograf® may be confused with Gengraf®

**Synonyms** FK506

**U.S./Canadian Brand Names** Prograf® [US/Can]; Protopic® [US/Can]

**Therapeutic Category** Immunosuppressant Agent

**Use**

Oral/injection: Potent immunosuppressive drug used in liver or kidney transplant recipients

Topical: Moderate to severe atopic dermatitis in patients not responsive to conventional therapy or when conventional therapy is not appropriate

**Usual Dosage**

Children:

Liver transplant: Patients without pre-existing renal or hepatic dysfunction have required and tolerated higher doses than adults to achieve similar blood concentrations. It is recommended that therapy be initiated at high end of the recommended adult I.V. and oral dosing ranges; dosage adjustments may be required.

Oral: Initial dose: 0.15-0.20 mg/kg/day in 2 divided doses, given every 12 hours; begin oral dose no sooner than 6 hours post-transplant; adjunctive therapy with corticosteroids is recommended; if switching from I.V. to oral, the oral dose should be started 8-12 hours after stopping the infusion

Typical whole blood trough concentrations: Months 1-12: 5-20 ng/mL

I.V.: **Note:** I.V. route should only be used in patients not able to take oral medications, anaphylaxis has been reported. Initial dose: 0.03-0.05 mg/kg/day as a continuous infusion; begin no sooner than 6 hours post-transplant; adjunctive therapy with corticosteroids is recommended; continue only until oral medication can be tolerated

Children ≥2 years: Moderate to severe atopic dermatitis: Topical: Apply 0.03% ointment to affected area twice daily; rub in gently and completely; continue applications for 1 week after symptoms have cleared

Adults:

Kidney transplant:

Oral: Initial dose: 0.2 mg/kg/day in 2 divided doses, given every 12 hours; initial dose may be given within 24 hours of transplant, but should be delayed until renal function has recovered; African-American patients may require larger doses to maintain trough concentration

Typical whole blood trough concentrations: Months 1-3: 7- 20 ng/mL; months 4-12: 5-15 ng/mL

I.V.: **Note:** I.V. route should only be used in patients not able to take oral medications, anaphylaxis has been reported. Initial dose: 0.03-0.05 mg/kg/day as a continuous infusion; begin no sooner than 6 hours post-transplant, starting at lower end of the dosage range; adjunctive therapy with corticosteroids is recommended; continue only until oral medication can be tolerated

Liver transplant:

Oral: Initial dose: 0.1-0.15 mg/kg/day in 2 divided doses, given every 12 hours; begin oral dose no sooner than 6 hours post-transplant; adjunctive therapy with corticosteroids is recommended; if switching from I.V. to oral, the oral dose should be started 8-12 hours after stopping the infusion

Typical whole blood trough concentrations: Months 1-12: 5-20 ng/mL

I.V.: **Note:** I.V. route should only be used in patients not able to take oral medications, anaphylaxis has been reported. Initial dose: 0.03-0.05 mg/kg/day as a continuous infusion; begin no sooner than 6 hours post-transplant starting at lower end of the dosage range; adjunctive therapy with corticosteroids is recommended; continue only until oral medication can be tolerated

Prevention of graft-vs-host disease: I.V.: 0.03 mg/kg/day as continuous infusion

Atopic dermatitis (moderate to severe): Topical: Apply 0.03% or 0.1% ointment to affected area twice daily; rub in gently and completely; continue applications for 1 week after symptoms have cleared

**Dosage Forms**

Capsule (Prograf®): 0.5 mg, 1 mg, 5 mg

Injection, solution (Prograf®): 5 mg/mL (1 mL) [contains dehydrated alcohol 80% and polyoxyl 60 hydrogenated castor oil]

Ointment, topical (Protopic®): 0.03% (30 g, 60 g, 100 g); 0.1% (30 g, 60 g, 100 g)

# tadalafil (tah DA la fil)

**Synonyms** GF196960

**U.S./Canadian Brand Names** Cialis® [US/Can]

**Therapeutic Category** Phosphodiesterase-5 Enzyme Inhibitor

**Use** Treatment of erectile dysfunction

**Usual Dosage** Oral: Adults: Erectile dysfunction: 10 mg prior to anticipated sexual activity (dosing range: 5-20 mg); to be given as one single dose and not given more than once daily. **Note:** Erectile function may be improved for up to 36 hours following a single dose; adjust dose.

(Continued)

## tadalafil (Continued)

**Dosing adjustment with concomitant medications:**

Alpha blockers: If stabilized on either alpha blockers or tadalafil therapy, initiate new therapy with the other agent at the lowest possible dose.

CYP3A4 inhibitors: Dose reduction of tadalafil is recommended with strong CYP3A4 inhibitors. The dose of tadalafil should not exceed 10 mg, and tadalafil should not be taken more frequently than once every 72 hours. Examples of such inhibitors include azole antifungals, clarithromycin, diclofenac, doxycycline, erythromycin, grapefruit juice, imatinib, isoniazid, nefazodone, nicardipine, propofol, protease inhibitors, quinidine, and verapamil.

**Dosage Forms** Tablet: 5 mg, 10 mg, 20 mg

**Tagamet® [US]** see cimetidine on page 183

**Tagamet® 800 mg (Discontinued)** see cimetidine on page 183

**Tagamet® HB [Can]** see cimetidine on page 183

**Tagamet® HB 200 [US-OTC]** see cimetidine on page 183

**Talwin® [US/Can]** see pentazocine on page 631

**Talwin® NX [US]** see pentazocine on page 631

**TAM** see tamoxifen on this page

**Tambocor™ [US/Can]** see flecainide on page 340

**Tamiflu® [US/Can]** see oseltamivir on page 603

**Tamofen® [Can]** see tamoxifen on this page

## tamoxifen (ta MOKS i fen)

**Sound-Alike/Look-Alike Issues**

tamoxifen may be confused with pentoxifylline, Tambocor™

**Synonyms** ICI-46474; NSC-180973; TAM; tamoxifen citrate

**U.S./Canadian Brand Names** Apo-Tamox® [Can]; Gen-Tamoxifen [Can]; Nolvadex® [US/Can]; Nolvadex®-D [Can]; Novo-Tamoxifen [Can]; Tamofen® [Can]

**Therapeutic Category** Antineoplastic Agent

**Use** Palliative or adjunctive treatment of advanced breast cancer; reduce the incidence of breast cancer in women at high risk; reduce risk of invasive breast cancer in women with ductal carcinoma in situ (DCIS); metastatic female and male breast cancer; treatment of melanoma, desmoid tumors

**Usual Dosage** Oral (refer to individual protocols):

Adults: Breast cancer:

Metastatic (males and females) or adjuvant therapy (females): 20-40 mg/day; daily doses >20 mg should be given in 2 divided doses (morning and evening)

Prevention (high-risk females): 20 mg/day for 5 years

DCIS (females): 20 mg once daily for 5 years

**Note:** Higher dosages (up to 700 mg/day) have been investigated for use in modulation of multidrug resistance (MDR), but are not routinely used in clinical practice

**Dosage Forms** Tablet: 10 mg, 20 mg

**tamoxifen citrate** see tamoxifen on this page

## tamsulosin (tam SOO loe sin)

**Sound-Alike/Look-Alike Issues**

Flomax® may be confused with Fosamax®, Volmax®

**Synonyms** tamsulosin hydrochloride

**U.S./Canadian Brand Names** Flomax® [US/Can]

**Therapeutic Category** Alpha-Adrenergic Blocking Agent

**Use** Treatment of signs and symptoms of benign prostatic hyperplasia (BPH)

**Usual Dosage** Oral: Adults: 0.4 mg once daily ~30 minutes after the same meal each day; dose may be increased after 2-4 weeks to 0.8 mg once daily in patients who fail to respond. If therapy is interrupted for several days, restart with 0.4 mg once daily.

**Dosage Forms** Capsule, as hydrochloride: 0.4 mg

**tamsulosin hydrochloride** see tamsulosin on this page

**Tanac® (Discontinued)** see benzocaine on page 95

Tanafed® *(Discontinued)* *see* chlorpheniramine and pseudoephedrine *on page 172*

Tanafed DMX™ [US] *see* chlorpheniramine, pseudoephedrine, and dextromethorphan *on page 177*

Tannate 12 S [US] *see* carbetapentane and chlorpheniramine *on page 142*

Tannic-12 [US] *see* carbetapentane and chlorpheniramine *on page 142*

Tannic-12 S [US] *see* carbetapentane and chlorpheniramine *on page 142*

Tannihist-12 RF [US] *see* carbetapentane and chlorpheniramine *on page 142*

Tantum® [Can] *see* benzydamine *(Canada only)* *on page 100*

Tao® [US] *see* troleandomycin *on page 829*

TAP-144 *see* leuprolide acetate *on page 471*

Tapazole® [US/Can] *see* methimazole *on page 523*

Tarabine® PFS *(Discontinued)* *see* cytarabine *on page 219*

Tarceva™ [US] *see* erlotinib *on page 294*

Targel® [Can] *see* coal tar *on page 201*

Targretin® [US/Can] *see* bexarotene *on page 105*

Tarka® [US/Can] *see* trandolapril and verapamil *on page 815*

Taro-Carbamazepine Chewable [Can] *see* carbamazepine *on page 140*

Taro-Desoximetasone [Can] *see* desoximetasone *on page 232*

Taro-Sone® [Can] *see* betamethasone (topical) *on page 103*

Taro-Warfarin [Can] *see* warfarin *on page 854*

Tarsum® [US-OTC] *see* coal tar and salicylic acid *on page 202*

Tasmar® [US] *see* tolcapone *on page 809*

TAT *see* tetanus antitoxin *on page 789*

Tavist® Allergy [US-OTC] *see* clemastine *on page 191*

Tavist® ND [US-OTC] *see* loratadine *on page 491*

Taxol® [US/Can] *see* paclitaxel *on page 612*

Taxotere® [US/Can] *see* docetaxel *on page 263*

## tazarotene (taz AR oh teen)

**U.S./Canadian Brand Names** Avage™ [US]; Tazorac® [US/Can]

**Therapeutic Category** Keratolytic Agent

**Use** Topical treatment of facial acne vulgaris; topical treatment of stable plaque psoriasis of up to 20% body surface area involvement; mitigation (palliation) of facial skin wrinkling, facial mottled hyper/hypopigmentation, and benign facial lentigines

**Usual Dosage** Topical: **Note:** In patients experiencing excessive pruritus, burning, skin redness, or peeling, discontinue until integrity of the skin is restored, or reduce dosing to an interval the patient is able to tolerate.

Children ≥12 years and Adults:

Acne: Tazorac® cream/gel 0.1%: Cleanse the face gently. After the skin is dry, apply a thin film of tazarotene (2 mg/cm$^2$) once daily, in the evening, to the skin where the acne lesions appear; use enough to cover the entire affected area

Psoriasis: Tazorac® gel 0.05% or 0.1%: Apply once daily, in the evening, to psoriatic lesions using enough (2 mg/cm$^2$) to cover only the lesion with a thin film to no more than 20% of body surface area. If a bath or shower is taken prior to application, dry the skin before applying. Unaffected skin may be more susceptible to irritation, avoid application to these areas.

Children ≥17 years and Adults: Palliation of fine facial wrinkles, facial mottled hyper/hypopigmentation, benign facial lentigines: Avage™: Apply a pea-sized amount once daily to clean dry face at bedtime; lightly cover entire face including eyelids if desired. Emollients or moisturizers may be applied before or after; if applied before tazarotene, ensure cream or lotion has absorbed into the skin and has dried completely.

Adults: Psoriasis: Tazorac® cream 0.05% or 0.1%: Apply once daily, in the evening, to psoriatic lesions using enough (2 mg/cm$^2$) to cover only the lesion with a thin film to no more than 20% of body surface area. If a bath or shower is taken prior to application, dry the skin before applying. Unaffected skin may be more susceptible to irritation, avoid application to these areas.

(Continued)

## tazarotene *(Continued)*

Dosage Forms
Cream:
Avage™: 0.1% (30 g) [contains benzyl alcohol]
Tazorac®: 0.05% (30 g, 60 g); 0.1% (30 g, 60 g) [contains benzyl alcohol]
Gel (Tazorac®): 0.05% (30 g, 100 g); 0.1% (30 g, 100 g) [contains benzyl alcohol]

**Tazicef® [US]** *see* ceftazidime *on page 157*

**Tazocin® [Can]** *see* piperacillin and tazobactam sodium *on page 649*

**Tazorac® [US/Can]** *see* tazarotene *on previous page*

**Taztia XT™ [US]** *see* diltiazem *on page 251*

**3TC** *see* lamivudine *on page 464*

**3TC, abacavir, and zidovudine** *see* abacavir, lamivudine, and zidovudine *on page 2*

**T-cell growth factor** *see* aldesleukin *on page 25*

**TCGF** *see* aldesleukin *on page 25*

**TCN** *see* tetracycline *on page 791*

**Td** *see* diphtheria and tetanus toxoid *on page 257*

**Tdap** *see* diphtheria, tetanus toxoids, and acellular pertussis vaccine *on page 259*

**TDF** *see* tenofovir *on page 786*

**Teardrops® [Can]** *see* artificial tears *on page 71*

**Tear Drop® Solution *(Discontinued)*** *see* artificial tears *on page 71*

**TearGard® Ophthalmic Solution *(Discontinued)*** *see* artificial tears *on page 71*

**Teargen® [US-OTC]** *see* artificial tears *on page 71*

**Teargen® II [US-OTC]** *see* artificial tears *on page 71*

**Tearisol® [US-OTC]** *see* artificial tears *on page 71*

**Tears Again® [US-OTC]** *see* artificial tears *on page 71*

**Tears Again® MC [US-OTC]** *see* hydroxypropyl methylcellulose *on page 422*

**Tears Again® Gel Drops™ [US-OTC]** *see* carboxymethylcellulose *on page 148*

**Tears Again® Night and Day™ [US-OTC]** *see* carboxymethylcellulose *on page 148*

**Tears Naturale® [US-OTC]** *see* artificial tears *on page 71*

**Tears Naturale® II [US-OTC]** *see* artificial tears *on page 71*

**Tears Naturale® Free [US-OTC]** *see* artificial tears *on page 71*

**Tears Plus® [US-OTC]** *see* artificial tears *on page 71*

**Tears Renewed® [US-OTC]** *see* artificial tears *on page 71*

**TEAS** *see* triethanolamine salicylate *on page 823*

**Tebamide™ [US]** *see* trimethobenzamide *on page 825*

**Tebrazid™ [Can]** *see* pyrazinamide *on page 698*

**Tecnal C 1/2 [Can]** *see* butalbital, aspirin, caffeine, and codeine *on page 125*

**Tecnal C 1/4 [Can]** *see* butalbital, aspirin, caffeine, and codeine *on page 125*

## tegaserod *(teg a SER od)*

Synonyms HTF919; tegaserod maleate
U.S./Canadian Brand Names Zelnorm® [US/Can]
Therapeutic Category Serotonin 5-HT$_4$ Receptor Agonist
Use Short-term treatment of constipation-predominate irritable bowel syndrome (IBS) in women; treatment of chronic idiopathic constipation
Usual Dosage Oral: Adults:
IBS with constipation (females): 6 mg twice daily, before meals, for 4-6 weeks; may consider continuing treatment for an additional 4-6 weeks in patients who respond initially
Chronic idiopathic constipation: 6 mg twice daily, before meals; the need for continued therapy should be reassessed periodically
Dosage Forms Tablet: 2 mg, 6 mg

**tegaserod maleate** *see* tegaserod *on previous page*

**Tega-Vert**® Oral *(Discontinued)* *see* dimenhydrinate *on page 252*

**Tegretol**® **[US/Can]** *see* carbamazepine *on page 140*

**Tegretol**®**-XR [US]** *see* carbamazepine *on page 140*

**Tegrin**® **[US-OTC]** *see* coal tar *on page 201*

**Telachlor**® Oral *(Discontinued)* *see* chlorpheniramine *on page 171*

**Teladar**® Topical *(Discontinued)*

**Teldrin**® **HBP [US-OTC]** *see* chlorpheniramine *on page 171*

**Teldrin**® Oral *(Discontinued)* *see* chlorpheniramine *on page 171*

**Telepaque**® **[US]** *see* radiological/contrast media (ionic) *on page 707*


**telithromycin** (tel ith roe MYE sin)
Synonyms HMR 3647
U.S./Canadian Brand Names Ketek® [US/Can]
Therapeutic Category Antibiotic, Ketolide
Use Treatment of community-acquired pneumonia (mild-to-moderate) caused by susceptible strains of *Streptococcus pneumoniae* (including multidrug-resistant isolates), *Haemophilus influenzae*, *Chlamydia pneumoniae*, *Moraxella catarrhalis*, and *Mycoplasma pneumoniae*; treatment of bacterial exacerbation of chronic bronchitis caused by susceptible strains of *S. pneumoniae*, *H. influenzae* and *Moraxella catarrhalis*; treatment of acute bacterial sinusitis caused by *Streptococcus pneumoniae*, *Haemophilus influenzae*, *Moraxella catarrhalis*, and *Staphylococcus aureus*
Usual Dosage Oral: Adults:
Acute exacerbation of chronic bronchitis, acute bacterial sinusitis: 800 mg once daily for 5 days
Community-acquired pneumonia: 800 mg once daily for 7-10 days
Dosage Forms
Tablet [film coated]: 300 mg [not available in Canada], 400 mg
Ketek Pak™ [blister pack]: 400 mg (10s) [packaged as 10 tablets/card; 2 tablets/blister]


**telmisartan** (tel mi SAR tan)
U.S./Canadian Brand Names Micardis® [US/Can]
Therapeutic Category Angiotensin II Receptor Antagonist
Use Treatment of hypertension; may be used alone or in combination with other antihypertensive agents
Usual Dosage Adults: Oral: Initial: 40 mg once daily; usual maintenance dose range: 20-80 mg/day. Patients with volume depletion should be initiated on the lower dosage with close supervision.
Dosage Forms Tablet: 20 mg, 40 mg, 80 mg


**telmisartan and hydrochlorothiazide** (tel mi SAR tan & hye droe klor oh THYE a zide)
Synonyms hydrochlorothiazide and telmisartan
U.S./Canadian Brand Names Micardis® HCT [US]; Micardis® Plus [Can]
Therapeutic Category Antihypertensive Agent, Combination
Use Treatment of hypertension; combination product should not be used for initial therapy
Usual Dosage Adults: Oral: Replacement therapy: Combination product can be substituted for individual titrated agents. Initiation of combination therapy when monotherapy has failed to achieve desired effects:
**Patients currently on telmisartan:** Initial dose if blood pressure is not currently controlled on monotherapy of 80 mg telmisartan: Telmisartan 80 mg/hydrochlorothiazide 12.5 mg once daily; may titrate up to telmisartan 160 mg/hydrochlorothiazide 25 mg if needed
**Patients currently on HCTZ:** Initial dose if blood pressure is not currently controlled on monotherapy of 25 mg once daily: Telmisartan 80 mg/hydrochlorothiazide 12.5 mg once daily or telmisartan 80 mg/hydrochlorothiazide 25 mg once daily; may titrate up to telmisartan 160 mg/hydrochlorothiazide 25 mg if blood pressure remains uncontrolled after 2-4 weeks of therapy. Patients who develop hypokalemia may be switched to telmisartan 80 mg/hydrochlorothiazide 12.5 mg.
Dosage Forms Tablet:
40/12.5: Telmisartan 40 mg and hydrochlorothiazide 12.5 mg
80/12.5: Telmisartan 80 mg and hydrochlorothiazide 12.5 mg
80/25: Telmisartan 80 mg and hydrochlorothiazide 25 mg

**Telzir**® **[Can]** *see* fosamprenavir *on page 360*

## temazepam (te MAZ e pam)

**Sound-Alike/Look-Alike Issues**
temazepam may be confused with flurazepam, lorazepam
Restoril® may be confused with Vistaril®, Zestril®

**U.S./Canadian Brand Names** Apo-Temazepam® [Can]; CO Temazepam [Can]; Gen-Temazepam [Can]; Novo-Temazepam [Can]; Nu-Temazepam [Can]; PMS-Temazepam [Can]; ratio-Temazepam [Can]; Restoril® [US/Can]

**Therapeutic Category** Benzodiazepine

**Controlled Substance** C-IV

**Use** Short-term treatment of insomnia

**Usual Dosage** Oral: Adults: 15-30 mg at bedtime

**Dosage Forms**
Capsule: 15 mg, 30 mg
Restoril®: 7.5 mg, 15 mg, 30 mg

**Temodal**™ **[Can]** *see* temozolomide *on this page*

**Temodar**® **[US/Can]** *see* temozolomide *on this page*

**Temovate**® **[US]** *see* clobetasol *on page 194*

**Temovate E**® **[US]** *see* clobetasol *on page 194*

## temozolomide (te moe ZOE loe mide)

**Synonyms** NSC-362856; TMZ

**U.S./Canadian Brand Names** Temodal™ [Can]; Temodar® [US/Can]

**Therapeutic Category** Antineoplastic Agent, Alkylating Agent

**Use** Treatment of adult patients with refractory (first relapse) anaplastic astrocytoma who have experienced disease progression on nitrosourea and procarbazine; newly-diagnosed glioblastoma multiforme

**Usual Dosage** Oral (refer to individual protocols): Adults:
**Anaplastic astrocytoma (refractory):** Initial dose: 150 mg/m$^2$/day for 5 days; repeat every 28 days. Subsequent doses of 100-200 mg/m$^2$/day; based upon hematologic tolerance. This monthly-cycle regimen may be preceded by a 6- to 7-week regimen of 75 mg/m$^2$/day.
ANC <1000/mm$^3$ or platelets <50,000/mm$^3$ on day 22 or day 29 (day 1 of next cycle): Postpone therapy until ANC >1500/mm$^3$ and platelets >100,000/mm$^3$; reduce dose by 50 mg/m$^2$/day for subsequent cycle
ANC 1000-1500/mm$^3$ or platelets 50,000-100,000/mm$^3$ on day 22 or day 29 (day 1 of next cycle): Postpone therapy until ANC >1500/mm$^3$ and platelets >100,000/mm$^3$; maintain initial dose
ANC >1500/mm$^3$ and platelets >100,000/mm$^3$ on day 22 or day 29 (day 1 of next cycle): Increase dose to or maintain dose at 200 mg/m$^2$/day for 5 days for subsequent cycle

**Glioblastoma multiforme (high-grade glioma):**
**Concomitant phase:** 75 mg/m$^2$/day for 42 days with radiotherapy (60Gy administered in 30 fractions). **Note:** PCP prophylaxis is required during concomitant phase and should continue in patients who develop lymphocytopenia until recovery (common toxicity criteria [CTC] ≤1). Obtain weekly CBC.
ANC ≥1500/mm$^3$, platelet count ≥100,000/mm$^3$, and nonhematologic CTC ≤grade 1 (excludes alopecia, nausea/vomiting): Temodar® 75 mg/m$^2$/day may be continued throughout the 42-day concomitant period up to 49 days
*Dosage modification:*
ANC ≥500/mm$^3$ but <1500/mm$^3$ **or** platelet count ≥10,000/mm$^3$ but <100,000/mm$^3$ **or** nonhematologic CTC grade 2 (excludes alopecia, nausea/vomiting): Interrupt therapy
ANC <500/mm$^3$ **or** platelet count <10,000/mm$^3$ **or** nonhematologic CTC grade 3/4 (excludes alopecia, nausea/vomiting): Discontinue therapy
**Maintenance phase (consists of 6 treatment cycles):** Begin 4 weeks after concomitant phase completion. **Note:** Each subsequent cycle is 28 days (consisting of 5 days of drug treatment followed by 23 days without treatment). Draw CBC within 48 hours of day 22; hold next cycle and do weekly CBC until ANC >1500/mm$^3$ and platelet count >100,000/mm$^3$; dosing modification should be based on lowest blood counts and worst nonhematologic toxicity during the previous cycle.
Cycle 1: 150 mg/m$^2$/day for 5 days

*Dosage modification for next cycle:*

ANC <1000/mm$^3$, platelet count <50,000/mm$^3$, or nonhematologic CTC grade 3 (excludes for alopecia, nausea/vomiting) during previous cycle: Decrease dose by 50 mg/m$^2$/day for 5 days, unless dose has already been lowered to 100 mg/m$^2$/day, then discontinue therapy.

If dose reduction <100 mg/m$^2$/day is required or nonhematologic CTC grade 4 (excludes for alopecia, nausea/vomiting), or if the same grade 3 nonhematologic toxicity occurs after dose reduction: Discontinue therapy

Cycle 2: 200 mg/m$^2$/day for 5 days unless prior toxicity, then refer to Dosage Modifications under "Cycle 1" and give adjusted dose for 5 days

Cycles 3-6: Continue with previous cycle's dose for 5 days unless toxicity has occurred then, refer to Dosage Modifications under "Cycle 1" and give adjusted dose for 5 days

**Dosage Forms** Capsule: 5 mg, 20 mg, 100 mg, 250 mg

**Tempra**® **[Can]** *see* acetaminophen *on page 4*

**Tempra**® *(Discontinued)* *see* acetaminophen *on page 4*

## tenecteplase (ten EK te plase)

**Sound-Alike/Look-Alike Issues**

TNKase™ may be confused with t-PA

TNK (occasional abbreviation for TNKase™) is an error-prone abbreviation (mistaken as TPA)

**U.S./Canadian Brand Names** TNKase™ [US/Can]

**Therapeutic Category** Thrombolytic Agent

**Use** Thrombolytic agent used in the management of acute myocardial infarction for the lysis of thrombi in the coronary vasculature to restore perfusion and reduce mortality.

**Usual Dosage** I.V.:

Adult: Recommended total dose should not exceed 50 mg and is based on patient's weight; administer as a bolus over 5 seconds

If patient's weight:

<60 kg, dose: 30 mg

≥60 to <70 kg, dose: 35 mg

≥70 to <80 kg, dose: 40 mg

≥80 to <90 kg, dose: 45 mg

≥90 kg, dose: 50 mg

All patients received 150-325 mg of aspirin as soon as possible and then daily. Intravenous heparin was initiated as soon as possible and aPTT was maintained between 50-70 seconds.

**Dosage Forms** Injection, powder for reconstitution, recombinant: 50 mg [packaged with diluent and syringe]

**Tenex**® **[US/Can]** *see* guanfacine *on page 393*

## teniposide (ten i POE side)

**Sound-Alike/Look-Alike Issues**

teniposide may be confused with etoposide

**Synonyms** EPT; VM-26

**U.S./Canadian Brand Names** Vumon® [US/Can]

**Therapeutic Category** Antineoplastic Agent

**Use** Treatment of acute lymphocytic leukemia, small cell lung cancer

**Usual Dosage** I.V.:

Children: 130 mg/m$^2$/week, increasing to 150 mg/m$^2$ after 3 weeks and up to 180 mg/m$^2$ after 6 weeks

Acute lymphoblastic leukemia (ALL): 165 mg/m$^2$ twice weekly for 8-9 doses **or** 250 mg/m$^2$ weekly for 4-8 weeks

Adults: 50-180 mg/m$^2$ once or twice weekly for 4-6 weeks or 20-60 mg/m$^2$/day for 5 days

Small cell lung cancer: 80-90 mg/m$^2$/day for 5 days every 4-6 weeks

**Dosage Forms** Injection, solution: 10 mg/mL (5 mL) [contains benzyl alcohol, dehydrated alcohol, and polyoxyethylated castor oil]

**Ten-K**® *(Discontinued)* *see* potassium chloride *on page 663*

# tenofovir (te NOE fo veer)

**Synonyms** PMPA; TDF; tenofovir disoproxil fumarate
**U.S./Canadian Brand Names** Viread® [US/Can]
**Therapeutic Category** Antiretroviral Agent, Reverse Transcriptase Inhibitor (Nucleotide)
**Use** Management of HIV infections in combination with at least two other antiretroviral agents
**Usual Dosage** Oral: Adults: HIV infection: 300 mg once daily
**Dosage Forms** Tablet, as disoproxil fumarate: 300 mg [equivalent to 245 mg tenofovir disoproxil]

**tenofovir and emtricitabine** *see* emtricitabine and tenofovir *on page 283*

**tenofovir disoproxil fumarate** *see* tenofovir *on this page*

**Tenolin [Can]** *see* atenolol *on page 76*

**Tenoretic® [US/Can]** *see* atenolol and chlorthalidone *on page 77*

**Tenormin® [US/Can]** *see* atenolol *on page 76*

**Tenuate® [US/Can]** *see* diethylpropion *on page 246*

**Tenuate® Dospan® [US/Can]** *see* diethylpropion *on page 246*

**Tequin® [US/Can]** *see* gatifloxacin *on page 367*

**Terak™ [US]** *see* oxytetracycline and polymyxin B *on page 612*

**Terazol® [Can]** *see* terconazole *on next page*

**Terazol® 3 [US]** *see* terconazole *on next page*

**Terazol® 7 [US]** *see* terconazole *on next page*

# terazosin (ter AY zoe sin)

**U.S./Canadian Brand Names** Alti-Terazosin [Can]; Apo-Terazosin® [Can]; Hytrin® [US/Can]; Novo-Terazosin [Can]; Nu-Terazosin [Can]; PMS-Terazosin [Can]
**Therapeutic Category** Alpha-Adrenergic Blocking Agent
**Use** Management of mild to moderate hypertension; alone or in combination with other agents such as diuretics or beta-blockers; benign prostate hyperplasia (BPH)
**Usual Dosage** Oral: Adults:
Hypertension: Initial: 1 mg at bedtime; slowly increase dose to achieve desired blood pressure, up to 20 mg/day; usual dose range (JNC 7): 1-20 mg once daily
Dosage reduction may be needed when adding a diuretic or other antihypertensive agent; if drug is discontinued for greater than several days, consider beginning with initial dose and retitrate as needed; dosage may be given on a twice daily regimen if response is diminished at 24 hours and hypotensive is observed at 2-4 hours following a dose
Benign prostatic hyperplasia: Initial: 1 mg at bedtime, increasing as needed; most patients require 10 mg day; if no response after 4-6 weeks of 10 mg/day, may increase to 20 mg/day
**Dosage Forms** Capsule: 1 mg, 2 mg, 5 mg, 10 mg

# terbinafine (oral) (TER bin a feen OR al)

**U.S./Canadian Brand Names** Lamisil® Oral [US/Can]
**Therapeutic Category** Antifungal Agent
**Use** Treatment of onychomycosis infections of the toenail or fingernail
**Usual Dosage** Adults: Oral:
Fingernail onychomycosis: 250 mg once daily for 6 weeks
Toenail onychomycosis: 250 mg once daily for 12 weeks
**Dosage Forms** Tablet: 250 mg

# terbinafine (topical) (TER bin a feen TOP i kal)

**U.S./Canadian Brand Names** Lamisil® Topical [US/Can]
**Therapeutic Category** Antifungal Agent
**Use** Topical antifungal for the treatment of tinea pedis (athlete's foot), tinea cruris (jock itch), and tinea corporis (ring worm); tinea versicolor (lotion)
**Usual Dosage** Adults: Topical:
Athlete's foot: Apply to affected area twice daily for at least 1 week, not to exceed 4 weeks
Ringworm and jock itch: Apply to affected area once or twice daily for at least 1 week, not to exceed 4 weeks

**Dosage Forms**
Cream: 1% (15 g, 30 g)
Lotion: 1%

# terbutaline (ter BYOO ta leen)

**Sound-Alike/Look-Alike Issues**
terbutaline may be confused with terbinafine, TOLBUTamide
**U.S./Canadian Brand Names** Brethine® [US]; Bricanyl® [Can]
**Therapeutic Category** Adrenergic Agonist Agent
**Use** Bronchodilator in reversible airway obstruction and bronchial asthma; tocolytic agent
**Usual Dosage**
Children <12 years: Bronchoconstriction:
Oral: Initial: 0.05 mg/kg/dose 3 times/day, increased gradually as required; maximum: 0.15 mg/kg/dose 3-4 times/day or a total of 5 mg/24 hours
SubQ: 0.005-0.01 mg/kg/dose to a maximum of 0.3 mg/dose every 15-20 minutes for 3 doses
Children ≥6 years and Adults: Bronchospasm (acute): Inhalation (Bricanyl® [CAN] MDI: 500 mcg/puff, *not labeled for use in the U.S.*): One puff as needed; may repeat with 1 inhalation (after 5 minutes); more than 6 inhalations should not be necessary in any 24 hour period. **Note:** If a previously effective dosage regimen fails to provide the usual relief, or the effects of a dose last for >3 hours, medical advice should be sought immediately; this is a sign of seriously worsening asthma that requires reassessment of therapy.
Children >12 years and Adults: Bronchoconstriction:
Oral:
12-15 years: 2.5 mg every 6 hours 3 times/day; not to exceed 7.5 mg in 24 hours
>15 years: 5 mg/dose every 6 hours 3 times/day; if side effects occur, reduce dose to 2.5 mg every 6 hours; not to exceed 15 mg in 24 hours
SubQ: 0.25 mg/dose repeated in 15-30 minutes for one time only; a total dose of 0.5 mg should not be exceeded within a 4-hour period inhalations
**Dosage Forms**
Injection, solution, as sulfate: 1 mg/mL (1 mL)
Tablet, as sulfate: 2.5 mg, 5 mg

Additional dosage forms available in Canada: Powder for oral inhalation (Bricanyl® Turbuhaler): 500 mcg/actuation [50 or 200 metered doses]

# terconazole (ter KONE a zole)

**Sound-Alike/Look-Alike Issues**
terconazole may be confused with tioconazole
**Synonyms** triaconazole
**U.S./Canadian Brand Names** Terazol® 3 [US]; Terazol® 7 [US]; Terazol® [Can]
**Therapeutic Category** Antifungal Agent
**Use** Local treatment of vulvovaginal candidiasis
**Usual Dosage** Adults: Female:
Terazol® 3 vaginal cream: Insert 1 applicatorful intravaginally at bedtime for 3 consecutive days
Terazol® 7 vaginal cream: Insert 1 applicatorful intravaginally at bedtime for 7 consecutive days
Terazol® 3 vaginal suppository: Insert 1 suppository intravaginally at bedtime for 3 consecutive days
**Dosage Forms**
Cream, vaginal:
Terazol® 7: 0.4% (45 g) [packaged with measured-dose applicator]
Terazol® 3: 0.8% (20 g) [packaged with measured-dose applicator]
Suppository, vaginal (Terazol® 3): 80 mg (3s) [may contain coconut and/or palm kernel oil]

# Terfluzine [Can] *see* trifluoperazine *on page 823*

# teriparatide (ter i PAR a tide)

**Synonyms** parathyroid hormone (1-34); recombinant human parathyroid hormone (1-34); rhPTH(1-34)
**U.S./Canadian Brand Names** Forteo™ [US/Can]
**Therapeutic Category** Diagnostic Agent
**Use** Treatment of osteoporosis in postmenopausal women at high risk of fracture; treatment of primary or hypogonadal osteoporosis in men at high risk of fracture
**Usual Dosage** SubQ: Adults: 20 mcg once daily; **Note:** Initial administration should occur under circumstances in which the patient may sit or lie down, in the event of orthostasis.
(Continued)

## teriparatide *(Continued)*

**Dosage Forms** Injection, solution: 250 mcg/mL (3 mL) [prefilled syringe, delivers teriparatide 20 mcg/dose]

**terpin hydrate** *(Discontinued)*

**Terra-Cortril® Ophthalmic Suspension** *(Discontinued)*

**Terramycin® [Can]** *see* oxytetracycline *on page 611*

**Terramycin® I.M. [US]** *see* oxytetracycline *on page 611*

**Terramycin® Oral** *(Discontinued)* *see* oxytetracycline *on page 611*

**Tesamone® Injection** *(Discontinued)* *see* testosterone *on this page*

**Teslac® [US/Can]** *see* testolactone *on this page*

**TESPA** *see* thiotepa *on page 799*

**Tessalon® [US/Can]** *see* benzonatate *on page 98*

**Testim® [US]** *see* testosterone *on this page*

**Testoderm®** *(Discontinued)* *see* testosterone *on this page*

**Testoderm® TTS** *(Discontinued)* *see* testosterone *on this page*

**Testoderm® With Adhesive** *(Discontinued)* *see* testosterone *on this page*

## testolactone (tes toe LAK tone)

**Sound-Alike/Look-Alike Issues**
testolactone may be confused with testosterone
**U.S./Canadian Brand Names** Teslac® [US/Can]
**Therapeutic Category** Androgen
**Controlled Substance** C-III
**Use** Palliative treatment of advanced or disseminated breast carcinoma
**Usual Dosage** Adults: Female: Oral: 250 mg 4 times/day for at least 3 months; desired response may take as long as 3 months
**Dosage Forms** Tablet: 50 mg

**Testomar®** *(Discontinued)* *see* yohimbine *on page 857*

**Testopel® [US]** *see* testosterone *on this page*

**Testopel® Pellet** *(Discontinued)* *see* testosterone *on this page*

## testosterone (tes TOS ter one)

**Sound-Alike/Look-Alike Issues**
testosterone may be confused with testolactone
Testoderm® may be confused with Estraderm®
**Synonyms** testosterone cypionate; testosterone enanthate
**U.S./Canadian Brand Names** Andriol® [Can]; Androderm® [US/Can]; AndroGel® [US/Can]; Andropository [Can]; Delatestryl® [US/Can]; Depotest® 100 [Can]; Depo®-Testosterone [US]; Everone® 200 [Can]; First® Testosterone MC [US]; First® Testosterone [US]; Striant® [US]; Testim® [US]; Testopel® [US]; Virilon® IM [Can]
**Therapeutic Category** Androgen
**Controlled Substance** C-III
**Use**
Injection: Androgen replacement therapy in the treatment of delayed male puberty; male hypogonadism (primary or hypogonadotropic); inoperable female breast cancer (enanthate only)
Pellet: Androgen replacement therapy in the treatment of delayed male puberty; male hypogonadism (primary or hypogonadotropic)
Buccal, topical: Male hypogonadism (primary or hypogonadotropic)
**Usual Dosage**
Adolescents: I.M.:
Male hypogonadism:
Initiation of pubertal growth: 40-50 mg/m$^2$/dose (cypionate or enanthate ester) monthly until the growth rate falls to prepubertal levels
Terminal growth phase: 100 mg/m$^2$/dose (cypionate or enanthate ester) monthly until growth ceases

Maintenance virilizing dose: 100 mg/m$^2$/dose (cypionate or enanthate ester) twice monthly

Delayed male puberty: 40-50 mg/m$^2$/dose monthly (cypionate or enanthate ester) for 6 months

Adolescents and Adults: Pellet (for subcutaneous implantation): Delayed male puberty, male hypogonadism: 150-450 mg every 3-6 months

Adults:

I.M.:

Female: Inoperable breast cancer: Testosterone enanthate: 200-400 mg every 2-4 weeks

Male: Long-acting formulations: Testosterone enanthate (in oil)/testosterone cypionate (in oil):

Hypogonadism: 50-400 mg every 2-4 weeks

Delayed puberty: 50-200 mg every 2-4 weeks for a limited duration

Transdermal: Primary male hypogonadism **or** hypogonadotropic hypogonadism:

Androderm®: Initial: Apply 5 mg/day once nightly to clean, dry area on the back, abdomen, upper arms, or thighs (do **not** apply to scrotum); dosing range: 2.5-7.5 mg/day; in nonvirilized patients, dose may be initiated at 2.5 mg/day

AndroGel®, Testim®: 5 g (to deliver 50 mg of testosterone with 5 mg systemically absorbed) applied once daily (preferably in the morning) to clean, dry, intact skin of the shoulder and upper arms. AndroGel® may also be applied to the abdomen. Dosage may be increased to a maximum of 10 g (100 mg). **Do not apply testosterone gel to the genitals**.

Oral (buccal): Hypogonadism or hypogonadotropic hypogonadism: 30 mg twice daily (every 12 hours) applied to the gum region above the incisor tooth

**Dosage Forms**

Gel, topical:

AndroGel®:

1.25 g/actuation (75 g) [1% metered-dose pump; delivers 5 g/4 actuations; provides 60 1.25 g actuations; contains ethanol]

2.5 g (30s) [1% unit dose packets; contains ethanol]

5 g (30s) [1% unit dose packets; contains ethanol]

Testim®: 5 g (30s) [1% unit-dose tube; contains ethanol]

Injection, in oil, as cypionate: 200 mg/mL (10 mL)

Depo®-Testosterone: 100 mg/mL (10 mL); 200 mg/mL (1 mL, 10 mL) [contains benzyl alcohol, benzyl benzoate, and cottonseed oil]

Injection, in oil, as enanthate: 200 mg/mL (5 mL)

Delatestryl®: 200 mg/mL (1 mL) [prefilled syringe; contains sesame oil]; (5 mL) [multidose vial; contains sesame oil]

Kit [for prescription compounding testosterone 2%; kits also contain mixing jar and stirrer]:

First® Testosterone:

Injection, in oil: Testosterone propionate 100 mg/mL (12 mL) [contains sesame oil and benzyl alcohol]

Ointment: White petroleum (48 g)

First® Testosterone MC:

Injection, in oil: Testosterone propionate 100 mg/mL (12 mL) [contains sesame oil and benzyl alcohol]

Cream: Moisturizing cream (48 g)

Mucoadhesive, for buccal application [buccal system] (Striant®): 30 mg (10s)

Pellet, for subcutaneous implantation (Testopel®): 75 mg (1 pellet/vial)

Transdermal system (Androderm®): 2.5 mg/day (60s); 5 mg/day (30s) [contains ethanol]

**testosterone cypionate** *see* testosterone *on previous page*

**testosterone enanthate** *see* testosterone *on previous page*

**Testred® [US]** *see* methyltestosterone *on page 533*

**tetanus and diphtheria toxoid** *see* diphtheria and tetanus toxoid *on page 257*

# tetanus antitoxin (TET a nus an tee TOKS in)

**Synonyms** TAT

**Therapeutic Category** Antitoxin

**Use** Tetanus prophylaxis or treatment of active tetanus only when tetanus immune globulin (TIG) is not available; tetanus immune globulin (Hyper-Tet®) is the preferred tetanus immunoglobulin for the treatment of active tetanus; may be given concomitantly with tetanus toxoid adsorbed when immediate treatment is required, but active immunization is desirable

**Usual Dosage**

Prophylaxis: I.M., SubQ:

Children <30 kg: 1500 units

Children and Adults ≥30 kg: 3000-5000 units

(Continued)

## tetanus antitoxin *(Continued)*

Treatment: Children and Adults: Inject 10,000-40,000 units into wound; administer 40,000-100,000 units
**Dosage Forms** Injection, equine: Not less than 400 units/mL (12.5 mL, 50 mL)

## tetanus immune globulin (human) (TET a nus i MYUN GLOB yoo lin HYU man)

**Synonyms** TIG
**U.S./Canadian Brand Names** BayTet™ [US/Can]
**Therapeutic Category** Immune Globulin
**Use** Passive immunization against tetanus; tetanus immune globulin is preferred over tetanus antitoxin for treatment of active tetanus; part of the management of an unclean, wound in a person whose history of previous receipt of tetanus toxoid is unknown or who has received less than three doses of tetanus toxoid
**Usual Dosage** I.M.:
Prophylaxis of tetanus:
  Children: 4 units/kg; some recommend administering 250 units to small children
  Adults: 250 units
Treatment of tetanus:
  Children: 500-3000 units; some should infiltrate locally around the wound
  Adults: 3000-6000 units
**Dosage Forms** Injection, solution [preservative free]: 250 units/mL (1 mL) [prefilled syringe]

## tetanus toxoid (adsorbed) (TET a nus TOKS oyd, ad SORBED)

**Therapeutic Category** Toxoid
**Use** Active immunization against tetanus when combination antigen preparations are not indicated. **Note:** Tetanus and diphtheria toxoids for adult use (Td) is the preferred immunizing agent for most adults and for children after their seventh birthday. Young children should receive trivalent DTaP (diphtheria/ tetanus/acellular pertussis), as part of their childhood immunization program, unless pertussis is contra- indicated, then TD is warranted.
**Usual Dosage** Children ≥7 years and Adults: I.M.:
Primary immunization: 0.5 mL; repeat 0.5 mL at 4-8 weeks after first dose and at 6-12 months after second dose
Routine booster dose: Recommended every 10 years
**Note:** In most patients, Td is the recommended product for primary immunization, booster doses, and tetanus immunization in wound management (refer to Diphtheria and Tetanus Toxoid *on page 257* monograph)
**Dosage Forms** Injection, suspension: Tetanus 5 Lf units per 0.5 mL (0.5 mL) [contains trace amounts of thimerosal]; (5 mL) [contains thimerosal; vial stopper contains latex]

## tetanus toxoid (fluid) (TET a nus TOKS oyd FLOO id)

**Synonyms** tetanus toxoid plain
**Therapeutic Category** Toxoid
**Use** Indicated as booster dose in the active immunization against tetanus in the rare adult or child who is allergic to the aluminum adjuvant (a product containing adsorbed tetanus toxoid is preferred); not indicated for primary immunization
**Usual Dosage**
Primary immunization: Not indicated for this use.
Booster doses: I.M., SubQ: 0.5 mL every 10 years
**Dosage Forms** Injection, solution: Tetanus 4 Lf units per 0.5 mL (7.5 mL) [contains thimerosal; vial stopper contains dry natural latex rubber]

**tetanus toxoid plain** *see* tetanus toxoid (fluid) *on this page*

**tetanus toxoid, reduced diphtheria toxoid, and acellular pertussis, adsorbed** *see* diph- theria, tetanus toxoids, and acellular pertussis vaccine *on page 259*

## tetrabenazine *(Canada only)* (tet ra BEN a zeen)

**U.S./Canadian Brand Names** Nitoman™ [Can]
**Therapeutic Category** Monoamine Depleting Agent
**Use** Treatment of hyperkinetic movement disorders, including Huntington chorea, hemiballismus, senile chorea, Tourette syndrome, and tardive dyskinesia

**Usual Dosage** Oral:

Children (limited data): Consider initiation at $^1/_2$ recommended adult dosage; must be titrated slowly to individualize dosage

Adults: Initial: 12.5 mg twice daily (may be given 3 times/day); may be increased by 12.5 mg/day every 3-5 days; should be titrated slowly to maximal tolerated and effective dose (dose is individualized)

Usual maximum tolerated dosage: 25 mg 3 times/day; maximum recommended dose:. 200 mg/day

**Note:** If there is no improvement at the maximum tolerated dose after 7 days, improvement is unlikely; discontinuation should be considered.

**Dosage Forms** Tablet: 25 mg

## tetracaine (TET ra kane)

**Synonyms** amethocaine hydrochloride; tetracaine hydrochloride

**U.S./Canadian Brand Names** Ametop™ [Can]; Pontocaine® Niphanoid® [US]; Pontocaine® [US/Can]

**Therapeutic Category** Local Anesthetic

**Use** Spinal anesthesia; local anesthesia in the eye for various diagnostic and examination purposes; topically applied to nose and throat for various diagnostic procedures

**Usual Dosage** Adults:

Ophthalmic: Short-term anesthesia of the eye: 0.5% solution: Instill 1-2 drops; prolonged use (especially for at-home self-medication) is not recommended

Injection: Spinal anesthesia: **Note:** Dosage varies with the anesthetic procedure, the degree of anesthesia required, and the individual patient response; it is administered by subarachnoid injection for spinal anesthesia.

Perineal anesthesia: 5 mg

Perineal and lower extremities: 10 mg

Anesthesia extending up to costal margin: 15 mg; doses up to 20 mg may be given, but are reserved for exceptional cases

Low spinal anesthesia (saddle block): 2-5 mg

Topical mucous membranes (rhinolaryngology): Used as a 0.25% or 0.5% solution by direct application or nebulization; total dose should not exceed 20 mg

**Dosage Forms** [DSC] = Discontinued product

Injection, solution, as hydrochloride [preservative free] (Pontocaine®): 1% [10 mg/mL] (2 mL) [contains sodium bisulfite]

Injection, solution, as hydrochloride [premixed in dextrose 6%] (Pontocaine®): 0.3% [3 mg/mL] (5 mL) [DSC]

Injection, powder for reconstitution, as hydrochloride [preservative free] (Pontocaine® Niphanoid®): 20 mg

Solution, ophthalmic, as hydrochloride: 0.5% [5 mg/mL] (15 mL)

Solution, topical, as hydrochloride (Pontocaine®): 2% [20 mg/mL] (30 mL, 118 mL) [for rhinolaryngology]

## tetracaine and dextrose (TET ra kane & DEKS trose)

**Synonyms** dextrose and tetracaine

**U.S./Canadian Brand Names** Pontocaine® With Dextrose [US]

**Therapeutic Category** Local Anesthetic

**Use** Spinal anesthesia (saddle block)

**Usual Dosage** Dose varies with procedure, depth of anesthesia, duration desired and physical condition of patient

**Dosage Forms** Injection, as hydrochloride [premixed in dextrose 6%]: Tetracaine hydrochloride 0.3% and dextrose 6% (5 mL)

**tetracaine hydrochloride** *see* tetracaine *on this page*

**tetracaine hydrochloride, benzocaine butyl aminobenzoate, and benzalkonium chloride** *see* benzocaine, butyl aminobenzoate, tetracaine, and benzalkonium chloride *on page 97*

**Tetracap® *(Discontinued)*** *see* tetracycline *on this page*

**tetracosactide** *see* cosyntropin *on page 210*

## tetracycline (tet ra SYE kleen)

**Sound-Alike/Look-Alike Issues**

tetracycline may be confused with tetradecyl sulfate

achromycin may be confused with actinomycin, Adriamycin PFS®

*(Continued)*

## tetracycline *(Continued)*

**Synonyms** achromycin; TCN; tetracycline hydrochloride

**U.S./Canadian Brand Names** Apo-Tetra® [Can]; Nu-Tetra [Can]; Sumycin® [US]

**Therapeutic Category** Antibiotic, Ophthalmic; Antibiotic, Topical; Tetracycline Derivative

**Use** Treatment of susceptible bacterial infections of both gram-positive and gram-negative organisms; also infections due to *Mycoplasma*, *Chlamydia*, and *Rickettsia*; indicated for acne, exacerbations of chronic bronchitis, and treatment of gonorrhea and syphilis in patients that are allergic to penicillin; as part of a multidrug regimen for *H. pylori* eradication to reduce the risk of duodenal ulcer recurrence

**Usual Dosage** Oral:

Children >8 years: 25-50 mg/kg/day in divided doses every 6 hours

Adults: 250-500 mg/dose every 6 hours

*Helicobacter pylori* eradication: 500 mg 2-4 times/day depending on regimen; requires combination therapy with at least one other antibiotic and an acid-suppressing agent (proton pump inhibitor or $H_2$ blocker)

**Dosage Forms**

Capsule, as hydrochloride: 250 mg, 500 mg

Suspension, oral, as hydrochloride (Sumycin®): 125 mg/5 mL (480 mL) [contains sodium benzoate and sodium metabisulfite; fruit flavor]

Tablet, as hydrochloride (Sumycin®): 250 mg, 500 mg

**tetracycline, bismuth subsalicylate, and metronidazole** *see* bismuth subsalicylate, metronidazole, and tetracycline *on page 108*

**tetracycline hydrochloride** *see* tetracycline *on previous page*

**tetracycline, metronidazole, and bismuth subsalicylate** *see* bismuth subsalicylate, metronidazole, and tetracycline *on page 108*

**tetrahydroaminoacrine** *see* tacrine *on page 778*

**tetrahydrocannabinol** *see* dronabinol *on page 274*

## tetrahydrozoline *(tet ra hye DROZ a leen)*

**Sound-Alike/Look-Alike Issues**

Visine® may be confused with Visken®

**Synonyms** tetrahydrozoline hydrochloride; tetryzoline

**U.S./Canadian Brand Names** Eye-Sine™ [US-OTC]; Geneye® [US-OTC]; Murine® Tears Plus [US-OTC]; Optigene® 3 [US-OTC]; Tyzine® Pediatric [US]; Tyzine® [US]; Visine® Advanced Relief [US-OTC]; Visine® Original [US-OTC]

**Therapeutic Category** Adrenergic Agonist Agent

**Use** Symptomatic relief of nasal congestion and conjunctival congestion

**Usual Dosage**

Nasal congestion: Intranasal:

Children 2-6 years: Instill 2-3 drops of 0.05% solution every 4-6 hours as needed, no more frequent than every 3 hours

Children >6 years and Adults: Instill 2-4 drops or 3-4 sprays of 0.1% solution every 3-4 hours as needed, no more frequent than every 3 hours

Conjunctival congestion: Ophthalmic: Adults: Instill 1-2 drops in each eye 2-4 times/day

**Dosage Forms**

Solution, intranasal, as hydrochloride:

Tyzine®: 0.1% (15 mL) [spray bottle; contains benzalkonium chloride]; (30 mL) [dropper bottle; contains benzalkonium chloride]

Tyzine® Pediatric: 0.05% (15 mL) [spray bottle; contains benzalkonium chloride]

Solution, ophthalmic, as hydrochloride: 0.05% (15 mL)

Eye-Sine™, Geneye®, Optigene® 3: 0.05% (15 mL) [may contain benzalkonium chloride]

Murine® Tears Plus: 0.05% (15 mL, 30 mL) [contains benzalkonium chloride]

Visine® Advanced Relief: 0.05% (30 mL) [contains benzalkonium chloride and polyethylene glycol]

Visine® Original: 0.05% (15 mL, 30 mL) [contains benzalkonium chloride; 15 mL size also available with dropper]

**tetrahydrozoline hydrochloride** *see* tetrahydrozoline *on this page*

**Tetramune® *(Discontinued)***

**Tetrasine® Extra Ophthalmic *(Discontinued)*** *see* tetrahydrozoline *on this page*

**Tetrasine**® **Ophthalmic** *(Discontinued)* *see* tetrahydrozoline *on previous page*

**Tetra Tannate Pediatric [US]** *see* chlorpheniramine, ephedrine, phenylephrine, and carbetapentane *on page 173*

**tetryzoline** *see* tetrahydrozoline *on previous page*

**Teveten**® **[US/Can]** *see* eprosartan *on page 291*

**Teveten**® **HCT [US/Can]** *see* eprosartan and hydrochlorothiazide *on page 292*

**Teveten**® **Plus [Can]** *see* eprosartan and hydrochlorothiazide *on page 292*

**Tev-Tropin**™ **[US]** *see* somatropin *on page 760*

**Texacort**® **[US]** *see* hydrocortisone (topical) *on page 417*

**TG** *see* thioguanine *on page 797*

**T-Gen**® *(Discontinued)* *see* trimethobenzamide *on page 825*

**THA** *see* tacrine *on page 778*

## thalidomide (tha LI doe mide)

**Sound-Alike/Look-Alike Issues**
thalidomide may be confused with flutamide
**U.S./Canadian Brand Names** Thalomid® [US/Can]
**Therapeutic Category** Immunosuppressant Agent
**Use** Treatment and maintenance of cutaneous manifestations of erythema nodosum leprosum
**Usual Dosage** Oral: Cutaneous ENL:
Initiate dosing at 100-300 mg/day taken once daily at bedtime with water (at least 1 hour after evening meal)
Patients weighing <50 kg: Initiate at lower end of the dosing range
Severe cutaneous reaction or previously requiring high dose may be initiated at 400 mg/day; doses may be divided, but taken 1 hour after meals
Dosing should continue until active reaction subsides (usually at least 2 weeks), then tapered in 50 mg decrements every 2-4 weeks
Patients who flare during tapering or with a history or requiring prolonged maintenance should be maintained on the minimum dosage necessary to control the reaction. Efforts to taper should be repeated every 3-6 months, in increments of 50 mg every 2-4 weeks.
**Dosage Forms** Capsule: 50 mg, 100 mg, 200 mg

**Thalitone**® **[US]** *see* chlorthalidone *on page 179*

**Thalomid**® **[US/Can]** *see* thalidomide *on this page*

**THAM**® **[US]** *see* tromethamine *on page 829*

**THC** *see* dronabinol *on page 274*

**Theo-X**® *(Discontinued)* *see* theophylline *on this page*

**Theo-24**® **[US]** *see* theophylline *on this page*

**Theobid**® *(Discontinued)* *see* theophylline *on this page*

**Theochron**® **[US]** *see* theophylline *on this page*

**Theochron**® **SR [Can]** *see* theophylline *on this page*

**Theoclear-80**® *(Discontinued)* *see* theophylline *on this page*

**Theoclear**®-**L.A.** *(Discontinued)* *see* theophylline *on this page*

**Theo-Dur**® **(all products)** *(Discontinued)* *see* theophylline *on this page*

**Theolair**™ **[US/Can]** *see* theophylline *on this page*

**Theolair-SR**® *(Discontinued)* *see* theophylline *on this page*

**Theolate** *(Discontinued)* *see* theophylline and guaifenesin *on page 795*

## theophylline (thee OFF i lin)

**Sound-Alike/Look-Alike Issues**
Theolair™ may be confused with Thiola®, Thyrolar®
**Synonyms** theophylline anhydrous
**U.S./Canadian Brand Names** Apo-Theo LA® [Can]; Elixophyllin® [US]; Novo-Theophyl SR [Can]; PMS-Theophylline [Can]; Pulmophylline [Can]; Quibron®-T [US]; Quibron®-T/SR [US]; ratio-Theo-Bronc *(Continued)*

## theophylline *(Continued)*

[Can]; T-Phyl® [US]; Theo-24® [US]; Theochron® SR [Can]; Theochron® [US]; Theolair™ [US/Can]; Uniphyl® SRT [Can]; Uniphyl® [US]

**Therapeutic Category** Theophylline Derivative

**Use** Treatment of symptoms and reversible airway obstruction due to chronic asthma, chronic bronchitis, or COPD

**Usual Dosage** Use ideal body weight for obese patients

I.V.: Initial: Maintenance infusion rates:

Children:

6 weeks to 6 months: 0.5 mg/kg/hour
6 months to 1 year: 0.6-0.7 mg/kg/hour

Children >1 year and Adults:

**Acute bronchospasm:** Approximate I.V. theophylline dosage for treatment of acute bronchospasm: **Note:** Equivalent hydrousaminophylline dosage is indicated in parentheses.

Infants 6 weeks to 6 months: 0.5 mg/kg/hour for next 12 hours
Children 6 months to 1 year: 0.6-0.7 mg/kg/hour for next 12 hours
Children 1-9 years: 0.95 mg/kg/hour (1.2 mg/kg/hour) for next 12 hours; 0.79 mg/kg/hour (1 mg/kg/hour) after 12 hours
Children 9-16 years and young adult smokers: 0.79 mg/kg/hour (1 mg/kg/hour) for next 12 hours;0.63 mg/kg/hour (0.8 mg/kg/hour) after 12 hours
Healthy, nonsmoking adults: 0.55 mg/kg/hour (0.7 mg/kg/hour) for next 12 hours; 0.39 mg/kg/hour (0.5 mg/kg/hour) after 12 hours
Older patients and patients with corpulmonale: 0.47 mg/kg/hour (0.6 mg/kg/hour) for next 12 hours;0.24 mg/kg/hour (0.3 mg/kg/hour) after 12 hours
Patients with congestive heart failure or liver failure: 0.39 mg/kg/hour (0.5 mg/kg/hour) for next 12 hours; 0.08-0.16 mg/kg/hour (0.1-0.2 mg/kg/hour) after 12 hours

**Approximate I.V. maintenance dosages are based upon continuous infusions**; bolus dosing (often used in children <6 months of age) may be determined by multiplying the hourly infusion rate by 24 hours and dividing by the desired number of doses/day. See the following: Maintenance dose for acute symptoms:

Premature infant or newborn to 6 weeks (for apnea/bradycardia):
Oral theophylline: 4 mg/kg/day
I.V. aminophylline: 5 mg/kg/day
6 weeks to 6 months:
Oral theophylline: 10 mg/kg/day
I.V. aminophylline: 12 mg/kg/day or continuous I.V. infusion[1]
Infants 6 months to 1 year:
Oral theophylline: 12-18 mg/kg/day
I.V. aminophylline: 15 mg/kg/day or continuous I.V. infusion[1]
Children 1-9 years:
Oral theophylline: 20-24 mg/kg/day
I.V. aminophylline: 1 mg/kg/hour
Children 9-12 years, and adolescent daily smokers of cigarettes or marijuana, and otherwise healthy adult smokers <50 years:
Oral theophylline: 16 mg/kg/day
I.V. aminophylline: 0.9 mg/kg/hour
Adolescents 12-16 years (nonsmokers):
Oral theophylline: 13 mg/kg/day
I.V. aminophylline: 0.7 mg/kg/hour
Otherwise healthy nonsmoking adults:
Oral theophylline: 10 mg/kg/day (not to exceed 900 mg/day)
I.V. aminophylline: 0.5 mg/kg/hour
Cardiac decompensation, corpulmonale, and/or liver dysfunction:
Oral theophylline: 5 mg/kg/day (not to exceed 400 mg/day)
I.V. aminophylline: 0.25 mg/kg/hour
[1]For continuous I.V. infusion, divide total daily dose by 24 = mg/kg/hour.

**Oral theophylline dosage for bronchial asthma** (by age):
<1 year:
Initial 3 days and second 3 days: 0.2 x (age in weeks) + 5 = mg/kg/24 hours of theophylline
Steady-state maintenance: 0.3 x (age in weeks) + 8 = mg/kg/24 hours of theophylline

1-9 years:
Initial 3 days: 16 mg/kg/24 hours of theophylline, up to a maximum of 400 mg/24 hours
Second 3 days: 20 mg/kg/24 hours of theophylline
Steady-state maintenance: 22 mg/kg/24 hours of theophylline
9-12 years:
Initial 3 days: 16 mg/kg/24 hours of theophylline, up to a maximum of 400 mg/24 hours
Second 3 days: 16 mg/kg/24 hours of theophylline, up to a maximum of 600 mg/24 hours
Steady-state maintenance: 20 mg/kg/24 hours of theophylline, up to a maximum of 800 mg/24 hours
12-16 years:
Initial 3 days: 16 mg/kg/24 hours of theophylline, up to a maximum of 400 mg/24 hours
Second 3 days: 16 mg/kg/24 hours of theophylline, up to a maximum of 600 mg/24 hours
Steady-state maintenance: 18 mg/kg/24 hours of theophylline, up to a maximum of 900 mg/24 hours
Adults:
Initial 3 days: 400 mg/24 hours
Second 3 days: 600 mg/24 hours
Steady-state maintenance: 900 mg/24 hours
**Increasing dose:** The dosage may be increased in approximately 25% increments at 2- to 3-day intervals so long as the drug is tolerated or until the maximum dose is reached
**Maintenance dose:** In children and healthy adults, a slow-release product can be used; the total daily dose can be divided every 8-12 hours
Dosage Forms [DSC] = Discontinued product
Capsule, extended release (Theo-24®): 100 mg, 200 mg, 300 mg, 400 mg [24 hours]
Elixir (Elixophyllin®): 80 mg/15 mL (480 mL) [contains alcohol 20%; fruit flavor]
Infusion [premixed in D₅W]: 0.8 mg/mL (500 mL, 1000 mL); 1.6 mg/mL (250 mL, 500 mL); 2 mg/mL (100 mL); 3.2 mg/mL (250 mL); 4 mg/mL (50 mL, 100 mL)
Solution, oral: 80 mg/15 mL (15 mL, 18.75 mL, 500 mL) [dye free, sugar free; contains alcohol 0.4% and benzoic acid; orange flavor]
Tablet, controlled release:
T-Phyl®: 200 mg [12 hours; contains cetostearyl alcohol]
Uniphyl®: 400 mg, 600 mg [24 hours; contains cetostearyl alcohol]
Tablet, extended release: 100 mg, 200 mg, 300 mg, 450 mg
Theochron®: 100 mg, 200 mg, 300 mg [12-24 hours]
Tablet, immediate release:
Quibron®-T: 300 mg
Theolair™: 125 mg, 250 mg
Tablet, sustained release (Quibron®-T/SR): 300 mg [8-12 hours]
Tablet, timed release (Theolair™-SR [DSC]): 300 mg, 500 mg

## theophylline and guaifenesin (thee OFF i lin & gwye FEN e sin)

Synonyms guaifenesin and theophylline
U.S./Canadian Brand Names Elixophyllin-GG® [US]; Quibron® [US]
Therapeutic Category Theophylline Derivative
Use Symptomatic treatment of bronchospasm associated with bronchial asthma, chronic bronchitis, and pulmonary emphysema
Usual Dosage Adults: Oral: 16 mg/kg/day or 400 mg theophylline/day, in divided doses, every 6-8 hours
Dosage Forms [DSC] = Discontinued product
Capsule (Quibron®): Theophylline 150 mg and guaifenesin 90 mg
Liquid:
Elixophyllin-GG®: Theophylline 100 mg and guaifenesin 100 mg per 15 mL (240 mL, 480 mL) [alcohol free, dye free, sugar free; cherry-berry flavor]
Theolate: Theophylline 150 mg and guaifenesin 90 mg per 15 mL (480 mL) [alcohol free, dye free] [DSC]

**theophylline anhydrous** *see* theophylline *on page 793*

**theophylline ethylenediamine** *see* aminophylline *on page 41*

**Theo-Sav® *(Discontinued)*** *see* theophylline *on page 793*

**Theospan®-SR *(Discontinued)*** *see* theophylline *on page 793*

**Theostat-80® *(Discontinued)*** *see* theophylline *on page 793*

**Theovent® *(Discontinued)*** *see* theophylline *on page 793*

**Therabid® *(Discontinued)***

**TheraCys® [US]** *see* BCG vaccine *on page 90*

**Thera-Flu® Cold and Sore Throat Night Time [US-OTC]** *see* acetaminophen, chlorphenira-mine, and pseudoephedrine *on page 10*

**Thera-Flur® (Discontinued)** *see* fluoride *on page 347*

**Thera-Flur-N® [US]** *see* fluoride *on page 347*

**Thera-Flu® Severe Cold Non-Drowsy (Discontinued)** *see* acetaminophen, dextromethorphan, and pseudoephedrine *on page 11*

**Theragran-M® Advanced Formula (Discontinued)** *see* vitamins (multiple/oral) *on page 852*

**Theragran® Heart Right™ (Discontinued)** *see* vitamins (multiple/oral) *on page 852*

**Theramycin Z® [US]** *see* erythromycin *on page 295*

**TheraPatch® Warm (Discontinued)** *see* capsaicin *on page 138*

**therapeutic multivitamins** *see* vitamins (multiple/oral) *on page 852*

**Theratears® [US]** *see* carboxymethylcellulose *on page 148*

**Thermazene® [US]** *see* silver sulfadiazine *on page 747*

## thiabendazole (thye a BEN da zole)

**Synonyms** tiabendazole
**U.S./Canadian Brand Names** Mintezol® [US]
**Therapeutic Category** Anthelmintic
**Use** Treatment of strongyloidiasis, cutaneous larva migrans, visceral larva migrans, dracunculiasis, trichinosis, and mixed helminthic infections
**Usual Dosage** Purgation is not required prior to use; drinking of fruit juice aids in expulsion of worms by removing the mucous to which the intestinal tapeworms attach themselves.

Children and Adults: Oral: 50 mg/kg/day divided every 12 hours (if >68 kg: 1.5 g/dose); maximum dose: 3 g/day
Treatment duration:
Strongyloidiasis, ascariasis, uncinariasis: For 2 consecutive days
Cutaneous larva migrans: For 2 consecutive days; if active lesions are still present 2 days after completion, a second course of treatment is recommended.
Visceral larva migrans: For 7 consecutive days
Trichinosis: For 2-4 consecutive days; optimal dosage not established
Dracunculosis: 50-75 mg/kg/day divided every 12 hours for 3 days
**Dosage Forms** [DSC] = Discontinued product
Suspension, oral: 500 mg/5 mL (120 mL) [DSC]
Tablet, chewable: 500 mg [orange flavor]

**thiamazole** *see* methimazole *on page 523*

## thiamine (THYE a min)

**Sound-Alike/Look-Alike Issues**
thiamine may be confused with Tenormin®, Thorazine®
**Synonyms** aneurine hydrochloride; thiamine hydrochloride; thiaminium chloride hydrochloride; vitamin B₁
**U.S./Canadian Brand Names** Betaxin® [Can]
**Therapeutic Category** Vitamin, Water Soluble
**Use** Treatment of thiamine deficiency including beriberi, Wernicke encephalopathy syndrome, and periph-eral neuritis associated with pellagra, alcoholic patients with altered sensorium; various genetic meta-bolic disorders
**Usual Dosage**
Recommended daily allowance:
<6 months: 0.3 mg
6 months to 1 year: 0.4 mg
1-3 years: 0.7 mg
4-6 years: 0.9 mg
7-10 years: 1 mg
11-14 years: 1.1-1.3 mg
>14 years: 1-1.5 mg

Thiamine deficiency (beriberi):
Children: 10-25 mg/dose I.M. or I.V. daily (if critically ill), or 10-50 mg/dose orally every day for 2 weeks, then 5-10 mg/dose orally daily for 1 month
Adults: 5-30 mg/dose I.M. or I.V. 3 times/day (if critically ill); then orally 5-30 mg/day in single or divided doses 3 times/day for 1 month
Wernicke's encephalopathy: Adults: Initial: 100 mg I.V., then 50-100 mg/day I.M. or I.V. until consuming a regular, balanced diet
Dietary supplement (depends on caloric or carbohydrate content of the diet):
Infants: 0.3-0.5 mg/day
Children: 0.5-1 mg/day
Adults: 1-2 mg/day
**Note:** The above doses can be found in multivitamin preparations
Metabolic disorders: Oral: Adults: 10-20 mg/day (dosages up to 4 g/day in divided doses have been used)
**Dosage Forms**
Injection, solution, as hydrochloride: 100 mg/mL (2 mL)
Tablet, as hydrochloride: 50 mg, 100 mg, 250 mg, 500 mg

**thiamine hydrochloride** see thiamine on previous page

**thiaminium chloride hydrochloride** see thiamine on previous page

## thimerosal (thye MER oh sal)
**U.S./Canadian Brand Names** Mersol® [US-OTC]; Merthiolate® [US-OTC]
**Therapeutic Category** Antibacterial, Topical
**Use** Organomercurial antiseptic with sustained bacteriostatic and fungistatic activity
**Usual Dosage** Apply 1-3 times/day
**Dosage Forms**
Solution, topical (Merthiolate®): 0.1% [1 mg/mL = 1:1000] (30 mL)
Solution, topical spray (Merthiolate®): 0.1% [1 mg/mL = 1:1000] (60 g)
Tincture, topical (Mersol®): 0.1% [1 mg/mL = 1:1000] (120 mL, 480 mL, 4000 mL)

## thioguanine (thye oh GWAH neen)
**Sound-Alike/Look-Alike Issues**
6-thioguanine and 6-TG are error-prone abbreviations (associated with six-fold overdoses of thioguanine)
**Synonyms** 2-amino-6-mercaptopurine; NSC-752; TG; tioguanine
**U.S./Canadian Brand Names** Lanvis® [Can]; Tabloid® [US]
**Therapeutic Category** Antineoplastic Agent
**Use** Treatment of acute myelogenous (nonlymphocytic) leukemia; treatment of chronic myelogenous leukemia and granulocytic leukemia
**Usual Dosage** Total daily dose can be given at one time.
Oral (refer to individual protocols):
Infants and Children <3 years: Combination drug therapy for acute nonlymphocytic leukemia: 3.3 mg/kg/day in divided doses twice daily for 4 days
Children and Adults: 2-3 mg/kg/day calculated to nearest 20 mg or 75-200 mg/m$^2$/day in 1-2 divided doses for 5-7 days or until remission is attained
**Dosage Forms**
Injection, powder for reconstitution: 75 mg [investigational in U.S.]
Tablet [scored]: 40 mg

**Thiola® [US/Can]** see tiopronin on page 805

## thiopental (thye oh PEN tal)
**Synonyms** thiopental sodium
**U.S./Canadian Brand Names** Pentothal® [US/Can]
**Therapeutic Category** Barbiturate
**Controlled Substance** C-III
**Use** Induction of anesthesia; adjunct for intubation in head injury patients; control of convulsive states; treatment of elevated intracranial pressure
(Continued)

# thiopental *(Continued)*

Usual Dosage I.V.:
  Induction anesthesia:
    Infants: 5-8 mg/kg
    Children 1-12 years: 5-6 mg/kg
    Adults: 3-5 mg/kg
  Maintenance anesthesia:
    Children: 1 mg/kg as needed
    Adults: 25-100 mg as needed
  Increased intracranial pressure: Children and Adults: 1.5-5 mg/kg/dose; repeat as needed to control intracranial pressure
  Seizures:
    Children: 2-3 mg/kg/dose; repeat as needed
    Adults: 75-250 mg/dose; repeat as needed
Dosage Forms Injection, powder for reconstitution, as sodium: 250 mg, 400 mg, 500 mg, 1 g

**thiopental sodium** *see thiopental on previous page*

**thiophosphoramide** *see thiotepa on next page*

**Thioplex®** *(Discontinued) see thiotepa on next page*

# thioproperazine *(Canada only)* (thye oh pro PER a zeen)

U.S./Canadian Brand Names Majeptil® [Can]

Therapeutic Category Neuroleptic Agent

Use All types of acute and chronic schizophrenia, including those which did not respond to the usual neuroleptics; manic syndromes.

Usual Dosage Initial treatment: Adults: It is recommended to start treatment at a low dosage of about 5 mg/day in a single dose or in divided doses. This initial dosage is gradually increased by the same amount every 2-3 days until the usual effective dosage of 30-40 mg/day is reached. In some cases, higher dosages of 90 mg or more per day, are necessary to control the psychotic manifestations.
  Children >10 years of age: Start treatment with a daily dosage of 1-3 mg following the method of treatment described for adults
  Maintenance therapy: Adults and Children: Dosage should be reduced gradually to the lowest effective level, which may be as low as a few mg per day and maintained as long as necessary
Dosage Forms Tablet, as mesylate: 10 mg

# thioridazine (thye oh RID a zeen)

Sound-Alike/Look-Alike Issues
  thioridazine may be confused with thiothixene, Thorazine®
  Mellaril® may be confused with Elavil®, Mebaral®
Synonyms thioridazine hydrochloride
U.S./Canadian Brand Names Apo-Thioridazine® [Can]; Mellaril® [Can]
Therapeutic Category Phenothiazine Derivative
Use Management of schizophrenic patients who fail to respond adequately to treatment with other antipsychotic drugs, either because of insufficient effectiveness or the inability to achieve an effective dose due to intolerable adverse effects from those medications
Usual Dosage Oral:
  Children >2-12 years: Range: 0.5-3 mg/kg/day in 2-3 divided doses; usual: 1 mg/kg/day; maximum: 3 mg/kg/day
    Behavior problems: Initial: 10 mg 2-3 times/day, increase gradually
    Severe psychoses: Initial: 25 mg 2-3 times/day, increase gradually
  Children >12 years and Adults:
    Schizophrenia/psychoses: Initial: 50-100 mg 3 times/day with gradual increments as needed and tolerated; maximum: 800 mg/day in 2-4 divided doses
    Depressive disorders/dementia: Initial: 25 mg 3 times/day; maintenance dose: 20-200 mg/day
Dosage Forms Tablet, as hydrochloride: 10 mg, 15 mg, 25 mg, 50 mg, 100 mg, 150 mg, 200 mg

**thioridazine hydrochloride** *see thioridazine on this page*

**thiosulfuric acid disodium salt** *see sodium thiosulfate on page 758*

# thiotepa (thye oh TEP a)
**Synonyms** TESPA; thiophosphoramide; triethylenethiophosphoramide; TSPA
**Therapeutic Category** Antineoplastic Agent
**Use** Treatment of superficial tumors of the bladder; palliative treatment of adenocarcinoma of breast or ovary; lymphomas and sarcomas; controlling intracavitary effusions caused by metastatic tumors; I.T. use: CNS leukemia/lymphoma, CNS metastases
**Usual Dosage** Refer to individual protocols.
  Children: Sarcomas: I.V.: 25-65 mg/m$^2$ as a single dose every 21 days
  Adults:
    I.M., I.V., SubQ: 30-60 mg/m$^2$ once weekly
    I.V.: 0.3-0.4 mg/kg by rapid I.V. administration every 1-4 weeks, **or** 0.2 mg/kg or 6-8 mg/m$^2$/day for 4-5 days every 2-4 weeks
    High-dose therapy for bone marrow transplant: I.V.: 500 mg/m$^2$, up to 900 mg/m$^2$
    I.M.: 15-30 mg in various schedules have been given
    Intracavitary: 0.6-0.8 mg/kg or 30-60 mg weekly
    Intrapericardial: 15-30 mg
    Intrathecal: 10-15 mg or 5-11.5 mg/m$^2$
**Dosage Forms** Injection, powder for reconstitution: 15 mg, 30 mg

# thiothixene (thye oh THIKS een)
**Sound-Alike/Look-Alike Issues**
  thiothixene may be confused with thioridazine
  Navane® may be confused with Norvasc®, Nubain®
**Synonyms** tiotixene
**U.S./Canadian Brand Names** Navane® [US/Can]
**Therapeutic Category** Thioxanthene Derivative
**Use** Management of schizophrenia
**Usual Dosage** Oral: Children >12 years and Adults:
  Mild to moderate psychosis: 2 mg 3 times/day, up to 20-30 mg/day; more severe psychosis: Initial: 5 mg 2 times/day, may increase gradually, if necessary; maximum: 60 mg/day
  Rapid tranquilization of the agitated patient (administered every 30-60 minutes): 5-10 mg; average total dose for tranquilization: 15-30 mg
**Dosage Forms** [DSC] = Discontinued product
  Capsule: 1 mg, 2 mg, 5 mg, 10 mg
  Navane®: 1 mg [DSC], 2 mg, 5 mg, 10 mg, 20 mg

**thonzonium, neomycin, colistin, and hydrocortisone** *see* neomycin, colistin, hydrocortisone, and thonzonium *on page 567*

**Thorazine® *(Discontinued)*** *see* chlorpromazine *on page 178*

**Thorets [US-OTC]** *see* benzocaine *on page 95*

**Thrombate III® [US/Can]** *see* antithrombin III *on page 58*

**Thrombinar® *(Discontinued)*** *see* thrombin (topical) *on this page*

**Thrombin-JMI® [US]** *see* thrombin (topical) *on this page*

# thrombin (topical) (THROM bin, TOP i kal)
**U.S./Canadian Brand Names** Thrombin-JMI® [US]
**Therapeutic Category** Hemostatic Agent
**Use** Hemostasis whenever minor bleeding from capillaries and small venules is accessible
**Usual Dosage** Use 1000-2000 units/mL of solution where bleeding is profuse; apply powder directly to the site of bleeding or on oozing surfaces; use 100 units/mL for bleeding from skin or mucosal surfaces
**Dosage Forms** Powder for reconstitution, topical
  Thrombin-JMI®: 5000 units, 20,000 units [packaged with diluent]
  Thrombin-JMI® Spray Kit: 20,000 units [packaged with diluent and spray pump]
  Thrombin-JMI® Syringe Spray Kit: 20,000 units [packaged with diluent, spray tip, and syringe]

**Thrombostat® *(Discontinued)*** *see* thrombin (topical) *on this page*

**thymocyte stimulating factor** *see* aldesleukin *on page 25*

**Thymoglobulin® [US]** *see* antithymocyte globulin (rabbit) *on page 59*

**Thyrar**® *(Discontinued)* *see* thyroid *on this page*

**Thyro-Block**® *(Discontinued)* *see* potassium iodide *on page 665*

**Thyrogen**® **[US/Can]** *see* thyrotropin alpha *on this page*

## thyroid (THYE roid)

**Synonyms** desiccated thyroid; thyroid extract; thyroid USP

**U.S./Canadian Brand Names** Armour® Thyroid [US]; Nature-Throid® NT [US]; Westhroid® [US]

**Therapeutic Category** Thyroid Product

**Use** Replacement or supplemental therapy in hypothyroidism; pituitary TSH suppressants (thyroid nodules, thyroiditis, multinodular goiter, thyroid cancer), thyrotoxicosis, diagnostic suppression tests

**Usual Dosage** Oral:

Children: Recommended pediatric dosage for congenital hypothyroidism:

0-6 months: 15-30 mg/day; 4.8-6 mg/kg/day
6-12 months: 30-45 mg/day; 3.6-4.8 mg/kg/day
1-5 years: 45-60 mg/day; 3-3.6 mg/kg/day
6-12 years: 60-90 mg/day; 2.4-3 mg/kg/day
>12 years: >90 mg/day; 1.2-1.8 mg/kg/day

Adults: Initial: 15-30 mg; increase with 15 mg increments every 2-4 weeks; use 15 mg in patients with cardiovascular disease or myxedema. Maintenance dose: Usually 60-120 mg/day; monitor TSH and clinical symptoms.

Thyroid cancer: Requires larger amounts than replacement therapy

**Dosage Forms**

Tablet: 30 mg, 32.5 mg, 60 mg, 65 mg, 90 mg, 120 mg, 130 mg, 180 mg, 240 mg, 300 mg
Armour® Thyroid: 15 mg, 30 mg, 60 mg, 90 mg, 120 mg, 180 mg, 240 mg, 300 mg
Nature-Throid® NT, Westhroid®: 32.5 mg, 65 mg, 130 mg, 195 mg

**thyroid extract** *see* thyroid *on this page*

**Thyroid Strong**® *(Discontinued)* *see* thyroid *on this page*

**thyroid USP** *see* thyroid *on this page*

**Thyrolar**® **[US/Can]** *see* liotrix *on page 484*

**ThyroSafe**™ **[US-OTC]** *see* potassium iodide *on page 665*

**ThyroShield**™ **[US-OTC]** *see* potassium iodide *on page 665*

## thyrotropin alpha (thye roe TROH pin AL fa)

**Sound-Alike/Look-Alike Issues**

Thyrogen® may be confused with Thyrolar®

**Synonyms** human thyroid stimulating hormone; TSH

**U.S./Canadian Brand Names** Thyrogen® [US/Can]

**Therapeutic Category** Diagnostic Agent

**Use** As an adjunctive diagnostic tool for serum thyroglobulin (Tg) testing with or without radioiodine imaging in the follow-up of patients with well-differentiated thyroid cancer

Potential clinical use:

1. Patients with an undetectable Tg on thyroid hormone suppressive therapy to exclude the diagnosis of residual or recurrent thyroid cancer
2. Patients requiring serum Tg testing and radioiodine imaging who are unwilling to undergo thyroid hormone withdrawal testing and whose treating physician believes that use of a less sensitive test is justified
3. Patients who are either unable to mount an adequate endogenous TSH response to thyroid hormone withdrawal or in whom withdrawal is medically contraindicated

**Usual Dosage** Children >16 years and Adults: I.M.: 0.9 mg every 24 hours for 2 doses or every 72 hours for 3 doses

For radioiodine imaging, radioiodine administration should be given 24 hours following the final Thyrogen® injection. Scanning should be performed 48 hours after radioiodine administration (72 hours after the final injection of Thyrogen®).

For serum testing, serum Tg should be obtained 72 hours after final injection.

**Dosage Forms** Injection, powder for reconstitution: Four-vial kit: 1.1 mg [supplied as two vials of Thyrogen® and two 10 mL vials of SWFI]

*L*-**thyroxine sodium** *see* levothyroxine *on page 477*

**tiabendazole** *see* thiabendazole *on page 796*

**tiagabine** (tye AG a been)
**Sound-Alike/Look-Alike Issues**
tiagabine may be confused with tizanidine
**Synonyms** tiagabine hydrochloride
**U.S./Canadian Brand Names** Gabitril® [US/Can]
**Therapeutic Category** Anticonvulsant
**Use** Adjunctive therapy in adults and children ≥12 years of age in the treatment of partial seizures
**Usual Dosage** Oral (administer with food):
Patients receiving enzyme-inducing AED regimens:
Children 12-18 years: 4 mg once daily for 1 week; may increase to 8 mg daily in 2 divided doses for 1 week; then may increase by 4-8 mg weekly to response or up to 32 mg daily in 2-4 divided doses
Adults: 4 mg once daily for 1 week; may increase by 4-8 mg weekly to response or up to 56 mg daily in 2-4 divided doses
Patients **not** receiving enzyme-inducing AED regimens: The estimated plasma concentrations of tiagabine in patients not taking enzyme-inducing medications is twice that of patients receiving enzyme-inducing AEDs. Lower doses are required; slower titration may be necessary.
**Dosage Forms** Tablet, as hydrochloride: 2 mg, 4 mg, 12 mg, 16 mg

**tiagabine hydrochloride** *see* tiagabine *on this page*

**Tiamate®** *(Discontinued)* *see* diltiazem *on page 251*

**Tiamol®** **[Can]** *see* fluocinonide *on page 345*

**Tiaprofenic-200 [Can]** *see* tiaprofenic acid *(Canada only)* *on this page*

**Tiaprofenic-300 [Can]** *see* tiaprofenic acid *(Canada only)* *on this page*

**tiaprofenic acid** *(Canada only)* (tye ah PRO fen ik AS id)
**U.S./Canadian Brand Names** Albert® Tiafen [Can]; Apo-Tiaprofenic® [Can]; Dom-Tiaprofenic® [Can]; Novo-Tiaprofenic [Can]; Nu-Tiaprofenic [Can]; PMS-Tiaprofenic [Can]; Surgam® SR [Can]; Surgam® [Can]; Tiaprofenic-200 [Can]; Tiaprofenic-300 [Can]
**Therapeutic Category** Nonsteroidal Antiinflammatory Drug (NSAID)
**Use** Relief of signs and symptoms of rheumatoid arthritis and osteoarthritis (degenerative joint disease)
**Usual Dosage** Oral: Adults:
Rheumatoid arthritis:
Tablet: Usual initial and maintenance dose: 600 mg/day in 3 divided doses; some patients may do well on 300 mg twice daily; maximum daily dose: 600 mg
Sustained release capsule: Initial and maintenance dose: 2 sustained release capsules of 300 mg once daily; Surgam® SR capsules should be swallowed whole
Osteoarthritis:
Tablet: Usual initial and maintenance dose: 600 mg/day in 2 or 3 divided doses; in rare instances patients may be maintained on 300 mg/day in divided doses; maximum daily dose: 600 mg
Sustained release capsule: Initial and maintenance dose: 2 sustained release capsules of 300 mg once daily; Surgam® SR capsules should be swallowed whole
**Dosage Forms**
Capsule, sustained release: 300 mg
Tablet: 200 mg, 300 mg

**Tiazac®** **[US/Can]** *see* diltiazem *on page 251*

**Tiazac®** **XC [Can]** *see* diltiazem *on page 251*

**Ticar®** **[US]** *see* ticarcillin *on this page*

**ticarcillin** (tye kar SIL in)
**Sound-Alike/Look-Alike Issues**
Ticar® may be confused with Tigan®
(Continued)

## ticarcillin *(Continued)*

**Synonyms** ticarcillin disodium

**U.S./Canadian Brand Names** Ticar® [US]

**Therapeutic Category** Penicillin

**Use** Treatment of susceptible infections such as septicemia, acute and chronic respiratory tract infections, skin and soft tissue infections, and urinary tract infections due to susceptible strains of *Pseudomonas*, and other gram-negative bacteria

**Usual Dosage** Ticarcillin is generally given I.V., I.M. injection is only for the treatment of uncomplicated urinary tract infections and dose should not exceed 2 g/injection when administered I.M.

Neonates: I.M., I.V.:
 Postnatal age <7 days:
  <2000 g: 75 mg/kg/dose every 12 hours
  >2000 g: 75 mg/kg/dose every 8 hours
 Postnatal age >7 days:
  <1200 g: 75 mg/kg/dose every 12 hours
  1200-2000 g: 75 mg/kg/dose every 8 hours
  >2000 g: 75 mg/kg/dose every 6 hours
Infants and Children:
 Systemic infections: I.V.: 200-300 mg/kg/day in divided doses every 4-6 hours
 Urinary tract infections: I.M., I.V.: 50-100 mg/kg/day in divided doses every 6-8 hours
 Maximum dose: 24 g/day
Adults: I.M., I.V.: 1-4 g every 4-6 hours, usual dose: 3 g I.V. every 4-6 hours

**Dosage Forms** Injection, powder for reconstitution, as disodium: 3 g

## ticarcillin and clavulanate potassium

(tye kar SIL in & klav yoo LAN ate poe TASS ee um)

**Synonyms** ticarcillin and clavulanic acid

**U.S./Canadian Brand Names** Timentin® [US/Can]

**Therapeutic Category** Penicillin

**Use** Treatment of infections of lower respiratory tract, urinary tract, skin and skin structures, bone and joint, and septicemia caused by susceptible organisms. Clavulanate expands activity of ticarcillin to include beta-lactamase producing strains of *S. aureus*, *H. influenzae*, *Bacteroides* species, and some other gram-negative bacilli

**Usual Dosage** I.V.:
Children and Adults <60 kg: 200-300 mg of ticarcillin component/kg/day in divided doses every 4-6 hours
Children >60 kg and Adults: 3.1 g (ticarcillin 3 g plus clavulanic acid 0.1 g) every 4-6 hours; maximum: 24 g/day
Urinary tract infections: 3.1 g every 6-8 hours

**Dosage Forms**
Infusion [premixed, frozen]: Ticarcillin 3 g and clavulanic acid 0.1 g (100 mL) [contains sodium 4.51 mEq and potassium 0.15 mEq per g]
Injection, powder for reconstitution: Ticarcillin 3 g and clavulanic acid 0.1 g (3.1 g, 31 g) [contains sodium 4.51 mEq and potassium 0.15 mEq per g]

**ticarcillin and clavulanic acid** *see* ticarcillin and clavulanate potassium *on this page*

**ticarcillin disodium** *see* ticarcillin *on previous page*

**TICE® BCG [US]** *see* BCG vaccine *on page 90*

**Ticlid® [US/Can]** *see* ticlopidine *on this page*

## ticlopidine (tye KLOE pi deen)

**Synonyms** ticlopidine hydrochloride

**U.S./Canadian Brand Names** Alti-Ticlopidine [Can]; Apo-Ticlopidine® [Can]; Gen-Ticlopidine [Can]; Novo-Ticlopidine [Can]; Nu-Ticlopidine [Can]; Rhoxal-ticlopidine [Can]; Ticlid® [US/Can]

**Therapeutic Category** Antiplatelet Agent

**Use** Platelet aggregation inhibitor that reduces the risk of thrombotic stroke in patients who have had a stroke or stroke precursors. **Note:** Due to its association with life-threatening hematologic disorders, ticlopidine should be reserved for patients who are intolerant to aspirin, or who have failed aspirin therapy. Adjunctive therapy (with aspirin) following successful coronary stent implantation to reduce the incidence of subacute stent thrombosis.

**Usual Dosage** Oral: Adults:
Stroke prevention: 250 mg twice daily with food
Coronary artery stenting (initiate after successful implantation): 250 mg twice daily with food (in combination with antiplatelet doses of aspirin) for up to 30 days
**Dosage Forms** Tablet, as hydrochloride: 250 mg

**ticlopidine hydrochloride** see ticlopidine on previous page

**Ticon® (Discontinued)** see trimethobenzamide on page 825

**TIG** see tetanus immune globulin (human) on page 790

**Tigan® [US/Can]** see trimethobenzamide on page 825

## tigecycline (tye ge SYE kleen)
**Synonyms** GAR-936
**U.S./Canadian Brand Names** Tygacil™ [US]
**Therapeutic Category** Antibiotic, Glycylcycline
**Use** Treatment of complicated skin and skin structure infections caused by susceptible organisms, including methicillin-resistant *Staphylococcus aureus* and vancomycin-sensitive *Enterococcus faecalis*; treatment of complicated intra-abdominal infections
**Usual Dosage** I.V.: Adults:
Initial: 100 mg as a single dose
Maintenance dose: 50 mg every 12 hours
Recommended duration of therapy: Intra-abdominal infections or complicated skin/skin structure infections: 5-14 days.
**Dosage Forms** Injection, powder for reconstitution: 50 mg

**Tikosyn™ [US/Can]** see dofetilide on page 264

**Tilade® [US/Can]** see nedocromil (inhalation) on page 565

## tiludronate (tye LOO droe nate)
**Synonyms** tiludronate disodium
**U.S./Canadian Brand Names** Skelid® [US]
**Therapeutic Category** Bisphosphonate Derivative
**Use** Treatment of Paget disease of the bone in patients who have a level of serum alkaline phosphatase (SAP) at least twice the upper limit of normal, or who are symptomatic, or who are at risk for future complications of their disease
**Usual Dosage** Tiludronate should be taken with 6-8 oz of plain water and not taken within 2 hours of food
Adults: Oral: 400 mg (2 tablets of tiludronic acid) daily for a period of 3 months; allow an interval of 3 months to assess response
**Dosage Forms** Tablet, tiludronic acid: 200 mg [equivalent to 240 mg tiludronate disodium]

**tiludronate disodium** see tiludronate on this page

**Tim-AK [Can]** see timolol on this page

**Timecelles® (Discontinued)** see ascorbic acid on page 71

**Timentin® [US/Can]** see ticarcillin and clavulanate potassium on previous page

## timolol (TYE moe lole)
**Sound-Alike/Look-Alike Issues**
timolol may be confused with atenolol, Tylenol®
Timoptic® may be confused with Talacen®, Viroptic®
**Synonyms** timolol hemihydrate; timolol maleate
**U.S./Canadian Brand Names** Alti-Timolol [Can]; Apo-Timol® [Can]; Apo-Timop® [Can]; Betimol® [US]; Blocadren® [US]; Gen-Timolol [Can]; Istalol™ [US]; Nu-Timolol [Can]; Phoxal-timolol [Can]; PMS-Timolol [Can]; Tim-AK [Can]; Timoptic-XE® [US/Can]; Timoptic® OcuDose® [US]; Timoptic® [US/Can]
**Therapeutic Category** Beta-Adrenergic Blocker
**Use** Ophthalmic dosage form used in treatment of elevated intraocular pressure such as glaucoma or ocular hypertension; oral dosage form used for treatment of hypertension and angina, to reduce mortality following myocardial infarction, and for prophylaxis of migraine
(Continued)

# timolol *(Continued)*

## Usual Dosage
Ophthalmic:
Children and Adults:
Solution: Initial: Instill 1 drop (0.25% solution) twice daily; increase to 0.5% solution if response not adequate; decrease to 1 drop/day if controlled; do not exceed 1 drop twice daily of 0.5% solution
Gel-forming solution (Timoptic-XE®): Instill 1 drop (either 0.25% or 0.5% solution) once daily
Adults: Solution (Istalol®): Instill 1 drop (0.5% solution) once daily in the morning
Oral: Adults:
Hypertension: Initial: 10 mg twice daily, increase gradually every 7 days, usual dosage: 20-40 mg/day in 2 divided doses; maximum: 60 mg/day
Prevention of myocardial infarction: 10 mg twice daily initiated within 1-4 weeks after infarction
Migraine headache: Initial: 10 mg twice daily, increase to maximum of 30 mg/day

## Dosage Forms Note: Strength expressed as base.
Gel-forming solution, ophthalmic, as maleate: 0.25% (5 mL); 0.5% (2.5 mL, 5 mL)
Timoptic-XE®: 0.25% (5 mL); 0.5% (5 mL)
Solution, ophthalmic, as hemihydrate (Betimol®): 0.25% (5 mL, 10 mL, 15 mL); 0.5% (5 mL, 10 mL, 15 mL) [contains benzalkonium chloride]
Solution, ophthalmic, as maleate: 0.25% (5 mL, 10 mL, 15 mL); 0.5% (5 mL, 10 mL, 15 mL) [contains benzalkonium chloride]
Istalol™: 0.5% (10 mL) [contains benzalkonium chloride and potassium sorbate]
Timoptic®: 0.25% (5 mL, 10 mL); 0.5% (5 mL, 10 mL) [contains benzalkonium chloride]
Solution, ophthalmic, as maleate [preservative free] (Timoptic® OcuDose®): 0.25% (0.2 mL); 0.5% (0.2 mL) [single use]
Tablet, as maleate: 5 mg, 10 mg, 20 mg
Blocadren®: 20 mg

**timolol and dorzolamide** *see* dorzolamide and timolol *on page 267*

**timolol hemihydrate** *see* timolol *on previous page*

**timolol maleate** *see* timolol *on previous page*

**Timoptic® [US/Can]** *see* timolol *on previous page*

**Timoptic® OcuDose® [US]** *see* timolol *on previous page*

**Timoptic-XE® [US/Can]** *see* timolol *on previous page*

**Tinactin® Antifungal [US-OTC]** *see* tolnaftate *on page 809*

**Tinactin® Antifungal Jock Itch [US-OTC]** *see* tolnaftate *on page 809*

**Tinaderm [US-OTC]** *see* tolnaftate *on page 809*

**Tinamed® [US-OTC]** *see* salicylic acid *on page 734*

**TinBen® *(Discontinued)*** *see* benzoin *on page 98*

**Tindamax™ [US]** *see* tinidazole *on this page*

**tine test** *see* tuberculin tests *on page 830*

**Ting® Cream [US-OTC]** *see* tolnaftate *on page 809*

# tinidazole (tye NI da zole)

**U.S./Canadian Brand Names** Tindamax™ [US]
**Therapeutic Category** Amebicide; Antibiotic, Miscellaneous; Antiprotozoal, Nitroimidazole
**Use** Treatment of trichomoniasis caused by *T. vaginalis*; treatment of giardiasis caused by *G. duodenalis* (*G. lamblia*); treatment of intestinal amebiasis and amebic liver abscess caused by *E. histolytica*
**Usual Dosage** Oral:
Children >3 years:
Amebiasis, intestinal: 50 mg/kg/day for 3 days (maximum dose: 2 g/day)
Amebiasis, liver abscess: 50 mg/kg/day for 3-5 days (maximum dose: 2 g/day)
Giardiasis: 50 mg/kg as a single dose (maximum dose: 2 g)
Adults:
Amebiasis, intestinal: 2 g/day for 3 days
Amebiasis, liver abscess: 2 g/day for 3-5 days
Giardiasis: 2 g as a single dose
Trichomoniasis: Oral: 2 g as a single dose; sexual partners should be treated at the same time
**Dosage Forms** Tablet, scored: 250 mg, 500 mg

Tinver® *(Discontinued)* *see* sodium thiosulfate *on page 758*

# tinzaparin (tin ZA pa rin)
**Synonyms** tinzaparin sodium
**U.S./Canadian Brand Names** Innohep® [US/Can]
**Therapeutic Category** Anticoagulant (Other)
**Use** Treatment of acute symptomatic deep vein thrombosis, with or without pulmonary embolism, in conjunction with warfarin sodium
**Usual Dosage** SubQ:
Adults: 175 anti-Xa int. units/kg of body weight once daily. Warfarin sodium should be started when appropriate. Administer tinzaparin for at least 6 days and until patient is adequately anticoagulated with warfarin.
**Note:** To calculate the volume of solution to administer per dose: Volume to be administered (mL) = patient weight (kg) x 0.00875 mL/kg (may be rounded off to the nearest 0.05 mL)
**Dosage Forms** Injection, solution, as sodium: 20,000 anti-Xa int. units/mL (2 mL) [contains benzyl alcohol and sodium metabisulfite]

**tinzaparin sodium** *see* tinzaparin *on this page*

# tioconazole (tye oh KONE a zole)
**Sound-Alike/Look-Alike Issues**
tioconazole may be confused with terconazole
**U.S./Canadian Brand Names** 1-Day™ [US-OTC]; Vagistat®-1 [US-OTC]
**Therapeutic Category** Antifungal Agent
**Use** Local treatment of vulvovaginal candidiasis
**Usual Dosage** Adults: Vaginal: Insert 1 applicatorful in vagina, just prior to bedtime, as a single dose
**Dosage Forms** Ointment, vaginal: 6.5% (4.6 g) [with applicator]

**tioguanine** *see* thioguanine *on page 797*

# tiopronin (tye oh PROE nin)
**Sound-Alike/Look-Alike Issues**
Thiola® may be confused with Theolair™
**U.S./Canadian Brand Names** Thiola® [US/Can]
**Therapeutic Category** Urinary Tract Product
**Use** Prevention of kidney stone (cystine) formation in patients with severe homozygous cystinuric who have urinary cystine >500 mg/day who are resistant to treatment with high fluid intake, alkali, and diet modification, or who have had adverse reactions to penicillamine
**Usual Dosage** Adults: Initial dose is 800 mg/day, average dose is 1000 mg/day
**Dosage Forms** Tablet: 100 mg

**tiotixene** *see* thiothixene *on page 799*

# tiotropium (ty oh TRO pee um)
**Sound-Alike/Look-Alike Issues**
Spiriva® may be confused with Inspra™
**Synonyms** tiotropium bromide monohydrate
**U.S./Canadian Brand Names** Spiriva® [US/Can]
**Therapeutic Category** Anticholinergic Agent
**Use** Maintenance treatment of bronchospasm associated with COPD (bronchitis and emphysema)
**Usual Dosage** Oral inhalation: Adults: Contents of 1 capsule (18 mcg) inhaled once daily using HandiHaler® device
**Dosage Forms** Powder for oral inhalation [capsule]: 18 mcg/capsule [contains lactose; packaged in 6s or 30s with HandiHaler® device]

**tiotropium bromide monohydrate** *see* tiotropium *on this page*

## tipranavir (tip RA na veer)
**Synonyms** PNU-140690E; TPV
**U.S./Canadian Brand Names** Aptivus® [US]
**Therapeutic Category** Antiretroviral Agent, Protease Inhibitor
**Use** Treatment of HIV-1 infections in combination with ritonavir and other antiretroviral agents; limited to highly treatment experienced or multi-protease inhibitor resistant patients.
**Usual Dosage** Oral: Adults: 500 mg twice daily with a high-fat meal. **Note:** Coadministration with ritonavir (200 mg twice daily) is required.
**Dosage Forms** Capsule, gelatin: 250 mg [contains dehydrated ethanol 7% per capsule]

**TipTapToe** *(Discontinued)* *see* tolnaftate *on page 809*

## tirofiban (tye roe FYE ban)
**Sound-Alike/Look-Alike Issues**
   Aggrastat® may be confused with Aggrenox®, argatroban
**Synonyms** MK383; tirofiban hydrochloride
**U.S./Canadian Brand Names** Aggrastat® [US/Can]
**Therapeutic Category** Antiplatelet Agent
**Use** In combination with heparin, is indicated for the treatment of acute coronary syndrome, including patients who are to be managed medically and those undergoing PTCA or atherectomy. In this setting, it has been shown to decrease the rate of a combined endpoint of death, new myocardial infarction or refractory ischemia/repeat cardiac procedure.
**Usual Dosage** Adults: I.V.: Initial rate of 0.4 mcg/kg/minute for 30 minutes and then continued at 0.1 mcg/kg/minute; dosing should be continued through angiography and for 12-24 hours after angioplasty or atherectomy.
**Dosage Forms**
   Infusion [premixed in sodium chloride]: 50 mcg/mL (100 mL, 250 mL)
   Injection, solution: 250 mcg/mL (50 mL)

**tirofiban hydrochloride** *see* tirofiban *on this page*

**Ti-Screen®** **[US-OTC]** *see* methoxycinnamate and oxybenzone *on page 527*

**Tiseb®** **[US-OTC]** *see* salicylic acid *on page 734*

**Tisit®** **[US-OTC]** *see* pyrethrins and piperonyl butoxide *on page 699*

**Tisit®** **Blue Gel [US-OTC]** *see* pyrethrins and piperonyl butoxide *on page 699*

**Tisseel®** **VH [US/Can]** *see* fibrin sealant kit *on page 337*

**Titralac™** **[US-OTC]** *see* calcium carbonate *on page 130*

**Titralac™** **Extra Strength [US-OTC]** *see* calcium carbonate *on page 130*

**Titralac®** **Plus [US-OTC]** *see* calcium carbonate and simethicone *on page 132*

**Ti-U-Lac®** **H [Can]** *see* urea and hydrocortisone *on page 835*

## tizanidine (tye ZAN i deen)
**Sound-Alike/Look-Alike Issues**
   tizanidine may be confused with tiagabine
**U.S./Canadian Brand Names** Apo-Tizanidine® [Can]; Zanaflex® [US/Can]
**Therapeutic Category** Alpha$_2$-Adrenergic Agonist Agent
**Use** Skeletal muscle relaxant used for treatment of muscle spasticity
**Usual Dosage** Adults: 2-4 mg 3 times/day
   Usual initial dose: 4 mg, may increase by 2-4 mg as needed for satisfactory reduction of muscle tone every 6-8 hours to a maximum of three doses in any 24 hour period
   Maximum dose: 36 mg/day
**Dosage Forms**
   Capsule: 2 mg, 4 mg, 6 mg
   Tablet: 2 mg, 4 mg

**TMP** *see* trimethoprim *on page 825*

**TMP-SMZ** *see* sulfamethoxazole and trimethoprim *on page 773*

**TMZ** *see* temozolomide *on page 784*

T.N. Dickinson's® **Hazelets [US-OTC]** *see* witch hazel *on page 855*

TNKase™ **[US/Can]** *see* tenecteplase *on page 785*

TOBI® **[US/Can]** *see* tobramycin *on this page*

TobraDex® **[US/Can]** *see* tobramycin and dexamethasone *on next page*

# tobramycin (toe bra MYE sin)

## Sound-Alike/Look-Alike Issues
tobramycin may be confused with Trobicin®
AKTob® may be confused with AK-Trol®
Nebcin® may be confused with Inapsine®, Naprosyn®, Nubain®
Tobrex® may be confused with TobraDex®

**Synonyms** tobramycin sulfate

**U.S./Canadian Brand Names** AKTob® [US]; Apo-Tobramycin® [Can]; PMS-Tobramycin [Can]; TOBI® [US/Can]; Tobrex® [US/Can]

**Therapeutic Category** Aminoglycoside (Antibiotic); Antibiotic, Ophthalmic

**Use** Treatment of documented or suspected infections caused by susceptible gram-negative bacilli including *Pseudomonas aeruginosa*; topically used to treat superficial ophthalmic infections caused by susceptible bacteria. Tobramycin solution for inhalation is indicated for the management of cystic fibrosis patients (>6 years of age) with *Pseudomonas aeruginosa*.

**Usual Dosage** Individualization is **critical** because of the low therapeutic index.

**Use of ideal body weight (IBW) for determining the mg/kg/dose appears to be more accurate than dosing on the basis of total body weight (TBW).** In morbid obesity, dosage requirement may best be estimated using a dosing weight of IBW + 0.4 (TBW - IBW).

Initial and periodic plasma drug levels (eg, peak and trough with conventional dosing) should be determined, particularly in critically-ill patients with serious infections or in disease states known to significantly alter aminoglycoside pharmacokinetics (eg, cystic fibrosis, burns, or major surgery).

I.M., I.V.:
Infants and Children <5 years: 2.5 mg/kg/dose every 8 hours
Children >5 years: 2-2.5 mg/kg/dose every 8 hours
Cystic fibrosis: 2.5-3.3 mg/kg every 6-8 hours
**Note:** Some patients may require larger or more frequent doses if serum levels document the need (eg, cystic fibrosis or febrile granulocytopenic patients). Also see "Note" on monitoring and adjustment.
Adults:
Severe life-threatening infections:
Conventional dosing: 2-2.5 mg/kg/dose every 8-12 hours; to ensure adequate peak concentrations early in therapy, higher initial dosages may be considered in selected patients (eg, edema, septic shock, postsurgery, and/or trauma).
Once-daily dosing: Some clinicians suggest a daily dose of 4-7 mg/kg for all patients with normal renal function; this dose is at least as efficacious with similar, if not less, toxicity than conventional dosing.
Urinary tract infection: 1.5 mg/kg/dose
Synergy (for gram-positive infections): 1 mg/kg/dose

Ophthalmic: Children ≥2 months and Adults:
Ointment: Apply 2-3 times/day; for severe infections, apply every 3-4 hours
Solution: Instill 1-2 drops every 4 hours; for severe infections, instill 2 drops every 30-60 minutes initially, then reduce to less frequent intervals
Inhalation: Pulmonary infections:
Standard aerosolized tobramycin:
Children: 40-80 mg 2-3 times/day
Adults: 60-80 mg 3 times/day
High-dose regimen: Children ≥6 years and Adults: 300 mg every 12 hours (do not administer doses <6 hours apart); administer in repeated cycles of 28 days on drug followed by 28 days off drug

## Dosage Forms
Infusion [premixed in NS]: 60 mg (50 mL); 80 mg (100 mL)
Injection, powder for reconstitution: 1.2 g
Injection, solution: 10 mg/mL (2 mL, 8 mL); 40 mg/mL (2 mL, 30 mL, 50 mL) [may contain sodium metabisulfite]
Ointment, ophthalmic (Tobrex®): 0.3% (3.5 g)
Solution for nebulization [preservative free] (TOBI®): 60 mg/mL (5 mL)
Solution, ophthalmic (AKTob®, Tobrex®): 0.3% (5 mL) [contains benzalkonium chloride]

## tobramycin and dexamethasone (toe bra MYE sin & deks a METH a sone)

**Sound-Alike/Look-Alike Issues**
TobraDex® may be confused with Tobrex®

**Synonyms** dexamethasone and tobramycin

**U.S./Canadian Brand Names** TobraDex® [US/Can]

**Therapeutic Category** Antibiotic/Corticosteroid, Ophthalmic

**Use** Treatment of external ocular infection caused by susceptible gram-negative bacteria and steroid responsive inflammatory conditions of the palpebral and bulbar conjunctiva, lid, cornea, and anterior segment of the globe

**Usual Dosage** Children and Adults: Ophthalmic: Instill 1-2 drops of solution every 4 hours; apply ointment 2-3 times/day; for severe infections apply ointment every 3-4 hours, or solution 2 drops every 30-60 minutes initially, then reduce to less frequent intervals

**Dosage Forms**
Ointment, ophthalmic: Tobramycin 0.3% and dexamethasone 0.1% (3.5 g)
Suspension, ophthalmic: Tobramycin 0.3% and dexamethasone 0.1% (2.5 mL, 5 mL, 10 mL) [contains benzalkonium chloride]

**tobramycin sulfate** *see* tobramycin *on previous page*

**Tobrex® [US/Can]** *see* tobramycin *on previous page*

**tocophersolan** *(Discontinued)*

**Today® Sponge [US-OTC]** *see* nonoxynol 9 *on page 580*

**Tofranil® [US/Can]** *see* imipramine *on page 432*

**Tofranil-PM® [US]** *see* imipramine *on page 432*

## tolazamide (tole AZ a mide)

**Sound-Alike/Look-Alike Issues**
TOLAZamide may be confused with tolazoline, TOLBUTamide
Tolinase® may be confused with Orinase®

**Tall-Man TOLAZ**amide

**U.S./Canadian Brand Names** Tolinase® [Can]

**Therapeutic Category** Antidiabetic Agent, Oral

**Use** Adjunct to diet for the management of mild to moderately severe, stable, type 2 diabetes mellitus (noninsulin dependent, NIDDM)

**Usual Dosage** Oral (doses >1000 mg/day normally do not improve diabetic control):
Adults:
Initial: 100-250 mg/day with breakfast or the first main meal of the day
Fasting blood sugar <200 mg/dL: 100 mg/day
Fasting blood sugar >200 mg/dL: 250 mg/day
Patient is malnourished, underweight, elderly, or not eating properly: 100 mg/day
Adjust dose in increments of 100-250 mg/day at weekly intervals to response. If >500 mg/day is required, give in divided doses twice daily; maximum daily dose: 1 g (doses >1 g/day are not likely to improve control)
**Conversion from insulin to tolazamide**
10 units day = 100 mg/day
20-40 units/day = 250 mg/day
>40 units/day = 250 mg/day and 50% of insulin dose
Doses >500 mg/day should be given in 2 divided doses

**Dosage Forms** [DSC] = Discontinued product
Tablet: 100 mg, 250 mg, 500 mg
Tolinase® [DSC]: 100 mg, 250 mg

## tolbutamide (tole BYOO ta mide)

**Sound-Alike/Look-Alike Issues**
TOLBUTamide may be confused with terbutaline, TOLAZamide
Orinase® may be confused with Orabase®, Ornex®, Tolinase®

**Synonyms** tolbutamide sodium

**Tall-Man TOLBUT**amide

**U.S./Canadian Brand Names** Apo-Tolbutamide® [Can]

**Therapeutic Category** Antidiabetic Agent, Oral

**Use** Adjunct to diet for the management of mild to moderately severe, stable, type 2 diabetes mellitus (noninsulin dependent, NIDDM)

**Usual Dosage** Divided doses may improve gastrointestinal tolerance

Adults: Oral: Initial: 1-2 g/day as a single dose in the morning or in divided doses throughout the day. Total doses may be taken in the morning; however, divided doses may allow increased gastrointestinal tolerance. Maintenance dose: 0.25-3 g/day; however, a maintenance dose >2 g/day is seldom required.

**Dosage Forms** Tablet: 500 mg

**tolbutamide sodium** *see* tolbutamide *on previous page*

## tolcapone (TOLE ka pone)

**U.S./Canadian Brand Names** Tasmar® [US]

**Therapeutic Category** Anti-Parkinson Agent

**Use** Adjunct to levodopa and carbidopa for the treatment of signs and symptoms of idiopathic Parkinson disease

**Usual Dosage** Adults: Oral: Initial: 100-200 mg 3 times/day; levodopa therapy may need to be decreased upon initiation of tolcapone

**Dosage Forms** Tablet: 100 mg, 200 mg

**Tolectin® [US/Can]** *see* tolmetin *on this page*

**Tolectin® DS *(Discontinued)*** *see* tolmetin *on this page*

**Tolinase® [Can]** *see* tolazamide *on previous page*

**Tolinase® *(Discontinued)*** *see* tolazamide *on previous page*

## tolmetin (TOLE met in)

**Synonyms** tolmetin sodium

**U.S./Canadian Brand Names** Tolectin® [US/Can]

**Therapeutic Category** Analgesic, Nonnarcotic; Nonsteroidal Antiinflammatory Drug (NSAID)

**Use** Treatment of rheumatoid arthritis and osteoarthritis, juvenile rheumatoid arthritis

**Usual Dosage** Oral:

Children ≥2 years:

Antiinflammatory: Initial: 20 mg/kg/day in 3 divided doses, then 15-30 mg/kg/day in 3 divided doses

Analgesic: 5-7 mg/kg/dose every 6-8 hours

Adults: 400 mg 3 times/day; usual dose: 600 mg to 1.8 g/day; maximum: 2 g/day

**Dosage Forms**

Capsule: 400 mg

Tablet: 200 mg, 600 mg

Tolectin®: 600 mg [contains sodium 54 mg (2.35 mEq)]

**tolmetin sodium** *see* tolmetin *on this page*

## tolnaftate (tole NAF tate)

**Sound-Alike/Look-Alike Issues**

tolnaftate may be confused with Tornalate®

Tinactin® may be confused with Talacen®

**U.S./Canadian Brand Names** Aftate® Antifungal [US-OTC]; Blis-To-Sol® [US-OTC]; Fungi-Guard [US-OTC]; Gold Bond® Antifungal [US-OTC]; Pitrex [Can]; Podactin Powder [US-OTC]; Q-Naftate [US-OTC]; Tinactin® Antifungal Jock Itch [US-OTC]; Tinactin® Antifungal [US-OTC]; Tinaderm [US-OTC]; Ting® Cream [US-OTC]

**Therapeutic Category** Antifungal Agent

**Use** Treatment of tinea pedis, tinea cruris, tinea corporis

**Usual Dosage** Children ≥2 years and Adults: Topical: Wash and dry affected area; spray aerosol or apply 1-3 drops of solution or a small amount of cream, or powder and rub into the affected areas 2 times/day

**Note:** May use for up to 4 weeks for tinea pedis or tinea corporis, and up to 2 weeks for tinea cruris

(Continued)

## tolnaftate *(Continued)*

### Dosage Forms
Aerosol, liquid, topical:
  Aftate®: 1% (120 mL) [contains alcohol]
  Tinactin® Antifungal: 1% (60 mL, 150 mL) [contains alcohol]
Aerosol, powder, topical:
  Aftate®: 1% (105 g) [contains alcohol]
  Tinactin® Antifungal: 1% (133 g) [contains alcohol]
  Tinactin® Antifungal Jock Itch: 1% (100 g, 133 g) [contains alcohol]
Cream, topical: 1% (15 g, 30 g)
  Fungi-Guard, Tinactin® Antifungal Jock Itch, Ting®: 1% (15 g)
  Q-Naftate, Tinactin® Antifungal: 1% (15 g, 30 g)
Liquid, topical:
  Blis-To-Sol®: 1% (30 mL, 55 mL)
  Fungi-Guard: 1% (30 mL) [contains vitamin E and aloe; brush applicator provided]
Powder, topical: 1% (45 g)
  Podactin: 1% (45 g)
  Tinactin® Antifungal: 1% (108 g)
Solution, topical: 1% (10 mL)
  Tinaderm: 1% (10 mL)
Swab, topical [liquid-filled swabstick]: 1% (36s)
  Gold Bond® Antifungal: 1% (24s)
  TipTapToe: 1% (72s) [DSC]

## tolterodine (tole TER oh deen)
### Sound-Alike/Look-Alike Issues
Detrol® may be confused with Ditropan®
**Synonyms** tolterodine tartrate
**U.S./Canadian Brand Names** Detrol® LA [US]; Detrol® [US/Can]; Unidet® [Can]
**Therapeutic Category** Anticholinergic Agent
**Use** Treatment of patients with an overactive bladder with symptoms of urinary frequency, urgency, or urge incontinence
### Usual Dosage
Children: Safety and efficacy in pediatric patients have not been established
Adults: Treatment of overactive bladder: Oral:
  Immediate release tablet: 2 mg twice daily; the dose may be lowered to 1 mg twice daily based on individual response and tolerability
    Dosing adjustment in patients concurrently taking CYP3A4 inhibitors: 1 mg twice daily
  Extended release capsule: 4 mg once a day; dose may be lowered to 2 mg daily based on individual response and tolerability
    Dosing adjustment in patients concurrently taking CYP3A4 inhibitors: 2 mg daily
### Dosage Forms
Capsule, extended release, as tartrate (Detrol® LA): 2 mg, 4 mg
Tablet, as tartrate (Detrol®): 1 mg, 2 mg

**tolterodine tartrate** *see* tolterodine *on this page*

**Tomocat® [US]** *see* radiological/contrast media (ionic) *on page 707*

**tomoxetine** *see* atomoxetine *on page 77*

**Tomudex® [Can]** *see* raltitrexed *(Canada only) on page 710*

**Tomycine® *(Discontinued)*** *see* tobramycin *on page 807*

**Tonopaque® [US]** *see* radiological/contrast media (ionic) *on page 707*

**Topamax® [US/Can]** *see* topiramate *on next page*

**Topicaine® [US-OTC]** *see* lidocaine *on page 479*

**Topicort® [US/Can]** *see* desoximetasone *on page 232*

**Topicort®-LP [US]** *see* desoximetasone *on page 232*

**Topicycline® Topical *(Discontinued)*** *see* tetracycline *on page 791*

**Topilene® [Can]** *see* betamethasone (topical) *on page 103*

# topiramate (toe PYRE a mate)

**Sound-Alike/Look-Alike Issues**
Topamax® may be confused with Toprol-XL®

**U.S./Canadian Brand Names** Topamax® [US/Can]

**Therapeutic Category** Anticonvulsant

**Use** Monotherapy or adjunctive therapy for partial onset seizures and primary generalized tonic-clonic seizures; adjunctive treatment of seizures associated with Lennox-Gastaut syndrome; prophylaxis of migraine headache

**Usual Dosage** Oral: **Note:** Do not abruptly discontinue therapy; taper dosage gradually to prevent rebound seizure.

Monotherapy: Children ≥10 years and Adults: Partial onset seizure and primary generalized tonic-clonic seizure: Initial: 25 mg twice daily; may increase weekly by 50 mg/day up to 100 mg twice daily (week 4 dose); thereafter, may further increase weekly by 100 mg/day up to the recommended maximum of 200 mg twice daily.

Adjunctive therapy:

Children 2-16 years:

Partial onset seizure or seizure associated with Lennox-Gastaut syndrome: Initial dose titration should begin at 25 mg (or less, based on a range of 1-3 mg/kg/day) nightly for the first week; dosage may be increased in increments of 1-3 mg/kg/day (administered in 2 divided doses) at 1- or 2-week intervals to a total daily dose of 5-9 mg/kg/day

Primary generalized tonic-clonic seizure: Use initial dose listed above, but use slower initial titration rate; titrate to recommended maintenance dose by the end of 8 weeks

Adolescents ≥17 years and Adults:

Partial onset seizures: Initial: 25-50 mg/day (given in 2 divided doses) for 1 week; increase at weekly intervals by 25-50 mg/day until response; usual maintenance dose: 100-200 mg twice daily. Doses >1600 mg/day have not been studied.

Primary generalized tonic-clonic seizures: Use initial dose as listed above for partial onset seizures, but use slower initial titration rate; titrate upwards to recommended dose by the end of 8 weeks; usual maintenance dose: 200 mg twice daily. Doses >1600 mg/day have not been studied.

Adults: Migraine prophylaxis: Initial: 25 mg/day (in the evening), titrated at weekly intervals in 25 mg increments, up to the recommended total daily dose of 100 mg/day given in 2 divided doses

**Dosage Forms**
Capsule, sprinkle: 15 mg, 25 mg
Tablet: 25 mg, 50 mg, 100 mg, 200 mg

**Topisone® [Can]** *see* betamethasone (topical) *on page 103*

**TOPO** *see* topotecan *on this page*

**Toposar® [US]** *see* etoposide *on page 322*

# topotecan (toe poe TEE kan)

**Sound-Alike/Look-Alike Issues**
Hycamtin® may be confused with Hycomine®

**Synonyms** hycamptamine; NSC-609699; SK and F 104864; SKF 104864-A; SKF 104864; TOPO; topotecan hydrochloride; TPT

**U.S./Canadian Brand Names** Hycamtin® [US/Can]

**Therapeutic Category** Antineoplastic Agent

**Use** Treatment of ovarian cancer, small cell lung cancer

**Usual Dosage** Adults (refer to individual protocols):

Metastatic ovarian cancer and small cell lung cancer:

IVPB: 1.5 mg/m$^2$/day for 5 days; repeated every 21 days (neutrophil count should be >1500/mm$^3$ and platelet count should be >100,000/mm$^3$)

I.V. continuous infusion: 0.2-0.7 mg/m$^2$/day for 7-21 days

Dosage adjustment for hematological effects: If neutrophil count <1500/mm$^3$, reduce dose by 0.25 mg/m$^2$/day for 5 days for next cycle

**Dosage Forms** Injection, powder for reconstitution, as hydrochloride: 4 mg [base]

**topotecan hydrochloride** *see* topotecan *on this page*

**Toprol-XL® [US/Can]** *see* metoprolol *on page 534*

**Topsyn® [Can]** *see* fluocinonide *on page 345*

**Toradol® [US/Can]** *see* ketorolac *on page 458*

Toradol® IM [Can] *see* ketorolac *on page 458*

# toremifene (TORE em i feen)

**Synonyms** FC1157a; toremifene citrate
**U.S./Canadian Brand Names** Fareston® [US/Can]
**Therapeutic Category** Antineoplastic Agent
**Use** Treatment of advanced breast cancer; management of desmoid tumors and endometrial carcinoma
**Usual Dosage** Refer to individual protocols.
  Adults: Oral: 60 mg once daily, generally continued until disease progression is observed
**Dosage Forms** Tablet: 60 mg

**toremifene citrate** *see* toremifene *on this page*

# torsemide (TORE se mide)

**Sound-Alike/Look-Alike Issues**
  torsemide may be confused with furosemide
  Demadex® may be confused with Denorex®
**U.S./Canadian Brand Names** Demadex® [US]
**Therapeutic Category** Diuretic, Loop
**Use** Management of edema associated with congestive heart failure and hepatic or renal disease; used alone or in combination with antihypertensives in treatment of hypertension; I.V. form is indicated when rapid onset is desired
**Usual Dosage** Adults: Oral, I.V.:
  Congestive heart failure: 10-20 mg once daily; may increase gradually for chronic treatment by doubling dose until the diuretic response is apparent (for acute treatment, I.V. dose may be repeated every 2 hours with double the dose as needed)
  Chronic renal failure: 20 mg once daily; increase as described above
  Hepatic cirrhosis: 5-10 mg once daily with an aldosterone antagonist or a potassium-sparing diuretic; increase as described above
  Hypertension: 2.5-5 mg once daily; increase to 10 mg after 4-6 weeks if an adequate hypotensive response is not apparent; if still not effective, an additional antihypertensive agent may be added
**Dosage Forms**
  Injection, solution: 10 mg/mL (2 mL, 5 mL)
  Tablet: 5 mg, 10 mg, 20 mg, 100 mg

**tositumomab I-131** *see* tositumomab and iodine I 131 tositumomab *on this page*

# tositumomab and iodine I 131 tositumomab

  (toe si TYOO mo mab & EYE oh dyne eye one THUR tee one toe si TYOO mo mab)
**Synonyms** 131 I anti-B1 antibody; 131 I-anti-B1 monoclonal antibody; anti-CD20-murine monoclonal antibody I-131; B1 antibody; B1; iodine I 131 tositumomab and tositumomab; tositumomab I-131
**U.S./Canadian Brand Names** Bexxar® [US]
**Therapeutic Category** Antineoplastic Agent, Monoclonal Antibody; Radiopharmaceutical
**Use** Treatment of relapsed or refractory CD20 positive, low-grade, follicular, or transformed non-Hodgkin's lymphoma
**Usual Dosage** I.V.: Adults: Dosing consists of four components administered in 2 steps. Thyroid protective agents (SSKI, Lugol's solution or potassium iodide), acetaminophen and diphenhydramine should be given prior to or with treatment.
  Step 1: Dosimetric step (Day 0):
    Tositumomab 450 mg in NS 50 mL administered over 60 minutes
    Iodine I 131 tositumomab (containing I-131 5.0 mCi and tositumomab 35mg) in NS 30 mL administered over 20 minutes
    **Note:** Whole body dosimetry and biodistribution should be determined on Day 0; days 2, 3, or 4; and day 6 or 7 prior to administration of Step 2. If biodistribution is not acceptable, do not administer the therapeutic step. On day 6 or 7, calculate the patient specific activity of iodine I 131 tositumomab to deliver 75 cGy TBD or 65 cGy TBD (in mCi).
  Step 2: Therapeutic step (Day 7):
    Tositumomab 450 mg in NS 50 mL administered over 60 minutes
    Iodine I 131 tositumomab:
    Platelets $\geq$150,000/mm$^3$: Iodine I 131 calculated to deliver 75 cGy total body irradiation and tositumomab 35 mg over 20 minutes

Platelets ≥100,000/mm³ and <150,000/mm³: Iodine I 131 calculated to deliver 65 cGy total body irradiation and tositumomab 35 mg over 20 minutes

**Dosage Forms Note:** Not all components are shipped from the same facility. When ordering, ensure that all will arrive on the same day.

Kit [dosimetric package]: Tositumomab 225 mg/16.1 mL [2 vials], tositumomab 35 mg/2.5 mL [1 vial], and iodine I 131 tositumomab 0.1 mg/mL and 0.61mCi/mL (20 mL) [1 vial]

Kit [therapeutic package]: Tositumomab 225 mg/16.1 mL [2 vials], tositumomab 35 mg/2.5 mL [1 vial], and iodine I 131 tositumomab 1.1 mg/mL and 5.6 mCi/mL (20 mL) [1 or 2 vials]

**Totacillin**® *(Discontinued)* see ampicillin *on page 50*

**Touro**™ **CC [US]** *see* guaifenesin, pseudoephedrine, and dextromethorphan *on page 391*

**Touro**™ **Allergy [US]** *see* brompheniramine and pseudoephedrine *on page 115*

**Touro**® **DM [US]** *see* guaifenesin and dextromethorphan *on page 385*

**Touro Ex**® *(Discontinued)* see guaifenesin *on page 383*

**Touro LA**® **[US]** *see* guaifenesin and pseudoephedrine *on page 388*

**tPA** *see* alteplase *on page 32*

**T-Phyl**® **[US]** *see* theophylline *on page 793*

**TPT** *see* topotecan *on page 811*

**TPV** *see* tipranavir *on page 806*

**tRA** *see* tretinoin (oral) *on page 817*

## trace metals (trase MET als)

**Synonyms** chromium; copper; iodine; manganese; molybdenum; neonatal trace metals; selenium; zinc

**U.S./Canadian Brand Names** Iodopen® [US]; M.T.E.-4® [US]; M.T.E.-5® [US]; M.T.E.-6® [US]; M.T.E.-7® [US]; Molypen® [US]; Multitrace™-4 Neonatal [US]; Multitrace™-4 Pediatric [US]; Multitrace™-4 [US]; Multitrace™-5 [US]; Neotrace-4® [US]; P.T.E.-4® [US]; P.T.E.-5® [US]; Pedtrace-4® [US]; Selepen® [US]

**Therapeutic Category** Trace Element

**Use** Prevention and correction of trace metal deficiencies

**Usual Dosage Recommended daily parenteral dosage:**

Chromium:[1]
Infants: 0.2 mcg/kg
Children: 0.2 mcg/kg (maximum: 5 mcg)
Adults: 10-15 mcg

Copper:[2]
Infants: 20 mcg/kg
Children: 20 mcg/kg (maximum: 300 mcg)
Adults: 0.5-1.5 mg

Manganese:[2,3]
Infants: 1 mcg/kg
Children: 1 mcg/kg (maximum: 50 mcg)
Adults: 150-800 mcg

Molybdenum:[1,4]
Infants: 0.25 mcg/kg
Children: 0.25 mcg/kg (maximum: 5 mcg)
Adults: 20-120 mcg

Selenium:[1,4]
Infants: 2 mcg/kg
Children: 2 mcg/kg (maximum: 30 mcg)
Adults: 20-40 mcg

Zinc:
Infants, preterm: 400 mcg/kg
Infants, term <3 months: 250 mcg/kg
Infants, term >3 months: 100 mcg/kg
Children: 50 mcg/kg (maximum: 5 mg)
Adults: 2.5-4 mg

[1]Omit in patients with renal dysfunction.

[2]Omit in patients with obstructive jaundice.

[3]Current available commercial products are not in appropriate ratios to maintain this recommendation; doses of up to 10 mcg/kg have been used.

[4]Indicated for use in long-term parenteral nutrition patients.

(Continued)

# trace metals *(Continued)*

## Dosage Forms

Injection, solution [combination products]:

M.T.E.-4®: Chromium 4 mcg, copper 0.4 mg, manganese 0.1 mg, and zinc 1 mg per mL (3 mL, 10 mL, 30 mL) [30 mL contains benzyl alcohol]

M.T.E.-4® Concentrate: Chromium 10 mcg, copper 1 mg, manganese 0.5 mg, and zinc 5 mg per mL (1 mL, 10 mL) [10 mL contains benzyl alcohol]

M.T.E.-5® [preservative free]: Chromium 4 mcg, copper 0.4 mg, manganese 0.1 mg, selenium 20 mcg, and zinc 1 mg per mL (10 mL)

M.T.E.-5® Concentrate: Chromium 10 mcg, copper 1 mg, manganese 0.5 mg, selenium 60 mcg, and zinc 5 mg per mL (1 mL, 10 mL) [10 mL contains benzyl alcohol]

M.T.E.-6® [preservative free]: Chromium 4 mcg, copper 0.4 mg, iodide 25 mcg, manganese 0.1 mg, selenium 20 mcg, and zinc 1 mg per mL (10 mL)

M.T.E.-6® Concentrate: Chromium 10 mcg, copper 1 mg, iodide 75 mcg, manganese 0.5 mg, selenium 60 mcg, and zinc 5 mg per mL (10 mL) [contains benzyl alcohol]

M.T.E.-7® [preservative free]: Chromium 4 mcg, copper 0.4 mg, iodide 25 mcg, manganese 0.1 mg, molybdenum 25 mcg, selenium 20 mcg, and zinc 1 mg per mL (10 mL)

Multitrace™-4: Chromium 4 mcg, copper 0.4 mg, manganese 0.1 mg, and zinc 1 mg per mL (10 mL) [contains benzyl alcohol]

Multitrace™-4 Neonatal: Chromium 0.85 mcg, copper 0.1 mg, manganese 0.025 mg, and zinc 1.5 mg per mL (2 mL)

Multitrace™-4 Pediatric: Chromium 1 mcg, copper 0.1 mg, manganese 0.025 mg, and zinc 1 mg per mL (3 mL)

Multitrace™-4 Concentrate: Chromium 10 mcg, copper 1 mg, manganese 0.5 mg, and zinc 5 mg per mL (1 mL, 10 mL) [10 mL contains benzyl alcohol]

Multitrace™-5: Chromium 4 mcg, copper 0.4 mg, manganese 0.1 mg, selenium 20 mcg, and zinc 1 mg per mL (10 mL) [contains benzyl alcohol]

Multitrace™-5 Concentrate: Chromium 10 mcg, copper 1 mg, manganese 0.5 mg, selenium 60 mcg, and zinc 5 mg per mL (1 mL, 10 mL) [10 mL contains benzyl alcohol]

Neotrace-4® [preservative free]: Chromium 0.85 mcg, copper 0.1 mg, manganese 0.025 mg, and zinc 1.5 mg per mL (2 mL)

Pedtrace-4® [preservative free]: Chromium 0.85 mcg, copper 0.1 mg, manganese 0.025 mg, and zinc 0.5 mg per mL (3 mL, 10 mL)

P.T.E.-4® [preservative free]: Chromium 1 mcg, copper 0.1 mg, manganese 0.025 mg, and zinc 1 mg per mL (3 mL)

P.T.E.-5® [preservative free]: Chromium 1 mcg, copper 0.1 mg, manganese 0.025 mg, selenium 15 mcg, and zinc 1 mg per mL (3 mL)

Trace elements pediatric: Chromium 1 mcg, copper 0.1 mg, manganese 0.03 mg, and zinc 0.5 mg per mL (10 mL) [contains benzyl alcohol]

Injection, solution [elemental equivalence]:

Chromium, as chromic chloride (hexahydrate) [preservative free]: 0.0205 mg/mL [0.004 mg/mL] (10 mL)

Copper, as cupric chloride: 1.07 mg/mL [0.4 mg/mL] (10 mL)

Iodine, as iodine sodium (Iodopen®): 0.118 mg/mL [0.1 mg/mL] (10 mL)

Manganese:

As chloride: 0.36 mg/mL [0.1 mg/mL] (10 mL)

As sulfate [preservative free]: 0.31 mg/mL [0.1 mg/mL] (10 mL)

Molybdenum, as ammonium molybdate (tetrahydrate) (Molypen®): 46 mcg/mL [25 mcg/mL] (10 mL)

Selenium, as selenious acid: 0.0654 mg/mL [0.04 mg/mL] (10 mL)

Selepen®: 0.0654 mg/mL [0.04 mg/mL] (10 mL, 30 mL) [30 mL contains benzyl alcohol]

Zinc:

As chloride: 2.09 mg/mL [1 mg/mL] (10 mL, 50 mL)

As sulfate, anhydrous [preservative free]: 2.46 mg/mL [1 mg/mL] (10 mL)

As sulfate, anhydrous, concentrate [preservative free]: 12.32 mg/mL [5 mg/mL] (5 mL)

**Tracleer® [US/Can]** *see* bosentan *on page 111*

**Tracrium® [US]** *see* atracurium *on page 79*

**Tramacet [Can]** *see* acetaminophen and tramadol *on page 9*

# tramadol (TRA ma dole)

**Sound-Alike/Look-Alike Issues**
tramadol may be confused with Toradol®, Trandate®, Voltaren®
Ultram® may be confused with Ultane®, Voltaren®

**Synonyms** tramadol hydrochloride

**U.S./Canadian Brand Names** Ultram® [US/Can]

**Therapeutic Category** Analgesic, Nonnarcotic

**Use** Relief of moderate to moderately-severe pain

**Usual Dosage** Oral: Adults: Moderate to severe chronic pain: 50-100 mg every 4-6 hours, not to exceed
400 mg/day
For patients not requiring rapid onset of effect, tolerability may be improved by starting dose at 25 mg/
day and titrating dose by 25 mg every 3 days, until reaching 25 mg 4 times/day. Dose may then be
increased by 50 mg every 3 days as tolerated, to reach dose of 50 mg 4 times/day.

**Dosage Forms** Tablet, as hydrochloride: 50 mg

**tramadol hydrochloride** *see* tramadol *on this page*

**tramadol hydrochloride and acetaminophen** *see* acetaminophen and tramadol *on page 9*

**Trandate® [US/Can]** *see* labetalol *on page 460*

# trandolapril (tran DOE la pril)

**U.S./Canadian Brand Names** Mavik® [US/Can]

**Therapeutic Category** Angiotensin-Converting Enzyme (ACE) Inhibitor

**Use** Management of hypertension alone or in combination with other antihypertensive agents; treatment
of left ventricular dysfunction after myocardial infarction

**Usual Dosage** Adults: Oral:
Hypertension: Initial dose in patients not receiving a diuretic: 1 mg/day (2 mg/day in black patients).
Adjust dosage according to the blood pressure response. Make dosage adjustments at intervals of ≥1
week. Most patients have required dosages of 2-4 mg/day. There is a little experience with doses >8
mg/day. Patients inadequately treated with once daily dosing at 4 mg may be treated with twice daily
dosing. If blood pressure is not adequately controlled with trandolapril monotherapy, a diuretic may be
added.
Usual dose range (JNC 7): 1-4 mg once daily
Heart failure postmyocardial infarction or left ventricular dysfunction postmyocardial infarction: Initial: 1
mg/day; titrate patients (as tolerated) towards the target dose of 4 mg/day. If a 4 mg dose is not
tolerated, patients can continue therapy with the greatest tolerated dose.

**Dosage Forms** Tablet: 1 mg, 2 mg, 4 mg

# trandolapril and verapamil (tran DOE la pril & ver AP a mil)

**Synonyms** verapamil and trandolapril

**U.S./Canadian Brand Names** Tarka® [US/Can]

**Therapeutic Category** Antihypertensive Agent, Combination

**Use** Combination drug for the treatment of hypertension, however, not indicated for initial treatment of
hypertension; replacement therapy in patients receiving separate dosage forms (for patient convenience); when monotherapy with one component fails to achieve desired antihypertensive effect, or
when dose-limiting adverse effects limit upward titration of monotherapy

**Usual Dosage** Dose is individualized.

**Dosage Forms** Tablet, variable release:
1/240: Trandolapril 1 mg [immediate release] and verapamil hydrochloride 240 mg [sustained release]
2/180: Trandolapril 2 mg [immediate release] and verapamil hydrochloride 180 mg [sustained release]
2/240: Trandolapril 2 mg [immediate release] and verapamil hydrochloride 240 mg [sustained release]
4/240: Trandolapril 4 mg [immediate release] and verapamil hydrochloride 240 mg [sustained release]

# tranexamic acid (tran eks AM ik AS id)

**Sound-Alike/Look-Alike Issues**
Cyklokapron® may be confused with cycloSPORINE

**U.S./Canadian Brand Names** Cyklokapron® [US/Can]

**Therapeutic Category** Antihemophilic Agent

**Use** Short-term use (2-8 days) in hemophilia patients during and following tooth extraction to reduce or
prevent hemorrhage
(Continued)

# tranexamic acid *(Continued)*

**Usual Dosage** Children and Adults: I.V.: 10 mg/kg immediately before surgery, then 25 mg/kg/dose orally 3-4 times/day for 2-8 days

Alternatively:
Oral: 25 mg/kg 3-4 times/day beginning 1 day prior to surgery
I.V.: 10 mg/kg 3-4 times/day in patients who are unable to take oral

**Dosage Forms**
Injection, solution: 100 mg/mL (10 mL)
Tablet: 500 mg [Not marketed in U.S.; available from manufacturer for select cases]

**transamine sulphate** *see* tranylcypromine *on this page*

**Transderm-V® [Can]** *see* scopolamine derivatives *on page 740*

**Transdermal-NTG® Patch *(Discontinued)*** *see* nitroglycerin *on page 578*

**Transderm-Nitro® [Can]** *see* nitroglycerin *on page 578*

**Transderm Scōp® [US]** *see* scopolamine derivatives *on page 740*

**Trans-Plantar® [Can]** *see* salicylic acid *on page 734*

**Trans-Plantar® Transdermal Patch *(Discontinued)*** *see* salicylic acid *on page 734*

***trans*-retinoic acid** *see* tretinoin (topical) *on page 818*

**Trans-Ver-Sal® [US-OTC/Can]** *see* salicylic acid *on page 734*

**Tranxene® [US]** *see* clorazepate *on page 199*

**Tranxene® SD™ [US]** *see* clorazepate *on page 199*

**Tranxene® SD™-Half Strength [US]** *see* clorazepate *on page 199*

**Tranxene T-Tab®** *see* clorazepate *on page 199*

# tranylcypromine (tran il SIP roe meen)

**Synonyms** transamine sulphate; tranylcypromine sulfate
**U.S./Canadian Brand Names** Parnate® [US/Can]
**Therapeutic Category** Antidepressant, Monoamine Oxidase Inhibitor
**Use** Treatment of major depressive episode without melancholia
**Usual Dosage** Adults: Oral: 10 mg twice daily, increase by 10 mg increments at 1- to 3-week intervals; maximum: 60 mg/day
**Dosage Forms** Tablet: 10 mg

**tranylcypromine sulfate** *see* tranylcypromine *on this page*

**Trasicor® [Can]** *see* oxprenolol *(Canada only) on page 607*

# trastuzumab (tras TU zoo mab)

**U.S./Canadian Brand Names** Herceptin® [US/Can]
**Therapeutic Category** Antineoplastic Agent
**Use**
Treatment of metastatic breast cancer whose tumors overexpress the HER-2/*neu* protein
**Usual Dosage** I.V. infusion: Adults:
Initial loading dose: 4 mg/kg intravenous infusion over 90 minutes
Maintenance dose: 2 mg/kg intravenous infusion over 90 minutes (can be administered over 30 minutes if prior infusions are well tolerated) weekly until disease progression
**Dosage Forms** Injection, powder for reconstitution: 440 mg [packaged with bacteriostatic water for injection; diluent contains benzyl alcohol]

**Trasylol® [US/Can]** *see* aprotinin *on page 67*

**Travatan® [US/Can]** *see* travoprost *on this page*

# travoprost (TRA voe prost)

**Sound-Alike/Look-Alike Issues**
Travatan® may be confused with Xalatan®

U.S./Canadian Brand Names Travatan® [US/Can]

Therapeutic Category Prostaglandin, Ophthalmic

Use Reduction of elevated intraocular pressure in patients with open-angle glaucoma or ocular hypertension who are intolerant of the other IOP-lowering medications or insufficiently responsive (failed to achieve target IOP determined after multiple measurements over time) to another IOP-lowering medication

Usual Dosage Ophthalmic: Adults: Glaucoma (open angle) or ocular hypertension: Instill 1 drop into affected eye(s) once daily in the evening; do not exceed once-daily dosing (may decrease IOP-lowering effect). If used with other topical ophthalmic agents, separate administration by at least 5 minutes.

Dosage Forms Solution, ophthalmic: 0.004% (2.5 mL, 5 mL) [contains benzalkonium chloride]

## trazodone (TRAZ oh done)

Sound-Alike/Look-Alike Issues

Desyrel® may be confused with Demerol®, Delsym®, Zestril®

Synonyms trazodone hydrochloride

U.S./Canadian Brand Names Alti-Trazodone [Can]; Apo-Trazodone D® [Can]; Apo-Trazodone® [Can]; Desyrel® [US/Can]; Gen-Trazodone [Can]; Novo-Trazodone [Can]; Nu-Trazodone [Can]; PMS-Trazodone [Can]

Therapeutic Category Antidepressant, Triazolopyridine

Use Treatment of depression

Usual Dosage Oral: Therapeutic effects may take up to 6 weeks to occur; therapy is normally maintained for 6-12 months after optimum response is reached to prevent recurrence of depression

Adults: Depression: Initial: 150 mg/day in 3 divided doses (may increase by 50 mg/day every 3-7 days); maximum: 600 mg/day

Dosage Forms Tablet, as hydrochloride: 50 mg, 100 mg, 150 mg, 300 mg

trazodone hydrochloride see trazodone on this page

Trecator® [US/Can] see ethionamide on page 319

Trelstar™ Depot [US/Can] see triptorelin on page 828

Trelstar™ LA [US] see triptorelin on page 828

Trendar® (Discontinued) see ibuprofen on page 427

Trental® [US/Can] see pentoxifylline on page 632

## treprostinil (tre PROST in il)

Synonyms treprostinil sodium

U.S./Canadian Brand Names Remodulin® [US]

Therapeutic Category Vasodilator

Use Treatment of pulmonary arterial hypertension (PAH) in patients with NYHA Class II-IV symptoms to decrease exercise-associated symptoms

Usual Dosage SubQ or I.V. infusion: Adults: PAH: Initial: 1.25 ng/kg/minute continuous; if dose cannot be tolerated, reduce to 0.625 ng/kg/minute. Increase at rate not >1.25 ng/kg/minute per week for first 4 weeks, and not >2.5 ng/kg/minute per week for remainder of therapy. Limited experience with doses >40 ng/kg/minute.

Note: Dose must be carefully and individually titrated (symptom improvement with minimal adverse effects). Avoid abrupt withdrawal.

Dosage Forms Injection, solution: 1 mg/mL (20 mL) [contains sodium chloride 5.3 mg/mL]; 2.5 mg/mL (20 mL) [contains sodium chloride 5.3 mg/mL]; 5 mg/mL (20 mL) [contains sodium chloride 5.3 mg/mL]; 10 mg/mL (20 mL) [contains sodium chloride 4 mg/mL]

treprostinil sodium see treprostinil on this page

tretinoin and mequinol see mequinol and tretinoin on page 514

tretinoin, fluocinolone acetonide, and hydroquinone see fluocinolone, hydroquinone, and tretinoin on page 345

## tretinoin (oral) (TRET i noyn, oral)

Sound-Alike/Look-Alike Issues

tretinoin may be confused with trientine

(Continued)

# tretinoin (oral) *(Continued)*

**Synonyms** all-*trans*-retinoic acid; ATRA; NSC-122758; Ro 5488; tRA
**U.S./Canadian Brand Names** Vesanoid® [US/Can]
**Therapeutic Category** Antineoplastic Agent
**Use** Induction of remission in patients with acute promyelocytic leukemia (APL), French American British (FAB) classification M3 (including the M3 variant)
**Usual Dosage** Oral: Children and Adults:
Remission induction: 45 mg/m$^2$/day in 2-3 divided doses for up to 30 days after complete remission (maximum duration of treatment: 90 days)
Remission maintenance: 45-200 mg/m$^2$/day in 2-3 divided doses for up to 12 months.
**Dosage Forms** Capsule: 10 mg [contains soybean oil and parabens]

# tretinoin (topical) (TRET i noyn TOP i kal)

**Sound-Alike/Look-Alike Issues**
tretinoin may be confused with trientine
**Synonyms** *trans*-retinoic acid; retinoic acid; vitamin A acid
**U.S./Canadian Brand Names** Avita® [US]; Rejuva-A® [Can]; Renova® [US]; Retin-A® Micro [US/Can]; Retin-A® [US/Can]; Retinova® [Can]
**Therapeutic Category** Retinoic Acid Derivative
**Use** Treatment of acne vulgaris; photodamaged skin; palliation of fine wrinkles, mottled hyperpigmentation, and tactile roughness of facial skin as part of a comprehensive skin care and sun avoidance program
**Usual Dosage** Topical:
Children >12 years and Adults: Acne vulgaris: Begin therapy with a weaker formulation of tretinoin (0.025% cream, 0.04% microsphere gel, or 0.01% gel) and increase the concentration as tolerated; apply once daily to acne lesions before retiring or on alternate days; if stinging or irritation develop, decrease frequency of application
Adults ≥18: Palliation of fine wrinkles, mottled hyperpigmentation, and tactile roughness of facial skin: Pea-sized amount of the 0.02% or 0.05% cream applied to entire face once daily in the evening
**Dosage Forms**
Cream, topical: 0.025% (20 g, 45 g); 0.05% (20 g, 45 g); 0.1% (20 g, 45 g)
Altinac™: 0.025% (20 g, 45 g); 0.05% (20 g, 45 g); 0.1% (20 g, 45 g)
Avita®: 0.025% (20 g, 45 g)
Renova®: 0.02% (40 g); 0.05% (40 g, 60 g)
Retin-A®: 0.025% (20 g, 45 g); 0.05% (20 g, 45 g); 0.1% (20 g, 45 g)
Gel, topical: 0.025% (15 g, 45 g)
Avita®: 0.025% (15 g, 45 g)
Retin-A®: 0.01% (15 g, 45 g); 0.025% (15 g, 45 g)
Retin-A® Micro [microsphere gel]: 0.04% (20 g, 45 g); 0.1% (20 g, 45 g)
Liquid, topical (Retin-A®): 0.05% (28 mL)

**Trexall™ [US]** *see* methotrexate *on page 524*

# triacetin (trye a SEE tin)

**Sound-Alike/Look-Alike Issues**
triacetin may be confused with Triacin®
**Synonyms** glycerol triacetate
**U.S./Canadian Brand Names** Myco-Nail [US-OTC]
**Therapeutic Category** Antifungal Agent
**Use** Fungistat for athlete's foot and other superficial fungal infections
**Usual Dosage** Apply twice daily, cleanse areas with dilute alcohol or mild soap and water before application; continue treatment for 7 days after symptoms have disappeared
**Dosage Forms** Liquid, topical: 25% (30 mL)

**triacetyloleandomycin** *see* troleandomycin *on page 829*

**Triacin-C® *(Discontinued)*** *see* triprolidine, pseudoephedrine, and codeine *(Canada only)* on page 827

**triaconazole** *see* terconazole *on page 787*

**Triafed® *(Discontinued)*** *see* triprolidine and pseudoephedrine *on page 827*

**triamcinolone acetonide, parenteral** *see* triamcinolone (systemic) *on next page*

**triamcinolone and nystatin** *see* nystatin and triamcinolone *on page 592*

**triamcinolone diacetate, oral** *see* triamcinolone (systemic) *on this page*

**triamcinolone diacetate, parenteral** *see* triamcinolone (systemic) *on this page*

**triamcinolone hexacetonide** *see* triamcinolone (systemic) *on this page*

# triamcinolone (inhalation, nasal) (trye am SIN oh lone in hil LA shun, NAY sal)

### Sound-Alike/Look-Alike Issues
Nasacort® may be confused with NasalCrom®

**U.S./Canadian Brand Names** Nasacort® AQ [US/Can]; Nasacort® HFA [US]; Tri-Nasal® [US/Can]

**Therapeutic Category** Corticosteroid, Topical

**Use** Nasal inhalation: Management of seasonal and perennial allergic rhinitis in patients ≥6 years of age

**Usual Dosage** Intranasal: Perennial allergic rhinitis, seasonal allergic rhinitis:

Nasal spray:

Children 6-11 years: 110 mcg/day as 1 spray in each nostril once daily.

Children ≥12 years and Adults: 220 mcg/day as 2 sprays in each nostril once daily

Nasal inhaler:

Children 6-11 years: Initial: 220 mcg/day as 2 sprays in each nostril once daily

Children ≥12 years and Adults: Initial: 220 mcg/day as 2 sprays in each nostril once daily; may increase dose to 440 mcg/day (given once daily or divided and given 2 or 4 times/day)

### Dosage Forms

Aerosol for nasal inhalation, as acetonide [CFC free] (Nasacort® [HFA]): 55 mcg/inhalation (9.3 g) [100 doses]

Solution, spray for nasal inhalation, as acetonide (Tri-Nasal®): 50 mcg/inhalation (15 mL) [120 doses]

Suspension, spray for nasal inhalation, as acetonide (Nasacort® AQ): 55 mcg/inhalation (16.5 g) [120 doses]

# triamcinolone (inhalation, oral) (trye am SIN oh lone in hil LA shun, OR al)

**U.S./Canadian Brand Names** Azmacort® [US/Can]

**Therapeutic Category** Adrenal Corticosteroid

**Use**

Oral inhalation: Control of bronchial asthma and related bronchospastic conditions

**Usual Dosage** Oral inhalation: Asthma:

Children 6-12 years: 100-200 mcg 3-4 times/day **or** 200-400 mcg twice daily; maximum dose: 1200 mg/day

Children >12 years and Adults: 200 mcg 3-4 times/day **or** 400 mcg twice daily; maximum dose: 1600 mcg/day

**Dosage Forms** Aerosol for oral inhalation, as acetonide (Azmacort®): 100 mcg per actuation (20 g) [240 actuations]

**triamcinolone, oral** *see* triamcinolone (systemic) *on this page*

# triamcinolone (systemic) (trye am SIN oh lone sis TEM ik)

### Sound-Alike/Look-Alike Issues
Kenalog® may be confused with Ketalar®

**Synonyms** triamcinolone acetonide, parenteral; triamcinolone diacetate, oral; triamcinolone diacetate, parenteral; triamcinolone hexacetonide; triamcinolone, oral

**U.S./Canadian Brand Names** Aristocort® [US/Can]; Aristospan® [US/Can]; Kenalog-10® [US]; Kenalog-40® [US]; Kenalog® [US/Can]

**Therapeutic Category** Adrenal Corticosteroid

**Use** Systemic: Adrenocortical insufficiency, rheumatic disorders, allergic states, respiratory diseases, systemic lupus erythematosus (SLE), and other diseases requiring anti-inflammatory or immunosuppressive effects

**Usual Dosage** The lowest possible dose should be used to control the condition; when dose reduction is possible, the dose should be reduced gradually. Parenteral dose is usually $\frac{1}{3}$ to $\frac{1}{2}$ the oral dose given every 12 hours. In life-threatening situations, parenteral doses larger than the oral dose may be needed.

#### Injection:

Acetonide:

Intra-articular: Large joints: 5-15 mg; small joints: 2.5-5mg

Intradermal: 1 mg per injection site

(Continued)

## triamcinolone (systemic) *(Continued)*

Intralesional or sublesional: 1-30 mg (usually 1 mg per injection site); 10 mg/mL suspension usually used

Intrasynovial: 2.5-40 mg

Systemic (I.M.): Usual adult dose: 60 mg; may repeat with 20-100 mg dose when symptoms recur

Tendon sheath: 2.5-10 mg

Hexacetonide:

Intra-articular: Large joints: 10-20 mg; small joints: 2-6 mg

Intralesional or sublesional: Up to 0.5 mg per square inch of affected area

**Oral: Adults:**

Acute rheumatic carditis: Initial: 20-60 mg/day; reduce dose during maintenance therapy

Acute seasonal or perennial allergic rhinitis: 8-12 mg/day

Adrenocortical insufficiency: Range 4-12 mg/day

Bronchial asthma: 8-16 mg/day

Dermatological disorders, contact/atopic dermatitis: Initial: 8-16 mg/day

Ophthalmic disorders: 12-40 mg/day

Rheumatic disorders: Range: 8-16 mg/day

SLE: Initial: 20-32 mg/day, some patients may need initial doses ≥48 mg; reduce dose during maintenance therapy

**Dosage Forms**

Injection, suspension, as acetonide:

Kenalog-10®: 10 mg/mL (5 mL) [contains benzyl alcohol; not for I.V. or I.M. use]

Kenalog-40®: 40 mg/mL (1 mL, 5 mL, 10 mL) [contains benzyl alcohol; not for I.V. or intradermal use]

Injection, suspension, as hexacetonide (Aristospan®): 5 mg/mL (5 mL); 20 mg/mL (1 mL, 5 mL) [contains benzyl alcohol; not for I.V. use]

Tablet (Aristocort®): 4 mg [contains lactose and sodium benzoate]

## triamcinolone (topical) (trye am SIN oh lone TOP i kal)

**Sound-Alike/Look-Alike Issues**

Kenalog® may be confused with Ketalar®

**U.S./Canadian Brand Names** Aristocort® A [US]; Aristocort® [US/Can]; Kenalog® in Orabase [Can]; Kenalog® [US/Can]; Triderm® [US]

**Therapeutic Category** Corticosteroid, Topical

**Use**

Oral topical: Adjunctive treatment and temporary relief of symptoms associated with oral inflammatory lesions and ulcerative lesions resulting from trauma

Topical: Inflammatory dermatoses responsive to steroids

**Usual Dosage**

**Oral topical:** Oral inflammatory lesions/ulcers: Press a small dab (about ¼ inch) to the lesion until a thin film develops. A larger quantity may be required for coverage of some lesions. For optimal results use only enough to coat the lesion with a thin film; do not rub in.

**Topical:**

Cream, Ointment: Apply thin film to affected areas 2-4 times/day

Spray: Apply to affected area 3-4 times/day

**Dosage Forms**

Cream, as acetonide: 0.025% (15 g, 80 g, 454 g); 0.1% (15 g, 80 g, 454 g, 2270 g); 0.5% (15 g)

Aristocort® A: 0.025% (15 g, 60 g); 0.1% (15 g, 60 g); 0.5% (15 g) [contains benzyl alcohol]

Triderm®: 0.1% (30 g, 85 g)

Lotion, as acetonide: 0.025% (60 mL); 0.1% (60 mL)

Ointment, topical, as acetonide: 0.025% (15g, 80 g, 454 g); 0.1% (15 g, 80 g, 454 g); 0.5% (15 g )

Aristocort® A: 0.1% (15 g, 60 g)

Paste, oral, topical, as acetonide: 0.1% (5 g)

**Triaminic® Cold and Allergy [US-OTC/Can]** *see* chlorpheniramine and pseudoephedrine *on* page 172

**Triaminic® Cold and Cough [US-OTC]** *see* chlorpheniramine, pseudoephedrine, and dextromethorphan on page 177

**Triaminic® Cough [US-OTC]** *see* pseudoephedrine and dextromethorphan on page 693

**Triaminic® Cough and Sore Throat Formula [US-OTC]** *see* acetaminophen, dextromethorphan, and pseudoephedrine on page 11

**Triaminic® Cough & Nasal Congestion [US-OTC]** *see* pseudoephedrine and dextromethorphan *on page 693*

**Triaminic® Expectorant *(Discontinued)***

**Triaminic® Night Time Cough and Cold [US-OTC]** *see* chlorpheniramine, pseudoephedrine, and dextromethorphan *on page 177*

**Triaminic® Thin Strips™ Cough and Runny Nose [US-OTC]** *see* diphenhydramine *on page 254*

**Triaminic® Thin Strips™ Long Acting Cough [US-OTC]** *see* dextromethorphan *on page 238*

**Triamonide® Injection *(Discontinued)***

**triamterene** (trye AM ter een)
**Sound-Alike/Look-Alike Issues**
triamterene may be confused with trimipramine
Dyrenium® may be confused with Pyridium®
**U.S./Canadian Brand Names** Dyrenium® [US]
**Therapeutic Category** Diuretic, Potassium Sparing
**Use** Alone or in combination with other diuretics in treatment of edema and hypertension; decreases potassium excretion caused by kaliuretic diuretics
**Usual Dosage** Adults: Oral: 100-300 mg/day in 1-2 divided doses; maximum dose: 300 mg/day; usual dosage range (JNC 7): 50-100 mg/day
**Dosage Forms** Capsule: 50 mg, 100 mg [contains benzyl alcohol]

**triamterene and hydrochlorothiazide** *see* hydrochlorothiazide and triamterene *on page 410*

**Triapin® *(Discontinued)***

**Triatec-8 [Can]** *see* acetaminophen and codeine *on page 6*

**Triatec-8 Strong [Can]** *see* acetaminophen and codeine *on page 6*

**Triatec-30 [Can]** *see* acetaminophen and codeine *on page 6*

**Triavil® [US]** *see* amitriptyline and perphenazine *on page 43*

**Triavil® 4-50 *(Discontinued)*** *see* amitriptyline and perphenazine *on page 43*

**Triaz® [US]** *see* benzoyl peroxide *on page 98*

**Triaz® Cleanser [US]** *see* benzoyl peroxide *on page 98*

**triazolam** (trye AY zoe lam)
**Sound-Alike/Look-Alike Issues**
triazolam may be confused with alprazolam
Halcion® may be confused with halcinonide, Haldol®
**U.S./Canadian Brand Names** Apo-Triazo® [Can]; Gen-Triazolam [Can]; Halcion® [US/Can]
**Therapeutic Category** Benzodiazepine
**Controlled Substance** C-IV
**Use** Short-term treatment of insomnia
**Usual Dosage** Oral (onset of action is rapid, patient should be in bed when taking medication):
Children <18 years: Dosage not established
Adults:
Hypnotic: 0.125-0.25 mg at bedtime (maximum dose: 0.5 mg/day)
Preprocedure sedation (dental): 0.25 mg taken the evening before oral surgery; or 0.25 mg 1 hour before procedure
**Dosage Forms** Tablet: 0.125 mg, 0.25 mg [contains sodium benzoate]

**tribavirin** *see* ribavirin *on page 720*

**tricalcium phosphate** *see* calcium phosphate (tribasic) *on page 135*

**Tricardio B [US]** *see* folic acid, cyanocobalamin, and pyridoxine *on page 357*

**Tri-Chlor® [US]** *see* trichloroacetic acid *on next page*

**Trichlorex® [Can]** *see* trichlormethiazide *on next page*

## trichlormethiazide (trye klor meth EYE a zide)
**U.S./Canadian Brand Names** Metahydrin® [Can]; Metatensin® [Can]; Naqua® [Can]; Trichlorex® [Can]
**Therapeutic Category** Diuretic, Thiazide
**Use** Management of mild to moderate hypertension; treatment of edema in congestive heart failure and nephrotic syndrome
**Usual Dosage** Adults: Oral: 1-4 mg/day; initially doses may be given twice daily.
**Dosage Forms** Tablet: 4 mg

**trichloroacetaldehyde monohydrate** *see* chloral hydrate *on page 166*

## trichloroacetic acid (trye klor oh a SEE tik AS id)
**U.S./Canadian Brand Names** Tri-Chlor® [US]
**Therapeutic Category** Keratolytic Agent
**Use** Debride callous tissue
**Usual Dosage** Topical: Apply to verruca, cover with bandage for 5-6 days, remove verruca, reapply as needed
**Dosage Forms** Liquid: 80% (15 mL)

**trichloromonofluoromethane and dichlorodifluoromethane** *see* dichlorodifluoromethane and trichloromonofluoromethane *on page 243*

## *Trichophyton* skin test (trye koe FYE ton skin test)
**Therapeutic Category** Diagnostic Agent
**Use** Assess cell-mediated immunity
**Usual Dosage** 0.1 mL intradermally, examine reaction site in 24-48 hours; induration of ≥5 mm in diameter is a positive reaction
**Dosage Forms** Injection, solution: 1:500 (1 mL)

**Tri-Clear® Expectorant** *(Discontinued)*

**TriCor® [US/Can]** *see* fenofibrate *on page 330*

**tricosal** *see* choline magnesium trisalicylate *on page 180*

**Tri-Cyclen® [Can]** *see* ethinyl estradiol and norgestimate *on page 317*

**Tri-Cyclen® Lo [Can]** *see* ethinyl estradiol and norgestimate *on page 317*

**Triderm® [US]** *see* triamcinolone (topical) *on page 820*

**Tridesilon® [US]** *see* desonide *on page 231*

**Tridil® Injection** *(Discontinued)* *see* nitroglycerin *on page 578*

## trientine (TRYE en teen)
**Sound-Alike/Look-Alike Issues**
    trientine may be confused with Trental®, tretinoin
**Synonyms** trientine hydrochloride
**U.S./Canadian Brand Names** Syprine® [US/Can]
**Therapeutic Category** Chelating Agent
**Use** Treatment of Wilson disease in patients intolerant to penicillamine
**Usual Dosage** Oral (administer on an empty stomach):
    Children <12 years: 500-750 mg/day in divided doses 2-4 times/day; maximum: 1.5 g/day
    Adults: 750-1250 mg/day in divided doses 2-4 times/day; maximum dose: 2 g/day
**Dosage Forms** Capsule, as hydrochloride: 250 mg

**trientine hydrochloride** *see* trientine *on this page*

## triethanolamine polypeptide oleate-condensate
(trye eth a NOLE a meen pol i PEP tide OH lee ate-KON den sate)
**U.S./Canadian Brand Names** Cerumenex® [Can]
**Therapeutic Category** Otic Agent, Ceruminolytic
**Use** Removal of ear wax (cerumen)

Usual Dosage Children and Adults: Otic: Fill ear canal, insert cotton plug; allow to remain 15-30 minutes; flush ear with lukewarm water as a single treatment; if a second application is needed for unusually hard impactions, repeat the procedure

Dosage Forms [DSC] = Discontinued product

Solution, otic: 10% (6 mL, 12 mL) [DSC]

## triethanolamine salicylate (trye eth a NOLE a meen sa LIS i late)

Sound-Alike/Look-Alike Issues

Myoflex® may be confused with Mycelex®

Synonyms TEAS; trolamine

U.S./Canadian Brand Names Antiphlogistine Rub A-535 No Odour [Can]; Aspercreme® [US-OTC]; Flex-Power [US-OTC]; Mobisyl® [US-OTC]; Myoflex® [US-OTC/Can]; Sportscreme® [US-OTC]

Therapeutic Category Analgesic, Topical

Use Relief of pain of muscular aches, rheumatism, neuralgia, sprains, arthritis on intact skin

Usual Dosage Topical: Apply to area as needed

Dosage Forms

Cream, topical: 10% (90 g)

Aspercreme®: 10% (5 g, 35 g, 142 g) [odorless]

Flex-Power: 10% (113 g) [clean or light scent; contains sodium metabisulfite and tartrazine]

Mobisyl®: 10% (100 g, 227 g) [odorless; contains sweet almond oil]

Myoflex®: 10% (60 g, 120 g) [odorless]

Sportscreme®: 10% (40 g, 90 g) [odorless fresh scent; contains tartrazine]

Lotion, topical (Aspercreme®): 10% (180 mL) [odorless]

## triethylenethiophosphoramide see thiotepa on page 799

## Trifed-C® (Discontinued) see triprolidine, pseudoephedrine, and codeine (Canada only) on page 827

## trifluoperazine (trye floo oh PER a zeen)

Sound-Alike/Look-Alike Issues

trifluoperazine may be confused with triflupromazine, trihexyphenidyl

Stelazine® may be confused with selegiline

Synonyms trifluoperazine hydrochloride

U.S./Canadian Brand Names Apo-Trifluoperazine® [Can]; Novo-Trifluzine [Can]; PMS-Trifluoperazine [Can]; Terfluzine [Can]

Therapeutic Category Phenothiazine Derivative

Use Treatment of schizophrenia

Usual Dosage

Children 6-12 years: Schizophrenia/psychoses: Oral: Hospitalized or well-supervised patients: Initial: 1 mg 1-2 times/day, gradually increase until symptoms are controlled or adverse effects become troublesome; maximum: 15 mg/day

Adults:

Schizophrenia/psychoses:

Outpatients: Oral: 1-2 mg twice daily

Hospitalized or well-supervised patients: Initial: 2-5 mg twice daily with optimum response in the 15-20 mg/day range; do not exceed 40 mg/day

Nonpsychotic anxiety: Oral: 1-2 mg twice daily; maximum: 6 mg/day; therapy for anxiety should not exceed 12 weeks; do not exceed 6 mg/day for longer than 12 weeks when treating anxiety; agitation, jitteriness, or insomnia may be confused with original neurotic or psychotic symptoms

Dosage Forms Tablet: 1 mg, 2 mg, 5 mg, 10 mg

## trifluoperazine hydrochloride see trifluoperazine on this page

## trifluorothymidine see trifluridine on this page

## trifluridine (trye FLURE i deen)

Sound-Alike/Look-Alike Issues

Viroptic® may be confused with Timoptic®

(Continued)

## trifluridine *(Continued)*

**Synonyms** F$_3$T; trifluorothymidine

**U.S./Canadian Brand Names** SAB-Trifluridine [Can]; Viroptic® [US/Can]

**Therapeutic Category** Antiviral Agent

**Use** Treatment of primary keratoconjunctivitis and recurrent epithelial keratitis caused by herpes simplex virus types I and II

**Usual Dosage** Adults: Instill 1 drop into affected eye every 2 hours while awake, to a maximum of 9 drops/day, until re-epithelialization of corneal ulcer occurs; then use 1 drop every 4 hours for another 7 days; do **not** exceed 21 days of treatment; if improvement has not taken place in 7-14 days, consider another form of therapy

**Dosage Forms** Solution, ophthalmic: 1% (7.5 mL)

**Triglide**™ **[US]** *see* fenofibrate *on page 330*

**triglycerides, medium chain** *see* medium chain triglycerides *on page 507*

## trihexyphenidyl (trye heks ee FEN i dil)

**Sound-Alike/Look-Alike Issues**

trihexyphenidyl may be confused with trifluoperazine

Artane® may be confused with Altace®, Anturane®, Aramine®

**Synonyms** benzhexol hydrochloride; trihexyphenidyl hydrochloride

**U.S./Canadian Brand Names** Apo-Trihex® [Can]

**Therapeutic Category** Anti-Parkinson Agent; Anticholinergic Agent

**Use** Adjunctive treatment of Parkinson's disease; treatment of drug-induced extrapyramidal symptoms

**Usual Dosage** Adults: Oral: Initial: 1-2 mg/day, increase by 2 mg increments at intervals of 3-5 days; usual dose: 5-15 mg/day in 3-4 divided doses

**Dosage Forms**

Elixir, as hydrochloride: 2 mg/5 mL (480 mL)

Tablet, as hydrochloride: 2 mg, 5 mg

**trihexyphenidyl hydrochloride** *see* trihexyphenidyl *on this page*

**TriHIBit® [US]** *see* diphtheria, tetanus toxoids, and acellular pertussis vaccine and *Haemophilus* b conjugate vaccine *on page 259*

**Tri-K® [US]** *see* potassium acetate, potassium bicarbonate, and potassium citrate *on page 662*

**Trikacide [Can]** *see* metronidazole *on page 535*

**TRIKOF-D® *(Discontinued)***

**Tri-Kort® Injection *(Discontinued)***

**Trilafon® *(Discontinued)*** *see* perphenazine *on page 635*

**Trileptal® [US/Can]** *see* oxcarbazepine *on page 606*

**Tri-Levlen® [US]** *see* ethinyl estradiol and levonorgestrel *on page 312*

**Trilisate® *(Discontinued)*** *see* choline magnesium trisalicylate *on page 180*

**Trilog® Injection *(Discontinued)***

**Trilone® Injection *(Discontinued)***

**Tri-Luma**™ **[US]** *see* fluocinolone, hydroquinone, and tretinoin *on page 345*

**TriLyte**™ **[US]** *see* polyethylene glycol-electrolyte solution *on page 658*

**Trimazide® *(Discontinued)*** *see* trimethobenzamide *on next page*

## trimebutine *(Canada only)* (trye me BYOO teen)

**Synonyms** trimebutine maleate

**U.S./Canadian Brand Names** Apo-Trimebutine® [Can]; Modulon® [Can]

**Therapeutic Category** Antispasmodic Agent, Gastrointestinal

**Use** Treatment and relief of symptoms associated with irritable bowel syndrome (IBS) (spastic colon). In postoperative paralytic ileus in order to accelerate the resumption of the intestinal transit following abdominal surgery.

**Usual Dosage** Children ≥12 years and Adults: Oral: 200 mg 3 times/day before meals

**Dosage Forms** Tablet, as maleate: 100 mg, 200 mg

**trimebutine maleate** *see* trimebutine *(Canada only)* *on previous page*

# trimeprazine *(Canada only)* (trye MEP re zeen)
**U.S./Canadian Brand Names** Panectyl® [Can]
**Therapeutic Category** Antihistamine
**Use** Perennial and seasonal allergic rhinitis and other allergic symptoms including urticaria
**Usual Dosage** Oral:
  Children:
    6 months to 3 years: 1.25 mg at bedtime or 3 times/day if needed
    >3 years: 2.5 mg at bedtime or 3 times/day if needed
    >6 years: 5 mg/day
  Adults: 2.5 mg 4 times/day
**Dosage Forms** Tablet, as tartrate: 2.5 mg, 5 mg

# trimethobenzamide (trye meth oh BEN za mide)
**Sound-Alike/Look-Alike Issues**
  Tigan® may be confused with Tiazac®, Ticar®
**Synonyms** trimethobenzamide hydrochloride
**U.S./Canadian Brand Names** Tebamide™ [US]; Tigan® [US/Can]
**Therapeutic Category** Anticholinergic Agent; Antiemetic
**Use** Treatment of nausea and vomiting
**Usual Dosage** Rectal use is contraindicated in neonates and premature infants
  Children:
    <14 kg: Oral, rectal: 100 mg 3-4 times/day
    14-40 kg: Oral, rectal: 100-200 mg 3-4 times/day
  Adults:
    Oral: 250-300 mg 3-4 times/day
    I.M., rectal: 200 mg 3-4 times/day
**Dosage Forms**
  Capsule, as hydrochloride (Tigan®): 300 mg
  Injection, solution, as hydrochloride: 100 mg/mL (2 mL)
    Tigan®: 100 mg/mL (2 mL [preservative free], 20 mL)
  Suppository, rectal, as hydrochloride: 100 mg, 200 mg
    Tebamide™: 100 mg, 200 mg [contains benzocaine]
    Tigan®, Trimazide [DSC]: 200 mg [contains benzocaine]

**trimethobenzamide hydrochloride** *see* trimethobenzamide *on this page*

# trimethoprim (trye METH oh prim)
**Sound-Alike/Look-Alike Issues**
  trimethoprim may be confused with trimethaphan
  Proloprim® may be confused with Prolixin®, Protropin®
**Synonyms** TMP
**U.S./Canadian Brand Names** Apo-Trimethoprim® [Can]; Primsol® [US]; Proloprim® [US]
**Therapeutic Category** Antibiotic, Miscellaneous
**Use** Treatment of urinary tract infections due to susceptible strains of *E. coli*, *P. mirabilis*, *K. pneumoniae*, *Enterobacter* sp and coagulase-negative *Staphylococcus* including *S. saprophyticus*; acute otitis media in children; acute exacerbations of chronic bronchitis in adults; in combination with other agents for treatment of toxoplasmosis, *Pneumocystis carinii*; treatment of superficial ocular infections involving the conjunctiva and cornea
**Usual Dosage** Oral:
  Children: 4 mg/kg/day in divided doses every 12 hours
  Adults: 100 mg every 12 hours or 200 mg every 24 hours for 10 days; longer treatment periods may be necessary for prostatitis (ie, 4-16 weeks); in the treatment of *Pneumocystis carinii* pneumonia; dose may be as high as 15-20 mg/kg/day in 3-4 divided doses
**Dosage Forms** [DSC] = Discontinued product
  Solution, oral (Primsol®): 50 mg (base)/5 mL (480 mL) [contains sodium benzoate; bubble gum flavor]
  Tablet: 100 mg
    Proloprim®: 100 mg, 200 mg [DSC]

## trimethoprim and polymyxin B (trye METH oh prim & pol i MIKS in bee)
**Synonyms** polymyxin B and trimethoprim
**U.S./Canadian Brand Names** PMS-Polytrimethoprim [Can]; Polytrim® [US/Can]
**Therapeutic Category** Antibiotic, Ophthalmic
**Use** Treatment of surface ocular bacterial conjunctivitis and blepharoconjunctivitis
**Usual Dosage** Instill 1-2 drops in eye(s) every 4-6 hours
**Dosage Forms** Solution, ophthalmic: Trimethoprim 1 mg and polymyxin B sulfate 10,000 units per mL (10 mL) [contains benzalkonium chloride]

**trimethoprim and sulfamethoxazole** *see* sulfamethoxazole and trimethoprim *on page 773*

## trimetrexate glucuronate (tri me TREKS ate gloo KYOOR oh nate)
**Synonyms** NSC-352122
**U.S./Canadian Brand Names** NeuTrexin® [US]
**Therapeutic Category** Antibiotic, Miscellaneous
**Use** Alternative therapy for the treatment of moderate-to-severe *Pneumocystis carinii* pneumonia (PCP) in immunocompromised patients, including patients with acquired immunodeficiency syndrome (AIDS), who are intolerant of, or are refractory to, co-trimoxazole therapy or for whom co-trimoxazole and pentamidine are contraindicated. **Concurrent folinic acid (leucovorin) must always be administered.**
**Usual Dosage Note:** Concurrent leucovorin 20 mg/m$^2$ every 6 hours must be administered daily (oral or I.V.) during treatment and for 72 hours past the last dose of trimetrexate glucuronate.

Adults: I.V.:
*Pneumocystis carinii*: 45 mg/m$^2$ once daily for 21 days; **alternative dosing based on weight:**
<50 kg:Trimetrexate glucuronate 1.5 mg/kg/day; leucovorin 0.6 mg/kg 4 times/day
50-80 kg:Trimetrexate glucuronate 1.2 mg/kg/day; leucovorin 0.5 mg/kg/4 times/day
>80 kg: Trimetrexate glucuronate 1 mg/kg/day; leucovorin 0.5 mg/kg/4 times/day
**Note:** Oral doses of leucovorin should be rounded up to the next higher 25 mg increment.
**Dosage Forms** Injection, powder for reconstitution [preservative free]: 25 mg, 200 mg

## trimipramine (trye MI pra meen)
**Sound-Alike/Look-Alike Issues**
trimipramine may be confused with triamterene, trimeprazine
**Synonyms** trimipramine maleate
**U.S./Canadian Brand Names** Apo-Trimip® [Can]; Nu-Trimipramine [Can]; Rhotrimine® [Can]; Surmontil® [US/Can]
**Therapeutic Category** Antidepressant, Tricyclic (Tertiary Amine)
**Use** Treatment of depression
**Usual Dosage** Oral: Adults: 50-150 mg/day as a single bedtime dose up to a maximum of 200 mg/day outpatient and 300 mg/day inpatient
**Dosage Forms** Capsule: 25 mg, 50 mg, 100 mg

**trimipramine maleate** *see* trimipramine *on this page*

**Trimox® [US]** *see* amoxicillin *on page 46*

**Trimpex® *(Discontinued)*** *see* trimethoprim *on previous page*

**Trinalin® [US/Can]** *see* azatadine and pseudoephedrine *on page 83*

**Tri-Nasal® [US/Can]** *see* triamcinolone (inhalation, nasal) *on page 819*

**Trinate [US]** *see* vitamins (multiple/prenatal) *on page 852*

**TriNessa™ [US]** *see* ethinyl estradiol and norgestimate *on page 317*

**Tri-Norinyl® [US]** *see* ethinyl estradiol and norethindrone *on page 314*

**Trinsicon® [US]** *see* vitamin B complex combinations *on page 849*

**Triofed® Syrup *(Discontinued)*** *see* triprolidine and pseudoephedrine *on next page*

**Triostat® [US]** *see* liothyronine *on page 484*

**Tripedia® [US]** *see* diphtheria, tetanus toxoids, and acellular pertussis vaccine *on page 259*

**Triphasil® [US/Can]** *see* ethinyl estradiol and levonorgestrel *on page 312*

**Triphenyl® Expectorant *(Discontinued)***

**triple antibiotic** *see* bacitracin, neomycin, and polymyxin B *on page 87*

**triple sulfa** *see* sulfabenzamide, sulfacetamide, and sulfathiazole *on page 771*

**Triposed® Syrup *(Discontinued)*** *see* triprolidine and pseudoephedrine *on this page*

**Tri-Previfem™ [US]** *see* ethinyl estradiol and norgestimate *on page 317*

# triprolidine and pseudoephedrine (trye PROE li deen & soo doe e FED rin)

**Sound-Alike/Look-Alike Issues**
Aprodine® may be confused with Aphrodyne®

**Synonyms** pseudoephedrine and triprolidine

**U.S./Canadian Brand Names** Actifed® Cold and Allergy [US-OTC]; Actifed® [Can]; Allerfrim® [US-OTC]; Aphedrid™ [US-OTC]; Aprodine® [US-OTC]; Genac® [US-OTC]; Silafed® [US-OTC]; Sudafed® Sinus Nighttime [US-OTC]; Tri-Sudo® [US-OTC]

**Therapeutic Category** Antihistamine/Decongestant Combination

**Use** Temporary relief of nasal congestion, decongest sinus openings, running nose, sneezing, itching of nose or throat and itchy, watery eyes due to common cold, hay fever, or other upper respiratory allergies

**Usual Dosage** Oral:
Children:
Syrup:
4 months to 2 years: 1.25 mL 3-4 times/day
2-4 years: 2.5 mL 3-4 times/day
4-6 years: 3.75 mL 3-4 times/day
6-12 years: 5 mL every 4-6 hours; do not exceed 4 doses in 24 hours
Tablet: ½ every 4-6 hours; do not exceed 4 doses in 24 hours
Children >12 years and Adults:
Syrup: 10 mL every 4-6 hours; do not exceed 4 doses in 24 hours
Tablet: 1 every 4-6 hours; do not exceed 4 doses in 24 hours

**Dosage Forms**
Syrup: Triprolidine hydrochloride 1.25 mg and pseudoephedrine hydrochloride 30 mg per 5 mL (120 mL)
Allerfrim®: Triprolidine hydrochloride 1.25 mg and pseudoephedrine hydrochloride 30 mg per 5 mL (120 mL, 480 mL) [contains sodium benzoate]
Aprodine®: Triprolidine hydrochloride 1.25 mg and pseudoephedrine hydrochloride 30 mg per 5 mL (120 mL)
Silafed®: Triprolidine hydrochloride 1.25 mg and pseudoephedrine hydrochloride 30 mg per 5 mL (120 mL, 240 mL)
Tablet (Actifed® Cold and Allergy, Allerfrim®, Aphedrid™, Aprodine®, Genac®, Tri-Sudo®): Triprolidine hydrochloride 2.5 mg and pseudoephedrine hydrochloride 60 mg

**triprolidine, codeine, and pseudoephedrine** *see* triprolidine, pseudoephedrine, and codeine *(Canada only) on this page*

# triprolidine, pseudoephedrine, and codeine *(Canada only)*
(trye PROE li deen, soo doe e FED rin, & KOE deen)

**Sound-Alike/Look-Alike Issues**
Triacin-C® may be confused with triacetin

**Synonyms** codeine, pseudoephedrine, and triprolidine; codeine, triprolidine, and pseudoephedrine; pseudoephedrine, codeine, and triprolidine; pseudoephedrine, triprolidine, and codeine; triprolidine, codeine, and pseudoephedrine

**U.S./Canadian Brand Names** CoActifed® [Can]; Covan® [Can]; ratio-Cotridin [Can]

**Therapeutic Category** Antihistamine/Decongestant/Antitussive

**Controlled Substance** C-V (CDSA-I)

**Use** Symptomatic relief of upper respiratory symptoms and cough

**Usual Dosage** Oral:
Children:
2-6 years: 2.5 mL 4 times/day
7-12 years: 5 mL 4 times/day **or** ½ tablet 4 times/day
Children >12 years and Adults: 10 mL 4 times/day **or** 1 tablet 4 times/day

**Dosage Forms**
Syrup:
Triprolidine hydrochloride 1.25 mg, pseudoephedrine hydrochloride 30 mg, and codeine phosphate 10 mg per 5 mL [contains alcohol 4.3%]
(Continued)

## triprolidine, pseudoephedrine, and codeine *(Canada only)* *(Continued)*

CoActifed®, CoVan®, ratio-Cotridin: Triprolidine hydrochloride 2 mg, pseudoephedrine hydrochloride 30 mg, and codeine phosphate 10 mg per 5 mL [available in Canada; not available in U.S.]
Tablet (CoActifed®): Triprolidine hydrochloride 4 mg, pseudoephedrine hydrochloride 60 mg, and codeine phosphate 20 mg (50s) [available in Canada; not available in U.S.]

**Tri-Pseudo®** *(Discontinued)* *see* triprolidine and pseudoephedrine *on previous page*

**TripTone®** [US-OTC] *see* dimenhydrinate *on page 252*

**triptoraline** *see* triptorelin *on this page*

## triptorelin *(trip toe REL in)*

**Synonyms** AY-25650; CL-118,532; D-Trp(6)-LHRH; triptoraline; triptorelin pamoate; tryptoreline
**U.S./Canadian Brand Names** Trelstar™ Depot [US/Can]; Trelstar™ LA [US]
**Therapeutic Category** Luteinizing Hormone-Releasing Hormone Analog
**Use** Palliative treatment of advanced prostate cancer as an alternative to orchiectomy or estrogen administration
**Usual Dosage** I.M.: Adults: Prostate cancer:
Trelstar™ Depot: 3.75 mg once every 28 days
Trelstar™ LA: 11.25 mg once every 84 days
**Dosage Forms** Injection, powder for reconstitution, as pamoate [also available packaged with Debioclip™ (prefilled syringe containing sterile water)]:
Trelstar™ Depot: 3.75 mg
Trelstar™ LA: 11.25 mg

**triptorelin pamoate** *see* triptorelin *on this page*

**Triquilar®** [Can] *see* ethinyl estradiol and levonorgestrel *on page 312*

**tris buffer** *see* tromethamine *on next page*

**Trisenox™** [US] *see* arsenic trioxide *on page 70*

**tris(hydroxymethyl)aminomethane** *see* tromethamine *on next page*

**trisodium calcium diethylenetriaminepentaacetate (Ca-DTPA)** *see* diethylene triamine penta-acetic acid *on page 246*

**Tri-Sprintec™** [US] *see* ethinyl estradiol and norgestimate *on page 317*

**Tri-Statin®** II Topical *(Discontinued)* *see* nystatin and triamcinolone *on page 592*

**Tristoject®** Injection *(Discontinued)*

**Trisudex®** *(Discontinued)* *see* triprolidine and pseudoephedrine *on previous page*

**Tri-Sudo®** [US-OTC] *see* triprolidine and pseudoephedrine *on previous page*

**Tri-Tannate Plus®** *(Discontinued)* *see* chlorpheniramine, ephedrine, phenylephrine, and carbetapentane *on page 173*

**Trivagizole-3®** [Can] *see* clotrimazole *on page 199*

**Trivagizole-3®** *(Discontinued)* *see* clotrimazole *on page 199*

**trivalent inactivated influenza vaccine (TIV)** *see* influenza virus vaccine *on page 437*

**Tri-Vent™** DM [US] *see* guaifenesin, pseudoephedrine, and dextromethorphan *on page 391*

**Tri-Vent™** DPC [US] *see* chlorpheniramine, phenylephrine, and dextromethorphan *on page 174*

**Tri-Vent™** HC [US] *see* hydrocodone, carbinoxamine, and pseudoephedrine *on page 414*

**Tri-Vi-Flor®** [US] *see* vitamins (multiple/pediatric) *on page 852*

**Tri-Vi-Flor®** with Iron [US] *see* vitamins (multiple/pediatric) *on page 852*

**Tri-Vi-Sol®** [US-OTC] *see* vitamins (multiple/pediatric) *on page 852*

**Tri-Vi-Sol®** with Iron [US-OTC] *see* vitamins (multiple/pediatric) *on page 852*

**Trivora®** [US] *see* ethinyl estradiol and levonorgestrel *on page 312*

**Trizivir®** [US] *see* abacavir, lamivudine, and zidovudine *on page 2*

**Trobicin®** [US] *see* spectinomycin *on page 764*

**Trocaine®** [US-OTC] *see* benzocaine *on page 95*

**Trocal**® **(Discontinued)** *see* dextromethorphan *on page 238*

**trolamine** *see* triethanolamine salicylate *on page 823*

## troleandomycin (troe lee an doe MYE sin)
**Synonyms** triacetyloleandomycin
**U.S./Canadian Brand Names** Tao® [US]
**Therapeutic Category** Macrolide (Antibiotic)
**Use** Antibiotic with spectrum of activity similar to erythromycin
**Usual Dosage** Oral:
    Children 7-13 years: 25-40 mg/kg/day divided every 6 hours (125-250 mg every 6 hours)
    Adults: 250-500 mg 4 times/day (around-the-clock every 6 hours)
**Dosage Forms** Capsule: 250 mg

**Trombovar**® **[Can]** *see* sodium tetradecyl *on page 758*

## tromethamine (troe METH a meen)
**Synonyms** tris buffer; tris(hydroxymethyl)aminomethane
**U.S./Canadian Brand Names** THAM® [US]
**Therapeutic Category** Alkalinizing Agent
**Use** Correction of metabolic acidosis associated with cardiac bypass surgery or cardiac arrest; to correct excess acidity of stored blood that is preserved with acid citrate dextrose; to prime the pump-oxygenator during cardiac bypass surgery; indicated in infants needing alkalinization after receiving maximum sodium bicarbonate (8-10 mEq/kg/24 hours); (advantage of THAM® is that it alkalinizes without increasing $pCO_2$ and sodium)
**Usual Dosage**
    Neonates and Infants: Metabolic acidosis associated with RDS: Initial: Approximately 1 mL/kg for each pH unit below 7.4; additional dosess determined by changes in $PaO_2$, pH, and $pCO_2$; **Note:** Although THAM® solution does not raise $pCO_2$ when treating metabolic acidosis with concurrent respiratory acidosis, bicarbonate may be preferred because the osmotic effects of THAM® are greater.

    Adults: Dose depends on buffer base deficit; when deficit is known: tromethamine (mL of 0.3 M solution) = body weight (kg) x base deficit (mEq/L); when base deficit is not known: 3-6 mL/kg/dose I.V. (1-2 mEq/kg/dose)
    Metabolic acidosis with cardiac arrest:
      I.V.: 3.5-6 mL/kg (1-2 mEq/kg/dose) into large peripheral vein; 500-1000 mL if needed in adults
      I.V. continuous drip: Infuse slowly by syringe pump over 3-6 hours
    Acidosis associated with cardiac bypass surgery: Average dose: 9 mL/kg (2.7 mEq/kg); 500 mL is adequate for most adults; maximum dose: 500 mg/kg in ≤1 hour
    Excess acidity of acid citrate dextrose priming blood: 14-70 mL of 0.3 molar solution added to each 500 mL of blood
**Dosage Forms** Injection, solution: 18 g [0.3 molar] (500 mL)

**Tronolane**® **[US-OTC]** *see* pramoxine *on page 670*

**Tropicacyl**® **[US]** *see* tropicamide *on this page*

## tropicamide (troe PIK a mide)
**Synonyms** bistropamide
**U.S./Canadian Brand Names** Diotrope® [Can]; Mydral™ [US]; Mydriacyl® [US/Can]; Tropicacyl® [US]
**Therapeutic Category** Anticholinergic Agent
**Use** Short-acting mydriatic used in diagnostic procedures; as well as preoperatively and postoperatively; treatment of some cases of acute iritis, iridocyclitis, and keratitis
**Usual Dosage** Ophthalmic: Children and Adults (individuals with heavily pigmented eyes may require larger doses):
    Cycloplegia: Instill 1-2 drops (1%); may repeat in 5 minutes
    Exam must be performed within 30 minutes after the repeat dose; if the patient is not examined within 20-30 minutes, instill an additional drop
    Mydriasis: Instill 1-2 drops (0.5%) 15 20 minutes before exam; may repeat every 30 minutes as needed
**Dosage Forms**
    Solution, ophthalmic: 0.5% (15 mL); 1% (2 mL, 15 mL) [contains benzalkonium chloride]
    Mydriacyl®: 1% (3 mL, 15 mL) [contains benzalkonium chloride]
    Mydral™, Tropicacyl®: 0.5% (15 mL); 1% (15 mL) [contains benzalkonium chloride]

## trospium (TROSE pee um)
**Synonyms** trospium chloride
**U.S./Canadian Brand Names** Sanctura™ [US]
**Therapeutic Category** Anticholinergic Agent
**Use** Treatment of overactive bladder with symptoms of urgency, incontinence, and urinary frequency
**Usual Dosage** Oral: Adults: 20 mg twice daily
**Dosage Forms** Tablet, as chloride: 20 mg

**trospium chloride** *see* trospium *on this page*

**Truphylline® (Discontinued)** *see* aminophylline *on page 41*

**Trusopt® [US/Can]** *see* dorzolamide *on page 267*

**Truvada™ [US]** *see* emtricitabine and tenofovir *on page 283*

## trypsin, balsam peru, and castor oil (TRIP sin, BAL sam pe RUE, & KAS tor oyl)
**Sound-Alike/Look-Alike Issues**
Granulex® may be confused with Regranex®
**Synonyms** balsam peru, trypsin, and castor oil; castor oil, trypsin, and balsam peru
**U.S./Canadian Brand Names** Granulex® [US]; Xenaderm™ [US]
**Therapeutic Category** Protectant, Topical
**Use** Treatment of decubitus ulcers, varicose ulcers, debridement of eschar, dehiscent wounds and sunburn; promote wound healing; reduce odor from necrotic wounds
**Usual Dosage** Topical: Apply a minimum of twice daily or as often as necessary
**Dosage Forms**
Aerosol, topical: Trypsin 0.12 mg, balsam Peru 87 mg, and castor oil 788 mg per gram (120 g)
Granulex®: Trypsin 0.12 mg, balsam Peru 87 mg, and castor oil 788 mg per gram (60 g, 120 g)
Ointment, topical (Xenaderm™): Trypsin 90 USP units, balsam Peru 87 mg, and castor oil 788 mg per gram (60 g)

**tryptoreline** *see* triptorelin *on page 828*

**Trysul® (Discontinued)** *see* sulfabenzamide, sulfacetamide, and sulfathiazole *on page 771*

**TSH** *see* thyrotropin alpha *on page 800*

**TSPA** *see* thiotepa *on page 799*

**TST** *see* tuberculin tests *on this page*

**T-Stat® (Discontinued)**

**T-Tab® [US]** *see* clorazepate *on page 199*

**tuberculin purified protein eerivative** *see* tuberculin tests *on this page*

**tuberculin skin test** *see* tuberculin tests *on this page*

## tuberculin tests (too BER kyoo lin tests)
**Sound-Alike/Look-Alike Issues**
Aplisol® may be confused with Anusol®, A.P.L.®, Aplitest®, Atropisol®
Tuberculin products may be confused with tetanus toxoid products and influenza virus vaccine. Medication errors have occurred when tuberculin skin tests (PPD) have been inadvertently administered instead of tetanus toxoid products and influenza virus vaccine. These products are refrigerated and often stored in close proximity to each other.
**Synonyms** mantoux; PPD; tine test; TST; tuberculin purified protein eerivative; tuberculin skin test
**U.S./Canadian Brand Names** Aplisol® [US]; Tubersol® [US]
**Therapeutic Category** Diagnostic Agent
**Use** Skin test in diagnosis of tuberculosis, cell-mediated immunodeficiencies
**Usual Dosage** Children and Adults: Intradermal: 0.1 mL about 4" below elbow; use 1/4" to 1/2" or 26- or 27-gauge needle; significant reactions are ≥5 mm in diameter
Interpretation of induration of tuberculin skin test injections: Positive: ≥10 mm; inconclusive: 5-9 mm; negative: <5 mm
Interpretation of induration of Tine test injections: Positive: >2 mm and vesiculation present; inconclusive: <2 mm (give patient Mantoux test of 5 TU/0.1 mL - base decisions on results of Mantoux test); negative: <2 mm or erythema of any size (no need for retesting unless person is a contact of a patient with tuberculosis or there is clinical evidence suggestive of the disease)
**Dosage Forms** Injection, solution: 5 TU/0.1 mL (1 mL, 5 mL)

**Tubersol**® **[US]** *see* tuberculin tests *on previous page*

**Tucks**® **[US-OTC]** *see* witch hazel *on page 855*

**Tucks**® **Anti-Itch [US-OTC]** *see* hydrocortisone (topical) *on page 417*

**Tucks**® **Hemorrhoidal [US-OTC]** *see* pramoxine *on page 670*

**Tuinal**® *(Discontinued) see* amobarbital and secobarbital *on page 45*

**Tums**® **[US-OTC]** *see* calcium carbonate *on page 130*

**Tums**® **500 [US-OTC]** *see* calcium carbonate *on page 130*

**Tums**® **E-X [US-OTC]** *see* calcium carbonate *on page 130*

**Tums**® **Extra Strength Sugar Free [US-OTC]** *see* calcium carbonate *on page 130*

**Tums**® **Smooth Dissolve [US-OTC]** *see* calcium carbonate *on page 130*

**Tums**® **Ultra [US-OTC]** *see* calcium carbonate *on page 130*

**Tusal**® *(Discontinued)*

**Tusibron**® *(Discontinued) see* guaifenesin *on page 383*

**Tusibron-DM**® *(Discontinued) see* guaifenesin and dextromethorphan *on page 385*

**Tussafed**® **[US]** *see* carbinoxamine, pseudoephedrine, and dextromethorphan *on page 145*

**Tussafin**® **Expectorant** *(Discontinued) see* hydrocodone, pseudoephedrine, and guaifenesin *on page 415*

**Tussend**® **Expectorant [US]** *see* hydrocodone, pseudoephedrine, and guaifenesin *on page 415*

**Tussend**® **Syrup [US]** *see* pseudoephedrine, hydrocodone, and chlorpheniramine *on page 695*

**Tussend**® **Tablet [US]** *see* pseudoephedrine, hydrocodone, and chlorpheniramine *on page 695*

**Tussi-12**® **[US]** *see* carbetapentane and chlorpheniramine *on page 142*

**Tussi-12 S**™ **[US]** *see* carbetapentane and chlorpheniramine *on page 142*

**Tussigon**® **[US]** *see* hydrocodone and homatropine *on page 413*

**Tussin [US-OTC]** *see* guaifenesin *on page 383*

**TussiNate**™ **[US]** *see* hydrocodone, phenylephrine, and diphenhydramine *on page 414*

**Tussionex**® **[US]** *see* hydrocodone and chlorpheniramine *on page 412*

**Tussi-Organidin**® **DM NR** *(Discontinued) see* guaifenesin and dextromethorphan *on page 385*

**Tussi-Organidin**® **NR [US]** *see* guaifenesin and codeine *on page 384*

**Tussi-Organidin**® **S-NR [US]** *see* guaifenesin and codeine *on page 384*

**Tussizone-12 RF**™ **[US]** *see* carbetapentane and chlorpheniramine *on page 142*

**Tuss-LA**® *(Discontinued) see* guaifenesin and pseudoephedrine *on page 388*

**T-Vites [US-OTC]** *see* vitamins (multiple/oral) *on page 852*

**Twelve Resin-K [US]** *see* cyanocobalamin *on page 212*

**Twilite**® **[US-OTC]** *see* diphenhydramine *on page 254*

**Twinject**™ **[US]** *see* epinephrine *on page 287*

**Twin-K**® *(Discontinued)*

**Twinrix**® **[US/Can]** *see* hepatitis A inactivated and hepatitis B (recombinant) vaccine *on page 400*

**Two-Dyne**® *(Discontinued)*

**Tygacil**™ **[US]** *see* tigecycline *on page 803*

**Tylenol**® **[US-OTC/Can]** *see* acetaminophen *on page 4*

**Tylenol**® **8 Hour [US-OTC]** *see* acetaminophen *on page 4*

**Tylenol**® **Allergy Sinus [US-OTC/Can]** *see* acetaminophen, chlorpheniramine, and pseudoephedrine *on page 10*

**Tylenol**® **Arthritis Pain [US-OTC]** *see* acetaminophen *on page 4*

**Tylenol® Children's [US-OTC]** *see* acetaminophen *on page 4*

**Tylenol® Cold Day Non-Drowsy [US-OTC]** *see* acetaminophen, dextromethorphan, and pseudoephedrine *on page 11*

**Tylenol® Cold Daytime [Can]** *see* acetaminophen, dextromethorphan, and pseudoephedrine *on page 11*

**Tylenol® Cold, Infants [US-OTC]** *see* acetaminophen and pseudoephedrine *on page 8*

**Tylenol® Decongestant [Can]** *see* acetaminophen and pseudoephedrine *on page 8*

**Tylenol® Elixir with Codeine [Can]** *see* acetaminophen and codeine *on page 6*

**Tylenol® Extra Strength [US-OTC]** *see* acetaminophen *on page 4*

**Tylenol® Flu Non-Drowsy Maximum Strength [US-OTC]** *see* acetaminophen, dextromethorphan, and pseudoephedrine *on page 11*

**Tylenol® Infants [US-OTC]** *see* acetaminophen *on page 4*

**Tylenol® Junior Strength [US-OTC]** *see* acetaminophen *on page 4*

**Tylenol® No. 1 [Can]** *see* acetaminophen and codeine *on page 6*

**Tylenol® No. 1 Forte [Can]** *see* acetaminophen and codeine *on page 6*

**Tylenol® No. 2 with Codeine [Can]** *see* acetaminophen and codeine *on page 6*

**Tylenol® No. 3 with Codeine [Can]** *see* acetaminophen and codeine *on page 6*

**Tylenol® No. 4 with Codeine [Can]** *see* acetaminophen and codeine *on page 6*

**Tylenol® PM Extra Strength [US-OTC]** *see* acetaminophen and diphenhydramine *on page 7*

**Tylenol® Severe Allergy [US-OTC]** *see* acetaminophen and diphenhydramine *on page 7*

**Tylenol® Sinus [Can]** *see* acetaminophen and pseudoephedrine *on page 8*

**Tylenol® Sinus, Children's [US-OTC]** *see* acetaminophen and pseudoephedrine *on page 8*

**Tylenol® Sinus Day Non-Drowsy [US-OTC]** *see* acetaminophen and pseudoephedrine *on page 8*

**Tylenol® Sore Throat [US-OTC]** *see* acetaminophen *on page 4*

**Tylenol® With Codeine [US]** *see* acetaminophen and codeine *on page 6*

**Tylenol® with Codeine (Elixir) *(Discontinued)*** *see* acetaminophen and codeine *on page 6*

**Tylox® [US]** *see* oxycodone and acetaminophen *on page 609*

**Typherix™ [Can]** *see* Salmonella typhi Vi capsular polysaccharide vaccine *(Canada only) on page 738*

**Typhim Vi® [US]** *see* typhoid vaccine *on this page*

## typhoid vaccine (TYE foid vak SEEN)

**Synonyms** typhoid vaccine live oral Ty21a

**U.S./Canadian Brand Names** Typhim Vi® [US]; Vivotif Berna® [US]

**Therapeutic Category** Vaccine, Inactivated Bacteria

**Use** Typhoid vaccine: Live, attenuated Ty21a typhoid vaccine should not be administered to immunocompromised persons, including those known to be infected with HIV. Parenteral inactivated vaccine is a theoretically safer alternative for this group.

Parenteral: Promotes active immunity to typhoid fever for patients intimately exposed to a typhoid carrier or foreign travel to a typhoid fever endemic area

Oral: For immunization of children >6 years of age and adults who expect intimate exposure of or household contact with typhoid fever, travelers to areas of world with risk of exposure to typhoid fever, and workers in microbiology laboratories with expected frequent contact with *S. typhi*

**Usual Dosage** Immunization:

Oral: Children ≥6 years and Adults:

Primary immunization: One capsule on alternate days (day 1, 3, 5, and 7) for a total of 4 doses; all doses should be complete at least 1 week prior to potential exposure

Booster immunization: Repeat full course of primary immunization every 5 years

I.M. (Typhim Vi®): Children ≥2 years and Adults: 0.5 mL given at least 2 weeks prior to expected exposure

Reimmunization: 0.5 mL; optimal schedule has not been established; a single dose every 2 years is currently recommended for repeated or continued exposure

Dosage Forms
Capsule, enteric coated (Vivotif Berna®): Viable *S. typhi* Ty21a colony-forming units 2-6 x $10^9$ and nonviable *S. typhi* Ty21a colony-forming units 5-50 x $10^9$ [contains lactose]
Injection, solution (Typhim Vi®): Purified Vi capsular polysaccharide 25 mcg/0.5 mL (0.5 mL, 10 mL)

**typhoid vaccine live oral Ty21a** *see* typhoid vaccine *on previous page*

**Tyrodone® Liquid *(Discontinued)*** *see* hydrocodone and pseudoephedrine *on page 413*

**tyropanoate sodium** *see* radiological/contrast media (ionic) *on page 707*

**Tyzine® [US]** *see* tetrahydrozoline *on page 792*

**Tyzine® Pediatric [US]** *see* tetrahydrozoline *on page 792*

**U-90152S** *see* delavirdine *on page 227*

**UAA® [US]** *see* methenamine, phenyl salicylate, atropine, hyoscyamine, benzoic acid, and methylene blue *on page 523*

**UAD Otic® *(Discontinued)*** *see* neomycin, polymyxin B, and hydrocortisone *on page 568*

**UCB-P071** *see* cetirizine *on page 162*

**UK-88,525** *see* darifenacin *on page 225*

**UK109496** *see* voriconazole *on page 853*

**UK92480** *see* sildenafil *on page 746*

**Ulcerease® [US-OTC]** *see* phenol *on page 638*

**ULR-LA® *(Discontinued)***

**Ultane® [US]** *see* sevoflurane *on page 745*

**Ultiva® [US/Can]** *see* remifentanil *on page 714*

**Ultracet™ [US]** *see* acetaminophen and tramadol *on page 9*

**Ultra Freeda Iron Free [US-OTC]** *see* vitamins (multiple/oral) *on page 852*

**Ultra Freeda with Iron [US-OTC]** *see* vitamins (multiple/oral) *on page 852*

**Ultram® [US/Can]** *see* tramadol *on page 815*

**Ultra Mide® [US-OTC]** *see* urea *on next page*

**UltraMide 25™ [Can]** *see* urea *on next page*

**Ultramop™ [Can]** *see* methoxsalen *on page 527*

**Ultra NatalCare® [US]** *see* vitamins (multiple/prenatal) *on page 852*

**Ultraprin [US-OTC]** *see* ibuprofen *on page 427*

**Ultraquin™ [Can]** *see* hydroquinone *on page 420*

**Ultrase® [US/Can]** *see* pancrelipase *on page 615*

**Ultrase® MT [US/Can]** *see* pancrelipase *on page 615*

**Ultra Tears® [US-OTC]** *see* artificial tears *on page 71*

**Ultravate® [US/Can]** *see* halobetasol *on page 395*

**Unasyn® [US/Can]** *see* ampicillin and sulbactam *on page 51*

## undecylenic acid and derivatives (un de sil EN ik AS id & dah RIV ah tivs)

Synonyms zinc undecylenate
U.S./Canadian Brand Names Fungi-Nail® [US-OTC]
Therapeutic Category Antifungal Agent
Use Treatment of athlete's foot (tinea pedis); ringworm (except nails and scalp)
Usual Dosage Children and Adults: Topical: Apply twice daily to affected area for 4 weeks; apply to clean, dry area
Dosage Forms Solution, topical: Undecylenic acid 25% (29.57 mL)

**Unguentine® *(Discontinued)*** *see* benzocaine *on page 95*

**Uni-Bent® Cough Syrup *(Discontinued)*** *see* diphenhydramine *on page 254*

**Unicap M® [US-OTC]** *see* vitamins (multiple/oral) *on page 852*

**Unicap Sr® [US-OTC]** *see* vitamins (multiple/oral) *on page 852*

**Unicap T™ [US-OTC]** *see* vitamins (multiple/oral) *on page 852*

**Unidet® [Can]** *see* tolterodine *on page 810*

**Uni-Dur®** *(Discontinued) see* theophylline *on page 793*

**Unipen® [Can]** *see* nafcillin *on page 557*

**Uniphyl® [US]** *see* theophylline *on page 793*

**Uniphyl® SRT [Can]** *see* theophylline *on page 793*

**Uni-Pro®** *(Discontinued) see* ibuprofen *on page 427*

**Uniretic® [US/Can]** *see* moexipril and hydrochlorothiazide *on page 547*

**Uni-Senna [US-OTC]** *see* senna *on page 743*

**Unisom® [US-OTC]** *see* doxylamine *on page 273*

**Unisom® Maximum Strength SleepGels® [US-OTC]** *see* diphenhydramine *on page 254*

**Unithroid® [US]** *see* levothyroxine *on page 477*

**Uni-Tricof HC [US]** *see* phenylephrine, hydrocodone, and chlorpheniramine *on page 643*

**Unitrol®** *(Discontinued)*

**Uni-Tuss HC [US]** *see* phenylephrine, hydrocodone, and chlorpheniramine *on page 643*

**Uni-tussin®** *(Discontinued) see* guaifenesin *on page 383*

**Uni-tussin® DM** *(Discontinued) see* guaifenesin and dextromethorphan *on page 385*

**Univasc® [US]** *see* moexipril *on page 546*

**unna's boot** *see* zinc gelatin *on page 861*

**unna's paste** *see* zinc gelatin *on page 861*

**Urabeth®** *(Discontinued) see* bethanechol *on page 104*

**Uracel®** *(Discontinued) see* sodium salicylate *on page 758*

**Urasal® [Can]** *see* methenamine *on page 522*

**urea** (yoor EE a)

**Synonyms** carbamide

**U.S./Canadian Brand Names** Amino-Cerv™ [US]; Aquacare® [US-OTC]; Aquaphilic® With Carbamide [US-OTC]; Carmol® 10 [US-OTC]; Carmol® 20 [US-OTC]; Carmol® 40 [US]; Carmol® Deep Cleaning [US]; DPM™ [US-OTC]; Gormel® [US-OTC]; Kerlac® [US]; Lanaphilic® [US-OTC]; Nutraplus® [US-OTC]; Rea-Lo® [US-OTC]; Ultra Mide® [US-OTC]; UltraMide 25™ [Can]; Ureacin® [US-OTC]; Uremol® [Can]; Urisec® [Can]; Vanamide™ [US]

**Therapeutic Category** Diuretic, Osmotic; Topical Skin Product

**Use**

Topical: Keratolytic agent to soften nails or skin; OTC: Moisturizer for dry, rough skin

Vaginal: Treatment of cervicitis

**Usual Dosage** Adults:

Hyperkeratotic conditions, dry skin: Topical: Apply 1-3 times/day

Cervicitis: Vaginal: Insert 1 applicatorful in vagina at bedtime for 2-4 weeks

**Dosage Forms**

Cream: 40% (30 g, 85 g, 199 g)

Aquacare®: 10% (75 g)

Carmol® 20: 20% (90 g)

Carmol® 40: 40% (30 g, 90 g, 210 g)

DPM™: 20% (118 g) [contains menthol and peppermint oil]

Gormel®: 20% (75 g, 120 g, 454 g, 2270 g)

Nutraplus®: 10% (90 g, 454 g)

Rea-Lo®: 30% (60 g, 240 g)

Ureacin®-20: 20% (120 g)

Vanamide™: 40% (85 g, 199 g)

Cream, vaginal (Amino-Cerv™): 8.34% [83.4 mg/g] (82.5 g)

Gel: 40% (15 mL)

Carmol® 40: 40% (15 mL)

Kerlac®: 50% (18 mL) [contains lactic acid and zinc]

Lotion: 40% (240 mL)

Aquacare®: 10% (240 mL)
Carmol® 10: 10% (180 mL)
Carmol® 40: 40% (240 mL)
Kerlac®: 35% (207 mL, 325 mL) [contains lactic acid, vitamin E, and zinc]
Nutraplus®: 10% (240 mL, 480 mL)
Ultra Mide®: 25% (120 mL, 240 mL)
Ureacin®-10: 10% (240 mL)
Ointment:
Aquaphilic® with Carbamide: 10% (180 g, 480 g); 20% (480 g)
Lanaphilic®: 10% (454 g); 20% (454 g)
Shampoo: Carmol® Deep Cleaning: 10% (240 mL)

## urea and hydrocortisone (yoor EE a & hye droe KOR ti sone)

**Synonyms** hydrocortisone and urea
**U.S./Canadian Brand Names** Carmol-HC® [US]; Ti-U-Lac® H [Can]; Uremol® HC [Can]
**Therapeutic Category** Corticosteroid, Topical
**Use** Inflammation of corticosteroid-responsive dermatoses
**Usual Dosage** Apply thin film and rub in well 1-4 times/day. Therapy should be discontinued when control is achieved; if no improvement is seen, reassessment of diagnosis may be necessary.
**Dosage Forms** Cream: Urea 10% and hydrocortisone acetate 1% (30 g) [in water soluble vanishing cream base]

**Ureacin®** [US-OTC] *see* urea *on previous page*

**urea peroxide** *see* carbamide peroxide *on page 141*

**Urecholine®** [US] *see* bethanechol *on page 104*

**Uremol®** [Can] *see* urea *on previous page*

**Uremol® HC** [Can] *see* urea and hydrocortisone *on this page*

**Urex®** [US/Can] *see* methenamine *on page 522*

**Uridon Modified®** [US] *see* methenamine, phenyl salicylate, atropine, hyoscyamine, benzoic acid, and methylene blue *on page 523*

**Urisec®** [Can] *see* urea *on previous page*

**Urised®** [US] *see* methenamine, phenyl salicylate, atropine, hyoscyamine, benzoic acid, and methylene blue *on page 523*

**Urispas®** [US/Can] *see* flavoxate *on page 339*

**Uristat®** [US-OTC] *see* phenazopyridine *on page 636*

**Uritin®** [US] *see* methenamine, phenyl salicylate, atropine, hyoscyamine, benzoic acid, and methylene blue *on page 523*

**Urocit®-K** [US] *see* potassium citrate *on page 664*

**Urodine®** *(Discontinued)* *see* phenazopyridine *on page 636*

## urofollitropin (yoor oh fol li TROE pin)

**U.S./Canadian Brand Names** Fertinorm® H.P. [Can]
**Therapeutic Category** Ovulation Stimulator
**Use** Induction of ovulation in patients with polycystic ovarian disease and to stimulate the development of multiple oocytes
**Usual Dosage** Adults: Female: SubQ: 75 units/day for 7-12 days, used with hCG may repeat course of treatment 2 more times
**Dosage Forms** Injection: 0.83 mg [75 units FSH activity] (2 mL)

**Uro-KP-Neutral®** [US] *see* potassium phosphate and sodium phosphate *on page 667*

**Urolene Blue®** [US] *see* methylene blue *on page 530*

**Uro-Mag®** [US-OTC] *see* magnesium oxide *on page 499*

**Uromitexan** [Can] *see* mesna *on page 516*

**Uroplus® DS** *(Discontinued)*

**Uroplus® SS** *(Discontinued)*

**Urovist Cysto**® **[US]** *see* radiological/contrast media (ionic) *on page 707*

**Urovist**® **Meglumine [US]** *see* radiological/contrast media (ionic) *on page 707*

**Urovist**® **Sodium 300 [US]** *see* radiological/contrast media (ionic) *on page 707*

**Uroxatral**™ **[US]** *see* alfuzosin *on page 27*

**Urso**® **[Can]** *see* ursodiol *on this page*

**Urso 250**™ **[US]** *see* ursodiol *on this page*

**ursodeoxycholic acid** *see* ursodiol *on this page*

## ursodiol (ER soe dye ole)

**Synonyms** ursodeoxycholic acid

**U.S./Canadian Brand Names** Actigall® [US]; Urso 250™ [US]; Urso Forte™ [US]; Urso® [Can]

**Therapeutic Category** Gallstone Dissolution Agent

**Use** Actigall®: Gallbladder stone dissolution; prevention of gallstones in obese patients experiencing rapid weight loss; Urso®: Primary biliary cirrhosis

**Usual Dosage** Adults: Oral:

Gallstone dissolution: 8-10 mg/kg/day in 2-3 divided doses; use beyond 24 months is not established; obtain ultrasound images at 6-month intervals for the first year of therapy; 30% of patients have stone recurrence after dissolution

Gallstone prevention: 300 mg twice daily

Primary biliary cirrhosis: 13-15 mg/kg/day in 2-4 divided doses (with food)

**Dosage Forms**

Capsule (Actigall®): 300 mg

Tablet:

Urso 250™: 250 mg

Urso Forte™: 500 mg

**Urso Forte**™ **[US]** *see* ursodiol *on this page*

**UTI Relief**® **[US-OTC]** *see* phenazopyridine *on page 636*

**Utradol**™ **[Can]** *see* etodolac *on page 321*

**Uvadex**® **[US/Can]** *see* methoxsalen *on page 527*

**vaccinia vaccine** *see* smallpox vaccine *on page 751*

**Vagifem**® **[US/Can]** *see* estradiol *on page 299*

**Vagi-Gard**® **[US-OTC]** *see* povidone-iodine *on page 668*

**Vagistat**®-1 **[US-OTC]** *see* tioconazole *on page 805*

**Vagitrol**® *(Discontinued)*

## valacyclovir (val ay SYE kloe veer)

**Sound-Alike/Look-Alike Issues**

valacyclovir may be confused with valganciclovir

Valtrex® may be confused with Valcyte™

**Synonyms** valacyclovir hydrochloride

**U.S./Canadian Brand Names** Valtrex® [US/Can]

**Therapeutic Category** Antiviral Agent

**Use** Treatment of herpes zoster (shingles) in immunocompetent patients; treatment of first-episode genital herpes; episodic treatment of recurrent genital herpes; suppression of recurrent genital herpes and reduction of heterosexual transmission of genital herpes in immunocompetent patients; suppression of genital herpes in HIV-infected individuals; treatment of herpes labialis (cold sores)

**Usual Dosage** Oral:

Adolescents and Adults: Herpes labialis (cold sores): 2 g twice daily for 1 day (separate doses by ~12 hours)

Adults:

Herpes zoster (shingles): 1 g 3 times/day for 7 days

Genital herpes:

Initial episode: 1 g twice daily for 10 days

Recurrent episode: 500 mg twice daily for 3 days

Reduction of transmission: 500 mg once daily (source partner)

Suppressive therapy:
  Immunocompetent patients: 1000 mg once daily (500 mg once daily in patients with <9 recurrences per year)
  HIV-infected patients (CD4 ≥100 cells/mm$^3$): 500 mg twice daily
**Dosage Forms** Caplet: 500 mg, 1000 mg

**valacyclovir hydrochloride** *see* valacyclovir *on previous page*

**Valcyte™ [US/Can]** *see* valganciclovir *on this page*

## valdecoxib (val de KOKS ib)
**U.S./Canadian Brand Names** Bextra® [US]
**Therapeutic Category** Nonsteroidal Antiinflammatory Drug (NSAID), COX-2 Selective
**Use** Relief of signs and symptoms of osteoarthritis and adult rheumatoid arthritis; treatment of primary dysmenorrhea
**Usual Dosage** Oral: Adults:
  Osteoarthritis and rheumatoid arthritis: 10 mg once daily; **Note:** No additional benefits seen with 20 mg/day
  Primary dysmenorrhea: 20 mg twice daily as needed
**Dosage Forms** Tablet: 10 mg, 20 mg

**23-valent pneumococcal polysaccharide vaccine** *see* pneumococcal polysaccharide vaccine (polyvalent) *on page 655*

## valganciclovir (val gan SYE kloh veer)
**Sound-Alike/Look-Alike Issues**
  valganciclovir may be confused with valacyclovir
  Valcyte™ may be confused with Valium®, Valtrex®
**Synonyms** valganciclovir hydrochloride
**U.S./Canadian Brand Names** Valcyte™ [US/Can]
**Therapeutic Category** Antiviral Agent
**Use** Treatment of cytomegalovirus (CMV) retinitis in patients with acquired immunodeficiency syndrome (AIDS); prevention of CMV disease in high-risk patients (donor CMV positive/recipient CMV negative) undergoing kidney, heart, or kidney/pancreas transplantation
**Usual Dosage** Oral: Adults:
  CMV retinitis:
    Induction: 900 mg twice daily for 21 days (with food)
    Maintenance: Following induction treatment, or for patients with inactive CMV retinitis who require maintenance therapy: Recommended dose: 900 mg once daily (with food)
  Prevention of CMV disease following transplantation: 900 mg once daily (with food) beginning within 10 days of transplantation; continue therapy until 100 days post-transplantation
**Dosage Forms** Tablet, as hydrochloride: 450 mg [valganciclovir hydrochloride 496.3 mg equivalent to valganciclovir 450 mg]

**valganciclovir hydrochloride** *see* valganciclovir *on this page*

**Valisone® Scalp Lotion [Can]** *see* betamethasone (topical) *on page 103*

**Valisone® Topical** *(Discontinued)*

**Valium® [US/Can]** *see* diazepam *on page 241*

**Valorin [US-OTC]** *see* acetaminophen *on page 4*

**Valorin Extra [US-OTC]** *see* acetaminophen *on page 4*

**valproate semisodium** *see* valproic acid and derivatives *on this page*

**valproate sodium** *see* valproic acid and derivatives *on this page*

**valproic acid** *see* valproic acid and derivatives *on this page*

## valproic acid and derivatives (val PROE ik AS id & dah RIV ah tives)
**Sound-Alike/Look-Alike Issues**
  Depakene® may be confused with Depakote®
  Depakote® may be confused with Depakene®, Depakote® ER, Senokot®
**Synonyms** 2-propylpentanoic acid; 2-propylvaleric acid; dipropylacetic acid; divalproex sodium; DPA; valproate semisodium; valproate sodium; valproic acid
(Continued)

# valproic acid and derivatives *(Continued)*

**U.S./Canadian Brand Names** Alti-Divalproex [Can]; Apo-Divalproex® [Can]; Depacon® [US]; Depakene® [US/Can]; Depakote® Delayed Release [US]; Depakote® ER [US]; Depakote® Sprinkle® [US]; Epival® I.V. [Can]; Gen-Divalproex [Can]; Novo-Divalproex [Can]; Nu-Divalproex [Can]; PMS-Valproic Acid E.C. [Can]; PMS-Valproic Acid [Can]; Rhoxal-valproic [Can]

**Therapeutic Category** Anticonvulsant

**Use** Monotherapy and adjunctive therapy in the treatment of patients with complex partial seizures; monotherapy and adjunctive therapy of simple and complex absence seizures; adjunctive therapy patients with multiple seizure types that include absence seizures

Mania associated with bipolar disorder (Depakote®)

Migraine prophylaxis (Depakote®, Depakote® ER)

**Usual Dosage**

Seizures:

Children >10 years and Adults:

Oral: Initial: 10-15 mg/kg/day in 1-3 divided doses; increase by 5-10 mg/kg/day at weekly intervals until therapeutic levels are achieved; maintenance: 30-60 mg/kg/day. Adult usual dose: 1000-2500 mg/day. **Note:** Regular release and delayed release formulations are usually given in 2-4 divided doses/day, extended release formulation (Depakote® ER) is usually given once daily. Conversion to Depakote® ER from a stable dose of Depakote® may require an increase in the total daily dose between 8% and 20% to maintain similar serum concentrations.

Children receiving more than one anticonvulsant (ie, polytherapy) may require doses up to 100 mg/kg/day in 3-4 divided doses

I.V.: Administer as a 60-minute infusion (≤20 mg/minute) with the same frequency as oral products; switch patient to oral products as soon as possible. Alternatively, rapid infusions have been given: ≤15 mg/kg over 5-10 minutes (1.5-3 mg/kg/minute).

Mania: Adults: Oral: 750-1500 mg/day in divided doses; dose should be adjusted as rapidly as possible to desired clinical effect; a loading dose of 20 mg/kg may be used; maximum recommended dosage: 60 mg/kg/day

Migraine prophylaxis: Adults: Oral:

Extended release tablets: 500 mg once daily for 7 days, then increase to 1000 mg once daily; adjust dose based on patient response; usual dosage range 500-1000 mg/day

Delayed release tablets: 250 mg twice daily; adjust dose based on patient response, up to 1000 mg/day

**Dosage Forms Note:** Strength expressed as valproic acid

Capsule, as valproic acid (Depakene®): 250 mg

Capsule, sprinkles, as divalproex sodium (Depakote® Sprinkle®): 125 mg

Injection, solution, as valproate sodium (Depacon®): 100 mg/mL (5 mL) [contains edetate disodium]

Syrup, as valproic acid: 250 mg/5 mL (480 mL)

Depakene®: 250 mg/5 mL (480 mL)

Tablet, delayed release, as divalproex sodium (Depakote®): 125 mg, 250 mg, 500 mg

Tablet, extended release, as divalproex sodium (Depakote® ER): 250 mg, 500 mg

# valsartan *(val SAR tan)*

**Sound-Alike/Look-Alike Issues**

valsartan may be confused with losartan, Valstar™

Diovan® may be confused with Darvon®, Dioval®, Zyban®

**U.S./Canadian Brand Names** Diovan® [US/Can]

**Therapeutic Category** Angiotensin II Receptor Antagonist

**Use** Alone or in combination with other antihypertensive agents in the treatment of essential hypertension; treatment of heart failure (NYHA Class II-IV); reduction of cardiovascular mortality in patients with left ventricular dysfunction post-myocardial infarction

**Usual Dosage** Adults: Oral:

Hypertension: Initial: 80 mg or 160 mg once daily (in patients who are not volume depleted); dose may be increased to achieve desired effect; maximum recommended dose: 320 mg/day

Heart failure: Initial: 40 mg twice daily; titrate dose to 80-160 mg twice daily, as tolerated; maximum daily dose: 320 mg

Left ventricular dysfunction after MI: Initial: 20 mg twice daily; titrate dose to target of 160 mg twice daily as tolerated; may initiate ≥12 hours following MI

**Dosage Forms** Tablet: 40 mg, 80 mg, 160 mg, 320 mg

# valsartan and hydrochlorothiazide (val SAR tan & hye droe klor oh THYE a zide)
**Sound-Alike/Look-Alike Issues**
Diovan® may be confused with Darvon®, Dioval®, Zyban®
**Synonyms** hydrochlorothiazide and valsartan
**U.S./Canadian Brand Names** Diovan HCT® [US/Can]
**Therapeutic Category** Antihypertensive Agent, Combination
**Use** Treatment of hypertension (not indicated for initial therapy)
**Usual Dosage** Oral: Adults: Dose is individualized (combination substituted for individual components); dose may be titrated after 3-4 weeks of therapy.
Usual recommended starting dose of valsartan: 80 mg or 160 mg once daily when used as monotherapy in patients who are not volume depleted
**Dosage Forms** Tablet:
80 mg/12.5 mg: Valsartan 80 mg and hydrochlorothiazide 12.5 mg
160 mg/12.5 mg: Valsartan 160 mg and hydrochlorothiazide 12.5 mg
160 mg/25 mg: Valsartan 160 mg and hydrochlorothiazide 25 mg

**Valstar®** *(Discontinued)*

**Valtrex® [US/Can]** *see* valacyclovir *on page 836*

**Vamate® Oral** *(Discontinued) see* hydroxyzine *on page 423*

**Vanamide™ [US]** *see* urea *on page 834*

**Vanatrip®** *(Discontinued) see* amitriptyline *on page 42*

**Vancenase® AQ 84 mcg** *(Discontinued) see* beclomethasone *on page 91*

**Vancenase® Pockethaler®** *(Discontinued) see* beclomethasone *on page 91*

**Vanceril® AEM [Can]** *see* beclomethasone *on page 91*

**Vanceril®** *(Discontinued) see* beclomethasone *on page 91*

**Vancocin® [US/Can]** *see* vancomycin *on this page*

# vancomycin (van koe MYE sin)
**Sound-Alike/Look-Alike Issues**
vancomycin may be confused with vecuronium
I.V. vancomycin may be confused with Invanz®
**Synonyms** vancomycin hydrochloride
**U.S./Canadian Brand Names** Vancocin® [US/Can]
**Therapeutic Category** Antibiotic, Miscellaneous
**Use** Treatment of patients with infections caused by staphylococcal species and streptococcal species; used orally for staphylococcal enterocolitis or for antibiotic-associated pseudomembranous colitis produced by *C. difficile*
**Usual Dosage** Initial dosage recommendation:
Neonates: I.V.:
Postnatal age ≤7 days:
<1200 g: 15 mg/kg/dose every 24 hours
1200-2000 g: 10 mg/kg/dose every 12 hours
>2000 g: 15 mg/kg/dose every 12 hours
Postnatal age >7 days:
<1200 g: 15 mg/kg/dose every 24 hours
≥1200 g: 10 mg/kg/dose divided every 8 hours
Infants >1 month and Children: I.V.:
40 mg/kg/day in divided doses every 6 hours
Prophylaxis for bacterial endocarditis:
Dental, oral, or upper respiratory tract surgery: 20 mg/kg 1 hour prior to the procedure
GI/GU procedure: 20 mg/kg plus gentamicin 2 mg/kg 1 hour prior to surgery
Infants >1 month and Children with staphylococcal central nervous system infection: I.V.: 60 mg/kg/day in divided doses every 6 hours
Adults: I.V.:
With normal renal function: 1 g **or** 10-15 mg/kg/dose every 12 hours
Prophylaxis for bacterial endocarditis:
Dental, oral, or upper respiratory tract surgery: 1 g 1 hour before surgery
GI/GU procedure: 1 g plus 1.5 mg/kg gentamicin 1 hour prior to surgery
(Continued)

## vancomycin *(Continued)*

**Antibiotic lock technique (for catheter infections):** 2 mg/mL in SWI/NS or $D_5W$; instill 3-5 mL into catheter port as a flush solution instead of heparin lock (**Note:** Do not mix with any other solutions)

**Intrathecal:** Vancomycin is available as a powder for injection and may be diluted to 1-5 mg/mL concentration in preservative-free 0.9% sodium chloride for administration into the CSF

Neonates: 5-10 mg/day

Children: 5-20 mg/day

Adults: Up to 20 mg/day

Oral: Pseudomembranous colitis produced by *C. difficile*:

Neonates: 10 mg/kg/day in divided doses

Children: 40 mg/kg/day in divided doses, added to fluids

Adults: 125 mg 4 times/day for 10 days

**Dosage Forms**

Capsule (Vancocin®): 125 mg, 250 mg

Infusion [premixed in iso-osmotic dextrose] (Vancocin®): 500 mg (100 mL); 1 g (200 mL)

Injection, powder for reconstitution: 500 mg, 1 g, 5 g, 10 g

**vancomycin hydrochloride** *see vancomycin on previous page*

**Vanex Forte™-D** *(Discontinued)* *see chlorpheniramine, phenylephrine, and methscopolamine on page 175*

**Vanex-HD®** [US] *see phenylephrine, hydrocodone, and chlorpheniramine on page 643*

**Vaniqa™** [US] *see eflornithine on page 281*

**Vanos™** [US] *see fluocinonide on page 345*

**Vanoxide®** *(Discontinued)* *see benzoyl peroxide on page 98*

**Vanoxide-HC®** [US/Can] *see benzoyl peroxide and hydrocortisone on page 99*

**Vanquish® Extra Strength Pain Reliever [US-OTC]** *see acetaminophen, aspirin, and caffeine on page 9*

**Vansil™** *(Discontinued)*

**Vantin®** [US/Can] *see cefpodoxime on page 156*

**Vaponefrin®** [Can] *see epinephrine on page 287*

**Vaponefrin®** *(Discontinued)* *see epinephrine on page 287*

**VAQTA®** [US/Can] *see hepatitis A vaccine on page 400*

## vardenafil *(var DEN a fil)*

**Sound-Alike/Look-Alike Issues**

Levitra® may be confused with Lexiva™

**Synonyms** vardenafil hydrochloride

**U.S./Canadian Brand Names** Levitra® [US/Can]

**Therapeutic Category** Phosphodiesterase (Type 5) Enzyme Inhibitor

**Use** Treatment of erectile dysfunction

**Usual Dosage** Oral: Adults: Erectile dysfunction: 10 mg 60 minutes prior to sexual activity; dosing range: 5-20 mg; to be given as one single dose and not given more than once daily

Dosing adjustment with concomitant medications:

Alpha blocker (dose should be stable at time of vardenafil initiation): Initial vardenafil dose: 5 mg/24 hours; if an alpha blocker is added to vardenafil therapy, it should be initiated at the smallest possible dose, and titrated carefully.

Erythromycin: Maximum vardenafil dose: 5 mg/24 hours

Indinavir: Maximum vardenafil dose: 2.5 mg/24 hours

Itraconazole:

200 mg/day: Maximum vardenafil dose: 5 mg/24 hours

400 mg/day: Maximum vardenafil dose: 2.5 mg/24 hours

Ketoconazole:

200 mg/day: Maximum vardenafil dose: 5 mg/24 hours

400 mg/day: Maximum vardenafil dose: 2.5 mg/24 hours

Ritonavir: Maximum vardenafil dose: 2.5 mg/72 hours

**Dosage Forms** Tablet [film-coated]: 2.5 mg, 5 mg, 10 mg, 20 mg

**vardenafil hydrochloride** *see vardenafil on this page*

## varicella virus vaccine (var i SEL a VYE rus vak SEEN)

**Sound-Alike/Look-Alike Issues**
varicella virus vaccine has been given in error (instead of the indicated varicella immune globulin) to pregnant women exposed to varicella

**Synonyms** chicken pox vaccine; varicella-zoster virus (VZV) vaccine

**U.S./Canadian Brand Names** Varilrix® [Can]; Varivax® [US/Can]

**Therapeutic Category** Vaccine, Live Virus

**Use** Immunization against varicella in children ≥12 months of age and adults

**Usual Dosage** SubQ:
Children 12 months to 12 years: 0.5 mL; a second dose may be administered ≥3 months later
Children ≥13 years to Adults: 2 doses of 0.5 mL separated by 4-8 weeks

**Dosage Forms** Injection, powder for reconstitution [preservative free; single-dose vial]: 1350 plaque-forming units (PFU) [contains gelatin and trace amounts of neomycin]

## varicella-zoster immune globulin (human)
(var i SEL a- ZOS ter i MYUN GLOB yoo lin HYU man)

**Sound-Alike/Look-Alike Issues**
varicella virus vaccine has been given in error (instead of the indicated varicella immune globulin) to pregnant women exposed to varicella

**Synonyms** VZIG

**Therapeutic Category** Immune Globulin

**Use** Passive immunization of susceptible  patients who are at a greater risk of complications following significant exposure to varicella

**Restrict administration to those patients meeting the following criteria:**
Immunocompromised children including those with neoplastic disease (eg, leukemia or lymphoma); congenital or acquired immunodeficiency; immunosuppressive therapy with steroids, antimetabolites or other immunosuppressive treatment regimens
Newborn of mother who had onset of varicella (chickenpox) within 5 days before delivery or within 48 hours after delivery (not indicated if the mother has zoster)
Premature infants (≥28 weeks gestation) whose mother has no history of chickenpox
Premature infants (<28 weeks gestation or ≤1000 g) regardless of maternal history
Immunocompromised adults

**Significant exposure includes:**
Continuous household contact
Playmate contact (>1 hour play indoors)
Hospital contact (in same 2-4 bedroom or adjacent beds in a large ward or prolonged face-to-face contact with an infectious staff member or patient)

**Usual Dosage Note:** High risk susceptible patients who are exposed again more than 3 weeks after a prior dose of VZIG should receive another full dose.
I.M.: 125 units/10 kg (22 lb); maximum dose: 625 units (5 vials); minimum dose: 125 units; do not administer fractional doses

**Dosage Forms** Injection, solution [preservative free]: 125 units (1.25 mL); 625 units (6.25 mL)

**varicella-zoster virus (VZV) vaccine** *see* varicella virus vaccine *on this page*

**Varilrix®** **[Can]** *see* varicella virus vaccine *on this page*

**Varivax®** **[US/Can]** *see* varicella virus vaccine *on this page*

**Vascor®** **[Can]** *see* bepridil *on page 101*

**Vascoray®** **[US]** *see* radiological/contrast media (ionic) *on page 707*

**Vascor®** ***(Discontinued)*** *see* bepridil *on page 101*

**Vaseretic®** **[US/Can]** *see* enalapril and hydrochlorothiazide *on page 284*

**VasoClear®** ***(Discontinued)*** *see* naphazoline *on page 561*

**Vasocon®** **[Can]** *see* naphazoline *on page 561*

**Vasocon®-A [Can]** *see* naphazoline and antazoline *on page 561*

**Vasocon®-A** ***(Discontinued)*** *see* naphazoline and antazoline *on page 561*

**Vasocon Regular®** **Ophthalmic** ***(Discontinued)*** *see* naphazoline *on page 561*

**Vasodilan®** ***(Discontinued)*** *see* isoxsuprine *on page 452*

**Vasophrinic DH [Can]** *see* pseudoephedrine, hydrocodone, and chlorpheniramine *on page 695*

# vasopressin (vay soe PRES in)

**Sound-Alike/Look-Alike Issues**
Pitressin® may be confused with Pitocin®
**Synonyms** 8-arginine vasopressin; ADH; antidiuretic hormone
**U.S./Canadian Brand Names** Pitressin® [US]; Pressyn® AR [Can]; Pressyn® [Can]
**Therapeutic Category** Hormone, Posterior Pituitary
**Use** Treatment of diabetes insipidus; prevention and treatment of postoperative abdominal distention; differential diagnosis of diabetes insipidus
**Usual Dosage**
Diabetes insipidus (highly variable dosage; titrated based on serum and urine sodium and osmolality in addition to fluid balance and urine output):
I.M., SubQ:
Children: 2.5-10 units 2-4 times/day as needed
Adults: 5-10 units 2-4 times/day as needed (dosage range 5-60 units/day)
Continuous I.V. infusion: Children and Adults: 0.5 milliunit/kg/hour (0.0005 unit/kg/hour); double dosage as needed every 30 minutes to a maximum of 0.01 unit/kg/hour
Intranasal: Administer on cotton pledget, as nasal spray, or by dropper
Abdominal distention: Adults: I.M.: 5 units stat, 10 units every 3-4 hours
Pulseless VT/VF (ACLS protocol): I.V.: 40 units (as a single dose only); if no I.V. access, administer 40 units diluted with NS (to a total volume of 10 mL) endotracheally
**Dosage Forms**
Injection, solution: 20 units/mL (0.5 mL, 1 mL, 10 mL)
Pitressin®: 20 units/mL (1 mL)

**Vasotec® [US/Can]** *see* enalapril *on page 283*

**Vaxigrip® [Can]** *see* influenza virus vaccine *on page 437*

**VCF™ [US-OTC]** *see* nonoxynol 9 *on page 580*

**VCR** *see* vincristine *on page 846*

**Vectrin® (Discontinued)** *see* minocycline *on page 542*

# vecuronium (ve KYOO roe ni um)

**Sound-Alike/Look-Alike Issues**
vecuronium may be confused with vancomycin
Norcuron® may be confused with Narcan®
**Synonyms** ORG NC 45
**U.S./Canadian Brand Names** Norcuron® [Can]
**Therapeutic Category** Skeletal Muscle Relaxant
**Use** Adjunct to general anesthesia to facilitate endotracheal intubation and to relax skeletal muscles during surgery; to facilitate mechanical ventilation in ICU patients; does not relieve pain or produce sedation
**Usual Dosage** Administer I.V.; dose to effect; doses will vary due to interpatient variability; use ideal body weight for obese patients
Surgery:
Neonates: 0.1 mg/kg/dose; maintenance: 0.03-0.15 mg/kg every 1-2 hours as needed
Infants >7 weeks to 1 year: Initial: 0.08-0.1 mg/kg/dose; maintenance: 0.05-0.1 mg/kg every 60 minutes as needed
Children >1 year and Adults: Initial: 0.08-0.1 mg/kg or 0.04-0.06 mg/kg after initial dose of succinylcholine for intubation; maintenance: 0.01-0.015 mg/kg 25-40 minutes after initial dose, then 0.01-0.015 mg/kg every 12-15 minutes (higher doses will allow less frequent maintenance doses); may be administered as a continuous infusion at 0.8-2 mcg/kg/minute
Pretreatment/priming: Adults: 10% of intubating dose given 3-5 minutes before initial dose
ICU: Adults: 0.05-0.1 mg/kg bolus followed by 0.8-1.7 mcg/kg/minute once initial recovery from bolus observed or 0.1-0.2 mg/kg/dose every 1 hour

**Note:** Children (1-10 years) may require slightly higher initial doses and slightly more frequent supplementation; infants >7 weeks to 1 year may be more sensitive to vecuronium and have a longer recovery time
**Dosage Forms** Injection, powder for reconstitution, as bromide: 10 mg, 20 mg [may be supplied with diluent containing benzyl alcohol]

**Veetids® [US]** *see* penicillin V potassium *on page 627*

**Velban**® *(Discontinued)* *see* vinblastine *on page 846*

**Velcade**™ **[US/Can]** *see* bortezomib *on page 110*

**Velivet**™ **[US]** *see* ethinyl estradiol and desogestrel *on page 309*

**Velosef**® **[US]** *see* cephradine *on page 162*

**Velosulin**® **BR (Buffered)** *(Discontinued)*

## venlafaxine (VEN la faks een)

**U.S./Canadian Brand Names** Effexor® XR [US/Can]; Effexor® [US]

**Therapeutic Category** Antidepressant, Phenethylamine

**Use** Treatment of major depressive disorder; generalized anxiety disorder (GAD), social anxiety disorder (social phobia)

**Usual Dosage** Oral: Adults:

Depression:

Immediate-release tablets: 75 mg/day, administered in 2 or 3 divided doses, taken with food; dose may be increased in 75 mg/day increments at intervals of at least 4 days, up to 225-375 mg/day

Extended-release capsules: 75 mg once daily taken with food; for some new patients, it may be desirable to start at 37.5 mg/day for 4-7 days before increasing to 75 mg once daily; dose may be increased by up to 75 mg/day increments every 4 days as tolerated, up to a maximum of 225 mg/day

GAD, social anxiety disorder: Extended-release capsules: 75 mg once daily taken with food; for some new patients, it may be desirable to start at 37.5 mg/day for 4-7 days before increasing to 75 mg once daily; dose may be increased by up to 75 mg/day increments every 4 days as tolerated, up to a maximum of 225 mg/day

**Note:** When discontinuing this medication after more than 1 week of treatment, it is generally recommended that the dose be tapered. If venlafaxine is used for 6 weeks or longer, the dose should be tapered over 2 weeks when discontinuing its use.

**Dosage Forms**

Capsule, extended release (Effexor® XR): 37.5 mg, 75 mg, 150 mg

Tablet (Effexor®): 25 mg, 37.5 mg, 50 mg, 75 mg, 100 mg

**Venofer**® **[US/Can]** *see* iron sucrose *on page 449*

**Venoglobulin**®**-I** *(Discontinued)* *see* immune globulin (intravenous) *on page 433*

**Venoglobulin**®**-S** *(Discontinued)* *see* immune globulin (intravenous) *on page 433*

**Ventolin**® **[Can]** *see* albuterol *on page 22*

**Ventolin**® *(Discontinued)* *see* albuterol *on page 22*

**Ventolin**® **Diskus [Can]** *see* albuterol *on page 22*

**Ventolin**® **HFA [US/Can]** *see* albuterol *on page 22*

**Ventolin**® **Inhaler Aerosol** *(Discontinued)* *see* albuterol *on page 22*

**Ventrodisk [Can]** *see* albuterol *on page 22*

**VePesid**® **[US/Can]** *see* etoposide *on page 322*

**Veracolate [US-OTC]** *see* bisacodyl *on page 107*

## verapamil (ver AP a mil)

**Sound-Alike/Look-Alike Issues**

verapamil may be confused with Verelan®

Calan® may be confused with Colace®

Covera-HS® may be confused with Provera®

Isoptin® may be confused with Isopto® Tears

Verelan® may be confused with verapamil, Virilon®, Voltaren®

**Synonyms** iproveratril hydrochloride; verapamil hydrochloride

**U.S./Canadian Brand Names** Alti-Verapamil [Can]; Apo-Verap® [Can]; Calan® SR [US]; Calan® [US/Can]; Chronovera® [Can]; Covera-HS® [US]; Covera® [Can]; Gen-Verapamil SR [Can]; Gen-Verapamil [Can]; Isoptin® SR [US/Can]; Novo-Veramil SR [Can]; Nu-Verap [Can]; Verelan® PM [US]; Verelan® [US]

**Therapeutic Category** Antiarrhythmic Agent, Class IV; Calcium Channel Blocker

**Use** Orally for treatment of angina pectoris (vasospastic, chronic stable, unstable) and hypertension; I.V. for supraventricular tachyarrhythmias (PSVT, atrial fibrillation, atrial flutter)

(Continued)

## verapamil *(Continued)*

### Usual Dosage
Children: SVT:
I.V.:
<1 year: 0.1-0.2 mg/kg over 2 minutes; repeat every 30 minutes as needed
1-15 years: 0.1-0.3 mg/kg over 2 minutes; maximum: 5 mg/dose, may repeat dose in 15 minutes if adequate response not achieved; maximum for second dose: 10 mg/dose
Oral (dose not well established):
1-5 years: 4-8 mg/kg/day in 3 divided doses **or** 40-80 mg every 8 hours
>5 years: 80 mg every 6-8 hours
Adults:
SVT: I.V.: 2.5-5 mg (over 2 minutes); second dose of 5-10 mg (~0.15 mg/kg) may be given 15-30 minutes after the initial dose if patient tolerates, but does not respond to initial dose; maximum total dose: 20 mg
Angina: Oral: Initial dose: 80-120 mg 3 times/day (elderly or small stature: 40 mg 3 times/day); range: 240-480 mg/day in 3-4 divided doses
Hypertension: Oral:
Immediate release: 80 mg 3 times/day; usual dose range (JNC 7): 80-320 mg/day in 2 divided doses
Sustained release: 240 mg/day; usual dose range (JNC 7): 120-360 mg/day in 1-2 divided doses; 120 mg/day in the elderly or small patients (no evidence of additional benefit in doses >360 mg/day).
Extended release:
Covera-HS®: Usual dose range (JNC 7): 120-360 mg once daily (once-daily dosing is recommended at bedtime)
Verelan® PM: Usual dose range: 200-400 mg once daily at bedtime

### Dosage Forms
Caplet, sustained release (Calan® SR): 120 mg, 180 mg, 240 mg
Capsule, extended release, controlled onset (Verelan® PM): 100 mg, 200 mg, 300 mg
Capsule, sustained release, as hydrochloride (Verelan®): 120 mg, 180 mg, 240 mg, 360 mg
Injection, solution, as hydrochloride: 2.5 mg/mL (2 mL, 4 mL)
Tablet, as hydrochloride: 80 mg, 120 mg
Calan®: 40 mg, 80 mg, 120 mg
Tablet, extended release: 120 mg, 180 mg, 240 mg
Tablet, extended release, controlled onset (Covera-HS®): 180 mg, 240 mg
Tablet, sustained release, as hydrochloride (Isoptin® SR): 120 mg, 180 mg, 240 mg

**verapamil and trandolapril** *see* trandolapril and verapamil *on page 815*

**verapamil hydrochloride** *see* verapamil *on previous page*

**Verazinc® Oral *(Discontinued)*** *see* zinc sulfate *on page 861*

**Verelan® [US]** *see* verapamil *on previous page*

**Verelan® PM [US]** *see* verapamil *on previous page*

**Vergogel® Gel *(Discontinued)*** *see* salicylic acid *on page 734*

**Vergon® *(Discontinued)*** *see* meclizine *on page 506*

**Vermox® [Can]** *see* mebendazole *on page 505*

**Vermox® *(Discontinued)*** *see* mebendazole *on page 505*

**Versed® *(Discontinued)*** *see* midazolam *on page 539*

**Versel® [Can]** *see* selenium sulfide *on page 742*

**Versiclear™ [US]** *see* sodium thiosulfate *on page 758*

## verteporfin (ver te POR fin)

**U.S./Canadian Brand Names** Visudyne® [US/Can]
**Therapeutic Category** Ophthalmic Agent
**Use** Treatment of predominantly classic subfoveal choroidal neovascularization due to macular degeneration, presumed ocular histoplasmosis, or pathologic myopia
**Usual Dosage** Therapy is a two-step process; first the infusion of verteporfin, then the activation of verteporfin with a nonthermal diode laser.
Adults: I.V.: 6 mg/m² body surface area
**Note:** Treatment in more than one eye: Patients who have lesions in both eyes should be evaluated and treatment should first be done to the more aggressive lesion. Following safe and acceptable

treatment, the second eye can be treated one week later. Patients who have had previous verteporfin therapy, with an acceptable safety profile, may then have both eyes treated concurrently. Treat the more aggressive lesion followed immediately with the second eye. The light treatment to the second eye should begin no later than 20 minutes from the start of the infusion.

**Dosage Forms** Injection, powder for reconstitution: 15 mg   [contains egg phosphatidylglycerol]

**Verukan**® **Solution** *(Discontinued)* *see* salicylic acid *on page 734*

**Vesanoid**® **[US/Can]** *see* tretinoin (oral) *on page 817*

**VESIcare**® **[US]** *see* solifenacin *on page 759*

**Vexol**® **[US/Can]** *see* rimexolone *on page 724*

**VFEND**® **[US/Can]** *see* voriconazole *on page 853*

**Viactiv**® **Multivitamin [US-OTC]** *see* vitamins (multiple/oral) *on page 852*

**Viadur**® **[US/Can]** *see* leuprolide acetate *on page 471*

**Viagra**® **[US/Can]** *see* sildenafil *on page 746*

**Vibramycin**® **[US]** *see* doxycycline *on page 271*

**Vibramycin**® **I.V.** *(Discontinued)* *see* doxycycline *on page 271*

**Vibra-Tabs**® **[US/Can]** *see* doxycycline *on page 271*

**Vicks**® **44**® **Cough Relief [US-OTC]** *see* dextromethorphan *on page 238*

**Vicks**® **44D Cough & Head Congestion [US-OTC]** *see* pseudoephedrine and dextromethorphan *on page 693*

**Vicks**® **44E [US-OTC]** *see* guaifenesin and dextromethorphan *on page 385*

**Vicks**® **44**® **Non-Drowsy Cold & Cough Liqui-Caps** *(Discontinued)* *see* pseudoephedrine and dextromethorphan *on page 693*

**Vicks**® **Children's Chloraseptic**® *(Discontinued)* *see* benzocaine *on page 95*

**Vicks**® **Children's NyQuil**® **[US-OTC]** *see* chlorpheniramine, pseudoephedrine, and dextromethorphan *on page 177*

**Vicks**® **Chloraseptic**® **Sore Throat** *(Discontinued)* *see* benzocaine *on page 95*

**Vicks**® **DayQuil**® **Multi-Symptom Cold and Flu [US-OTC]** *see* acetaminophen, dextromethorphan, and pseudoephedrine *on page 11*

**Vicks**® **DayQuil**® **Sinus Pressure & Congestion Relief** *(Discontinued)*

**Vicks**® **Formula 44**® *(Discontinued)* *see* dextromethorphan *on page 238*

**Vicks**® **Formula 44**® **Pediatric Formula** *(Discontinued)* *see* dextromethorphan *on page 238*

**Vicks**® **Pediatric 44**®**m [US-OTC]** *see* chlorpheniramine, pseudoephedrine, and dextromethorphan *on page 177*

**Vicks**® **Pediatric Formula 44E [US-OTC]** *see* guaifenesin and dextromethorphan *on page 385*

**Vicks**® **Sinex**® **12 Hour [US-OTC]** *see* oxymetazoline *on page 610*

**Vicks**® **Sinex**® **12 Hour Ultrafine Mist [US-OTC]** *see* oxymetazoline *on page 610*

**Vicks**® **Sinex**® **Nasal Spray [US-OTC]** *see* phenylephrine *on page 640*

**Vicks**® **Sinex**® **UltraFine Mist [US-OTC]** *see* phenylephrine *on page 640*

**Vicodin**® **[US]** *see* hydrocodone and acetaminophen *on page 411*

**Vicodin**® **ES [US]** *see* hydrocodone and acetaminophen *on page 411*

**Vicodin**® **HP [US]** *see* hydrocodone and acetaminophen *on page 411*

**Vicon-C**® **[US-OTC]** *see* vitamin B complex with vitamin C *on page 850*

**Vicon Forte**® **[US]** *see* vitamins (multiple/oral) *on page 852*

**Vicoprofen**® **[US/Can]** *see* hydrocodone and ibuprofen *on page 413*

**Vi-Daylin**® **ADC** *(Discontinued)* *see* vitamins (multiple/pediatric) *on page 852*

**Vi-Daylin**® **ADC + Iron** *(Discontinued)* *see* vitamins (multiple/pediatric) *on page 852*

**Vi-Daylin**® **Drops** *(Discontinued)* *see* vitamins (multiple/pediatric) *on page 852*

**Vi-Daylin**®**/F ADC** *(Discontinued)* *see* vitamins (multiple/pediatric) *on page 852*

**Vi-Daylin®/F ADC + Iron** *(Discontinued)* see vitamins (multiple/pediatric) *on page 852*

**Vi-Daylin®/F** *(Discontinued)* see vitamins (multiple/pediatric) *on page 852*

**Vi-Daylin®/F + Iron** *(Discontinued)* see vitamins (multiple/pediatric) *on page 852*

**Vi-Daylin® + Iron Drops** *(Discontinued)* see vitamins (multiple/pediatric) *on page 852*

**Vi-Daylin® + Iron Liquid** *(Discontinued)* see vitamins (multiple/oral) *on page 852*

**Vi-Daylin® Liquid** *(Discontinued)* see vitamins (multiple/oral) *on page 852*

**Vidaza™ [US]** see azacitidine *on page 82*

**Videx® [US/Can]** see didanosine *on page 245*

**Videx® EC [US/Can]** see didanosine *on page 245*

## vigabatrin *(Canada only)* (vye GA ba trin)
**U.S./Canadian Brand Names** Sabril® [Can]
**Therapeutic Category** Anticonvulsant
**Use** Active management of partial or secondary generalized seizures not controlled by usual treatments; treatment of infantile spasms
**Usual Dosage** Oral:
Children: **Note:** Administer daily dose in 2 divided doses, especially in the higher dosage ranges:
Adjunctive treatment of seizures: Initial: 40 mg/kg/day; maintenance dosages based on patient weight:
10-15 kg: 0.5-1 g/day
16-30 kg: 1-1.5 g/day
31-50 kg: 1.5-3 g/day
>50 kg: 2-3 g/day
Infantile spasms: 50-100 mg/kg/day, depending on severity of symptoms; higher doses (up to 150 mg/kg/day) have been used in some cases.
Adults: Adjunctive treatment of seizures: Initial: 1 g/day (severe manifestations may require 2 g/day); dose may be given as a single daily dose or divided into 2 equal doses. Increase daily dose by 0.5 g based on response and tolerability. Optimal dose range: 2-3 g/day (maximum dose: 3 g/day)
**Dosage Forms**
Powder for oral suspension [sachets]: 0.5 g [contains povidone]
Tablet: 500 mg

**Vigamox™ [US/Can]** see moxifloxacin *on page 552*

## vinblastine (vin BLAS teen)
**Sound-Alike/Look-Alike Issues**
vinBLAStine may be confused with vinCRIStine, vinorelbine
**Synonyms** NSC-49842; vinblastine sulfate; VLB
**Tall-Man** vin**BLAS**tine
**Therapeutic Category** Antineoplastic Agent
**Use** Treatment of Hodgkin's and non-Hodgkin's lymphoma, testicular, lung, head and neck, breast, and renal carcinomas, Mycosis fungoides, Kaposi's sarcoma, histiocytosis, choriocarcinoma, and idiopathic thrombocytopenic purpura
**Usual Dosage** Refer to individual protocols.
Children and Adults: I.V.: 4-20 mg/m$^2$ (0.1-0.5 mg/kg) every 7-10 days **or** 5-day continuous infusion of 1.5-2 mg/m$^2$/day **or** 0.1-0.5 mg/kg/week
**Dosage Forms**
Injection, powder for reconstitution, as sulfate: 10 mg
Injection, solution, as sulfate: 1 mg/mL (10 mL) [contains benzyl alcohol]

**vinblastine sulfate** see vinblastine *on this page*

**Vincasar PFS® [US/Can]** see vincristine *on this page*

## vincristine (vin KRIS teen)
**Sound-Alike/Look-Alike Issues**
vinCRIStine may be confused with vinBLAStine
Oncovin® may be confused with Ancobon®
**Synonyms** LCR; leurocristine sulfate; NSC-67574; VCR; vincristine sulfate
**Tall-Man** vin**CRIS**tine

**U.S./Canadian Brand Names** Vincasar PFS® [US/Can]

**Therapeutic Category** Antineoplastic Agent

**Use** Treatment of leukemias, Hodgkin disease, non-Hodgkin lymphomas, Wilms tumor, neuroblastoma, rhabdomyosarcoma

**Usual Dosage Note:** Doses are often capped at 2 mg; however, this may reduce the efficacy of the therapy and may not be advisable. Refer to individual protocols; orders for single doses >2.5 mg or >5 mg/treatment cycle should be verified with the specific treatment regimen and/or an experienced oncologist prior to dispensing. I.V.:

Children ≤10 kg or BSA <1 m$^2$: Initial therapy: 0.05 mg/kg once weekly then titrate dose; maximum single dose: 2 mg

Children >10 kg or BSA ≥1 m$^2$: 1-2 mg/m$^2$, may repeat once weekly for 3-6 weeks; maximum single dose: 2 mg

Neuroblastoma: I.V. continuous infusion with doxorubicin: 1 mg/m$^2$/day for 72 hours

Adults: 0.4-1.4 mg/m$^2$, may repeat every week **or**

0.4-0.5 mg/day continuous infusion for 4 days every 4 weeks **or**

0.25-0.5 mg/m$^2$/day for 5 days every 4 weeks

**Dosage Forms** Injection, solution, as sulfate: 1 mg/mL (1 mL, 2 mL)

**vincristine sulfate** *see* vincristine *on previous page*

# vinorelbine (vi NOR el been)

**Sound-Alike/Look-Alike Issues**

vinorelbine may be confused with vinBLAStine

**Synonyms** dihydroxydeoxynorvinkaleukoblastine; NVB; vinorelbine tartrate

**U.S./Canadian Brand Names** Navelbine® [US/Can]

**Therapeutic Category** Antineoplastic Agent

**Use** Treatment of nonsmall cell lung cancer

**Usual Dosage** Refer to individual protocols.

Adults: I.V.:

Single-agent therapy: 30 mg/m$^2$ every 7 days

Combination therapy with cisplatin: 25 mg/m$^2$ every 7 days (with cisplatin 100 mg/m$^2$ every 4 weeks); **Alternatively:** 30 mg/m$^2$ in combination with cisplatin 120 mg/m$^2$ on days 1 and 29, then every 6 weeks

**Dosage Forms** Injection, solution [preservative free]: 10 mg/mL (1 mL, 5 mL)

**vinorelbine tartrate** *see* vinorelbine *on this page*

**Vioform® *(Discontinued)*** *see* clioquinol *on page 193*

**Viokase® [US/Can]** *see* pancrelipase *on page 615*

**viosterol** *see* ergocalciferol *on page 292*

**Vioxx® *(Discontinued)*** *see* rofecoxib *on page 729*

**Viracept® [US/Can]** *see* nelfinavir *on page 565*

**Viramune® [US/Can]** *see* nevirapine *on page 571*

**Viravan® [US]** *see* phenylephrine and pyrilamine *on page 641*

**Viravan®-DM [US]** *see* phenylephrine, pyrilamine, and dextromethorphan *on page 644*

**Virazole® [US/Can]** *see* ribavirin *on page 720*

**Viread® [US/Can]** *see* tenofovir *on page 786*

**Virilon® [US]** *see* methyltestosterone *on page 533*

**Virilon® IM [Can]** *see* testosterone *on page 788*

**Viroptic® [US/Can]** *see* trifluridine *on page 823*

**Viscoat® [US]** *see* chondroitin sulfate and sodium hyaluronate *on page 180*

**Visicol® [US]** *see* sodium phosphates *on page 756*

**Visine-A**™ **[US-OTC]** *see* naphazoline and pheniramine *on page 561*

**Visine® Advanced Allergy [Can]** *see* naphazoline and pheniramine *on page 561*

**Visine® Advanced Relief [US-OTC]** *see* tetrahydrozoline *on page 792*

**Visine® L.R. [US-OTC]** *see* oxymetazoline *on page 610*

**Visine® Original [US-OTC]** *see* tetrahydrozoline *on page 792*

**Visken® [Can]** *see* pindolol *on page 648*

**Visken® (Discontinued)** *see* pindolol *on page 648*

**Vistacon-50® Injection (Discontinued)** *see* hydroxyzine *on page 423*

**Vistaquel® Injection (Discontinued)** *see* hydroxyzine *on page 423*

**Vistaril® [US/Can]** *see* hydroxyzine *on page 423*

**Vistazine® Injection (Discontinued)** *see* hydroxyzine *on page 423*

**Vistide® [US]** *see* cidofovir *on page 182*

**Visudyne® [US/Can]** *see* verteporfin *on page 844*

**Vita 3B+C [Can]** *see* vitamin B complex with vitamin C *on page 850*

**Vita-C® [US-OTC]** *see* ascorbic acid *on page 71*

**Vitaball® [US-OTC]** *see* vitamins (multiple/pediatric) *on page 852*

**Vitaball® Wild 'N Fruity [US-OTC]** *see* vitamins (multiple/pediatric) *on page 852*

**VitaCarn® Oral (Discontinued)** *see* levocarnitine *on page 474*

**Vitacon Forte [US]** *see* vitamins (multiple/oral) *on page 852*

**Vital HN® [US-OTC]** *see* nutritional formula, enteral/oral *on page 591*

**vitamin C** *see* ascorbic acid *on page 71*

**vitamin D$_2$** *see* ergocalciferol *on page 292*

## vitamin A (VYE ta min aye)

**Sound-Alike/Look-Alike Issues**
Aquasol® may be confused with Anusol®

**Synonyms** oleovitamin A

**U.S./Canadian Brand Names** Aquasol A® [US]; Palmitate-A® [US-OTC]

**Therapeutic Category** Vitamin, Fat Soluble

**Use** Treatment and prevention of vitamin A deficiency; parenteral (I.M.) route is indicated when oral administration is not feasible or when absorption is insufficient (malabsorption syndrome)

**Usual Dosage**
RDA:
<1 year: 375 mcg
1-3 years: 400 mcg
4-6 years: 500 mcg*
7-10 years: 700 mcg*
>10 years: 800-1000 mcg*
Male: 1000 mcg
Female: 800 mcg
* mcg retinol equivalent (0.3 mcg retinol = 1 unit vitamin A)
Vitamin A supplementation in measles (recommendation of the World Health Organization): Children: Oral: Administer as a single dose; repeat the next day and at 4 weeks for children with ophthalmologic evidence of vitamin A deficiency:
6 months to 1 year: 100,000 units
>1 year: 200,000 units
**Note:** Use of vitamin A in measles is recommended only for patients 6 months to 2 years of age hospitalized with measles and its complications **or** patients >6 months of age who have any of the following risk factors and who are not already receiving vitamin A: immunodeficiency, ophthalmologic evidence of vitamin A deficiency including night blindness, Bitot's spots or evidence of xerophthalmia, impaired intestinal absorption, moderate to severe malnutrition including that associated with eating disorders, or recent immigration from areas where high mortality rates from measles have been observed
**Note:** Monitor patients closely; dosages >25,000 units/kg have been associated with toxicity
Severe deficiency with xerophthalmia: Oral:
Children 1-8 years: 5000-10,000 units/kg/day for 5 days or until recovery occurs
Children >8 years and Adults: 500,000 units/day for 3 days, then 50,000 units/day for 14 days, then 10,000-20,000 units/day for 2 months
Deficiency (without corneal changes): Oral:
Infants <1 year: 100,000 units every 4-6 months

Children 1-8 years: 200,000 units every 4-6 months

Children >8 years and Adults: 100,000 units/day for 3 days then 50,000 units/day for 14 days

Deficiency: I.M.: **Note:** I.M. route is indicated when oral administration is not feasible or when absorption is insufficient (malabsorption syndrome):

Infants: 7500-15,000 units/day for 10 days

Children 1-8 years: 17,500-35,000 units/day for 10 days

Children >8 years and Adults: 100,000 units/day for 3 days, followed by 50,000 units/day for 2 weeks

**Note:** Follow-up therapy with an oral therapeutic multivitamin (containing additional vitamin A) is recommended:

Low Birth Weight Infants: Additional vitamin A is recommended, however, no dosage amount has been established

Children ≤8 years: 5000-10,000 units/day

Children >8 years and Adults: 10,000-20,000 units/day

Malabsorption syndrome (prophylaxis): Children >8 years and Adults: Oral: 10,000-50,000 units/day of water miscible product

Dietary supplement: Oral:

Infants up to 6 months: 1500 units/day

Children:

6 months to 3 years: 1500-2000 units/day

4-6 years: 2500 units/day

7-10 years: 3300-3500 units/day

Children >10 years and Adults: 4000-5000 units/day

**Dosage Forms**

Capsule [softgel]: 10,000 units; 25,000 units

Injection, solution (Aquasol A®): 50,000 units/mL (2 mL) [contains polysorbate 80]

Tablet (Palmitate-A®): 5000 units, 15,000 units

**vitamin A acid** *see* tretinoin (topical) *on page 818*

# vitamin A and vitamin D (VYE ta min aye & VYE ta min dee)

**Synonyms** cod liver oil

**U.S./Canadian Brand Names** A and D® Ointment [US-OTC]; Baza® Clear [US-OTC]; Clocream® [US-OTC]; Sween Cream® [US-OTC]

**Therapeutic Category** Protectant, Topical

**Use** Temporary relief of discomfort due to chapped skin, diaper rash, minor burns, abrasions, as well as irritations associated with ostomy skin care

**Usual Dosage** Topical: Apply locally with gentle massage as needed

**Dosage Forms**

Capsule: Vitamin A 1250 int. units and vitamin D 135 int. units; Vitamin A 5000 int. units and vitamin D 400 int. units; Vitamin A 10,000 int. units and vitamin D 400 int. units; Vitamin A 25,000 int. units and vitamin D 400 int. units

Cream:

Sween Cream® [original]: 14 g, 57 g, 142 g, 255 g

Sween Cream®: 14 g, 57 g, 142 g [fresh scent]

Sween Cream®: 57 g [fragrance free]

Ointment: 5 g, 60 g, 120 g, 454 g [in lanolin-petrolatum base]

A and D® Ointment: 45 g, 120 g, 454 g

Baza® Clear: 15 g, 50 g, 150 g, 240 g

Clocream®: 30 g

**vitamin B₁** *see* thiamine *on page 796*

**vitamin B₂** *see* riboflavin *on page 721*

**vitamin B₃** *see* niacin *on page 571*

**vitamin B₅** *see* pantothenic acid *on page 618*

**vitamin B₆** *see* pyridoxine *on page 701*

**vitamin B₁₂** *see* cyanocobalamin *on page 212*

# vitamin B complex combinations (VYE ta min bee KOM pleks kom bi NAY shuns)

**Sound-Alike/Look-Alike Issues**

Nephrocaps® may be confused with Nephro-Calci®

(Continued)

# vitamin B complex combinations *(Continued)*

Surbex® may be confused with Sebex®, Suprax®, Surfak®

**Synonyms** B complex combinations; B vitamin combinations

**U.S./Canadian Brand Names** Allbee® C-800 + Iron [US-OTC]; Allbee® C-800 [US-OTC]; Allbee® with C [US-OTC]; Apatate® [US-OTC]; DiatxFe™ [US]; Diatx™ [US]; Gevrabon® [US-OTC]; NephPlex® Rx [US]; Nephro-Vite® Rx [US]; Nephro-Vite® [US]; Nephrocaps® [US]; Nephron FA® [US]; Stresstabs® B-Complex + Iron [US-OTC]; Stresstabs® B-Complex + Zinc [US-OTC]; Stresstabs® B-Complex [US-OTC]; Surbex-T® [US-OTC]; Trinsicon® [US]; Z-Bec® [US-OTC]

**Therapeutic Category** Vitamin, Water Soluble

**Use** Supplement for use in the wasting syndrome in chronic renal failure, uremia, impaired metabolic functions of the kidney, dialysis; labeled for OTC use as a dietary supplement

**Usual Dosage** Oral: Adults:

Dietary supplement: One tablet daily

Apatate® liquid: One teaspoonful daily, 1 hour prior to mid-day meal

Gevrabon® liquid: Two tablespoonsful (30 mL) once daily; shake well before use

Renal patients: One tablet or capsule daily between meals; take after treatment if on dialysis

Nephron FA®: Two tablets once daily, between meals

**Dosage Forms** Content varies depending on product used. For more detailed information on ingredients in these and other multivitamins, please refer to Vitamin Products on page 986 in the Appendix.

# vitamin B complex with vitamin C *(VYE ta min bee KOM pleks with VYE ta min see)*

**U.S./Canadian Brand Names** Allbee® With C [US-OTC]; Penta/3B®+C [Can]; Surbex-T® Filmtabs® [US-OTC]; Surbex® With C Filmtabs® [US-OTC]; Vicon-C® [US-OTC]; Vita 3B+C [Can]

**Therapeutic Category** Vitamin, Water Soluble

**Use** Supportive nutritional supplementation in conditions in which water-soluble vitamins are required like GI disorders, chronic alcoholism, pregnancy, severe burns, and recovery from surgery

**Usual Dosage** Adults: Oral: 1 tablet/capsule daily

**Dosage Forms** Content varies depending on product used. For more detailed information on ingredients see Vitamin Products on page 986 in the Appendix.

# vitamin B complex with vitamin C and folic acid

*(VYE ta min bee KOM pleks with VYE ta min see & FOE lik AS id)*

**U.S./Canadian Brand Names** Nephrocaps® [US]

**Therapeutic Category** Vitamin, Water Soluble

**Use** Supportive nutritional supplementation in conditions in which water-soluble vitamins are required like GI disorders, chronic alcoholism, pregnancy, severe burns, and recovery from surgery

**Usual Dosage** Adults: Oral: 1 capsule/day

**Dosage Forms** Content varies depending on product used. For more detailed information on ingredients see Vitamin Products on page 986 in the Appendix.

**vitamin D3** *see* alendronate and cholecalciferol *on page 26*

# vitamin E *(VYE ta min ee)*

**Sound-Alike/Look-Alike Issues**

Aquasol E® may be confused with Anusol®

**Synonyms** *d*-alpha tocopherol; *dl*-alpha tocopherol

**U.S./Canadian Brand Names** Aqua Gem E® [US-OTC]; Aquasol E® [US-OTC]; E-Gems® [US-OTC]; Key-E® Kaps [US-OTC]; Key-E® [US-OTC]

**Therapeutic Category** Vitamin, Fat Soluble; Vitamin, Topical

**Use** Prevention and treatment of hemolytic anemia secondary to vitamin E deficiency; dietary supplement

**Usual Dosage** One unit of vitamin E = 1 mg *dl*-alpha-tocopherol acetate. Oral:

Recommended daily allowance (RDA):

Premature infants ≤3 months: 17 mg (25 units)

Infants:

≤6 months: 3 mg (4.5 units)

7-12 months: 4 mg (6 units)

Children:

1-3 years: 6 mg (9 units); upper limit of intake should not exceed 200 mg/day

4-8 years: 7 mg (10.5 units); upper limit of intake should not exceed 300 mg/day

9-13 years: 11 mg (16.5 units); upper limit of intake should not exceed 600 mg/day

14-18 years: 15 mg (22.5 units); upper limit of intake should not exceed 800 mg/day
Adults: 15 mg (22.5 units); upper limit of intake should not exceed 1000 mg/day
Pregnant female:
≤18 years: 15 mg (22.5 units); upper level of intake should not exceed 800 mg/day
19-50 years: 15 mg (22.5 units); upper level of intake should not exceed 1000 mg/day
Lactating female:
≤18 years: 19 mg (28.5 units); upper level of intake should not exceed 800 mg/day
19-50 years: 19 mg (28.5 units); upper level of intake should not exceed 1000 mg/day

Vitamin E deficiency:
Children (with malabsorption syndrome): 1 unit/kg/day of water miscible vitamin E (to raise plasma tocopherol concentrations to the normal range within 2 months and to maintain normal plasma concentrations)
Adults: 60-75 units/day
Prevention of vitamin E deficiency: Adults: 30 units/day
Prevention of retinopathy of prematurity or BPD secondary to $O_2$ therapy (AAP considers this use investigational and routine use is not recommended):
Retinopathy prophylaxis: 15-30 units/kg/day to maintain plasma levels between 1.5-2 mcg/mL (may need as high as 100 units/kg/day)
Cystic fibrosis, beta-thalassemia, sickle cell anemia may require higher daily maintenance doses:
Children:
Cystic fibrosis: 100-400 units/day
Beta-thalassemia: 750 units/day
Adults:
Sickle cell: 450 units/day
Alzheimer's disease: 1000 units twice daily
Tardive dyskinesia: 1600 units/day

**Dosage Forms**
Capsule: 100 units, 200 units, 400 units, 500 units, 600 units, 1000 units
Aqua Gem E®: 200 units, 400 units
E-Gems®: 30 units, 100 units, 600 units, 800 units, 1000 units, 1200 units
Key-E® Kaps: 200 units, 400 units
Cream: 100 units/g (60 g)
Key-E®: 30 units/g (60 g, 120 g, 480 g)
Oil: 100 units/0.25 mL (60 mL); 1150 units/0.25 mL (30 mL, 60 mL, 120 mL)
E-Gems®: 100 units/10 drops (15 mL, 60 mL)
Ointment, topical (Key-E®): 30 units/g (60 g, 120 g, 480 g)
Powder (Key-E®): 700 units/dose (15 g, 75 g, 1000 g)
Solution, oral drops (Aquasol E®): 15 units/0.3 mL (12 mL, 30 mL)
Spray (Key-E®): 30 units/3 seconds (105 g)
Suppository (Key-E®): 30 units (12s, 24s)
Tablet: 100 units, 200 units, 400 units, 500 units, 800 units
Key-E®: 100 units, 200 units, 400 units

**vitamin G** *see* riboflavin *on page 721*

**vitamin K$_1$** *see* phytonadione *on page 646*

# vitamins (multiple/injectable) (VYE ta mins, MUL ti pul/in JEK ti bal)

**U.S./Canadian Brand Names** Infuvite® Adult [US]; Infuvite® Pediatric [US]; M.V.I. Adult™ [US]; M.V.I® Pediatric [US]

**Therapeutic Category** Vitamin

**Use** Nutritional supplement in patients receiving parenteral nutrition or requiring intravenous administration

**Usual Dosage** I.V.: Not for direct infusion
Children: ≥3 kg to 11 years: Pediatric formulation: 5 mL/day added to TPN or ≥100 mL of appropriate solution
Children >11 years and Adults: Adult formulation: 10 mL/day added to TPN or ≥500 mL of appropriate solution

**Dosage Forms** Content varies depending on product used. For more detailed information on ingredients in these and other multivitamins, please refer to Vitamin Products on page 986 in the Appendix.

## vitamins (multiple/oral) (VYE ta mins, MUL ti pul/OR al)

**Sound-Alike/Look-Alike Issues**
Theragran® may be confused with Phenergan®

**Synonyms** multiple vitamins; therapeutic multivitamins; vitamins, multiple (oral); vitamins, multiple (therapeutic); vitamins, multiple with iron

**U.S./Canadian Brand Names** Centrum® Performance™ [US-OTC]; Centrum® Silver® [US-OTC]; Centrum® [US-OTC]; Geriation [US-OTC]; Geritol Complete® [US-OTC]; Geritol Extend® [US-OTC]; Geritol® Tonic [US-OTC]; Glutofac®-MX [US]; Glutofac®-ZX [US]; Gynovite® Plus [US-OTC]; Hemocyte Plus® [US]; Hi-Kovite [US-OTC]; Iberet® [US-OTC]; Iberet®-500 [US-OTC]; Monocaps [US-OTC]; Multiret Folic 500 [US]; Ocuvite® Extra® [US-OTC]; Ocuvite® Lutein [US-OTC]; Ocuvite® [US-OTC]; Olay® Vitamins Complete Women's 50+ [US-OTC]; Olay® Vitamins Complete Women's [US-OTC]; Olay® Vitamins Even Complexion [US-OTC]; One-A-Day® 50 Plus Formula [US-OTC]; One-A-Day® Active Formula [US-OTC]; One-A-Day® Carb Smart [US-OTC]; One-A-Day® Cholesterol Plus™ [US-OTC]; One-A-Day® Essential Formula [US-OTC]; One-A-Day® Maximum Formula [US-OTC]; One-A-Day® Men's Formula [US-OTC]; One-A-Day® Today [US-OTC]; One-A-Day® Weight Smart [US-OTC] ; One-A-Day® Women's Formula [US-OTC]; Optivite® P.M.T. [US-OTC]; PreserVision® AREDS [US-OTC]; PreserVision® Lutein [US-OTC]; Quintabs [US-OTC]; Quintabs-M [US-OTC]; Replace with Iron [US-OTC]; Replace [US-OTC]; Strovite® Forte [US]; T-Vites [US-OTC]; Ultra Freeda Iron Free [US-OTC]; Ultra Freeda with Iron [US-OTC]; Unicap M® [US-OTC]; Unicap Sr® [US-OTC]; Unicap T™ [US-OTC]; Viactiv® Multivitamin [US-OTC]; Vicon Forte® [US]; Vitacon Forte [US]; Xtramins [US-OTC]

**Therapeutic Category** Vitamin

**Use** Prevention/treatment of vitamin and mineral deficiencies; labeled for OTC use as a dietary supplement

**Usual Dosage** Oral: Adults: Daily dose of adult preparations varies by product. Generally, 1 tablet or capsule or 5-15 mL of liquid per day. Consult package labeling. Prescription doses may be higher for burn or cystic fibrosis patients.

**Dosage Forms** Content varies depending on product used. For more detailed information on ingredients in these and other multivitamins, please refer to Vitamin Products on page 986 in the Appendix.

## vitamins (multiple/pediatric) (VYE ta mins, MUL ti pul/pe de AT rik)

**Synonyms** children's vitamins; multivitamins/fluoride

**U.S./Canadian Brand Names** ADEKs [US-OTC]; Centrum® Kids Jimmy Neutron® Complete [US-OTC]; Centrum® Kids Jimmy Neutron® Extra C [US-OTC]; Centrum® Kids Rugrats™ Complete [US-OTC]; Centrum® Kids Rugrats™ Extra C [US-OTC]; Centrum® Kids Rugrats™ Extra Calcium [US-OTC]; Flintstones® Complete [US-OTC]; Flintstones® Plus Calcium [US-OTC]; Flintstones® Plus Extra C [US-OTC]; Flintstones® Plus Iron [US-OTC]; My First Flintstones® [US-OTC]; One-A-Day® Kids Bugs Bunny and Friends Complete [US-OTC]; One-A-Day® Kids Bugs Bunny and Friends Plus Extra C [US-OTC]; One-A-Day® Kids Extreme Sports [US-OTC]; One-A-Day® Kids Scooby-Doo! Complete [US-OTC]; One-A-Day® Kids Scooby-Doo! Fizzy Vites [US-OTC]; One-A-Day® Kids Scooby-Doo! Plus Calcium [US-OTC]; Poly-Vi-Flor® With Iron [US]; Poly-Vi-Flor® [US]; Poly-Vi-Sol® with Iron [US-OTC]; Poly-Vi-Sol® [US-OTC]; Soluvite-F [US]; Tri-Vi-Flor® with Iron [US]; Tri-Vi-Flor® [US]; Tri-Vi-Sol® with Iron [US-OTC]; Tri-Vi-Sol® [US-OTC]; Vitaball® Wild 'N Fruity [US-OTC]; Vitaball® [US-OTC]

**Therapeutic Category** Vitamin

**Use** Prevention/treatment of vitamin deficiency; products containing fluoride are used to prevent dental caries; labeled for OTC use as a dietary supplement

**Usual Dosage** Daily dose varies by product; refer to package insert for specific product labeling

**Dosage Forms** Content varies depending on product used. For more detailed information on ingredients in these and other multivitamins, please refer to Vitamin Products on page 986 in the Appendix.

## vitamins (multiple/prenatal) (VYE ta mins, MUL ti pul/pree NAY tal)

**Sound-Alike/Look-Alike Issues**
Niferex® may be confused with Nephrox®
PreCare® may be confused with Precose®

**Synonyms** prenatal vitamins

**U.S./Canadian Brand Names** A-Free Prenatal [US]; Advanced NatalCare® [US]; Aminate Fe-90 [US]; Anemagen™ OB [US]; Cal-Nate™ [US]; CareNate™ 600 [US]; Chromagen® OB [US]; Citracal® Prenatal Rx [US]; Duet® [US]; Duet™ DHA [US]; KPN Prenatal [US]; NataChew™ [US]; NataFort® [US]; Natal-Care® GlossTabs™ [US]; NatalCare® PIC Forte [US]; NatalCare® PIC [US]; NatalCare® Plus [US]; NatalCare® Rx [US]; NatalCare® Three [US]; NataTab™ CFe [US]; NataTab™ FA [US]; NataTab™ Rx [US]; Nestabs® CBF [US]; Nestabs® FA [US]; Nestabs® RX [US]; Niferex®-PN Forte [US]; Niferex®-PN [US]; NutriNate® [US]; OB-20 [US]; Obegyn® [US]; PreCare® Conceive™ [US]; PreCare® Prenatal [US];

PreCare® [US]; Prenatal 1-A-Day [US]; Prenatal AD [US]; Prenatal H [US]; Prenatal MR 90 Fe™ [US]; Prenatal MTR with Selenium [US]; Prenatal Plus [US]; Prenatal Rx 1 [US]; Prenatal U [US]; Prenatal Z [US]; Prenate Elite™ [US]; Prenate GT™ [US]; StrongStart™ [US]; Stuart Prenatal® [US-OTC]; Stuart-natal® Plus 3™ [US-OTC]; Trinate [US]; Ultra NatalCare® [US]

**Therapeutic Category** Vitamin

**Use** Nutritional supplement for use prior to conception, during pregnancy, and postnatal (in lactating and nonlactating women)

**Usual Dosage** Oral: Adults:
Capsule, tablet: One daily
Powder: 4 teaspoonfuls/day; given once daily or in divided doses; mix 1 teaspoonful in 1 ounce of water

**Dosage Forms** Content varies depending on product used. For more detailed information on ingredients in these and other multivitamins, please refer to Vitamin Products on page 986 in the Appendix.

**vitamins, multiple (therapeutic)** *see* vitamins (multiple/oral) *on previous page*

**vitamins, multiple with iron** *see* vitamins (multiple/oral) *on previous page*

**Vitaneed™ [US-OTC]** *see* nutritional formula, enteral/oral *on page 591*

**Vitelle™ Irospan® *(Discontinued)*** *see* ferrous sulfate and ascorbic acid *on page 335*

**Vitrase® [US]** *see* hyaluronidase *on page 407*

**Vitrasert® [US/Can]** *see* ganciclovir *on page 366*

**Vitravene™ [Can]** *see* fomivirsen *(Canada only)* *on page 358*

**Vitravene™ *(Discontinued)*** *see* fomivirsen *(Canada only)* *on page 358*

**Vitrax® [US]** *see* hyaluronate and derivatives *on page 406*

**Vitussin [US]** *see* hydrocodone and guaifenesin *on page 412*

**Vivactil® [US]** *see* protriptyline *on page 691*

**Viva-Drops® [US-OTC]** *see* artificial tears *on page 71*

**Vivelle® [US]** *see* estradiol *on page 299*

**Vivelle-Dot® [US]** *see* estradiol *on page 299*

**Vivonex® [US-OTC]** *see* nutritional formula, enteral/oral *on page 591*

**Vivonex® T.E.N. [US-OTC]** *see* nutritional formula, enteral/oral *on page 591*

**Vivotif Berna® [US]** *see* typhoid vaccine *on page 832*

**VLB** *see* vinblastine *on page 846*

**VM-26** *see* teniposide *on page 785*

**Volmax® *(Discontinued)*** *see* albuterol *on page 22*

**Voltaren® [US/Can]** *see* diclofenac *on page 243*

**Voltaren Ophtha® [Can]** *see* diclofenac *on page 243*

**Voltaren Ophthalmic® [US]** *see* diclofenac *on page 243*

**Voltaren Rapide® [Can]** *see* diclofenac *on page 243*

**Voltaren®-XR [US]** *see* diclofenac *on page 243*

## voriconazole (vor i KOE na zole)

**Synonyms** UK109496

**U.S./Canadian Brand Names** VFEND® [US/Can]

**Therapeutic Category** Antifungal Agent

**Use** Treatment of invasive aspergillosis; treatment of esophageal candidiasis; treatment of candidemia (in non-neutropenic patients); treatment of *Candida* deep tissue infections; treatment of serious fungal infections caused by *Scedosporium apiospermum* and *Fusarium* spp (including *Fusarium solani*) in patients intolerant of, or refractory to, other therapy

**Usual Dosage**
Children <12 years: No data available
Children ≥12 years and Adults:
Invasive aspergillosis and other serious fungal infections: I.V.: Initial: Loading dose: 6 mg/kg every 12 hours for 2 doses; followed by maintenance dose of 4 mg/kg every 12 hours
Candidemia and other deep tissue *Candida* infections: I.V.: Initial: Loading dose 6 mg/kg every 12 hours for 2 doses; followed by maintenance dose of 3-4 mg/kg every 12 hours
(Continued)

## voriconazole *(Continued)*

**Note:** Conversion to oral dosing:

Patients <40 kg: 100 mg every 12 hours; increase to 150 mg every 12 hours in patients who fail to respond adequately

Patients ≥40 kg: 200 mg every 12 hours; increase to 300 mg every 12 hours in patients who fail to respond adequately

Esophageal candidiasis: Oral:

Patients <40 kg: 100 mg every 12 hours

Patients ≥40 kg: 200 mg every 12 hours

**Note:** Treatment should continue for a minimum of 14 days, and for at least 7 days following resolution of symptoms.

**Dosage adjustment in patients unable to tolerate treatment:**

I.V.: Dose may be reduced to 3 mg/kg every 12 hours

Oral: Dose may be reduced in 50 mg increments to a minimum dosage of 200 mg every 12 hours in patients weighing ≥40 kg (100 mg every 12 hours in patients <40 kg)

**Dosage adjustment in patients receiving concomitant phenytoin:**

I.V.: Increase maintenance dosage to 5 mg/kg every 12 hours

Oral: Increase dose from 200 mg to 400 mg every 12 hours in patients ≥40 kg (100 mg to 200 mg every 12 hours in patients <40 kg)

**Dosage Forms**

Injection, powder for reconstitution: 200 mg [contains SBECD 3200 mg]

Powder for oral suspension: 200 mg/5 mL (70 mL) [contains sodium benzoate and sucrose; orange flavor]

Tablet: 50 mg, 200 mg [contains lactose]

**VoSol® [US]** *see* acetic acid *on page 13*

**VoSol® HC [US]** *see* acetic acid, propylene glycol diacetate, and hydrocortisone *on page 14*

**VoSpire ER™ [US]** *see* albuterol *on page 22*

**VP-16** *see* etoposide *on page 322*

**VP-16-213** *see* etoposide *on page 322*

**V-Tann [US]** *see* phenylephrine and pyrilamine *on page 641*

**Vumon® [US/Can]** *see* teniposide *on page 785*

**V.V.S.® [US]** *see* sulfabenzamide, sulfacetamide, and sulfathiazole *on page 771*

**Vytone® [US]** *see* iodoquinol and hydrocortisone *on page 445*

**Vytorin™ [US]** *see* ezetimibe and simvastatin *on page 324*

**VZIG** *see* varicella-zoster immune globulin (human) *on page 841*

## warfarin *(WAR far in)*

**Sound-Alike/Look-Alike Issues**

Coumadin® may be confused with Avandia®, Cardura®, Compazine®, Kemadrin®

**Synonyms** warfarin sodium

**U.S./Canadian Brand Names** Apo-Warfarin® [Can]; Coumadin® [US/Can]; Gen-Warfarin [Can]; Jantoven™ [US]; Taro-Warfarin [Can]

**Therapeutic Category** Anticoagulant (Other)

**Use** Prophylaxis and treatment of venous thrombosis, pulmonary embolism and thromboembolic disorders; atrial fibrillation with risk of embolism and as an adjunct in the prophylaxis of systemic embolism after myocardial infarction

**Usual Dosage**

Oral:

Infants and Children: 0.05-0.34 mg/kg/day; infants <12 months of age may require doses at or near the high end of this range; consistent anticoagulation may be difficult to maintain in children <5 years of age

Adults: Initial dosing must be individualized. Consider the patient (hepatic function, cardiac function, age, nutritional status, concurrent therapy, risk of bleeding) in addition to prior dose response (if available) and the clinical situation. Start 5-10 mg daily for 2 days. Adjust dose according to INR results; usual maintenance dose ranges from 2-10 mg daily (individual patients may require loading and maintenance doses outside these general guidelines).

**Note**: Lower starting doses may be required for patients with hepatic impairment, poor nutrition, CHF, elderly, or a high risk of bleeding. Higher initial doses may be reasonable in selected patients (ie, receiving enzyme-inducing agents and with low risk of bleeding).

I.V. (administer as a slow bolus injection): 2-5 mg/day

**Dosage Forms**

Injection, powder for reconstitution, as sodium (Coumadin®): 5 mg

Tablet, as sodium (Coumadin®, Jantoven™): 1 mg, 2 mg, 2.5 mg, 3 mg, 4 mg, 5 mg, 6 mg, 7.5 mg, 10 mg

**warfarin sodium** *see* warfarin *on previous page*

**Wartec® [Can]** *see* podofilox *on page 656*

**Wart-Off® Maximum Strength [US-OTC]** *see* salicylic acid *on page 734*

**4-Way® 12 Hour [US-OTC]** *see* oxymetazoline *on page 610*

**WelChol® [US/Can]** *see* colesevelam *on page 205*

**Wellbutrin® [US/Can]** *see* bupropion *on page 122*

**Wellbutrin XL™ [US]** *see* bupropion *on page 122*

**Wellbutrin SR® [US]** *see* bupropion *on page 122*

**Wellcovorin® *(Discontinued)*** *see* leucovorin *on page 470*

**Westcort® [US/Can]** *see* hydrocortisone (topical) *on page 417*

**Westhroid® [US]** *see* thyroid *on page 800*

**40 Winks® *(Discontinued)*** *see* diphenhydramine *on page 254*

**Winpred™ [Can]** *see* prednisone *on page 674*

**WinRho SD® *(Discontinued)***

**WinRho SDF® [US]** *see* Rh$_o$(D) immune globulin *on page 717*

**Winstrol® [US]** *see* stanozolol *on page 765*

**witch hazel** (witch HAY zel)

**Synonyms** hamamelis water

**U.S./Canadian Brand Names** Dickinson's® Witch Hazel [US-OTC]; Preparation H® Cleansing Pads [Can]; Preparation H® Medicated Wipes [US-OTC]; T.N. Dickinson's® Hazelets [US-OTC]; Tucks® [US-OTC]

**Therapeutic Category** Astringent

**Use** After-stool wipe to remove most causes of local irritation; temporary management of vulvitis, pruritus ani and vulva; help relieve the discomfort of simple hemorrhoids, anorectal surgical wounds, and episiotomies

**Usual Dosage** Apply to anorectal area as needed

**Dosage Forms**

Liquid, topical: 100% (120 mL, 480 mL)

Dickinson's® Witch Hazel: 100% (60 mL, 240 mL, 480 mL)

Pads: 50% (100s)

Dickinson's® Witch Hazel: 50% (20s) [towelettes]; (50s) [contains aloe]; (100s) [hemorrhoidal]

Preparation H® Medicated Wipes: 50% (8s, 48s) [contains aloe]

T.N. Dickinson's® Hazelets: 50% (50s) [contains aloe]; (60s)

Tucks®: 50% (12s, 40s, 100s)

**Wolfina® *(Discontinued)***

**wood sugar** *see* d-xylose *on page 276*

**Wound Wash Saline™ [US-OTC]** *see* sodium chloride *on page 752*

**WR-139007** *see* dacarbazine *on page 220*

**WR-139013** *see* chlorambucil *on page 166*

**WR-139021** *see* carmustine *on page 149*

**WR-2721** *see* amifostine *on page 38*

**Wycillin® [Can]** *see* penicillin G procaine *on page 629*

**Wycillin *(Discontinued)*** *see* penicillin G procaine *on page 629*

**Wydase**® *(Discontinued)* *see* hyaluronidase *on page 407*

**Wygesic**® *(Discontinued)* *see* propoxyphene and acetaminophen *on page 687*

**Wymox**® *(Discontinued)* *see* amoxicillin *on page 46*

**Wytensin**® **[Can]** *see* guanabenz *on page 393*

**Wytensin**® *(Discontinued)* *see* guanabenz *on page 393*

**Xalatan**® **[US/Can]** *see* latanoprost *on page 469*

**Xanax**® **[US/Can]** *see* alprazolam *on page 30*

**Xanax TS**™ **[Can]** *see* alprazolam *on page 30*

**Xanax XR**® **[US]** *see* alprazolam *on page 30*

**Xatral [Can]** *see* alfuzosin *on page 27*

**Xeloda**® **[US/Can]** *see* capecitabine *on page 138*

**Xenaderm**™ **[US]** *see* trypsin, balsam peru, and castor oil *on page 830*

**Xenical**® **[US/Can]** *see* orlistat *on page 602*

**Xerac AC**™ **[US]** *see* aluminum chloride hexahydrate *on page 34*

**Xibrom**™ **[US]** *see* bromfenac *on page 114*

**Xifaxan**™ **[US]** *see* rifaximin *on page 723*

**Xigris**® **[US/Can]** *see* drotrecogin alfa *on page 274*

**XiraTuss [US]** *see* carbetapentane, phenylephrine, and chlorpheniramine *on page 142*

**Xolair**® **[US/Can]** *see* omalizumab *on page 597*

**Xopenex**® **[US/Can]** *see* levalbuterol *on page 472*

**Xopenex HFA**™ **[US]** *see* levalbuterol *on page 472*

**X-Prep**® **[US-OTC]** *see* senna *on page 743*

**X-Seb T**® **Pearl [US-OTC]** *see* coal tar and salicylic acid *on page 202*

**X-Seb T**® **Plus [US-OTC]** *see* coal tar and salicylic acid *on page 202*

**Xtramins [US-OTC]** *see* vitamins (multiple/oral) *on page 852*

**Xylocaine**® **[US/Can]** *see* lidocaine *on page 479*

**Xylocaine**® **MPF [US]** *see* lidocaine *on page 479*

**Xylocaine**® **MPF With Epinephrine [US]** *see* lidocaine and epinephrine *on page 480*

**Xylocaine**® **Viscous [US]** *see* lidocaine *on page 479*

**Xylocaine**® **With Epinephrine [US/Can]** *see* lidocaine and epinephrine *on page 480*

**Xylocard**® **[Can]** *see* lidocaine *on page 479*

**Xyrem**® **[US]** *see* sodium oxybate *on page 755*

**Y-90 zevalin** *see* ibritumomab *on page 427*

**Yasmin**® **[US/Can]** *see* ethinyl estradiol and drospirenone *on page 310*

## yellow fever vaccine (YEL oh FEE ver vak SEEN)

**U.S./Canadian Brand Names** YF-VAX® [US/Can]

**Therapeutic Category** Vaccine, Live Virus

**Use** Induction of active immunity against yellow fever virus, primarily among persons traveling or living in areas where yellow fever infection exists

**Usual Dosage** Children ≥9 months and Adults: SubQ: One dose (0.5 mL) ≥10 days before travel; Booster: Every 10 years

**Dosage Forms** Injection, powder for reconstitution [17D-204 strain]: ≥4.74 $Log_{10}$ plaque-forming units (PFU) per 0.5 mL dose  [single-dose or 5-dose vial; produced in chicken embryos; packaged with diluent; vial stopper contains latex]

**yellow mercuric oxide** *see* mercuric oxide *on page 515*

**YF-VAX**® **[US/Can]** *see* yellow fever vaccine *on this page*

**YM-08310** *see* amifostine *on page 38*

**Yocon**® **[US/Can]** *see* yohimbine *on next page*

**Yodoxin**® **[US]** *see* iodoquinol *on page 445*

# yohimbine (yo HIM bine)

**Sound-Alike/Look-Alike Issues**
Aphrodyne® may be confused with Aprodine®
Yocon® may be confused with Zocor®
**Synonyms** yohimbine hydrochloride
**U.S./Canadian Brand Names** Aphrodyne® [US]; PMS-Yohimbine [Can]; Yocon® [US/Can]
**Therapeutic Category** Miscellaneous Product
**Usual Dosage** Adults: Oral:
Male erectile impotence: 5.4 mg tablet 3 times/day have been used. If side effects occur, reduce to 1/2 tablet (2.7 mg) 3 times/day followed by gradual increases to 1 tablet 3 times/day. Results of therapy >10 weeks are not known.
Orthostatic hypotension: Doses of 12.5 mg/day have been utilized; however, more research is necessary
**Dosage Forms** Tablet, as hydrochloride: 5.4 mg

**yohimbine hydrochloride** *see* yohimbine *on this page*

**Yohimex**™ *(Discontinued)* *see* yohimbine *on this page*

**Z4942** *see* ifosfamide *on page 430*

**Zaditen**® **[Can]** *see* ketotifen *on page 458*

**Zaditor**™ **[US/Can]** *see* ketotifen *on page 458*

# zafirlukast (za FIR loo kast)

**Sound-Alike/Look-Alike Issues**
Accolate® may be confused with Accupril®, Accutane®, Aclovate®
**Synonyms** ICI-204,219
**U.S./Canadian Brand Names** Accolate® [US/Can]
**Therapeutic Category** Leukotriene Receptor Antagonist
**Use** Prophylaxis and chronic treatment of asthma in adults and children ≥5 years of age
**Usual Dosage** Oral:
Children <5 years: Safety and effectiveness have not been established
Children 5-11 years: 10 mg twice daily
Children ≥12 years and Adults: 20 mg twice daily
**Dosage Forms** Tablet: 10 mg, 20 mg

**Zagam**® *(Discontinued)* *see* sparfloxacin *on page 763*

# zalcitabine (zal SITE a been)

**Synonyms** ddC; dideoxycytidine
**U.S./Canadian Brand Names** Hivid® [US/Can]
**Therapeutic Category** Antiviral Agent
**Use** In combination with at least two other antiretrovirals in the treatment of patients with HIV infection; it is not recommended that zalcitabine be given in combination with didanosine, stavudine, or lamivudine due to overlapping toxicities, virologic interactions, or lack of clinical data
**Usual Dosage** Oral:
Neonates: Dose unknown
Infants and Children <13 years: Safety and efficacy have not been established; suggested usual dose: 0.01 mg/kg every 8 hours; range: 0.005-0.01 mg/kg every 8 hours
Adolescents and Adults: 0.75 mg 3 times/day
**Dosage Forms** Tablet: 0.375 mg, 0.75 mg

# zaleplon (ZAL e plon)

**U.S./Canadian Brand Names** Sonata® [US/Can]; Starnoc® [Can]
**Therapeutic Category** Hypnotic, Nonbenzodiazepine (Pyrazolopyrimidine)
**Controlled Substance** C-IV
**Use** Short-term (7-10 days) treatment of insomnia (has been demonstrated to be effective for up to 5 weeks in controlled trial)
(Continued)

## zaleplon (Continued)

**Usual Dosage** Oral: Adults: 10 mg at bedtime (range: 5-20 mg); has been used for up to 5 weeks of treatment in controlled trial setting

**Dosage Forms** Capsule: 5 mg, 10 mg [contains tartrazine]

**Zanaflex**® **[US/Can]** see tizanidine on page 806

## zanamivir (za NA mi veer)

**U.S./Canadian Brand Names** Relenza® [US/Can]

**Therapeutic Category** Antiviral Agent, Inhalation Therapy

**Use** Treatment of uncomplicated acute illness due to influenza virus A and B in adults and children ≥7 years of age; should not be used in patients with underlying airway disease. Treatment should only be initiated in patients who have been symptomatic for no more than 2 days.

**Usual Dosage** Children ≥7 years and Adults: 2 inhalations (10 mg total) twice daily for 5 days. Two doses should be taken on the first day of dosing, regardless of interval, while doses should be spaced by approximately 12 hours on subsequent days.

**Dosage Forms** Powder for oral inhalation: 5 mg/blister (20s) [4 blisters per Rotadisk® foil pack, 5 Rotadisk® per package; packaged with Diskhaler® inhalation device; contains lactose]

**Zanosar**® **[US/Can]** see streptozocin on page 767

**Zantac**® **[US/Can]** see ranitidine hydrochloride on page 710

**Zantac 75**® **[US-OTC/Can]** see ranitidine hydrochloride on page 710

**Zantac 150**™ **[US-OTC]** see ranitidine hydrochloride on page 710

**Zantac**® **EFFERdose**® **[US]** see ranitidine hydrochloride on page 710

**Zantryl**® **(Discontinued)** see phentermine on page 639

**Zapzyt**® **[US-OTC]** see benzoyl peroxide on page 98

**Zapzyt**® **Acne Wash [US-OTC]** see salicylic acid on page 734

**Zapzyt**® **Pore Treatment [US-OTC]** see salicylic acid on page 734

**Zarontin**® **[US/Can]** see ethosuximide on page 320

**Zaroxolyn**® **[US/Can]** see metolazone on page 534

**Zartan**® **(Discontinued)** see cephalexin on page 161

**Zavesca**® **[US/Can]** see miglustat on page 541

**Z-Bec**® **[US-OTC]** see vitamin B complex combinations on page 849

**Z-chlopenthixol** see zuclopenthixol (Canada only) on page 864

**Z-Cof DM [US]** see guaifenesin, pseudoephedrine, and dextromethorphan on page 391

**Z-Cof HC [US]** see phenylephrine, hydrocodone, and chlorpheniramine on page 643

**Z-Cof LA**™ **[US]** see guaifenesin and dextromethorphan on page 385

**ZD1033** see anastrozole on page 53

**ZD1694** see raltitrexed (Canada only) on page 710

**ZD1839** see gefitinib on page 368

**ZDV** see zidovudine on next page

**ZDV, abacavir, and lamivudine** see abacavir, lamivudine, and zidovudine on page 2

**Zeasorb**®**-AF [US-OTC]** see miconazole on page 537

**Zebeta**® **[US/Can]** see bisoprolol on page 108

**Zebutal**™ **[US]** see butalbital, acetaminophen, and caffeine on page 124

**Zefazone**® **(Discontinued)**

**Zegerid**™ **[US]** see omeprazole on page 598

**zeldox** see ziprasidone on page 862

**Zelnorm**® **[US/Can]** see tegaserod on page 782

**Zemaira**™ **[US]** see alpha₁-proteinase inhibitor on page 30

**Zemplar**® **[US/Can]** see paricalcitol on page 619

**Zemuron**® **[US/Can]** *see* rocuronium *on page 728*

**Zenapax**® **[US/Can]** *see* daclizumab *on page 221*

**zeneca 182,780** *see* fulvestrant *on page 363*

**Zephiran**® **[US-OTC]** *see* benzalkonium chloride *on page 95*

**Zephrex**® **[US]** *see* guaifenesin and pseudoephedrine *on page 388*

**Zephrex LA**® **[US]** *see* guaifenesin and pseudoephedrine *on page 388*

**Zerit**® **[US/Can]** *see* stavudine *on page 765*

**Zestoretic**® **[US/Can]** *see* lisinopril and hydrochlorothiazide *on page 486*

**Zestril**® **[US/Can]** *see* lisinopril *on page 485*

**Zetacet**® **[US]** *see* sulfur and sulfacetamide *on page 776*

**Zetar**® **[US-OTC]** *see* coal tar *on page 201*

**Zetia**™ **[US]** *see* ezetimibe *on page 324*

**Zevalin**™ **[US]** *see* ibritumomab *on page 427*

**Ziac**® **[US/Can]** *see* bisoprolol and hydrochlorothiazide *on page 109*

**Ziagen**® **[US/Can]** *see* abacavir *on page 2*

## ziconotide (zi KOE no tide)

**U.S./Canadian Brand Names** Prialt® [US]

**Therapeutic Category** Analgesic, Nonnarcotic; Calcium Channel Blocker, N-Type

**Use** Management of severe chronic pain in patients requiring intrathecal (I.T.) therapy and are intolerant or refractory to other therapies

**Usual Dosage** I.T.: Adults: Chronic pain: Initial dose: 2.4 mcg/day (0.1 mcg/hour)
Dose may be titrated by ≤2.4 mcg/day (0.1 mcg/hour) at intervals ≥2-3 times/week to a maximum dose of 19.2 mcg/day (0.8 mcg/hour) by day 21; average dose at day 21: 6.9 mcg/day (0.29 mcg/hour). A faster titration should be used only if the urgent need for analgesia outweighs the possible risk to patient safety.

**Dosage Forms** Injection, solution, as acetate [preservative free]: 25 mcg/mL (20 mL); 100 mcg/mL (1 mL, 2 mL, 5 mL)

## zidovudine (zye DOE vyoo deen)

**Sound-Alike/Look-Alike Issues**
azidothymidine may be confused with azathioprine, aztreonam
Retrovir® may be confused with ritonavir
AZT is an error-prone abbreviation (mistaken as azathioprine, aztreonam)

**Synonyms** azidothymidine; compound S; ZDV

**U.S./Canadian Brand Names** AZT™ [Can]; Retrovir® [US/Can]

**Therapeutic Category** Antiviral Agent

**Use** Management of patients with HIV infections in combination with at least two other antiretroviral agents; for prevention of maternal/fetal HIV transmission as monotherapy

**Usual Dosage**
Prevention of maternal-fetal HIV transmission:
Neonatal: **Note:** Dosing should begin 8-12 hours after birth and continue for the first 6 weeks of life.
Oral:
Full-term infants: 2 mg/kg/dose every 6 hours
Infants ≥30 weeks and <35 weeks gestation at birth: 2 mg/kg/dose every 12 hours; at 2 weeks of age, advance to 2 mg/kg/dose every 8 hours
Infants <30 weeks gestation at birth: 2 mg/kg/dose every 12 hours; at 4 weeks of age, advance to 2 mg/kg/dose every 8 hours
I.V.: Infants unable to receive oral dosing:
Full term: 1.5 mg/kg/dose every 6 hours
Infants ≥30 weeks and <35 weeks gestation at birth: 1.5 mg/kg/dose every 12 hours; at 2 weeks of age, advance to 1.5 mg/kg/dose every 8 hours
Infants <30 weeks gestation at birth: 1.5 mg/kg/dose every 12 hours; at 4 weeks of age, advance to 1.5 mg/kg/dose every 8 hours
Maternal: Oral (per AIDSinfo guidelines): 100 mg 5 times/day **or** 200 mg 3 times/day **or** 300 mg twice daily. Begin at 14-34 weeks gestation and continue until start of labor.
(Continued)

## zidovudine *(Continued)*

During labor and delivery, administer zidovudine I.V. at 2 mg/kg over 1 hour followed by a continuous I.V. infusion of 1 mg/kg/hour until the umbilical cord is clamped

Treatment of HIV infection:

Children 3 months to 12 years:

Oral: 160 mg/m$^2$/dose every 8 hours; dosage range: 90 mg/m$^2$/dose to 180 mg/m$^2$/dose every 6-8 hours; some Working Group members use a dose of 180 mg/m$^2$ to 240 mg/m$^2$ every 12 hours when using in drug combinations with other antiretroviral compounds, but data on this dosing in children is limited

I.V. continuous infusion: 20 mg/m$^2$/hour

I.V. intermittent infusion: 120 mg/m$^2$/dose every 6 hours

Adults:

Oral: 300 mg twice daily or 200 mg 3 times/day

I.V.: 1-2 mg/kg/dose (infused over 1 hour) administered every 4 hours around-the-clock (6 doses/day)

**Dosage Forms**

Capsule (Retrovir®): 100 mg

Injection, solution [preservative free] (Retrovir®): 10 mg/mL (20 mL)

Syrup (Retrovir®): 50 mg/5 mL (240 mL) [contains sodium benzoate; strawberry flavor]

Tablet (Retrovir®): 300 mg

**zidovudine, abacavir, and lamivudine** *see* abacavir, lamivudine, and zidovudine *on page 2*

## zidovudine and lamivudine (zye DOE vyoo deen & la MI vyoo deen)

**Sound-Alike/Look-Alike Issues**

Combivir® may be confused with Combivent®, Epivir®

AZT is an error-prone abbreviation (mistaken as azathioprine, aztreonam)

**Synonyms** lamivudine and zidovudine

**U.S./Canadian Brand Names** Combivir® [US/Can]

**Therapeutic Category** Antiviral Agent

**Use** Treatment of HIV infection when therapy is warranted based on clinical and/or immunological evidence of disease progression. Combivir® given twice daily, provides an alternative regimen to lamivudine 150 mg twice daily plus zidovudine 600 mg/day in divided doses; this drug form reduces capsule/tablet intake for these two drugs to 2 per day instead of up to 8.

**Usual Dosage** Children >12 years and Adults: Oral: One tablet twice daily

**Note:** Because this is a fixed-dose combination product, avoid use in patients requiring dosage reduction including children <12 years of age, renally impaired patients with a creatinine clearance ≤50 mL/minute, patients with low body weight (<50 kg or 110 pounds), or those experiencing dose-limiting adverse effects.

**Dosage Forms** Tablet: Zidovudine 300 mg and lamivudine 150 mg

**Zilactin® [Can]** *see* lidocaine *on page 479*

**Zilactin-L®  [US-OTC]** *see* lidocaine *on page 479*

**Zilactin®-B [US-OTC/Can]** *see* benzocaine *on page 95*

**Zilactin® Baby [US-OTC/Can]** *see* benzocaine *on page 95*

**Zinacef® [US/Can]** *see* cefuroxime *on page 158*

**zinc** *see* trace metals *on page 813*

**Zincate® [US]** *see* zinc sulfate *on next page*

## zinc chloride (zink KLOR ide)

**Therapeutic Category** Trace Element

**Use** Cofactor for replacement therapy to different enzymes helps maintain normal growth rates, normal skin hydration and senses of taste and smell

**Usual Dosage** Clinical response may not occur for up to 6-8 weeks

Supplemental to I.V. solutions:

Premature Infants <1500 g, up to 3 kg: 300 mcg/kg/day

Full-term Infants and Children ≤5 years: 100 mcg/kg/day

Adults:
  Stable with fluid loss from small bowel: 12.2 mg zinc/liter TPN or 17.1 mg zinc/kg (added to 1000 mL I.V. fluids) of stool or ileostomy output
  Metabolically stable: 2.5-4 mg/day, add 2 mg/day for acute catabolic states
**Dosage Forms** Injection, solution: 1 mg/mL (10 mL, 50 mL)

**zinc diethylenetriaminepentaacetate (Zn-DTPA)** *see* diethylene triamine penta-acetic acid *on page 246*

**Zincfrin® [US-OTC/Can]** *see* phenylephrine and zinc sulfate *on page 642*

## zinc gelatin (zink JEL ah tin)
**Synonyms** dome paste bandage; unna's boot; unna's paste; zinc gelatin boot
**U.S./Canadian Brand Names** Gelucast® [US]
**Therapeutic Category** Protectant, Topical
**Use** As a protectant and to support varicosities and similar lesions of the lower limbs
**Usual Dosage** Apply externally as an occlusive boot
**Dosage Forms** Bandage: 3" x 10 yards; 4" x 10 yards

**zinc gelatin boot** *see* zinc gelatin *on this page*

**Zincofax® [Can]** *see* zinc oxide *on this page*

**Zincon® [US-OTC]** *see* pyrithione zinc *on page 702*

## zinc oxide (zink OKS ide)
**Synonyms** base ointment; lassar's zinc paste
**U.S./Canadian Brand Names** Ammens® Medicated Deodorant [US-OTC]; Balmex® [US-OTC]; Boudreaux's® Butt Paste [US-OTC]; Critic-Aid Skin Care® [US-OTC]; Desitin® Creamy [US-OTC]; Desitin® [US-OTC]; Zincofax® [Can]
**Therapeutic Category** Topical Skin Product
**Use** Protective coating for mild skin irritations and abrasions, soothing and protective ointment to promote healing of chapped skin, diaper rash
**Usual Dosage** Infants, Children, and Adults: Topical: Apply as required for affected areas several times daily
**Dosage Forms**
  Ointment, topical: 20% (30 g, 60 g, 480 g)
    Balmex®: 11.3% (60 g, 120 g, 480 g)
    Desitin®: 40% (30 g, 60 g, 90 g, 120 g, 270 g, 480 g) [contains cod liver oil and lanolin]
    Desitin® Creamy: 10% (60 g, 120 g)
  Paste, topical:
    Boudreaux's® Butt Paste: 16% (30 g, 60 g, 120 g, 480 g) [contains castor oil, boric acid, mineral oil, and Peruvian balsam]
    Critic-Aid Skin Care®: 20% (71 g, 170 g)
  Powder, topical (Ammens® Medicated Deodorant): 9.1% (187.5 g, 330 g) [original and shower fresh scent]

## zinc sulfate (zink SUL fate)
**Sound-Alike/Look-Alike Issues**
  $ZnSO_4$ is an error-prone abbreviation (mistaken as morphine sulfate)
**U.S./Canadian Brand Names** Anuzinc [Can]; Orazinc® [US-OTC]; Rivasol [Can]; Zincate® [US]
**Therapeutic Category** Electrolyte Supplement, Oral
**Use** Zinc supplement (oral and parenteral); may improve wound healing in those who are deficient
**Usual Dosage**
  RDA: Oral:
  Birth to 6 months: 3 mg elemental zinc/day
  6-12 months: 5 mg elemental zinc/day
  1-10 years: 10 mg elemental zinc/day
  ≥11 years: 15 mg elemental zinc/day

  Zinc deficiency: Oral:
  Infants and Children: 0.5-1 mg elemental zinc/kg/day divided 1-3 times/day; somewhat larger quantities may be needed if there is impaired intestinal absorption or an excessive loss of zinc
  Adults: 110-220 mg zinc sulfate (25-50 mg elemental zinc)/dose 3 times/day
  (Continued)

# zinc sulfate *(Continued)*

Parenteral TPN: I.V.:

Infants (premature, birth weight <1500 g up to 3 kg): 300 mcg/kg/day

Infants (full-term) and Children ≤5 years: 100 mcg/kg/day

Adults:

Acute metabolic states: 4.5-6 mg/day

Metabolically stable: 2.5-4 mg/day

Stable with fluid loss from the small bowel: 12.2 mg zinc/L of TPN solution, or an additional 17.1 mg zinc (added to 1000 mL I.V. fluids) per kg of stool or ileostomy output

**Dosage Forms**

Capsule (Orazinc®, Zincate®): 220 mg [elemental zinc 50 mg]

Injection, solution [preservative free]: 1 mg elemental zinc/mL (10 mL); 5 mg elemental zinc/mL (5 mL)

Tablet (Orazinc®): 110 mg [elemental zinc 25 mg]

**zinc sulfate and phenylephrine** *see* phenylephrine and zinc sulfate *on page 642*

**zinc undecylenate** *see* undecylenic acid and derivatives *on page 833*

**Zinecard® [US/Can]** *see* dexrazoxane *on page 236*

# ziprasidone (zi PRAY si done)

**Synonyms** zeldox; ziprasidone hydrochloride; ziprasidone mesylate

**U.S./Canadian Brand Names** Geodon® [US]

**Therapeutic Category** Antipsychotic Agent

**Use** Treatment of schizophrenia; treatment of acute manic or mixed episodes associated with bipolar disorder with or without psychosis; acute agitation in patients with schizophrenia

**Usual Dosage** Adults:

Bipolar mania: Oral: Initial: 40 mg twice daily (with food)

Adjustment: May increase to 60 or 80 mg twice daily on second day of treatment; average dose 40-80 mg twice daily

Schizophrenia: Oral: Initial: 20 mg twice daily (with food)

Adjustment: Increases (if indicated) should be made no more frequently than every 2 days; ordinarily patients should be observed for improvement over several weeks before adjusting the dose

Maintenance: Range 20-100 mg twice daily; however, dosages >80 mg twice daily are generally not recommended

Acute agitation (schizophrenia): I.M.: 10 mg every 2 hours **or** 20 mg every 4 hours; maximum: 40 mg/day; oral therapy should replace I.M. administration as soon as possible

**Dosage Forms**

Capsule, as hydrochloride: 20 mg, 40 mg, 60 mg, 80 mg

Injection, powder for reconstitution, as mesylate: 20 mg

**ziprasidone hydrochloride** *see* ziprasidone *on this page*

**ziprasidone mesylate** *see* ziprasidone *on this page*

**Zithromax® [US/Can]** *see* azithromycin *on page 84*

**Zithromax® TRI-PAK™** *see* azithromycin *on page 84*

**Zithromax® Z-PAK®** *see* azithromycin *on page 84*

**ZM-182,780** *see* fulvestrant *on page 363*

**Zmax™ [US]** *see* azithromycin *on page 84*

**Zn-DTPA** *see* diethylene triamine penta-acetic acid *on page 246*

**ZNP® Bar [US-OTC]** *see* pyrithione zinc *on page 702*

**Zocor® [US/Can]** *see* simvastatin *on page 748*

**Zofran® [US/Can]** *see* ondansetron *on page 599*

**Zofran® ODT [US/Can]** *see* ondansetron *on page 599*

**Zoladex® [US/Can]** *see* goserelin *on page 381*

**Zoladex® LA [Can]** *see* goserelin *on page 381*

**zoledronate** *see* zoledronic acid *on next page*

## zoledronic acid (ZOE le dron ik AS id)

**Synonyms** CGP-42446; zoledronate
**U.S./Canadian Brand Names** Aclasta® [Can]; Zometa® [US/Can]
**Therapeutic Category** Bisphosphonate Derivative
**Use** Treatment of hypercalcemia of malignancy, multiple myeloma, bone metastases of solid tumors
**Usual Dosage** I.V.: Adults:

Hypercalcemia of malignancy (albumin-corrected serum calcium ≥12 mg/dL): 4 mg (maximum) given as a single dose. Wait at least 7 days before considering retreatment. Dosage adjustment may be needed in patients with decreased renal function following treatment.

Multiple myeloma or metastatic bone lesions from solid tumors: 4 mg every 3-4 weeks

**Note:** Patients should receive a daily calcium supplement and multivitamin containing vitamin D

Paget's disease (Aclasta®, not available in U.S.): 5 mg infused over at least 15 minutes. **Note:** Data concerning retreatment is not available.

**Dosage Forms**

Injection, solution: 4 mg/5 mL (5 mL) [as monohydrate 4.264 mg]

Additional dosage form available in Canada: Infusion, solution [premixed] (Aclasta® [CAN]): 5 mg (100 mL)

**Zolicef®** *(Discontinued)* see cefazolin on page 153

## zolmitriptan (zohl mi TRIP tan)

**Sound-Alike/Look-Alike Issues**

zolmitriptan may be confused with sumatriptan

**Synonyms** 311C90
**U.S./Canadian Brand Names** Zomig-ZMT™ [US]; Zomig® Rapimelt [Can]; Zomig® [US/Can]
**Therapeutic Category** Antimigraine Agent; Serotonin Agonist
**Use** Acute treatment of migraine with or without aura
**Usual Dosage** Oral:

Children: Safety and efficacy have not been established

Adults: Migraine:

Tablet: Initial: ≤2.5 mg at the onset of migraine headache; may break 2.5 mg tablet in half

Orally-disintegrating tablet: Initial: 2.5 mg at the onset of migraine headache

Nasal spray: Initial: 1 spray (5 mg) at the onset of migraine headache

**Note:** Use the lowest possible dose to minimize adverse events. If the headache returns, the dose may be repeated after 2 hours; do not exceed 10 mg within a 24-hour period. Controlled trials have not established the effectiveness of a second dose if the initial one was ineffective

**Dosage Forms**

Solution, nasal spray [single dose] (Zomig®): 5 mg/0.1 mL (0.1 mL)

Tablet (Zomig®): 2.5 mg, 5 mg

Tablet, orally-disintegrating (Zomig-ZMT™): 2.5 mg [contains phenylalanine 2.81 mg/tablet; orange flavor]; 5 mg [contains phenylalanine 5.62 mg/tablet; orange flavor]

**Zoloft® [US/Can]** *see* sertraline *on page 744*

## zolpidem (zole PI dem)

**Sound-Alike/Look-Alike Issues**

Ambien® may be confused with Ambi 10®

**Synonyms** zolpidem tartrate
**U.S./Canadian Brand Names** Ambien CR™ [US]; Ambien® [US]
**Therapeutic Category** Hypnotic, Nonbarbiturate
**Controlled Substance** C-IV
**Use** Short-term treatment of insomnia (sleep onset and/or sleep maintenance)
**Usual Dosage** Oral:

Ambien®: 10 mg immediately before bedtime; maximum dose: 10 mg

Ambien CR™: 12.5 mg immediately before bedtime

**Dosage Forms**

Tablet, as tartrate:

Ambien®: 5 mg, 10 mg

Ambien® PAK™ [dose pack]: 5 mg (30s), 10 mg (30s)

Tablet, as tartrate, extended release (Ambien CR™): 6.25 mg, 12.5 mg

**zolpidem tartrate** *see* zolpidem *on previous page*

**Zometa**® **[US/Can]** *see* zoledronic acid *on previous page*

**Zomig**® **[US/Can]** *see* zolmitriptan *on previous page*

**Zomig**® **Rapimelt [Can]** *see* zolmitriptan *on previous page*

**Zomig-ZMT**™ **[US]** *see* zolmitriptan *on previous page*

**Zonalon**® **[US/Can]** *see* doxepin *on page 269*

**Zone-A**® **[US]** *see* pramoxine and hydrocortisone *on page 671*

**Zone-A Forte**® **[US]** *see* pramoxine and hydrocortisone *on page 671*

**Zonegran**® **[US/Can]** *see* zonisamide *on this page*

**zonisamide** (zoe NIS a mide)
   U.S./Canadian Brand Names Zonegran® [US/Can]
   Therapeutic Category Anticonvulsant, Sulfonamide
   Use Adjunct treatment of partial seizures in children >16 years of age and adults with epilepsy
   Usual Dosage Oral: Children >16 years and Adults: Adjunctive treatment of partial seizures: Initial: 100 mg/day; dose may be increased to 200 mg/day after 2 weeks. Further dosage increases to 300 mg/day and 400 mg/day can then be made with a minimum of 2 weeks between adjustments, in order to reach steady state at each dosage level. Doses of up to 600 mg/day have been studied, however, there is no evidence of increased response with doses above 400 mg/day.
   Dosage Forms Capsule: 25 mg, 50 mg, 100 mg

**zopiclone** *(Canada only)* (ZOE pi clone)
   U.S./Canadian Brand Names Alti-Zopiclone [Can]; Apo-Zopiclone® [Can]; Gen-Zopiclone [Can]; Imovane® [Can]; Novo-Zopiclone [Can]; Nu-Zopiclone [Can]; PMS-Zopiclone [Can]; Rhovane® [Can]; Rhoxal-zopiclone [Can]
   Therapeutic Category Hypnotic
   Use Symptomatic relief of transient and short-term insomnia
   Usual Dosage Administer just before bedtime: Oral: Adults: 5-7.5 mg
      Patients with chronic respiratory insufficiency: 3.75 mg; may increase up to 7.5 mg with caution in appropriate cases
   Dosage Forms Tablet: 5 mg, 7.5 mg

**Zorbtive**™ **[US]** *see* somatropin *on page 760*

**ZORprin**® **[US]** *see* aspirin *on page 73*

**Zostrix**® **[US-OTC/Can]** *see* capsaicin *on page 138*

**Zostrix**®**-HP [US-OTC/Can]** *see* capsaicin *on page 138*

**Zosyn**® **[US]** *see* piperacillin and tazobactam sodium *on page 649*

**Zovia**™ **[US]** *see* ethinyl estradiol and ethynodiol diacetate *on page 310*

**Zovirax**® **[US/Can]** *see* acyclovir *on page 17*

**Ztuss**™ **Tablet [US]** *see* hydrocodone, pseudoephedrine, and guaifenesin *on page 415*

**zuclopenthixol acetate** *see* zuclopenthixol *(Canada only)* *on this page*

**zuclopenthixol** *(Canada only)* (zoo kloe pen THIX ol)
   Synonyms Z-chlopenthixol; zuclopenthixol acetate; zuclopenthixol decanoate; zuclopenthixol dihydro-chloride
   U.S./Canadian Brand Names Clopixol-Acuphase® [Can]; Clopixol® Depot [Can]; Clopixol® [Can]
   Therapeutic Category Antipsychotic Agent
   Use Management of schizophrenia; acetate injection is intended for short-term acute treatment; deca-noate injection is for long-term management; dihydrochloride tablets may be used in either phase
   Usual Dosage Adults:
      Oral: Zuclopenthixol dihydrochloride: Initial: 20-30 mg/day in 2-3 divided doses; usual maintenance dose: 20-40 mg/day; maximum daily dose: 100 mg
      I.M.:
         Zuclopenthixol acetate: 50-150 mg; may be repeated in 2-3 days; no more than 4 injections should be given in the course of treatment; maximum dose during course of treatment: 400 mg (maximum treatment period: 2 weeks)

Transfer of patients from I.M. acetate (Acuphase®) to oral (tablets):
50 mg = 20 mg daily
100 mg = 40 mg daily
150 mg = 60 mg daily
Zuclopenthixol decanoate: 100 mg by deep I.M. injection; additional I.M. doses of 100-200 mg may be given over the following 1-4 weeks; maximum weekly dose: 600 mg; usual maintenance dose: 150-300 mg every 2 weeks
Transfer of patients from oral (tablets) to I.M. decanoate (depot):
≤20 mg daily = 100 mg every 2 weeks
25-40 mg daily = 200 mg every 2 weeks
50-75 mg daily = 300 mg every 2 weeks
>75 mg/day = 400 mg every 2 weeks
Transfer of patients from I.M. acetate (Acuphase®) to I.M. decanoate (depot):
50 mg every 2-3 days = 100 mg every 2 weeks
100 mg every 2-3 days = 200 mg every 2 weeks
150 mg every 2-3 days = 300 mg every 2 weeks

**Dosage Forms**
Injection:
Clopixol Acuphase®, as acetate: 50 mg/mL [zuclopenthixol 42.5 mg/mL] (1 mL, 2 mL)
Clopixol® Depot, as decanoate: 200 mg/mL [zuclopenthixol 144.4 mg/mL] (10 mL)
Tablet, as dihydrochloride (Clopixol®): 10 mg, 25 mg, 40 mg

**zuclopenthixol decanoate** *see* zuclopenthixol *(Canada only)* on previous page

**zuclopenthixol dihydrochloride** *see* zuclopenthixol *(Canada only)* on previous page

**Zyban® [US/Can]** *see* bupropion on page 122

**Zydone® [US]** *see* hydrocodone and acetaminophen on page 411

**Zyloprim® [US/Can]** *see* allopurinol on page 28

**Zymar™ [US/Can]** *see* gatifloxacin on page 367

**Zymase® *(Discontinued)*** *see* pancrelipase on page 615

**Zyprexa® [US/Can]** *see* olanzapine on page 595

**Zyprexa® Zydis® [US/Can]** *see* olanzapine on page 595

**Zyrtec® [US]** *see* cetirizine on page 162

**Zyrtec-D 12 Hour™ [US]** *see* cetirizine and pseudoephedrine on page 163

**Zyvox™ [US]** *see* linezolid on page 483

**Zyvoxam® [Can]** *see* linezolid on page 483

# APPENDIX

# ABBREVIATIONS & SYMBOLS COMMONLY USED IN MEDICAL ORDERS

| Abbreviation | From | Meaning |
| --- | --- | --- |
| < | | less than |
| > | | greater than |
| ≤ | | less than or equal to |
| ≥ | | greater than or equal to |
| a̅a̅, aa | ana | of each |
| AA | | Alcoholics Anonymous |
| ABG | | arterial blood gases |
| ac | ante cibum | before meals or food |
| ACA | | Adult Children of Alcoholics |
| ACLS | | advanced cardiac life support |
| ad | ad | to, up to |
| a.d. | aurio dextra | right ear |
| ADHD | | attention-deficit/hyperactivity disorder |
| ADLs | | activities of daily living |
| ad lib | ad libitum | at pleasure |
| AIDS | | acquired immune deficiency syndrome |
| AIMS | | Abnormal Involuntary Movement Scale |
| a.l. | aurio laeva | left ear |
| ALS | | amyotrophic lateral sclerosis |
| AM | ante meridiem | morning |
| AMA | | against medical advice |
| amp | | ampul |
| amt | | amount |
| aq | aqua | water |
| aq. dest. | aqua destillata | distilled water |
| ARC | | AIDS-related complex |
| ARDS | | adult respiratory distress syndrome |
| ARF | | acute renal failure |
| a.s. | aurio sinister | left ear |
| ASAP | | as soon as possible |
| a.u. | aures utrae | each ear |
| AUC | | area under the curve |
| BDI | | Beck Depression Inventory |
| bid | bis in die | twice daily |
| BLS | | basic life support |
| bm | | bowel movement |
| BMI | | body mass index |
| bp | | blood pressure |
| BPH | | benign prostatic hyperplasia |
| BPRS | | Brief Psychiatric Rating Scale |
| BSA | | body surface area |
| c | cong | a gallon |
| c̄ | cum | with |
| CA | | cancer |
| CABG | | coronary artery bypass graft |
| CAD | | coronary artery disease |
| cal | | calorie |
| cap | capsula | capsule |
| CBT | | cognitive behavioral therapy |
| cc | | cubic centimeter |
| CCL | | creatinine clearance |
| CF | | cystic fibrosis |
| CGI | | Clinical Global Impression |
| CIE | | chemotherapy-induced emesis |
| CIV | | continuous I.V. infusion |
| cm | | centimeter |
| CNS | | central nervous system |
| comp | compositus | compound |
| cont | | continue |
| COPD | | chronic obstructive pulmonary disease |
| CRF | | chronic renal failure |
| CT | | computed tomography |

*(continued)*

| Abbreviation | From | Meaning |
| --- | --- | --- |
| d | dies | day |
| DBP | | diastolic blood pressure |
| d/c | | discontinue |
| dil | dilue | dilute |
| disp | dispensa | dispense |
| div | divide | divide |
| DOE | | dyspnea on exertion |
| DSM-IV | | Diagnostic and Statistical Manual |
| DTs | | delirium tremens |
| dtd | dentur tales doses | give of such a dose |
| DVT | | deep vein thrombosis |
| Dx | | diagnosis |
| ECG | | electrocardiogram |
| ECT | | electroconvulsive therapy |
| EEG | | electroencephalogram |
| elix, el | elixir | elixir |
| emp | | as directed |
| EPS | | extrapyramidal side effects |
| ESRD | | end stage renal disease |
| et | et | and |
| EtOH | | alcohol |
| ex aq | | in water |
| f, ft | fac, fiat, fiant | make, let be made |
| FDA | | Food and Drug Administration |
| FMS | | fibromyalgia syndrome |
| g | gramma | gram |
| GA | | Gamblers Anonymous |
| GABA | | gamma-aminobutyric acid |
| GAD | | generalized anxiety disorder |
| GAF | | Global Assessment of Functioning Scale |
| GERD | | gastroesophageal reflux disease |
| GFR | | glomerular filtration rate |
| GITS | | gastrointestinal therapeutic system |
| gr | granum | grain |
| gtt | gutta | a drop |
| GVHD | | graft versus host disease |
| h | hora | hour |
| HAM-A | | Hamilton Anxiety Scale |
| HAM-D | | Hamilton Depression Scale |
| hs | hora somni | at bedtime |
| HSV | | herpes simplex virus |
| HTN | | hypertension |
| IBD | | inflammatory bowel disease |
| IBS | | irritable bowel syndrome |
| ICH | | intracranial hemorrhage |
| IHSS | | idiopathic hypertrophic subaortic stenosis |
| I.M. | | intramuscular |
| IOP | | intraocular pressure |
| IU | | international unit |
| I.V. | | intravenous |
| kcal | | kilocalorie |
| kg | | kilogram |
| KIU | | kallikrein inhibitor unit |
| L | | liter |
| LAMM | | L-$\alpha$-acetyl methadol |
| liq | liquor | a liquor, solution |
| LVH | | left ventricular hypertrophy |
| M | misce | mix; Molar |
| MADRS | | Montgomery Asbery Depression Rating Scale |
| MAOIs | | monoamine oxidase inhibitors |
| mcg | | microgram |
| MDEA | | 3.4-methylene-dioxy amphetamine |
| m. dict | more dictor | as directed |
| MDMA | | 3,4-methylene-dioxy methamphetamine |
| mEq | | milliequivalent |

| Abbreviation | From | Meaning |
|---|---|---|
| mg | | milligram |
| mixt | mixtura | a mixture |
| mL | | milliliter |
| mm | | millimeter |
| mM | | millimolar |
| MMSE | | Mini-Mental State Examination |
| MPPP | | l-methyl-4-proprionoxy-4-phenyl pyridine |
| MR | | mental retardation |
| MRI | | magnetic resonance image |
| MS | | multiple sclerosis |
| NF | | National Formulary |
| NKA | | no known allergies |
| NMS | | neuroleptic malignant syndrome |
| no. | numerus | number |
| noc | nocturnal | in the night |
| non rep | non repetatur | do not repeat, no refills |
| NPO | | nothing by mouth |
| NSAID | | nonsteroidal antiinflammatory drug |
| NV | | nausea and vomiting |
| O, Oct | octarius | a pint |
| OA | | osteoarthritis |
| OCD | | obsessive-compulsive disorder |
| o.d. | oculus dexter | right eye |
| o.l. | oculus laevus | left eye |
| o.s. | oculus sinister | left eye |
| o.u. | oculo uterque | each eye |
| PANSS | | Positive and Negative Symptom Scale |
| PAT | | paroxysmal artrial tachycardia |
| pc, post cib | post cibos | after meals |
| PCP | | phencyclidine |
| PD | | Parkinson disease |
| PE | | pulmonary embolus |
| per | | through or by |
| PID | | pelvic inflammatory disease |
| PM | post meridiem | afternoon or evening |
| P.O. | per os | by mouth |
| PONV | | postoperative nausea and vomiting |
| P.R. | per rectum | rectally |
| prn | pro re nata | as needed |
| PSVT | | paroxysmal supraventricular tachycardia |
| PTA | | prior to admission |
| PTSD | | post-traumatic stress disorder |
| PUD | | peptic ulcer disease |
| pulv | pulvis | a powder |
| PVD | | peripheral vascular disease |
| q | | every |
| qad | quoque alternis die | every other day |
| qd | | every day, daily |
| qh | quiaque hora | every hour |
| qid | quater in die | four times a day |
| qod | | every other day |
| qs | quantum sufficiat | a sufficient quantity |
| qs ad | | a sufficient quantity to make |
| qty | | quantity |
| qv | quam volueris | as much as you wish |
| RA | | rheumatoid arthritis |
| REM | | rapid eye movement |
| Rx | recipe | take, a recipe |
| rep | repetatur | let it be repeated |
| s̄ | sine | without |
| sa | secundum artem | according to art |
| SAH | | subarachnoid hemorrhage |
| sat | sataratus | saturated |
| SBE | | subacute bacterial endocarditis |
| SBP | | systolic blood pressure |

*(continued)*

| Abbreviation | From | Meaning |
|---|---|---|
| SIADH | | syndrome of inappropriate antidiuretic hormone secretion |
| sig | signa | label, or let it be printed |
| SL | | sublingual |
| SLE | | systemic lupus erythematosus |
| SOB | | shortness of breath |
| sol | solutio | solution |
| solv | | dissolve |
| s̄s, ss | semis | one-half |
| sos | si opus sit | if there is need |
| SSKI | | saturated solution of potassium iodide |
| SSRIs | | selective serotonin reuptake inhibitors |
| stat | statim | at once, immediately |
| STD | | sexually transmitted disease |
| SubQ | | subcutaneous |
| supp | suppositorium | suppository |
| SVT | | supraventricular tachycardia |
| Sx | | symptom |
| syr | syrupus | syrup |
| tab | tabella | tablet |
| tal | | such |
| TCA | | tricyclic antidepressant |
| TD | | tardive dyskinesia |
| tid | ter in die | three times a day |
| TKO | | to keep open |
| TPN | | total parenteral nutrition |
| tr, tinct | tinctura | tincture |
| trit | | triturate |
| tsp | | teaspoonful |
| Tx | | treatment |
| u.d., ut dict | | as directed |
| ULN | | upper limits of normal |
| ung | unguentum | ointment |
| URI | | upper respiratory infection |
| USAN | | United States Adopted Names |
| USP | | United States Pharmacopeia |
| UTI | | urinary tract infection |
| v.o. | | verbal order |
| VTE | | venous thromboembolism |
| VZV | | varicella zoster virus |
| w.a. | | while awake |
| x3 | | 3 times |
| x4 | | 4 times |
| YBOC | | Yale Brown Obsessive-Compulsive Scale |
| YMRS | | Young Mania Rating Scale |

# NORMAL LABORATORY VALUES FOR ADULTS

## Automated Chemistry (CHEMISTRY A)

| Test | Values | Remarks |
|------|--------|---------|
| **SERUM / PLASMA** | | |
| Acetone | Negative | |
| Albumin | 3.2-5 g/dL | |
| Alcohol, ethyl | Negative | |
| Aldolase | 1.2-7.6 IU/L | |
| Ammonia | 20-70 mcg/dL | Specimen to be placed on ice as soon as collected |
| Amylase | 30-110 units/L | |
| Bilirubin, direct | 0-0.3 mg/dL | |
| Bilirubin, total | 0.1-1.2 mg/dL | |
| Calcium | 8.6-10.3 mg/dL | |
| Calcium, ionized | 2.24-2.46 mEq/L | |
| Chloride | 95-108 mEq/L | |
| Cholesterol, total | ≤200 mg/dL | Fasted blood required --- normal value affected by dietary habits<br>This reference range is for a general adult population |
|    HDL cholesterol | 40-60 mg/dL | Fasted blood required --- normal value affected by dietary habits |
|    LDL cholesterol | <160 mg/dL | If triglyceride is >400 mg/dL, LDL cannot be calculated accurately (Friedewald equation). Target LDL-C depends on patient's risk factors. |
| $CO_2$ | 23-30 mEq/L | |
| Creatine kinase (CK) isoenzymes | | |
|    CK-BB | 0% | |
|    CK-MB (cardiac) | 0%-3.9% | |
|    CK-MM (muscle) | 96%-100% | |

CK-MB levels must be both ≥4% and 10 IU/L to meet diagnostic criteria for CK-MB positive result consistent with myocardial injury.

| Test | Values | Remarks |
|------|--------|---------|
| Creatine phosphokinase (CPK) | 8-150 IU/L | |
| Creatinine | 0.5-1.4 mg/dL | |
| Ferritin | 13-300 ng/mL | |
| Folate | 3.6-20 ng/dL | |
| GGT (gamma-glutamyltranspeptidase) | | |
|    male | 11-63 IU/L | |
|    female | 8-35 IU/L | |
| GLDH | To be determined | |
| Glucose (preprandial) | <115 mg/dL | Goals different for diabetics |
| Glucose, fasting | 60-110 mg/dL | Goals different for diabetics |
| Glucose, nonfasting (2-h postprandial) | <120 mg/dL | Goals different for diabetics |
| Hemoglobin $A_{1c}$ | <8 | |
| Hemoglobin, plasma free | <2.5 mg/100 mL | |
| Hemoglobin, total glycosolated (Hb $A_1$) | 4%-8% | |
| Iron | 65-150 mcg/dL | |
| Iron binding capacity, total (TIBC) | 250-420 mcg/dL | |
| Lactic acid | 0.7-2.1 mEq/L | Specimen to be kept on ice and sent to lab as soon as possible |
| Lactate dehydrogenase (LDH) | 56-194 IU/L | |
| Lactate dehydrogenase (LDH) isoenzymes | | |
|    $LD_1$ | 20%-34% | |
|    $LD_2$ | 29%-41% | |
|    $LD_3$ | 15%-25% | |
|    $LD_4$ | 1%-12% | |
|    $LD_5$ | 1%-15% | |

| Test | Values | Remarks |
|---|---|---|
| Flipped $LD_1/LD_2$ ratios (>1 may be consistent with myocardial injury) particularly when considered in combination with a recent CK-MB positive result | | |
| Lipase | 23-208 units/L | |
| Magnesium | 1.6-2.5 mg/dL | Increased by slight hemolysis |
| Osmolality | 289-308 mOsm/kg | |
| Phosphatase, alkaline | | |
|     adults 25-60 y | 33-131 IU/L | |
|     adults 61 y or older | 51-153 IU/L | |
|     infancy-adolescence | Values range up to 3-5 times higher than adults | |
| Phosphate, inorganic | 2.8-4.2 mg/dL | |
| Potassium | 3.5-5.2 mEq/L | Increased by slight hemolysis |
| Prealbumin | >15 mg/dL | |
| Protein, total | 6.5-7.9 g/dL | |
| SGOT (AST) | <35 IU/L (20-48) | |
| SGPT (ALT) (10-35) | <35 IU/L | |
| Sodium | 134-149 mEq/L | |
| Transferrin | >200 mg/dL | |
| Triglycerides | 45-155 mg/dL | Fasted blood required |
| Troponin I | <1.5 ng/mL | |
| Urea nitrogen (BUN) | 7-20 mg/dL | |
| Uric acid | | |
|     male | 2-8 mg/dL | |
|     female | 2-7.5 mg/dL | |

# APPENDIX

| Test | Values | Remarks |
|---|---|---|
| **CEREBROSPINAL FLUID** | | |
| Glucose | 50-70 mg/dL | |
| Protein | | |
| adults and children | 15-45 mg/dL | CSF obtained by lumbar puncture |
| newborn infants | 60-90 mg/dL | |

On CSF obtained by cisternal puncture: About 25 mg/dL

On CSF obtained by ventricular puncture: About 10 mg/dL

**Note:** Bloody specimen gives erroneously high value due to contamination with blood proteins

### URINE

**(24-hour specimen is required for all these tests unless specified)**

| Test | Values | Remarks |
|---|---|---|
| Amylase | 32-641 units/L | The value is in units/L and **not** calculated for total volume |
| Amylase, fluid (random samples) | | Interpretation of value left for physician, depends on the nature of fluid |
| Calcium | Depends upon dietary intake | |
| Creatine | | |
| male | 150 mg/24 h | Higher value on children and during pregnancy |
| female | 250 mg/24 h | |
| Creatinine | 1000-2000 mg/24 h | |
| Creatinine clearance (endogenous) | | |
| male | 85-125 mL/min | A blood sample must accompany urine specimen |
| female | 75-115 mL/min | |
| Glucose | 1 g/24 h | |
| 5-hydroxyindoleacetic acid | 2-8 mg/24 h | |
| Iron | 0.15 mg/24 h | Acid washed container required |
| Magnesium | 146-209 mg/24 h | |
| Osmolality | 500-800 mOsm/kg | With normal fluid intake |
| Oxalate | 10-40 mg/24 h | |
| Phosphate | 400-1300 mg/24 h | |
| Potassium | 25-120 mEq/24 h | Varies with diet; the interpretation of urine electrolytes and osmolality should be left for the physician |
| Sodium | 40-220 mEq/24 h | |
| Porphobilinogen, qualitative | Negative | |
| Porphyrins, qualitative | Negative | |
| Proteins | 0.05-0.1 g/24 h | |
| Salicylate | Negative | |
| Urea clearance | 60-95 mL/min | A blood sample must accompany specimen |
| Urea N | 10-40 g/24 h | Dependent on protein intake |
| Uric acid | 250-750 mg/24 h | Dependent on diet and therapy |
| Urobilinogen | 0.5-3.5 mg/24 h | For qualitative determination on random urine, send sample to urinalysis section in Hematology Lab |
| Xylose absorption test | | |
| children | 16%-33% of ingested xylose | |
| **FECES** | | |
| Fat, 3-day collection | <5 g/d | Value depends on fat intake of 100 g/d for 3 days preceding and during collection |
| **GASTRIC ACIDITY** | | |
| Acidity, total, 12 h | 10-60 mEq/L | Titrated at pH 7 |

## BLOOD GASES

|  | Arterial | Capillary | Venous |
|---|---|---|---|
| pH | 7.35-7.45 | 7.35-7.45 | 7.32-7.42 |
| $pCO_2$ (mm Hg) | 35-45 | 35-45 | 38-52 |
| $pO_2$ (mm Hg) | 70-100 | 60-80 | 24-48 |
| $HCO_3$ (mEq/L) | 19-25 | 19-25 | 19-25 |
| $TCO_2$ (mEq/L) | 19-29 | 19-29 | 23-33 |
| $O_2$ saturation (%) | 90-95 | 90-95 | 40-70 |
| Base excess (mEq/L) | -5 to +5 | -5 to +5 | -5 to +5 |

## HEMATOLOGY

### Complete Blood Count

| Age | Hgb (g/dL) | Hct (%) | MCV (fL) | MCH (pg) | MCHC (%) | RBC (mill/mm$^3$) | RDW | PLTS (x 10$^3$/mm$^3$) |
|---|---|---|---|---|---|---|---|---|
| 0-3 d | 15.0-20.0 | 45-61 | 95-115 | 31-37 | 29-37 | 4.0-5.9 | <18.0 | 250-450 |
| 1-2 wk | 12.5-18.5 | 39-57 | 86-110 | 28-36 | 28-38 | 3.6-5.5 | <17.0 | 250-450 |
| 1-6 mo | 10.0-13.0 | 29-42 | 74-96 | 25-35 | 30-36 | 3.1-4.3 | <16.5 | 300-700 |
| 7 mo - 2 y | 10.5-13.0 | 33-38 | 70-84 | 23-30 | 31-37 | 3.7-4.9 | <16.0 | 250-600 |
| 2-5 y | 11.5-13.0 | 34-39 | 75-87 | 24-30 | 31-37 | 3.9-5.0 | <15.0 | 250-550 |
| 5-8 y | 11.5-14.5 | 35-42 | 77-95 | 25-33 | 31-37 | 4.0-4.9 | <15.0 | 250-550 |
| 13-18 y | 12.0-15.2 | 36-47 | 78-96 | 25-35 | 31-37 | 4.5-5.1 | <14.5 | 150-450 |
| Adult male | 13.5-16.5 | 41-50 | 80-100 | 26-34 | 31-37 | 4.5-5.5 | <14.5 | 150-450 |
| Adult female | 12.0-15.0 | 36-44 | 80-100 | 26-34 | 31-37 | 4.0-4.9 | <14.5 | 150-450 |

## WBC and Diff

| Age | WBC (x 10$^3$/mm$^3$) | Segs | Bands | Eos | Basos | Lymphs | Atypical Lymphs | Monos | # of NRBCs |
|---|---|---|---|---|---|---|---|---|---|
| 0-3 d | 9.0-35.0 | 32-62 | 10-18 | 0-2 | 0-1 | 19-29 | 0-8 | 5-7 | 0-2 |
| 1-2 wk | 5.0-20.0 | 14-34 | 6-14 | 0-2 | 0-1 | 36-45 | 0-8 | 6-10 | 0 |
| 1-6 mo | 6.0-17.5 | 13-33 | 4-12 | 0-3 | 0-1 | 41-71 | 0-8 | 4-7 | 0 |
| 7 mo - 2 y | 6.0-17.0 | 15-35 | 5-11 | 0-3 | 0-1 | 45-76 | 0-8 | 3-6 | 0 |
| 2-5 y | 5.5-15.5 | 23-45 | 5-11 | 0-3 | 0-1 | 35-65 | 0-8 | 3-6 | 0 |
| 5-8 y | 5.0-14.5 | 32-54 | 5-11 | 0-3 | 0-1 | 28-48 | 0-8 | 3-6 | 0 |
| 13-18 y | 4.5-13.0 | 34-64 | 5-11 | 0-3 | 0-1 | 25-45 | 0-8 | 3-6 | 0 |
| Adults | 4.5-11.0 | 35-66 | 5-11 | 0-3 | 0-1 | 24-44 | 0-8 | 3-6 | 0 |

## Erythrocyte Sedimentation Rates and Reticulocyte Counts

Sedimentation rate, Westergren

| | |
|---|---|
| Children | 0-20 mm/hour |
| Adult male | 0-15 mm/hour |
| Adult female | 0-20 mm/hour |

Sedimentation rate, Wintrobe

| | |
|---|---|
| Children | 0-13 mm/hour |
| Adult male | 0-10 mm/hour |
| Adult female | 0-15 mm/hour |

Reticulocyte count

| | |
|---|---|
| Newborns | 2%-6% |
| 1-6 mo | 0%-2.8% |
| Adults | 0.5%-1.5% |

# NORMAL LABORATORY VALUES FOR CHILDREN

| CHEMISTRY | | Normal Values |
|---|---|---|
| Albumin | 0-1 y | 2.0-4.0 g/dL |
| | 1 y - adult | 3.5-5.5 g/dL |
| Ammonia | Newborns | 90-150 mcg/dL |
| | Children | 40-120 mcg/dL |
| | Adults | 18-54 mcg/dL |
| Amylase | Newborns | 0-60 units/L |
| | Adults | 30-110 units/L |
| Bilirubin, conjugated, direct | Newborns | <1.5 mg/dL |
| | 1 mo - adult | 0-0.5 mg/dL |
| Bilirubin, total | 0-3 d | 2.0-10.0 mg/dL |
| | 1 mo - adult | 0-1.5 mg/dL |
| Bilirubin, unconjugated, indirect | | 0.6-10.5 mg/dL |
| Calcium | Newborns | 7.0-12.0 mg/dL |
| | 0-2 y | 8.8-11.2 mg/dL |
| | 2 y - adult | 9.0-11.0 mg/dL |
| Calcium, ionized, whole blood | | 4.4-5.4 mg/dL |
| Carbon dioxide, total | | 23-33 mEq/L |
| Chloride | | 95-105 mEq/L |
| Cholesterol | Newborns | 45-170 mg/dL |
| | 0-1 y | 65-175 mg/dL |
| | 1-20 y | 120-230 mg/dL |
| Creatinine | 0-1 y | ≤0.6 mg/dL |
| | 1 y - adult | 0.5-1.5 mg/dL |
| Glucose | Newborns | 30-90 mg/dL |
| | 0-2 y | 60-105 mg/dL |
| | Children to Adults | 70-110 mg/dL |
| Iron | Newborns | 110-270 mcg/dL |
| | Infants | 30-70 mcg/dL |
| | Children | 55-120 mcg/dL |
| | Adults | 70-180 mcg/dL |
| Iron binding | Newborns | 59-175 mcg/dL |
| | Infants | 100-400 mcg/dL |
| | Adults | 250-400 mcg/dL |
| Lactic acid, lactate | | 2-20 mg/dL |
| Lead, whole blood | | <10 mcg/dL |
| Lipase | Children | 20-140 units/L |
| | Adults | 0-190 units/L |
| Magnesium | | 1.5-2.5 mEq/L |
| Osmolality. serum | | 275-296 mOsm/kg |
| Osmolality, urine | | 50-1400 mOsm/kg |

| CHEMISTRY | | Normal Values |
|---|---|---|
| Phosphorus | Newborns | 4.2-9.0 mg/dL |
| | 6 wk to 19 mo | 3.8-6.7 mg/dL |
| | 19 mo to 3 y | 2.9-5.9 mg/dL |
| | 3-15 y | 3.6-5.6 mg/dL |
| | >15 y | 2.5-5.0 mg/dL |
| Potassium, plasma | Newborns | 4.5-7.2 mEq/L |
| | 2 d - 3 mo | 4.0-6.2 mEq/L |
| | 3 mo - 1 y | 3.7-5.6 mEq/L |
| | 1-16 y | 3.5-5.0 mEq/L |
| Protein, total | 0-2 y | 4.2-7.4 g/dL |
| | >2 y | 6.0-8.0 g/dL |
| Sodium | | 136-145 mEq/L |
| Triglycerides | Infants | 0-171 mg/dL |
| | Children | 20-130 mg/dL |
| | Adults | 30-200 mg/dL |
| Urea nitrogen, blood | 0-2 y | 4-15 mg/dL |
| | 2 y - adult | 5-20 mg/dL |
| Uric acid | Male | 3.0-7.0 mg/dL |
| | Female | 2.0-6.0 mg/dL |

## ENZYMES

| | | |
|---|---|---|
| Alanine aminotransferase (ALT) (SGPT) | 0-2 mo | 8-78 units/L |
| | >2 mo | 8-36 units/L |
| Alkaline phosphatase (ALKP) | Newborns | 60-130 units/L |
| | 0-16 y | 85-400 units/L |
| | >16 y | 30-115 units/L |
| Aspartate aminotransferase (AST) (SGOT) | Infants | 18-74 units/L |
| | Children | 15-46 units/L |
| | Adults | 5-35 units/L |
| Creatine kinase (CK) | Infants | 20-200 units/L |
| | Children | 10-90 units/L |
| | Adult Male | 0-206 units/L |
| | Adult Female | 0-175 units/L |
| Lactate dehydrogenase (LDH) | Newborns | 290-501 units/L |
| | 1 mo - 2 y | 110-144 units/L |
| | >16 y | 60-170 units/L |

## THYROID FUNCTION TESTS

| | | |
|---|---|---|
| $T_4$ (thyroxine) | 1-7 d | 10.1-20.9 mcg/dL |
| | 8-14 d | 9.8-16.6 mcg/dL |
| | 1 mo - 1 y | 5.5-16.0 mcg/dL |
| | >1 y | 4.0-12.0 mcg/dL |
| FTI | 1-3 d | 9.3-26.6 |
| | 1-4 wk | 7.6-20.8 |
| | 1-4 mo | 7.4-17.9 |
| | 4-12 mo | 5.1-14.5 |
| | 1-6 y | 5.7-13.3 |
| | >6 y | 4.8-14.0 |
| $T_3$ by RIA | Newborns | 100-470 ng/dL |
| | 1-5 y | 100-260 ng/dL |
| | 5-10 y | 90-240 ng/dL |
| | 10 y - adult | 70-210 ng/dL |
| $T_3$ uptake | | 35%-45% |
| TSH | Cord | 3-22 µIU/mL |
| | 1-3 d | <40 µIU/mL |
| | 3-7 d | <25 µIU/mL |
| | >7 d | 0-10 µIU/mL |

# APOTHECARY/METRIC CONVERSIONS

## Approximate Liquid Measures

Basic equivalent: 1 fluid ounce = 30 mL

Examples:

| | | | |
|---|---|---|---|
| 1 gallon | 3800 mL | 4 fluid oz | 120 mL |
| 1 quart | 960 mL | 15 minims | 1 mL |
| 1 pint | 480 mL | 10 minims | 0.6 mL |
| 8 fluid oz | 240 mL | | |

| | |
|---|---|
| 1 gallon | 128 fluid ounces |
| 1 quart | 32 fluid ounces |
| 1 pint | 16 fluid ounces |

## Approximate Household Equivalents

1 teaspoonful . . . . 5 mL          1 tablespoonful . . . 15 mL

## Weights

Basic equivalents:

1 oz = 30 g                    15 gr = 1 g

Examples:

| | | | |
|---|---|---|---|
| 4 oz | 120 g | 1 gr | 60 mg |
| 2 oz | 60 g | $1/100$ gr | 600 mcg |
| 10 gr | 600 mg | $1/150$ gr | 400 mcg |
| 7 $1/2$ gr | 500 mg | $1/200$ gr | 300 mcg |
| 16 oz | 1 pound | | |

## Metric Conversions

Basic equivalents:

1 g . . . . . . . . 1000 mg          1 mg . . . . . . . . 1000 mcg

Examples:

| | | | |
|---|---|---|---|
| 5 g | 5000 mg | 5 mg | 5000 mcg |
| 0.5 g | 500 mg | 0.5 mg | 500 mcg |
| 0.05 g | 50 mg | 0.05 mg | 50 mcg |

## Exact Equivalents

| | |
|---|---|
| 1 g = 15.43 grains | 0.1 mg = $1/600$ gr |
| 1 milliliter (mL) = 16.23 minims | 0.12 mg = $1/500$ gr |
| 1 minim = 0.06 milliliter | 0.15 mg = $1/400$ gr |
| 1 gr = 64.8 milligrams | 0.2 mg = $1/300$ gr |
| 1 pint (pt) = 473.2 milliliters | 0.3 mg = $1/200$ gr |
| 1 oz = 28.35 grams | 0.4 mg = $1/150$ gr |
| 1 lb = 453.6 grams | 0.5 mg = $1/120$ gr |
| 1 kg = 2.2 pounds | 0.6 mg = $1/100$ gr |
| 1 qt = 946.4 milliliters | 0.8 mg = $1/80$ gr |
| | 1 mg = $1/65$ gr |

## Solids*

$1/4$ grain = 15 mg
$1/2$ grain = 30 mg
1 grain = 60 mg
$1 1/2$ grains = 90 mg
5 grains = 300 mg
10 grains = 600 mg

*Use exact equivalents for compounding and calculations requiring a high degree of accuracy.

## POUNDS/KILOGRAMS CONVERSION

**1 pound = 0.45359 kilograms**
**1 kilogram = 2.2 pounds**

| lb | = | kg | lb | = | kg | lb | = | kg |
|---|---|---|---|---|---|---|---|---|
| 1 | | 0.45 | 70 | | 31.75 | 140 | | 63.50 |
| 5 | | 2.27 | 75 | | 34.02 | 145 | | 65.77 |
| 10 | | 4.54 | 80 | | 36.29 | 150 | | 68.04 |
| 15 | | 6.80 | 85 | | 38.56 | 155 | | 70.31 |
| 20 | | 9.07 | 90 | | 40.82 | 160 | | 72.58 |
| 25 | | 11.34 | 95 | | 43.09 | 165 | | 74.84 |
| 30 | | 13.61 | 100 | | 45.36 | 170 | | 77.11 |
| 35 | | 15.88 | 105 | | 47.63 | 175 | | 79.38 |
| 40 | | 18.14 | 110 | | 49.90 | 180 | | 81.65 |
| 45 | | 20.41 | 115 | | 52.16 | 185 | | 83.92 |
| 50 | | 22.68 | 120 | | 54.43 | 190 | | 86.18 |
| 55 | | 24.95 | 125 | | 56.70 | 195 | | 88.45 |
| 60 | | 27.22 | 130 | | 58.91 | 200 | | 90.72 |
| 65 | | 29.48 | 135 | | 61.24 | | | |

## TEMPERATURE CONVERSION

**Centigrade to Fahrenheit = ($°C \times 9/5$) + 32 = $°F$**
**Fahrenheit to Centigrade = ($°F - 32$) x 5/9 = $°C$**

| °C | = | °F | °C | = | °F | °C | = | °F |
|---|---|---|---|---|---|---|---|---|
| 100.0 | | 212.0 | 39.0 | | 102.2 | 36.8 | | 98.2 |
| 50.0 | | 122.0 | 38.8 | | 101.8 | 36.6 | | 97.9 |
| 41.0 | | 105.8 | 38.6 | | 101.5 | 36.4 | | 97.5 |
| 40.8 | | 105.4 | 38.4 | | 101.1 | 36.2 | | 97.2 |
| 40.6 | | 105.1 | 38.2 | | 100.8 | 36.0 | | 96.8 |
| 40.4 | | 104.7 | 38.0 | | 100.4 | 35.8 | | 96.4 |
| 40.2 | | 104.4 | 37.8 | | 100.1 | 35.6 | | 96.1 |
| 40.0 | | 104.0 | 37.6 | | 99.7 | 35.4 | | 95.7 |
| 39.8 | | 103.6 | 37.4 | | 99.3 | 35.2 | | 95.4 |
| 39.6 | | 103.3 | 37.2 | | 99.0 | 35.0 | | 95.0 |
| 39.4 | | 102.9 | 37.0 | | 98.6 | 0 | | 32.0 |
| 39.2 | | 102.6 | | | | | | |

# ACQUIRED IMMUNODEFICIENCY SYNDROME (AIDS) — LAB TESTS AND APPROVED DRUGS FOR HIV INFECTION AND AIDS-RELATED CONDITIONS

This list of tests is not intended in any way to suggest patterns of physician's orders, nor is it complete. These tests may support possible clinical diagnoses or rule out other diagnostic possibilities. Each laboratory test relevant to AIDS is listed and weighted. Two symbols (**) indicate that the test is diagnostic, that is, documents the diagnosis if the expected is found. A single symbol (*) indicates a test frequently used in the diagnosis or management of the disease. The other listed tests are useful on a selective basis with consideration of clinical factors and specific aspects of the case.

Acid-Fast Stain
Acid-Fast Stain, Modified, *Nocardia* Species
Antimicrobial Susceptibility Testing, Fungi
Antimicrobial Susceptibility Testing, Mycobacteria
Arthropod Identification
Babesiosis Serological Test
Bacteremia Detection, Buffy Coat Micromethod
Bacterial Culture, Blood
Bacterial Culture, Bronchoscopy Specimen
Bacterial Culture, Sputum
Bacterial Culture, Stool
Bacterial Culture, Throat
Bacterial Culture, Urine, Clean Catch
Beta$_2$-Microglobulin
Blood and Fluid Precautions, Specimen Collection
Bronchial Washings Cytology
Bronchoalveolar Lavage Cytology
Brushings Cytology
*Candida* Antigen
Candidiasis Serologic Test
Cat Scratch Disease Serology
CD4/CD8 Enumeration
Cerebrospinal Fluid Cytology
Cryptococcal Antigen Titer
*Cryptosporidium* Diagnostic Procedures
Cytomegalic Inclusion Disease Cytology
Cytomegalovirus Antibody
Cytomegalovirus Antigen Detection
Cytomegalovirus Culture
Cytomegalovirus DNA Detection
Darkfield Examination, Syphilis
Electron Microscopy
Folic Acid, Serum
Fungal Culture, Biopsy or Body Fluid
Fungal Culture, Blood
Fungal Culture, Cerebrospinal Fluid
Fungal Culture, Sputum
Fungal Culture, Stool
Fungal Culture, Urine
Hemoglobin A$_2$
Hepatitis B Surface Antigen
Herpes Cytology
Herpes Simplex Virus Antigen Detection
Herpes Simplex Virus Culture
Histopathology
Histoplasmosis Antibody
Histoplasmosis Antigen
**HIV-1/HIV-2 Serology
HTLV-I/II Antibody
*Human Immunodeficiency Virus Culture
*Human Immunodeficiency Virus DNA Amplification

India Ink Preparation
Inhibitor, Lupus, Phospholipid Type
KOH Preparation
Leishmaniasis Serological Test
Leukocyte Immunophenotyping
Lymphocyte Transformation Test
Microsporidia Diagnostic Procedures
Mycobacteria by DNA Probe
Mycobacterial Culture, Biopsy or Body Fluid
Mycobacterial Culture, Cerebrospinal Fluid
Mycobacterial Culture, Cutaneous and Subcutaneous Tissue
Mycobacterial Culture, Sputum
Mycobacterial Culture, Stool
*Neisseria gonorrhoeae* Culture and Smear
*Nocardia* Culture
Ova and Parasites, Stool
*p24 Antigen
Platelet Count
*Pneumocystis carinii* Preparation
*Pneumocystis* Immunofluorescence
Polymerase Chain Reaction
Red Blood Cell Indices
Risks of Transfusion
Skin Biopsy
Sputum Cytology
Toxoplasmosis Serology
VDRL, Serum
Viral Culture
Viral Culture, Blood
Viral Culture, Body Fluid
Viral Culture, Central Nervous System Symptoms
Viral Culture, Dermatological Symptoms
Viral Culture, Tissue
Virus, Direct Detection by Fluorescent Antibody
White Blood Count

## CURRENTLY APPROVED ANTIRETROVIRAL DRUGS

### Fusion Protein Inhibitors
enfuvirtide (Fuzeon™)

### Non-Nucleoside Reverse Transcriptase Inhibitors (NNRTIs)
delavirdine (Rescriptor®)
efavirenz (Sustiva®)
nevirapine (Viramune®)

### Nucleoside/Nucleotide Reverse Transcriptase Inhibitors (NRTIs)
abacavir (Ziagen®)
abacavir and lamivudine (Epzicom™)
abacavir, lamivudine, and zidovudine (Trizivir®)
adefovir (Hepsera™)
didanosine (Videx®)
emtricitabine (Emtriva™)
emtricitabine and tenofovir (Truvada™)
entecavir (Baraclude™)
lamivudine (Epivir®)
stavudine (Zerit®)
zalcitabine (Hivid®)
zidovudine (Retrovir®)
zidovudine and lamivudine (Combivir®)

### Protease Inhibitors (PIs)
amprenavir (Agenerase®)
atazanavir (Reyataz™)
fosamprenavir (Lexiva™)
indinavir (Crixivan®)
lopinavir and ritonavir (Kaletra®)
nelfinavir (Viracept®)
ritonavir (Norvir®)
saquinavir (Fortovase®, Invirase®)
tipranavir (Aptivus®)

# DRUGS USED TO TREAT COMPLICATIONS OF HIV / AIDS

| Generic Name (Synonym) | Brand Name | Use |
|---|---|---|
| alitretinoin gel 0.1% | Panretin® Gel | AIDS-related Kaposi sarcoma |
| amphotericin B, lipid complex (ABLC) | Abelcet®, AmBisome® | Antifungal for aspergillosis |
| atovaquone | Mepron® | Antiprotozoal antibiotic used to treat and prevent *Pneumocystis carinii* pneumonia |
| azithromycin | Zithromax® | Antibiotic used to treat *Mycobacterium avium* |
| cidofovir | Vistide® | Antiviral used to treat cytomegalovirus (CMV) |
| clarithromycin (Cla) | Biaxin® | Antibiotic used to treat and prevent *Mycobacterium avium* |
| daunorubicin citrate (liposomal) | DaunoXome® | Chemotherapy for Kaposi sarcoma |
| doxorubicin (liposomal) | Doxil® | Chemotherapy for Kaposi sarcoma |
| dronabinol | Marinol® | Treat loss of appetite |
| epoetin alfa (erythropoietin, EPO) | Procrit®, Epogen® | Treat anemia related to AZT therapy |
| famciclovir | Famvir® | Antiviral used to treat herpes |
| fluconazole | Diflucan® | Antifungal used to treat candidiasis and cryptococcal meningitis |
| fomivirsen sodium injection | Vitravene™ intravitreal injection | Antiviral used to treat CMV retinitis |
| foscarnet | Foscavir® | Antiviral used to treat herpes and CMV retinitis |
| ganciclovir insert | Vitrasert® Implant | Antiviral used to treat CMV retinitis |
| ganciclovir (DHPG) | Cytovene® | Antiviral used to treat CMV retinitis |
| immune globulin, intravenous (IVIG) | Gamimune® N | Immune booster used to prevent bacterial infections in children |
| interferon alfa-2a (IFLrA, rIFN-A) | Roferon-A® | Treat Kaposi sarcoma and hepatitis C |
| interferon alfa-2b (INF-alpha 2) | Intron®-A | Treat Kaposi sarcoma and hepatitis C |
| itraconazole | Sporanox® | Antifungal used to treat blastomycosis, histoplasmosis, aspergillosis, and candidiasis |
| megestrol acetate | Megace® | Treat loss of appetite and weight |
| paclitaxel | Taxol® | Kaposi sarcoma |
| pentamidine | NebuPent® | Antiprotozoal antibiotic used to prevent *Pneumocystis carinii* pneumonia |
| rifabutin (ansamycin) | Mycobutin® | Antimycobacterial used to prevent *Mycobacterium avium* |
| human growth hormone (somatrem, somatropin) | Serostim® | Treat weight loss |
| sulfamethoxazole and trimethoprim (co-trimoxazole) | Bactrim™, Septra® | Antiprotozoal antibiotic used to treat and prevent *Pneumocystis carinii* pneumonia |
| trimetrexate glucuronate | Neutrexin® | Antiprotozoal antibiotic used to treat *Pneumocystis carinii* pneumonia |
| valganciclovir | Valcyte™ | Antiviral used to treat CMV retinitis |

# CHEMOTHERAPY REGIMENS

## 5 + 2

**Use:** Leukemia, acute myeloid (induction)
**Regimen:**

    Cytarabine: I.V.: 100-200 mg/m$^2$/day continuous infusion days 1-5
        [total dose/cycle = 500-1000 mg/m$^2$]
    **with**
    Daunorubicin: I.V.: 45 mg/m$^2$/day days 1 and 2  [total dose/cycle = 90 mg/m$^2$]
    **or**
    Mitoxantrone: I.V.: 12 mg/m$^2$/day days 1 and 2  [total dose/cycle = 24 mg/m$^2$]

## 7 + 3 (Daunorubicin)

**Use:** Leukemia, acute myeloid (induction)
**Regimen:**

    Cytarabine: I.V.: 100 mg/m$^2$/day continuous infusion days 1-7  [total dose/cycle = 700 mg/m$^2$]
    Daunorubicin: I.V.: 45 mg/m$^2$/day days 1-3 [total dose/cycle = 135 mg/m$^2$]
    Administer one cycle only

## 7 + 3 (Idarubicin)

**Use:** Leukemia, acute myeloid (induction)
**Regimen:**

    Cytarabine: I.V.: 100-200 mg/m$^2$/day continuous infusion days 1-7
        [total dose/cycle = 700-1400 mg/m$^2$]
    Idarubicin: I.V.: 12 mg/m$^2$/day days 1-3 [total dose/cycle = 36 mg/m$^2$]
    Administer one cycle only

## 7 + 3 (Mitoxantrone)

**Use:** Leukemia, acute myeloid (induction)
**Regimen:**

    Cytarabine: I.V.: 100-200 mg/m$^2$/day continuous infusion days 1-7
        [total dose/cycle = 700-1400 mg/m$^2$]
    Mitoxantrone: I.V.: 12 mg/m$^2$/day days 1-3  [total dose/cycle = 36 mg/m$^2$]
    Administer one cycle only

## 7 + 3 + 7

**Use:** Leukemia, acute myeloid
**Regimen:**

    Cytarabine: I.V.: 100 mg/m$^2$/day continuous infusion days 1-7  [total dose/cycle = 700 mg/m$^2$]
    Daunorubicin: I.V.: 50 mg/m$^2$/day days 1-3 [total dose/cycle = 150 mg/m$^2$]
    Etoposide: I.V.: 75 mg/m$^2$/day days 1-7 [total dose/cycle = 525 mg/m$^2$]
    Repeat cycle every 21 days; up to 3 cycles may be given based on individual response

# 8 in 1 (Brain Tumors)

**Use:** Brain tumors

**Regimen: Note:** Multiple variations are listed below.

### Variation 1:

Methylprednisolone: I.V.: 300 mg/m$^2$ every 6 hours day 1 (3 doses)
[total dose/cycle = 900 mg/m$^2$]

Vincristine: I.V.: 1.5 mg/m$^2$ (maximum 2 mg) day 1 [total dose/cycle = 1.5 mg/m$^2$]

Lomustine: Oral: 75 mg/m$^2$ day 1 [total dose/cycle = 75 mg/m$^2$]

Procarbazine: Oral: 75 mg/m$^2$ day 1; 1 hour after methylprednisolone and vincristine
[total dose/cycle = 75 mg/m$^2$]

Hydroxyurea: Oral: 3000 mg/m$^2$ day 1; 2 hours after methylprednisolone and vincristine
[total dose/cycle = 3000 mg/m$^2$]

Cisplatin: I.V.: 90 mg/m$^2$ day 1; 3 hours after methylprednisolone and vincristine
[total dose/cycle = 90 mg/m$^2$]

Cytarabine: I.V.: 300 mg/m$^2$ day 1; 9 hours after methylprednisolone and vincristine
[total dose/cycle = 300 mg/m$^2$]

Dacarbazine: I.V.: 150 mg/m$^2$ day 1; 12 hours after methylprednisolone and vincristine
[total dose/cycle = 150 mg/m$^2$]

Repeat cycle every 14 days

### Variation 2:

Methylprednisolone: I.V.: 300 mg/m$^2$ every 6 hours day 1 (3 doses)
[total dose/cycle = 900 mg/m$^2$]

Vincristine: I.V.: 1.5 mg/m$^2$ (maximum 2 mg) day 1 [total dose/cycle = 1.5 mg/m$^2$]

Lomustine: Oral: 75 mg/m$^2$ day 1 [total dose/cycle = 75 mg/m$^2$]

Procarbazine: Oral: 75 mg/m$^2$ day 1; 1 hour after methylprednisolone and vincristine
[total dose/cycle = 75 mg/m$^2$]

Hydroxyurea: Oral: 3000 mg/m$^2$ day 1; 2 hours after methylprednisolone and vincristine
[total dose/cycle = 3000 mg/m$^2$]

Cisplatin: I.V.: 60 mg/m$^2$ day 1; 3 hours after methylprednisolone and vincristine
[total dose/cycle = 60 mg/m$^2$]

Cytarabine: I.V.: 300 mg/m$^2$ day 1; 9 hours after methylprednisolone and vincristine
[total dose/cycle = 300 mg/m$^2$]

Cyclophosphamide: I.V.: 300 mg/m$^2$ day 1; 12 hours after methylprednisolone and vincristine
[total dose/cycle = 300 mg/m$^2$]

Repeat cycle every 14 days

# 8 in 1 (Retinoblastoma)

**Use:** Retinoblastoma

**Regimen:**

Vincristine: I.V.: 1.5 mg/m$^2$ day 1 [total dose/cycle = 1.5 mg/m$^2$]

Methylprednisolone: I.V.: 300 mg/m$^2$ day 1 [total dose/cycle = 300 mg/m$^2$]

Lomustine: Oral: 75 mg/m$^2$ day 1 [total dose/cycle = 75 mg/m$^2$]

Procarbazine: Oral: 75 mg/m$^2$ day 1 [total dose/cycle = 75 mg/m$^2$]

Hydroxyurea: Oral: 1500 mg/m$^2$ day 1 [total dose/cycle = 1500 mg/m$^2$]

Cisplatin: I.V.: 60 mg/m$^2$ day 1 [total dose/cycle = 60 mg/m$^2$]

Cytarabine: I.V.: 300 mg/m$^2$ day 1 [total dose/cycle = 300 mg/m$^2$]

Repeat cycle every 28 days

# AAV (DD)

**Use:** Wilms Tumor

**Regimen:**

Dactinomycin: I.V.: 15 mcg/kg/day days 1-5 of weeks 0, 13, 26, 39, 52, 65
[total dose/cycle = 450 mcg/kg]

Doxorubicin: I.V.: 20 mg/m$^2$/day days 1-3 of weeks 6, 19, 32, 45, 58
[total dose/cycle = 300 mg/m$^2$]

Vincristine: I.V.: 1.5 mg/m$^2$ day 1 of weeks 0-10, 13, 14, 26, 27, 39, 40, 52, 53, 65, 66
[total dose/cycle = 31.5 mg/m$^2$]

# ABVD
**Use:** Lymphoma, Hodgkin disease
**Regimen:**
Doxorubicin: I.V.: 25 mg/m$^2$/day days 1 and 15 [total dose/cycle = 50 mg/m$^2$]
Bleomycin: I.V.: 10 units/m$^2$/day days 1 and 15 [total dose/cycle = 20 units/m$^2$]
Vinblastine: I.V.: 6 mg/m$^2$/day days 1 and 15 [total dose/cycle = 12 mg/m$^2$]
Dacarbazine: I.V.: 375 mg/m$^2$/day days 1 and 15 [total dose/cycle = 750 mg/m$^2$]
Repeat cycle every 28 days

# AC
**Use:** Breast cancer
**Regimen: Note:** Multiple variations are listed below.
**Variation 1: AC (conventional):**
Doxorubicin: I.V.: 60 mg/m$^2$ day 1 [total dose/cycle = 60 mg/m$^2$]
Cyclophosphamide: I.V.: 600 mg/m$^2$ day 1 [total dose/cycle = 600 mg/m$^2$]
Repeat cycle every 21 days
**Variation 2: AC, Paclitaxel (conventional):**
Doxorubicin: I.V.: 60 mg/m$^2$ day 1 [total dose/cycle = 60 mg/m$^2$]
Cyclophosphamide: I.V.: 600 mg/m$^2$ day 1 [total dose/cycle = 60 mg/m$^2$]
Repeat cycle every 21 days for 4 cycles, then:
Paclitaxel: I.V.: 175 mg/m$^2$ day 1 [total dose/cycle = 175 mg/m$^2$]
Repeat cycle every 21 days for 4 cycles
**Variation 3: AC + Paclitaxel (dose dense):**
Doxorubicin: I.V.: 60 mg/m$^2$ day 1 [total dose/cycle = 60 mg/m$^2$]
Cyclophosphamide: I.V.: 600 mg/m$^2$ day 1 [total dose/cycle = 600 mg/m$^2$]
Filgrastim: SubQ: 5 mcg/kg for 7 days, beginning day 3 [total dose/cycle = 35-50 mcg/kg]
Repeat cycle every 14 days for 4 cycles
**then**
Paclitaxel: I.V.: 175 mg/m$^2$ day 1 [total dose/cycle = 175 mg/m$^2$]
Filgrastim: SubQ: 5 mcg/kg/day for 7 days, beginning day 3 [total dose/cycle = 350 mcg/kg]
Repeat cycle every 14 days for 4 cycles

# ACAV (J)
**Use:** Wilms tumor
**Regimen:**
Dactinomycin: I.V.: 15 mcg/kg/day days 1-5 of weeks 0, 13, 26, 39, 52, 65
[total dose/cycle = 450 mcg/kg]
Cyclophosphamide: I.V.: 10 mg/kg/day days 1-3 of weeks 0, 6, 13, 19, 26, 32, 39, 45, 52, 58, 65
[total dose/cycle = 330 mg/kg]
Doxorubicin: I.V.: 20 mg/m$^2$/day days 1-3 of weeks 6, 19, 32, 45, 58
[total dose/cycle = 300 mg/m$^2$]
Vincristine: I.V.: 1.5 mg/m$^2$ day 1 of weeks 0-10, 13, 14, 19, 20, 26, 27, 32, 33, 39, 40, 45, 52, 53, 56, 57, 65, 66
[total dose/cycle = 42 mg/m$^2$]

# AD
**Use:** Soft tissue sarcoma
**Regimen:**
Doxorubicin: I.V.: 60 mg/m$^2$/day day 1 [total dose/cycle = 60 mg/m$^2$]
Dacarbazine: I.V.: 250 mg/m$^2$ days 1-5 [total dose/cycle = 1250 mg/m$^2$]
Repeat cycle every 21 days

# AP
**Use:** Endometrial Cancer
**Regimen:**
Doxorubicin: I.V.: 60 mg/m$^2$ day 1 [total dose/cycle = 60 mg/m$^2$]
Cisplatin: I.V.: 60 mg/m$^2$ day 1 [total dose/cycle = 60 mg/m$^2$]
Repeat cycle every 21 days

## AV (EE)
**Use:** Wilms Tumor
**Regimen:**
Dactinomycin: I.V.: 15 mcg/kg/day days 1-5 of weeks 0, 5, 13, 26 [total dose/cycle = 300 mcg/kg]
Vincristine: I.V.: 1.5 mg/m$^2$/dose day 1 of weeks 0-10, 13, 14, 16, 17
[total dose/cycle = 22.5 mg/m$^2$]

## AV (K)
**Use:** Wilms tumor
**Regimen:**
Dactinomycin: I.V.: 15 mcg/kg/day days 1-5 of weeks 0, 5, 13, 22, 31, 40, 49, 58
[total dose/cycle = 600 mcg/kg]
Vincristine: I.V.: 1.5 mg/m$^2$/dose day 1 of weeks 0-10, 15-20, 24-29, 33-38, 42-47, 51-56, 60-65
[total dose/cycle = 70.5 mg/m$^2$]

## AV (L)
**Use:** Wilms tumor
**Regimen:**
Dactinomycin: I.V.: 15 mcg/kg/day days 1-5 of weeks 0 and 5 [total dose/cycle = 450 mcg/kg]
Vincristine: I.V.: 1.5 mg/m$^2$ day 1 of weeks 0-10 [total dose/cycle = 16.5 mg/m$^2$]

## AV (Wilms tumor)
**Use:** Wilms tumor
**Regimen:**
Dactinomycin: I.V.: 15 mcg/kg/day days 1-5 of weeks 0, 13, 26, 39, 52, 65
[total dose/cycle = 450 mcg/kg]
Vincristine: I.V.: 1.5 mg/m$^2$/dose day 1 of weeks 0-8, 13, 14, 26, 27, 39, 40, 52, 53, 65, 66
[total dose/cycle = 28.5 mg/m$^2$]

## AVD
**Use:** Wilms tumor
**Regimen:**
Dactinomycin: I.V.: 15 mcg/kg/day days 1-5 of weeks 0, 13, 26, 39, 52, 65
[total dose/cycle = 450 mcg/kg]
Doxorubicin: I.V.: 20 mg/m$^2$/day days 1-3 of weeks 6, 19, 32, 45, 58
[total dose/cycle = 300 mg/m$^2$]
Vincristine: I.V.: 1.5 mg/m$^2$ day 1 of weeks 0-8, 13, 14, 26, 27, 39, 40, 52, 53, 65, 66
[total dose/cycle = 28.5 mg/m$^2$]

## BEACOPP
**Use:** Lymphoma, Hodgkin disease
**Regimen:**
Bleomycin: I.V.: 10 units/m$^2$ day 8 [total dose/cycle = 10 units/m$^2$]
Etoposide: I.V.: 100 mg/m$^2$/day days 1-3 [total dose/cycle = 300 mg/m$^2$]
Doxorubicin: I.V.: 25 mg/m$^2$ day 1 [total dose/cycle = 25 mg/m$^2$]
Cyclophosphamide: I.V.: 650 mg/m$^2$ day 1 [total dose/cycle = 650 mg/m$^2$]
Vincristine: I.V.: 1.4 mg/m$^2$ (maximum 2 mg) day 1 [total dose/cycle = 1.4 mg/m$^2$]
Procarbazine: Oral: 100 mg/m$^2$/day days 1-7 [total dose/cycle = 700 mg/m$^2$]
Prednisone: Oral: 40 mg/m$^2$/day days 1-14 [total dose/cycle = 560 mg/m$^2$]
Repeat cycle every 21 days

## BEP (Ovarian)
**Use:** Ovarian cancer
**Regimen:**
Bleomycin: I.V.: 20 units/m$^2$ day 1 [total dose/cycle = 20 units/m$^2$]
Etoposide: I.V.: 75 mg/m$^2$/day days 1-5 [total dose/cycle = 375 mg/m$^2$]
Cisplatin: I.V.: 20 mg/m$^2$/day days 1-5 [total dose/cycle = 100 mg/m$^2$]
Repeat cycle every 3 weeks

## BEP (Ovarian, Testicular)

**Use:** Ovarian cancer; Testicular cancer
**Regimen:**

Bleomycin: I.V.: 30 units days 2, 9, 16  [total dose/cycle = 90 units]
Etoposide: I.V.: 100 mg/m$^2$/day days 1-5  [total dose/cycle = 500 mg/m$^2$]
**or** 120 mg/m$^2$/day days 1-3
Cisplatin: I.V.: 20 mg/m$^2$/day days 1-5  [total dose/cycle = 100 mg/m$^2$]
Repeat cycle every 21 days

## BEP (Testicular)

**Use:** Testicular cancer
**Regimen: Note:** Multiple variations are listed below.

**Variation 1:**
Bleomycin: I.V.: 30 units/day days 2, 9, 16  [total dose/cycle = 90 units]
Etoposide: I.V.: 100 mg/m$^2$/day days 1-5  [total dose/cycle = 500 mg/m$^2$]
Cisplatin: I.V.: 20 mg/m$^2$/day days 1-5  [total dose/cycle = 100 mg/m$^2$]
Repeat cycle every 21 days

**Variation 2:**
Bleomycin: I.V.: 30 units once weekly  [total dose/cycle = 90 units]
Etoposide: I.V.: 120 mg/m$^2$/day days 1, 3, 5  [total dose/cycle = 360 mg/m$^2$]
Cisplatin: I.V.: 20 mg/m$^2$/day days 1-5  [total dose/cycle = 100 mg/m$^2$]
Repeat cycle every 21 days

**Variation 3:**
Bleomycin: I.V.: 30 units/day days 1, 8, 15  [total dose/cycle = 90 units]
Etoposide: I.V.: 165 mg/m$^2$/day days 1-3  [total dose/cycle = 495 mg/m$^2$]
Cisplatin: I.V.: 50 mg/m$^2$/day days 1, 2  [total dose/cycle = 100 mg/m$^2$]
Repeat cycle every 21 days

## Bicalutamide + LHRH-A

**Use:** Prostate Cancer
**Regimen:**

Bicalutamide: Oral: 50 mg/day   [total dose/cycle = 50 mg] **with**
Goserelin acetate: SubQ: 3.6 mg day 1  [total dose/cycle = 3.6 mg] **or**
Leuprolide depot: I.M.: 7.5 mg day 1  [total dose/cycle = 7.5 mg]
Repeat cycle every 28 days

## BOLD

**Use:** Melanoma
**Regimen:**

Dacarbazine: I.V.: 200 mg/m$^2$/day days 1-5  [total dose/cycle = 1000 mg/m$^2$]
Vincristine: I.V.: 1 mg/m$^2$/day days 1 and 4  [total dose/cycle = 2 mg/m$^2$]
Bleomycin: I.V.: 15 units/day days 2 and 5  [total dose/cycle = 30 units]
Lomustine: Oral: 80 mg day 1  [total dose/cycle = 80 mg]
Repeat cycle every 4 weeks

## CA

**Use:** Leukemia, acute myeloid
**Regimen:**

Cytarabine: I.V.: 3000 mg/m$^2$ every 12 hours days 1 and 2 (4 doses)
[total dose/cycle = 12,000 mg/m$^2$]
Asparaginase: I.M.: 6000 units/m$^2$ at hour 42  [total dose/cycle = 6000 units/m$^2$]
Repeat cycle every 7 days for 2 or 3 cycles

# CABO
**Use:** Head and neck cancer
**Regimen:**
Cisplatin: I.V.: 50 mg/m$^2$ day 4  [total dose/cycle = 50 mg/m$^2$]
Methotrexate: I.V.: 40 mg/m$^2$/day days 1 and 15  [total dose/cycle = 80 mg/m$^2$]
Bleomycin: I.V.: 10 units/day days 1, 8, and 15  [total dose/cycle = 30 units]
Vincristine: I.V.: 2 mg/day days 1, 8, and 15  [total dose/cycle = 6 mg]
Repeat cycle every 21 days

# CAD/MOPP/ABV
**Use:** Lymphoma, Hodgkin disease
**Regimen:**
### CAD:
Lomustine: Oral: 100 mg/m$^2$ day 1  [total dose/cycle = 100 mg/m$^2$]
Melphalan: Oral: 6 mg/m$^2$/day days 1-4  [total dose/cycle = 24 mg/m$^2$]
Vindesine: I.V.: 3 mg/m$^2$/day days 1 and 8
### MOPP:
Mechlorethamine: I.V.: 6 mg/m$^2$/day days 1 and 8  [total dose/cycle = 12 mg/m$^2$]
Vincristine: I.V.: 1.4 mg/m$^2$/day days 1 and 8  [total dose/cycle = 2.8 mg/m$^2$]
Procarbazine: Oral: 100 mg/m$^2$/day days 1-14  [total dose/cycle = 1400 mg/m$^2$]
Prednisone: Oral: 40 mg/m$^2$/day days 1-14  [total dose/cycle = 560 mg/m$^2$]
### ABV:
Doxorubicin: I.V.: 25 mg/m$^2$/day days 1 and 14  [total dose/cycle = 50 mg/m$^2$]
Bleomycin: SubQ: 6 units/m$^2$/day days 1 and 14  [total dose/cycle = 12 units/m$^2$]
Vinblastine: I.V.: 2 mg/m$^2$ continuous infusion days 4-12 and 18-26
CAD is administered first, then MOPP begins on day 29 or day 37 following CAD. ABV is administered on day 29 following MOPP; CAD recycles on day 29 following ABV.

# CAF
**Use:** Breast cancer
**Regimen: Note:** Multiple variations are listed below.
### Variation 1:
Cyclophosphamide: Oral: 100 mg/m$^2$/day days 1-14  [total dose/cycle = 1400 mg/m$^2$]
Doxorubicin: I.V.: 30 mg/m$^2$/day days 1 and 8  [total dose/cycle = 60 mg/m$^2$]
Fluorouracil: I.V.: 500 mg/m$^2$/day days 1 and 8  [total dose/cycle = 1000 mg/m$^2$]
Repeat cycle every 28 days
### Variation 2:
Cyclophosphamide: Oral: 100 mg/m$^2$/day days 1-14  [total dose/cycle = 1400 mg/m$^2$]
Doxorubicin: I.V.: 25 mg/m$^2$/day days 1 and 8  [total dose/cycle = 50 mg/m$^2$]
Fluorouracil: I.V.: 500 mg/m$^2$/day days 1 and 8  [total dose/cycle = 1000 mg/m$^2$]
Repeat cycle every 28 days

# CAP
**Use:** Bladder Cancer
**Regimen:**
Cyclophosphamide: I.V.: 400 mg/m$^2$ day 1  [total dose = 400 mg/m$^2$]
Doxorubicin: I.V.: 40 mg/m$^2$ day 1  [total dose = 40 mg/m$^2$]
Cisplatin: I.V.: 60 mg/m$^2$ day 1  [total dose = 60 mg/m$^2$]
Repeat cycle every 21 days

# Carbo-Tax (Adenocarcinoma)
**Use:** Adenocarcinoma, unknown primary
**Regimen:**
Paclitaxel: I.V.: 135 mg/m$^2$ infused over 24 hours day 1  [total dose = 135 mg/m$^2$]
**followed by:**
Carboplatin: I.V.: Target AUC 7.5  [total dose = AUC = 7.5]
Repeat cycle every 21 days

# Carbo-Tax (Nonsmall Cell Lung Cancer)

**Use:** Lung cancer, nonsmall cell
**Regimen:**

Paclitaxel: I.V.: 135-215 mg/m$^2$ infused over 24 hours day 1  [total dose/cycle = 135-215 mg/m$^2$] **or** 175 mg/m$^2$ infused over 3 hours day 1  [total dose/cycle = 175 mg/m$^2$] **followed by:**
Carboplatin: I.V.: Target AUC 7.5  [total dose/cycle = AUC = 7.5]
Repeat cycle every 21 days

# Carbo-Tax (Ovarian Cancer)

**Use:** Ovarian cancer
**Regimen: Note:** Multiple variations are listed below.

**Variation 1:**
Paclitaxel: I.V.: 135 mg/m$^2$ infused over 24 hours day 1  [total dose/cycle = 135 mg/m$^2$] **or** 175 mg/m$^2$ over 3 hours day 1  [total dose/cycle = 175 mg/m$^2$]
**followed by:**
Carboplatin: I.V.: Target AUC 5  [total dose/cycle = AUC = 5]
Repeat cycle every 21 days
**Variation 2:**
Paclitaxel: I.V.: 175 mg/m$^2$ day 1  [total dose/cycle = 175 mg/m$^2$]
Carboplatin: I.V.: AUC 7.5 day 1  [total dose/cycle = AUC = 7.5]
Repeat cycle every 21 days
**Variation 3:**
Paclitaxel: I.V.: 185 mg/m$^2$ day 1  [total dose/cycle = 185 mg/m$^2$]
Carboplatin: I.V.: AUC 6 day 1  [total dose/cycle = AUC = 6]
Repeat cycle every 21 days

# CaT (Nonsmall Cell Lung Cancer)

**Use:** Lung cancer, nonsmall cell
**Regimen: Note:** Multiple variations are listed below.

**Variation 1:**
Paclitaxel: I.V.: 175 mg/m$^2$ day 1  [total dose/cycle = 175 mg/m$^2$] **or** 135 mg/m$^2$ continuous infusion day 1  [total dose/cycle = 135 mg/m$^2$]
Carboplatin: I.V.: AUC 7.5 day 1 or 2  [total dose/cycle = AUC = 7.5]
Repeat cycle every 21 days
**Variation 2:**
Paclitaxel: I.V.: 225 mg/m$^2$ day 1  [total dose/cycle = 225 mg/m$^2$]
Carboplatin: I.V.: AUC 6 day 1  [total dose/cycle = AUC = 6]
Repeat cycle every 21 days

# CaT (Ovarian Cancer)

**Use:** Ovarian cancer
**Regimen:**

Paclitaxel: I.V.: 175 mg/m$^2$ day 1  [total dose/cycle = 175 mg/m$^2$] **or** 135 mg/m$^2$ continuous infusion day 1  [total dose/cycle = 135 mg/m$^2$]
Carboplatin: I.V.: AUC 7.5 day 1 or 2  [total dose/cycle = AUC = 7.5]
Repeat cycle every 21 days

# CAVE

**Use:** Lung cancer, small cell
**Regimen:**

Cyclophosphamide: I.V.: 750 mg/m$^2$ day 1  [total dose/cycle = 750 mg/m$^2$]
Doxorubicin: I.V.: 50 mg/m$^2$ day 1  [total dose/cycle = 50 mg/m$^2$]
Vincristine: I.V.: 1.4 mg/m$^2$ (maximum 2 mg) day 1  [total dose/cycle = 1.4 mg/m$^2$]
Etoposide: I.V.: 60-100 mg/m$^2$/day days 1-3  [total dose/cycle = 180-300 mg/m$^2$]
Repeat cycle every 21 days

## CAV-P/VP
**Use:** Neuroblastomas
**Regimen:**

### Course 1, 2, 4, 6:
Cyclophosphamide: I.V.: 70 mg/kg/day days 1 and 2  [total dose/cycle = 140 mg/kg]
Doxorubicin: I.V.: 25 mg/m$^2$/day continuous infusion days 1-3  [total dose/cycle = 75 mg/m$^2$]
Vincristine: I.V.: 0.033 mg/kg/day continuous infusion days 1-3  [total dose/cycle = .099 mg/kg]
Vincristine: I.V.: 1.5 mg/m$^2$ day 9

### Course 3, 5, 7:
Etoposide: I.V.: 200 mg/m$^2$/day days 1-3  [total dose/cycle = 600 mg/m$^2$]
Cisplatin: I.V.: 50 mg/m$^2$/day days 1-4  [total dose/cycle = 200 mg/m$^2$]

## CC
**Use:** Ovarian cancer
**Regimen:**

Carboplatin: I.V.: Target AUC 5-7.5 day 1  [total dose/cycle = AUC = 5-7.5]
Cyclophosphamide: I.V.: 600 mg/m$^2$ day 1  [total dose/cycle = 600 mg/m$^2$]
Repeat cycle every 28 days

## CCCDE (Retinoblastoma)
**Use:** Retinoblastoma
**Regimen:**

Cyclophosphamide: I.V.: 150 mg/m$^2$/day days 1-7  [total dose/cycle = 1050 mg/m$^2$]
Cyclophosphamide: Oral: 150 mg/m$^2$/day days 22-28, 43-49  [total dose/cycle = 2100 mg/m$^2$]
Doxorubicin: I.V.: 35 mg/m$^2$/day days 10 and 52  [total dose/cycle = 70 mg/m$^2$]
Cisplatin: I.V.: 90 mg/m$^2$/day days 8, 50, 71  [total dose/cycle = 270 mg/m$^2$]
Etoposide: I.V.: 150 mg/m$^2$/day continuous infusion days 29-31, 73-75
    [total dose/cycle = 900 mg/m$^2$]

## CCDDT (Neuroblastomas)
**Use:** Neuroblastomas
**Regimen:**

Cyclophosphamide: I.V.: 40 mg/kg/day days 1 and 2  [total dose/cycle = 80 mg/kg]
Cisplatin: I.V.: 20 mg/m$^2$/day days 1-5  [total dose/cycle = 100 mg/m$^2$]
Teniposide: I.V.: 100 mg/m$^2$ day 7  [total dose/cycle = 100 mg/m$^2$]
Doxorubicin: I.V.: 60 mg/m$^2$ day 1  [total dose/cycle = 60 mg/m$^2$]
Dacarbazine: I.V.: 250 mg/m$^2$/day days 1-5  [total dose/cycle = 1250 mg/m$^2$]
Repeat cycle every 21-28 days

## CCDT (Melanoma)
**Use:** Melanoma
**Regimen:**

Dacarbazine: I.V.: 220 mg/m$^2$/day days 1-3, every 21-28 days  [total dose/cycle = 660 mg/m$^2$]
Carmustine: I.V.: 150 mg/m$^2$ day 1, every 42-56 days  [total dose/cycle = 150 mg/m$^2$]
Cisplatin: I.V.: 25 mg/m$^2$/day days 1-3, every 21-28 days  [total dose/cycle = 75 mg/m$^2$]
Tamoxifen: Oral: 20 mg/day (use of tamoxifen is optional)

## CCT (Neuroblastomas)
**Use:** Neuroblastomas
**Regimen:**

Cyclophosphamide: I.V.: 40 mg/kg/day days 1 and 2  [total dose/cycle = 80 mg/kg]
Cisplatin: I.V.: 20 mg/m$^2$/day days 22-26  [total dose/cycle = 100 mg/m$^2$]
Teniposide: I.V.: 100 mg/m$^2$ day 28  [total dose/cycle = 100 mg/m$^2$]
Repeat every 42 days for 3 cycles

## CD (Rhabdomyosarcoma)
**Use:** Rhabdomyosarcoma
**Regimen:**
Doxorubicin: I.V.: 35-60 mg/m$^2$ day 1
Cyclophosphamide: I.V.: 500-1500 mg/m$^2$ day 1
Repeat cycle every 21-28 days

## CDDP/VP-16
**Use:** Brain tumors
**Regimen:**
Cisplatin: I.V.: 90 mg/m$^2$ day 1  [total dose/cycle = 90 mg/m$^2$]
Etoposide: I.V.: 150 mg/m$^2$/day days 3 and 4  [total dose/cycle = 300 mg/m$^2$]
Repeat cycle every 21 days

## CE (Neuroblastomas)
**Use:** Neuroblastomas
**Regimen:**
Carboplatin: I.V.: 500 mg/m$^2$/day days 1 and 2  [total dose/cycle = 1000 mg/m$^2$]
Etoposide: I.V.: 100 mg/m$^2$/day days 1-3  [total dose/cycle = 300 mg/m$^2$]
Repeat cycle every 21-28 days

## CE (Retinoblastoma)
**Use:** Retinoblastoma
**Regimen:**
Etoposide: I.V.: 100 mg/m$^2$/day days 1-5  [total dose/cycle = 500 mg/m$^2$]
Carboplatin: I.V.: 160 mg/m$^2$/day days 1-5  [total dose/cycle = 800 mg/m$^2$]
Repeat cycle every 21 days

## CE-CAdO
**Use:** Neuroblastomas
**Regimen:**
Carboplatin: I.V.: 160 mg/m$^2$/day days 1-5  [total dose/cycle = 800 mg/m$^2$]
Etoposide: I.V.: 100 mg/m$^2$/day days 1-5  [total dose/cycle = 500 mg/m$^2$] **or**
Carboplatin: I.V.: 200 mg/m$^2$/day days 1-3  [total dose/cycle = 600 mg/m$^2$]
Etoposide: I.V.: 150 mg/m$^2$/day days 1-3  [total dose/cycle = 450 mg/m$^2$] **and**
Cyclophosphamide: I.V.: 300 mg/m$^2$/day days 1-5  [total dose/cycle = 1500 mg/m$^2$]
Doxorubicin: I.V.: 60 mg/m$^2$ day 5  [total dose/cycle = 60 mg/m$^2$]
Vincristine: I.V.: 1.5 mg/m$^2$/day days 1 and 5  [total dose/cycle = 3 mg/m$^2$]
Repeat cycle every 21 days

## CEF
**Use:** Breast cancer
**Regimen:**
Cyclophosphamide: Oral: 75 mg/m$^2$/day days 1-14  [total dose/cycle = 1050 mg/m$^2$]
Epirubicin: I.V.: 60 mg/m$^2$/day days 1 and 8  [total dose/cycle = 120 mg/m$^2$]
Fluorouracil: I.V.: 500 mg/m$^2$/day days 1 and 8  [total dose/cycle = 1000 mg/m$^2$]
Repeat cycle every 28 days

## CEPP(B)
**Use:** Lymphoma, non-Hodgkin
**Regimen:**
Cyclophosphamide: I.V.: 600-650 mg/m$^2$/day days 1-8  [total dose/cycle = 1200-1300 mg/m$^2$]
Etoposide: I.V.: 70-85 mg/m$^2$/day days 1-3   [total dose/cycle = 210-255 mg/m$^2$]
Procarbazine: Oral: 60 mg/m$^2$/day days 1-10  [total dose/cycle = 600 mg/m$^2$]
Prednisone: Oral: 60 mg/m$^2$/day days 1-10  [total dose/cycle = 600 mg/m$^2$]
Bleomycin: I.V.: 15 units/m$^2$/day days 1-15 (bleomycin is sometimes omitted)
    [total dose/cycle = 30 units/m$^2$]
Repeat cycle every 28 days

# CEV

**Use:** Rhabdomyosarcoma
**Regimen:**
Carboplatin: I.V.: 500 mg/m$^2$ day 1  [total dose/cycle = 500 mg/m$^2$]
Epirubicin: I.V.: 150 mg/m$^2$ day 1  [total dose/cycle = 150 mg/m$^2$]
Vincristine: I.V.: 1.5 mg/m$^2$/day days 1 and 7  [total dose/cycle = 3 mg/m$^2$]
Repeat cycle every 21 days

# CF

**Use:** Head and neck cancer
**Regimen:**
Cisplatin: I.V.: 100 mg/m$^2$ day 1  [total dose/cycle = 100 mg/m$^2$]
Fluorouracil: I.V.: 1000 mg/m$^2$/day continuous infusion days 1-4  [total dose/cycle = 4000 mg/m$^2$] **or**
Fluorouracil: I.V.: 1000 mg/m$^2$/day continuous infusion days 1-5  [total dose/cycle = 5000 mg/m$^2$]
Repeat cycle every 21-28 days

# CHAMOCA

**Use:** Gestational trophoblastic tumor
**Regimen:**
Hydroxyurea: Oral: 500 mg every 6 hours for 4 doses, day 1 (start at 6 AM)
[total dose/cycle = 2000 mg]
Dactinomycin: I.V.: 0.2 mg/day days 1-3 (give at 7 PM)  [total dose/cycle = 0.6 mg]
**followed by** 0.5 mg days 4 and 5 (give at 7 PM)  [total dose/cycle = 1 mg]
Cyclophosphamide: I.V.: 500 mg/m$^2$/day days 3 and 8 (give at 7 PM)
[total dose/cycle = 1000 mg/m$^2$]
Vincristine: I.V.: 1 mg/m$^2$ (maximum 2 mg) day 2 (give at 7 AM)  [total dose/cycle = 1 mg/m$^2$]
Methotrexate: I.V. push: 100 mg/m$^2$ day 2 (give at 7 PM)  [total dose/cycle = 100 mg/m$^2$]
**followed by** 200 mg/m$^2$ over 12 hours day 2  [total dose/cycle = 200 mg/m$^2$]
Leucovorin: I.M.: 14 mg/day every 6 hours for 6 doses days 3-5 (begin at 7 PM on day 3)
[total dose/cycle = 84 mg]
Doxorubicin: I.V.: 30 mg/m$^2$ day 8 (give at 7 PM)  [total dose/cycle = 30 mg/m$^2$]
Repeat cycle every 18 days or as toxicity permits

# ChIVPP

**Use:** Lymphoma, Hodgkin disease
**Regimen:**
Chlorambucil: Oral: 6 mg/m$^2$/day (maximum 10 mg) days 1-14  [total dose/cycle = 84 mg/m$^2$]
Vinblastine: I.V.: 6 mg/m$^2$/day (maximum 10 mg) days 1 and 8  [total dose/cycle = 12 mg/m$^2$]
Procarbazine: Oral: 100 mg/m$^2$/day (maximum 150 mg) days 1-14
[total dose/cycle = 1400 mg/m$^2$]
Prednisone: Oral: 40-50 mg/m$^2$/day days 1-14  [total dose/cycle = 560-700 mg]
Repeat cycle every 28 days

# CHL + PRED

**Use:** Leukemia, chronic lymphocytic
**Regimen:**
Chlorambucil: Oral: 0.4 mg/kg/day for 1 day every other week; increase initial dose of 0.4 mg/kg by 0.1 mg/kg every
2 weeks until toxicity or disease control is achieved
Prednisone: Oral: 100 mg/day for 2 days every other week

# CHOP

**Use:** Lymphoma, non-Hodgkin

**Regimen: Note:** Multiple variations are listed below.

**Variation 1:**

Cyclophosphamide: I.V.: 750 mg/m$^2$ day 1  [total dose/cycle = 750 mg/m$^2$]

Doxorubicin: I.V.: 50 mg/m$^2$ day 1  [total dose/cycle = 50 mg/m$^2$]

Vincristine: I.V.: 1.4 mg/m$^2$ (maximum 2 mg) day 1  [total dose/cycle = 1.4 mg/m$^2$]

Prednisone: Oral: 100 mg/day days 1-5  [total dose/cycle = 500 mg]

**or** 50 mg/m$^2$/day days 1-5  [total dose/cycle = 250 mg/m$^2$]

**or** 100 mg/m$^2$/day days 1-5  [total dose/cycle = 500 mg/m$^2$]

Repeat cycle every 21 days

**Variation 2:**

Cyclophosphamide: I.V.: 750 mg/m$^2$ day 1  [total dose/cycle = 750 mg/m$^2$]

Doxorubicin: I.V.: 50 mg/m$^2$ day 1  [total dose/cycle = 50 mg/m$^2$]

Vincristine: I.V.: 2 mg day 1  [total dose/cycle = 2 mg]

Prednisone: Oral: 75 mg/day days 1-5  [total dose/cycle = 375 mg]

Repeat cycle every 21 days

**Variation 3:**

Cyclophosphamide: I.V.: 750 mg/m$^2$/day days 1-8  [total dose/cycle = 1500 mg/m$^2$]

Doxorubicin: I.V.: 25 mg/m$^2$/day days 1-8  [total dose/cycle = 50 mg/m$^2$]

Vincristine: I.V.: 1.4 mg/m$^2$/day (maximum 2 mg) days 1-8  [total dose/cycle = 2.8 mg/m$^2$]

Prednisone: Oral: 50 mg/m$^2$/day days 1-8  [total dose/cycle = 400 mg/m$^2$]

Repeat cycle every 28 days

**Variation 4 (mini-CHOP):**

Cyclophosphamide: I.V.: 250 mg/m$^2$/day days 1, 8, 15  [total dose/cycle = 750 mg/m$^2$]

Doxorubicin: I.V.: 16.7 mg/m$^2$/day days 1, 8, 15  [total dose/cycle = 50.1 mg/m$^2$]

Vincristine: I.V.: 0.67 mg/day days 1, 8, 15  [total dose/cycle = 2.01 mg]

Prednisone: Oral: 75 mg/day days 1-5  [total dose/cycle = 375 mg]

Repeat cycle every 21 days

# CI (Neuroblastomas)

**Use:** Neuroblastomas

**Regimen:**

Ifosfamide: I.V.: 1500 mg/m$^2$/day days 1-3  [total dose/cycle = 4500 mg/m$^2$]

Carboplatin: I.V.: 400 mg/m$^2$ day 4  [total dose/cycle = 400 mg/m$^2$]

Repeat cycle every 21-28 days

# CISCA

**Use:** Bladder cancer

**Regimen:**

Cyclophosphamide: I.V.: 650 mg/m$^2$ day 1  [total dose = 650 mg/m$^2$]

Doxorubicin: I.V.: 50 mg/m$^2$ day 1  [total dose = 50 mg/m$^2$]

Cisplatin: I.V.: 100 mg/m$^2$ day 2  [total dose = 100 mg/m$^2$]

Repeat cycle every 21-28 days

# Cisplatin-Docetaxel

**Use:** Bladder cancer

**Regimen:**

Cisplatin: I.V.: 30 mg/m$^2$ day 1  [total dose/cycle = 30 mg/m$^2$]

Docetaxel: I.V.: 40 mg/m$^2$ day 4  [total dose/cycle = 40 mg/m$^2$]

Repeat cycle weekly for 8 weeks

# Cisplatin-Fluorouracil

**Use:** Cervical cancer
**Regimen: Note:** Multiple variations are listed below.
   **Variation 1:**
   Cisplatin: I.V.: 75 mg/m$^2$ day 1  [total dose/cycle = 75 mg/m$^2$]
   Fluorouracil: I.V.: 1000 mg/m$^2$/day continuous infusion days 1-4 (96 hours)
      [total dose/cycle = 4000 mg/m$^2$]
   Repeat cycle every 21 days
   **Variation 2:**
   Cisplatin: I.V.: 50 mg/m$^2$ day 1 starting 4 hours before radiotherapy  [total dose/cycle = 50 mg/m$^2$]
   Fluorouracil: I.V.: 1000 mg/m$^2$/day continuous infusion days 2-5 (96 hours)
      [total dose/cycle = 4000 mg/m$^2$]
   Repeat cycle every 28 days

# Cisplatin + Pemetrexed

**Use:** Malignant pleural mesothelioma
**Regimen:**
   Pemetrexed: I.V.: 500 mg/m$^2$ infused over 10 minutes day 1  [total dose/cycle = 500 mg/m$^2$]
   Cisplatin: I.V.: 75 mg/m$^2$ infused over 2 hours (start 30 minutes after pemetrexed)
      [total dose/cycle = 75 mg/m$^2$]
   Repeat cycle every 21 days

# Cisplatin-Vinorelbine

**Use:** Cervical cancer
**Regimen:**
   Cisplatin: I.V.: 80 mg/m$^2$ day 1  [total dose/cycle = 80 mg/m$^2$]
   Vinorelbine: I.V.: 25 mg/m$^2$/day days 1 and 8  [total dose/cycle = 50 mg/m$^2$]
   Repeat cycle every 21 days

# CMF

**Use:** Breast cancer
**Regimen: Note:** Multiple variations are listed below.
   **Variation 1:**
   Methotrexate: I.V.: 40 mg/m$^2$/day days 1 and 8  [total dose/cycle = 80 mg/m$^2$]
   Fluorouracil: I.V.: 600 mg/m$^2$/day days 1 and 8  [total dose/cycle = 1200 mg/m$^2$]
   Cyclophosphamide: Oral: 100 mg/m$^2$/day days 1-14  [total dose/cycle = 1400 mg/m$^2$]
   Repeat cycle every 28 days
   **Variation 2 (older than 60 years):**
   Methotrexate: I.V.: 30 mg/m$^2$ days 1 and 8  [total dose/cycle = 60 mg/m$^2$]
   Fluorouracil: I.V.: 400 mg/m$^2$ days 1 and 8  [total dose/cycle = 800 mg/m$^2$]
   Cyclophosphamide: Oral: 100 mg/m$^2$ days 1-14  [total dose/cycle = 1400 mg/m$^2$]
   Repeat cycle every 28 days

# CMF-IV

**Use:** Breast cancer
**Regimen:**
   Cyclophosphamide: I.V.: 600 mg/m$^2$ day 1  [total dose/cycle = 600 mg/m$^2$]
   Methotrexate: I.V.: 40 mg/m$^2$ day 1  [total dose/cycle = 40 mg/m$^2$]
   Fluorouracil: I.V.: 600 mg/m$^2$ day 1  [total dose/cycle = 600 mg/m$^2$]
   Repeat cycle every 21 or 28 days

# CMV

**Use:** Bladder cancer
**Regimen:**
   Cisplatin: I.V.: 100 mg/m$^2$ infused over 4 hours (start 12 hours after methotrexate) day 2
      [total dose = 100 mg/m$^2$]
   Methotrexate: I.V.: 30 mg/m$^2$/day days 1 and 8  [total dose = 60 mg/m$^2$]
   Vinblastine: I.V.: 4 mg/m$^2$/day days 1 and 8  [total dose = 8 mg/m$^2$]
   Repeat cycle every 21 days

# CNF
**Use:** Breast cancer
**Regimen: Note:** Multiple variations are listed below.
### Variation 1:
Cyclophosphamide: I.V: 500 mg/m$^2$ day 1  [total dose/cycle = 500 mg/m$^2$]
Mitoxantrone: I.V.: 10 mg/m$^2$ day 1  [total dose/cycle = 10 mg/m$^2$]
Fluorouracil: I.V.: 500 mg/m$^2$ day 1  [total dose/cycle = 500 mg/m$^2$]
Repeat cycle every 21 days
### Variation 2:
Cyclophosphamide: I.V.: 500-600 mg/m$^2$ day 1  [total dose/cycle = 500-600 mg/m$^2$]
Fluorouracil: I.V.: 500-600 mg/m$^2$ day 1  [total dose/cycle = 500-600 mg/m$^2$]
Mitoxantrone: I.V.: 10-12 mg/m$^2$ day 1  [total dose/cycle = 10-12 mg/m$^2$]
Repeat cycle every 21 days

# CNOP
**Use:** Lymphoma, non-Hodgkin
**Regimen:**
Cyclophosphamide: I.V.: 750 mg/m$^2$ day 1  [total dose/cycle = 750 mg/m$^2$]
Mitoxantrone: I.V.: 10-12 mg/m$^2$ day 1  [total dose/cycle = 10-12 mg/m$^2$]
Vincristine: I.V.: 1.4 mg/m$^2$ day 1  [total dose/cycle = 1.4 mg/m$^2$]
Prednisone: Oral: 50 mg/m$^2$/day days 1-5  [total dose/cycle = 250 mg/m$^2$]
Repeat cycle every 21 days

# CO
**Use:** Retinoblastoma
**Regimen:**
Cyclophosphamide: I.V.: 10 mg/kg/day days 1-3  [total dose/cycle = 30 mg/kg]
Vincristine: I.V.: 1.5 mg/m$^2$ day 1  [total dose/cycle = 1.5 mg/m$^2$]
Repeat cycle every 21 days

# CODOX-M
**Use:** Lymphoma, non-Hodgkin
**Regimen:**
Cytarabine: I.T.: 70 mg/day days 1 and 3  [total dose/cycle = 140 mg]
Cyclophosphamide: I.V.: 800 mg/m$^2$ day 1, then 200 mg/m$^2$ days 2-5
    [total dose/cycle = 1600 mg/m$^2$]
Vincristine: I.V.: 1.5 mg/m$^2$/day days 1, 8, 15  [total dose/cycle = 4.5 mg/m$^2$]
Doxorubicin: I.V.: 40 mg/m$^2$ day 1  [total dose/cycle = 40 mg/m$^2$]
Methotrexate:
I.T.: 12 mg day 15  [total dose/cycle = 12 mg]
I.V.: 1200 mg/m$^2$ loading dose then 240 mg/m$^2$/hour for 23 hours day 10
    [total dose/cycle = 6720 mg/m$^2$]
Leucovorin: I.V.: 192 mg/m$^2$ day 11 then 6 mg/m$^2$ every 6 hours until MTX level <10$^{-8}$M
Sargramostim: SubQ: 7.5 mcg/kg day 13 until ANC >1000 cells/mm$^3$ [total dose/cycle = ANC = >1000 cells/mm$^3$]
Repeat cycle when ANC >1000 cells/mm$^3$

# COMLA
**Use:** Lymphoma, non-Hodgkin
**Regimen:**
Cyclophosphamide: I.V.: 1500 mg/m$^2$ day 1  [total dose/cycle = 1500 mg/m$^2$]
Vincristine: I.V.: 1.4 mg/m$^2$/day (maximum 2 mg) days 1, 8, 15  [total dose/cycle = 4.2 mg/m$^2$]
Methotrexate: I.V.: 120 mg/m$^2$/day days 22, 29, 36, 43, 50, 57, 64, 71
    [total dose/cycle = 960 mg/m$^2$]
Leucovorin: Oral: 25 mg/m$^2$ every 6 hours for 4 doses (beginning 24 hours after each methotrexate dose)
    [total dose/cycle = 800 mg/m$^2$]
Cytarabine: I.V.: 300 mg/m$^2$/day days 22, 29, 36, 43, 50, 57, 64, 71
    [total dose/cycle = 2400 mg/m$^2$]
Repeat cycle every 85 days

# COMP

**Use:** Lymphoma, Hodgkin disease; Lymphoma, non-Hodgkin disease
**Regimen:**
Cyclophosphamide: I.V.: 1200 mg/m$^2$ day 1, cycle 1 [total dose/cycle = 1200 mg/m$^2$]
**followed by** 1000 mg/m$^2$ day 1 on subsequent cycles [total dose/cycle = 1000 mg/m$^2$]
Vincristine: I.V.: 2 mg/m$^2$/day (maximum 2 mg) days 3, 10, 17, 24, cycle 1
[total dose/cycle = 8 mg/m$^2$] **followed by** 1.5 mg/m$^2$/day days 1 and 4, on subsequent cycles
[total dose/cycle = 3 mg/m$^2$]
Methotrexate: I.V.: 300 mg/m$^2$ day 12 [total dose/cycle = 300 mg/m$^2$]
Prednisone: Oral: 60 mg/m$^2$/day (maximum 60 mg) days 3-30 then taper for 7 days, cycle 1
[total dose/cycle = 1680 mg/m$^2$ + taper dose over 7 days]
**followed by** 60 mg/m$^2$ (maximum 60 mg) days 1-5, on subsequent cycles [total dose/cycle = 300 mg/m$^2$]
Maintenance cycles repeat every 28 days

# COP-BLAM

**Use:** Lymphoma, non-Hodgkin
**Regimen:**
Cyclophosphamide: I.V.: 400 mg/m$^2$ day 1 [total dose/cycle = 400 mg/m$^2$]
Vincristine: I.V.: 1 mg/m$^2$ day 1 [total dose/cycle = 1 mg/m$^2$]
Prednisone: Oral: 40 mg/m$^2$/day days 1-10 [total dose/cycle = 400 mg/m$^2$]
Bleomycin: I.V.: 15 mg day 14 [total dose/cycle = 15 mg]
Doxorubicin: I.V.: 40 mg/m$^2$ day 1 [total dose/cycle = 40 mg/m$^2$]
Procarbazine: Oral: 100 mg/m$^2$/day days 1-10 [total dose/cycle = 1000 mg/m$^2$]

# COPE or Baby Brain I

**Use:** Brain tumors
**Regimen:**
**Cycle A:**
Vincristine: I.V.: 0.065 mg/kg/day (maximum 1.5 mg) days 1, 8 [total dose/cycle = 0.13 mg/kg]
Cyclophosphamide: I.V.: 65 mg/kg day 1 [total dose/cycle = 65 mg/kg]
**Cycle B:**
Cisplatin: I.V.: 4 mg/m$^2$ day 1 [total dose/cycle = 4 mg/kg]
Etoposide: I.V.: 6.5 mg/kg/day days 3, 4 [total dose/cycle = 13 mg/kg]
Repeat cycle every 28 days in the following sequence: AABAAB

# COPP (C MOPP)

**Use:** Lymphoma, non-Hodgkin
**Regimen:**
Cyclophosphamide: I.V.: 450-650 mg/m$^2$/day days 1 and 8 [total dose/cycle = 900-1300 mg/m$^2$]
Vincristine: I.V.: 1.4-2 mg/m$^2$/day (maximum 2 mg) days 1 and 8 [total dose/cycle = 2.8-4 mg/m$^2$]
Procarbazine: Oral: 100 mg/m$^2$/day days 1-14 [total dose/cycle = 1400 mg/m$^2$]
Prednisone: Oral: 40 mg/m$^2$/day days 1-14 [total dose/cycle = 560 mg/m$^2$]
Repeat cycle every 3 to 4 weeks

# CP (Leukemia)

**Use:** Leukemia, chronic lymphocytic
**Regimen:**
Chlorambucil: Oral: 30 mg/m$^2$ day 1 [total dose/cycle = 30 mg/m$^2$]
Prednisone: Oral: 80 mg days 1-5 [total dose/cycle = 400 mg]
Repeat cycle every 14 days

# CP (Ovarian Cancer)

**Use:** Ovarian cancer
**Regimen:**
Cyclophosphamide: I.V.: 750 mg/m$^2$ day 1 [total dose/cycle = 750 mg/m$^2$]
Cisplatin: I.V.: 75 mg/m$^2$ day 1 [total dose/cycle = 75 mg/m$^2$]
Repeat cycle every 21 days

# CT
**Use:** Ovarian cancer
**Regimen:**
    Cisplatin: I.V.: 75 mg/m$^2$ day 2  [total dose/cycle = 75 mg/m$^2$]
    Paclitaxel: I.V.: 135 mg/m$^2$ continuous infusion day 1  [total dose/cycle = 135 mg/m$^2$]
    Repeat cycle every 21 days

# CV
**Use:** Retinoblastoma
**Regimen:**
    Cyclophosphamide: I.V.: 300 mg/m$^2$ [total dose/cycle = 300 mg/m$^2$]
    Vincristine: I.V.: 1.5 mg/m$^2$  [total dose/cycle = 1.5 mg/m$^2$]
    Repeat weekly for 6 weeks
    **followed by:**
    Cyclophosphamide: I.V.: 200 mg/m$^2$  [total dose/cycle = 200 mg/m$^2$]
    Vincristine: I.V.: 1.5 mg/m$^2$ [total dose/cycle = 1.5 mg/m$^2$]
    Repeat weekly for 42 weeks

# CVD
**Use:** Melanoma
**Regimen:**
    Cisplatin: I.V.: 20 mg/m$^2$/day days 2-5  [total dose/cycle = 80 mg/m$^2$]
    Vinblastine: I.V.: 1.6 mg/m$^2$/day days 1-5  [total dose/cycle = 8 mg/m$^2$]
    Dacarbazine: I.V.: 800 mg/m$^2$ day 1  [total dose/cycle = 800 mg/m$^2$]
    Repeat cycle every 21 days

# CVP (Leukemia)
**Use:** Leukemia, chronic lymphocytic
**Regimen: Note:** Multiple variations are listed below.
    **Variation 1:**
    Cyclophosphamide: Oral: 400 or 300 mg/m$^2$/day days 1-5
        [total dose/cycle = 2000 or 1500 mg/m$^2$]
    Vincristine: I.V.: 1.4 mg/m$^2$ (maximum 2 mg) day 1  [total dose/cycle = 1.4 mg/m$^2$]
    Prednisone: Oral: 100 mg/m$^2$/day days 1-5
    Repeat cycle every 21 days
    **Variation 2:**
    Cyclophosphamide: I.V.: 800 mg/m$^2$ day 1  [total dose/cycle = 800 mg/m$^2$]
    Vincristine: I.V.: 1.4 mg/m$^2$ (maximum 2 mg) day 1  [total dose/cycle = 1.4 mg/m$^2$]
    Prednisone: Oral: 100 mg/m$^2$/day days 1-5  [total dose/cycle = 500 mg/m$^2$]
    Repeat cycle every 21 days

# CVP (Lymphoma, non-Hodgkin)
**Use:** Lymphoma, non-Hodgkin
**Regimen:**
    Cyclophosphamide: Oral: 400 mg/m$^2$/day days 1-5  [total dose/cycle = 2000 mg/m$^2$]
    Vincristine: I.V.: 1.4 mg/m$^2$ day 1  [total dose/cycle = 1.4 mg/m$^2$]
    Prednisone: Oral: 100 mg/m$^2$/day days 1-5
    Repeat cycle every 21 days

# Cyclophosphamide + Doxorubicin
**Use:** Prostate cancer
**Regimen:**
    Doxorubicin: I.V.: 40 mg/m$^2$ day 1  [total dose/cycle = 40 mg/m$^2$]
    Cyclophosphamide: I.V.: 800-2000 mg/m$^2$ day 1  [total dose/cycle = 800-2000 mg/m$^2$]
    Filgrastim: SubQ: 5 mcg/kg/day days 2-10 (or until ANC >10,000 cells/μL)
        [total dose/cycle = 45 mcg/kg or ANC = >10,000 cells/μL]
    Repeat cycle every 21 days

## Cyclophosphamide + Estramustine
**Use:** Prostate cancer
**Regimen:**
Cyclophosphamide: Oral: 2 mg/kg/day days 1-14 [total dose/cycle = 28 mg/kg]
Estramustine: Oral: 10 mg/kg/day days 1-14 [total dose/cycle = 140 mg/kg]
Repeat cycle every 28 days

## Cyclophosphamide + Etoposide
**Use:** Prostate cancer
**Regimen:**
Cyclophosphamide: Oral: 100 mg/day days 1-14 [total dose/cycle = 1400 mg]
Etoposide: Oral: 50 mg/day days 1-14 [total dose/cycle = 700 mg]
Repeat cycle every 28 days

## Cyclophosphamide + Vincristine + Dexamethasone
**Use:** Prostate cancer
**Regimen:**
Cyclophosphamide: Oral: 250 mg/day days 1-14 [total dose/cycle = 3500 mg]
Vincristine: I.V.: 1 mg/day days 1, 8, and 15 [total dose/cycle = 3 mg]
Dexamethasone: Oral: 0.75 mg twice daily days 1-14 [total dose/cycle = 21 mg]
Repeat cycle every 28 days

## CYVADIC
**Use:** Sarcoma
**Regimen:**
Cyclophosphamide: I.V.: 500 mg/m$^2$ day 1 [total dose/cycle = 500 mg/m$^2$]
Vincristine: I.V.: 1.4 mg/m$^2$/day days 1 and 5 [total dose/cycle = 2.8 mg/m$^2$]
Doxorubicin: I.V.: 50 mg/m$^2$ day 1 [total dose/cycle = 50 mg/m$^2$]
Dacarbazine: I.V.: 250 mg/m$^2$/day days 1-5 [total dose/cycle = 1250 mg/m$^2$]
Repeat cycle every 21 days

## DA
**Use:** Leukemia, acute myeloid (induction)
**Regimen:** Induction:
Daunorubicin: I.V.: 45 mg/m$^2$/day days 1-3 [total dose/cycle = 135 mg/m$^2$]
Cytarabine: I.V.: 100 mg/m$^2$/day continuous infusion days 1-7 [total dose/cycle = 700 mg/m$^2$]

## Dacarbazine-Carboplatin-Aldesleukin-Interferon
**Use:** Melanoma
**Regimen:**
Dacarbazine: I.V.: 750 mg/m$^2$/day days 1 and 22 [total dose/cycle = 1500 mg/m$^2$]
Carboplatin: I.V.: 400 mg/m$^2$/day days 1 and 22 [total dose/cycle = 800 mg/m$^2$]
Aldesleukin: SubQ: 4,800,000 units every 8 hours days 36 and 57
[total dose/cycle = 28,800,000 units]
**then** 4,800,000 units every 12 hours days 37 and 58 [total dose/cycle = 19,200,000 units]
**then** 4,800,000 units/day days 38 to 40, 43 to 47, 50 to 54, 59 to 61, 65 to 68, 71 to 75
[total dose/cycle = 86,400,000 units]
Interferon alpha-2a: SubQ: 6,000,000 units days 38, 40, 43, 45, 47, 50, 52, 54, 59, 61, 64, 66, 68, 71, 73, and 75
[total dose/cycle = 96,000,000 units]
Repeat cycle every 78 days for 3 cycles

## Dacarbazine/Tamoxifen
**Use:** Melanoma
**Regimen:**
Dacarbazine: I.V.: 250 mg/m$^2$/day days 1-5, every 21 days [total dose/cycle = 1250 mg/m$^2$]
Tamoxifen: Oral: 20 mg/day (use of tamoxifen is optional) [total dose/cycle = 20 mg]

# Dartmouth Regimen

**Use:** Melanoma
**Regimen:**
 Cisplatin: I.V.: 25 mg/m$^2$/day days 1-3 [total dose/cycle = 75 mg/m$^2$]
 Dacarbazine: I.V.: 220 mg/m$^2$/day days 1-3 [total dose/cycle = 660 mg/m$^2$]
 Carmustine: I.V.: 150 mg/m$^2$ day 1 (every other cycle) [total dose/cycle = 150 mg/m$^2$]
 Repeat cycle every 21 days

# DAT

**Use:** Leukemia, acute myeloid (induction)
**Regimen:** Induction:
 Daunorubicin: I.V. bolus: 45 mg/m$^2$/day days 1-3 [total dose/cycle = 135 mg/m$^2$]
 Cytarabine: I.V. bolus: 200 mg/m$^2$ [total dose/cycle = 200 mg/m$^2$]
 Thioguanine: Oral: 100 mg/m$^2$/day days 1-7 [total dose/cycle = 700 mg/m$^2$]

# DAV

**Use:** Leukemia, acute myeloid
**Regimen:**
 Daunorubicin: I.V.: 60 mg/m$^2$/day days 3-5 [total dose/cycle = 180 mg/m$^2$]
 Cytarabine: I.V.: 100 mg/m$^2$/day continuous infusion days 1-2
  [total dose/cycle = 200 mg/m$^2$] **followed by** 100 mg/m$^2$ every 12 hours days 3-8 (12 doses)
  [total dose/cycle = 1200 mg/m$^2$]
 Etoposide: I.V.: 150 mg/m$^2$/day days 6-8 [total dose/cycle = 450 mg/m$^2$]
 Administer one cycle only

# DHAP

**Use:** Lymphoma, non-Hodgkin
**Regimen: Note:** Multiple variations are listed below.
 **Variation 1:**
 Dexamethasone: I.V. or Oral: 40 mg/day days 1-4 [total dose/cycle = 160 mg]
 Cisplatin: I.V.: 100 mg/m$^2$ day 1 [total dose/cycle = 100 mg/m$^2$]
 Cytarabine: I.V.: 2000 mg/m$^2$ every 12 hours for 2 doses day 2 (begins at the end of the cisplatin infusion)
  [total dose/cycle = 4000 mg/m$^2$]
 Repeat cycle every 3-4 weeks for 6-10 cycles (salvage therapy) or 1-2 cycles (mobilization prior to high-dose
  therapy with peripheral hematopoietic progenitor cell support)
 **Variation 2:**
 Dexamethasone: I.V. or Oral: 40 mg/day days 1-4 [total dose/cycle = 160 mg]
 Oxaliplatin: I.V.: 130 mg/m$^2$ day 1 [total dose/cycle = 130 mg/m$^2$]
 Cytarabine: I.V.: 2000 mg/m$^2$ every 12 hours for 2 doses day 2 [total dose/cycle = 4000 mg/m$^2$]
 Repeat cycle every 3 weeks

# Docetaxel-Cisplatin

**Use:** Lung cancer, nonsmall cell
**Regimen:**
 Docetaxel: I.V.: 75 mg/m$^2$ day 1 [total dose/cycle = 75 mg/m$^2$]
 Cisplatin: I.V.: 75 mg/m$^2$ day 1 [total dose/cycle = 75 mg/m$^2$]
 Repeat cycle every 21 days

# Doxorubicin + Ketoconazole

**Use:** Prostate cancer
**Regimen:**
 Doxorubicin: I.V.: 20 mg/m$^2$ continuous infusion day 1 [total dose/cycle = 20 mg/m$^2$]
 Ketoconazole: Oral: 400 mg 3 times/day days 1-7 [total dose/cycle = 8400 mg]
 Repeat cycle every 7 days

## Doxorubicin + Ketoconazole/Estramustine + Vinblastine

**Use:** Prostate cancer
**Regimen:**
Doxorubicin: I.V.: 20 mg/m$^2$/day days 1, 15, and 29  [total dose/cycle = 60 mg/m$^2$]
Ketoconazole: Oral: 400 mg 3 times/day days 1-7, 15-21, and 29-35
[total dose/cycle = 25,200 mg]
Estramustine: Oral: 140 mg 3 times/day days 8-14, 22-28, and 36-42
[total dose/cycle = 8820 mg]
Vinblastine: I.V.: 5 mg/m$^2$/day days 8, 22, and 36  [total dose/cycle = 15 mg/m$^2$]
Repeat cycle every 8 weeks

## DTPACE

**Use:** Multiple myeloma
**Regimen:**
Dexamethasone: Oral: 40 mg/day days 1-4  [total dose/cycle = 160 mg]
Thalidomide: Oral: 400 mg/day  [total dose/cycle = 11,200-16,800 mg]
Cisplatin: I.V.: 10 mg/m$^2$/day continuous infusion days 1-4  [total dose/cycle = 40 mg/m$^2$]
Doxorubicin: I.V.: 10 mg/m$^2$/day continuous infusion days 1-4  [total dose/cycle = 40 mg/m$^2$]
Cyclophosphamide: I.V.: 400 mg/m$^2$ continuous infusion days 1-4
[total dose/cycle = 1600 mg/m$^2$]
Etoposide: I.V.: 40 mg/m$^2$ continuous infusion days 1-4  [total dose/cycle = 160 mg/m$^2$]
Repeat cycle every 4-6 weeks

## DVD

**Use:** Multiple myeloma
**Regimen:**
Doxorubicin, liposomal: I.V.: 40 mg/m$^2$ day 1  [total dose/cycle = 40 mg/m$^2$]
Vincristine: I.V.: 2 mg day 1  [total dose/cycle = 2 mg]
Dexamethasone: Oral or I.V.: 40 mg/day days 1-4  [total dose/cycle = 160 mg]
Repeat cycle every 4 weeks

## DVP

**Use:** Leukemia, acute lymphocytic
**Regimen:** Induction:
Daunorubicin: I.V.: 25 mg/m$^2$/day days 1, 8, and 15  [total dose/cycle = 75 mg/m$^2$]
Vincristine: I.V.: 1.5 mg/m$^2$/day (maximum 2 mg) days 1, 8, 15, and 22
[total dose/cycle = 6 mg/m$^2$]
Prednisone: Oral: 60 mg/m$^2$/day days 1-28 then taper over next 14 days
[total dose/cycle = 1680 mg/m$^2$ + taper over next 14 days]
Administer single cycle; used in conjunction with intrathecal chemotherapy

## EAP

**Use:** Gastric cancer
**Regimen:**
Etoposide: I.V.: 120 mg/m$^2$/day days 4-6  [total dose/cycle = 360 mg/m$^2$]
Doxorubicin: I.V.: 20 mg/m$^2$/day days 1 and 7  [total dose/cycle = 40 mg/m$^2$]
Cisplatin: I.V.: 40 mg/m$^2$/day days 2 and 8  [total dose/cycle = 80 mg/m$^2$]
Repeat cycle every 28 days

## ECF

**Use:** Gastric cancer
**Regimen:**
Epirubicin: I.V.: 50 mg/m$^2$ day 1  [total dose/cycle – 50 mg/m$^2$]
Cisplatin: I.V.: 60 mg/m$^2$ day 1  [total dose/cycle = 60 mg/m$^2$]
Repeat cycle every 3 weeks
Fluorouracil: I.V.: 200 mg/m$^2$/day continuous infusion for up to 6 months
[total dose/cycle = 36,000 mg/m$^2$]

# EC (Nonsmall Cell Lung Cancer)
**Use:** Lung cancer, nonsmall cell
**Regimen:**
> Etoposide: I.V.: 120 mg/m$^2$/day days 1-3  [total dose/cycle = 360 mg/m$^2$]
> Carboplatin: I.V.: AUC 6 day 1  [total dose/cycle = AUC = 6]
> Repeat cycle every 21-28 days

# EC (Small Cell Lung Cancer)
**Use:** Lung cancer, small cell
**Regimen: Note:** Multiple variations are listed below.
> **Variation 1:**
> Etoposide: I.V.: 100-120 mg/m$^2$/day days 1-3  [total dose/cycle = 300-360 mg/m$^2$]
> Carboplatin: I.V.: 325-400 mg/m$^2$ day 1  [total dose/cycle = 325-400 mg/m$^2$]
> Repeat cycle every 28 days
> **Variation 2:**
> Etoposide: I.V.: 120 mg/m$^2$/day days 1-3  [total dose/cycle = 360 mg/m$^2$]
> Carboplatin: I.V.: AUC 6 day 1  [total dose/cycle = AUC = 6]
> Repeat cycle every 21-28 days

# EE
**Use:** Wilms tumor
**Regimen:**
> Dactinomycin: I.V.: 15 mcg/kg/day days 1-5 of weeks 0, 5, 13, 24  [total dose/cycle = 300 mcg/kg]
> Vincristine: I.V.: 1.5 mg/m$^2$ day 1 of weeks 1-10, 13, 14, 24, 25  [total dose/cycle = 21 mg/m$^2$]

# EE-4A
**Use:** Wilms tumor
**Regimen:**
> Dactinomycin: I.V.: 45 mcg/kg day 1 of weeks 0, 3, 6, 9, 12, 15, 18
> [total dose/cycle = 315 mcg/kg]
> Vincristine: I.V.: 2 mg/m$^2$ day 1 of weeks 1-10, 12, 15, 18  [total dose/cycle = 26 mg/m$^2$]

# ELF
**Use:** Gastric cancer
**Regimen:**
> Leucovorin calcium: I.V.: 300 mg/m$^2$/day days 1-3, **followed by:**  [total dose/cycle = 900 mg/m$^2$]
> Etoposide: I.V.: 120 mg/m$^2$/day days 1-3, **followed by:**  [total dose/cycle = 360 mg/m$^2$]
> Fluorouracil: I.V.: 500 mg/m$^2$/day days 1-3  [total dose/cycle = 1500 mg/m$^2$]
> Repeat cycle every 21-28 days

# EMA 86
**Use:** Leukemia, acute myeloid
**Regimen:**
> Mitoxantrone: I.V.: 12 mg/m$^2$/day days 1-3  [total dose/cycle = 36 mg/m$^2$]
> Etoposide: I.V.: 200 mg/m$^2$/day continuous infusion days 8-10  [total dose/cycle = 600 mg/m$^2$]
> Cytarabine: I.V.: 500 mg/m$^2$/day continuous infusion days 1-3 and 8-10
> [total dose/cycle = 3000 mg/m$^2$]
> Administer one cycle only

# EMA/CO
**Use:** Gestational trophoblastic tumor
**Regimen:**
   Etoposide: I.V.: 100 mg/m$^2$/day days 1 and 2  [total dose/cycle = 200 mg/m$^2$]
   Methotrexate: I.V.: 300 mg/m$^2$ infused over 12 hours day 1  [total dose/cycle = 300 mg/m$^2$]
   Dactinomycin: I.V. push: 0.5 mg/day days 1 and 2  [total dose/cycle = 1 mg]
   Leucovorin: Oral, I.M.: 15 mg twice daily for 2 days (start 24 hours after the start of methotrexate) days 2, 3
      [total dose/cycle = 60 mg]
**Alternate weekly with:**
   Cyclophosphamide: I.V.: 600 mg/m$^2$ infused over 30 minutes day 1
      [total dose/cycle = 600 mg/m$^2$]
   Vincristine: I.V. push: 0.8 mg/m$^2$ (maximum 2 mg) day 1  [total dose/cycle = 0.8 mg/m$^2$]

# EP (Adenocarcinoma)
**Use:** Adenocarcinoma, unknown primary
**Regimen:**
   Cisplatin: I.V.: 60-100 mg/m$^2$ day 1  [total dose = 60-100 mg/m$^2$]
   Etoposide: I.V.: 80-100 mg/m$^2$/day days 1-3  [total dose = 240-300 mg/m$^2$]
   Repeat cycle every 21 days

# EP (Nonsmall Cell Lung Cancer)
**Use:** Lung cancer, nonsmall cell
**Regimen:**
   Etoposide: I.V.: 80-120 mg/m$^2$/day days 1-3  [total dose/cycle = 240-360 mg/m$^2$]
   Cisplatin: I.V.: 80-100 mg/m$^2$ day 1  [total dose/cycle = 80-100 mg/m$^2$]
   Repeat cycle every 21-28 days

# EP (Small Cell Lung Cancer)
**Use:** Lung cancer, small cell
**Regimen: Note:** Multiple variations are listed below.
   **Variation 1:**
   Etoposide: I.V.: 100 mg/m$^2$/day days 1-3  [total dose/cycle = 300 mg/m$^2$]
   Cisplatin: I.V.: 100 mg/m$^2$ day 1  [total dose/cycle = 100 mg/m$^2$]
   Repeat cycle every 21 days
   **Variation 2:**
   Etoposide: I.V.: 80 mg/m$^2$/day days 1-3  [total dose/cycle = 240 mg/m$^2$]
   Cisplatin: I.V.: 80 mg/m$^2$ day 1 [total dose/cycle = 80 mg/m$^2$]
   Repeat cycle every 21-28 days

# EP (Testicular Cancer)
**Use:** Testicular cancer
**Regimen: Note:** Multiple variations are listed below.
   **Variation 1:**
   Etoposide: I.V.: 100 mg/m$^2$/day days 1-5  [total dose/cycle = 500 mg/m$^2$]
   Cisplatin: I.V.: 20 mg/m$^2$/day days 1-5  [total dose/cycle = 100 mg/m$^2$]
   Repeat cycle every 21 days
   **Variation 2:**
   Etoposide: I.V.: 120 mg/m$^2$/day days 1-3  [total dose/cycle = 360 mg/m$^2$]
   Cisplatin: I.V.: 20 mg/m$^2$/day days 1-5
   Repeat cycle every 3 or 4 weeks
   **Variation 3:**
   Etoposide: I.V.: 120 mg/m$^2$/day days 1, 3, and 5  [total dose/cycle = 360 mg/m$^2$]
   Cisplatin: I.V.: 20 mg/m$^2$/day days 1-5  [total dose/cycle = 100 mg/m$^2$]
   Repeat cycle every 3 or 4 weeks

# EP/EMA

**Use:** Gestational trophoblastic tumor

**Regimen:**

> Etoposide: I.V.: 150 mg/m$^2$ day 1  [total dose/cycle = 150 mg/m$^2$]
>
> Cisplatin: I.V.: 25 mg/m$^2$ infused over 4 hours for 3 consecutive doses, day 1
> [total dose/cycle = 75 mg/m$^2$]
>
> **Alternate weekly with:**
>
> Etoposide: I.V.: 100 mg/m$^2$ day 1  [total dose/cycle = 100 mg/m$^2$]
>
> Methotrexate: I.V.: 300 mg/m$^2$ infused over 12 hours day 1  [total dose/cycle = 300 mg/m$^2$]
>
> Dactinomycin: I.V. push: 0.5 mg day 1  [total dose/cycle = 0.5 mg]
>
> Leucovorin: Oral, I.M.: 15 mg twice daily for 2 days (start 24 hours after the start of methotrexate) days 2, 3
> [total dose/cycle = 60 mg]

# EP/PE

**Use:** Lung cancer, nonsmall cell

**Regimen:**

> Etoposide: I.V.: 120 mg/m$^2$/day days 1-3  [total dose/cycle = 360 mg/m$^2$]
>
> Cisplatin: I.V.: 60-120 mg/m$^2$ day 1  [total dose/cycle = 60-120 mg/m$^2$]
>
> Repeat cycle every 21-28 days

# EPOCH

**Use:** Lymphoma, non-Hodgkin

**Regimen:**

> Etoposide: I.V.: 50 mg/m$^2$/day continuous infusion days 1-4  [total dose/cycle = 200 mg/m$^2$]
>
> Vincristine: I.V.: 0.4 mg/m$^2$/day continuous infusion days 1-4  [total dose/cycle = 1.6 mg/m$^2$]
>
> Doxorubicin: I.V.: 10 mg/m$^2$/day continuous infusion days 1-4  [total dose/cycle = 40 mg/m$^2$]
>
> Cyclophosphamide: I.V.: 750 mg/m$^2$ day 6  [total dose/cycle = 750 mg/m$^2$]
>
> Prednisone: Oral: 60 mg/m$^2$/day days 1-6  [total dose/cycle = 360 mg/m$^2$]
>
> Repeat cycle every 21 days

# ESHAP

**Use:** Lymphoma, non-Hodgkin

**Regimen: Note:** Multiple variations are listed below.

> **Variation 1:**
>
> Etoposide: I.V.: 40 mg/m$^2$/day days 1-4  [total dose/cycle = 160 mg/m$^2$]
>
> Methylprednisolone: I.V.: 500 mg/day days 1-5  [total dose/cycle = 2500 mg]
>
> Cytarabine: I.V.: 2000 mg/m$^2$ day 1  [total dose/cycle = 2000 mg/m$^2$]
>
> Cisplatin: I.V.: 25 mg/m$^2$/day continuous infusion days 1-4  [total dose/cycle = 100 mg/m$^2$]
>
> Repeat cycle every 21-28 days
>
> **Variation 2:**
>
> Etoposide: I.V.: 40 mg/m$^2$/day days 1-4  [total dose/cycle = 160 mg/m$^2$]
>
> Methylprednisolone: I.V.: 500 mg/day days 1-5  [total dose/cycle = 2500 mg]
>
> Cytarabine: I.V.: 2000 mg/m$^2$ day 5  [total dose/cycle = 2000 mg/m$^2$]
>
> Cisplatin: I.V.: 25 mg/m$^2$/day continuous infusion days 1-4  [total dose/cycle = 100 mg/m$^2$]
>
> Repeat cycle every 21-28 days
>
> **Variation 3:**
>
> Etoposide: I.V.: 60 mg/m$^2$/day days 1-4  [total dose/cycle = 240 mg/m$^2$]
>
> Methylprednisolone: I.V.: 500 mg/day days 1-4  [total dose/cycle = 2000 mg]
>
> Cytarabine: I.V.: 2000 mg/m$^2$ day 5  [total dose/cycle = 2000 mg/m$^2$]
>
> Cisplatin: I.V.: 25 mg/m$^2$/day continuous infusion days 1-4  [total dose/cycle = 100 mg/m$^2$]
>
> Repeat cycle every 21 days

# Estramustine + Docetaxel

**Use:** Prostate cancer
**Regimen: Note:** Multiple variations are listed below.

**Variation 1:**
Docetaxel: I.V.: 20-80 mg/m$^2$ day 2 [total dose/cycle = 20-80 mg/m$^2$]
Estramustine: Oral: 280 mg 3 times/day days 1-5 [total dose/cycle = 4200 mg]
Repeat cycle every 21 days

**Variation 2:**
Docetaxel: I.V.: 20-80 mg/m$^2$ day 2 [total dose/cycle = 20-80 mg/m$^2$]
Estramustine: Oral: 14 mg/kg/day days 1-21 [total dose/cycle = 294 mg/kg]
Repeat cycle every 21 days

**Variation 3:**
Docetaxel: I.V.: 35 mg/m$^2$/day days 2 and 9 [total dose/cycle = 70 mg/m$^2$]
Estramustine: Oral: 420 mg 3 times/day for 4 doses, then 280 mg 3 times/day for 5 doses days 1, 2, 3, 8, 9, and 10 [total dose/cycle = 6160 mg]
Repeat cycle every 21 days

# Estramustine + Docetaxel + Carboplatin

**Use:** Prostate cancer
**Regimen:**
Docetaxel: I.V.: 70 mg/m$^2$ day 2 [total dose/cycle = 70 mg/m$^2$]
Estramustine: Oral: 280 mg 3 times/day days 1-5 [total dose/cycle = 4200 mg]
Carboplatin: I.V.: Target AUC 5 day 2 [total dose/cycle = AUC = 5]
Repeat cycle every 3 weeks

# Estramustine + Docetaxel + Hydrocortisone

**Use:** Prostate cancer
**Regimen:**
Docetaxel: I.V.: 70 mg/m$^2$ day 2 [total dose/cycle = 70 mg/m$^2$]
Estramustine: Oral: 10 mg/kg/day days 1-5 [total dose/cycle = 50 mg/kg]
Hydrocortisone: Oral: 40 mg daily [total dose/cycle = 840 mg]
Repeat cycle every 3 weeks

# Estramustine + Etoposide

**Use:** Prostate cancer
**Regimen: Note:** Multiple variations are listed below.

**Variation 1:**
Estramustine: Oral: 15 mg/kg/day days 1-21 [total dose/cycle = 315 mg/kg]
Etoposide: Oral: 50 mg/m$^2$/day days 1-21 [total dose/cycle = 1050 mg/m$^2$]
Repeat cycle every 4 weeks

**Variation 2:**
Estramustine: Oral: 10 mg/kg/day days 1-21 [total dose/cycle = 210 mg/kg]
Etoposide: Oral: 50 mg/m$^2$/day days 1-21 [total dose/cycle = 1050 mg/m$^2$]
Repeat cycle every 4 weeks

**Variation 3:**
Estramustine: Oral: 140 mg 3 times/day days 1-21 [total dose/cycle = 8820 mg]
Etoposide: Oral: 50 mg/m$^2$/day days 1-21 [total dose/cycle = 1050 mg/m$^2$]
Repeat cycle every 4 weeks

# Estramustine + Vinorelbine

**Use:** Prostate cancer
**Regimen:**
Estramustine: Oral: 140 mg 3 times/day days 1-14 [total dose/cycle = 5880 mg]
Vinorelbine: I.V.: 25 mg/m$^2$/day days 1 and 8 [total dose/cycle = 50 mg/m$^2$]
Repeat cycle every 21 days

# EV
**Use:** Prostate cancer
**Regimen: Note:** Multiple variations are listed below.
**Variation 1:**
Estramustine: Oral: 10 mg/kg/day days 1-42 (given in 3 divided doses)
[total dose/cycle = 420 mg/kg]
Vinblastine: I.V.: 4 mg/m$^2$/day days 1, 8, 15, 22, 29, and 36 (weekly for 6 weeks)
[total dose/cycle = 24 mg/m$^2$]
Repeat cycle every 8 weeks
**Variation 2:**
Estramustine: Oral: 600 mg/m$^2$/day days 1-42 (given in 3 divided doses)
[total dose/cycle = 25,200 mg/m$^2$]
Vinblastine: I.V.: 4 mg/m$^2$/day days 1, 8, 15, 22, 29, and 36 [total dose/cycle = 24 mg/m$^2$]
Repeat cycle every 8 weeks

# EVA
**Use:** Lymphoma, Hodgkin disease
**Regimen:**
Etoposide: I.V.: 100 mg/m$^2$/day days 1-3 [total dose/cycle = 300 mg/m$^2$]
Vinblastine: I.V.: 6 mg/m$^2$ day 1 [total dose/cycle = 6 mg/m$^2$]
Doxorubicin: I.V.: 50 mg/m$^2$ day 1 [total dose/cycle = 50 mg/m$^2$]
Repeat cycle every 28 days

# FAC
**Use:** Breast cancer
**Regimen: Note:** Multiple variations are listed below.
**Variation 1:**
Fluorouracil: I.V.: 500 mg/m$^2$/day days 1 and 8 [total dose/cycle = 1000 mg/m$^2$]
or 500 mg/m$^2$ day 1 [total dose/cycle = 500 mg/m$^2$]
Doxorubicin: I.V.: 50 mg/m$^2$ day 1 [total dose/cycle = 50 mg/m$^2$]
Cyclophosphamide: I.V.: 500 mg/m$^2$ day 1 [total dose/cycle = 500 mg/m$^2$]
Repeat cycle every 21-28 days
**Variation 2:**
Fluorouracil: I.V.: 200 mg/m$^2$/day days 1-3 [total dose/cycle = 600 mg/m$^2$]
Doxorubicin: I.V.: 40 mg/m$^2$ day 1 [total dose/cycle = 40 mg/m$^2$]
Cyclophosphamide: I.V.: 400 mg/m$^2$ day 1 [total dose/cycle = 400 mg/m$^2$]
Repeat cycle every 28 days
**Variation 3:**
Fluorouracil: I.V.: 400 mg/m$^2$/day days 1 and 8 [total dose/cycle = 800 mg/m$^2$]
Doxorubicin: I.V.: 40 mg/m$^2$ day 1 [total dose/cycle = 40 mg/m$^2$]
Cyclophosphamide: I.V.: 400 mg/m$^2$ day 1 [total dose/cycle = 400 mg/m$^2$]
Repeat cycle every 28 days
**Variation 4:**
Fluorouracil: I.V.: 600 mg/m$^2$/day days 1 and 8 [total dose/cycle = 1200 mg/m$^2$]
Doxorubicin: I.V.: 60 mg/m$^2$ day 1 [total dose/cycle = 60 mg/m$^2$]
Cyclophosphamide: I.V.: 600 mg/m$^2$ day 1 [total dose/cycle = 600 mg/m$^2$]
Repeat cycle every 28 days
**Variation 5:**
Fluorouracil: I.V.: 300 mg/m$^2$/day days 1 and 8 [total dose/cycle = 600 mg/m$^2$]
Doxorubicin: I.V.: 30 mg/m$^2$ day 1 [total dose/cycle = 30 mg/m$^2$]
Cyclophosphamide: I.V.: 300 mg/m$^2$ day 1 [total dose/cycle = 300 mg/m$^2$]
Repeat cycle every 28 days

# FAM
**Use:** Gastric cancer; Pancreatic cancer
**Regimen:**
Fluorouracil: I.V.: 600 mg/m$^2$/day days 1, 8, 29, 36 [total dose/cycle = 2400 mg/m$^2$]
Doxorubicin: I.V.: 30 mg/m$^2$/day days 1 and 29 [total dose/cycle = 60 mg/m$^2$]
Mitomycin C: I.V.: 10 mg/m$^2$ day 1 [total dose/cycle = 10 mg/m$^2$]
Repeat cycle every 8 weeks

# FAMTX

**Use:** Gastric cancer
**Regimen:**
Methotrexate: I.V.: 1500 mg/m$^2$ day 1  [total dose/cycle = 1500 mg/m$^2$]
Fluorouracil: I.V.: 1500 mg/m$^2$ day 1  [total dose/cycle = 1500 mg/m$^2$]
Leucovorin: Oral: 15 mg/m$^2$ every 6 hours for 8 doses (start 24 hours after methotrexate)
    [total dose/cycle = 120 mg/m$^2$]
**followed by** 30 mg/m$^2$ every 6 hours for 8 more doses if 24-hour methotrexate level >2.5 mol/L (start 24 hours after methotrexate)
Doxorubicin: I.V.: 30 mg/m$^2$ day 15  [total dose/cycle = 30 mg/m$^2$]
Repeat cycle every 28 days

# F-CL

**Use:** Colorectal cancer
**Regimen: Note:** Multiple variations are listed below.
  **Variation 1 (Mayo Regimen):**
  Fluorouracil: I.V.: 425 mg/m$^2$/day days 1-5  [total dose/cycle = 2125 mg/m$^2$]
  Leucovorin: I.V.: 20 mg/m$^2$/day days 1-5  [total dose/cycle = 100 mg/m$^2$]
  Repeat cycle every 28 days
  **Variation 2:**
  Fluorouracil: I.V.: 400 mg/m$^2$/day days 1-5  [total dose/cycle = 2000 mg/m$^2$]
  Leucovorin: I.V.: 20 mg/m$^2$/day days 1-5  [total dose/cycle = 100 mg/m$^2$]
  Repeat cycle every 28 days
  **Variation 3:**
  Fluorouracil: I.V.: 500 mg/m$^2$ day 1  [total dose/cycle = 500 mg/m$^2$]
  Leucovorin: I.V.: 20 mg/m$^2$ (2-hour infusion) day 1
    [total dose/cycle = 20 mg/m$^2$] **or** 500 mg/m$^2$ (2-hour infusion) day 1 [total dose/cycle = 500 mg/m$^2$]
  Repeat cycle weekly
  **Variation 4:**
  Fluorouracil: I.V.: 600 mg/m$^2$ weekly for 6 weeks  [total dose/cycle = 3600 mg/m$^2$]
  Leucovorin: I.V.: 500 mg/m$^2$ (3-hour infusion) weekly for 6 weeks  [total dose/cycle = 3000 mg/m$_2$]
  Repeat cycle every 8 weeks
  **Variation 5:**
  Fluorouracil: I.V.: 600 mg/m$^2$ weekly for 6 weeks  [total dose/cycle = 3600 mg/m$^2$]
  Leucovorin: I.V.: 500 mg/m$^2$ weekly for 6 weeks  [total dose/cycle = 3000 mg/m$^2$]
  Repeat cycle every 8 weeks
  **Variation 6:**
  Fluorouracil: I.V.: 600 mg/m$^2$ weekly
  Leucovorin: I.V.: 500 mg/m$^2$ (2-hour infusion) weekly
  Repeat cycle weekly
  **Variation 7:**
  Fluorouracil: I.V.: 2600 mg/m$^2$ continuous infusion day 1  [total dose/cycle = 2600 mg/m$^2$]
  Leucovorin: I.V.: 500 mg/m$^2$ continuous infusion day 1  [total dose/cycle = 500 mg/m$^2$]
  Repeat cycle weekly
  **Variation 8:**
  Fluorouracil: I.V.: 2600 mg/m$^2$ continuous infusion day 1  [total dose/cycle = 2600 mg/m$^2$]
  Leucovorin: I.V.: 300 mg/m$^2$ (maximum 500 mg) continuous infusion day 1
    [total dose/cycle = 300 mg/m$^2$]
  Repeat cycle weekly
  **Variation 9:**
  Fluorouracil: I.V.: 2600 mg/m$^2$ continuous infusion once weekly for 6 weeks
    [total dose/cycle = 15,600 mg/m$^2$]
  Leucovorin: I.V.: 500 mg/m$^2$ weekly for 6 weeks  [total dose/cycle = 3000 mg/m$^2$]
  Repeat cycle every 8 weeks
  **Variation 10:**
  Fluorouracil: I.V.: 2300 mg/m$^2$ continuous infusion day 1  [total dose/cycle = 2300 mg/m$^2$]
  Leucovorin: I.V.: 50 mg/m$^2$ continuous infusion day 1  [total dose/cycle = 50 mg/m$^2$]
  Repeat cycle weekly
  **Variation 11:**
  Fluorouracil: I.V.: 200 mg/m$^2$/day continuous infusion days 1-14  [total dose/cycle = 2800 mg/m$_2$]
  Leucovorin: I.V.: 5 mg/m$^2$/day days 1-14  [total dose/cycle = 70 mg/m$^2$]
  Repeat cycle every 28 days
  **Variation 12:**
  Fluorouracil: I.V.: 200 mg/m$^2$ continuous infusion daily for 4 weeks
    **followed by (starting week 5):** 200 mg/m$^2$ continuous infusion days 1-21
    [total dose/cycle = 4200 mg/m$^2$]
  Leucovorin: I.V.: 20 mg/m$^2$/day days 1, 8, and 15  [total dose/cycle = 60 mg/m$^2$]
  Repeat cycle every 4 weeks

# FEC

**Use:** Breast cancer
**Regimen:**
Fluorouracil: I.V.: 500 mg/m$^2$ day 1   [total dose/cycle = 500 mg/m$^2$]
Cyclophosphamide: I.V.: 500 mg/m$^2$ day 1   [total dose/cycle = 500 mg/m$^2$]
Epirubicin: I.V.: 100 mg/m$^2$ day 1   [total dose/cycle = 100 mg/m$^2$]
Repeat cycle every 21 days

# FIS-HAM

**Use:** Leukemia, acute lymphocytic; Leukemia, acute myeloid
**Regimen:**
Fludarabine: I.V.: 15 mg/m$^2$/day every 12 hours days 1, 2, 8, and 9 [total dose/cycle = 120 mg/m$^2$]
Cytarabine: I.V.: 750 mg/m$^2$/day every 3 hours days 1, 2, 8, and 9 [total dose/cycle = 24,000 mg/m$^2$]
Mitoxantrone: I.V.: 10 mg/m$^2$/day days 3, 4, 10, and 11   [total dose/cycle = 40 mg/m$^2$]

# FL

**Use:** Prostate cancer
**Regimen: Note:** Multiple variations are listed below.
**Variation 1:**
Flutamide: Oral: 250 mg every 8 hours   [total dose/cycle = 21,000 mg]
Leuprolide acetate: SubQ: 1 mg/day   [total dose/cycle = 28 mg]
**or**
Leuprolide depot: I.M.: 7.5 mg day 1   [total dose/cycle = 7.5 mg]
Repeat cycle every 28 days
**Variation 2:**
Flutamide: Oral: 250 mg every 8 hours   [total dose/cycle = 67,500 mg]
Leuprolide acetate depot: I.M.: 22.5 mg day 1   [total dose/cycle = 22.5 mg]
Repeat cycle every 3 months

# FLAG

**Use:** Leukemia, acute myeloid
**Regimen:**
Fludarabine: I.V.: 30 mg/m$^2$/day days 1-5   [total dose/cycle = 150 mg/m$^2$]
Cytarabine: I.V.: 2000 mg/m$^2$/day days 1-5 (3.5 hours after end of fludarabine infusion)
[total dose/cycle = 10,000 mg/m$^2$]
Filgrastim: SubQ: 5 mcg/kg day 1
[total dose/cycle = 5 mcg/kg] **followed by** 300 mcg daily until ANC >500-1000 cells/mcL postnadir
[total dose/cycle = 40-7800 mcg/kg]
Repeat cycle every 3-4 weeks

# FLe

**Use:** Colorectal cancer
**Regimen:**
Fluorouracil: I.V.: 450 mg/m$^2$/day for 5 days   [total dose/cycle = 2250 mg/m$^2$]
After a pause of 4 weeks: 450 mg/m$^2$/week for 48 weeks   [total dose/cycle = 21.6 g/m$^2$]
Levamisole: Oral: 50 mg 3 times/day for 3 days, repeated every 2 weeks for 1 year [total dose/cycle = 11.7 g/m$^2$]

# Fludarabine-Rituximab

**Use:** Leukemia, chronic lymphocytic
**Regimen:**

Rituximab: I.V.: 375 mg/m$^2$/day days 1 and 4 (cycle 1)  [total dose/cycle 1 = 750 mg/m$^2$]
Rituximab: I.V.: 375 mg/m$^2$/day day 1 (cycles 2-6)  [total dose/cycle = 375 mg/m$^2$]
Fludarabine: I.V.: 25 mg/m$^2$/day days 1-5  [total dose/cycle = 125 mg/m$^2$]
Repeat cycle every 4 weeks

# FOIL

**Use:** Colorectal cancer
**Regimen:**

Irinotecan: I.V.: 175 mg/m$^2$ day 1  [total dose/cycle = 175 mg/m$^2$]
Oxaliplatin: I.V.: 100 mg/m$^2$ day 1  [total dose/cycle = 100 mg/m$^2$]
Leucovorin: I.V.: 200 mg/m$^2$ day 1  [total dose/cycle = 200 mg/m$^2$]
Fluorouracil: I.V.: 3800 mg/m$^2$/day continuous infusion days 1 and 2 [total dose/cycle = 7600 mg/m$^2$]
Repeat cycle every 14 days

# FOLFOX 1

**Use:** Colorectal cancer
**Regimen:**

Oxaliplatin: I.V.: 130 mg/m$^2$ day 1 (every other cycle)  [total dose/cycle = 130 mg/m$^2$]
Leucovorin: I.V.: 500 mg/m$^2$/day days 1 and 2  [total dose/cycle = 1000 mg/m$^2$]
Fluorouracil: I.V.: 1.5-2 g/m$^2$/day continuous infusion days 1 and 2  [total dose/cycle = 3-4 g/m$^2$]
Repeat cycle every 14 days

# FOLFOX 2

**Use:** Colorectal cancer
**Regimen:**

Oxaliplatin: I.V.: 100 mg/m$^2$ day 1  [total dose/cycle = 100 mg/m$^2$]
Leucovorin: I.V.: 500 mg/m$^2$/day days 1 and 2  [total dose/cycle = 1000 mg/m$^2$]
Fluorouracil: I.V.: 1.5-2 g/m$^2$/day continuous infusion days 1 and 2  [total dose/cycle = 3-4 g/m$^2$]
Repeat cycle every 14 days

# FOLFOX 3

**Use:** Colorectal cancer
**Regimen:**

Oxaliplatin: I.V.: 85 mg/m$^2$ day 1  [total dose/cycle = 85 mg/m$^2$]
Leucovorin: I.V.: 500 mg/m$^2$/day days 1 and 2  [total dose/cycle = 1000 mg/m$^2$]
Fluorouracil: I.V.: 1.5-2 g/m$^2$/day continuous infusion days 1 and 2  [total dose/cycle = 3-4 g/m$^2$]
Repeat cycle every 14 days

# FOLFOX 4

**Use:** Colorectal cancer
**Regimen:**

Oxaliplatin: I.V.: 85 mg/m$^2$ day 1  [total dose/cycle = 85 mg/m$^2$]
Leucovorin: I.V.: 200 mg/m$^2$/day days 1 and 2  [total dose/cycle = 400 mg/m$^2$]
Fluorouracil: I.V. bolus: 400 mg/m$^2$/day days 1 and 2
   [total dose/cycle = 800 mg/m$^2$] **followed by** 600 mg/m$^2$ CIVI (over 22-hour) days 1 and 2
   [total dose/cycle = 1200 mg/m$^2$]
**Note:** Bolus fluorouracil and CIVI are both given on each day.
Repeat cycle every 14 days

# FOLFOX 6

**Use:** Colorectal cancer
**Regimen:**

Oxaliplatin: I.V.: 100 mg/m$^2$ day 1  [total dose/cycle = 100 mg/m$^2$]
Leucovorin: I.V.: 400 mg/m$^2$ day 1  [total dose/cycle = 400 mg/m$^2$]
Fluorouracil: I.V. bolus: 400 mg/m$^2$ day 1  [total dose/cycle = 400 mg/m$^2$] **followed by** 2.4-3 g/m$^2$ CIVI (46 hours)
    continuous infusion extending over days 1 and 2   [total dose/cycle = 2.4-3 g/m$^2$]
Repeat cycle every 14 days

# FOLFOX 7

**Use:** Colorectal cancer
**Regimen:**

Oxaliplatin: I.V.: 130 mg/m$^2$ day 1  [total dose/cycle = 130 mg/m$^2$]
Leucovorin: I.V.: 400 mg/m$^2$ day 1  [total dose/cycle = 400 mg/m$^2$]
Fluorouracil: I.V. bolus: 400 mg/m$^2$ day 1
    [total dose/cycle = 400 mg/m$^2$] **followed by** 2.4 g/m$^2$ CIVI (46 hours) continuous infusion extending over days 1
    and 2  [total dose/cycle = 2.4 g/m$^2$]
Repeat cycle every 14 days

# FU HURT

**Use:** Head and neck cancer
**Regimen:**

Hydroxyurea: Oral: 1000 mg every 12 hours for 11 doses days 0-5  [total dose/cycle = 11,000 mg]
Fluorouracil: I.V.: 800 mg/m$^2$/day continuous infusion (start AM after admission) days 1-5
    [total dose/cycle = 4000 mg/m$^2$]
Paclitaxel: I.V.: 5-25 mg/m$^2$/day continuous infusion days 1-5  [total dose/cycle = 25-125 mg/m$^2$]
5-7 cycles may be administered

# FU/LV/CPT-11

**Use:** Colorectal cancer
**Regimen: Note:** Multiple variations are listed below.

**Variation: 1:**
Irinotecan: I.V.: 350 mg/m$^2$ day 1  [total dose/cycle = 350 mg/m$^2$]
Leucovorin: I.V.: 20 mg/m$^2$/day days 22-26  [total dose/cycle = 100 mg/m$^2$]
Fluorouracil: I.V.: 425 mg/m$^2$/day days 22-26  [total dose/cycle = 2125 mg/m$^2$]
Repeat cycle every 6 weeks

**Variation: 2:**
Irinotecan: I.V.: 80 mg/m$^2$ day 1  [total dose/cycle = 80 mg/m$^2$]
Fluorouracil: I.V.: 2300 mg/m$^2$ continuous infusion day 1  [total dose/cycle = 2300 mg/m$^2$]
Leucovorin: I.V.: 500 mg/m$^2$ day 1  [total dose/cycle = 500 mg/m$^2$]
Repeat cycle weekly **or**
Irinotecan: I.V.: 180 mg/m$^2$ day 1  [total dose/cycle = 180 mg/m$^2$]
Leucovorin: I.V.: 200 mg/m$^2$/day days 1 and 2  [total dose/cycle = 400 mg/m$^2$]
Fluorouracil: I.V.: 400 mg/m$^2$/day days 1 and 2  [total dose/cycle = 800 mg/m$^2$]
**followed by** 600 mg/m$^2$/day continuous infusion days 1 and 2  [total dose/cycle = 1200 mg/m$^2$]
Repeat cycle every 2 weeks

**Variation 3:**
Irinotecan: I.V.: 175 mg/m$^2$ day 1  [total dose/cycle = 175 mg/m$^2$]
Leucovorin: I.V.: 250 mg/m$^2$ day 2  [total dose/cycle = 250 mg/m$^2$]
Fluorouracil: I.V.: 950 mg/m$^2$ day 2  [total dose/cycle = 950 mg/m$^2$] **or**
Irinotecan: I.V.: 200 mg/m$^2$ day 1  [total dose/cycle = 200 mg/m$^2$]
Leucovorin: I.V.: 250 mg/m$^2$ day 2  [total dose/cycle = 250 mg/m$^2$]
Fluorouracil: I.V.: 850 mg/m$^2$ day 2  [total dose/cycle = 850 mg/m$^2$]
Repeat cycle every other week

## FU/LV/CPT-11 (Saltz Regimen)

**Use:** Colorectal cancer
**Regimen:**
Fluorouracil: I.V.: 500 mg/m$^2$/day days 1, 8, 15, and 22  [total dose/cycle = 2000 mg/m$^2$]
Leucovorin: I.V.: 20 mg/m$^2$/day days 1, 8, 15, and 22  [total dose/cycle = 80 mg/m$^2$]
Irinotecan: I.V.: 125 mg/m$^2$/day days 1, 8, 15, and 22  [total dose/cycle = 500 mg/m$^2$]
Repeat cycle every 42 days

## FUP

**Use:** Gastric cancer
**Regimen:**
Fluorouracil: I.V.: 1000 mg/m$^2$/day continuous infusion days 1-5  [total dose/cycle = 5000 mg/m$^2$]
Cisplatin: I.V.: 100 mg/m$^2$ day 2  [total dose/cycle = 100 mg/m$^2$]
Repeat cycle every 28 days

## FZ

**Use:** Prostate cancer
**Regimen: Note:** Multiple variations are listed below.
**Variation 1:**
Flutamide: Oral: 250 mg every 8 hours  [total dose/cycle = 21,000 mg]
Goserelin acetate: SubQ: 3.6 mg day 1  [total dose/cycle = 3.6 mg]
Repeat cycle every 28 days
**Variation 2:**
Flutamide: Oral: 250 mg every 8 hours  [total dose/cycle = 67,500 mg]
Goserelin acetate: SubQ: 10.8 mg day 1  [total dose/cycle = 10.8 mg]
Repeat cycle every 3 months

## GC

**Use:** Lung cancer, nonsmall cell
**Regimen:**
Gemcitabine: I.V.: 1000 mg/m$^2$/day days 1, 8, 15  [total dose/cycle = 3000 mg/m$^2$]
Cisplatin: I.V.: 100 mg/m$^2$ day 1 **or** 2 **or** 15  [total dose/cycle = 100 mg/m$^2$]
Repeat cycle every 28 days for 2-6 cycles

## Gemcitabine/Capecitabine

**Use:** Pancreatic cancer
**Regimen:**
Gemcitabine: I.V.: 1000 mg/m$^2$/day days 1 and 8  [total dose/cycle = 2000 mg/m$^2$]
Capecitabine: Oral: 650 mg/m$^2$ twice daily days 1-14  [total dose/cycle = 18,200 mg/m$^2$]
Repeat cycle every 21 days

## Gemcitabine-Carboplatin

**Use:** Lung cancer, nonsmall cell
**Regimen:**
Gemcitabine: I.V.: 1000 or 1100 mg/m$^2$/day days 1 and 8
    [total dose/cycle = 2000 or 2200 mg/m$^2$]
Carboplatin: I.V.: AUC 5 day 8  [total dose/cycle = AUC = 5]
Repeat cycle every 28 days

## Gemcitabine-Cis

**Use:** Lung cancer, nonsmall cell
**Regimen:**
Gemcitabine: I.V.: 1000-1200 mg/m$^2$/day days 1, 8, and 15  [total dose/cycle = 3000-3600 mg/m$^2$]
Cisplatin: I.V.: 100 mg/m$^2$ day 1 **or** 2 **or** 15  [total dose/cycle = 100 mg/m$^2$]
Repeat cycle every 28 days

# Gemcitabine-Cisplatin
**Use:** Bladder cancer
**Regimen:**
>Gemcitabine: I.V.: 1000 mg/m$^2$/day days 1, 8, and 15  [total dose/cycle = 3000 mg/m$^2$]
>Cisplatin: I.V.: 70 mg/m$^2$ day 2  [total dose/cycle = 70 mg/m$^2$]
>Repeat cycle every 28 days for 6 cycles

# Gemcitabine-Docetaxel
**Use:** Bony sarcoma; Soft tissue sarcoma
**Regimen:**
>Gemcitabine: I.V.: 675 mg/m$^2$/day days 1 and 8  [total dose/cycle = 1350 mg/m$^2$]
>Docetaxel: I.V.: 100 mg/m$^2$ day 8  [total dose/cycle = 100 mg/m$^2$]
>Repeat cycle every 21 days

# Gemcitabine/Irinotecan
**Use:** Pancreatic cancer
**Regimen:**
>Gemcitabine: I.V.: 1000 mg/m$^2$/day days 1 and 8  [total dose/cycle = 2000 mg/m$^2$]
>Irinotecan: I.V.: 100 mg/m$^2$/day days 1 and 8  [total dose/cycle = 200 mg/m$^2$]
>Repeat cycle every 21 days

# Gemcitabine-Paclitaxel
**Use:** Ovarian cancer
**Regimen:**
>Paclitaxel: I.V.: 80 mg/m$^2$ infused over 60 minutes days 1, 8, and 15
>    [total dose/cycle = 240 mg/m$^2$]
>Gemcitabine: I.V.: 1000 mg/m$^2$/day (start at end of paclitaxel infusion) days 1, 8, and 15
>    [total dose/cycle = 3000 mg/m$^2$]
>Repeat cycle every 4 weeks

# Gemcitabine-Vinorelbine
**Use:** Lung cancer, nonsmall cell
**Regimen: Note:** Multiple variations are listed below.
>**Variation 1:**
>Gemcitabine: I.V.: 1200 mg/m$^2$/day days 1 and 8  [total dose/cycle = 2400 mg/m$^2$]
>Vinorelbine: I.V.: 30 mg/m$^2$/day days 1 and 8  [total dose/cycle = 60 mg/m$^2$]
>Repeat cycle every 21 days for 6 cycles
>**Variation 2:**
>Gemcitabine: I.V.: 1000 mg/m$^2$/day days 1, 8, and 15  [total dose/cycle = 3000 mg/m$^2$]
>Vinorelbine: I.V.: 20 mg/m$^2$/day days 1, 8, and 15  [total dose/cycle = 60 mg/m$^2$]
>Repeat cycle every 28 days for 6 cycles

# HDMTX (Osteosarcoma)
**Use:** Osteosarcoma
**Regimen:**
>Methotrexate: I.V.: 12 g/m$^2$/week for 2-12 weeks  [total dose/cycle = 24-144 g/m$^2$]
>Leucovorin calcium rescue: Oral, I.V.: 15 mg/m$^2$ every 6 hours (beginning 30 hours after the beginning of the 4-hour methotrexate infusion) for 10 doses; **serum methotrexate levels must be monitored** [total dose/cycle = 150 mg/m$^2$]

# HIPE-IVAD

**Use:** Neuroblastomas
**Regimen:**

Cisplatin: I.V.: 40 mg/m$^2$/day days 1-5 [total dose/cycle = 200 mg/m$^2$]
Etoposide: I.V.: 100 mg/m$^2$/day days 1-5 [total dose/cycle = 500 mg/m$^2$]
Ifosfamide: I.V.: 3 g/m$^2$/day days 21-23 [total dose/cycle = 9 g/m$^2$]
Mesna: I.V.: 3 g/m$^2$/day continuous infusion days 21-23 [total dose/cycle = 9 g/m$^2$]
Vincristine: I.V.: 1.5 mg/m$^2$ day 21 [total dose/cycle = 1.5 mg/m$^2$]
Doxorubicin: I.V.: 60 mg/m$^2$ day 23 [total dose/cycle = 60 mg/m$^2$]
Repeat cycle every 28 days

# Hyper-CVAD

**Use:** Multiple myeloma; Lymphoma, non-Hodgkin (Burkitt); Leukemia, acute lymphocytic
**Regimen:**

**Course 1, 3, 5, and 7:**
Cyclophosphamide: I.V.: 300 mg/m$^2$/day every 12 hours days 1-3 [total dose/cycle = 1.8 g/m$^2$]
Mesna: I.V.: 3600 mg/m$^2$/day continuous infusion days 1-3 [total dose/cycle = 10,800 mg/m$^2$]
Methotrexate: I.T.: 12 mg day 2 [total dose/cycle = 12 mg]
Vincristine: I.V.: 2 mg/day days 4 and 11 [total dose/cycle = 4 mg]
Doxorubicin: I.V.: 50 mg/m$^2$ day 4 [total dose/cycle = 50 mg/m$^2$]
Cytarabine: I.T.: 100 mg day 8 [total dose/cycle = 100 mg]
Dexamethasone: Oral or I.V.: 40 mg/day days 1-4 and 11-14 [total dose/cycle = 320 mg]
**Course 2, 4, 6, and 8:**
Methotrexate: I.V.: 200 mg/m$^2$ day 1
[total dose/cycle = 200 mg/m$^2$] **followed by** 800 mg/m$^2$ continuous infusion day 1
[total dose/cycle = 800 mg/m$^2$]
Cytarabine: I.V.: 3 g/m$^2$ every 12 hours days 2 and 3 [total dose/cycle = 12 g/m$^2$]
Methotrexate: I.T.: 12 mg day 2 [total dose/cycle = 12 mg]
Leucovorin: I.V.: 15 mg every 6 hours days 3 and 4 [total dose/cycle = 120 mg]
Methylprednisolone: I.V.: 50 mg twice daily days 1-3 [total dose/cycle = 300 mg]
Cytarabine: I.T.: 100 mg day 8 [total dose/cycle = 100 mg]
Cycles are given when WBC is ≥3000 mm$^3$, Plt ≥60,000 mm$^3$

# ICE (Lymphoma, non-Hodgkin)

**Use:** Lymphoma, non-Hodgkin
**Regimen:**

Etoposide: I.V.: 100 mg/m$^2$/day days 1-3 [total dose/cycle = 300 mg/m$^2$]
Carboplatin: I.V.: AUC 5 day 2 (maximum 800 mg) [total dose/cycle = AUC = 5]
Ifosfamide: I.V.: 5000 mg/m$^2$ continuous infusion day 2 [total dose/cycle = 5000 mg/m$^2$]
Mesna: I.V.: 5000 mg/m$^2$ continuous infusion day 2 [total dose/cycle = 5000 mg/m$^2$]
Filgrastim: SubQ: 5 mcg/kg days 5 and 12 [total dose/cycle = 10 mcg/kg]
Repeat cycle every 2 weeks

# ICE (Sarcoma)

**Use:** Osteosarcoma; Soft tissue sarcoma
**Regimen:**

Ifosfamide: I.V.: 1250-1500 mg/m$^2$/day days 1-3 [total dose/cycle = 3750-4500 mg/m$^2$]
Carboplatin: I.V.: 300-635 mg/m$^2$ day 3 [total dose/cycle = 300-635 mg/m$^2$]
Etopside: I.V.: 80-100 mg/m$^2$/day days 1-3 [total dose/cycle = 240-300 mg/m$^2$]
Mesna: I.V.: 1250 mg/m$^2$/day days 1-3 [total dose/cycle = 3750 mg/m$^2$]
**or** 20% of ifosfamide dose before, 4 and 8 hours after each ifosfamide infusion
[total dose/cycle = 60% of ifosfamide dose]
Repeat cycle every 21-28 days

## ICE-T
**Use:** Soft tissue sarcoma
**Regimen:**

Ifosfamide: I.V.: 1250 mg/m$^2$/day days 1, 2, and 3  [total dose/cycle = 3750 mg/m$^2$]
Carboplatin: I.V.: 300 mg/m$^2$ day 1  [total dose/cycle = 300 mg/m$^2$]
Etopside: I.V.: 80 mg/m$^2$/day days 1, 2, and 3  [total dose/cycle = 240 mg/m$^2$]
Paclitaxel: I.V.: 175 mg/m$^2$ day 4  [total dose/cycle = 175 mg/m$^2$]
Mesna: I.V.: 20% of ifosfamide dose before
**followed by:** Oral: 40% of ifosfamide dose 4 and 8 hours after ifosfamide
[total dose/cycle = 100% of ifosfamide dose] **or**
Mesna: I.V.: 1250 mg/m$^2$/day days 1, 2, and 3  [total dose/cycle = 3750 mg/m$^2$]
Repeat cycle every 28 days

## Idarubicin, Cytarabine, Etoposide (ICE Protocol)
**Use:** Leukemia, acute myeloid
**Regimen:**

Idarubicin: I.V.: 6 mg/m$^2$/day days 1-5  [total dose/cycle = 30 mg/m$^2$]
Cytarabine: I.V.: 600 mg/m$^2$/day days 1-5  [total dose/cycle = 3000 mg/m$^2$]
Etoposide: I.V.: 150 mg/m$^2$/day days 1-3  [total dose/cycle = 450 mg/m$^2$]
Administer one cycle only

## Idarubicin, Cytarabine, Etoposide (IDA-Based BF12)
**Use:** Leukemia, acute myeloid
**Regimen:** Induction:

Idarubicin: I.V.: 5 mg/m$^2$/day days 1-5  [total dose/cycle = 25 mg/m$^2$]
Cytarabine: I.V.: 2000 mg/m$^2$ every 12 hours days 1-5 (10 doses)
[total dose/cycle = 20,000 mg/m$^2$]
Etoposide: I.V.: 100 mg/m$^2$/day days 1-5  [total dose/cycle = 500 mg/m$^2$]
Second cycle may be given based on individual respone; time between cycles not specified

## IDMTX/6-MP
**Use:** Leukemia, acute lymphocytic
**Regimen:** Intensification:

**Week 1:**
Methotrexate: I.V.: 200 mg/m$^2$
[total dose/cycle = 200 mg/m$^2$] **followed by** 800 mg/m$^2$ continuous infusion day 1
[total dose/cycle = 800 mg/m$^2$]
Mercaptopurine: I.V.: 200 mg/m$^2$
[total dose/cycle = 200 mg/m$^2$] **followed by** 800 mg/m$^2$ over 8 hours day 1  [total dose/cycle = 800 mg/m$^2$]
Leucovorin: Oral or I.V.: 5 mg/m$^2$ every 6 hours for 5-13 doses beginning 24 hours after end of methotrexate
infusion  [total dose/cycle = 30-65 mg/m$^2$]
**Week 2:**
Methotrexate: I.M.: 20 mg/m$^2$ day 8  [total dose/cycle = 20 mg/m$^2$]
Mercaptopurine: Oral: 50 mg/m$^2$/day days 8-14  [total dose/cycle = 350 mg/m$^2$]
Repeat cycle every 2 weeks up to 12 cycles

## IE
**Use:** Soft tissue sarcoma
**Regimen:**

Etoposide: I.V.: 100 mg/m$^2$/day days 1-3  [total dose/cycle = 300 mg/m$^2$]
Ifosfamide: I.V.: 2500 mg/m$^2$/day days 1-3  [total dose/cycle = 7500 mg/m$^2$]
Mesna: I.V.: 20% of ifosfamide dose prior to and at 4-, 8-, and 12 hours after ifosfamide administration
[total dose/cycle = 80% ifosfamide dose]
Repeat cycle every 28 days

## IL-2 + IFN

**Use:** Melanoma
**Regimen:**

Cisplatin: I.V.: 20 mg/m$^2$/day days 1-4  [total dose/cycle = 80 mg/m$^2$]
Vinblastine: I.V.: 1.6 mg/m$^2$/day days 1-4  [total dose/cycle = 6.4 mg/m$^2$]
Dacarbazine: I.V.: 800 mg/m$^2$ day 1  [total dose/cycle = 800 mg/m$^2$]
Aldesleukin: I.V.: 9 million units/m$^2$/day continuous infusion days 1-4
    [total dose/cycle = 36 million units/m$^2$]
Interferon alfa-2b: SubQ: 5 million units/m$^2$/day days 1-5, 7, 9, 11, 13
    [total dose/cycle = 45 million units/m$^2$]
Repeat cycle every 21 days

## IMVP-16

**Use:** Lymphoma, non-Hodgkin
**Regimen:**

Ifosfamide: I.V.: 4 g/m$^2$ continuous infusion over 24 hours day 1  [total dose/cycle = 4 g/m$^2$]
Mesna: I.V.: 800 mg/m$^2$ bolus prior to ifosfamide, then 4 g/m$^2$ continuous infusion over 12 hours concurrent with ifosfamide; then 2.4 g/m$^2$ continuous infusion over 12 hours after ifosfamide infusion day 1
    [total dose/cycle = 7.2 g/m$^2$]
Methotrexate: I.V.: 30 mg/m$^2$/day days 3 and 10  [total dose/cycle = 60 mg/m$^2$]
Etoposide: I.V.: 100 mg/m$^2$/day days 1-3  [total dose/cycle = 300 mg/m$^2$]
Repeat cycle every 21-28 days

## Interleukin 2-Interferon Alfa 2

**Use:** Renal cell cancer
**Regimen:**

**Weeks 1 and 4:**
Aldesleukin: SubQ: 20 million units/m$^2$ 3 times weekly  [total dose/cycle = 120 million units/m$^2$]
Interferon alfa: SubQ: 6 million units/m$^2$ once weekly  [total dose/cycle = 12 million units/m$^2$]
**Weeks 2, 3, 5, and 6:**
Aldesleukin: SubQ: 5 million units/m$^2$ 3 times weekly  [total dose/cycle = 60 million units/m$^2$]
Interferon alfa: SubQ: 6 million units/m$^2$ 3 times weekly  [total dose/cycle = 72 million units/m$^2$]
Repeat cycle every 56 days

## Interleukin 2-Interferon Alfa 2-Fluorouracil

**Use:** Renal cell cancer
**Regimen:**

**Weeks 1 and 4:**
Aldesleukin: SubQ: 20 million units/m$^2$ 3 times weekly  [total dose/cycle = 120 million units/m$^2$]
Interferon alfa: SubQ: 6 million units/m$^2$ once weekly  [total dose/cycle = 12 million units/m$^2$]
**Weeks 2 and 3:**
Aldesleukin: SubQ: 5 million units/m$^2$ 3 times weekly  [total dose/cycle = 30 million units/m$^2$]
**Weeks 5-8:**
Interferon alfa: SubQ: 9 million units/m$^2$ 3 times weekly  [total dose/cycle = 108 million units/m$^2$]
Fluorouracil: I.V.: 750 mg/m$^2$ once weekly  [total dose/cycle = 3000 mg/m$^2$]
Repeat cycle every 56 days

## IPA

**Use:** Hepatoblastoma
**Regimen:**

Ifosfamide: I.V.: 500 mg/m$^2$ day 1   [total dose/cycle = 500 mg/m$^2$] **followed by**
1000 mg/m$^2$/day continuous infusion days 1-3  [total dose/cycle = 3000 mg/m$^2$]
Cisplatin: I.V.: 20 mg/m$^2$/day days 4-8   [total dose/cycle = 100 mg/m$^2$]
Doxorubicin: I.V.: 30 mg/m$^2$/day continuous infusion days 9 and 10  [total dose/cycle = 60 mg/m$^2$]
Repeat cycle every 21 days

# Irinotecan/Cisplatin
**Use:** Esophageal cancer
**Regimen:**
    Cisplatin: I.V.: 30 mg/m$^2$/day days 1, 8, 15 and 22  [total dose/cycle = 120 mg/m$^2$]
    Irinotecan: I.V.: 65 mg/m$^2$/day days 1, 8, 15 and 22  [total dose/cycle = 260 mg/m$^2$]
    Repeat cycle every 6 weeks

# IVAC
**Use:** Lymphoma, non-Hodgkin
**Regimen:**
    Ifosfamide: I.V.: 1500 mg/m$^2$/day days 1-5  [total dose/cycle = 7500 mg/m$^2$]
    Etoposide: I.V.: 60 mg/m$^2$/day days 1-5 [total dose/cycle = 300 mg/m$^2$]
    Cytarabine: I.V.: 2000 mg/m$^2$ every 12 hours days 1 and 2  [total dose/cycle = 8000 mg/m$^2$]
    Mesna: I.V.: 360 mg/m$^2$ every 3 hours days 1-5 [total dose/cycle = 14,400 mg/m$^2$]
    Methotrexate: I.T.: 12 mg day 5 [total dose/cycle = 12 mg]
    Repeat when ANC >1000 cells/mm$^3$

# Larson Regimen
**Use:** Leukemia, acute lymphocytic
**Regimen:** Induction:
    Cyclophosphamide: I.V.: 1200 mg/m$^2$ day 1 [total dose/cycle = 1200 mg/m$^2$]
    Daunorubicin: I.V.: 45 mg/m$^2$/day days 1-3 [total dose/cycle = 135 mg/m$^2$]
    Vincristine: I.V.: 2 mg/day days 1, 8, 15, and 22 [total dose/cycle = 8 mg]
    Prednisone: Oral or I.V.: 60 mg/m$^2$/day days 1-21 [total dose/cycle = 1260 mg/m$^2$]
    Asparaginase: SubQ: 6000 units/m$^2$/day days 5, 8, 11, 15, 18, and 22
        [total dose/cycle = 36,000 units/m$^2$]
    Administer one cycle only

# Linker Protocol
**Use:** Leukemia, acute lymphocytic
**Regimen:**
    **Remission induction:**
    Daunorubicin: I.V.: 50 mg/m$^2$/day days 1-3 [total dose/cycle = 150 mg/m$^2$]
    Vincristine: I.V.: 2 mg/day days 1, 8, 15, and 22 [total dose/cycle = 8 mg]
    Prednisone: Oral: 60 mg/m$^2$/day days 1-28 [total dose/cycle = 1680 mg/m$^2$]
    Asparaginase: I.M.: 6000 units/m$^2$/day days 17-28 [total dose/cycle = 72,000 units/m$^2$]
    **If residual leukemia in bone marrow on day 14:**
    Daunorubicin: I.V.: 50 mg/m$^2$ day 15 [total dose/cycle = 50 mg/m$^2$]
    **If residual leukemia in bone marrow on day 28:**
    Daunorubicin: I.V.: 50 mg/m$^2$ days 29 and 30 [total dose/cycle = 100 mg/m$^2$]
    Vincristine: I.V.: 2 mg/day days 29 and 36 [total dose/cycle = 4 mg]
    Prednisone: Oral: 60 mg/m$^2$/day days 29-42 [total dose/cycle = 840 mg/m$^2$]
    Asparaginase: I.M.: 6000 units/m$^2$/day days 29-35
    **Consolidation therapy:**
    **Treatment A (cycles 1, 3, 5, and 7)**
    Daunorubicin: I.V.: 50 mg/m$^2$/day days 1 and 2 [total dose/cycle = 100 mg/m$^2$]
    Vincristine: I.V.: 2 mg/day days 1 and 8 [total dose/cycle = 4 mg]
    Prednisone: Oral: 60 mg/m$^2$/day days 1-14 [total dose/cycle = 840 mg/m$^2$]
    Asparaginase: I.M.: 12,000 units/m$^2$/day days 2, 4, 7, 9, 11, and 14
        [total dose/cycle = 72,000 units/m$^2$]
    **Treatment B (cycles 2, 4, 6, and 8)**
    Teniposide: I.V.: 165 mg/m$^2$/day days 1, 4, 8, and 11 [total dose/cycle = 660 mg/m$^2$]
    Cytarabine: I.V.: 300 mg/m$^2$/day days 1, 4, 8, and 11 [total dose/cycle = 1200 mg/m$^2$]
    **Treatment C (cycle 9)**
    Methotrexate: I.V.: 690 mg/m$^2$ continuous infusion day 1 (over 42 hours)
        [total dose/cycle = 690 mg/m$^2$]
    Leucovorin: I.V.: 15 mg/m$^2$ every 6 hours for 12 doses (start at end of methotrexate infusion)
        [total dose/cycle = 180 mg/m$^2$]
    Administer remission induction regimen for one cycle only. Repeat consolidation cycle every 28 days

# LOPP
**Use:** Lymphoma, Hodgkin disease
**Regimen:**
Chlorambucil: Oral: 10 mg/day days 1-10  [total dose/cycle = 100 mg]
Vincristine: I.V.: 1.4 mg/m$^2$/day (maximum 2 mg) days 1 and 8  [total dose/cycle = 2.8 mg/m$^2$]
Procarbazine: Oral: 100 mg/m$^2$/day days 1-10  [total dose/cycle = 1000 mg/m$^2$]
Prednisone: Oral: 25 mg/m$^2$/day (maximum 60 mg) days 1-14
    [total dose/cycle = 350 mg/m$^2$] **or**
Prednisolone: Oral: 25 mg/m$^2$/day (maximum 60 mg) days 1-14  [total dose/cycle = 350 mg/m$^2$]
Repeat cycle every 28 days

# M-2
**Use:** Multiple myeloma
**Regimen:**
Vincristine: I.V.: 0.03 mg/kg (maximum 2 mg) day 1  [total dose/cycle = 0.03 mg/kg]
Carmustine: I.V.: 0.5 mg/kg day 1  [total dose/cycle = 0.5 mg/kg]
Cyclophosphamide: I.V.: 10 mg/kg day 1  [total dose/cycle = 10 mg/kg]
Melphalan: Oral: 0.25 mg/kg/day days 1-4  [total dose/cycle = 1 mg/kg] **or** 0.1 mg/kg/day days 1-7
    **or** 1-10  [total dose/cycle = 0.7 or 1 mg/kg]
Prednisone: Oral: 1 mg/kg/day days 1-7 (taper over 14 days)
    [total dose/cycle = 7 mg/kg + taper over 14 days]
Repeat cycle every 5 weeks

# M-3
**Use:** Leukemia, acute promyelocytic
**Regimen: Note:** Multiple variations are listed below.
**Induction:**
**Variation 1:**
Tretinoin: Oral: 45 mg/m$^2$/day day 1 up to 90 days  [total dose/cycle = 45-4050 mg/m$^2$]
≤20 years: 25 mg/m$^2$/day day 1 up to 90 days  [total dose/cycle = 25-2250 mg/m$^2$]
Idarubicin: I.V.: 12 mg/m$^2$/day days 2, 4, 6, and 8  [total dose/cycle = 48 mg/m$^2$]
**Consolidation:**
**Course 1:**
Idarubicin: I.V.: 5 mg/m$^2$/day days 1-4  [total dose/cycle = 20 mg/m$^2$]
**or** 7 mg/m$^2$/day days 1-4  [total dose/cycle = 28 mg/m$^2$]
Tretinoin: Oral: 45 mg/m$^2$/day days 1-15  [total dose/cycle = 675 mg/m$^2$]
**Course 2:**
Mitoxantrone: I.V.: 10 mg/m$^2$/day days 1-5  [total dose/cycle = 50 mg/m$^2$]
**or** 10 mg/m$^2$/day days 1-5  [total dose/cycle = 50 mg/m$^2$]
Tretinoin: Oral: 45 mg/m$^2$/day days 1-15  [total dose/cycle = 675 mg/m$^2$]
**Course 3:**
Idarubicin: I.V.: 12 mg/m$^2$ on day 1  [total dose/cycle = 12 mg/m$^2$]
**or** 12 mg/m$^2$/day on days 1 and 2  [total dose/cycle = 24 mg/m$^2$]
Tretinoin: Oral: 45 mg/m$^2$/day days 1-15  [total dose/cycle = 675 mg/m$^2$]
Repeat course at one month intervals.
**Maintenance:**
Mercaptopurine: Oral: 50 mg/m$^2$ daily  [total dose/cycle = 4.5 g/m$^2$]
Methotrexate: I.M.: 15 mg/m$^2$ weekly  [total dose/cycle = 180 mg/m$^2$]
Tretinoin: Oral: 45 mg/m$^2$/day days 1-15  [total dose/cycle = 675 mg/m$^2$]
Repeat cycle every 3 months for 2 years
**Variation 2:**
**Induction:**
Tretinoin: Oral: 45 mg/m$^2$/day day 1 up to 90 days  [total dose/cycle = 45-4050 mg/m$^2$]
≤15 years: 25 mg/m$^2$/day day 1 up to 90 days  [total dose/cycle = 25-2250 mg/m$^2$]
Idarubicin: I.V.: 12 mg/m$^2$/day days 2, 4, 6, and 8  [total dose/cycle = 48 mg/m$^2$]
**Consolidation:**
**Course 1:**
Idarubicin: I.V.: 5 mg/m$^2$/day days 1-4  [total dose/cycle = 20 mg/m$^2$]
**Course 2:**
Mitoxantrone: I.V.: 10 mg/m$^2$/day days 1-5  [total dose/cycle = 50 mg/m$^2$]
**Course 3:**
Idarubicin: I.V.: 12 mg/m$^2$ day 1  [total dose/cycle = 12 mg/m$^2$]
Repeat course at one month intervals
**Maintenance:**
Mercaptopurine: Oral: 90 mg/m$^2$ daily  [total dose/cycle = 8.1 g/m$^2$]
Methotrexate: I.M.: 15 mg/m$^2$ weekly  [total dose/cycle = 60 mg/m$^2$]
Tretinoin: Oral: 45 mg/m$^2$/day days 1-15  [total dose/cycle = 675 mg/m$^2$]
Repeat cycle every 3 months for 2 years

# MACOP-B

**Use:** Lymphoma, non-Hodgkin

**Regimen:**

Methotrexate: I.V.: 400 mg/m$^2$ weeks 2, 6, 10  [total dose/cycle = 1200 mg/m$^2$]

Doxorubicin: I.V.: 50 mg/m$^2$ weeks 1, 3, 5, 7, 9, 11  [total dose/cycle = 300 mg/m$^2$]

Cyclophosphamide: I.V.: 350 mg/m$^2$ weeks 1, 3, 5, 7, 9, 11  [total dose/cycle = 2100 mg/m$^2$]

Vincristine: I.V.: 1.4 mg/m$^2$ (maximum 2 mg) weeks 2, 4, 8, 10, 12  [total dose/cycle = 7 mg/m$^2$]

Bleomycin: I.V.: 10 units/m$^2$ weeks 4, 8, 12  [total dose/cycle = 30 units/m$^2$]

Prednisone: Oral: 75 mg/day for 12 weeks, taper over last 2 weeks

Leucovorin calcium: Oral: 15 mg/m$^2$ every 6 hours for 6 doses (beginning 24 hours after methotrexate) weeks 2, 6, 10  [total dose/cycle = 270 mg/m$^2$]

Administer one cycle

# MAID

**Use:** Soft tissue sarcoma

**Regimen:**

Mesna: I.V.: 2500 mg/m$^2$/day continuous infusion days 1-4  [total dose/cycle = 10,000 mg/m$^2$]

Doxorubicin: I.V.: 20 mg/m$^2$/day continuous infusion days 1-3  [total dose/cycle = 60 mg/m$^2$]

Ifosfamide: I.V.: 2500 mg/m$^2$/day continuous infusion days 1-3  [total dose/cycle = 7500 mg/m$^2$]

Dacarbazine: I.V.: 300 mg/m$^2$/day continuous infusion days 1-3  [total dose/cycle = 900 mg/m$^2$]

Repeat cycle every 21-28 days

# m-BACOD

**Use:** Lymphoma, non-Hodgkin

**Regimen:**

Methotrexate: I.V.: 200 mg/m$^2$/day days 8 and 15  [total dose/cycle = 400 mg/m$^2$]

Leucovorin calcium: Oral: 10 mg/m$^2$ every 6 hours for 8 doses (beginning 24 hours after each methotrexate dose) days 9 and 16  [total dose/cycle = 160 mg/m$^2$]

Bleomycin: I.V.: 4 units/m$^2$ day 1  [total dose/cycle = 4 units/m$^2$]

Doxorubicin: I.V.: 45 mg/m$^2$ day 1  [total dose/cycle = 45 mg/m$^2$]

Cyclophosphamide: I.V.: 600 mg/m$^2$ day 1  [total dose/cycle = 600 mg/m$^2$]

Vincristine: I.V.: 1 mg/m$^2$ day 1  [total dose/cycle = 1 mg/m$^2$]

Dexamethasone: Oral: 6 mg/m$^2$/day days 1-5  [total dose/cycle = 30 mg/m$^2$]

Repeat cycle every 21 days

# MINE

**Use:** Lymphoma, non-Hodgkin

**Regimen:**

Mesna: I.V.: 1.33 g/m$^2$/day concurrent with ifosfamide dose, then 500 mg orally (4 hours after each ifosfamide infusion) days 1-3  [total dose/cycle = 3.99 g/m$^2$/1500 mg]

Ifosfamide: I.V.: 1.33 g/m$^2$/day days 1-3  [total dose/cycle = 3.99 mg/m$^2$]

Mitoxantrone: I.V.: 8 mg/m$^2$ day 1  [total dose/cycle = 8 mg/m$^2$]

Etoposide: I.V.: 65 mg/m$^2$/day days 1-3  [total dose/cycle = 195 mg/m$^2$]

Repeat cycle every 28 days

# MINE-ESHAP

**Use:** Lymphoma, non-Hodgkin

**Regimen:**

    Mesna: I.V.: 1.33 g/m$^2$ concurrent with ifosfamide dose, then 500 mg orally (4 hours after ifosfamide) days 1-3
        [total dose/cycle = 3.99 g/m$^2$/1500 mg]

    Ifosfamide: I.V.: 1.33 g/m$^2$/day days 1-3  [total dose/cycle = 3.99 mg/m$^2$]

    Mitoxantrone: I.V.: 8 mg/m$^2$ day 1  [total dose/cycle = 8 mg/m$^2$]

    Etoposide: I.V.: 65 mg/m$^2$/day days 1-3  [total dose/cycle = 195 mg/m$^2$]

    Repeat cycle every 21 days for 6 cycles, **followed by**
        3-6 cycles of ESHAP

# mini-BEAM

**Use:** Lymphoma, Hodgkin disease

**Regimen:**

    Carmustine: I.V.: 60 mg/m$^2$ day 1  [total dose/cycle = 60 mg/m$^2$]

    Etoposide: I.V.: 75 mg/m$^2$/day days 2-5  [total dose/cycle = 300 mg/m$^2$]

    Cytarabine: I.V.: 100 mg/m$^2$ every 12 hours days 2-5 (8 doses)  [total dose/cycle = 800 mg/m$^2$]

    Melphalan: I.V.: 30 mg/m$^2$ day 6  [total dose/cycle = 30 mg/m$^2$]

    Repeat cycle every 4-6 weeks

# Mitoxantrone + Hydrocortisone

**Use:** Prostate cancer

**Regimen:**

    Mitoxantrone: I.V.: 14 mg/m$^2$ day 1  [total dose/cycle = 14 mg/m$^2$]

    Hydrocortisone: Oral: 40 mg daily  [total dose/cycle = 840 mg]

    Repeat cycle every 3 weeks

# MM

**Use:** Leukemia, acute lymphocytic (maintenance)

**Regimen:**

    Mercaptopurine: Oral: 50-75 mg/m$^2$/day days 1-7  [total dose/cycle = 350-525 mg/m$^2$]

    Methotrexate: Oral, I.V.: 20 mg/m$^2$ day 1  [total dose/cycle = 20 mg/m$^2$]

    Repeat cycle every 7 days

# MOP

**Use:** Brain tumors

**Regimen:**

    Mechlorethamine: I.V.: 6 mg/m$^2$/day days 1 and 8  [total dose/cycle = 12 mg/m$^2$]

    Vincristine: I.V.: 1.5 mg/m$^2$/day (maximum 2 mg) days 1 and 8  [total dose/cycle = 3 mg/m$^2$]

    Procarbazine: Oral: 100 mg/m$^2$/day days 1-14  [total dose/cycle = 1400 mg/m$^2$]

    Repeat cycle every 28 days

## MOPP (Lymphoma, Hodgkin Disease)

**Use:** Lymphoma, Hodgkin disease
**Regimen: Note:** Multiple variations are listed below.

### Variation 1:
Mechlorethamine: I.V.: 6 mg/m$^2$/day days 1 and 8  [total dose/cycle = 12 mg/m$^2$]
Vincristine: I.V.: 1.4 mg/m$^2$/day days 1 and 8  [total dose/cycle = 2.8 mg/m$^2$]
Procarbazine: Oral: 100 mg/m$^2$/day days 1-14  [total dose/cycle = 1400 mg/m$^2$]
Prednisone: Oral: 40 mg/m$^2$/day days 1-14 (cycles 1 and 4)  [total dose/cycle = 560 mg/m$^2$]
Repeat cycle every 28 days for 6-8 cycles

### Variation 2:
Mechlorethamine: I.V.: 6 mg/m$^2$/day (maximum 15 mg) days 1 and 8
 [total dose/cycle = 12 mg/m$^2$]
Vincristine: I.V.: 1.4 mg/m$^2$/day (maximum 2 mg) days 1 and 8  [total dose/cycle = 2.8 mg/m$^2$]
Procarbazine: Oral: 100 mg/m$^2$/day days 1-10  [total dose/cycle = 1000 mg/m$^2$]
Prednisone: Oral: 25 mg/m$^2$/day (maximum 60 mg) days 1-14
 [total dose/cycle = 350 mg/m$^2$] **or**
Prednisolone: Oral: 25 mg/m$^2$/day (maximum 60 mg) days 1-14  [total dose/cycle = 350 mg/m$^2$]
Repeat cycle every 28 days

### Variation 3:
Mechlorethamine: I.V.: 6 mg/m$^2$/day days 1 and 8  [total dose/cycle = 12 mg/m$^2$]
Vincristine: I.V.: 1.4 mg/m$^2$/day days 1 and 8  [total dose/cycle = 2.8 mg/m$^2$]
Procarbazine: Oral: 50 mg day 1, 100 mg day 2, 100 mg/m$^2$/day days 3-14
 [total dose/cycle = 150 mg / 1200 mg/m$^2$]
Prednisone: Oral: 40 mg/m$^2$/day days 1-14  [total dose/cycle = 560 mg/m$^2$]
Repeat cycle every 28 days

### Variation 4:
Mechlorethamine: I.V.: 6 mg/m$^2$/day days 1 and 8  [total dose/cycle = 12 mg/m$^2$]
Vincristine: I.V.: 1.4 mg/m$^2$/day days 1 and 8  [total dose/cycle = 2.8 mg/m$^2$]
Procarbazine: Oral: 50 mg day 1, 100 mg day 2, 100 mg/m$^2$/day days 3-10
 [total dose/cycle = 150 mg / 800 mg/m$^2$]
Prednisone: Oral: 40 mg/m$^2$/day days 1-14  [total dose/cycle = 560 mg/m$^2$]
Repeat cycle every 28 days

### Variation 5:
Mechlorethamine: I.V.: 6 mg/m$^2$/day days 1 and 8  [total dose/cycle = 12 mg/m$^2$]
Vincristine: I.V.: 1.4 mg/m$^2$/day days 1 and 8  [total dose/cycle = 2.8 mg/m$^2$]
Procarbazine: Oral: 50 mg/m$^2$ day 1, then 100 mg/m$^2$/day days 2-14
 [total dose/cycle = 1350 mg/m$^2$]
Prednisone: Oral: 40 mg/m$^2$/day days 1-14  [total dose/cycle = 560 mg/m$^2$]
Repeat cycle every 28 days

## MOPP (Medulloblastoma)

**Use:** Brain tumors
**Regimen:**
Mechlorethamine: I.V.: 3 mg/m$^2$/day days 1 and 8  [total dose/cycle = 6 mg/m$^2$]
Vincristine: I.V.: 1.4 mg/m$^2$/day (maximum 2 mg) days 1 and 8  [total dose/cycle = 2.8 mg/m$^2$]
Prednisone: Oral: 40 mg/m$^2$/day days 1-10  [total dose/cycle = 400 mg/m$^2$]
Procarbazine: Oral: 50 mg day 1  [total dose = 50 mg] **followed by**
100 mg day 2  [total dose = 100 mg] **followed by**
100 mg/m$^2$/day days 3-10  [total dose = 800 mg/m$^2$]
Repeat cycle every 28 days

## MOPP/ABV Hybrid

**Use:** Lymphoma, Hodgkin disease
**Regimen:**
Mechlorethamine: I.V.: 6 mg/m$^2$ day 1  [total dose/cycle = 6 mg/m$^2$]
Vincristine: I.V.: 1.4 mg/m$^2$ (maximum 2 mg) day 1  [total dose/cycle = 1.4 mg/m$^2$]
Procarbazine: Oral: 100 mg/m$^2$/day days 1-7  [total dose/cycle = 700 mg/m$^2$]
Prednisone: Oral: 40 mg/m$^2$/day days 1-14  [total dose/cycle = 560 mg/m$^2$]
Doxorubicin: I.V.: 35 mg/m$^2$ day 8  [total dose/cycle = 35 mg/m$^2$]
Bleomycin: I.V.: 10 units/m$^2$ day 8  [total dose/cycle = 10 units/m$^2$]
Vinblastine: I.V.: 6 mg/m$^2$ day 8  [total dose/cycle = 6 mg/m$^2$]
Repeat cycle every 28 days

# MOPP/ABVD

**Use:** Lymphoma, Hodgkin disease
**Regimen: Note:** Multiple variations are listed below.
### Variation 1:
Mechlorethamine: I.V.: 6 mg/m$^2$/day days 1 and 8  [total dose/cycle = 12 mg/m$^2$]
Vincristine: I.V.: 1.4 mg/m$^2$/day (maximum 2 mg) days 1 and 8  [total dose/cycle = 2.8 mg/m$^2$]
Procarbazine: I.V.: 100 mg/m$^2$/day days 1-14  [total dose/cycle = 1400 mg/m$^2$]
Prednisone: Oral: 40 mg/m$^2$/day days 1-14 (during cycles 1, 4, 7, and 10 only)
    [total dose/cycle = 560 mg/m$^2$]
Doxorubicin: Oral: 25 mg/m$^2$/day days 29 and 43  [total dose/cycle = 50 mg/m$^2$]
Bleomycin: I.V.: 10 units/m$^2$/day day 29 and 43  [total dose/cycle = 20 units/m$^2$]
Vinblastine: I.V.: 6 mg/m$^2$/day days 29 and 43  [total dose/cycle = 12 mg/m$^2$]
Dacarbazine: I.V.: 375 mg/m$^2$/day days 29 and 43  [total dose/cycle = 750 mg/m$^2$]
Repeat cycle every 56 days
### Variation 2:
Mechlorethamine: I.V.: 6 mg/m$^2$/day days 1 and 8  [total dose/cycle = 12 mg/m$^2$]
Vincristine: I.V.: 1.4 mg/m$^2$/day (maximum 2 mg) days 1 and 8  [total dose/cycle = 2.8 mg/m$^2$]
Procarbazine: I.V.: 100 mg/m$^2$/day days 1-14  [total dose/cycle = 1400 mg/m$^2$]
Prednisone: Oral: 40 mg/m$^2$/day days 1-14 (during cycles 1 and 7 only)
    [total dose/cycle = 560 mg/m$^2$]
Doxorubicin: Oral: 25 mg/m$^2$/day days 29 and 43  [total dose/cycle = 50 mg/m$^2$]
Bleomycin: I.V.: 10 units/m$^2$/day days 29 and 43  [total dose/cycle = 20 units/m$^2$]
Vinblastine: I.V.: 6 mg/m$^2$/day days 29 and 43  [total dose/cycle = 12 mg/m$^2$]
Dacarbazine: I.V.: 375 mg/m$^2$/day days 29 and 43  [total dose/cycle = 750 mg/m$^2$]
Repeat cycle every 56 days
### Variation 3:
Mechlorethamine: I.V.: 6 mg/m$^2$/day days 1 and 8  [total dose/cycle = 12 mg/m$^2$]
Vincristine: I.V.: 1.4 mg/m$^2$/day (maximum 2 mg) days 1 and 8  [total dose/cycle = 2.8 mg/m$^2$]
Procarbazine: I.V.: 100 mg/m$^2$/day days 1-14  [total dose/cycle = 1400 mg/m$^2$]
Prednisone: Oral: 40 mg/m$^2$/day days 1-14 (every cycle)  [total dose/cycle = 560 mg/m$^2$]
Doxorubicin: Oral: 25 mg/m$^2$/day days 29 and 43  [total dose/cycle = 50 mg/m$^2$]
Bleomycin: I.V.: 10 units/m$^2$/day days 29 and 43  [total dose/cycle = 20 units/m$^2$]
Vinblastine: I.V.: 6 mg/m$^2$/day days 29 and 43  [total dose/cycle = 12 mg/m$^2$]
Dacarbazine: I.V.: 375 mg/m$^2$/day days 29 and 43  [total dose/cycle = 750 mg/m$^2$]
Repeat cycle every 56 days
### Variation 4:
**MOPP Regimen:**
Mechlorethamine: I.V.: 6 mg/m$^2$/day days 1 and 8  [total dose/cycle = 12 mg/m$^2$]
Vincristine: I.V.: 1.4 mg/m$^2$/day (maximum 2 mg) days 1 and 8  [total dose/cycle = 2.8 mg/m$^2$]
Procarbazine: I.V.: 100 mg/m$^2$/day days 1-14  [total dose/cycle = 1400 mg/m$^2$]
Prednisone: Oral: 25 mg/m$^2$/day days 1-14  [total dose/cycle = 350 mg/m$^2$]
**ABVD Regimen:**
Doxorubicin: Oral: 25 mg/m$^2$/day days 1 and 15  [total dose/cycle = 50 mg/m$^2$]
Bleomycin: I.V.: 6 units/m$^2$/day days 1 and 15  [total dose/cycle = 12 units/m$^2$]
Vinblastine: I.V.: 6 mg/m$^2$/day days 1 and 15  [total dose/cycle = 12 mg/m$^2$]
Dacarbazine: I.V.: 250 mg/m$^2$/day days 1 and 15  [total dose/cycle = 500 mg/m$^2$]
Each regimen cycle is 28 days. Administer regimens in alternating fashion as follows: 2 cycles of MOPP alternating
    with 2 cycles of ABVD for a total of 8 cycles
### Variation 5 (pediatrics):
Mechlorethamine: I.V.: 6 mg/m$^2$/day days 1 and 8  [total dose/cycle = 12 mg/m$^2$]
Vincristine: I.V.: 1.4 mg/m$^2$/day days 1 and 8  [total dose/cycle = 2.8 mg/m$^2$]
Procarbazine: Oral: 100 mg/m$^2$/day days 1-14  [total dose/cycle = 1400 mg/m$^2$]
Prednisone: Oral: 40 mg/m$^2$/day days 1-14  [total dose/cycle = 560 mg/m$^2$]
Doxorubicin: Oral: 25 mg/m$^2$/day days 29 and 42  [total dose/cycle = 50 mg/m$^2$]
Bleomycin: I.V.: 10 units/m$^2$/day days 29 and 42  [total dose/cycle = 20 units/m$^2$]
Vinblastine: I.V.: 6 mg/m$^2$/day days 29 and 42  [total dose/cycle = 12 mg/m$^2$]
Dacarbazine: I.V.: 150 mg/m$^2$/day days 29-33  [total dose/cycle = 750 mg/m$^2$]
Repeat cycle evey 56 days for 4 cycles
### Variation 6 (pediatrics):
Mechlorethamine: I.V.: 6 mg/m$^2$/day days 1 and 8  [total dose/cycle = 12 mg/m$^2$]
Vincristine: I.V.: 1.4 mg/m$^2$/day days 1 and 8  [total dose/cycle = 2.8 mg/m$^2$]
Procarbazine: Oral: 100 mg/m$^2$/day days 1-14  [total dose/cycle = 1400 mg/m$^2$]
Prednisone: Oral: 40 mg/m$^2$/day days 1-14  [total dose/cycle = 560 mg/m$^2$]
Doxorubicin: Oral: 25 mg/m$^2$/day days 29 and 42  [total dose/cycle = 50 mg/m$^2$]
Bleomycin: I.V.: 10 units/m$^2$/day days 29 and 42  [total dose/cycle = 20 units/m$^2$]
Vinblastine: I.V.: 6 mg/m$^2$/day days 29 and 42  [total dose/cycle = 12 mg/m$^2$]
Dacarbazine: I.V.: 375 mg/m$^2$/day days 29 and 43  [total dose/cycle = 750 mg/m$^2$]
Repeat cycle evey 56 days for 4 cycles

## MP (Multiple Myeloma)
**Use:** Multiple myeloma
**Regimen:**
   Melphalan: Oral: 8-10 mg/m$^2$/day days 1-4  [total dose/cycle = 32-40 mg/m$^2$]
   Prednisone: Oral: 40-60 mg/m$^2$/day days 1-4  [total dose/cycle = 160-240 mg/m$^2$]
   Repeat cycle every 28-42 days

## MP (Prostate Cancer)
**Use:** Prostate cancer
**Regimen:**
   Mitoxantrone: I.V.: 12 mg/m$^2$ day 1  [total dose/cycle = 12 mg/m$^2$]
   Prednisone: Oral: 5 mg twice daily  [total dose/cycle = 210 mg]
   Repeat cycle every 21 days

## MTX/6-MP/VP (Maintenance)
**Use:** Leukemia, acute lymphocytic
**Regimen:**
   Methotrexate: Oral: 20 mg/m$^2$ weekly  [total dose/cycle = 80 mg/m$^2$]
   Mercaptopurine: Oral: 75 mg/m$^2$/day  [total dose/cycle = 2250 mg/m$^2$]
   Vincristine: I.V.: 1.5 mg/m$^2$ day 1  [total dose/cycle = 1.5 mg/m$^2$]
   Prednisone: Oral: 40 mg/m$^2$/day days 1-5  [total dose/cycle = 200 mg/m$^2$]
   Repeat monthly for 2-3 years

## MTX-CDDPAdr
**Use:** Osteosarcoma
**Regimen:**
   Cisplatin: I.V.: 75 mg/m$^2$ day 1 of cycles 1-7  [total dose/cycle = 75 mg/m$^2$]
   Cisplatin: I.V.: 120 mg/m$^2$ day 1 cycles 8-10  [total dose/cycle = 120 mg/m$^2$]
   Doxorubicin: I.V.: 25 mg/m$^2$/day days 1-3 of cycles 1-7  [total dose/cycle = 75 mg/m$^2$]
   Methotrexate: I.V.: 12 g/m$^2$/day days 21 and 28  [total dose/cycle = 24 g/m$^2$]
   Leucovorin calcium rescue: I.V.: 20 mg/m$^2$ every 3 hours (beginning 16 hours after completion of methotrexate) for
      8 doses, then orally every 6 hours for 8 doses  [total dose/cycle = 640 mg/m$^2$]

## MV
**Use:** Leukemia, acute myeloid
**Regimen:**
   Mitoxantrone: I.V.: 10 mg/m$^2$/day days 1-5  [total dose/cycle = 50 mg/m$^2$]
   Etoposide: I.V.: 100 mg/m$^2$/day days 1-5  [total dose/cycle = 500 mg/m$^2$]
   Second cycle may be given based on individual respone; time between cycles not specified

## M-VAC (Bladder Cancer)
**Use:** Bladder cancer
**Regimen: Note:** Multiple variations are listed below.
   **Variation 1:**
   Methotrexate: I.V.: 30 mg/m$^2$/day days 1, 15, 22  [total dose/cycle = 90 mg/m$^2$]
   Vinblastine: I.V.: 3 mg/m$^2$/day days 2, 15, 22  [total dose/cycle = 9 mg/m$^2$]
   Doxorubicin: I.V.: 30 mg/m$^2$ day 2  [total dose/cycle = 30 mg/m$^2$]
   Cisplatin: I.V.: 70 mg/m$^2$ day 2  [total dose/cycle = 70 mg/m$^2$]
   Repeat cycle every 4 weeks
   **Variation 2:**
   Methotrexate: I.V.: 40 or 50 mg/m$^2$/day days 1, 15, and 22  [total dose/cycle = 120 or 150 mg/m$^2$]
   Vinblastine: I.V.: 4 or 5 mg/m$^2$/day days 2, 15, and 22  [total dose/cycle = 12 or 15 mg/m$^2$]
   Doxorubicin: I.V.: 40 or 50 mg/m$^2$ day 2  [total dose/cycle = 40 or 50 mg/m$^2$]
   Cisplatin: I.V.: 100 mg/m$^2$ day 2  [total dose/cycle = 100 mg/m$^2$]
   Repeat cycle every 4 weeks
   **Variation 3:**
   Methotrexate: I.V.: 30 mg/m$^2$/day days 1, 15, and 22  [total dose/cycle = 90 mg/m$^2$]
   Vinblastine: I.V.: 3 mg/m$^2$ day 2  [total dose/cycle = 3 mg/m$^2$]
   Doxorubicin: I.V.: 30 mg/m$^2$ day 2  [total dose/cycle = 30 mg/m$^2$]
   Cisplatin: I.V.: 70 mg/m$^2$ day 2  [total dose/cycle = 70 mg/m$^2$]
   Repeat cycle every 4 weeks

## M-VAC (Bladder Cancer) *(continued)*

**Variation 4:**
Methotrexate: I.V.: 60 mg/m$^2$ day 1  [total dose/cycle = 60 mg/m$^2$]
**followed by** 30 mg/m$^2$ day 16  [total dose/cycle = 30 mg/m$^2$]
Vinblastine: I.V.: 4 mg/m$^2$/day days 2 and 16  [total dose/cycle = 8 mg/m$^2$]
Doxorubicin: I.V.: 60 mg/m$^2$ day 2  [total dose/cycle = 60 mg/m$^2$]
Cisplatin: I.V.: 100 mg/m$^2$ day 2  [total dose/cycle = 100 mg/m$^2$]
Repeat cycle every 23 days

**Variation 5:**
Methotrexate: I.V.: 30 mg/m$^2$/day days 1, 16, and 23  [total dose/cycle = 90 mg/m$^2$]
Vinblastine: I.V.: 4 mg/m$^2$/day days 1, 16, and 23  [total dose/cycle = 12 mg/m$^2$]
Doxorubicin: I.V.: 60 mg/m$^2$ day 2  [total dose/cycle = 60 mg/m$^2$]
Cisplatin: I.V.: 100 mg/m$^2$ day 2  [total dose/cycle = 100 mg/m$^2$]
Repeat cycle every 23 days

**Variation 6:**
Methotrexate: I.V.: 30 or 35 mg/m$^2$ day 1  [total dose/cycle = 30 or 35 mg/m$^2$]
Vinblastine: I.V.: 3 or 3.5 mg/m$^2$ day 2  [total dose/cycle = 3 or 3.5 mg/m$^2$]
Doxorubicin: I.V.: 30 or 35 mg/m$^2$ day 2  [total dose/cycle = 30 or 35 mg/m$^2$]
Cisplatin: I.V.: 70 or 80 mg/m$^2$ day 2  [total dose/cycle = 70 or 80 mg/m$^2$]
Repeat cycle every 2 weeks

**Variation 7:**
Methotrexate: I.V.: 30 mg/m$^2$ day 1  [total dose/cycle = 30 mg/m$^2$]
Vinblastine: I.V.: 3 mg/m$^2$ day 2  [total dose/cycle = 3 mg/m$^2$]
Doxorubicin: I.V.: 30 mg/m$^2$ day 2  [total dose/cycle = 30 mg/m$^2$]
Cisplatin: I.V.: 70 mg/m$^2$ day 2  [total dose/cycle = 70 mg/m$^2$]
Repeat cycle every 14 days

**Variation 8:**
Methotrexate: I.V.: 30 mg/m$^2$/day days 1, 15, and 22  [total dose/cycle = 90 mg/m$^2$]
Vinblastine: I.V.: 3 mg/m$^2$/day days 1, 15, and 22  [total dose/cycle = 9 mg/m$^2$]
Doxorubicin: I.V.: 45 mg/m$^2$ day 2  [total dose/cycle = 45 mg/m$^2$]
Cisplatin: I.V.: 70 mg/m$^2$ day 2  [total dose/cycle = 70 mg/m$^2$]
Repeat cycle every 4 weeks

**Variation 9:**
Methotrexate: I.V.: 40 mg/m$^2$/day days 1 and 15  [total dose/cycle = 80 mg/m$^2$]
Vinblastine: I.V.: 4 mg/m$^2$/day days 1, 16, and 23  [total dose/cycle = 12 mg/m$^2$]
Doxorubicin: I.V.: 60 mg/m$^2$ day 2  [total dose/cycle = 60 mg/m$^2$]
Cisplatin: I.V.: 100 mg/m$^2$ day 2  [total dose/cycle = 100 mg/m$^2$]
Repeat cycle every 23 days

**Variation 10:**
Methotrexate: I.V.: 30 mg/m$^2$/day days 1, 15, and 22  [total dose/cycle = 90 mg/m$^2$]
Vinblastine: I.V.: 3 mg/m$^2$/day days 1, 16, and 22  [total dose/cycle = 9 mg/m$^2$]
Doxorubicin: I.V.: 30 mg/m$^2$ day 1  [total dose/cycle = 30 mg/m$^2$]
Cisplatin: I.V.: 70 mg/m$^2$ day 1  [total dose/cycle = 70 mg/m$^2$]
Repeat cycle every 4 weeks

**Variation 11:**
Methotrexate: I.V.: 30 mg/m$^2$/day days 1, 15, and 22  [total dose/cycle = 90 mg/m$^2$]
Vinblastine: I.V.: 3 mg/m$^2$/day days 2, 15, and 22  [total dose/cycle = 9 mg/m$^2$]
Doxorubicin: I.V.: 30 mg/m$^2$ day 2  [total dose/cycle = 30 mg/m$^2$]
Cisplatin: I.V.: 70 mg/m$^2$ day 2  [total dose/cycle = 70 mg/m$^2$]
Leucovorin: Oral: 15 mg every 6 hours for 4 doses, days 2, 16, and 23
   [total dose/cycle = 180 mg]
Repeat cycle every 4 weeks

**Variation 12:**
Methotrexate: I.V.: 30 mg/m$^2$/day days 1 and 15  [total dose/cycle = 60 mg/m$^2$]
Vinblastine: I.V.: 3 mg/m$^2$/day days 2 and 15  [total dose/cycle = 6 mg/m$^2$]
Doxorubicin: I.V.: 30 or 40 mg/m$^2$ day 3  [total dose/cycle = 30 or 40 mg/m$^2$]
Cisplatin: I.V.: 70 mg/m$^2$ day 2  [total dose/cycle = 70 mg/m$^2$]
Repeat cycle every 4 weeks

**Variation 13:**
Methotrexate: I.V.: 30 mg/m$^2$/day days 1 and 15  [total dose/cycle = 60 mg/m$^2$]
Vinblastine: I.V.: 3 mg/m$^2$/day days 2 and 15  [total dose/cycle = 6 mg/m$^2$]
Doxorubicin: I.V.: 30 or 40 mg/m$^2$ day 2  [total dose/cycle = 30 or 40 mg/m$^2$]
Cisplatin: I.V.: 70 mg/m$^2$ day 2  [total dose/cycle = 70 mg/m$^2$]
Repeat cycle every 4 weeks

# M-VAC (Breast Cancer)

**Use:** Breast cancer
**Regimen:**
> Methotrexate: I.V.: 30 mg/m$^2$/day days 1, 15, and 22 [total dose/cycle = 90 mg/m$^2$]
> Vinblastine: I.V.: 3 mg/m$^2$/day days 2, 15, and 22 [total dose/cycle = 9 mg/m$^2$]
> Doxorubicin: I.V.: 30 mg/m$^2$ day 2 [total dose/cycle = 30 mg/m$^2$]
> Cisplatin: I.V.: 70 mg/m$^2$ day 2 [total dose/cycle = 70 mg/m$^2$]
> Leucovorin: Oral: 10 mg every 6 hours for 6 doses days 2, 16, and 23
> [total dose/cycle = 180 mg]
> Repeat cycle every 4 weeks

# M-VAC (Cervical Cancer)

**Use:** Cervical cancer
**Regimen:**
> Methotrexate: I.V.: 30 mg/m$^2$/day days 1, 15, and 22 [total dose/cycle = 90 mg/m$^2$]
> Vinblastine: I.V.: 3 mg/m$^2$/day days 2, 15, and 22 [total dose/cycle = 9 mg/m$^2$]
> Doxorubicin: I.V.: 30 mg/m$^2$ day 2 [total dose/cycle = 30 mg/m$^2$]
> Cisplatin: I.V.: 70 mg/m$^2$ day 2 [total dose/cycle = 70 mg/m$^2$]
> Repeat cycle every 4 weeks

# M-VAC (Endometrial Cancer)

**Use:** Endometrial cancer
**Regimen:**
> Methotrexate: I.V.: 30 mg/m$^2$/day days 1, 15, and 22 [total dose/cycle = 90 mg/m$^2$]
> Vinblastine: I.V.: 3 mg/m$^2$/day days 2, 15, and 22 [total dose/cycle = 9 mg/m$^2$]
> Doxorubicin: I.V.: 30 mg/m$^2$/day day 2 [total dose/cycle = 30 mg/m$^2$]
> Cisplatin: I.V.: 70 mg/m$^2$/day day 2 [total dose/cycle = 70 mg/m$^2$]
> Repeat cycle every 4 weeks

# M-VAC (Head and Neck Cancer)

**Use:** Head and neck cancer
**Regimen:**
> Methotrexate: I.V.: 30 mg/m$^2$/day days 1, 15, and 22 [total dose/cycle = 90 mg/m$^2$]
> Vinblastine: I.V.: 3 mg/m$^2$/day days 2, 15, and 22 [total dose/cycle = 9 mg/m$^2$]
> Doxorubicin: I.V.: 30 mg/m$^2$ day 2 [total dose/cycle = 30 mg/m$^2$]
> Cisplatin: I.V.: 70 mg/m$^2$ day 2 [total dose/cycle = 70 mg/m$^2$]
> Repeat cycle every 4 weeks

# MVPP

**Use:** Lymphoma, Hodgkin disease
**Regimen:**
> **Variation 1:**
> Mechlorethamine: I.V.: 6 mg/m$^2$/day days 1 and 8 [total dose/cycle = 12 mg/m$^2$]
> Vinblastine: I.V.: 4 mg/m$^2$/day days 1 and 8 [total dose/cycle = 8 mg/m$^2$]
> Procarbazine: Oral: 100 mg/m$^2$/day days 1-14 [total dose/cycle = 1400 mg/m$^2$]
> Prednisone: Oral: 40 mg/m$^2$/day days 1-14 [total dose/cycle = 560 mg/m$^2$]
> Repeat cycle every 4-6 weeks

# N4SE Protocol

**Use:** Neuroblastomas
**Regimen:**
> Vincristine: I.V.: 0.05 mg/kg/day days 1 and 2 [total dose/cycle = 0.1 mg/kg]
> Doxorubicin: I.V.: 15 mg/m$^2$/day days 1 and 2 [total dose/cycle = 30 mg/m$^2$]
> Cyclophosphamide: I.V.: 30 mg/kg/day days 1 and 2 [total dose/cycle = 60 mg/kg]
> Fluorouracil: I.V.: 1 mg/kg/day days 3, 8, and 9 [total dose/cycle = 3 mg/kg]
> Cytarabine: I.V.: 3 mg/kg/day days 3, 8, and 9 [total dose/cycle = 9 mg/kg]
> Hydroxyurea: Oral: 40 mg/kg/day days 3, 8, and 9 [total dose/cycle = 120 mg/kg]
> Repeat cycle every 21-28 days

## N6 Protocol

**Use:** Neuroblastomas

**Regimen:**

### Course 1, 2, 4, 6
Cyclophosphamide: I.V.: 70 mg/kg/day days 1 and 2  [total dose/cycle = 140 mg/kg]
Doxorubicin: I.V.: 25 mg/m$^2$/day continuous infusion days 1-3  [total dose/cycle = 75 mg/m$^2$]
Vincristine: I.V.: 0.033 mg/kg/day continuous infusion days 1-3  [total dose/cycle = 0.099 mg/kg]
Vincristine: I.V.: 1.5 mg/m$^2$ day 9  [total dose/cycle = 1.5 mg/m$^2$]

### Course 3, 5, 7
Etoposide: I.V.: 200 mg/m$^2$/day days 1-3  [total dose/cycle = 600 mg/m$^2$]
Cisplatin: I.V.: 50 mg/m$^2$/day days 1-4  [total dose/cycle = 200 mg/m$^2$]

## NFL

**Use:** Breast cancer

**Regimen: Note:** Multiple variations are listed below.

### Variation 1:
Mitoxantrone: I.V.: 12 mg/m$^2$ day 1  [total dose/cycle = 12 mg/m$^2$]
Fluorouracil: I.V.: 350 mg/m$^2$/day days 1-3  [total dose/cycle = 1050 mg/m$^2$]
Leucovorin: I.V.: 300 mg/m$^2$/day days 1-3  [total dose/cycle = 900 mg/m$^2$]

### Variation 2:
Mitoxantrone: I.V.: 10 mg/m$^2$ day 1  [total dose/cycle = 10 mg/m$^2$]
Fluorouracil: I.V.: 1000 mg/m$^2$/day continuous infusion days 1-3  [total dose/cycle = 3000 mg/m$^2$]
Leucovorin: I.V.: 100 mg/m$^2$/day days 1-3  [total dose/cycle = 300 mg/m$^2$]
Repeat cycle every 21 days

## OPA

**Use:** Lymphoma, Hodgkin disease

**Regimen:**

Vincristine: I.V.: 1.5 mg/m$^2$/day (maximum 2 mg) days 1, 8, and 15  [total dose/cycle = 4.5 mg/m$^2$]
Prednisone: Oral: 60 mg/m$^2$/day days 1-15 in 3 divided doses  [total dose/cycle = 900 mg/m$^2$]
Doxorubicin: I.V.: 40 mg/m$^2$/day days 1 and 15  [total dose/cycle = 80 mg/m$^2$]
Second cycle may be given based on individual response; time between cycles not specified

## OPEC

**Use:** Neuroblastomas

**Regimen:**

Vincristine: I.V.: 1.5 mg/m$^2$ day 1  [total dose/cycle = 1.5 mg/m$^2$]
Cyclophosphamide: I.V.: 600 mg/m$^2$ day 1  [total dose/cycle = 600 mg/m$^2$]
Cisplatin: I.V.: 100 mg/m$^2$ day 2  [total dose/cycle = 100 mg/m$^2$]
Teniposide: I.V.: 150 mg/m$^2$ day 4  [total dose/cycle = 150 mg/m$^2$]
Repeat cycle every 21 days

## OPEC-D

**Use:** Neuroblastomas

**Regimen:**

Vincristine: I.V.: 1.5 mg/m$^2$ day 1  [total dose/cycle = 1.5 mg/m$^2$]
Cyclophosphamide: I.V.: 600 mg/m$^2$ day 1  [total dose/cycle = 600 mg/m$^2$]
Doxorubicin: I.V.: 40 mg/m$^2$ day 1  [total dose/cycle = 40 mg/m$^2$]
Cisplatin: I.V.: 100 mg/m$^2$ day 2  [total dose/cycle = 100 mg/m$^2$]
Teniposide: I.V.: 150 mg/m$^2$ day 4  [total dose/cycle = 150 mg/m$^2$]
Repeat cycle every 21 days

# OPPA

**Use:** Lymphoma, Hodgkin disease
**Regimen:**

Vincristine: I.V.: 1.5 mg/m$^2$/day (maximum 2 mg) days 1, 8, and 15  [total dose/cycle = 4.5 mg/m$^2$]
Prednisone: Oral: 60 mg/m$^2$/day days 1-15 in 3 divided doses  [total dose/cycle = 900 mg/m$^2$]
Doxorubicin: I.V.: 40 mg/m$^2$/day days 1 and 15  [total dose/cycle = 80 mg/m$^2$]
Procarbazine: Oral: 100 mg/m$^2$/day days 1-15 in 2 or 3 divided doses
    [total dose/cycle = 1500 mg/m$^2$]
Second cycle may be given based on individual response; time between cycles not specified

# PAC (CAP)

**Use:** Ovarian cancer
**Regimen:**

Cisplatin: I.V.: 50 mg/m$^2$ day 1  [total dose/cycle = 50 mg/m$^2$]
Doxorubicin: I.V.: 50 mg/m$^2$ day 1  [total dose/cycle = 50 mg/m$^2$]
Cyclophosphamide: I.V.: 1000 mg/m$^2$ day 1  [total dose/cycle = 1000 mg/m$^2$]
Repeat cycle every 21 days for 8 cycles

# PA-CI

**Use:** Hepatoblastoma
**Regimen: Note:** Multiple variations are listed below.

**Variation 1:**
Cisplatin: I.V.: 90 mg/m$^2$ day 1  [total dose/cycle = 90 mg/m$^2$]
Doxorubicin: I.V.: 20 mg/m$^2$/day continuous infusion days 2-5  [total dose/cycle = 80 mg/m$^2$]
Repeat cycle every 21 days
**Variation 2:**
Cisplatin: I.V.: 20 mg/m$^2$/day days 1-4  [total dose/cycle = 80 mg/m$^2$]
Doxorubicin: I.V.: 100 mg/m$^2$ continuous infusion day 1  [total dose/cycle = 100 mg/m$^2$]
Repeat cycle every 21-28 days

# Paclitaxel, Carboplatin, Etoposide

**Use:** Adenocarcinoma, unknown primary
**Regimen:**

Paclitaxel: I.V.: 200 mg/m$^2$ infused over 1 hour day 1  [total dose/cycle = 200 mg/m$^2$] **followed by:**
Carboplatin: I.V.: Target AUC 6  [total dose/cycle = AUC = 6]
Etoposide: Oral: 50 mg/day, alternate with 100 mg/day, days 1-10  [total dose/cycle = 750 mg/day]
Repeat cycle every 21 days

# Paclitaxel + Estramustine + Carboplatin

**Use:** Prostate cancer
**Regimen:**

Paclitaxel: I.V.: 100 mg/m$^2$ day 3 each week  [total dose/cycle = 400 mg/m$^2$]
Estramustine: Oral: 10 mg/kg/day days 1-5 each week  [total dose/cycle = 200 mg/kg]
Carboplatin: I.V.: Target AUC 6 day 3  [total dose/cycle = AUC = 6]
Repeat cycle every 28 days

# Paclitaxel + Estramustine + Etoposide

**Use:** Prostate cancer
**Regimen:**

Paclitaxel: I.V.: 135 mg/m$^2$ day 2  [total dose/cycle = 135 mg/m$^2$]
Estramustine: Oral: 280 mg 3 times/day days 1-14  [total dose/cycle = 11,760 mg]
Etoposide: Oral: 100 mg/day days 1-14  [total dose/cycle = 1400 mg]
Repeat cycle every 21 days

# Paclitaxel-Vinorelbine

**Use:** Breast cancer
**Regimen:**
    Paclitaxel: I.V.: 135 mg/m$^2$ day 1 [total dose/cycle = 135 mg/m$^2$]
    Vinorelbine: I.V.: 30 mg/m$^2$/day days 1 and 8 [total dose/cycle = 60 mg/m$^2$]
    Repeat cycle every 28 days

# PC (Bladder Cancer)

**Use:** Bladder cancer
**Regimen:**
    Paclitaxel: I.V.: 200 mg/m$^2$ or 225 mg/m$^2$ day 1 [total dose/cycle = 200 or 225 mg/m$^2$]
    Carboplatin: I.V.: AUC 5-6 day 1 [total dose/cycle = AUC = 5-6]
    Repeat cycle every 21 days

# PC (Nonsmall Cell Lung Cancer)

**Use:** Lung cancer, nonsmall cell
**Regimen: Note:** Multiple variations are listed below.
    **Variation 1:**
    Paclitaxel: I.V.: 175-225 mg/m$^2$ day 1 [total dose/cycle = 175-225 mg/m$^2$]
    Carboplatin: I.V.: Target AUC 5-7 day 1 [total dose/cycle = AUC = 5-7]
    Repeat cycle every 21 days for 2-8 cycles
    **Variation 2:**
    Paclitaxel: I.V.: 175 mg/m$^2$ day 1 [total dose/cycle = 175 mg/m$^2$]
    Cisplatin: I.V.: 80 mg/m$^2$ day 1 [total dose/cycle = 80 mg/m$^2$]
    Repeat cycle every 21 days
    **Variation 3:**
    Paclitaxel: I.V.: 135 mg/m$^2$ continuous infusion day 1 [total dose/cycle = 135 mg/m$^2$]
    Carboplatin: I.V.: AUC 7.5 day 2 [total dose/cycle = AUC = 7.5]
    Repeat cycle every 21 days
    **Variation 4:**
    Paclitaxel: I.V.: 135 mg/m$^2$ continuous infusion day 1 [total dose/cycle = 135 mg/m$^2$]
    Cisplatin: I.V.: 75 mg/m$^2$ day 2 [total dose/cycle = 75 mg/m$^2$]
    Repeat cycle every 21 days

# PCV

**Use:** Brain tumors
**Regimen:**
    Lomustine: Oral: 110 mg/m$^2$ day 1 [total dose/cycle = 110 mg/m$^2$]
    Procarbazine: Oral: 60 mg/m$^2$/day days 8-21 [total dose/cycle = 840 mg/m$^2$]
    Vincristine: I.V.: 1.4 mg/m$^2$/day (maximum 2 mg) days 8 and 29 [total dose/cycle = 2.8 mg/m$^2$]
    Repeat cycle every 6-8 weeks

# PE

**Use:** Prostate cancer
**Regimen: Note:** Multiple variations are listed below.
    **Variation 1:**
    Paclitaxel: I.V.: 30-35 mg/m$^2$/day continuous infusion days 2-5 (given in 2-3 divided doses daily)
        [total dose/cycle = 120-140 mg/m$^2$]
    Estramustine: Oral: 600 mg/m$^2$/day days 1-21 [total dose/cycle = 12,600 mg/m$^2$]
    Repeat cycle every 21 days
    **Variation 2:**
    Paclitaxel: I.V.: 60-107 mg/m$^2$ infused over 3 hours weekly [total dose/cycle = 180-321 mg/m$^2$]
    Estramustine: Oral: 280 mg twice daily 3 days/week [total dose/cycle = 5040 mg]
    **Variation 3:**
    Paclitaxel: I.V.: 150 mg/m$^2$ weekly [total dose/cycle = 450 mg/m$^2$]
    Estramustine: Oral: 280 mg 3 times/day 3 days/week [total dose/week = 7560 mg/m$^2$]
    **Variation 4:**
    Paclitaxel: I.V.: 100 mg/m$^2$/day days 1, 8, and 15 [total dose/cycle = 300 mg/m$^2$]
    Estramustine: Oral: 280 mg 3 times/day days 1, 2, and 3 every week
        [total dose/cycle = 10,080 mg]
    Repeat cycle every 4 weeks

## PE-CAdO
**Use:** Neuroblastomas
**Regimen:**
>Cisplatin: I.V.: 100 mg/m$^2$ day 1  [total dose/cycle = 100 mg/m$^2$]
>Teniposide: I.V.: 160 mg/m$^2$ day 3  [total dose/cycle = 160 mg/m$^2$]
>**alternating with**
>Cyclophosphamide: I.V.: 300 mg/m$^2$/day days 1-5  [total dose/cycle = 1500 mg/m$^2$]
>Doxorubicin: I.V.: 60 mg/m$^2$ day 5  [total dose/cycle = 60 mg/m$^2$]
>Vincristine: I.V.: 1.5 mg/m$^2$/day days 1 and 5  [total dose/cycle = 3 mg/m$^2$]
>Repeat cycle every 21 days

## PFL (Colorectal Cancer)
**Use:** Colorectal cancer
**Regimen:**
>Cisplatin: I.V.: 25 mg/m$^2$/day continuous infusion days 1-5  [total dose/cycle = 125 mg/m$^2$]
>Fluorouracil: I.V.: 800 mg/m$^2$/day continuous infusion days 2-5  [total dose/cycle = 3200 mg/m$^2$]
>Leucovorin calcium: I.V.: 500 mg/m$^2$/day continuous infusion days 1-5
>    [total dose/cycle = 2500 mg/m$^2$]
>Repeat cycle every 28 days

## PFL (Head and Neck Cancer)
**Use:** Head and neck cancer
**Regimen: Note:** Multiple variations are listed below.
>**Variation 1:**
>Cisplatin: I.V.: 25 mg/m$^2$/day continuous infusion days 1-5  [total dose/cycle = 125 mg/m$^2$]
>Fluorouracil: I.V.: 800 mg/m$^2$/day continuous infusion days 2-6  [total dose/cycle = 4000 mg/m$^2$]
>Leucovorin: I.V.: 500 mg/m$^2$/day continuous infusion days 1-6  [total dose/cycle = 3000 mg/m$^2$]
>Repeat cycle every 28 days
>**Variation 2:**
>Cisplatin: I.V.: 100 mg/m$^2$ day 1  [total dose/cycle = 100 mg/m$^2$]
>Fluorouracil: I.V.: 600-1000 mg/m$^2$/day continuous infusion days 1-5
>    [total dose/cycle = 3000-5000 mg/m$^2$]
>Leucovorin: Oral: 50 mg/m$^2$ every 4-6 hours days 1-6  [total dose/cycle = 1200-1800 mg/m$^2$]
>Repeat cycle every 21 days

## PFL + IFN
**Use:** Head and neck cancer
**Regimen:**
>Cisplatin: I.V.: 100 mg/m$^2$ day 1  [total dose/cycle = 100 mg/m$^2$]
>Fluorouracil: I.V.: 640 mg/m$^2$/day continuous infusion days 1-5  [total dose/cycle = 3200 mg/m$^2$]
>Leucovorin calcium: Oral: 100 mg every 4 hours days 1-5  [total dose/cycle = 3000 mg/m$^2$]
>Interferon alfa-2b: SubQ: 2 x 10$^6$ units/m$^2$ days 1-6  [total dose/cycle = 12 x 10$^6$ units/m$^2$]

## POC
**Use:** Brain tumors
**Regimen:**
>Prednisone: Oral: 40 mg/m$^2$/day days 1-14  [total dose/cycle = 560 mg/m$^2$]
>Vincristine: I.V.: 1.5 mg/m$^2$/day (maximum 2 mg) days 1, 8, and 15  [total dose/cycle = 4.5 mg/m$^2$]
>Lomustine: Oral: 100 mg/m$^2$ day 1  [total dose/cycle = 100 mg/m$^2$]
>Repeat cycle every 6 weeks

# POMP

**Use:** Leukemia, acute lymphocytic
**Regimen:** Maintenance:

Mercaptopurine: Oral: 50 mg 3 times a day  [total dose/cycle = 4.5 g]
Methotrexate: Oral: 20 mg/m$^2$ once weekly  [total dose/cycle = 80 mg/m$^2$]
Vincristine: I.V.: 2 mg day 1  [total dose/cycle = 2 mg]
Prednisone: Oral: 200 mg/day days 1-5  [total dose/cycle = 1000 mg]
Repeat cycle monthly for 2 years

# Pro-MACE-CytaBOM

**Use:** Lymphoma, non-Hodgkin
**Regimen:**

Prednisone: Oral: 60 mg/m$^2$/day days 1-14  [total dose/cycle = 840 mg/m$^2$]
Doxorubicin: I.V.: 25 mg/m$^2$ day 1  [total dose/cycle = 25 mg/m$^2$]
Cyclophosphamide: I.V.: 650 mg/m$^2$ day 1  [total dose/cycle = 650 mg/m$^2$]
Etoposide: I.V.: 120 mg/m$^2$ day 1  [total dose/cycle = 120 mg/m$^2$]
Cytarabine: I.V.: 300 mg/m$^2$ day 8  [total dose/cycle = 300 mg/m$^2$]
Bleomycin: I.V.: 5 units/m$^2$ day 8  [total dose/cycle = 5 units/m$^2$]
Vincristine: I.V.: 1.4 mg/m$^2$ (maximum 2 mg) day 8  [total dose/cycle = 1.4 mg/m$^2$]
Methotrexate: I.V.: 120 mg/m$^2$ day 8  [total dose/cycle = 120 mg/m$^2$]
Leucovorin: Oral: 25 mg/m$^2$ every 6 hours (start 24 hours after methotrexate) for 4 doses day 9
  [total dose/cycle = 100 mg/m$^2$]
Repeat cycle every 21 days

# PV

**Use:** Breast cancer
**Regimen: Note:** Multiple variations are listed below.

**Variation 1:**
Paclitaxel: I.V.: 135 mg/m$^2$ day 1  [total dose/cycle = 135 mg/m$^2$]
Vinorelbine: I.V.: 30 mg/m$^2$ day 1  [total dose/cycle = 30 mg/m$^2$]
Repeat cycle every 21 days

**Variation 2:**
Paclitaxel: I.V.: 150 mg/m$^2$ day 1  [total dose/cycle = 150 mg/m$^2$]
Vinorelbine: I.V.: 25 mg/m$^2$ day 1  [total dose/cycle = 25 mg/m$^2$]
Repeat cycle every 21 days

# PVA (POG 8602)

**Use:** Leukemia, acute lymphocytic
**Regimen:**

**Induction:**
Prednisone: Oral: 40 mg/m$^2$/day (maximum 60 mg) days 0-28 (given in 3 divided doses)
  [total dose/cycle = 1160 mg/m$^2$]
Vincristine: I.V.: 1.5 mg/m$^2$/day (maximum 2 mg) days 0, 7, 14, and 21
  [total dose/cycle = 6 mg/m$^2$]
Asparaginase: I.M.: 6000 units/m$^2$ 3 times per week for 2 weeks
  [total dose/cycle = 36,000/units/m$^2$]
Intrathecal therapy: Days 0 and 22
Administer one cycle only

**CNS consolidation:**
Mercaptopurine: Oral: 75 mg/m$^2$/day days 29-42  [total dose/cycle = 1050 mg/m$^2$]
Intrathecal therapy: Days 29 and 36
Administer one cycle only

## PVA (POG 8602) *(continued)*

### Intensification:
### Regimen A:
Methotrexate: I.V.: 1000 mg/m$^2$ continuous infusion day 1 [total dose/cycle = 1000 mg/m$^2$]

Cytarabine: I.V.: 1000 mg/m$^2$ continuous infusion day 1 (start 12 hours after methotrexate)
[total dose/cycle = 1000 mg/m$^2$]

Leucovorin: I.M., I.V., or Oral: 30 mg/m$^2$ 24 and 36 hours after the **start** of methotrexate
[total dose/cycle = 60 mg/m$^2$]

**followed by** 3 mg/m$^2$ 48, 60, and 72 hours after the **start** of methotrexate
[total dose/cycle = 9 mg/m$^2$]

Intrathecal therapy: Weeks 9, 12, 15, and 18

Repeat cycle every 3 weeks for 6 cycles **or**


### Regimen B:
Methotrexate: I.V.: 1000 mg/m$^2$ continuous infusion day 1 [total dose/cycle = 1000 mg/m$^2$]

Cytarabine: I.V.: 1000 mg/m$^2$ continuous infusion day 1 (start 12 hours after methotrexate)
[total dose/cycle = 1000 mg/m$^2$]

Leucovorin: I.M., I.V., or Oral: 30 mg/m$^2$ 24 and 36 hours after the **start** of methotrexate
[total dose/cycle = 60 mg/m$^2$]

**followed by** 3 mg/m$^2$ 48, 60, and 72 hours after the **start** of methotrexate
[total dose/cycle = 9 mg/m$^2$]

Intrathecal therapy: Weeks 9, 12, 15, and 18

Repeat cycle every 12 weeks for 6 cycles


### Maintenance:
### Regimen A:
Methotrexate: I.M.: 20 mg/m$^2$ weekly   [total dose/cycle = 2640 mg/m$^2$]

Mercaptopurine: Oral: 75 mg/m$^2$ daily   [total dose/cycle = 69,300 mg/m$^2$]

Intrathecal therapy: Day 1 every 8 weeks for 10 doses

Weeks 25-156

Prednisone: Oral: 40 mg/m$^2$/day (maximum 60 mg) days 1-7 (given in 3 divided doses)
[total dose/cycle = 2240 mg/m$^2$]

Vincristine: I.V.: 1.5 mg/m$^2$/day (maximum 2 mg) days 1 and 8
[total dose/cycle = 24 mg/m$^2$]

Weeks 8, 17, 25, 41, 57, 73, 89, 105 **or**


### Regimen B:
Methotrexate: I.M.: 20 mg/m$^2$ weekly for 7 weeks   [total dose/cycle = 140 mg/m$^2$]

Mercaptopurine: Oral: 75 mg/m$^2$ daily for 7 weeks   [total dose/cycle = 3675 mg/m$^2$]

Repeat cycle every 12 weeks for 4 cycles (begins weeks 22, 34, 46, 58, 70)

**followed by**

Methotrexate: I.M.: 20 mg/m$^2$ weekly   [total dose/cycle = 1720 mg/m$^2$]

Mercaptopurine: Oral: 75 mg/m$^2$ daily   [total dose/cycle = 45,150 mg/m$^2$]

Weeks 70-156

Intrathecal therapy: Day 1 every 8 weeks for 10 doses

Weeks 25-156

Prednisone: Oral: 40 mg/m$^2$/day (maximum 60 mg) days 1-7 (given in 3 divided doses)
[total dose/cycle = 2240 mg/m$^2$]

Vincristine: I.V.: 1.5 mg/m$^2$/day (maximum 2 mg) days 1 and 8 [total dose/cycle = 24 mg/m$^2$]

Weeks 8, 17, 25, 41, 57, 73, 89, and 105

## PVA (POG 9005)

**Use:** Leukemia, acute lymphocytic

**Regimen:**

### Induction:

Prednisone: Oral: 40 mg/m$^2$/day (maximum 60 mg) days 1-28 (given in 3 divided doses)
[total dose/cycle = 1120 mg/m$^2$]

Vincristine: I.V.: 1.5 mg/m$^2$/day (maximum 2 mg) days 1, 8, 15, and 22
[total dose/cycle = 6 mg/m$^2$]

Asparaginase: I.M.: 6000 units/m$^2$/day days 2, 5, 8, 12, 15, 19
[total dose/cycle = 36,000 units/m$^2$]

Intrathecal therapy: Day 1

Administer one cycle only

### Intensification:

#### Regimen A:

Methotrexate: I.V: 1000 mg/m$^2$ continuous infusion day 1 [total dose/cycle = 1000 mg/m$^2$]

Mercaptopurine: I.V.: 1000 mg/m$^2$ day 2 [total dose/cycle = 1000 mg/m$^2$]

Leucovorin: I.M., I.V., or Oral: 5 mg/m$^2$ every 6 hours for 5 doses day 3 (**start** 48 hours after the start of methotrexate) [total dose/cycle = 25 mg/m$^2$]

Repeat cycle every 2 weeks for 12 cycles **or**

#### Regimen B:

Methotrexate: Oral: 30 mg/m$^2$ every 6 hours for 6 doses day 1 [total dose/cycle = 180 mg/m$^2$]

Mercaptopurine: I.V.: 1000 mg/m$^2$ day 2 (start after last methotrexate dose)
[total dose/cycle = 1000 mg/m$^2$]

Leucovorin: I.M., I.V., or Oral: 5 mg/m$^2$ every 6 hours for 5 doses day 3 (start 48 hours after the **start** of methotrexate)

Repeat cycle every 2 weeks for 12 cycles

### Maintenance:

Methotrexate: I.M.: 20 mg/m$^2$ weekly [total dose/cycle = 2120 mg/m$^2$]

Mercaptopurine: Oral: 50 mg/m$^2$ daily [total dose/cycle = 37,100 mg/m$^2$]

Intrathecal therapy: Day 1 every 12 weeks weeks 25-130

## PVB

**Use:** Testicular cancer

**Regimen: Note:** Multiple variations are listed below.

### Variation 1:

Cisplatin: I.V.: 20 mg/m$^2$/day days 1-5 [total dose/cycle = 100 mg/m$^2$]

Vinblastine: I.V.: 0.2 mg/m$^2$/day days 1 and 2 [total dose/cycle = 0.4 mg/kg]

Bleomycin: I.V.: 30 units/day days 2, 9, and 16 [total dose/cycle = 90 units]

Repeat cycle every 3 weeks

### Variation 2:

Cisplatin: I.V.: 20 mg/m$^2$/day days 1-5 [total dose/cycle = 100 mg/m$^2$]

Vinblastine: I.V.: 0.15 mg/kg/day days 1 and 2 [total dose/cycle = 0.3 mg/kg]

Bleomycin: I.V.: 30 units days 2, 9, and 16 [total dose/cycle = 90 units]

Repeat cycle every 3 weeks

### Variation 3:

Cisplatin: I.V.: 20 mg/m$^2$/day days 1-5 [total dose/cycle = 100 mg/m$^2$]

Vinblastine: I.V.: 6 mg/m$^2$/day days 1 and 2 [total dose/cycle = 12 mg/m$^2$]

Bleomycin: I.M.: 30 units days 2, 9, and 16 [total dose/cycle = 90 units]

Repeat cycle every 3 weeks

## PVDA

**Use:** Leukemia, acute lymphocytic

**Regimen:**

Prednisone: Oral: 60 mg/m$^2$/day days 1-28 [total dose/cycle = 1680 mg/m$^2$]

Vincristine: I.V.: 1.5 mg/m$^2$/day days 1, 8, 15, and 22 [total dose/cycle = 6 mg/m$^2$]

Daunorubicin: I.V.: 25 mg/m$^2$/day days 1, 8, 15, and 22 [total dose/cycle = 100 mg/m$^2$]

Asparaginase: I.M., SubQ, or I.V.: 5000 units/m$^2$/day days 1-14
[total dose/cycle = 70,000 units/m$^2$]

Administer one cycle only; used in conjuction with intrathecal chemotherapy

## R-CHOP
**Use:** Lymphoma, non-Hodgkin
**Regimen:**
Rituximab: I.V.: 375 mg/m$^2$ day 1  [total dose/cycle = 375 mg/m$^2$]
Cyclophosphamide: I.V.: 750 mg/m$^2$ day 3  [total dose/cycle = 750 mg/m$^2$]
Doxorubicin: I.V.: 50 mg/m$^2$ day 3   [total dose/cycle = 50 mg/m$^2$]
Vincristine: I.V.: 1.4 mg/m$^2$ (maximum 2 mg) day 3  [total dose/cycle = 1.4 mg/m$^2$]
Prednisone: Oral: 40 mg/m$^2$/day days 1-5  [total dose/cycle = 200 mg/m$^2$]
Repeat cycle every 21 days

## R-CVP
**Use:** Lymphoma, non-Hodgkin
**Regimen:**
Rituximab: I.V.: 375 mg/m$^2$ day 1  [total dose/cycle = 375 mg/m$^2$]
Cyclophosphamide: I.V.: 750 mg/m$^2$ day 1  [total dose/cycle = 750 mg/m$^2$]
Vincristine: I.V.: 1.4 mg/m$^2$ day 1  [total dose/cycle = 1.4 mg/m$^2$]
Prednisolone: Oral: 40 mg/m$^2$/day days 1 to 5  [total dose/cycle = 200 mg/m$^2$]
Repeat cycle every 21 days

## Regimen A1
**Use:** Neuroblastomas
**Regimen:**
Cyclophosphamide: I.V.: 1.2 g/m$^2$ day 1  [total dose/cycle = 1.2 g/m$^2$]
Vincristine: I.V.: 1.5 mg/m$^2$ day 1  [total dose/cycle = 1.5 mg/m$^2$]
Doxorubicin: I.V.: 40 mg/m$^2$ day 3  [total dose/cycle = 40 mg/m$^2$]
Cisplatin: I.V.: 90 mg/m$^2$ day 5  [total dose/cycle = 90 mg/m$^2$]
Repeat cycle every 28 days

## Regimen A2
**Use:** Neuroblastomas
**Regimen:**
Cyclophosphamide: I.V.: 1.2 g/m$^2$ day 1  [total dose/cycle = 1.2 g/m$^2$]
Etoposide: I.V.: 100 mg/m$^2$/day days 1-5  [total dose/cycle = 500 mg/m$^2$]
Doxorubicin: I.V.: 40 mg/m$^2$ day 3  [total dose/cycle = 40 mg/m$^2$]
Cisplatin: I.V.: 90 mg/m$^2$ day 5  [total dose/cycle = 90 mg/m$^2$]
Repeat cycle every 28 days

## Sequential Dox-CMF
**Use:** Breast cancer
**Regimen:**
Doxorubicin: I.V.: 75 mg/m$^2$ every 21 days for 4 cycles followed by 21- or 28-day CMF for 8 cycles

## Stanford V
**Use:** Lymphoma, Hodgkin disease
**Regimen:**
Mechlorethamine: I.V.: 6 mg/m$^2$ day 1  [total dose/cycle = 6 mg/m$^2$]
Doxorubicin: I.V.: 25 mg/m$^2$/day days 1 and 15  [total dose/cycle = 50 mg/m$^2$]
Vinblastine: I.V.: 6 mg/m$^2$/day days 1 and 15  [total dose/cycle = 12 mg/m$^2$]
Vincristine: I.V.: 1.4 mg/m$^2$/day (maximum 2 mg) days 8 and 22  [total dose/cycle = 2.8 mg/m$^2$]
Bleomycin: I.V.: 5 units/m$^2$/day days 8 and 22  [total dose/cycle = 10 units/m$^2$]
Etoposide: I.V.: 60 mg/m$^2$/day days 15 and 16  [total dose/cycle = 120 mg/m$^2$]
Prednisone: Oral: 40 mg/m$^2$ every other day for 10 weeks
  [total dose/cycle = 1400 mg/m$^2$] **followed by** tapering of dose by 10 mg every other day for next 14 days
Repeat cycle every 28 days

# TAC
**Use:** Breast cancer
**Regimen:**
Docetaxel: I.V.: 75 mg/m$^2$ day 1  [total dose/cycle = 75 mg/m$^2$]
Doxorubicin: I.V.: 50 mg/m$^2$ day 1  [total dose/cycle = 50 mg/m$^2$]
Cyclophosphamide: I.V.: 500 mg/m$^2$ day 1  [total dose/cycle = 500 mg/m$^2$]
Repeat cycle every 3 weeks

# TAD
**Use:** Leukemia, acute myeloid
**Regimen:**
Daunorubicin: I.V.: 60 mg/m$^2$/day days 3-5  [total dose/cycle = 180 mg/m$^2$]
Cytarabine: I.V.: 100 mg/m$^2$/day continuous infusion days 1 and 2
　　　[total dose/cycle = 200 mg/m$^2$] **followed by** 100 mg/m$^2$/day every 12 hours days 3-8
　　　[total dose/cycle = 1200 mg/m$^2$]
Thioguanine: Oral: 100 mg/m$^2$/day every 12 hours days 3-9  [total dose/cycle = 1400 mg/m$^2$]
Administer one cycle only

# Tamoxifen-Epirubicin
**Use:** Breast cancer
**Regimen:**
Tamoxifen: Oral: 20 mg daily  [total dose/cycle = 560 mg]
Epirubicin: I.V.: 50 mg/m$^2$/day days 1 and 8  [total dose/cycle = 100 mg/m$^2$]
Repeat epirubicin cycle every 28 days for 6 cycles; continue tamoxifen for 4 years

# TCF
**Use:** Esophageal cancer
**Regimen:**
Paclitaxel: I.V.: 175 mg/m$^2$ day 1  [total dose/cycle = 175 mg/m$^2$]
Cisplatin: I.V.: 20 mg/m$^2$/day days 1-5  [total dose/cycle = 100 mg/m$^2$]
Fluorouracil: I.V.: 750 mg/m$^2$/day continuous infusion days 1-5   [total dose/cycle = 3750 mg/m$^2$]
Repeat cycle every 28 days

# Thalidomide + Dexamethasone
**Use:** Multiple myeloma
**Regimen: Note:** Multiple variation are listed below.
　**Variation 1:**
　Thalidomide: Oral: 100 mg/day days 1-28  [total dose/cycle = 2800 mg]
　Dexamethasone: Oral: 40 mg/day days 1-4  [total dose/cycle = 160 mg]
　Repeat cycle every 28 days
　**Variation 2:**
　Thalidomide: Oral: 200 mg/day days 1-14 cycle 1
　**followed by** 400 mg/day days 15-28 cycle 1  [total dose/cycle = 8400 mg]
　Thalidomide: Oral: 400 mg/day days 1-28 (subsequent cycles)  [total dose/cycle = 11,200 mg]
　Dexamethasone: Oral: 20 mg/m$^2$/day days 1-4, 9-12, and 17 to 20 cycle 1
　　　[total dose/cycle = 240 mg/m$^2$]
　Dexamethasone: Oral: 20 mg/m$^2$/day days 1-4 (subsequent cycles)  [total dose/cycle = 80 mg/m$^2$]
　Repeat cycle every 28 days
　**Variation 3:**
　Thalidomide: Oral: 100 mg/day days 1-7, 150 mg/day days 8-14, 200 mg/day days 15-21,  250 mg/day days 22-28,
　　　and 300 mg/day days 29-35 (cycle 1)  [total dose/cycle = 7000 mg]
　Thalidomide: Oral: 300 mg/day days 1-35 (subsequent cycles)  [total dose/cycle = 10,500 mg]
　Dexamethasone: Oral: 20 mg/m$^2$/day days 1-4, 9-12, and 17-20  [total dose/cycle = 240 mg/m$^2$]
　Repeat cycle every 35 days
　**Variation 4:**
　Thalidomide: Oral: 200 mg/day days 1-28  [total dose/cycle = 5600 mg]
　Dexamethasone: Oral: 40 mg/day days 1-4, 9-12, and 17-20 (odd cycles)
　　　[total dose/cycle = 480 mg]
　Dexamethasone: Oral: 40 mg/day days 1-4 (even cycles)  [total dose/cycle = 160 mg]

# TIP
**Use:** Esophageal cancer; Head and neck cancer
**Regimen:**
    Paclitaxel: I.V.: 175 mg/m$^2$ day 1  [total dose/cycle = 175 mg/m$^2$]
    Ifosfamide: I.V.: 1000 mg/m$^2$/day days 1-3  [total dose/cycle = 3000 mg/m$^2$]
    Mesna: I.V.: 400 mg/m$^2$/day before ifosfamide days 1-3  [total dose/cycle = 1200 mg/m$^2$]
    **followed by:** 200 mg/m$^2$ 4 hours after ifosfamide days 1-3  [total dose/cycle = 600 mg/m$^2$]
    Cisplatin: I.V.: 60 mg/m$^2$ day 1  [total dose/cycle = 60 mg/m$^2$]
    Repeat cycle every 21-28 days

# Trastuzumab-Paclitaxel
**Use:** Breast cancer
**Regimen:**
    Paclitaxel: I.V.: 175 mg/m$^2$ day 1  [total dose/cycle = 175 mg/m$^2$]
    Trastuzumab: I.V.: 4 mg/kg (loading dose) day 1 cycle 1
        [total dose/cycle = 4 mg/kg] **followed by** 2 mg/kg/day days 1, 8, and 15 (subsequent cycles)
        [total dose/cycle = 6 mg/kg]
    Repeat cycle every 21 days for at least 6 cycles

# Tretinoin/Idarubicin
**Use:** Leukemia, acute promyelocytic
**Regimen:**
    **Variation 1: Induction:**
    Tretinoin: Oral: >20 years: 45 mg/m$^2$/day day 1 up to 90 days  [total dose/cycle = 4050 mg/m$^2$]
    Tretinoin Oral: ≤20 years: 25 mg/m$^2$/day day 1 up to 90 days  [total dose/cycle = 2250 mg/m$^2$]
    Idarubicin: I.V.: 12 mg/m$^2$/day days 2, 4, 6, and 8  [total dose/cycle = 48 mg/m$^2$]
    **Consolidation Course 1:**
    Idarubicin: I.V.: 5 mg/m$^2$/day days 1-4  [total dose/cycle = 20 mg/m$^2$] **or**
    Idarubicin: I.V.: 7 mg/m$^2$/day days 1-4  [total dose/cycle = 28 mg/m$^2$]
    Tretinoin: Oral: 45 mg/m$^2$/day days 1-15  [total dose/cycle = 675 mg/m$^2$]
    **Consolidation Course 2:**
    Mitoxantrone: I.V.: 10 mg/m$^2$/day days 1-5  [total dose/cycle = 50 mg/m$^2$]
    Tretinoin: Oral: 45 mg/m$^2$/day days 1-15  [total dose/cycle = 675 mg/m$^2$]
    **Consolidation Course 3:**
    Idarubicin: I.V.: 12 mg/m$^2$ day 1  [total dose/cycle = 12 mg/m$^2$] **or**
    Idarubicin: I.V.: 12 mg/m$^2$/day days 1-2  [total dose/cycle = 24 mg/m$^2$]
    Tretinoin: Oral: 45 mg/m$^2$/day days 1-15  [total dose/cycle = 675 mg/m$^2$]
    Given at 1 month intervals
    **Maintenance:**
    Mercaptopurine: Oral: 50 mg/m$^2$ daily  [total dose/cycle = 4200 mg/m$^2$]
    Methotrexate: I.M.: 15 mg/m$^2$ weekly  [total dose/cycle = 180 mg/m$^2$]
    Tretinoin: Oral: 45 mg/m$^2$/day days 1-15  [total dose/cycle = 675 mg/m$^2$]
    Repeat every 3 months for 2 years

# TVTG
**Use:** Leukemia, acute lymphocytic; Leukemia, acute myeloid
**Regimen:**
    Topotecan: I.V.: 1 mg/m$^2$/day continuous infusion days 1-5  [total dose/cycle = 5 mg/m$^2$]
    Vinorelbine: I.V.: 20 mg/m$^2$/day days 0, 7, 14, and 21  [total dose/cycle = 80 mg/m$^2$]
    Thiotepa: I.V.: 15 mg/m$^2$ day 2  [total dose/cycle = 15 mg/m$^2$]
    Gemcitabine: I.V.: 3600 mg/m$^2$ day 7  [total dose/cycle = 3600 mg/m$^2$]
    Dexamethasone: Oral or I.V.: 45 mg/m$^2$/day days 7-14 (given in 3 divided doses)
        [total dose/cycle = 315 mg/m$^2$]
    Repeat cycle when ANC >500 cells/mcL and platelet count >75,000 cells/mcL

# VAC (Ovarian Cancer)

**Use:** Ovarian cancer

**Regimen:**

Vincristine: I.V.: 1.2-1.5 mg/m$^2$ (maximum 2 mg) weekly for 10-12 weeks
[total dose/cycle = 12-15 mg/m$^2$ to 14.4-18]

**or** every 2 weeks for 12 doses  [total dose/cycle = 14.4-18 mg/m$^2$]

Dactinomycin: I.V.: 0.3-0.4 mg/m$^2$/day days 1-5  [total dose/cycle = 1.5-2 mg/m$^2$]

Cyclophosphamide: I.V.: 150 mg/m$^2$/day days 1-5  [total dose/cycle = 750 mg/m$^2$]

Repeat every 28 days

# VAC (Retinoblastoma)

**Use:** Retinoblastoma

**Regimen:**

Vincristine: I.V.: 1.5 mg/m$^2$ day 1  [total dose/cycle = 1.5 mg/m$^2$]

Dactinomycin: I.V.: 0.015 mg/kg/day days 1-5  [total dose/cycle = 0.075 mg/kg]

Cyclophosphamide: I.V.: 200 mg/m$^2$/day days 1-5  [total dose/cycle = 1000 mg/m$^2$]

# VAC (Rhabdomyosarcoma)

**Use:** Rhabdomyosarcoma

**Regimen:**

**Induction:**

Vincristine: I.V. push: 1.5 mg/m$^2$ (maximum 2 mg) weekly for 12 weeks, then at week 16
[total dose/cycle = 19.5 mg/m$^2$]

Dactinomycin: I.V. push: 0.015 mg/kg/day (maximum 0.5 mg) days 1-5, repeat every 3 weeks for 3 cycles, then stop
for 2 cycles; repeat at week 16

Cyclophosphamide: I.V.: 10 mg/kg/day days 1-3 (alternately: 2.2 g/m$^2$ day 1), repeat every 3 weeks for 5 cycles;
then at week 16

**Continuation:**

Vincristine: I.V. push: 1.5 mg/m$^2$ (maximum 2 mg) weeks 20-25, 29-34, 38-43
[total dose/cycle = 27 mg/m$^2$]

Dactinomycin: I.V. push: 0.015 mg/kg (maximum 0.5 mg) weeks 20 and 23, 29 and 32, 38 and 41
[total dose/cycle = .18 mg/kg]

Cyclophosphamide: I.V.: 2.2 mg/m$^2$ weeks 20 and 23, 29 and 32, 38 and 41
[total dose/cycle = 26.4 g/m$^2$]

# VAC Pulse

**Use:** Rhabdomyosarcoma

**Regimen:**

Vincristine: I.V.: 2 mg/m$^2$/dose (maximum 2 mg/dose) every 7 days for 12 weeks
[total dose/cycle = 24 mg/m$^2$]

Dactinomycin: I.V.: 0.015 mg/kg/day (maximum 0.5 mg/day) days 1-5, weeks 1 and 13
[total dose/cycle = 0.15 mg/kg]

Cyclophosphamide: Oral, I.V.: 10 mg/kg/day for 7 days, repeat every 6 weeks

# VAD

**Use:** Multiple myeloma

**Regimen:**

Vincristine: I.V.: 0.4 mg/day continuous infusion days 1-4  [total dose/cycle = 1.6 mg]

Doxorubicin. I.V.: 9 mg/m$^2$/day continuous infusion days 1-4  [total dose/cycle = 36 mg/m$^2$]

Dexamethasone: Oral: 40 mg/day days 1-4, 9-12, 17-20

Repeat cycle every 28-35 days

## VAD/CVAD
**Use:** Leukemia, acute lymphocytic
**Regimen:**
**Induction:**
Vincristine: I.V.: 0.4 mg continuous infusion/day days 1-4 and 24-27  [total dose/cycle = 3.2 mg]
Doxorubicin: I.V.: 12 mg/m$^2$/day continuous infusion days 1-4 and 24-27
   [total dose/cycle = 96 mg/m$^2$]
Dexamethasone: Oral: 40 mg/day days 1-4, 9-12 and 17-20  [total dose/cycle = 480 mg]
Cyclophosphamide: I.V.: 1 g/m$^2$ day 24  [total dose/cycle = 1 g/m$^2$]
Dexamethasone: Oral: 40 mg/day days 24-27, 32-35 and 40-43  [total dose/cycle ≐ 480 mg]
Administer one cycle only

## VATH
**Use:** Breast cancer
**Regimen:**
Vinblastine: I.V.: 4.5 mg/m$^2$ day 1  [total dose/cycle = 4.5 mg/m$^2$]
Doxorubicin: I.V.: 45 mg/m$^2$ day 1  [total dose/cycle = 45 mg/m$^2$]
Thiotepa: I.V.: 12 mg/m$^2$ day 1  [total dose/cycle = 12 mg/m$^2$]
Fluoxymesterone: Oral: 10 mg 3 times/day days 1-21  [total dose/cycle = 630 mg]
Repeat cycle every 21 days

## VBAP
**Use:** Multiple myeloma
**Regimen:**
Vincristine: I.V.: 1 mg day 1  [total dose/cycle = 1 mg]
Carmustine: I.V.: 30 mg/m$^2$ day 1  [total dose/cycle = 30 mg/m$^2$]
Doxorubicin: I.V.: 30 mg/m$^2$ day 1  [total dose/cycle = 30 mg/m$^2$]
Prednisone: Oral: 100 mg/day days 1-4  [total dose/cycle = 400 mg]
Repeat cycle every 21 days

## VBMCP
**Use:** Multiple myeloma
**Regimen:**
Vincristine: I.V.: 1.2 mg/m$^2$ (maximum 2 mg) day 1  [total dose/cycle = 1.2 mg/m$^2$]
Carmustine: I.V.: 20 mg/m$^2$ day 1  [total dose/cycle = 20 mg/m$^2$]
Melphalan: Oral: 8 mg/m$^2$/day days 1-4  [total dose/cycle = 32 mg/m$^2$]
Cyclophosphamide: I.V.: 400 mg/m$^2$ day 1  [total dose/cycle = 400 mg/m$^2$]
Prednisone: Oral: 40 mg/m$^2$/day days 1-7 (all cycles)  [total dose/cycle = 280 mg/m$^2$]
**followed by** 20 mg/m$^2$/day days 8-14 (first 3 cycles only)  [total dose/cycle = 140 mg/m$^2$]
Repeat cycle every 35 days

## VBP (PVB)
**Use:** Testicular cancer
**Regimen:**
Vinblastine: I.V.: 6 mg/m$^2$/day days 1 and 2  [total dose/cycle = 12 mg/m$^2$]
Bleomycin: I.V.: 30 units/day days 1, 8, 15, (22)  [total dose/cycle = 120 units]
Cisplatin: I.V.: 20 mg/m$^2$/day days 1-5  [total dose/cycle = 100 mg/m$^2$]
Repeat cycle every 21-28 days

## VC
**Use:** Lung cancer, nonsmall cell
**Regimen:**
Vinorelbine: I.V.: 30 mg/m$^2$ weekly  [total dose/cycle = 180 mg/m$^2$]
Cisplatin: I.V.: 120 mg/m$^2$/day days 1 and 29 (cycle 1); day 1 only on subsequent cycles
   [total dose/cycle = 240 mg/m$^2$ cycle 1 only, 120 mg/m$^2$ (subsequent cycles)]
Repeat cycle every 6 weeks

## VCAP

**Use:** Multiple myeloma
**Regimen:**
Vincristine: I.V.: 1 mg day 1 [total dose/cycle = 1 mg]
Cyclophosphamide: Oral: 100 mg/m$^2$/day days 1-4 [total dose/cycle = 400 mg/m$^2$]
Doxorubicin: I.V.: 25 mg/m$^2$ day 2 [total dose/cycle = 25 mg/m$^2$]
Prednisone: Oral: 60 mg/m$^2$/day days 1-4 [total dose/cycle = 240 mg/m$^2$]
Repeat cycle every 28 days

## Vinorelbine-Cis

**Use:** Lung cancer, nonsmall cell
**Regimen:**
Vinorelbine: I.V.: 30 mg/m$^2$ every 7 days
Cisplatin: I.V.: 120 mg/m$^2$/day day 1 and 29, then every 6 weeks

## Vinorelbine-Gemcitabine

**Use:** Lung cancer, nonsmall cell
**Regimen:**
Vinorelbine: I.V.: 20 mg/m$^2$/day days 1, 8, and 15 [total dose/cycle = 60 mg/m$^2$]
Gemcitabine: I.V.: 800 mg/m$^2$/day days 1, 8, and 15 [total dose/cycle = 2400 mg/m$^2$]
Repeat cycle every 28 days

## VIP (Etoposide) (Testicular Cancer)

**Use:** Testicular cancer
**Regimen: Note:** Multiple variations are listed below.
**Variation 1:**
Etoposide: I.V.: 75 mg/m$^2$/day days 1-5 [total dose/cycle = 375 mg/m$^2$]
Ifosfamide: I.V.: 1200 mg/m$^2$/day days 1-5 [total dose/cycle = 6000 mg/m$^2$]
Cisplatin: I.V.: 20 mg/m$^2$/day days 1-5 [total dose/cycle = 100 mg/m$^2$]
Repeat cycle every 21 days
**Variation 2:**
Etoposide: I.V.: 100 mg/m$^2$/day days 1-5 [total dose/cycle = 500 mg/m$^2$]
Ifosfamide: I.V.: 1200 mg/m$^2$/day days 1-5
Cisplatin: I.V.: 20 mg/m$^2$/day days 1-5 [total dose/cycle = 100 mg/m$^2$]
Repeat cycle every 21 days
**Variation 3:**
Ifosfamide: I.V.: 2500 mg/m$^2$/day days 1 and 2 [total dose/cycle = 5000 mg/m$^2$]
Mesna: I.V.: 2400 mg/m$^2$/day days 1 and 2 [total dose/cycle = 4800 mg/m$^2$]
Etoposide: I.V.: 100 mg/m$^2$/day days 3, 4, and 5 [total dose/cycle = 300 mg/m$^2$]
Cisplatin: I.V.: 40 mg/m$^2$/day days 3, 4, and 5 [total dose/cycle = 120 mg/m$^2$]
Repeat cycle every 21 days
**Variation 4:**
Etoposide: I.V.: 75 mg/m$^2$/day days 1-5 [total dose/cycle = 375 mg/m$^2$]
Ifosfamide: I.V.: 1200 mg/m$^2$/day days 1-5 [total dose/cycle = 6000 mg/m$^2$]
Cisplatin: I.V.: 20 mg/m$^2$/day days 1-5 [total dose/cycle = 100 mg/m$^2$]
Mesna: I.V.: 120 mg/m$^2$ day 1 only, then 1200 mg/m$^2$ continuous infusion days 1-5
Repeat cycle every 21 days

## VIP (Small Cell Lung Cancer)

**Use:** Lung cancer, small cell
**Regimen:**
Etoposide: I.V.: 75 mg/m$^2$/day days 1-4 [total dose/cycle = 300 mg/m$^2$]
Ifosfamide: I.V.: 1200 mg/m$^2$/day days 1-4 [total dose/cycle = 4800 mg/m$^2$]
Cisplatin: I.V.: 20 mg/m$^2$/day days 1-4 [total dose/cycle = 80 mg/m$^2$]
Mesna: I.V.: 300 mg/m$^2$ day 1 [total dose/cycle = 300 mg/m$^2$] **followed by**
1200 mg/m$^2$/day continuous infusion days 1-4 [total dose/cycle = 4800 mg/m$^2$]
Repeat cycle every 21 days

# VIP (Vinblastine) (Testicular Cancer)

**Use:** Testicular Cancer
**Regimen: Note:** Multiple variations are listed below.

    **Variation 1:**
    Vinblastine: I.V.: 0.11 mg/kg/day days 1 and 2  [total dose/cycle = 0.22 mg/kg]
    Ifosfamide: I.V.: 1200 mg/m$^2$/day days 1-5  [total dose/cycle = 6000 mg/m$^2$]
    Cisplatin: I.V.: 20 mg/m$^2$/day days 1-5  [total dose/cycle = 100 mg/m$^2$]
    Repeat cycle every 21 days

    **Variation 2:**
    Vinblastine: I.V.: 6 mg/m$^2$/day days 1 and 2  [total dose/cycle = 12 mg/m$^2$]
    Ifosfamide: I.V.: 1500 mg/m$^2$/day days 1-5  [total dose/cycle = 7500 mg/m$^2$]
    Cisplatin: I.V.: 20 mg/m$^2$/day days 1-5  [total dose/cycle = 100 mg/m$^2$]
    Repeat cycle every 21 days

# VP (Small Cell Lung Cancer)

**Use:** Lung cancer, small cell
**Regimen:**

    Etoposide: I.V.: 100 mg/m$^2$/day days 1-4  [total dose/cycle = 400 mg/m$^2$]
    Cisplatin: I.V.: 20 mg/m$^2$/day days 1-4  [total dose/cycle = 80 mg/m$^2$]
    Repeat cycle every 21 days

# V-TAD

**Use:** Leukemia, acute myeloid
**Regimen:**

    **Induction:**
    Etoposide: I.V.: 50 mg/m$^2$/day days 1-3  [total dose/cycle = 150 mg/m$^2$]
    Thioguanine: Oral: 75 mg/m$^2$/day every 12 hours days 1-5  [total dose/cycle = 750 mg/m$^2$]
    Daunorubicin: I.V.: 20 mg/m$^2$/day days 1 and 2  [total dose/cycle = 40 mg/m$^2$]
    Cytarabine: I.V.: 75 mg/m$^2$/day continuous infusion days 1-5  [total dose/cycle = 375 mg/m$^2$]
    Up to 3 cycles may be given based on individual response; time between cycles not specified

# XelOx

**Use:** Colorectal cancer
**Regimen: Note:** Multiple variations are listed below.

    **Variation 1:**
    Oxaliplatin: I.V.: 130 mg/m$^2$ day 1   [total dose/cycle = 130 mg/m$^2$]
    Capecitabine: Oral: 2500 mg/m$^2$/day days 1-14   [total dose/cycle = 35,000 mg/m$^2$]
    Repeat cycle every 21 days

    **Variation 2:**
    Oxaliplatin: I.V.: 85 mg/m$^2$/day days 1 and 14  [total dose/cycle = 170 mg/m$^2$]
    Capecitabine: Oral: 3500 mg/m$^2$/day days 1-7 and 14-21  [total dose/cycle = 52,500 mg/m$^2$]
    Repeat cycle every 28 days

    **Variation 3:**
    Oxaliplatin: I.V.: 50 mg/m$^2$/day days 1, 8, 22, and 29  [total dose/cycle = 200 mg/m$^2$]
    Capecitabine: Oral: 1650 mg/m$^2$/day days 1-14 and 22-35  [total dose/cycle = 46,200 mg/m$^2$]

    **Variation 4:**
    Oxaliplatin: I.V.: 70 mg/m$^2$/day days 1 and 8  [total dose/cycle = 140 mg/m$^2$]
    Capecitabine: Oral: 2000 mg/m$^2$/day days 1-14  [total dose/cycle = 28,000 mg/m$^2$]

    **Variation 5:**
    Oxaliplatin: I.V.: 120 mg/m$^2$ day 1  [total dose/cycle = 120 mg/m$^2$]
    Capecitabine: Oral: 2500 mg/m$^2$/day days 1-14  [total dose/cycle = 35,000 mg/m$^2$]

    **Variation 6:**
    Oxaliplatin: I.V.: 85 mg/m$^2$ day 1  [total dose/cycle = 85 mg/m$^2$]
    Capecitabine: Oral: 2500 mg/m$^2$/day days 1-7  [total dose/cycle = 17,500 mg/m$^2$] **or**
    Capecitabine: Oral: 3000 mg/m$^2$/day days 1-7  [total dose/cycle = 21,000 mg/m$^2$] **or**
    Capecitabine: Oral: 3500 mg/m$^2$/day days 1-7  [total dose/cycle = 24,500 mg/m$^2$] **or**
    Capecitabine: Oral: 4000 mg/m$^2$/day days 1-7  [total dose/cycle = 28,00 mg/m$^2$]
    Repeat cycle every 14 days

# CHEMOTHERAPY REGIMEN INDEX

# Gastrointestinal

# Genitourinary

# Head and Neck Cancer

# Hematologic/Leukemia

### Lymphoid Tissue (Lymphoma) *(continued)*

### Lymphoma, Non-Hodgkin

### Lymphoma, Non-Hodgkin (Burkitt)

## Malignant Pleural Mesothelioma

## Myeloma
### Multiple Myeloma

## Sarcoma

### Osteosarcoma

## Sarcoma *(continued)*

**Rhabdomyosarcoma**

**Soft Tissue Sarcoma**

# Skin

**Melanoma**

# HERBS AND COMMON NATURAL AGENTS

The authors have chosen to include this list of natural products and their reported uses. Due to limited scientific evidence to support these uses, the information provided here is not intended as a cure for any disease, and should not be construed as curative or healing. In addition, the reader is strongly encouraged to seek other references that discuss this information in more detail, and that discuss important issues such as contraindications, warnings, precautions, adverse reactions, and interactions.

## PROPOSED CLAIMS

| Herb | Reported Uses |
| --- | --- |
| Acetyl-L-carnitine (ALC) | Alzheimer disease; depression; diabetic peripheral neuropathy; Parkinson disease |
| Adrenal extract | Depression; fatigue; stress; fibromylagia |
| Aloe (*Aloe supp*) | Gingivitis; healing agent for wounds, minor burns, and other minor skin irritations |
| Alpha-Lipoic acid | Diabetes, diabetic peripheral neuropathy; glaucoma; prevention of cataracts; prevention of neurologic disorders, including stroke; chemotherapy and radiation (adjunct); circulation; multiple sclerosis; hypertension |
| Androstenedione | Athletic performance (enhancement) |
| Aortic extract | Circulation structure, function, and integrity (arteries and veins); prevention of vascular disease including atherosclerosis, cerebral and peripheral arterial insufficiency, varicose veins, hemorrhoids, and vascular retinopathies such as macular degeneration |
| Arabinoxylane | Chemotherapy-induced leukopenia; immune system enhancement (antiviral and anticancer activity); HIV infection |
| Arginine | Cardiovascular disease; chronic heart failure; hypercholesterolemia; circulation; increases lean body mass; inflammatory bowel disease; immune support; male infertility; sexual vitality and enhancement; wound healing |
| Artichoke (*Cynara scolymus*) | Eczema and other dermatologic problems; hepatic protection/stimulation; hypercholesterolemia; bile flow; indigestion |
| Ashwagandha (*Withania somnifera*) | Adaptogen/tonic (promote wellness); chemotherapy and radiation (adjunct); stress, fatigue, nervous exhaustion |
| Astragalus (*Astragalus membranaceus*) [Milk Vetch] | Adaptogen/tonic (promote wellness); chemotherapy and radiation (adjunct); immune support; multiple sclerosis; otitis media; tissue oxygenation |
| Bacopa (*Bacopa monniera*) | Alzheimer disease/senility; memory enhancement and improvement of cognitive function |
| Beta-Carotene | Asthma; cervical dysplasia; coronary heart disease (risk reduction; in combination); immune support; photoprotection (erythropoietic protoporphyria); prevention of lung cancer |
| Betaine hydrochloride | Digestive aid (hypochlorhydria and achlorhydria); rosacea |
| *Bifidobacterium bifidum* (*bifidus*) | Crohn disease; diarrhea; gastrointestinal microflora recolonization (anaerobic); ulcerative colitis |
| Bilberry (*Vaccinium myrtillus*) | Diarrhea; hemorrhoids; ophthalmologic disorders (antioxidant) including myopia, diminished acuity, glaucoma; dark adaptation, macular degeneration, night blindness, diabetic retinopathy, cataracts; scleroderma; vascular disorders including varicose veins, capillary permeability/stability, phlebitis |
| Biotin (Vitamin H) | Brittle nails; diabetes; diabetic peripheral neuropathy; seborrheic dermatitis; uncombable hair syndrome |
| Bismuth | Ulcers |
| Bitter melon (*Momordica charantia*) | Antiviral; diabetes, including impaired glucose tolerance (IGT) |
| Black cohosh (*Cimicifuga racemosa*) | Arthritis; menopause symptoms (including vasomotor); premenstrual syndrome (PMS); mild depression |
| Bladderwrack (*Fucus vesiculosus*) | Fibrocystic breast disease; hypothyroidism; nutrient (rich source of iodine, potassium, magnesium, calcium, and iron) |
| Boron | Osteoarthritis; osteoporosis; rheumatoid arthritis |

*(continued)*

| Herb | Reported Uses |
|---|---|
| Boswellia (*Boswellia serrata*) | Antiinflammatory; arthritis; ulcerative colitis |
| Branched-chain amino acids (BCAAs) | Muscle development and lean body mass (increase) |
| Bromelain (*Anas comosus*) | Arthritis (antiinflammatory; proteolytic); cervical dysplasia; digestive enzyme; sinusitis |
| Bupleurum (*Bupleurum falcatum*) | Chronic inflammatory disease; fatigue; hepatic protection; systemic lupus erythematosus (SLE) |
| Calcium | Blood pressure regulation; cancer prevention; hypercholesterolemia; hypertension; kidney stones; poison ivy (topical; lactate form); premenstrual syndrome (PMS); pregnancy; prevention of osteoporosis |
| Calendula (*Calendula officinalis*) | Antibacterial, antifungal, antiviral, antiprotozoal; vulnerary; wound-healing (immune stimulant) |
| Caprylic acid | Antifungal/antiyeast; candidiasis; Crohn disease; dysbiosis |
| Carnitine | Athletic performance (enhancement); congestive heart failure (CHF); hypercholesterolemia; male infertility; weight loss |
| Cascara (*Rhamnus purshiana*) | Laxative |
| Cat's claw (*Uncaria tomentosa*) | Antiinflammatory; antimicrobial (antibacterial, antifungal, antiviral); antioxidant; cervical dysplasia; Crohn disease; diverticulitis; endometriosis; fibromyalgia; immune support; multiple sclerosis; rosacea; systemic lupus erythematosus (SLE) |
| Cayenne (*Capsicum annuum, Capsicum frutescens*) | Antiinflammatory and analgesic (topical); cardiovascular circulatory support; digestive stimulant |
| Chamomile, German (*Matricaria chamomilla, Matricaria recutita*) | Minor injury (topical antiinflammatory); carminative, antispasmodic; insomnia (mild sedative); anxiolytic; colic; diaper rash; indigestion; nausea/vomiting; oral health (as mouth rinse/gargle); stress/anxiety; teething; uterine tonic |
| Chasteberry (*Vitex agnus-castus*) | Acne vulgaris; cervical dysplasia; corpus luteum insufficiency; hyperprolactinemia and insufficient lactation; menopause; menorrhagia; menstrual disorders including amenorrhea, endometriosis, premenstrual syndrome (PMS); rosacea |
| Chitosan | Weight reduction |
| Chlorophyll | Antiinflammatory, antioxidant, and wound-healing properties; bacteriostatic; odor absorbent/suppressant (breath freshener, toothpaste, mouthwash, and deodorant); protectant |
| Chondroitin sulfate | Osteoarthritis |
| Chromium | Atherosclerosis; diabetes, type 1; diabetes, type 2; glaucoma; hypercholesterolemia; hypertriglyceridemia; hypothyroidism; premenstrual syndrome (PMS); weight loss |
| Clove (*Syzygium aromaticum*) | Antiseptic; analgesic (toothache and teething) |
| Coenzyme Q$_{10}$ | Angina; cancer (preventive); chemotherapy (adjunct); chronic fatigue syndrome; congestive heart failure (CHF); fibromyalgia; gingivitis; hypercholesterolemia; hypertension; HMG-CoA reductase inhibitors may cause depletion of this nutraceutical; multiple sclerosis; muscular dystrophy; periodontal disease; weight loss |
| Coleus (*Coleus forskohlii*) | Asthma and allergies; eczema; hypertension and congestive heart failure (CHF); psoriasis |
| Collagen (Type II) | Arthritis (rheumatoid and osteo); burns (first- and second-degree); ulcers (pressure, venous stasis, diabetic); surgical and traumatic wounds; wound healing (topical) |
| Colostrum | Antiviral (mild); athletic performance (enhancement); diarrhea; immune support |
| Conjugated linoleic acid (CLA) | Muscle development and lean body mass (increase) |
| Copper | Anemia; osteoporosis; rheumatoid arthritis |
| Cordyceps (*Cordyceps sinensis*) | Adaptogen/tonic (promote wellness); antioxidant; chemotherapy and radiation (adjunct); endurance and stamina; fibromyalgia; hepatoprotection; lung, liver, and kidney function (general support); sexual vitality (males and females); tissue oxygenation; fatigue; immunomodulator |

*(continued)*

| Herb | Reported Uses |
|---|---|
| Cranberry (*Vaccinium macrocarpon*) | Nephrolithiasis (preventive); urinary tract infection, including prevention |
| Creatine | Enhancement of athletic performance (energy production and protein synthesis for muscle building) |
| Cyclo-hispro | Diabetes, type 2; hypoglycemia |
| Dandelion (*Taraxacum officinale*) | Leaf used as a diuretic; root used for disorders of bile secretion (choleretic), appetite stimulation, dyspepsia |
| Dehydroepiandrosterone (DHEA) | Antiaging; depression; diabetes, type 2; fatigue; lupus |
| Devil's claw (*Harpagophytum procumbens*) | Antiinflammatory; back pain; osteoarthritis, gout, and other inflammatory conditions |
| Docosahexaenoic acid (DHA) | Alzheimer disease; attention deficit disorder (ADD) and attention deficit hyperactivity disorder (ADHD); coronary heart disease (risk reduction); Crohn disease; diabetes; eczema; hypertension; hypertriglyceridemia; psoriasis; rheumatoid arthritis; stroke (risk reduction) |
| Dong quai (*Angelica sinensis*) | Anemia; energy enhancement (particularly in females); hypertension; menopause, dysmenorrhea, premenstrual syndrome (PMS), and amenorrhea; menorrhagia; phytoestrogen |
| Echinacea (*Echinacea purpurea, Echinacea angustifolia*) | Antibacterial (topical; boils, abscesses, tonsillitis, poison ivy); antiviral; arthritis (*E. augustifolia*); immune support (cold and other upper respiratory infections); otitis media |
| Elder (*Sambucus nigra, Sambucus canadensis*) | Berry used as an antiviral, antioxidant, and for influenza; flower used as an antiinflammatory, colds and influenza, diaphoretic, diuretic, fever, sinusitis, and sore throat |
| Ephedra (*Ephedra sinica*) | Allergies, sinusitis, hay fever; asthma; weight loss |
| Evening primrose (*Oenothera biennis*) | Amenorrhea; attention deficit disorder (ADD); depression; diabetes; diabetic peripheral neuropathy; eczema, dermatitis, and psoriasis; endometriosis; fatigue; fibrocystic breast disease (FBD); hypercholesterolemia; irritable bowel syndrome; menorrhagia; multiple sclerosis; omega-6 fatty acid supplementation; premenstrual syndrome (PMS) and menopause; rheumatoid arthritis; rosacea; scleroderma |
| Eyebright (*Euphrasia officinalis*) | Eye fatigue; catarrh of the eyes |
| Fenugreek (*Trigonella foenum-graecum*) | Diabetes; hypercholesterolemia |
| Feverfew (*Tanacetum parthenium*) | Antiinflammatory, rheumatoid arthritis; migraine headache (preventive); muscle soreness |
| Fish oils | Acne vulgaris; asthma; cardiac death (sudden; preventive); cardiac support (general; proposed benefits); circulation; coronary heart disease (preventive); Crohn disease; diabetes; dysmenorrhea; eczema, psoriasis; fatigue; headache; heart disease and heart attack (risk reduction), including women; herpes simplex 2; hypertension; hypertriglyceridemia; memory enhancement; multiple sclerosis; premenstrual syndrome (PMS); rheumatoid arthritis; rosacea; scleroderma; stroke (risk reduction) |
| Flaxseed oil | Acne vulgaris; arthritis (rheumatoid); asthma; constipation; coronary heart disease (risk reduction); hemorrhoids; hypertension; multiple sclerosis; omega-3 essential fatty acid source (cell wall and cellular membrane structure; cholesterol transport and oxidation); premenstrual syndrome (PMS); prostaglandins production; psoriasis; stroke (risk reduction); systemic lupus erythematosus (SLE) |
| Folic acid | Alcoholism; anemia; atherosclerosis; cancer prevention (colon and breast); cervical dysplasia; coronary heart disease (risk reduction); coronary restenosis (rate reduction by decreasing plasma homocysteine levels); Crohn disease; dementia and Alzheimer disease (risk reduction); depression; gingivitis; osteoporosis; pregnancy (prevention of birth defects) and lactation; schizophrenia (risk reduction, by decreasing homocysteine levels), ulcer, aphthous |
| Garcinia (*Garcinia cambogia*) | Pancreatic function (supportive) and glucose regulation; weight loss |

*(continued)*

| Herb | Reported Uses |
|---|---|
| Garlic (*Allium sativum*) | Antimicrobial (bacterial and fungal); antioxidant (practitioners should be aware that aged garlic extracts have been reported to improve this benefit); coagulation (mild inhibitor of platelet-activating factor); hyperlipidemia; hypertension; immune support |
| Ginger (*Zingiber officinale*) | Antiemetic, for nausea and vomiting in pregnancy; motion sickness; antiinflammatory (musculoskeletal); diverticulitis; indigestion/heartburn; osteoarthritis |
| Ginkgo (*Ginkgo biloba*) | Alzheimer disease, dementia; asthma; depression; epilepsy; headaches; intermittent claudication; macular degeneration; memory enhancement; Parkinson disease; peripheral blood flow (cerebral vascular disease, peripheral vascular insufficiency, impotence, tinnitus, and depression); seizures; sexual dysfunction (antidepressant-induced) |
| Ginseng, Panax (*Panax ginseng*) | Adrenal tonic; diabetes; physical and mental performance, [energy enhancement], chemotherapy and radiation (adjunct); immune support |
| Ginseng, Siberian (*Eleutherococcus senticosus*) | Adaptogen/tonic (promote wellness); athletic performance (enhancement); stress (decreased fatigue); immune support |
| Glucosamine | Osteoarthritis and joint structure support; rheumatoid arthritis and other inflammatory conditions |
| Glutamine | Alcoholism; athletic performance (enhancement); cancer (adjunct); catabolic wasting; chemotherapy (prevention of adverse effects); fibromyalgia; HIV infection (adjunct); immune support; peptic ulcer disease; postsurgical healing; ulcerative colitis and other inflammatory bowel diseases |
| Glutathione | Hepatoprotection (alcohol-induced liver damage); immune support; peptic ulcer disease |
| Golden seal (*Hydrastis canadensis*) | Fever; gallbladder; mucous membrane tonifying (used in inflammation of mucosal membranes); gastritis; antimicrobial (antibacterial/antifungal); bronchitis, cystitis, and infectious diarrhea; sinusitis; sore throat; urinary tract infection (UTI) |
| Gotu kola (*Centella asiatica*) | Connective tissue (support); hemorrhoids (topical); macular degeneration; memory enhancement; psoriasis; venous insufficiency; wound healing (topical) |
| Grapefruit seed (*Citrus paradisi*) | Antifungal, antibacterial, antiparasitic; diarrhea; diverticulitis; eczema; endometriosis; irritable bowel syndrome (IBS); rosacea; sinusitis; sore throat; ulcerative colitis; urinary tract infection (UTI) |
| Grape seed (*Vitis vinifera*) | Allergies, antiinflammatory, asthma; antioxidant; circulation, platelet aggregation inhibitor, capillary fragility, arterial/venous insufficiency (intermittent claudification, varicose veins); gingivitis; glaucoma; macular degeneration; multiple sclerosis; Parkinson disease; scleroderma |
| Green tea (*Camellia sinensis*) | Antioxidant; cancer and cardiovascular disease (preventive); chemotherapy and radiation (adjunct); diarrhea; gingivitis; hypercholesterolemia; macular degeneration; platelet-aggregation inhibitor |
| Ground ivy (*Hedera helix*) | Croup; mucolytic; upper respiratory congestion and cough |
| Guggul (*Commiphora mukul*) | Hypercholesterolemia; hypothyroidism; osteoarthritis; weight loss |
| Gymnema (*Gymnema sylvestre*) | Diabetes, blood sugar regulation |
| Hawthorn (*Crataegus oxyacantha*) | Angina, hypotension, hypertension, peripheral vascular disease, tachycardia; cardiotonic; congestive heart failure |
| Hops (*Humulus lupulus*) | Sedative/hypnotic (mild) |
| Horse chestnut (*Aesculus hippocastanum*) | Scleroderma; venous insufficiency (varicose veins, hemorrhoids, deep venous thrombosis, lower extremity edema [oral and topical]) |
| Horsetail (*Equisetum arvense*) | Diuretic; high mineral content (including silicic acid); bone and connective tissue strengthening, including osteoporosis |
| Huperzine A (*Huperzia serrata*) | Senile dementia and Alzheimer disease |
| Hydroxymethyl butyrate (HMB) | Athletic performance (enhancement) |
| 5-Hydroxytryptophan (5-HTP) | Anxiety; depression; fibromyalgia; headache; migraine; sleep disorders, insomnia (stimulates the production of melatonin); weight loss |

*(continued)*

| Herb | Reported Uses |
| --- | --- |
| Inositol hexaphosphate (IP-6) | Cancer (preventive) |
| Iodine | Fibrocystic breast disease; goiter (preventive); hypothyroidism; mucolytic agent |
| Ipriflavone | Prevention of osteoporosis (men and women) |
| Iron | Anemia; menorrhagia; pregnancy; restless legs syndrome |
| Isoflavones (soy) | Benign prostatic hyperplasia (BPH); cancer (preventive); cervical dysplasia; chemotherapy (adjunct); endometriosis; hypercholesterolemia; menopausal symptoms; osteoarthritis; osteoporosis; premenstrual syndrome (PMS) |
| Kava kava (*Piper methysticum*) | Fibromyalgia; insomnia; anxiety/stress, skeletal muscle relaxation, postischemic episodes; muscle soreness |
| Lactobacillus acidophilus | Constipation; diarrhea (infantile); eczema (preventive); gastrointestinal microflora recolonization; hypercholesterolemia; immune support; lactose intolerance; vaginal candidiasis |
| Lavender (*Lavendula officinalis*) | Wound healing including minor burns (topical) |
| Lemon balm/Melissa (*Melissa officinalis*) | Antiviral (oral herpes virus); attention deficit hyperactivity disorder (ADHD); sedation (pediatrics); teething (topical) |
| Licorice (*Glycyrrhiza glabra*) | Adrenal insufficiency (licorice); Crohn disease; croup; expectorant and antitussive (licorice); gastrointestinal ulceration (DGL chewable products) |
| Liver extract | Liver tonic |
| Lutein | Cataracts; macular degeneration |
| Lycopene | Atherosclerosis; cancer (preventive; especially lung and prostate); macular degeneration |
| Lysine | Angina pectoris; herpes simplex; osteoporosis; ulcer, aphthous |
| Magnesium | Asthma; attention deficit hyperactivity disorder (ADHD); cardiovascular disease; circulation; colic (magnesium salt); congestive heart failure (CHF); diabetes; dysmenorrhea; epilepsy; fatigue; fibromyalgia (magnesium salt); gallbladder (magnesium salt); heart disease; hypertension; hypoglycemia; insomnia; kidney stones; migraine headache; mitral valve prolapse (MVP); muscle cramps; nervousness; osteoporosis; premenstrual syndrome (PMS); stress/anxiety; multiple sclerosis |
| Malic acid | Aluminum toxicity; fibromyalgia |
| Manganese | Diabetes; epilepsy; osteoporosis |
| Marshmallow (*Althaea officinalis*) | Cough; croup; mucilaginous, demulcent; peptic ulcer disease; sore throat |
| Mastic (*Pistacia lentiscus*) | *H. pylori* inhibitor; peptic ulcer disease |
| Melatonin | Insomnia; jet lag; oxidative stress in dialysis patients (preventive) |
| Methionine | Liver detoxification |
| Methyl sulfonyl methane (MSM) | Allergies; analgesic; arthritis (osteo and rheumatoid); interstitial cystitis; lupus |
| Milk thistle (*Silybum marianum*) | Antidote for poisoning by Death Cup mushroom; antioxidant (specifically hepatic cells), liver diseases including acute/chronic hepatitis, jaundice, and stimulation of bile secretion/cholagogue; chemotherapy and radiation (adjunct); constipation; eczema; gallbladder; halitosis; hepatoprotective, including drug toxicities (ie, phenothiazines, butyrophenones, ethanol, and acetaminophen); hyperthyroidism; psoriasis; rosacea |
| Modified citrus pectin (MCP) | Anticarcinogenic; hypercholesterolemia |
| Muira puama (*Ptychopetalum olacoides*) | Athletic performance (enhancement); sexual vitality (males) |
| N-Acetyl cysteine (NAC) | Acetaminophen toxicity; AIDS; asthma (mucolytic, antioxidant); bronchitis; cardioprotection (during chemotherapy); fatigue; glutathione production; heavy metal detoxification; hyperthyroidism; hypothyroidism; macular degeneration; multiple sclerosis; nephropathy (preventive); Parkinson disease; scleroderma; systemic lupus erythematosus (SLE) |
| Nicotinamide adenine dinucleotide (NADH) | Chronic fatigue; Parkinson disease; stamina and energy |
| Olive leaf (*Olea europaea*) | Acne vulgaris; antibacterial; antifungal, antiviral; Crohn disease; diabetes; diarrhea; diverticulitis; eczema; endometriosis; hypertension; multiple sclerosis; scleroderma; ulcerative colitis; urinary tract infection (UTI) |

# APPENDIX

*(continued)*

| Herb | Reported Uses |
| --- | --- |
| Pancreatic extract | Antiinflammatory; cancer (adjunct); celiac disease; digestive disturbances; food allergies; immune complex diseases |
| Para-Aminobenzoic acid (PABA) | Peyronie disease; scleroderma; vitiligo |
| Parsley (*Petroselinum crispum*) | Halitosis; antibacterial, antifungal |
| Passion flower (*Passiflora spp*) | Hyperthyroidism; insomnia (sedative) |
| Peppermint (*Mentha piperita*) | Carminative, spasmolytic; colic; indigestion; irritable bowel syndrome; motion sickness |
| Phenylalanine | Reward deficiency syndrome in addiction; analgesic; depression; vitiligo |
| Phosphatidyl choline (PC) | Alcohol-induced liver damage; Alzheimer disease; gallstones; hepatitis |
| Phosphatidyl serine (PS) | Alzheimer disease; depression; memory enhancement |
| Potassium | Cardiac arrhythmias; congestive heart failure (CHF); hypertension; kidney stones |
| Pregnenolone | Arthritis; hormone precursor (DHEA, cortisol, progesterone, estrogens, and testosterone); mental performance |
| Progesterone | Breast cancer (preventive); dysmenorrhea; endometriosis; menopause symptoms; osteoporosis; premenstrual syndromes (PMS) |
| Psyllium (*Plantago ovata, Plantago isphagula*) | Bulk-forming laxative (containing 10% to 30% mucilage); halitosis |
| Pygeum (*Pygeum africanum, Prunus africana*) | Benign prostatic hyperplasia (BPH) |
| Pyruvate | Athletic performance (enhancement); weight loss |
| Quercetin | Allergies; asthma; atherosclerosis; cataracts; peptic ulcer disease; sinusitis |
| Red clover (*Trifolium pratense*) | Endometriosis; liver and kidney detoxification (liquid extract); menopause symptoms (proprietary extract contains 4 phytoestrogens); menorrhagia |
| Red yeast rice (*Monascus purpureus*) | Hypercholesterolemia |
| Rehmannia (*Rehmannia glutinosa*) | Rheumatoid arthritis; systemic lupus erythematosus (SLE) |
| Reishi (*Ganoderma lucidum*) | Chemotherapy and radiation (adjunct); hypertension; seizure disorder; immune support; fatigue |
| SAMe (S-adenosyl methionine) | Cardiovascular disease; depression; fibromyalgia; headache; insomnia; liver disease; osteoarthritis; rheumatoid arthritis |
| Saw palmetto (*Serenoa repens*) | Benign prostatic hyperplasia (BPH) |
| Schisandra (*Schizandra chinensis*) | Adaptogen/tonic (to promote wellness); hepatic protection and detoxification; chemotherapy and radiation (adjunct); endurance, stamina, and work performance (enhancement); decreases fatigue |
| Selenium | Acne vulgaris (with vitamin E); AIDS; atherosclerosis; bronchial asthma; cancer (preventive); cardiomyopathy; cataracts; chemotherapy and radiation (adjunct); circulation; eczema; epilepsy; hemorrhoids; herpes simplex 1 and 2; hypothyroidism; macular degeneration; prostate cancer (preventive); ulcerative colitis |
| Senna (*Cassia senna*) | Laxative |
| Shark cartilage | Cancer; osteoarthritis, rheumatoid arthritis |
| Spleen extract | Chemotherapy and radiation (adjunct); cold/flu; fatigue; spleen function (supportive) |
| Stinging nettle (*Urtica dioica*) | Leaf used for allergic rhinitis, allergy and hay fever symptoms, uric acid excretion, and sinusitis; root used for benign prostatic hyperplasia (BPH) |
| St John's wort (*Hypericum perforatum*) | Antibacterial, antiinflammatory (topical: minor wounds, infections, bruises, muscle soreness, and sprains); mild to moderate depression, melancholia, stress and anxiety |
| Taurine | Congestive heart failure (CHF); diabetes; gallbladder; hypertension; seizure disorders |

*(continued)*

| Herb | Reported Uses |
|------|---------------|
| Tea tree (*Melaleuca alternifolia*) | **Not for ingestion**; acne vulgaris; antifungal, antibacterial; mouthwash for dental and oral health; burns, cuts, scrapes, insect bites |
| Thyme (*Thymus vulgaris*) | Antifungal; cough (upper respiratory origin); croup |
| Thymus extract | Fatigue; immune support; otitis media; sinusitis; systemic lupus erythematosus (SLE) |
| Thyroid extract | Fatigue; immune support; fibromyalgia |
| Tocotrienols | Cancer (preventive); heart disease; hypercholesterolemia; skin (supportive, protective) |
| Tribulus (*Tribulus terrestris*) | Athletic performance (enhancement), sexual vitality |
| Turmeric (*Curcuma longa*) | Antioxidant; antiinflammatory; antirheumatic; hypercholesterolemia; dysmenorrhea; muscle soreness |
| Tylophora (*Tylophora asthmatica*) | Allergies; asthma |
| Tyrosine | Alzheimer disease; depression; hypothyroidism; phenylketonuria (PKU); substance abuse |
| Uva-Ursi (*Arctostaphylos uva-ursi*) | Urinary tract infections and kidney stone prevention |
| Valerian (*Valeriana officinalis*) | Hyperthyroidism; insomnia (sedative/hypnotic); premenstrual syndrome (PMS), menopause; restless motor syndromes and muscle spasms |
| Vanadium | Diabetes, type 1; diabetes, type 2; hypoglycemia |
| Vinpocetine | Cognitive function; Alzheimer disease and senility |
| Vitamin A (Retinol) | Acne vulgaris; AIDS; cancer (preventive); cervical dysplasia; circulation; cold/flu; Crohn disease; diverticulitis; eczema; fibrocystic breast disease (FBD); glaucoma; hemorrhoids; measles; menorrhagia; night blindness; otitis media; premenstrual syndrome (PMS); psoriasis; rosacea; sore throat; ulcerative colitis; urinary tract infection (UTI) |
| Vitamin $B_1$ (Thiamine) | Alcoholism; Alzheimer disease; anemia (megaloblastic); congestive heart failure (CHF); diabetes; fibromyalgia; insomnia; neurological conditions (Bell palsy, trigeminal neuralgia, sciatica, sensory neuropathies); psychiatric illness |
| Vitamin $B_2$ | Cataracts; depression; migraine |
| Vitamin $B_3$ | Acne vulgaris (4% niacinamide topical gel); cataracts; coronary disease (preventive); diabetes, type 1; diabetes, type 2; hyperlipidemia (hypercholesterolemia, hypertriglyceridemia); impaired glucose tolerance; intermittent claudication; myocardial infarction (risk reduction); osteoarthritis; Raynaud syndrome; rheumatoid arthritis; schizophrenia; antioxidant |
| Vitamin $B_5$ (Pantothenic acid) | Adrenal support; allergies; arthritis; constipation; hyperlipidemia (pantethine, but not pantothenic acid, lowers cholesterol and triglycerides); rheumatoid arthritis; wound healing |
| Vitamin $B_6$ (Pyridoxine) | Arthritis; asthma; autism; cardiovascular disease; carpal tunnel syndrome; coronary heart disease (risk reduction); coronary restenosis (rate reduction by lowering plasma homocysteine levels); dementia and Alzheimer disease (risk reduction); depression (associated with oral contraceptives); diabetic peripheral neuropathy; epilepsy, $B_6$-dependant; headache; insomnia; kidney stones; monosodium glutamate (MSG) sensitivity; nausea and vomiting (in pregnancy); peptic ulcer disease; PMS |
| Vitamin $B_{12}$ (Cobalamin) | AIDS; asthma; atherosclerosis (due to homocysteine elevation); coronary restenosis (rate reduction by lowering plasma homocysteine levels); Crohn disease; dementia and Alzheimer disease (risk reduction); depression; diabetic peripheral neuropathy; male infertility; memory loss; multiple sclerosis; pernicious anemia; sulfite sensitivity |
| Vitamin B complex-25 | See individual B vitamins |
| Vitamin C | AIDS; allergies; antioxidant; asthma; atherosclerosis; cancer; cataracts; cervical dysplasia; circulation; cold; constipation; coronary heart disease (preventive, in patients taking lipid-lowering agents); Crohn disease; diabetes; diverticulitis; eczema; endometriosis; fatigue; fever; fibrocystic breast disease (FBD); fibromyalgia; gallbladder disease (risk reduction); gingivitis; glaucoma; herpes simplex virus 1 and 2; immune support; irritable bowel syndrome (IBS); multiple sclerosis; myocardial infarction (risk reduction); nitrate tolerance (preventive); osteoporosis; otitis media; Parkinson disease; peptic ulcer disease; psoriasis; reflex sympathetic dystrophy (preventive); sinusitis; sore throat; stress/anxiety; sunburn; ulcerative colitis; urinary tract infection (UTI); wound healing |
| Vitamin D | Crohn disease; epilepsy (during anticonvulsant therapy); hearing loss; osteoporosis; psoriasis; rickets; scleroderma |

*(continued)*

| Herb | Reported Uses |
|------|---------------|
| Vitamin E | Acne vulgaris (with selenium); Alzheimer disease; atherosclerosis; Benign prostatic hyperplasia (BPH); cancer (preventive); cataracts; cervical dysplasia; circulation; diabetes; dyslipidemias; eczema; endometriosis; epilepsy; fibrocystic breast disease (FBD); gallbladder; hemorrhoids; macular degeneration; multiple sclerosis; myocardial infarction (risk reduction); osteoarthritis; peptic ulcer disease; peripheral circulation; premenstrual syndrome (PMS); psoriasis; rheumatoid arthritis; scleroderma; sunburn; systemic lupus erythematosus; ulcerative colitis |
| Vitamin K | Osteoporosis; synthesis of blood clotting factors |
| White oak (*Quercus alba*) | Antiinflammatory (mild: throat and mouth as a soothing agent) |
| White willow (*Salix alba*) | Antipyretic; antiinflammatory |
| Wild yam (*Dioscorea villosa*) | Female vitality (conversion to progesterone in the body is poor) |
| Yohimbe (*Pausinystalia yohimbe*) | Sexual vitality (men and women); male erectile dysfunction |
| Zinc | Acne vulgaris; aphthous ulcers; benign prostatic hyperplasia (BPH); common cold; Crohn disease; diabetes; diaper rash; diverticulitis; gastric ulcer healing; immune support; macular degeneration; osteoporosis; otitis media; sexual vitality (men); skin conditions, eczema, psoriasis; sore throat; ulcerative colitis; wound healing |

# TOP 200 PRESCRIBED DRUGS*

| Brand Name (if appropriate) | Generic Name | Rank |
|---|---|---|
| Accupril® | quinapril | 48 |
| ---- | acetaminophen and codeine | 31 |
| Aciphex® | rabeprazole | 105 |
| Actonel® | risedronate | 187 |
| Actos® | pioglitazone | 82 |
| ---- | acyclovir | 160 |
| Adderall XR™ | dextroamphetamine and amphetamine | 164 |
| Advair™ Diskus® | fluticasone and salmeterol | 71 |
| ---- | albuterol (aerosol) | 12 |
| ---- | albuterol (sulfate) | 63 |
| Allegra® | fexofenadine | 24 |
| Allegra-D® | fexofenadine and pseudoephedrine | 107 |
| ---- | allopurinol | 79 |
| ---- | alprazolam | 11 |
| Altace® | ramipril | 78 |
| Amaryl® | glimepiride | 126 |
| Ambien® | zolpidem | 32 |
| ---- | amitriptyline | 39 |
| ---- | amoxicillin | 8 |
| ---- | amoxicillin and clavulanate potassium | 163 |
| Amoxil® | amoxicillin | 74 |
| Apri® | ethinyl estradiol and desogestrel | 195 |
| ---- | aspirin | 158 |
| ---- | atenolol | 3 |
| Augmentin® | amoxicillin and clavulanate potassium | 46 |
| Augmentin ES-600® | amoxicillin and clavulanate potassium | 198 |
| Avalide® | irbesartan and hydrochlorothiazide | 200 |
| Avandia® | rosiglitazone | 81 |
| Avapro® | irbesartan | 147 |
| Aviane™ | ethinyl estradiol and levonorgestrel | 186 |
| Bactroban® | mupirocin | 179 |
| Bextra® | valdecoxib | 146 |
| Biaxin® | clarithromycin | 173 |
| Biaxin® XL | clarithromycin | 165 |
| ---- | bisoprolol and hydrochlorothiazide | 138 |
| ---- | buspirone | 149 |
| ---- | captopril | 156 |
| ---- | levodopa and carbidopa | 199 |
| ---- | carisoprodol | 77 |
| Cartia® XT | diltiazem | 125 |
| Cefzil® | cefprozil | 168 |
| Celebrex® | celecoxib | 21 |
| Celexa™ | citalopram | 26 |
| ---- | cephalexin | 20 |
| Cipro® | ciprofloxacin | 58 |
| Clarinex® | desloratadine | 84 |
| Claritin® | loratadine | 29 |

*NDC Health, "The Top 200 Prescriptions for 2004 by Number of U.S. Prescriptions Dispensed," Available at: http://www.rxlist.com/top200.htm

*(continued)*

| Brand Name (if appropriate) | Generic Name | Rank |
|---|---|---|
| Claritin-D® 12 Hour | loratadine and pseudoephedrine | 162 |
| Claritin-D® 24 Hour | loratadine and pseudoephedrine | 124 |
| Claritin® Reditabs® | loratadine | 184 |
| ---- | clindamycin | 157 |
| ---- | clonazepam | 54 |
| ---- | clonidine | 92 |
| Combivent® | ipratropium and albuterol | 132 |
| Concerta™ | methylphenidate | 119 |
| Coreg® | carvedilol | 171 |
| Cotrim® | sulfamethoxazole and trimethoprim | 102 |
| Coumadin® | warfarin | 68 |
| Cozaar® | losartan | 89 |
| ---- | cyclobenzaprine | 60 |
| Depakote® | valproic acid and derivatives | 118 |
| Detrol® LA | tolterodine | 170 |
| ---- | diazepam | 66 |
| ---- | diclofenac | 197 |
| Diflucan® | fluconazole | 70 |
| Digitek® | digoxin | 94 |
| Dilantin® | phenytoin | 153 |
| ---- | diltiazem | 91 |
| Diovan® | valsartan | 75 |
| Diovan HCT® | valsartan and hydrochlorothiazide | 104 |
| Ditropan® XL | oxybutynin | 193 |
| ---- | doxazosin | 109 |
| ---- | doxycycline | 87 |
| Effexor® XR | venlafaxine | 50 |
| ---- | enalapril | 62 |
| Endocet® | oxycodone and acetaminophen | 178 |
| ---- | estradiol | 80 |
| Evista® | raloxifene | 96 |
| ---- | famotidine | 144 |
| Flomax® | tamsulosin | 112 |
| Flonase® | fluticasone | 59 |
| Flovent® | fluticasone | 100 |
| ---- | fluoxetine | 30 |
| ---- | folic acid | 97 |
| Fosamax® | alendronate | 35 |
| ---- | furosemide | 7 |
| ---- | gemfibrozil | 111 |
| ---- | glipizide | 148 |
| Glucophage® | metformin | 140 |
| Glucophage® XR | metformin | 98 |
| Glucotrol® XL | glipizide | 67 |
| Glucovance™ | glyburide and metformin | 121 |
| ---- | glyburide | 76 |
| Humalog® | insulin preparations | 176 |
| Humulin® 70/30 | insulin preparations | 169 |
| Humulin® N | insulin preparations | 117 |
| ---- | hydrochlorothiazide | 10 |
| ---- | hydrochlorothiazide and triamterene | 18 |
| ---- | hydrocodone and acetaminophen | 1 |

*(continued)*

| Brand Name (if appropriate) | Generic Name | Rank |
|---|---|---|
| ---- | hydroxyzine | 130 |
| Hyzaar® | losartan and hydrochlorothiazide | 115 |
| Imitrex® | sumatriptan | 122 |
| ---- | isosorbide mononitrate | 64 |
| Klor-Con® | potassium chloride | 120 |
| Klor-Con® M20 | potassium chloride | 135 |
| Lanoxin® | digoxin | 88 |
| ---- | ibuprofen | 17 |
| Levaquin™ | levofloxacin | 65 |
| Levothroid® | levothyroxine | 108 |
| Levoxyl® | levothyroxine | 23 |
| Lipitor® | atorvastatin | 2 |
| ---- | lisinopril | 49 |
| ---- | lorazepam | 34 |
| Lotensin® | benazepril | 83 |
| Lotrel® | amlodipine and benazepril | 73 |
| Macrobid® | nitrofurantoin | 161 |
| ---- | meclizine | 133 |
| ---- | medroxyprogesterone | 85 |
| ---- | metformin | 37 |
| ---- | methylprednisolone | 95 |
| ---- | metoclopramide | 136 |
| ---- | metoprolol | 33 |
| ---- | metronidazole | 145 |
| Microgestin™ Fe | ethinyl estradiol and norethindrone | 189 |
| ---- | minocycline | 137 |
| Mircette® | ethinyl estradiol and desogestrel | 191 |
| Monopril® | fosinopril | 131 |
| ---- | naproxen | 55 |
| Nasacort® AQ | triamcinolone | 175 |
| Nasonex® | mometasone | 90 |
| Necon® | ethinyl estradiol and norethindrone | 155 |
| Neurontin® | gabapentin | 43 |
| Nexium™ | esomeprazole | 47 |
| ---- | nifedipine | 192 |
| ---- | nortriptyline | 185 |
| Norvasc® | amlodipine | 9 |
| ---- | nystatin | 150 |
| Ortho-Cyclen® | ethinyl estradiol and norgestimate | 167 |
| Ortho-Novum® | ethinyl estradiol and norethindrone | 129 |
| Ortho Tri-Cyclen® | ethinyl estradiol and norgestimate | 25 |
| ---- | oxycodone and acetaminophen | 86 |
| Oxycontin® | oxycodone | 116 |
| Paxil® | paroxetine | 14 |
| ---- | penicillin V potassium | 99 |
| Plavix® | clopidogrel | 69 |
| ---- | potassium chloride | 53 |
| Pravachol® | pravastatin | 45 |
| ---- | prednisone | 27 |
| Premarin® | estrogens (conjugated) | 5 |
| Prempro™ | estrogens (conjugated/equine) and medroxyprogesterone | 41 |

*(continued)*

| Brand Name (if appropriate) | Generic Name | Rank |
|---|---|---|
| Prevacid® | lansoprazole | 16 |
| Prilosec® | omeprazole | 28 |
| Prinivil® | lisinopril | 93 |
| ---- | promethazine | 103 |
| ---- | promethazine and codeine | 154 |
| Propacet® | propoxyphene and acetaminophen | 141 |
| ---- | propoxyphene and acetaminophen | 36 |
| ---- | propranolol | 139 |
| Protonix® | pantoprazole | 72 |
| ---- | ranitidine | 38 |
| Remeron® | mirtazapine | 143 |
| Rhinocort® Aqua® | budesonide | 183 |
| Risperdal® | risperidone | 101 |
| Serevent® Diskus® | salmeterol | 152 |
| Seroquel® | quetiapine | 159 |
| Singulair® | montelukast | 51 |
| Skelaxin® | metaxalone | 151 |
| ---- | spironolactone | 127 |
| ---- | sulfamethoxazole and trimethoprim | 181 |
| Synthroid® | levothyroxine | 4 |
| ---- | tamoxifen | 190 |
| ---- | temazepam | 113 |
| ---- | terazosin | 123 |
| ---- | tetracycline | 194 |
| Tiazac® | diltiazem | 172 |
| ---- | timolol | 182 |
| Topamax® | topiramate | 188 |
| Toprol-XL® | metoprolol | 19 |
| ---- | tramadol | 174 |
| ---- | trazodone | 57 |
| ---- | triamcinolone | 134 |
| TriCor® | fenofibrate | 128 |
| Trimox® | amoxicillin | 42 |
| Trivora®-28 | ethinyl estradiol and levonorgestrel | 166 |
| Ultracet™ | acetaminophen and tramadol | 177 |
| Ultram® | tramadol | 114 |
| Valtrex® | valacyclovir | 142 |
| Veetids® | penicillin V potassium | 180 |
| ---- | verapamil | 61 |
| Viagra® | sildenafil | 40 |
| ---- | warfarin | 56 |
| Wellbutrin® SR | bupropion | 44 |
| Xalatan® | latanoprost | 110 |
| Zestoretic® | lisinopril and hydrochlorothiazide | 196 |
| Zestril® | lisinopril | 52 |
| Zithromax® | azithromycin | 6 |
| Zocor® | simvastatin | 15 |
| Zoloft® | sertraline | 13 |
| Zyprexa® | olanzapine | 106 |
| Zyrtec® | cetirizine | 22 |

# NEW DRUGS ADDED SINCE LAST EDITION

| Brand Name | Generic Name | Use |
|---|---|---|
| Abraxane™ | paclitaxel (protein bound) | Breast cancer |
| Aczone™ | dapsone | Acne vulgaris |
| Adacel™ | diphtheria, tetanus toxoids, and acellular pertussis vaccine | Booster vaccine |
| Ammonul® | sodium phenylacetate and sodium benzoate | Hyperammonemia |
| Amphadase™ | hyaluronidase | Increase dispersion and absorption of other drugs |
| Aptivus® | tipranavir | HIV infections |
| Asmanex® Twisthaler® | mometasone | Asthma |
| BiDil® | isosorbide dinitrate and hydralazine | Hypertension in African-Americans |
| Boniva® | ibandronate | Osteoporosis |
| Boostrix® | diphtheria, tetanus toxoids, and acellular pertussis vaccine | Booster vaccine |
| Byetta™ | exenatide | Type 2 diabetes |
| Ca-DTPA | diethylene triamine penta-acetic acid | Treating internal contamination from radioactive elements |
| Clolar™ | clofarabine | Acute lymphoblastic leukemia |
| Cymbalta® | duloxetine | Depression |
| Elestat® | epinastine | Allergic conjunctivitis |
| Enablex® | darifenacin | Symptoms of bladder overactivity |
| Focalin™ XR | dexmethylphenidate | Attention-deficit/hyperactivity disorder (ADHD) |
| Fosamax Plus D® | alendronate and cholecalciferol | Osteoporosis |
| Fosrenol™ | lanthanum | End-stage renal disease |
| Kepivance™ | palifermin | Oral mucositis |
| Lunesta™ | eszopiclone | Insomnia |
| Macugen® | pegaptanib | Macular degeneration |
| Menactra™ | meningococcal polysaccharide (Groups A/C/Y and W-135) diphtheria toxoid conjugate vaccine | Vaccine |
| Mycamine™ | micafungin | Antifungal |
| Naglazyme™ | galsulfase | Mucopolysaccharidosis |
| Omacor® | omega-3-acid ethyl esters | Hypertriglyceridemia |
| Pediarix™ | diphtheria, tetanus toxoids, acellular pertussis, hepatitis B (recombinant), and poliovirus (inactivated) vaccine | Vaccine |
| Prialt® | ziconotide | Chronic pain |
| Revatio™ | sildenafil | Pulmonary arterial hypertension |
| Symlin® | pramlintide | Diabetes |
| Tarceva™ | erlotinib | Lung cancer |
| Twinrix® | hepatitis A inactivated and hepatitis B (recombinant) vaccine | Vaccine |
| Tygacil™ | tigecycline | Antibiotic |
| Vitrase® | hyaluronidase | Increase dispersion and absorption of other drugs |
| Xibrom™ | bromfenac | Postoperative ophthalmic inflammation |

# PENDING DRUGS OR DRUGS IN CLINICAL TRIALS

| Proposed Brand Name or Synonym | Generic Name | Use |
|---|---|---|
| Alvesco™ | ciclesonide | Asthma |
| Alzhemed™ | NC-531 | Alzheimer's |
| Angeliq™ | estradiol and drospirenone | Menopausal symptoms |
| Ariflo™ | cilomilast | Chronic obstructive pulmonary disease |
| Bonefos™ | clodronate | Breast cancer |
| Certican™ | everolimus | Prevention of rejection after transplantation |
| Combidex™ | ferumoxtran-10 | Imaging aid |
| Extravan™ | travoprost and timolol | Glaucoma |
| Implanon™ | etonogestrel | Contraceptive |
| MT-1000 | naproxen and metoclopramide | Migraine headache |
| Orthovisc™ | hyaluronic acid | Osteoarthritis of knee |
| Oxyprim™ | oxypurinol | Allopurinol intolerant hyperuricemia |
| Ranexa™ | ranolazine | Angina |
| Retaane™ | anecortave | Wet age-related macular degeneration |
| Riquent™ | abetimus | Lupus |
| Rotateq™ | rotavirus vaccine | Prevention of rotavirus gastroenteritis |
| Sanvar IR™ | vapreotide | Acute esophageal variceal bleeding |
| Surfaxin™ | lucinactant | Infant respiratory distress syndrome |
| Vaprisol™ | conivaptan | Hyponatremia |
| Zarnestra™ | tipifarnib | Acute myeloid leukemia |
| Zostavax™ | zoster vaccine | Prevention of herpes zoster |

# PHARMACEUTICAL MANUFACTURERS AND DISTRIBUTORS

**AAI Development Services
(aaiPharma)**
2320 Scientific Park Drive
Wilmington, NC 28405
(800) 575-4224
www.aaiintl.com

**aaiPharma**
2320 Scientific Park Drive
Wilmington, NC 28405
(800) 575-4224
www.aaipharma.com

**Abbott Laboratories
(Pharmaceutical Products Division)**
100 Abbott Park Road
Abbott Park, IL 60064-3500
(800) 222-6883
www.abbott.com

**Adams Respiratory Therapeutics**
425 Main Street
Colonial Court
Chester, NJ 07930
(908) 879-1400
www.adamslabs.com

**Advanced Medical Optics**
1700 East Street Andrew Place
Santa Ana, CA 92705
(714) 247-8200
www.amo-inc.com

**Advanced Vision Research**
12 Alfred Street
Suite 200
Woburn, MA 01801
(800) 579-8327
www.theratears.com

**Aero Pharmaceuticals, Inc**
3848 FAU Boulevard
Suite 100
Boca Raton, FL 33431
(800) 223-6837
www.aeropharmaceuticals.com

**Akorn, Inc**
2500 Millbrook Drive
Buffalo Grove, IL 60089
(800) 535-7155
www.akorn.com

**AkPharma, Inc**
6840 Old Egg Harbor Road
Pleasantville, NJ 08232
(800) 994-4711
www.akpharma.com

**Alcon Laboratories, Inc**
6201 South Freeway
Fort Worth, TX 76134
(800) 451-3937
www.alconlabs.com

**Allen & Hanburys**
Five Moore Drive
Research Triangle Park, NC 27709
(800) 334-0089

**ALLERDERM Laboratories**
3400 East McDowell Road
Phoenix, AZ 85008-7899
(800) 365-6868
www.allerderm.com

**Allergan, Inc**
PO Box 19534
Irvine, CA 92623-9534
(714) 246-4500
www.allergan.com

**Alliance Pharmaceutical, Inc**
4660 LaJolla Village Drive
Suite 825
San Diego, CA 92122
(858) 410-5200
www.allp.com

**Allscripts, LLC**
2401 Commerce Avenue
Libertyville, IL 60048-4464
(800) 654-0889
www.allscripts.com

**Almay, Inc**
1501 Williamsboro Street
Oxford, NC 27565
(800) 992-5629
www.almay.com

**Alpharma, Inc**
One Executive Drive
Fort Lee, NJ 07024
(800) 645-4216
www.alpharma.com

**Alpharma USPD, Inc**
200 Elmora Avenue
Elizabeth, NJ 07207
(800) 432-8534
www.alpharmauspd.com

**Alpha Therapeutic** (see Grifols)

**Altaire Pharmaceuticals, Inc**
PO Box 849
West Lane
Aquebogue, NY 11931
(800) 258-2471
www.otcdruggist.com

**Alza Corp**
1900 Charleston Road
PO Box 7210
Mountain View, CA 94039-7210
(650) 564-5000
www.alza.com

**Amarin Pharmaceuticals, Inc**
(see Valeant Pharmaceuticals)

**Ambix Laboratories**
55 West End Road
Totowa, NJ 07512
(973) 890-9002
www.ambixlabs.com

**Amcon Laboratories**
40 North Rock Hill Road
St Louis, MO 63119
(800) 255-6161
www.amcon-labs.com

**American Lecithin Company**
115 Hurley Road
Unit 2B
Oxford, CT 06478
(800) 364-4416
www.americanlecithin.com

**American Medical Industries**
**Health Products**
330 East Third Street
Suite 2
Dell Rapids, SD 57022-1918
(605) 428-5501
www.ezhealthcare.com

**American Pharmaceutical Partners, Inc (APP)**
1501 East Woodfield Road
Suite 300 East
Schaumburg, IL 60173-5837
(888) 391-6300
www.appdrugs.com

**American Red Cross**
2025 E Street Northwest
Washington, DC 20006
(202) 303-4498
www.redcross.org

**American Regent Laboratories**
One Luitpold Drive
Shirley, NY 11967
(800) 645-1706
www.americanregent.com

**Amgen, Inc**
One Amgen Center Drive
Thousand Oaks, CA 91320-1799
(800) 772-6436
www.amgen.com

**AMSCO Scientific** (see Steris Corp)

**Amylin Pharmaceuticals, Inc**
9360 Towne Centre Drive
Suite 110
San Diego, California 92121
(858) 552-2200
www.amylin.com

**Andrew Jergens Company**
2535 Spring Grove Avenue
Cincinnati, OH 45214-1773
(800) 742-8798
www.jergens.com

**Andrx Corp**
4955 Orange Drive
Davie, FL 33314
(954) 584-0300
www.andrx.com

**Angelini Pharmaceuticals**
50 Tice Boulevard
Woodcliff Lake, NJ 07677
(201) 476-9000
www.angelinipharmaceuticals.com

**Antibodies, Inc**
PO Box 1560
Davis, CA 95617
(800) 824-8540
www.antibodiesinc.com

**Antigenics, Inc**
630 Fifth Avenue
Suite 2100
New York, NY 10111
(212) 994-8200
www.antigenic.com

**Apotex Corp**
2400 North Commerce Parkway
Suite 400
Weston, FL 33326
(800) 706-5575
www.apotexcorp.com

**Apothecary Products, Inc**
11750 12th Avenue South
Burnsville, MN 55337-1295
(800) 328-2742
www.apothecaryproducts.com

**Apothecon**
PO Box 4500
Princeton, NJ 08543-4500
(800) 321-1335

**Apothecus Pharmaceutical Corp**
220 Townsend Square
Oyster Bay, NY 11771-1532
(800) 227-2393
www.apothecus.com

**A P Pharma**
123 Saginaw Drive
Redwood City, CA 94063
(650) 366-2626
www.appharma.com

**Applied Genetics, Inc**
**Dermatics**
205 Buffalo Avenue
Freeport, NY 11520
(516) 868-9026
www.agiderm.com

**Astellas Pharma U.S., Inc**
Three Parkway North
Deerfield, IL 60015-2548
(800) 695-4321
www.astellas.com

**AstraZeneca Pharmaceuticals, LP**
1800 Concord Pike
PO Box 15437
Wilmington, DE 19850-5437
(800) 842-9920
www.astrazeneca-us.com

**Atley Pharmaceuticals, Inc**
10511 Old Ridge Road
Ashland, VA 23005
(804) 227-2250
www.atley.com

**Aventis Behring**
1020 First Avenue
PO Box 61501
King of Prussia, PA 19406-0901
(610) 878-4000
www.aventisbehring.com

**Axcan Scandipharm, Inc**
22 Inverness Center Parkway
Birmingham, AL 35242
(800) 472-2634
www.axcanscandipharm.com

**AXM Pharma**
7251 West Lake Mead Boulevard
Suite 300
Las Vegas, Nevada 89128
(702) 562-4155
www.axmpharma.com

**Bajamar Chemical Company, Inc**
9609 Dielman Rock Island
St Louis, MO 63132
(888) 242-3414
www.vesselvite.com

**Banner**
4100 Mendenhall Oaks Parkway
Suite 301
High Point, NC 27265
(336) 812-3442
www.banpharm.com

**Barr Laboratories, Inc**
2 Quaker Road
PO Box 2900
Pomona, NY 10970
(800) 222-0190
www.barrlabs.com

**Bausch & Lomb Pharmaceuticals (BD)**
8500 Hidden River Parkway
Tampa, FL 33637
(800) 323-0000
www.bausch.com

**Bausch & Lomb Surgical, Inc**
180 Via Verde
San Dimas, CA 91773
(800) 338-2020
www.bausch.com

**Baxa Corp**
13760 East Arapahoe Road
Englewood, CO 80112-3903
(800) 567-2292
www.baxa.com

**Baxter Healthcare Corp**
**Corp Headquarters**
One Baxter Parkway
Deerfield, IL 60015-4625
(800) 422-9837
www.baxter.com

**Baxter Pharmaceutical Solutions**
927 South Curry Pike
Bloomington, IN 47403
(800) 353-0887
www.baxterdrugdelivery.com

**Bayer Corp**
**(Pharmaceutical Division)**
400 Morgan Lane
West Haven, CT 06516-4175
(203) 812-2000
www.bayerus.com

**Bayer Corp**
**(Consumer Care Division)**
36 Columbia Road
PO Box 1910
Morristown, NJ 07962-1910
(800) 331-4536
www.bayercare.com

**Bayer Corp**
**(Diagnostic Division)**
511 Benedict Avenue
Tarrytown, NY 10591-5097
(914) 631-8000
www.bayerdiag.com

**Bayer, Inc**
77 Belfield Road
Etobicoke, Ontario, Canada M9W 1G6
(800) 268-1331
www.bayer.ca

**B Braun Medical**
824 Twelfth Avenue
Bethlehem, PA 18018
(610) 691-5400
www.bbraunusa.com

**BD Medical Pharmaceutical Systems**
One Becton Drive
Franklin Lakes, NJ 07417
(201) 847-4017
www.bd.com

**BD Biosciences**
2350 Qume Drive
San Jose, CA 95131-1807
(877) 232-8995
www.bdbiosciences.com

**Beckman Coulter, Inc**
4300 North Harbor Boulevard
PO Box 3100
Fullerton, CA 92834-3100
(800) 742-2345
www.beckman.com

**Bedford Laboratories**
300 Northfield Road
Bedford, OH 44146
(440) 232-3320
www.bedfordlabs.com

**Beiersdorf, Inc**
Wilton Corporate Center
187 Danbury Road
Wilton, CT 06897
(203) 563-5800
www.beiersdorf.com

**Berlex Laboratories, Inc**
340 Changebridge Road
PO Box 1000
Montville, NJ 07045-1000
(973) 487-2000
www.berlex.com

**Berna Products Corp**
4216 Ponce de Leon Boulevard
Coral Gables, FL 33146
(800) 533-5899
www.bernaproducts.com

**Bertek**
**Pharmaceuticals, Inc**
781 Chestnut Ridge Road
Morgantown, WV 26505
(304) 285-6420
www.bertek.com

**Beta Dermaceuticals, Inc**
PO Box 691106
San Antonio, TX 78269-1106
(210) 349-9326
www.beta-derm.com

**Beutlich Pharmaceuticals**
1541 Shields Drive
Waukegan, IL 60085
(800) 238-8542
www.beutlich.com

**B. F. Ascher & Company, Inc**
15501 West 109th Street
Lenexa, KS 66219-1308
(913) 888-1880
www.bfascher.com

**Biocraft Laboratories, Inc**
(see Teva Pharmaceuticals USA)

**BioCryst Pharmaceuticals, Inc**
2190 Parkway Lake Drive
Birmingham, AL 35244
(205) 444-4600
www.biocryst.com

**Biogen idec**
14 Cambridge Center
Cambridge, MA 02142
(617) 679-2000
www.biogen.com

**BioGenex**
4600 Norris Canyon Road
San Ramon, CA 94583
(800) 421-4149
www.biogenex.net

**Biomerica, Inc**
1533 Monrovia Avenue
Newport Beach, CA 92663
(949) 645-2111
www.biomerica.com

**Biomira USA, Inc**
70 South Main Street
Suite B and C
Cranbury, NJ 08512
(877) 234-0444
www.biomira.com

**Biopure Corp**
11 Hurley Street
Cambridge, MA 02141
(617) 234-6500
www.biopure.com

**BioScrip**
10900 Red Circle Drive
Minnetonka, MN 55343
(800) 444-5951
www.bioscrip.com

**Biospecifics Technologies Corp**
35 Wilbur Street
Lynbrook, NY 11563
(516) 593-7000
www.biospecifics.com

**BIO-TECH Pharmacal, Inc**
PO Box 1992
Fayetteville, AR 72702
(800) 345-1199
www.bio-tech-pharm.com

**Birchwood Laboratories, Inc**
7900 Fuller Road
Eden Prairie, MN 55344-2195
(800) 328-6156
www.birchlabs.com

**Blaine Pharmaceuticals**
1717 Dixie Highway
Suite 700
Fort Wright, KY 41011
(800) 633-9353
www.blainepharma.com

**Blairex Laboratories, Inc**
1600 Brian Drive
PO Box 2127
Columbus, IN 47202-2127
(800) 252-4739
www.blairex.com

**Blansett Pharmacal Company, Inc**
PO Box 638
North Little Rock, AR 72115
(800) 816-9695
www.blansett.com

**Blistex, Inc**
1800 Swift Drive
Oak Brook, IL 60523-1574
(800) 837-1800
www.blistex.com

**Block Drug Company, Inc**
(see GlaxoSmithKline)

**Bluco, Inc**
28350 Schoolcraft
Livonia, MI 48150
(800) 832-4464
www.blucoinc.com

**Boehringer Ingelheim Pharmaceuticals, Inc**
900 Ridgebury Road
PO Box 368
Ridgefield, CT 06877-0368
(203) 798-9988
www.us.boehringer-ingelheim.com

**Boehringer Mannheim** (see Roche Pharmaceuticals)

**Bone Care International**
(see Genzyme Corp)

**Bracco Diagnostics, Inc**
107 College Road East
Princeton, NJ 08540
(800) 631-5245
www.bracco.com

**Bradley Pharmaceuticals, Inc**
383 Route 46 West
Fairfield, NJ 07004-2402
(973) 882-1505
www.bradpharm.com

**Braintree Laboratories, Inc**
PO Box 850929
Braintree, MA 02185-0929
(800) 874-6756
www.braintreeLabs.com

**Breckenridge Pharmaceutical, Inc**
1141 South Rogers Circle
Suite 3
Boca Raton, FL 33487
(800) 367-3395
www.breckenridgepharma.com

**Bristol-Myers Squibb Company**
**(Pharmaceutical Division)**
PO Box 4500
Princeton, NJ 08543-4500
(800) 321-1335
www.bms.com

**Bristol-Myers Squibb OTC**
1350 Liberty Avenue
Hillside, NJ 07205
(800) 468-7746
www.bms.com

**Bryan Corp**
4 Plympton Street
Woburn, MA 01801
(800) 343-7711
www.bryancorporation.com

**Burroughs Wellcome Company**
(see GlaxoSmithKline)

**Calmoseptine, Inc**
16602 Burke Lane
Huntington Beach, CA 92647
(800) 800-3405
www.calmoseptineointment.com

**Capellon Pharmaceuticals, LTD**
7509 Flagstone Street
Fort Worth, TX 76118
(817) 595-5820
www.capellon.com

**Caraco Pharmaceutical Laboratories, LTD**
1150 Elijah McCoy Drive
Detroit, MI 48202
(800) 818-4555
www.caraco.com

**Cardinal Health, Inc**
7000 Cardinal Place
Dublin, OH 43017
(800) 234-8701
www.cardinal.com

**Cardinal Health, Inc**
**Nuclear Pharmacy Services**
6464 Canoga Avenue
Woodland Hills, CA 91367
(818) 737-4000
www.cardinal.com/nps

**Carma Laboratories, Inc**
5801 West Airways Avenue
Franklin, WI 53132
(414) 421-7707
www.carma-labs.com

**Carolina Medical Products Company**
PO Box 147
Farmville, NC 27828
(800) 227-6637
www.carolinamedical.com

**Carrington Laboratories**
2001 Walnut Hill Lane
Irving, TX 73038
(972) 518-1300
www.carringtonlabs.com

**C. B. Fleet Company, Inc**
4615 Murray Place
PO Box 11349
Lynchburg, VA 24506
(434) 528-4000
www.cbfleet.com

**CCA Industries, Inc**
200 Murray Hill Parkway
East Rutherford, NJ 07073
(201) 330-1400
www.ccaindustries.com

**Celgene Corp**
7 Powder Horn Drive
Warren, NJ 07059
(732) 271-1001
www.celgene.com

**Cellegy Pharmaceuticals, Inc**
349 Oyster Point Boulevard
Suite 200
South San Francisco, CA 94080
(650) 616-2200
www.cellegy.com

**Celltech Pharmaceuticals, Inc**
755 Jefferson Road
Rochester, NY 14623
(800) 234-5535
www.celltechgroup.com

**Centeon** (see Aventis Behring)

**Centers for Disease Control and Prevention**
1600 Clifton Road
Atlanta, GA 30333
(800) 311-3435
www.cdc.gov

**Centocor, Inc**
800/850 Ridgeview Drive
Horsham, PA 19044
(610) 651-6000
www.contocor.com

**Central Pharmaceuticals, Inc**
(see Schwarz Pharma, Inc)

**Cephalon, Inc**
41 Moores Road
Frazer, PA 19355
(610) 344-0200
www.cephalon.com

**Cetylite Industries, Inc**
9051 River Road
Pennsauken, NJ 08110
(800) 257-7740
www.cetylite.com

**Chesapeake Biological Laboratories, Inc**
1111 South Paca Street
Baltimore, MD 21230
(410) 843-5000
www.cblinc.com

**Chiron Corp**
4560 Horton Street
Emeryville, CA 94608-2916
(510) 655-8730
www.chiron.com

**Chronimed, Inc**
(see BioScrip)

**Chugai Pharma USA, LLC**
One Crossroads Drive
Building A, 2nd Floor
Bedminister, NJ 07921-2688
(212) 759-8812
www.chugai-pharm.com

**Ciba-Geigy Pharmaceuticals**
(see Novartis Pharmaceuticals Corp)

**CIBA Vision**
11460 Johns Creek Parkway
Duluth, GA 30097
(678) 415-3937
www.cibavision.com

**Circa Pharmaceuticals, Inc**
(see Watson Laboratories, Inc)

**Cirrus Healthcare Products, LLC**
60 Main Street
PO Box 220
Cold Spring Harbor, NY 11724
(800) 327-6151
www.earplanes.com

**CIS-US, Inc**
10 DeAngelo Drive
Bedford, MA 01730
(800) 221-7554
www.cisusinc.com

**Claragen, Inc**
387 Technology Drive
College Park, MD 20742
(301) 405-8593
www.claragen.com

**Clay-Park Labs, Inc**
1700 Bathgate Avenue
Bronx, NY 10457
(800) 933-5550
www.claypark.com

**C & M Pharmacal, Inc**
(see Genesis Pharmaceutical, Inc)

**CNS, Inc**
20 Troy Road
Whippany, NJ 07981
(800) 858-6673
www.cns.com

**Colgate Oral Pharmaceuticals**
One Colgate Way
Canton, MA 02021
(800) 226-5428
www.colgateprofessional.com

**Colgate-Palmolive Company**
300 Park Avenue
New York, NY 10022
(800) 468-6502
www.colgate.com

**CollaGenex Pharmaceuticals, Inc**
41 University Drive
Newtown, PA 18940
(888) 339-5678
www.collagenex.com

**Columbia Laboratories, Inc**
354 Eisenhower Parkway
Second Floor-Plaza 1
Livingston, NJ 07039
(973) 994-3999
www.columbialabs.com

**Combe, Inc**
1101 Westchester Avenue
White Plains, NY 10604
(800) 873-7400
www.combe.com

**CompliMed Medical Research Group**
1441 West Smith Road
Ferndale, WA 98248
(888) 977-8008
www.complimed.com

**Conair Interplak Division**
One Cummings Point Road
Stamford, CT 06902
(203) 351-9000
www.interplak.com

**Connaught Labs** (see Aventis Pasteur)

**Connetics Corp**
3160 Porter Drive
Palo Alto, CA 94304
(888) 969-2628
www.connetics.com

**Contract Pharmacal Corp**
135 Adams Avenue
Hauppauge, NY 11788
(631) 231-4610
www.contractpharmacal.com

**ConvaTec**
**(Bristol-Myers Squibb Company)**
PO Box 5254
Princeton, NJ 08543-5254
(800) 422-8811
www.convatec.com

**CooperVision**
370 Woodcliff Drive
Suite 200
Fairport, NY 14450
(800) 538-7850
www.coopervision.com

**Corixa**
1124 Columbia Street
Suite 200
Seattle, WA 98104
(206) 754-5711
www.corixa.com

**C. R. Bard, Inc**
8195 Industrial Boulevard
Covington, GA 30014
(800) 526-4455
www.bardmedical.com

**Cumberland Pharmaceuticals, Inc**
2525 West End Avenue
Suite 950
Nashville, TN 37203
(615) 255-0068
www.cumberlandpharma.com

**Cyanotech Corp**
73-4460 Queen Kaahamanu Highway
Suite 102
Kailua-Kona, HI 96740
(800) 395-1353
www.cyanotech.com

**Cygnus, Inc**
400 Penobscot Drive
Redwood City, CA 94063-4719
(650) 369-4300
www.cygn.com

**CYNACON/OCuSOFT**
5311 Avenue North
Rosenburg, TX 77471
(800) 233-5469
www.ocusoft.com

**Cypress Pharmaceutical, Inc**
135 Industrial Boulevard
Madison, MS 39110
(800) 856-4393
www.cypressrx.com

**CYTOGEN Corp**
650 College Road East
Suite 3100
Princeton, NJ 08540
(800) 833-3533
www.cytogen.com

**CytRx Corp**
11726 San Vicente Boulevard
Suite 650
Los Angeles, CA 90049
(310) 826-5648
www.cytrx.com

**Daiichi Pharmaceutical Corp**
11 Philips Parkway
Montvale, NJ 07645-1810
(877) 324-4244
www.daiichius.com

**Danco Labs, LLC**
PO Box 4816
New York, NY 10185
(877) 432-7596
www.earlyoptionpill.com

**Dartmouth Pharmaceuticals**
38 Church Avenue
Wareham, MA 02571
(508) 295-2200
www.ilovemynails.com

**Davol, Inc**
100 Sockanossett Crossroad
PO Box 8500
Cranston, RI 02920
(800) 556-6756
www.davol.com

**Del Laboratories, Inc**
726 EAB Plaza
Uniondale, NY 11553
(800) 952-5080
www.dellabs.com

**Delmont Laboratories, Inc**
715 Harvard Avenue
PO Box 269
Swarthmore, PA 19081
(800) 562-5541
www.delmont.com

**Den-Mat Corp**
2727 Skyway Drive
Santa Maria, CA 93455
(800) 445-0345
www.den-mat.com

**Derma Sciences**
214 Carnegie Center
Suite 100
Princeton, NJ 08540
(800) 825-4325
www.dermasciences.com

**Dermik Laboratories**
500 Arcola Road
PO Box 1200
Collegeville, PA 19426
(800) 340-7502
www.dermik.com

**DeRoyal Industries, Inc**
200 DeBusk Lane
Powell, TN 37849
(800) 337-6925
www.deroyal.com

**DexGen Pharmaceuticals, Inc**
PO Box 675
Manasquan, NJ 08736
(877) DEXGEN1
www.dexgen.com

**Dey LP**
2751 Napa Valley Corporate Drive
Napa, CA 94558
(707) 224-3200
www.deyinc.com

**DiaPharma Group, Inc**
8948 Beckett Road
West Chester, OH 45069
(800) 526-5224
www.diapharma.com

**Diatide, Inc**
9 Delta Drive
Londonderry, NH 03053
(603) 437-8970
www.diatide.com

**Dickinson Brands, Inc**
31 East High Street
East Hampton, CT 06424
(888) 860-2279
www.dickinsonbrands.com

**Digestive Care, Inc**
1120 Win Drive
Bethlehem, PA 18017-7059
(610) 882-5950
www.pancrecarb.com

**Discovery Laboratories, Inc**
350 South Main Street
Suite 307
Doylestown, PA 18901
(215) 340-4699
www.discoverylabs.com

**Discus Dental, Inc**
8550 Higuera Street
Culver City, CA 90232
(800) 422-9448
www.discusdental.com

**Dista Products Company**
(see Eli Lilly & Company)

**Doak Dermatologics**
383 Route 46 West
Fairfield, NJ 07004-2402
(800) 405-3625
www.bradpharm.com

**Dow Hickam, Inc**
(see Bertek Pharmaceuticals, Inc)

**Dreir Pharmaceuticals, Inc**
9602 North 122nd Place
Scottsdale, AZ 85259
(800) 541-4044
www.dreirpharmaceuticals.com

**Dr Reddy's Laboratories, Inc**
200 Somerset Corp Boulevard
Bridgewater, NJ 08807
(908) 203-4900
www.drreddys.com

**DuPont Pharmaceuticals**
Chestnut Run Plaza
974 Centre Road
Wilmington, DE 19805
(800) 474-2762
www.dupontpharma.com

**Duramed Pharmaceuticals**
5040 Duramed Drive
Cincinnati, OH 45213
(513) 731-9900
www.duramed.com

**Dura Pharmaceuticals**
(see Elan Pharmaceuticals)

**Durex Consumer Products**
3585 Engineering Drive
Suite 200
Norcross, GA 30092
(888) 566-3468
www.durex.com

**Durham Pharmacal Corp**
Route 145
Oak Hill, NY 12460
(888) 438-7426
www.cummingsadvertisingart.com/durham/index-dp2.htm

**DUSA Pharmaceuticals, Inc**
25 Upton Drive
Wilmington, MA 01887
(978) 657-7500
www.dusapharma.com

**Eagle Vison, Inc**
8500 Wolf Lake Drive
Suite 110
PO Box 34877
Memphis, TN 38133
(800) 222-7584
www.eaglevis.com

**ECR Pharmaceuticals**
PO Box 71600
Richmond, VA 23255
(804) 527-1950
www.ecrpharma.com

**Edwards Lifesciences**
One Edwards Way
Irvine, CA 92614
(949) 250-2500
www.edwards.com

**E. Fougera & Company**
60 Baylis Road
Melville, NY 11747
(800) 645-9833
www.fougera.com

**Eisai, Inc**
500 Frank W. Burr Boulevard
Teaneck, NJ 07666
(201) 692-1100
www.eisai.com

**Elan Corp**
800 Gateway Boulevard
South San Francisco, CA 94080
(650) 877-0900
www.elan.com

**Eli Lilly & Company**
Lilly Corporate Center
Indianapolis, IN 46285
(800) 545-5979
www.lilly.com

**Elkins-Sinn, Inc**
(see Wyeth Pharmaceuticals)

**EMD Chemicals, Inc**
480 South Democrat Road
Gibbstown, NJ 08027
(800) 222-0342
www.emdchemicals.com

**Endo Pharmaceuticals**
100 Endo Boulevard
Chadds Ford, PA 19317
(610) 558-9800
www.endo.com

**EnviroDerm Pharmaceuticals, Inc**
PO Box 32370
Louisville, KY 40232-2370
(800) 991-3376
www.enviroderm.com

**Enzon, Inc**
685 Route 202/206
Bridgewater, NJ 08807
(908) 541-8600
www.enzon.com

**Eon Labs Manufacturing, Inc**
227-15 North Conduit Avenue
Laurelton, NY 11413
(800) 526-0225
www.eonlabs.com

**Epien Medical, Inc**
4225 White Bear Parkway
Suite 600
St Paul, MN 55110-3389
(888) 884-4675
www.northernresearch.com

**E. R. Squibb & Sons, Inc**
(see Bristol-Myers Squibb Company)

**Ethex Corp**
10888 Metro Court
St Louis, MO 63043-2413
(800) 321-1705
www.ethex.com

**Ethicon, Inc**
**(Johnson & Johnson)**
US Route 22 West
PO Box 151
Somerville, NJ 08876-0151
(800) 255-2500
www.ethiconinc.com

**Everett Laboratories, Inc**
29 Spring Street
West Orange, NJ 07052
(973) 324-0200
www.everettlabs.com

**E-Z-EM**
717 Main Street
Westbury, NY 11590
(800) 544-4624
www.ezem.com

**Female Health Company**
515 North State Street
Suite 2225
Chicago, IL 60610
(312) 595-9123
www.femalehealth.com

**Ferndale Laboratories, Inc**
780 West Eight Mile Road
Ferndale, MI 48220
(800) 621-6003
www.ferndalelabs.com

**Ferring Pharmaceuticals, Inc**
400 Rella Boulevard
Suffern, NY 10901
(888) 337-7464
www.ferringusa.com

**Fidia Pharmaceutical Corp**
2000 K Street Northwest
Suite 700
Washington, DC 20006
(202) 371-9898
www.fidiapharma.com

**First Horizon Pharmaceutical Corp**
6195 Shiloh Road
Alpharetta, GA 30005
(770) 442-9707
www.horizonpharm.com

**Fischer Pharmaceuticals, Inc**
165 Gibraltar Court
Sunnyvale, CA 94089
(800) 782-0222
www.dr-fischer.com

**Fisons Corp** (see Celltech Pharmaceuticals, Inc)

**Fleming & Company**
1733 Gilsinn Lane
Fenton, MO 63026
(800) 343-0164
www.flemingcompany.com

**Forest Laboratories, Inc**
909 Third Avenue
New York, NY 10022
(800) 947-5227
www.frx.com

**Freeda Vitamins, Inc**
36 East 41st Street
New York, NY 10017
(800) 777-3737
www.freedavitamins.com

**Fujisawa Healthcare, Inc**
(see Astellas Pharma U.S., Inc)

**Galderma Laboratories, Inc**
14501 North Freeway
Fort Worth, TX 76177
(817) 961-5000
www.galdermausa.com

**Gallipot, Inc**
2020 Silver Bell Road
St Paul, MN 55122
(800) 423-6967
www.gallipot.com

**Gambro Renal Products, USA**
10810 West Collins Avenue
Lakewood, CO 80215-4498
(800) 525-2623
www.gambro.com

**Gate Pharmaceuticals**
PO Box 1090
North Wales, PA 19454-1090
(800) 292-4283
www.gatepharma.com

**Gebauer Company**
4444 East 153rd Street
Cleveland, OH 44128
(216) 581-3030
www.gebauerco.com

**Geigy Pharmaceuticals**
(see Novartis Pharmaceuticals Corp)

**Genaissance Pharmaceuticals, Inc**
Five Science Park
New Haven, CT 06511
(203) 773-1450
www.genaissance.com

**GenDerm Corp** (see Medicis
Pharmaceutical Corp)

**Gen-King** (see Kinray)

**Genentech, Inc**
One DNA Way
South San Francisco, CA 94080-4990
(650) 225-1000
www.gene.com

**General Injectables & Vaccines**
US Highway 52 South
PO Box 9
Bastian, VA 24314-0009
(800) 521-7468
www.giv.com

**General Nutrition, Inc**
300 6th Avenue
Pittsburgh, PA 15222
(888) 462-2548
www.gnc.com

**Genesis Nutrition**
1816 Wall Street
Florence, SC 29501
(800) 451-7933
www.genesisnutrition.com

**Genesis Pharmaceutical, Inc**
1721 Maplelane Avenue
Hazel Park, MI 48030
(800) 459-8663
www.genesispharm.com

**Geneva Pharmaceuticals, Inc**
(see Sandoz, Inc)

**GenPharm International, Inc**
(see Medarex)

**GensiaSicor Pharmaceuticals**
(see SICOR Pharmaceuticals, Inc)

**Genta, Inc**
Two Connell Drive
Berkeley Heights, New Jersey 07922
(908) 286-9800
www.genta.com

**GenVec, Inc**
65 West Watkins Mill Road
Gaithersburg. MD 20878
(240) 632-0740
www.genvec.com

**Genzyme Corp**
500 Kendall Street
Cambridge, MA 02142
(617) 252-7500
www.genzyme.com

**Geodesic MediTech, Inc**
2921 Sandy Pointe No. 3
Del Mar, CA 92014
(888) 357-9399
www.geodesicmeditech.com

**Gerber Products Company**
445 State Street
Fremont, MI 49413-0001
(800) 443-7237
www.gerber.com

**Geritrex Corp**
144 Kingsbridge Road East
Mount Vernon, NY 10550
(800) 736-3437
www.geritrex.com

**Geron Corp**
230 Constitution Drive
Menlo Park, CA 94025
(650) 473-7700
www.geron.com

**Gilead**
333 Lakeside Drive
Foster City, CA 94404
(800) 445-3235
www.gilead.com

**Glades Pharmaceuticals, LLC**
6340 Sugarloaf Parkway
Duluth, GA 30097
(888) 445-2337
www.glades.com

**GlaxoSmithKline**
Five Moore Drive
PO Box 13398
Research Triangle Park, NC 27709
(888) 825-5249
www.gsk.com

**GlaxoSmithKline**
One Franklin Plaza
Philadelphia, PA 19102
(888) 825-5249
www.gsk.com

**GlaxoSmithKline**
**Consumer Healthcare**
PO Box 1467
Pittsburgh, PA 15230
(412) 928-1000
www.gsk.com

**GlaxoWellcome, Inc** (see GlaxoSmithKline)

**Glenwood, LLC**
111 Cedar Lane
Englewood, NJ 07631
(800) 542-0772
www.glenwood-llc.com

**Global Pharmaceuticals, Inc**
3735 Castor Avenue
Philadelphia, PA 19124
(215) 289-2220
www.globalphar.com

**Gordon Laboratories**
6801 Ludlow Street
Upper Darby, PA 19082-2408
(800) 356-7870
www.gordonlabs.com

**GF Health Products, Inc**
2935 Northeast Parkway
Atlanta, GA 30360
(800) 347-5678
www.grahamfield.com

**Grandpa Brands Company**
1820 Airport Exchange Boulevard
Erlanger, KY 41018
(800) 684-1468
www.csdent.com

**Green Turtle Bay Vitamin Company**
56 High Street
Summit, NJ 07901
(800) 887-8535
www.energywave.com

**Greer Laboratories, Inc**
639 Nuway Circle
PO Box 800
Lenoir, NC 28645-0800
(800) 438-0088
www.greerlabs.com

**Grifols**
**(Bioscience Division)**
2410 Lillyvale Avenue
Los Angeles, CA 90032
(888) 474-3657
www.grifolsusa.com

**Guilford Pharmaceuticals, Inc**
6611 Tributary Street
Baltimore, MD 21224
(410) 631-6300
www.guilfordpharm.com

**Gynetics**
PO Box 8509
Somerville, NJ 08876
(800) 311-7378
www.gynetics.com

**Halocarbon Products Corp**
PO Box 661
River Edge, NJ 07661
(201) 262-8899
www.halocarbon.com

**Hart Health & Safety**
PO Box 94044
Seattle, WA 98124
(800) 234-4278
www.harthealth.com

**Harvard Drug Group, LLC**
31778 Enterprise Drive
Livonia, MI 48150
(800) 875-0123
www.harvarddrugs.com

**Hauser Pharmaceutical, Inc**
4401 East US Highway 30
Valparaiso, IN 46383
(800) 441-2309
www.hauserpharmaceutical.com

**Hawthorn Pharmaceuticals, Inc**
PO Box 2248
Madison, MS 39130
(888) 455-5253
www.hawthornrx.com

**HDC Corp**
628 Gibraltar Court
Milpitas, CA 95035
(800) 227-8162
www.hdccorp.com

**HealthAsure, Inc**
**(Rainbow Light Nutritional Systems)**
125 McPherson Street
Santa Cruz, CA 95060
(800) 635-1233
www.healthasure.com

**Healthfirst Corp**
22316 70th Avenue West
Unit A
Mountlake Terrace, WA 98043-2184
(425) 771-5733
www.healthfirst.com

**Helix BioPharma Corp**
305 Industrial Parkway South
Unit 3
Aurora, ON L4G 6X7
(905) 841-2300
www.helixbiopharma.com

**Hemacare Corp**
21101 Oxnard Street
Woodland HIlls, CA 91367
(877) 310-0717
www.hemacare.com

**Hemagen Diagnostics, Inc**
9033 Red Branch Road
Columbia, MD 21045
(800) 495-2180
www.hemagen.com

**Hemispherx Biopharma, Inc**
One Penn Center
1617 John F. Kennedy Boulevard
6th Floor
Philadelphia, PA 19103
(215) 988-0080
www.hemispherx.net

**Henry Schein, Inc**
135 Duryea Road
Melville, NY 11747
(631) 843-5500
www.henryschein.com

**Hill Dermaceuticals, Inc**
2650 South Mellonville Avenue
Sanford, FL 32773-9311
(800) 344-5707
www.hillderm.com

**Hi-Tech Pharmacal, Inc**
369 Bayview Avenue
Amityville, NY 11701
(631) 789-8228
www.hitechpharm.com

**Hoechst-Marion Roussel, Inc** (see Aventis)

**Hoffmann-LaRoche**
(see Roche Pharmaceuticals)

**Hogil Pharmaceutical Corp**
237 Mamaroneck Avenue
Suite 303
White Plains, NY 10605
(914) 681-1800
www.hogil.com

**Hollister-Stier Laboratories, LLC**
3525 North Regal Street
Spokane, WA 99207-5788
(800) 992-1120
www.hollister-stier.com

**Home Access Health Corp**
2401 West Hassell Road
Suite 1510
Hoffman Estates, IL 60195
(847) 781-2500
www.homeaccess.com

**Hope Pharmaceuticals**
8260 East Gelding Drive
Suite 104
Scottsdale, AZ 85260
(800) 755-9595
www.hopepharm.com

**Horizon Diagnostics, Inc**
2930 East Houston Street
San Antonio, TX 78202
(210) 222-2108
www.horizondiagnostics.com

**Horizon Pharmaceutical Corp**
(see First Horizon Pharmaceutical Corp)

**Hospira, Inc**
275 North Field Drive
Lake Forest, IL 60045
(877) 467-7472
www.hospira.com

**Hyland Immuno**
**(Baxter)**
550 North Brand Boulevard
Glendale, CA 91203
(800) 423-2090
http://baxdb1.baxter.com

**Hyland Laboratories, Inc**
**(Standard Homeopathic Company)**
210 West 131st Street
Los Angeles, CA 90061
(800) 624-9659
www.hylands.com

**ICN Pharmaceuticals, Inc**
(see Valeant Pharmaceuticals)

**IDEC Pharmaceuticals**
(see Bogen idec)

**Ilex Oncology, Inc**
(see Genzyme Corp)

**Immune Response Corp**
5931 Darwin Court
Carlsbad, CA 92008
(760) 431-7080
www.imnr.com

**ImmunoGen, Inc**
128 Sidney Street
Cambridge, MA 02139
(617) 995-2500
www.immunogen.com

**Immunomedics, Inc**
300 American Road
Morris Plains, NJ 07950
(973) 605-8200
www.immunomedics.com

**IMPAX Laboratories, Inc**
30831 Huntwood Avenue
Hayward, CA 94544
(510) 476-2000
www.impaxlabs.com

**Incyte Corp**
Experimental Station
Route 141 & Henry Clay Road
Building E336
Wilmington, DE 19880
(302) 498-6700
www.incyte.com

**Indevus Pharmaceuticals, Inc**
99 Hayden Avenue
Suite 200
Lexington, MA 02421
(781) 861-8444
www.interneuron.com

**InKine Pharmaceutical Company, Inc**
1787 Sentry Parkway
West Building 18
Suite 440
Blue Bell, PA 19422
(215) 283-6850
www.inkine.com

**INO Therapeutics**
6th State Route 173
Clinton, NJ 08809
(908) 238-6600
www.inotherapeutics.com

**Inspire Pharmaceuticals, Inc**
4222 Emperor Boulevard
Suite 200
Durham, NC 27703
(919) 941-9777
www.inspirepharm.com

**Interferon Sciences, Inc**
783 Jersey Avenue
New Brunswick, NJ 08901-3660
(888) 728-4372
www.interferonsciences.com

**InterMune Pharmaceuticals, Inc**
3280 Bayshore Boulevard
Brisbane, CA 94005
(415) 466-2200
www.intermune.com

**International Medication Systems, Limited (IMS)**
1886 Santa Anita Avenue
South El Monte, CA 91733
(800) 423-4136
www.ims-limited.com

**IntraBiotics Pharmaceuticals, Inc**
2483 East Bayshore Road
Suite 100
Palo Alto, CA 94303
(650) 526-6800
www.intrabiotics.com

**Introgen Therapeutics, Inc**
301 Congress Avenue
Suite 1850
Austin, TX 78701
(512) 708-9310
www.introgen.com

**Inveresk**
11000 Westen Parkway
Cary, NC 27513
(919) 460-9005
www.inveresk.com

**Inverness Medical Innovations**
51 Sawyer Road
Suite 200
Waltham, MA 02453-3448
(781) 647-3900
www.invernessmedical.com

**Inwood Laboratories (Forest)**
321 Prospect Street
Inwood, NY 11096
(800) 685-5227
www.frx.com

**Iomed, Inc**
2441 South 3850 West
Suite A
Salt Lake City, UT 84120
(800) 621-3347
www.iomed.com

**IOP, Inc**
3151 Airway Avenue
Costa Mesa, CA 92626
(800) 535-3545
www.iopinc.com

**Isis Pharmaceuticals**
2292 Faraday Avenue
Carlsbad, CA 92008
(760) 931-9200
www.isispharm.com

**Ivax Pharmaceuticals, Inc**
4400 Biscayne Boulevard
Miami, FL 33137
(800) 327-4114
www.ivaxpharmaceuticals.com

**IVPCARE**
7164 Technology Drive
Suite 100
Frisco, TX 75034
(800) 424-9002
www.ivpcare.com

**Janssen Pharmaceutica Products, LP**
1125 Trenton-Harbourton Road
PO Box 200
Titusville, NJ 08560-0200
(800) 526-7736
www.us.janssen.com

**Jerome Stevens Pharmaceuticals, Inc**
60 DaVinci Drive
Bohemia, NY 11716-2613
(631) 567-1113

**Johnson & Johnson**
One Johnson & Johnson Plaza
New Brunswick, NJ 08933
(732) 524-0400
www.jnj.com

**Jones Pharma**
(see King Pharmaceuticals, Inc)

**J. R. Carlson Laboratories, Inc**
15 College Drive
Arlington Heights, IL 60004-1985
(847) 255-1600
www.carlsonlabs.com

**J. T. Baker, Inc** (see Mallinckrodt Baker, Inc)

**Kendall Healthcare Products**
15 Hampshire Street
Mansfield, MA 02048
(800) 962-9888
www.kendallhq.com

**Key Pharmaceuticals** (see Schering-Plough Corp)

**Kimberly-Clark/Ballard Medical Products**
12050 Lone Peak Parkway
Draper, UT 84020
(800) 528-5591
www.kchealthcare.com

**King Pharmaceuticals, Inc**
501 Fifth Street
Bristol, TN 37620
(800) 776-3637
www.kingpharm.com

**Kingswood Laboratories, Inc**
10375 Hague Road
Indianapolis, IN 46256
(800) 968-7772
www.kingswood-labs.com

**Kinray**
152-35 10th Avenue
Whitestone, NY 11357
(800) 854-6729
www.kinray.com

**Kirkman Laboratories, Inc**
6400 Southwest Rosewood Street
Lake Oswego, OR 97035
(800) 245-8282
www.kirkmanlabs.com

**KLI Corp**
1119 Third Avenue Southwest
Carmel, IN 46032
(800) 308-7452
www.entertainers-secret.com

**Knoll Pharmaceuticals Company**
(see Abbott Laboratories)

**Konsyl Pharmaceuticals, Inc**
8050 Industrial Park Road
Easton, MD 21601
(800) 356-6795
www.konsyl.com

**Kos Pharmaceuticals, Inc**
One Cedar Brook Drive
Cranbury, New Jersey 08512-3618
(609) 495-0500
www.kospharm.com

**Kramer Laboratories, Inc**
8778 Southwest 8th Street
Miami, FL 33174
(800) 824-4894
www.kramerlabs.com

**K. V. Pharmaceutical Company**
2503 South Hanley Road
St Louis, MO 63144
(314) 645-6600
www.kvpharma.com

**Lacrimedics, Inc**
PO Box 1209
Eastsound, WA 98245
(800) 367-8327
www.lacrimedics.com

**Lactaid, Inc**
7050 Camp Hill Road
Fort Washington, PA 19034
(800) 522-8243
www.lactaid.com

**Lannett Company, Inc**
9000 State Road
Philadelphia, PA 19136
(800) 325-9994
www.lannett.com

**LecTec Corp**
5616 Lincoln Drive
Edina, MN 55436
(952) 933-2291
www.lectec.com

**Lee Laboratories**
1475 Athens Highway
Grayson, GA 30017
(770) 972-4450
www.leelabs.com

**Lee Pharmaceuticals**
1434 Santa Anita Avenue
South El Monte, CA 91733
(800) 950-5337
www.leepharmaceuticals.com

**Leiner Health Products**
901 East 233rd Street
Carson, CA 90745
(310) 835-8400
www.leiner.com

**LifeScan, Inc**
**(Johnson & Johnson Company)**
1000 Gibraltar Drive
Milpitas, CA 95035
(800) 227-8862
www.lifescan.com

**LifeSign LLC**
71 Veronica Avenue
PO Box 218
Somerset, NJ 08875-0218
(800) 526-2125
www.lifesignmed.com

**Ligand Pharmaceuticals**
10275 Science Center Drive
San Diego, CA 92121
(858) 550-7500
www.ligand.com

**Lilly & Company** (see Eli Lilly & Company)

**Lincoln Diagnostics**
PO Box 1128
Decatur, IL 62525
(217) 877-2531
www.lincolndiagnostics.com

**LSI America Corp**
4732 Twin Valley Drive
Austin, TX 78731-3537
(800) 720-5936
www.ondrox.com

**Lyne Laboratories**
10 Burke Drive
Brockton, MA 02301
(800) 525-0450
www.lyne.com

**3M Pharmaceuticals**
3M Center
Building 275-3W-01
PO Box 33275
St Paul, MN 55133
(800) 328-0255
3m.com/pharma

**Magno-Humphries Laboratories**
8800 Southwest Commercial Street
Tigard, OR 97223
(503) 684-5464
www.magno-humphries.com

**Mallinckrodt Baker, Inc**
222 Red School Lane
Phillipsburg, NJ 08865
(800) 582-2537
www.mallbaker.com

**Mallinckrodt, Inc**
**(Corp Headquarters)**
675 McDonnell Boulevard
Hazelwood, MO 63042
(314) 654-2000
www.mallinckrodt.com

**Martec Pharmaceutical, Inc**
1800 North Topping
Kansas City, MO 64120
(800) 822-6782
www.martec-kc.com

**Martek Biosciences Corp**
6480 Dobbin Road
Columbia, MD 21045
(410) 740-0081
www.martekbio.com

**Mason Vitamins, Inc**
5105 Northwest 159th Street
Miami Lakes, FL 33014-6370
(800) 327-6005
www.masonvitamins.com

**Mayne Pharma (USA), Inc**
650 From Road
(Mack-Cali Centre II)
Second Floor
Paramus, NJ 07652
(201) 225-5500
www.us.maynepharma.com

**McGuff Company, Inc**
3524 West Lake Center Drive
Santa Ana, CA 92704
(800) 854-7220
www.mcguffmedical.com

**McNeil Consumer & Specialty Pharmaceuticals
(Johnson & Johnson)**
Camp Hill Road
Mail Stop 278
Fort Washington, PA 19034-2292
(800) 962-5357
www.jnj.com

**Mead Johnson Laboratories**
(see Bristol-Myers Squibb Company)

**Medarex, Inc**
707 State Road
Princeton, NJ 08540-1437
(609) 430-2880
www.medarex.com

**Medco Lab, Inc**
716 West 7th Street
Sioux City, IA 51103
(712) 255-8770
www.medcolab.com

**Medeva Pharmaceuticals**
(see Celltech Pharmaceuticals, Inc)

**Medicis Pharmaceutical Corp**
8125 North Hayden Road
Scottsdale, AZ 85258-2463
(602) 808-8800
www.medicis.com

**Medi-Dose, Inc**
70 Industrial Drive
Ivyland, PA 18974
(800) 523-8966
www.medidose.com

**MedImmune, Inc**
One MedImmune Way
Gaithersburg, MD 20878
(877) 633-4411
www.medimmune.com

**Medisca, Inc**
661 Route 3, Unit C
Plattsburgh, NY 12901
(800) 932-1039
www.medisca.com

**MediSense, Inc
(Abbott Laboratories)**
4A Crosby Drive
Bedford, MA 01730
(800) 323-9100

**Medix Pharmaceuticals Americas, Inc (MPA)**
12505 Starkey Road
Suite M
Largo, FL 33773
(888) 242-3463
www.biafine.com

**MedPointe Pharmaceuticals**
265 Davidson Avenue
Suite 300
Somerset, NJ 08873-4120
(732) 564-2200
www.medpointeinc.com

**Medtronic, Inc**
710 Medtronic Parkway
Minneapolis, MN 55432-5604
(763) 514-4000
www.medtronic.com

**Menicon America, Inc**
1840 Gateway Drive
Second Floor
San Mateo, CA 94404
(650) 378-1424
www.menicon.com

**Mentholatum Company, Inc
(Rohto Pharmaceutical Company)**
707 Sterling Drive
Orchard Park, NY 14127
(716) 677-2500
www.mentholatum.com

**Merck & Company**
One Merck Drive
PO Box 100
Whitehouse Station, NJ 08889-0100
(908) 423-1000
www.merck.com

**Mericon Industries, Inc**
8819 North Pioneer Road
Peoria, IL 61615-1561
(800) 242-6464
www.mericon-industries.com

**Meridian Medical Technologies
(King Pharmaceuticals, Inc)**
10240 Old Columbia Road
Columbia, MD 21046
(800) 638-8093
www.meridianmeds.com

**Merit Pharmaceuticals**
2611 San Fernando Road
Los Angeles, CA 90065
(800) 696-3748
www.meritpharm.com

**Merz Pharmaceuticals**
4215 Tudor Lane
Greensboro, NC 27410
(800) 334-0514
www.merzusa.com

**Methapharm, Inc**
11772 West Sample Road
Suite 101
Coral Springs, FL 33065
(800) 287-7686
www.methapharm.com

**MGI Pharma, Inc**
5775 West Old Shakopee Road
Suite 100
Bloomington, MN 55437-3174
(800) 562-5580
www.mgipharma.com

**Mikart, Inc**
1750 Chattahoochee Avenue
Atlanta, GA 30318
(404) 351-4510
www.mikart.com

**Miles, Inc** (see Bayer Corp)

**Milex Products, Inc**
4311 North Normandy
Chicago, IL 60634-1403
(800) 621-1278
www.milexproducts.com

**Miller Pharmacal Group, Inc**
350 Randy Road
Suite 2
Carol Stream, IL 60188-1831
(800) 323-2935
www.millerpharmacal.com

**Mission Pharmacal Company**
10999 IH-10 West
Suite 1000
San Antonio, TX 78230
(210) 696-8400
www.missionpharmacal.com

**Monaghan Medical Corp**
5 Latour Avenue
Suite 1600
PO Box 2805
Plattsburgh, NY 12901
(800) 833-9653
www.monaghanmed.com

**Monarch Pharmaceuticals
(King Pharmaceuticals, Inc)**
355 Beecham Street
Bristol, TN 37620
(800) 776-3637
www.monarchpharm.com

**Monticello Drug Company**
1604 Stockton Street
Jacksonville, FL 32204
(800) 735-0666
www.monticellocompanies.com

**Moore Medical Corp**
PO Box 1500
New Britain, CT 06050-1500
(800) 234-1464
www.mooremedical.com

**Morton Grove Pharmaceuticals**
6451 West Main Street
Morton Grove, IL 60053
(800) 346-6854
www.mgp-online.com

**MotherSOY, Inc**
424 South Kentucky Avenue
Evansville, IN 47714
(888) 769-0769
www.mothersoy.com

**Mutual Pharmaceutical Company, Inc/United
Research Laboratories**
1100 Orthodox Street
Philadelphia, PA 19124
(800) 523-3684
www.urlmutual.com

**Mylan Laboratories, Inc**
1500 Corporate Drive
Suite 400
Canonsburg, PA 15317
(724) 514-1800
www.mylan.com

**Mylan Pharmaceuticals, Inc**
781 Chestnut Ridge Road
Morgantown, WV 26505
(800) 826-9526
www.mylanpharm.com

**Nabi
(Corp Headquarters)**
5800 Park of Commerce Boulevard Northwest
Boca Raton, FL 33487
(561) 989-5800
www.nabi.com

**Nagase Pharmaceuticals**
500 Fifth Avenue
Suite 840
New York, NY 10110
(212) 354-3140
www.nagase.com

**Nastech Pharmaceutical Company, Inc**
45 Adams Avenue
Hauppauge, NY 11788
(631) 273-0101
www.nastech.com

**NATREN, Inc**
3105 Willow Lane
Westlake Village, CA 91361
(800) 992-3323
www.natren.com

**Natrol, Inc**
21411 Prairie Street
Chatsworth, CA 91311
(800) 326-1520
www.natrol.com

**Naturally Vitamins
(Marlyn Nutraceuticals, Inc)**
4404 East Elwood
Phoenix, AZ 85040
(888) 766-4406
www.naturallyvitamins.com

**Natures Bounty, Inc
(NBTY, Inc)**
90 Orville Drive
Bohemia, NY 11716
(888) 465-6757
www.naturesbounty.com

**Nature's Sunshine Products, Inc**
75 East 1700 South
Provo, UT 84606
(800) 223-8225
www.nsponline.com

**NeoPharm, Inc**
150 Field Drive
Suite 195
Lake Forest, IL 60045
(847) 295-8678
www.neophrm.com

**NeoRx Corp**
300 Elliott Avenue West
Suite 500
Seattle, WA 98119-4007
(206) 281-7001
www.neorx.com

**Nephron Pharmaceuticals Corp**
4121 34th Street
Orlando, FL 32811
(800) 443-4313
www.nephronpharm.com

**Nestle Clinical Nutrition**
3 Parkway North
Suite 500
Deerfield, IL 60015
(800) 422-2752
www.nestleclinicalnutrition.com

**NeuroGenesis/Matrix Tech, Inc**
120 Park Avenue
League City, TX 77573
(800) 345-8912
www.neurogenesis.com

**Neutrogena Corp**
5760 West 96th Street
Los Angeles, CA 90045-5595
(800) 582-4048
www.neutrogena.com

**NeXstar Pharmaceuticals, Inc**
(see Gilead)

**Niche Pharmaceuticals, Inc**
209 North Oak Street
Roanoke, TX 76262
(800) 677-0355
www.niche-inc.com

**Nnodum Pharmaceuticals
(Zikspain)**
PO Box 19725
Cincinnati, OH 45219
(513) 861-2329
www.zikspain.com

**Nomax, Inc**
40 North Rock Hill Road
St Louis, MO 63119
(314) 961-2500
www.nomax.com

**Noramco, Inc
(Johnson & Johnson)**
1440 Olympic Drive
Athens, GA 30601
(706) 353-4400
www.noramco.com

**Norstar Consumer Products Company, Inc**
5517 95th Avenue
Kenosha, WI 53144
(262) 652-8505
www.norstarcpc.com

**Northern Research Laboratories, Inc**
(see Epien Medical, Inc)

**Nova Factor, Inc**
1620 Century Center Parkway
Suite 109
Memphis, TN 38134
(800) 235-8498
www.accredohealth.net/nova/

**Novartis Pharmaceuticals Corp**
One Health Plaza
East Hanover, NJ 07936-1080
(973) 781-8265
www.pharma.us.novartis.com

**Noven Pharmaceuticals, Inc**
11960 Southwest 144th Street
Miami, FL 33186
(305) 253-5099
www.noven.com

**Novocol**
(see Septodont, Inc)

**Novo Nordisk Pharmaceuticals, Inc**
100 College Road West
Princeton, NJ 08540
(800) 727-6500
www.novonordisk-us.com

**Novopharm USA, Inc**
165 East Commerce Drive
Suite 100
Schaumburg, IL 60173-5326
(800) 426-0769

**Numark Laboratories, Inc**
164 Northfield Avenue
Edison, NJ 08837
(800) 338-8079
www.numarklabs.com

**Nutraceutical Solutions, Inc**
6704 Ranger Avenue
Corpus Christi, TX 78415
(800) 856-7040
www.eliquidsolutions.com

**Nutramax Laboratories, Inc**
2208 Lakeside Boulevard
Edgewood, MD 21040
(800) 925-5187
www.nutramaxlabs.com

**NutriSoy International, Inc**
(see MotherSOY, Inc)

**Octamer, Inc**
392 Cecilia Way
Tiburon, CA 94920
(415) 381-1602
www.octamer.com

**Odyssey Pharmaceuticals, Inc**
200 Park Avenue
PO Box 683
Florham Park, NJ 07932
(973) 884-5300
www.odysseypharm.com

**Ohmeda Pharmaceuticals**
(see Baxter Pharmaceutical Products, Inc)

**Omnicell**
1201 Charleston Road
Mountain View, CA 94043-1337
(800) 850-6664
www.omnicell.com

**Omnii Products**
1500 North Florida Mango Road
Suite 1
West Palm Beach, FL 33409
(800) 445-3386
www.omniiproducts.com

**Onyx Pharmaceuticals, Inc**
2100 Powell Street
Emeryville, CA 94608
(510) 597-6500
www.onyx-pharm.com

**Optics Laboratory, Inc**
9480 Telstar Avenue #3
El Monte, CA 91731
(626) 350-1926
www.opticslab.com

**Optimox Corp**
PO Box 3378
Torrance, CA 90510-3378
(800) 223-1601
www.optimox.com

**Organogenesis, Inc**
150 Dan Road
Canton, MA 02021
(781) 575-0775
www.organogenesis.com

**Organon, Inc**
375 Mt Pleasant Avenue
West Orange, NJ 07052
(973) 325-4500
www.organon-usa.com

**Orphan Medical, Inc**
13911 Ridgedale Drive
Suite 250
Minnetonka, MN 55305
(888) 867-7426
www.orphan.com

**Ortho Biotech Products, LP**
430 Route 22 East
PO Box 6914
Bridgewater, NJ 08807-0914
(908) 541-4000
www.orthobiotech.com

**Ortho-Clinical Diagnostics
(Johnson & Johnson)**
100 Indigo Creek Drive
Rochester, NY 14626
(800) 828-6316
www.orthoclinical.com

**Ortho-McNeil Pharmaceutical, Inc**
1000 U.S. Route 202 South
Raritan, NJ 08869
(800) 682-6532
www.ortho-mcneil.com

**Oscient Pharmaceuticals**
1000 Winter Street
Suite 2200
Waltham, MA 02451
(781) 398-2300
www.oscient.com

**Otsuka America Pharmaceutical, Inc**
2440 Research Boulevard
Rockville, MD 20850
(800) 562-3974
www.otsuka.com

**Ovation Pharmaceuticals, Inc**
Four Parkway North
Deerfield, IL 60015
(847) 282-1000
www.ovationpharma.com

**Oxford Pharmaceutical Services, Inc**
One US Highway 46 West
Totowa, NJ 07512
(877) 284-9120
www.oxfordpharm.com

**OXIS International, Inc**
6040 North Cutter Circle
Suite 317
Portland, OR 97217
(503) 283-3911
www.oxis.com

**Paddock Laboratories, Inc**
3940 Quebec Avenue North
Minneapolis, MN 55427
(800) 328-5113
www.paddocklabs.com

**PamLab LLC
(Pan American Laboratories, LLC)**
PO Box 8950
Mandeville, LA 70470-8950
(985) 893-4097
www.panamericanlabs.com

**Parke-Davis**
(see Pfizer Pharmaceuticals Group PPG)

**Parnell Pharmaceuticals**
1525 Francisco Boulevard
San Rafael, CA 94901
(800) 457-4276
www.parnellpharm.com

**Par Pharmaceutical, Inc**
One Ram Ridge Road
Spring Valley, NY 10977
(800) 828-9393
www.parpharm.com

**Pasteur Merieux Connaught USA**
(see Sanofi Pasteur)

**PDRx Pharmaceuticals, Inc**
727 North Ann Arbor
Oklahoma City, OK 73127
(800) 299-7379
www.pdrx.com

**Pediatric Pharmaceuticals, Inc**
120 Wood Avenue South
Suite 300
Iselin, NJ 08830
(732) 603-7708
www.pediatricpharm.com

**Pedinol Pharmacal, Inc**
30 Banfi Plaza North
Farmingdale, NY 11735
(800) 733-4665
www.pedinol.com

**Perrigo Company**
515 Eastern Avenue
Allegan, MI 49010
(800) 719-9260
www.perrigo.com

**Person & Covey, Inc**
616 Allen Avenue
Glendale, CA 91201
(800) 423-2341
www.personandcovey.com

**Pfizer Pharmaceuticals Group (PPG)**
235 East 42nd Street
New York, NY 10017-5755
(800) 438-1985
www.pfizer.com

**Pharma 21, Inc**
1363 Shinly
Suite 100
Escondido, CA 92026
(760) 743-7441
www.pharma21.net

**Pharmaceutical Formulations, Inc**
PO Box 1904
Edison, NJ 08818-1904
(732) 985-7100
www.pfiotc.com

**Pharmaceutical Specialties, Inc**
PO Box 6298
Rochester, MN 55903-6298
(800) 325-8232
www.psico.com

**Pharmacia Corp**
(see Pfizer Pharmaceuticals Group (PPG))

**Pharmakon Labs**
6050 Jet Port Industrial Boulevard
Tampa, FL 33634
(800) 888-4045
www.pharmakonlabs.com

**Pharmanex**
75 West Center
Provo, UT 84601
(801) 345-9800
www.pharmanex.com

**Pharmatek Laboratories, Inc**
5626 Oberlin Drive
San Diego, CA 92121
(858) 587-8783
www.pharmatek.com

**Pharmics, Inc**
PO Box 27554
Salt Lake City, UT 84127
(801) 966-4138
www.pharmics.com

**PhytoPharmica, Inc**
825 Challenger Drive
Green Bay, WI 54311
(800) 553-2370
www.phytopharmica.com

**Plantex USA, Inc**
Two University Plaza
Suite 305
Hackensack, NJ 07601
(201) 343-4141
www.plantexusa.com

**Playtex Company**
74 Commerce Drive
Allendale, NJ 07401-1600
(800) 816-5742
www.playtex.com

**PLIVA, Inc**
72 Eagle Rock Avenue
East Hanover, NJ 07936
(973) 386-5566
www.plivainc.com

**Plough, Inc**
(see Schering-Plough Corp)

**PolyMedica Corp**
11 State Street
Woburn, MA 01801
(781) 933-2020
www.polymedica.com

**Procter & Gamble Pharmaceuticals, Inc**
One Proctor & Gamble Plaza
Cincinnati, OH 45201
(513) 983-1100
www.pg.com

**ProCyte Corp**
PO Box 808
Redmond, WA 98073-0808
(425) 869-1239
www.procyte.com

**Protein Design Labs, Inc**
34801 Campus Drive
Fremont, CA 94555
(510) 574-1400
www.pdl.com

**Protein Sciences Corp**
1000 Research Parkway
Meriden, CT 06450
(800) 488-7099
www.proteinsciences.com

**Protherics, Inc**
5214 Maryland Way
Suite 405
Brentwood, TN 37027
(615) 327-1027
www.protherics.com

**Psychemedics Corp**
1280 Massachusetts Avenue
Cambridge, MA 02138
(800) 628-8073
www.psychemedics.com

**Purdue Pharma, LP**
**(The Purdue Frederick Company)**
One Stamford Forum
201 Tresser Boulevard
Stamford, CT 06901-3431
(888) 726-7535
www.purduepharma.com

**Purepac Pharmaceuticals Company**
14 Commerce Drive
Suite 301
Cranford, NJ 07016
(800) 432-8534
www.purepac.com

**Puritan's Pride**
1233 Montauk Highway
PO Box 9001
Oakdale, NY 11769-9001
(800) 645-1030
www.puritanspride.com

**QLT, Inc**
887 Great Northern Way
Vancouver, BC
Canada V5T 4T5
(800) 663-5486
www.qlt-pdt.com

**Questcor Pharmaceuticals, Inc**
3260 Whipple Road
Union City, CA 94587
(510) 400-0700
www.questcor.com

**Quidel Corp**
10165 McKellar Court
San Diego, CA 92121
(800) 874-1517
www.quidel.com

**Ranbaxy Pharmaceuticals, Inc USA**
600 College Road East
Princeton, NJ 08540
(609) 720-9200
www.ranbaxyusa.com

**Reese Pharmaceutical Company, Inc**
10617 Frank Avenue
Cleveland, OH 44106
(800) 321-7178
www.reesechemical.com

**Regeneron Pharmaceuticals, Inc**
777 Old Saw Mill River Road
Tarrytown, NY 10591
(914) 345-7400
www.regeneron.com

**Remel, Inc**
12076 Santa Fe Drive
PO Box 14428
Lenexa, KS 66215
(800) 255-6730
www.remelinc.com

**Requa, Inc**
540 Barnum Avenue
PO Box 2384
Bridgeport, CT 06608
(800) 321-1085
www.requa.com

**Rexall Sundown, Inc**
**(Royal Numico, N.V.)**
6111 Broken Sound Parkway Northwest
Boca Raton, FL 33487
(800) 327-0908
www.rexallsundown.com

**Rhone-Poulenc Rorer Pharmaceuticals, Inc**
500 Arcola Road
PO Box 1200
Collegeville, PA 19426-0998
(800) 340-7502

**Richardson-Vicks, Inc**
(see Procter & Gamble Pharmaceuticals, Inc)

**Ricola, Inc**
51 Gibraltar Drive
Morris Plains, NJ 07950
(973) 984-6811
www.ricolausa.com

**R.I.D., Inc**
**(Bayer Consumer Care Division)**
36 Columbia Road
PO Box 1910
Morristown, NJ 07962-1910
(800) 331-4536
www.licerid.com

**Rite Aid Corp**
PO Box 3165
Harrisburg, PA 17105
(800) 748-3243
www.riteaid.com

**Roberts Pharmaceuticals Corp**
(see Shire Pharmaceuticals)

**Roche Pharmaceuticals**
340 Kingsland Street
Nutley, NJ 07110
(973) 235-5000
www.rocheusa.com

**Roerig**
(see Pfizer Pharmaceuticals Group PPG)

**Rorer** (see Rhone-Poulenc Rorer Pharmaceuticals, Inc)

**Ross Products Division**
**Abbott Labs**
625 Cleveland Avenue
Columbus, OH 43215
(800) 986-8510
www.ross.com

**Roxane Laboratories, Inc**
PO Box 16532
Columbus, OH 43216
(800) 962-8364
www.roxane.com

**R. P. Scherer, Inc**
(see Cardinal Health, Inc)

**RTI International**
**(Research Triangle Institute)**
PO Box 12194
Research Triangle Park, NC 27709-2194
(919) 485-6000
www.rti.org

**Salix Pharmaceuticals, Inc**
1700 Perimeter Park Drive
Morrisville, NC 27560-8404
(919) 862-1000
www.salix.com

**Sandoz, Inc**
**(Novartis Pharmaceuticals Corp)**
506 Carnegie Center
Suite 400
Princeton, NJ 08540
(800) 525-8747
www.us.sandoz.com

**SangStat, Inc**
(see Genzyme Corp)

**Sanofi-Aventis**
300 Somerset Corporate Boulevard
Bridgewater, NJ 08807-2854
(800) 981-2491
www.sanofi-aventis.us

**Sanofi Pasteur**
Discovery Drive
Box 187
Swiftwater, PA 18370-0187
(570) 839-7187
www.sanofipasteur.com

**Sanofi-Synthelabo, Inc**
90 Park Avenue
New York, NY 10016
(212) 551-4000
www.sanofi-synthelabous.com

**Santen, Inc**
555 Gateway Drive
Napa, CA 94558
(707) 254-1750
www.santeninc.com

**Savage Laboratories**
**(Altana Inc)**
60 Baylis Road
Melville, NY 11747-2006
(800) 231-0206
www.savagelabs.com

**Scandinavian Naturals**
13 North 7th Street
Perkasie, PA 18944
(800) 288-2844
www.scandinaviannaturals.com

**Scandipharm**
(see Axcan Pharma, Inc)

**Schaffer Laboratories**
1058 North Allen Avenue
Pasadena, CA 91104
(800) 231-6725
www.schafferlabs.com

**Schein Pharmaceutical, Inc**
(see Watson Laboratories, Inc)

**Schering-Plough Corp**
**(World Headquarters)**
2000 Galloping Hill Road
Kenilworth, NJ 07033-0530
(908) 298-4000
www.schering-plough.com

**Schwarz Pharma, Inc**
6140 West Executive Drive
Mequon, WI 53092
(800) 558-5114
www.schwarzusa.com

**SciClone Pharmaceuticals, Inc**
901 Mariner's Island Boulevard
Suite 205
San Mateo, CA 94404
(650) 358-3456
www.sciclone.com

**Scios**
**(Corp Headquarters)**
6500 Paseo Padre Parkway
Freemont, CA 94555
(510) 248-2500
www.sciosinc.com

**Sepracor**
**(Corp Headquarters)**
84 Waterford Drive
Marlborough, MA 01752
(877) SEPRACOR
www.sepracor.com

**Septodont, Inc**
PO Box 11926
Wilmington, DE 19850
(800) 872-8305
www.septodontinc.com

**Seres Laboratories, Inc**
3331-B Industrial Drive
Santa Rosa, CA 95403
(707) 526-4526
www.sereslabs.com

**Serono, Inc**
One Technology Place
Rockland, MA 02370
(800) 283-8088
www.seronousa.com

**Shaklee Corporation**
**(Corp Headquarters)**
4747 Willow Road
Pleasanton, CA 94588
(925) 924-2000
www.shaklee.com

**Sheffield Laboratories**
**(Faria Ltd LLC)**
170 Broad Street
New London, CT 06320
(800) 442-4451
www.sheffield-labs.com

**Sherwood Davis & Geck**
(see Kendall Healthcare Products)

**Sherwood Medical**
(see Kendall Healthcare Products)

**Shire Pharmaceuticals**
725 Chesterbrook Boulevard
Wayne, PA 19087-5637
(484) 595-8800
www.shire.com

**Shire Laboratories**
1550 East Gude Drive
Rockville, MD 20850
(301) 838-2500
www.shirelabs.com

**SHS North America**
PO Box 117
Gaithersburg, MD 20884-0117
(800) 365-7354
www.SHSNA.com

**SICOR Pharmaceuticals, Inc**
19 Hughes
Irvine, CA 92618
(800) 729-9991
www.gensiasicor.com

**Sigma-Tau, Inc**
800 South Frederick Avenue
Suite 300
Gaithersburg, MD 20877
(800) 447-0169
www.sigma-tau.com

**Silarx Pharmaceuticals, Inc**
19 West Street
Spring Valley, NY 10977
(845) 352-4020
www.silarx.com

**Sirius Laboratories, Inc**
100 Fairway Drive
Suite 130
Vernon Hills, IL 60061
(866) 292-2108
www.siriuslabs.com

**Sirna Therapeutics**
185 Berry Street
Suite 6504
San Francisco, CA 94107
(415) 512-7624
www.sirna.com

**SkyePharma US, Inc**
10 East 63rd Street
New York, NY 10021
(212) 753-5780
www.skyepharma.com

**Slim Fast Foods Company**
PO Box 3625
West Palm Beach, FL 33402
(561) 833-9920
www.slim-fast.com

**Smith & Nephew, Inc**
150 Minuteman Road
Andover, MA 01810
(978) 749-1000
www.smithnephew.com

**Snuva, Inc**
715 South Boulevard
Oak Park, IL 60302
(708) 848-4783
www.snuva.com

**Solvay Pharmaceuticals**
901 Sawyer Road
Marietta, GA 30062
(770) 578-9000
www.solvaypharmaceuticals-us.com

**Somerset Pharmaceuticals, Inc**
2202 Northwest Shore Boulevard
Suite 450
Tampa, FL 33607
(800) 892-8889
www.somersetpharm.com

**Sonus Pharmaceuticals**
22026 20th Avenue Southeast
Bothell, Washington 98021
(425) 487-9500
www.sonuspharma.com

**Spectrum Chemical
Manufacturing Corp**
14422 South San Pedro Street
Gardena, CA 90248-9985
(800) 813-1514
www.spectrumchemical.com

**St Jude Medical, Inc**
One Lillehei Plaza
St Paul, MN 55117-9983
(800) 328-9634
www.sjm.com

**Stada Pharmaceuticals**
5 Cedar Brook Drive
Cranbury, NJ 08512
(800) 542-6682
www.stadausa.com

**Star Pharmaceuticals, Inc**
1881 West State 84
Suite 101
Fort Lauderdale, FL 33315
(800) 845-7827
www.starpharm.com

**Squibb** (see Bristol-Myers Squibb Company)

**Steris Corp**
5960 Heisley Road
Mentor, OH 44060-1834
(440) 354-2600
www.americantable.com

**Sterling Health**
(see Bayer Corp Consumer Care Division)

**Sterling Winthrop**
(see Sanofi-Synthelabo, Inc)

**Stiefel Laboratories, Inc**
255 Alhambra Circle
Coral Gables, FL 33134
(305) 443-3800
www.stiefel.com

**Stratus Pharmaceuticals, Inc**
14377 Southwest 142nd Street
Miami, FL 33186
(800) 442-7882
www.stratuspharmaceuticals.com

**SummaRx Laboratories**
2940 FM 3028
Mineral Wells, TX 76067-9258
(800) 527-7319
www.summalabs.com

**Summers Laboratories, Inc**
103 G.P. Clement Drive
Collegeville, PA 19426-2044
(800) 533-7546
www.sumlab.com

**Summit Pharmaceuticals**
(see Novartis Pharmaceuticals Corp)

**SuperGen, Inc**
4140 Dublin Boulevard
Suite 200
Dublin, CA 94568
(925) 560-0100
www.supergen.com

**Superior Pharmaceutical Company**
1385 Kemper Meadow Drive
Cincinnati, OH 45240-1635
(800) 826-5035
www.superiorpharm.com

**Swiss-American Products, Inc**
4641 Nall Road
Dallas, TX 75244
(800) 633-8872
www.elta.net

**Syncor**
(see Cardinal Health, Inc)

**Syntex Laboratories** (see Roche Pharmaceuticals)

**Takeda Pharmaceuticals North America, Inc**
475 Half Day Road
Lincolnshire, IL 60069
(847) 383-3000
www.tpna.com

**Tanox, Inc**
10301 Stella Link
Houston, TX 77025-5445
(713) 578-4000
www.tanox.com

**TAP Pharmaceutical Products, Inc**
675 North Field Drive
Lake Forest, IL 60045
(800) 621-1020
www.tap.com

**Targeted Genetics Corp**
1100 Olive Way
Suite 100
Seattle, WA 98101
(206) 623-7612
www.targen.com

**Taro Pharmaceuticals USA, Inc**
5 Skyline Drive
Hawthorne, NY 10532
(914) 345-9001
www.tarousa.com

**Tec Laboratories, Inc**
7100 Tec Labs Way Southwest
Albany, OR 97321
(800) 482-4464
www.teclabsinc.com

**Telluride Pharmaceutical Corp**
300 Valley Road
Hillsborough, NJ 08844-4656
(908) 369-1800
www.tellpharm.com

**Teva Pharmaceuticals USA**
1090 Horsham Road
PO Box 1090
North Wales, PA 19454-1090
(215) 591-3000
www.tevapharmusa.com

**The Key Company**
1313 West Essex Avenue
St Louis, MO 63122
(800) 325-9592
www.thekeycompany.com

**The Medicines Company**
One Cambridge Center
Cambridge, MA 02142
(617) 225-9099
www.angiomax.com

**Therasense**
(see Abbott Laboratories)

**Tishcon Corp**
30 New York Avenue
Westbury, NY 11590-5910
(516) 333-3050
www.tishcon.com

**Tom's of Maine, Inc**
302 LaFayette Center
PO Box 710
Kennebunk, ME 04043
(800) 367-8667
www.tomsofmaine.com

**Triton Consumer Products, Inc**
561 West Golf Road
Arlington Heights, IL 60005-3904
(800) 942-2009
www.tritonconsumerproducts.com

**Tweezerman International**
2 Tri Harbor Court
Port Washington, NY 11050-4617
(800) 645-3340
www.tweezerman.com

**TwinLab Corporation**
150 Motor Parkway
Suite 210
Hauppauge, NY 11788
(800) 645-5626
www.twinlab.com

**UAD Laboratories, Inc**
(see Forest Laboratories, Inc)

**UCB Pharmaceuticals, Inc**
1950 Lake Park Drive
Smyrna, GA 30080
(770) 970-7500
www.ucb-pharma.com

**UDL Laboratories, Inc**
1718 Northrock Court
Rockford, IL 61103
(800) 848-0462
www.udllabs.com

**Unimed Pharmaceuticals**
(see Solvay Pharmaceuticals)

**Unipath Diagnostics, Inc**
51 Sawyer Road
Suite 200
Waltham, MA 02453
(781) 647-3900
www.unipath.com

**United Guardian, Inc**
230 Marcus Boulevard
PO Box 18050
Hauppauge, NY 11788
(800) 645-5566
www.u-g.com

**Upjohn** (see Pharmacia & Upjohn Company)

**Upsher-Smith Laboratories, Inc**
6701 Evenstad Drive
Maple Grove, MN 55369
(763) 315-2000
www.upsher-smith.com

**UroCor Labs**
800 Research Parkway
Oklahoma City, OK 73104
(800) 634-9330
www.urocor.com

**Urologix**
14405 21st Avenue North
Minneapolis, MN 55447
(800) 475-1403
www.urologix.com

**USA Nutritionals, Inc**
513 Commack Road
Deerpark, NY 11729
(631) 643-0600
www.USANutritionals.com

**US DenTek**
307 Excellence Way
Maryville, TN 37801
(800) 433-6835
www.usdentek.com

**US Surgical**
150 Glover Avenue
Norwalk, CT 06856
(800) 722-8772
www.ussurg.com

**Valeant Pharmaceuticals International**
**Valeant Plaza**
3300 Hyland Avenue
Costa Mesa, CA 92626
(800) 548-5100
www.valeant.com

**Value in Pharmaceuticals**
3000 Alt Boulevard
Grand Island, NY 14072
(800) 724-3784
www.vippharm.com

**Vertex Pharmaceuticals, Inc**
130 Waverly Street
Cambridge, MA 02139
(617) 444-6100
www.vpharm.com

**VHA, Inc**
220 East Las Colinas Boulevard
Irving, TX 75039
(972) 830-0000
www.vha.com

**Vicks Health Care Products**
(see Procter & Gamble Pharmaceuticals, Inc)

**Vicks Pharmacy Products**
(see Procter & Gamble Pharmaceuticals, Inc)

**ViRexx Medical Corp**
8223 Roper Road
Edmonton, Alberta Canada T6E 6S4
(780) 433-4411
www.virexx.com

**VISION Pharmaceuticals, Inc**
1022 North Main Street
PO Box 400
Mitchell, SD 57301
(800) 325-6789
www.visionpharm.com

**VistaPharm**
2224 Cahaba Valley Drive
Suite B3
Birmingham, AL 35242
(205) 981-1387
www.vistapharm.com

**Vitaline Formulary**
825 Challenger Drive
Green Bay, WI 54311
(800) 287-5972
www.vitalineformulary.com

**Vitamin Research Products**
4610 Arrowhead Drive
Carson City, NV 89706
(800) 877-2447
www.vrp.com

**VIVUS, Inc**
1172 Castro Street
Mountain View, CA 94040
(650) 934-5200
www.vivus.com

**Walgreen Company**
200 Wilmont Road
Dearfield, IL 60015
(847) 940-2500
www.walgreens.com

**Wallace Pharmaceuticals**
(see MedPointe Pharmaceuticals)

**Wal-Mart Stores, Inc**
702 Southwest 8th Street
Bentonville, AR 72716
(501) 273-4000
www.wal-mart.com

**Wampole Laboratories**
2 Research Way
Princeton, NJ 08540
(800) 257-9525
www.wampolelabs.com

**Warner Chilcott Laboratories**
100 Enterprise Drive
Rockaway, NJ 07866
(973) 442-3200
www.warnerchilcott.com

**Watson Laboratories, Inc**
311 Bonnie Circle
Corona, CA 92880
(800) 272-5525
www.watsonpharm.com

**Wellements**
3925 East Watkins Drive
Suite 200
Phoenix, AZ 85034
(800) 255-2690
www.mdlabs.com

**Westwood-Squibb Pharmaceuticals**
**(Bristol-Myers Squibb)**
100 Forest Avenue
Buffalo, NY 14213
(800) 332-2056

**W. F. Young, Inc**
PO Box 1990
East Longmeadow, MA 01028-5990
(800) 628-9653
www.absorbine.com

**Whitehall-Robins Healthcare**
(see Wyeth Pharmaceuticals)

**Winthrop Pharmaceuticals**
(see Sanofi-Synthelabo, Inc)

**Wisconsin Pharmacal Company**
**(WPC Brands)**
1 Pharmacal Way
Jackson, WI 53037
(800) 558-6614
www.pharmacalway.com

**Women First Healthcare, Inc**
5355 Mira Sorrento Place
Suite 700
San Diego, CA 92121
(858) 509-1171
www.womenfirst.com

**Woodward Laboratories, Inc**
125-B Columbia
Aliso Viejo, CA 92656-1458
(949) 362-4600
www.woodwardlabs.com

**Wyeth Pharmaceuticals**
5 Giralda Farms
Madison, NJ 07940
www.wyeth.com

**Xoma**
2910 7th Street
Berkeley, CA 94710
(510) 204-7200
www.xoma.com

**Xttrium Laboratories, Inc**
415 West Pershing Road
Chicago, IL 60609
(877) 988-2721
www.adultrashcreme.com

**Young Dental Manufacturing**
13705 Shoreline Court East
Earth City, MO 63045
(800) 325-1881
www.youngdental.com

**Zanfel Laboratories, Inc**
Morton, IL 61550
(800) 401-4002
www.zanfel.com

**Zeneca Pharmaceuticals**
(see AstraZeneca Pharmaceuticals, LP)

**Zenith Goldline Pharmaceuticals**
4400 Biscayne Boulevard
Miami, FL 33137-3227
(305) 575-6000

**Zila Pharmaceuticals, Inc**
5227 North 7th Street
Phoenix, AZ 85014-2800
(602) 266-6700
www.zila.com

**ZLB Behring**
1020 First Avenue
PO Box 61501
King of Prussia, PA 19406
(610) 878-4000
www.zlbbehring.com

**Zonagen, Inc**
2408 Timberloch Place, B-1
The Woodlands, TX 77380
(281) 719-3400
www.zonagen.com

**ZymeTx, Inc**
655 Research Parkway
Suite 554
Oklahoma City, OK 73104
(888) 817-1314
www.zymetx.com

**ZymoGenetics, Inc**
1201 Eastlake Avenue East
Seattle, WA 98102-3702
(206) 442-6600
www.zymogenetics.com

# VITAMIN PRODUCTS

## Injectable Formulations

| Product | A (int. units) | B₁ (mg) | B₂ (mg) | B₆ (mg) | B₁₂ (mcg) | C (mg) | D (int. units) | E (int. units) | K (mcg) | Additional Information |
|---|---|---|---|---|---|---|---|---|---|---|
| | | | | | | | Solution | | | |
| Infuvite® Adult (per 10 mL) | 3300 | 6 | 3.6 | 6 | 5 | 200 | 200 | 10 | 150 | Supplied as two 5 mL vials. Biotin 60 mcg, folic acid 600 mcg, niacinamide 40 mg, dexpanthenol 15 mg |
| Infuvite® Pediatric (per 5 mL) | 2300 | 1.6 | 1.4 | 1 | 1 | 80 | 400 | 7 | 200 | Supplied as one 4 mL vial and one 1 mL vial. Biotin 20 mcg, folic acid 140 mcg, niacinamide 17 mg, dexpanthenol 5 mg |
| M.V.I.®-12 [DSC] (per 10 mL) | 3300 | 3 | 3.6 | 4 | 12.5 | 100 | 200 | 10 | --- | Supplied as two 5 mL vials or a single 2-chambered 10 mL vial. Biotin 60 mcg, folic acid 400 mcg, niacinamide 40 mg, dexpanthenol 15 mg |
| M.V.I. Adult™ (per 10 mL) | 3300 | 6 | 3.6 | 6 | 5 | 200 | 200 | 10 | 150 | Supplied as two 5 mL vials or a single 2-chambered 10 mL vial. Also available in a pharmacy bulk package (two 50 mL vials). Biotin 60 mcg, folic acid 600 mcg, niacinamide 40 mg, dexpanthenol 15 mg |
| | | | | | | | Powder for Reconstitution | | | |
| M.V.I.® Pediatric | 2300 | 1.2 | 1.4 | 1 | 1 | 80 | 400 | 7 | 200 | Biotin 20 mcg, folic acid 140 mcg, niacinamide 17 mg, dexpanthenol 5 mg, aluminum, polysorbate 80 |

## Adult Formulations

| Product | A (int. units) | B₁ (mg) | B₂ (mg) | B₆ (mg) | B₁₂ (mcg) | C (mg) | D (int. units) | E (int. units) | Additional Information |
|---|---|---|---|---|---|---|---|---|---|
| **Liquid** | | | | | | | | | |
| Centrum® [OTC] (per 15 mL) | 2500 | 1.5 | 1.7 | 2 | 6 | 60 | 400 | 30 | Biotin 300 mcg, Cr 25 mcg, Fe 9 mg, iodine 150 mcg, Mn 2 mg, Mo 25 mg, niacin 20 mg, pantothenic acid 10 mg, Zn 3 mg; alcohol 5.4%, sodium benzoate (240 mL) |
| Geriation® [OTC] (per 30 mL) | | 5 | 2.5 | 1 | 1 | | | | Choline 100 mg, Fe 15 mg, iodine 100 mcg, Mg 2 mg, Mn 2 mg, niacinamide 50 mg, pantothenic acid 10 mg, Zn 2 mg; sherry flavor (480 mL) |
| Geritol® Tonic [OTC] (per 15 mL) | | 2.5 | 2.5 | 0.5 | | | | | Chlorine bitartrate 50 mg, Fe 18 mg, methionine 25 mg, niacin 50 mg, pantothenic acid 2 mg; sugars 7 g, alcohol 12%, benzoic acid (120 mL, 360 mL) |
| Strovite® Forte (per 15 mL) | 4000 | 15 | 17 | 20 | 20 | 300 | 400 | 30 | Biotin 150 mcg, Cr 50 mcg, Cu 3 mg, Fe 10 mg, folic acid 1 mg, Mg 50 mg, Mn 5 mg, niacinamide 100 mg, pantothenic acid 25 mg, Se 55 mcg, Zn 15 mg; contains aspartame |
| Vi-Daylin® [OTC] [DSC] (per 5 mL) | 2500 | 1.05 | 1.2 | 1.05 | 4.5 | 60 | 400 | 15 | Niacin 13.5 mg; alcohol <0.5%, benzoic acid; lemon/orange flavor (240 mL, 480 mL) |
| Vi-Daylin® + Iron [OTC] [DSC] (per 5 mL) | 2500 | 1.05 | 1.2 | 1.05 | 4.5 | 60 | 400 | 15 | Fe 10 mg, niacin 13.5 mg; alcohol <0.5%, benzoic acid; lemon/orange flavor (240 mL, 480 mL) |
| **Caplet** | | | | | | | | | |
| Glutofac®-MX (per 1 light purple caplet and 1 dark purple caplet) | | | | | 10 | | | | Ascorbic acid 100 mg, biotin 300 mcg, boron 150 mcg, Ca 425 mg, Cr 200 mcg, dioctyl sodium sulfosuccinate 10 mg, Fe 15 mg, folic acid 800 mcg, iodine 150 mcg, Mg 415 mg, Mn 5 mg, Mo 75 mcg, nickel 5 mcg, pantothenic acid 25 mg, phosphorus 130 mg, potassium 80 mg, Se 100 mcg, tin 10 mcg, vanadium 10 mcg, Zn 35 mg |
| Glutofac®-ZX | 5000 | 20 | 20 | 25 | 50 | 500 | 400 | 50 | Biotin 200 mcg, Ca 66 mg, Cr 200 mcg, Cu 2.5 mg, niacinamide 100 mg, folic acid 1000 mcg, Mg 50 mg, Mn 5 mg, pantothenic acid 25 mg, Se 50 mcg, Zn 20 mg |

(continued)

| Product | A (int. units) | B₁ (mg) | B₂ (mg) | B₆ (mg) | B₁₂ (mcg) | C (mg) | D (int. units) | E (int. units) | Additional Information |
|---|---|---|---|---|---|---|---|---|---|
| Theragran® Heart Right™ [OTC] [DSC] | 5000 | 3 | 3.4 | 16 | 30 | 120 | 400 | 400 | Alpha-carotene, beta-carotene, biotin 30 mcg, Ca 55 mg, Cr 50 mcg, cryptoxanthin, Cu 1.5 mg, Fe 4 mg, folic acid as folate 0.6 mg, iodine 150 mcg, lutein, lycopene, Mg 150 mg, Mn 2 mg, Mo 75 mcg, niacin 20 mg, pantothenic acid 10 mg, Se 70 mcg, vitamin K 14 mcg, zeaxanthin, Zn 15 mg |
| Theragran-M® Advanced Formula [OTC] [DSC] | 5000 | 3 | 3.4 | 6 | 12 | 90 | 400 | 60 | Biotin 30 mcg, boron 150 mcg, Ca 40 mg, chloride 7.5 mg, Cr 50 mcg, Cu 2 mg, Fe 9 mg, folic acid 0.4 mg, iodine 150 mcg, Mg 100 mg, Mn 2 mg, Mo 75 mcg, niacin 20 mg, nickel 5 mcg, pantothenic acid 10 mg, phosphorus 31 mg, potassium 7.5 mg, Se 70 mcg, silicon 2 mg, tin 10 mcg, vanadium 10 mcg, vitamin K 28 mcg, Zn 15 mg |
| Capsule | | | | | | | | | |
| Hemocyte Plus® | | 10 | 6 | 5 | 15 | 200 | | | Cu 0.8 mg, Fe 106 mg, folic acid 1 mg, Mg 6.9 mg, Mn 1.3 mg, niacinamide 30 mg, pantothenic acid 10 mg, Zn 18.2 mg |
| Multiret Folic 500 | | 6 | 6 | 5 | 25 | 500 | | | Calcium pantothenate 10 mg, Fe 525 mg (timed-release), niacinamide 30 mg |
| Ocuvite® Lutein | | | | | | 60 | | 30 | Cu 2 mg, lutein 6 mg, Zn 15 mg |
| Replace [OTC] (per 2 capsules) | 5000 | 25 | 25 | 25 | 25 | 60 | 75 | 30 | Betaine 20 mg, biotin 20 mcg, Ca 180 mg, choline 25 mg, Cr 50 mcg, Cu 0.1 mg, folic acid 400 mcg, inositol 25 mg, iodine 0.225 mg, lemon bioflavonoid complex 50 mg, Mg 90 mg, Mn 2.5 mg, Mo 20 mcg, niacin 40 mg, PABA 12.5 mg, pancreatin 50 mg, pantothenic acid 75 mg, potassium 20 mg, Se 50 mcg, Zn 10 mg |
| Replace With Iron [OTC] (per 2 capsules) | 5000 | 25 | 25 | 25 | 25 | 60 | 75 | 30 | Betaine 20 mg, biotin 20 mcg, Ca 180 mg, choline 25 mg, Cr 50 mcg, Cu 0.1 mg, Fe 10 mg, folic acid 400 mcg, inositol 25 mg, iodine 0.225 mg, lemon bioflavonoid complex 50 mg, Mg 90 mg, Mn 2.5 mg, Mo 20 mcg, niacin 40 mg, PABA 12.5 mg, pancreatin 50 mg, pantothenic acid 75 mg, potassium 20 mg, Se 50 mcg, Zn 10 mg |
| Vicon Forte® | 8000 | 10 | 5 | 2 | 10 | 150 | | 50 | Folic acid 1 mg, Mg 70 mg, Mn 4 mg, niacinamide 25 mg, Zn 80 mg |

*(continued)*

| Product | A (int. units) | $B_1$ (mg) | $B_2$ (mg) | $B_6$ (mg) | $B_{12}$ (mcg) | C (mg) | D (int. units) | E (int. units) | Additional Information |
|---|---|---|---|---|---|---|---|---|---|
| Vitacon Forte | 8000 | 10 | 5 | 2 | 10 | 150 | | 50 | Folic acid 1 mg, Mg 70 mg, Mn 4 mg, niacinamide 25 mg, Zn 80 mg |
| **Capsule, Softgel** | | | | | | | | | |
| PreserVision® Lutein [OTC] | | | | | | 226 | | 200 | Cu 0.8 mg, lutein 5 mg, Zn 34.8 mg |
| PreserVision® AREDS [OTC] | 14,320 | | | | | 226 | | 200 | Cu 0.8 mg, Zn 34.8 mg |
| **Tablet** | | | | | | | | | |
| Androvite® [OTC] (per 6 tablets) | 2500 | 50 | 50 | 100 | 125 | 1000 | 400 | 400 | Beta ne 100 mg, boron 3 mg, Cr 200 mcg, Cu 2 mg, Fe 13 mg, folic acid 400 mcg, hesperidin 35 mg, inositol 36 mg, iodine 150 mcg, Mg 500 mg, Mn 10 mg, niacinamide 50 mg, PABA 25 mg, pancreatin 4X 75 mg, pantothenic acid 100 mg, rutin 25 mg, Se 200 mcg, Zn 50 mg |
| Centrum® [OTC] | 3500 | 1.5 | 1.7 | 2 | 6 | 60 | 400 | 30 | Biotin 30 mcg, boron 150 mcg, Ca 162 mg, chloride 72 mg, Cr 120 mcg, Cu 2 mg, Fe 18 mg, folic acid 0.4 mg, iodine 150 mcg, lutein 250 mcg, lycopene 300 mcg, Mg 100 mg, Mn 2 mg, Mo 75 mcg, niacin 20 mg, nickel 5 mcg, pantothenic acid 10 mg, phosphorus 109 mg, potassium 80 mg, Se 20 mcg, silicon 2 mg, tin 10 mcg, vanadium 10 mcg, vitamin K 25 mcg, Zn 15 mg |
| Centrum® Carb Assist™ [OTC] | 3500 | 4.5 | 5.1 | 6 | 18 | 120 | 400 | 60 | Biotin 40 mcg, boron 60 mcg, Ca 100 mg, chloride 72 mg, Cr 120 mcg, Cu 2 mg, Fe 18 mg, folic acid 400 mcg, ginkgo biloba leaf 60 mg, ginseng root 50 mg, iodine 150 mcg, Mg 40 mg, Mo 75 mcg, niacin 40 mg, nickel 5 mcg, pantothenic acid 10 mg, phosphorus 48 mg, potassium 80 mg, Se 70 mcg, silicon 4 mg, tin 10 mcg, vanadium 10 mcg, vitamin K 25 mcg, Zn 15 mg |
| Centrum® Performance™ [OTC] | 3500 | 4.5 | 5.1 | 6 | 18 | 120 | 400 | 60 | Biotin 40 mcg, boron 60 mcg, chloride 72 mg, folic acid 0.4 mg, Ca 100 mg, Cr 120 mcg, Cu 2 mg, Fe 18 mg, ginkgo biloba leaf 60 mg, ginseng root 50 mg, iodine 150 mcg, Mg 40 mg, Mn 4 mg, Mo 75 mcg, niacin 40 mg, nickel 5 mcg, pantothenic acid 10 mg, phosphorus 48 mg, potassium 80 mg, Se 70 mcg, silicon 4 mg, tin 10 mcg, vanadium 10 mcg, vitamin K 25 mcg, Zn 15 mg |

*(continued)*

| Product | A (int. units) | B$_1$ (mg) | B$_2$ (mg) | B$_6$ (mg) | B$_{12}$ (mcg) | C (mg) | D (int. units) | E (int. units) | Additional Information |
|---|---|---|---|---|---|---|---|---|---|
| Centrum® Silver® [OTC] | 3500 | 1.5 | 1.7 | 3 | 25 | 60 | 400 | 45 | Biotin 30 mcg, boron 150 mcg, Ca 200 mg, chloride 72 mg, Cr 150 mcg, Cu 2 mg, folic acid 0.4 mg, iodine 150 mcg, lutein 250 mcg, lycopene 300 mcg, Mg 100 mg, Mn 2 mg, Mo 75 mcg, niacin 20 mg, nickel 5 mcg, pantothenic acid 10 mg, phosphorus 48 mg, potassium 80 mg, Se 20 mcg, silicon 2 mg, vanadium 10 mcg, vitamin K 10 mcg, Zn 15 mg |
| Diatx® ZN | | 1.5 | 1.5 | 2 | 2 | 60 | 400 | | Cu 1.5 mg, D-biotin 300 mcg, folic acid 5 mg, niacinamide 20 mg, pantothenic acid 10 mg, Zn 25 mg [gluten free, lactose free, sugar free, yeast free] |
| Freedavite [OTC] | 5000 | 1.5 | 1.7 | 2 | 6 | 60 | 400 | 30 | Biotin 30 mcg, Ca 20 mg, Cu 0.1 mg, Fe 1.8 mg, folic acid 400 mcg, iodine 75 mcg, Mg 8 mg, Mn 0.625 mg, niacinamide 20 mg, pantothenic acid 10 mg, Se 35 mcg, Zn 1.5 mg |
| Geri-Freeda [OTC] | 5000 | 15 | 15 | 15 | 15 | 150 | 400 | 15 | Betaine 10 mg, biotin 15 mcg, Ca 50 mg, choline 10 mg, Cr 60 mcg, Cu 0.5 mg, folic acid 400 mcg, hesperidin 10 mg, inositol 25 mg, iodine 150 mcg, L-lysine 25 mg, Mg 25 mg, Mn 1 mg, niacinamide 50 mg, PABA 10 mg, pantothenic acid 15 mg, Se 35 mcg, Zn 7.5 mg |
| Geritol Complete® [OTC] | 6100 | 1.5 | 1.7 | 2 | 6.7 | 57 | 400 | 30 | Biotin 44 mcg, Ca 148 mg, chloride 20 mg, Cr 12 mcg, Cu 1.8 mg, Fe 16 mg, folic acid 0.38 mg, iodine 120 mcg, Mg 86 mg, Mn 2.4 mg, Mo 1 mcg, niacin 20 mg, pantothenic acid 13 mg, phosphorous 118 mg, potassium 36 mg, vitamin K 24 mcg, Zn 13.5 mg |
| Geritol Extend® [OTC] | 3333 | 1.2 | 1.3 | 2 | 2.5 | 55 | 200 | 13 | Ca 120 mg, Fe 9.5 mg, folic acid 0.2 mg, iodine 130 mcg, Mg 32 mg, niacin 15 mg, phosphorous 98 mg, Se 35 mcg, vitamin K 80 mcg, Zn 14 mg |

(continued)

| Product | A (int. units) | B$_1$ (mg) | B$_2$ (mg) | B$_6$ (mg) | B$_{12}$ (mcg) | C (mg) | D (int. units) | E (int. units) | Additional Information |
|---|---|---|---|---|---|---|---|---|---|
| Gynovite® Plus [OTC] (per 6 tablets) | 5000 | 10 | 10 | 20 | 125 | 180 | 400 | 400 | Betaine 100 mg, biotin 125 mcg, boron 3 mg, Ca 500 mg, Cr 200 mcg, Cu 2 mg, Fe 18 mg, folic acid 400 mcg, hesperidin 35 mg, inositol 50 mg, iodine 150 mcg, Mg 600 mg, Mn 10 mg, niacin 20 mg, PABA 25 mg, pancreatin 4X 93 mg, pantothenic acid 10 mg, rutin 25 mg, Se 200 mcg, Zn 15 mg |
| Hemocyte Plus® | | 10 | 6 | 5 | 15 | 200 | | | Cu 0.3 mg, Fe 106 mg, folic acid 1 mg, Mg 6.9 mg, Mn 1.3 mg, niacinamide 30 mg, pantothenic acid 10 mg, Zn 18.2 mg |
| Hi-Kovite [OTC] (per contents of 1 vitamin tablet plus 1 mineral tablet) | 5000 | 10 | 10 | 10 | 10 | 200 | 400 | 30 | Bioflavonoids 10 mg, biotin 30 mcg, Ca 120 mg, Cu 0.5 mg, Fe 9 mg, folic acid 400 mcg, inositol 10 mg, iodine 9 mg, L-lysine 10 mg, Mg 60 mg, Mn 1 mg, niacinamide 100 mg, PABA 10 mg, pantothenic acid 10 mg, potassium 35 mg, Se 17.5 mg, Zn 7.5 mg |
| Iberet®-500 [OTC] | | 4.96 | 5.4 | 3.7 | 22.5 | 500 | | | Fe 95 mg (controlled release), niacin 27.2 mg, pantothenic acid 8.28 mg, sodium 65 mg |
| Iberet-Folic-500® [OTC] | | 6 | 6 | 5 | 25 | 500 | | | Fe 105 mg (controlled release), folic acid 0.8 mg, niacinamide 30 mg, calcium pantothenate 10 mg |
| Monocaps [OTC] | 5000 | 15 | 15 | 15 | 15 | 120 | 400 | 15 | Biotin 15 mcg, Ca 50 mg, Cu 0.1 mg, Fe 14 mg, folic acid 400 mcg, iodine 150 mcg, lecithin 10 mg, L-lysine 10 mg, Mg 30 mg, Mn 1 mg, niacinamide 40 mg, PABA 10 mg, pantothenic acid 15 mg, Se 35 mcg, Zn 3.75 mg |
| Ocuvite® [OTC] | 1000 | | | | | 200 | | 60 | Cu 2 mg, lutein 2 mg, Se 55 mg, Zn 40 mg |
| Ocuvite® Extra [OTC] | 1000 | | 3 | | | 300 | | 100 | Cu 2 mg, L-glutathione 5 mg, lutein 2 mg, Mn 5 mg, niacinamide 40 mg, Se 55 mg, Zn 40 mg |
| Olay® Vitamins Complete Women's [OTC] | 5000 | 1.5 | 1.7 | 2 | 6 | 120 | 400 | 50 | Biotin 30 mcg, boron 150 mcg, Ca 250 mg, chloride 36 mg, coenzyme Q$_{10}$ 2 mg, Cr 120 mcg, Cu 5 mg, Fe 18 mg, folic acid 0.4 mg, iodine 150 mcg, lutein 250 mg, Mg 100 mg, Mn 2 mg, Mo 25 mcg, niacin 20 mg, nickel 5 mcg, pantothenic acid 10 mg, phosphorus 77 mg, potassium 40 mg, Se 25 mcg, silicon 2 mg, vanadium 10 mcg, Zn 15 mg |

*(continued)*

| Product | A (int. units) | B₁ (mg) | B₂ (mg) | B₆ (mg) | B₁₂ (mcg) | C (mg) | D (int. units) | E (int. units) | Additional Information |
|---|---|---|---|---|---|---|---|---|---|
| Olay® Vitamins Complete Women's 50+ [OTC] | 5000 | 3 | 3.4 | 4 | 25 | | 400 | 60 | Biotin 30 mcg, boron 150 mcg, Ca 250 mg, chloride 72 mg, coenzyme Q₁₀ 2 mg, Cr 120 mcg, Cu 5 mg, folic acid 0.4 mg, iodine 150 mcg, lutein 250 mcg, Mg 120 mg, Mn 2 mg, Mo 25 mcg, niacin 20 mg, nickel 5 mcg, pantothenic acid 10 mg, phosphorus 48 mg, potassium 80 mg, Se 50 mcg, silicon 2 mg, vanadium 10 mcg, Zn 22 mg |
| Olay® Vitamins Even Complexion [OTC] | 5000 | | | | | 120 | 100 | 60 | Cu 2 mg, folic acid 200 mcg, Se 50 mcg, Zn 15 mg |
| One-A-Day® 50 Plus Formula [OTC] | 2500 | 4.5 | 3.4 | 6 | 25 | 120 | 400 | 33 | Biotin 30 mcg, Ca 120 mg, chloride 34 mg, Cr 180 mcg, Cu 2 mg, folic acid 0.4 mg, iodine 150 mcg, Mg 100 mg, Mn 4 mg, Mo 90 mcg, niacin 20 mg, pantothenic acid 15 mg, potassium 37.5 mg, Se 105 mcg, vitamin K 20 mcg, Zn 22.5 mg |
| One-A-Day® Active Formula [OTC] | 5000 | 4.5 | 5.1 | 6 | 18 | 120 | 400 | 60 | American ginseng 55 mg, biotin 40 mcg, boron 150 mcg, Ca 110 mg, chloride 180 mg, Cr 100 mcg, Cu 2 mg, Fe 9 mg, folic acid 0.4 mg, iodine 150 mcg, Mg 40 mg, Mn 2 mg, Mo 25 mcg, niacin 40 mg, nickel 5 mcg, pantothenic acid 10 mg, phosphorus 48 mg, potassium 200 mg, Se 45 mcg, silicon 6 mg, tin 10 mcg, vanadium 10 mcg, vitamin K 25 mcg, Zn 15 mg |
| One-A-Day® Carb Smart [OTC] | 2500 | 2.2 | 2.5 | 3 | 9 | 90 | 400 | 45 | Biotin 450 mcg, Ca 200 mg, Cr 200 mcg, Cu 2 mg, folic acid 400 mcg, Mg 100 mg, Mn 2 mg, Mo 75 mg, niacin 25 mg, pantothenic acid 15 mg, phosphorous 154 mg, potassium 99 mg, Se 105 mcg, vitamin K 25 mcg, Zn 22.5 mg |
| One-A-Day® Cholesterol Plus™ [OTC] | 2500 | 1.5 | 1.7 | 2 | 6 | 60 | 400 | 30 | Biotin 50 mcg, Ca 100 mg, Cr 120 mcg, Cu 2 mg, folic acid 400 mcg, iodine 150 mg, Mg 100 mg, Mn 2 mg, Mo 75 mg, niacin 20 mg, pantothenic acid 10 mg, policosanol 10 mg, potassium 99 mg, Se 70 mcg, Zn 15 mg |
| One-A-Day® Essential Formula [OTC] | 5000 | 1.5 | 1.7 | 2 | 6 | 60 | 400 | 30 | Folic acid 0.4 mg, niacin 20 mg, pantothenic acid 10 mg |

*(continued)*

| Product | A (int. units) | B₁ (mg) | B₂ (mg) | B₆ (mg) | B₁₂ (mcg) | C (mg) | D (int. units) | E (int. units) | Additional Information |
|---|---|---|---|---|---|---|---|---|---|
| One-A-Day® Maximum Formula [OTC] | 5000 | 1.5 | 1.7 | 2 | 6 | 60 | 400 | 30 | Biotin 30 mcg, boron 150 mcg, Ca 210 mg, chloride 72 mg, Cr 120 mcg, Cu 2 mg, Fe 18 mg, folic acid 0.4 mg, iodine 150 mcg, lycopene 600 mcg, Mg 120 mg, Mn 2 mg, Mo 160 mcg, niacin 20 mg, nicke 5 mcg, pantothenic acid 5 mg, phosphorus 109 mg, potassium 100 mg, Se 105 mcg, silicon 2 mg, tin 10 mcg, vanadium 10 mcg, vitamin K 25 mcg, Zn 15 mg |
| One-A-Day® Men's Formula [OTC] | 3500 | 1.2 | 1.7 | 3 | 18 | 90 | 400 | 45 | Biotin 30 mcg, chloride 34 mg, Cr 150 mcg, Cu 2 mg, folic acid 0.4 mg, iodine 150 mcg, Mg 100 mg, Mn 3.5 rrg, Mo 42 mcg, niacin 16 mg, pantothenic acid 10 mg, potassium 37.5 mg, Se 87.5 mcg, vitamin K 20 mcg, Zn 15 mg |
| One-A-Day® Today [OTC] | 3000 | 1.1 | 1.7 | 3 | 18 | 75 | 400 | 33 | Biotin 30 mcg, Ca 240 mg, Cr 120 mcg, Cu 2 mg, folic acid 0.4 mg, Mg 120 mg, Mn 2 mg, niacin 14 mg, pantothenic acid 5 mg, potassium 100 mg, Se 70 mcg, soy extract 10 mg, vitamin K 20 mcg, Zn 15 mg |
| One-A-Day® Weight Smart [OTC] | 2500 | 1.9 | 2.125 | 2.5 | 7.5 | 60 | 400 | 30 | Ca 300 mg, Cr 200 mcg, Cu 2 mg, EGCG 32 mcg, Fe 18 mg, folic acid 400 mcg, Mg 50 mg, Mn 2 mg, niacin 25 mg, pantothenic acid 12.5 mg, Se 70 mcg, vitamin K 80 mcg, Zn 15 mg |
| One-A-Day® Women's Formula [OTC] | 2500 | 1.5 | 1.7 | 2 | 6 | 60 | 400 | 30 | Ca 450 mg, Fe 18 mg, folic acid 0.4 mg, Mg 50 mg, niacin 10 mg, pantothenic acid 5 mg, Zn 15 mg |
| Optivite® P.M.T. [OTC] (per 6 tablets) | 125,000 | 25 | 25 | 300 | 60 | 1500 | 100 | 100 | Betaine 100 mg, biotin 60 mcg, Ca 125 mg, choline 313 mg, citrus bioflavonioids 250 mg, Cr 100 mcg, Fe 15 mg, folic acid 200 mcg, inositol 24 mg, iodine 75 mcg, Mg 250 mg, Mn 10 mg, niacinamide 25 mg, PABA 25 mg, pancreatin 4X 93 mg, pantothenic acid 25 mg, potassium 48 mg, rutin 25 mg, Se 100 mcg, Zn 25 mg |
| PreserVision® AREDS [OTC] | 14,320 | | | | | 226 | | 200 | Cu 0.8 mg, Zn 34.8 mg |
| Quintabs [OTC] | 5000 | 30 | 30 | 30 | 30 | 300 | 400 | 50 | Biotin 30 mcg, folic acid 400 mcg, niacinamide 100 mg, pantothenic acid 30 mg |

(continued)

| Product | A (int. units) | B$_1$ (mg) | B$_2$ (mg) | B$_6$ (mg) | B$_{12}$ (mcg) | C (mg) | D (int. units) | E (int. units) | Additional Information |
|---|---|---|---|---|---|---|---|---|---|
| Quintabs-M [OTC] | 5000 | 30 | 30 | 30 | 30 | 300 | 400 | 50 | Biotin 30 mcg, Ca 30 mg, Cu 0.2 mg, Fe 10 mg, folic acid 400 mcg, iodine 150 mcg, Mg 15 mg, Mn 2 mg, niacinamide 100 mg, PABA 10 mg, pantothenic acid 30 mg, Se 35 mcg, Zn 7.5 mg |
| T-Vites [OTC] | | 25 | 25 | 25 | 30 | 100 | 400 | | Biotin 30 mcg, folic acid 400 mcg, Mg 100 mg, Mn 0.5 mg, niacinamide 150 mg, pantothenic acid 25 mg, potassium 35 mg, Zn 3.75 mg |
| Ultra Freeda Iron Free [OTC] (per 3 tablets) | 12,500 | 50 | 50 | 50 | 100 | 1000 | 400 | 200 | Bioflavonoids 100 mg, biotin 300 mcg, Ca 250 mg, Cr 200 mcg, folic acid 800 mcg, Mg 100 mg, Mn 10 mg, Mo 12.5 mcg, niacinamide and niacin 100 mg, pantothenic acid 100 mg, potassium 35 mg, Se 100 mcg, Zn 22.5 mg |
| Ultra Freeda With Iron [OTC] (per 3 tablets) | 5000 | 50 | 50 | 50 | 100 | 1000 | 400 | 200 | Bioflavonoids 100 mg, biotin 300 mcg, Ca 250 mg, Cr 200 mcg, Fe 18 mg, folic acid 800 mcg, Mg 100 mg, Mn 10 mg, Mo 12.5 mcg, niacinamide and niacin 100 mg, pantothenic acid 100 mg, potassium 35 mg, Se 100 mcg, Zn 22.5 mg |
| Unicap Sr.® [OTC] | 5000 | 1.2 | 1.4 | 2.2 | 3 | 60 | 200 | 15 | Ca 100 mg, Cu 2 mg, Fe 10 mg, folic acid 400 mcg, iodine 150 mcg, Mg 30 mg, Mn 1 mg, niacin 16 mg, pantothenic acid 10 mg, phosphorus 77 mg, potassium 5 mg, Zn 15 mg |
| Unicap T® [OTC] | 5000 | 10 | 10 | 6 | 18 | 500 | 400 | 30 | Cu 2 mg, Fe 18 mg, folic acid 400 mcg, iodine 150 mcg, Mn 1 mg, niacin 100 mg, pantothenic acid 25 mg, potassium 5 mg, Se 10 mg, Zn 15 mg |
| Xtramins [OTC] | 1000 | 5 | 2 | 5 | 10 | 50 | 100 | 10 | Boron 1 mg, Ca 250 mg, Cr 40 mcg, Cu 0.5 mg, d-calcium pantothenate 5 mg, Fe 10 mg, folic acid 400 mcg, iodine 150 mcg, Mg 20 mg, Mn 2 mg, niacinamide 15 mg, PABA 5 mg, potassium 45 mg, Se 30 mcg, Zn 10 mg |
| **Tablet, Chewable** | | | | | | | | | |
| Centrum® [OTC] | 3500 | 1.5 | 1.7 | 2 | 6 | 60 | 400 | 30 | Biotin 45 mcg, Ca 108 mg, Cr 20 mcg, Cu 2 mg, Fe 18 mg, folic acid 0.4 mg, iodine 150 mcg, Mg 40 mg, Mn 1 mg, Mo 20 mcg, niacin 20 mg, pantothenic acid 10 mg, phosphorus 50 mg, vitamin K 10 mcg, Zn 15 mg |

*(continued)*

| Product | A (int. units) | B₁ (mg) | B₂ (mg) | B₆ (mg) | B₁₂ (mcg) | C (mg) | D (int. units) | E (int. units) | Additional Information |
|---|---|---|---|---|---|---|---|---|---|
| Viactiv® Multivitamin [OTC] (softchews) | 2500 | 1.5 | 1.7 | 2 | 6 | 60 | 400 | 33 | Biotin 30 mcg, Ca 200 mg, folic acid 400 mcg, niacin 15 mg, pantothenic acid 10 mg; sodium 25 mg; milk chocolate or tropical fruit splash flavors |

Key: Ca = calcium, Cr = chromium, Cu = copper, Fe = iron, Mg = magnesium, Mn = manganese, Mo = molybdenum, Se = selenium, Zn = zinc.

## Pediatric Formulations

| Product | A (int. units) | B₁ (mg) | B₂ (mg) | B₆ (mg) | B₁₂ (mcg) | C (mg) | D (int. units) | E (int. units) | Additional Information |
|---|---|---|---|---|---|---|---|---|---|
| | | | | | | Drops | | | |
| ADEKs [OTC] (per mL) | 3170 (50% as beta-carotene) | 0.5 | 0.6 | 0.6 | 4 | 45 | 400 | 40 | Biotin 15 mcg, niacin 6 mg, pantothenic acid 3 mg, vitamin K 0.1 mg, Zn 5 mg; alcohol free, dye free (60 mL) |
| Poly-Vi-Flor® 0.25 mg (per mL) | 1500 | 0.5 | 0.6 | 0.4 | 2 | 35 | 400 | 5 | **Fluoride 0.25 mg**, niacin 8 mg; fruit flavor (50 mL) |
| Poly-Vi-Flor® 0.5 mg (per mL) | 1500 | 0.5 | 0.6 | 0.4 | 2 | 35 | 400 | 5 | **Fluoride 0.5 mg**, niacin 8 mg; fruit flavor (50 mL) |
| Poly-Vi-Flor® With Iron 0.25 mg (per mL) | 1500 | 0.5 | 0.6 | 0.4 | | 35 | 400 | 5 | **Fluoride 0.25 mg**, iron 10 mg, niacin 8 mg; fruit flavor (50 mL) |
| Poly-Vi-Sol® [OTC] (per mL) | 1500 | 0.5 | 0.6 | 0.4 | 2 | 35 | 400 | 5 | Niacin 8 mg (50 mL) |
| Poly-Vi-Sol® With Iron [OTC] (per mL) | 1500 | 0.5 | 0.6 | 0.4 | | 35 | 400 | 5 | Iron 10 mg, niacin 8 mg (50 mL) |
| Soluvite-F® (per 0.6 mL) | 1500 | | | | 35 | 400 | | | **Fluoride 0.25 mg**; alcohol free, dye free, orange flavor (57 mL) |
| Tri-Vi-Flor® 0.25 mg (per mL) | 1500 | | | | | 35 | 400 | | **Fluoride 0.25 mg**; fruit flavor (50 mL) |
| Tri-Vi-Flor® With Iron 0.25 mg (per mL) | 1500 | | | | | 35 | 400 | | **Fluoride 0.25 mg**, iron 10 mg; fruit flavor (50 mL) |
| Tri-Vi-Sol® [OTC] (per mL) | 1500 | | | | | 35 | 400 | | Fruit flavor (50 mL) |
| Tri-Vi-Sol® With Iron [OTC] (per mL) | 1500 | | | | | 35 | 400 | | Iron 10 mg; fruit flavor (50 mL) |
| Vi-Daylin® [OTC] [DSC] (per mL) | 1500 | 0.5 | 0.6 | 0.4 | 1.5 | 35 | 400 | 5 | Niacin 8 mg; alcohol <0.5%, sugar free, fruit flavor (50 mL) |
| Vi-Daylin® + Iron [OTC] [DSC] (per mL) | 1500 | 0.5 | 0.6 | 0.4 | | 35 | 400 | 5 | Iron 10 mg, niacin 8 mg; alcohol <0.5%, sugar free, fruit flavor (50 mL) |
| Vi-Daylin® ADC [OTC] [DSC] (per mL) | 1500 | | | | | 35 | 400 | | Alcohol <0.5%, sugar free, fruit flavor (50 mL) |

*(continued)*

| Product | A (int. units) | B₁ (mg) | B₂ (mg) | B₆ (mg) | B₁₂ (mcg) | C (mg) | D (int. units) | E (int. units) | Additional Information |
|---|---|---|---|---|---|---|---|---|---|
| Vi-Daylin® ADC + Iron [OTC] [DSC] (per mL) | 1500 | | | | | 35 | 400 | | Iron 10 mg; benzoic acid, sugar free, fruit flavor (50 mL) |
| Vi-Daylin®/F [DSC] (per mL) | 1500 | 0.5 | 0.6 | 0.4 | | 35 | 400 | 5 | **Fluoride 0.25 mg**, niacin 8 mg; alcohol <0.1%, benzoic acid, sugar free, fruit flavor (50 mL) |
| Vi-Daylin®/F + Iron [DSC] (per mL) | 1500 | 0.5 | 0.6 | 0.4 | | 35 | 400 | 5 | **Fluoride 0.25 mg**, iron 10 mg, niacin 8 mg; alcohol <0.1%, benzoic acid, sugar free, fruit flavor (50 mL) |
| Vi-Daylin®/F ADC [DSC] (per mL) | 1500 | | | | | 35 | 400 | | **Fluoride 0.25 mg**; sugar free, fruit flavor (50 mL) |
| Vi-Daylin®/F ADC + Iron [DSC] (per mL) | 1500 | | | | | 35 | 400 | | **Fluoride 0.25 mg**, iron 10 mg; sugar free, fruit flavor (50 mL) |
| **Gum** | | | | | | | | | |
| Vitaball® | 5000 | 1.5 | 1.7 | 2 | 6 | 60 | 400 | 30 | Biotin 45 mcg, folic acid 400 mcg, niacinamide 20 mg, pantothenic acid 10 mg; bubble gum, cherry, grape, and watermelon (contains tartrazine) flavors |
| Vitaball® Wild 'N Fruity [OTC] | 5000 | 1.5 | 1.7 | 2 | 6 | 240 | 400 | 30 | Biotin 45 mcg, folic acid 400 mcg, niacinamide 20 mg, pantothenic acid 10 mg; berry, lemon (contains tartrazine), orange, and strawberry flavors |
| **Tablet, Chewable** | | | | | | | | | |
| ADEKs® [OTC] | 9000 (60% as beta-carotene) | 1.2 | 1.3 | 1.5 | 12 | 60 | 400 | 150 | Biotin 50 mcg, folic acid 0.2 mg, niacin 10 mg, pantothenic acid 10 mg, vit K 150 mcg, Zn 7.5 mg; dye free |
| Centrum Kids® Jimmy Neutron™ Complete | 5000 | 1.5 | 1.7 | 2 | 6 | 60 | 400 | 30 | Biotin 45 mcg, Ca 108 mg, Cr 20 mcg, Cu 2 mg, Fe 18 mcg, folic acid 0.4 mg, iodine 150 mcg, Mg 40 mg, Mn 1 mg, Mo 20 mcg, niacin 20 mg, pantothenic acid 10 mg, phosphorus 50 mg, vitamin K 10 mcg, Zn 15 mg; **contains phenylalanine**; cherry, fruit punch, and orange flavors |
| Centrum Kids® Jimmy Neutron™ Extra C | 5000 | 1.5 | 1.7 | 1 | 5 | 250 | 400 | 15 | Ca 108 mg, Cu 0.5 mg, folic acid 0.3 mg, niacin 13.5 mg, phosphorus 50 mg, sodium 16 mg, Zn 4 mg; **contains phenylalanine**; cherry, fruit punch, and orange flavors |
| Centrum® Kids Rugrats™ Complete [OTC] | 5000 | 1.5 | 1.7 | 2 | 6 | 60 | 400 | 30 | Biotin 45 mcg, Ca 108 mg, Cr 20 mcg, Cu 2 mg, Fe 18 mg, folic acid 0.4 mg, iodine 150 mcg, Mg 40 mg, Mn 1 mg, Mo 20 mcg, niacin 20 mg, pantothenic acid 10 mg, phosphorus 50 mg, vitamin K 10 mg, Zn 15 mg; **contains phenylalanine**; cherry, fruit punch, and orange flavors |

(continued)

| Product | A (int. units) | B₁ (mg) | B₂ (mg) | B₆ (mg) | B₁₂ (mcg) | C (mg) | D (int. units) | E (int. units) | Additional Information |
|---|---|---|---|---|---|---|---|---|---|
| Centrum® Kids Rugrats™ Extra C [OTC] | 5000 | 1.5 | 1.7 | 1 | 5 | 250 | 400 | 15 | Ca 108 mg, Cu 0.5 mg, folic acid 0.3 mg, niacin 13.5 mg, phosphorus 50 mg, sodium 15 mg, Zn 4 mg; **contains phenylalanine**; cherry, fruit punch, and orange flavors |
| Centrum® Kids Rugrats™ Extra Calcium [OTC] | 5000 | 1.5 | 1.7 | 1 | 5 | 60 | 400 | 15 | Ca 200 mg, Cu 0.5 mg, folic acid 0.3 mg, niacin 13.5 mg, phosphorus 50 mg, Zn 4 mg; **contains phenylalanine**; cherry, fruit punch, and orange flavors |
| Flintstones® Complete [OTC] | 5000 | 1.5 | 1.7 | 2 | 6 | 60 | 400 | 30 | Biotin 40 mcg, Ca 100 mg, Cu 2 mg, Fe 18 mg, folic acid 0.4 mg, iodine 150 mcg, Mg 20 mg, niacin 20 mg, pantothenic acid 10 mg, phosphorus 100 mg, Zn 15 mg; **phenylalanine 4.56 mg**; cherry, grape, and orange flavors |
| Flintstones® Plus Calcium [OTC] | 2500 | 1.05 | 1.2 | 1.05 | 4.5 | 60 | 400 | 15 | Ca 200 mg, folic acid 0.3 mg, niacin 13.5 mg; **phenylalanine <4 mg**: cherry, grape, and orange flavors |
| Flintstones® Plus Extra C [OTC] | 2500 | 1.05 | 1.2 | 1.05 | 4.5 | 250 | 400 | 15 | Folic acid 0.3 mg, niacin 13.5 mg; grape, orange, peach-apricot, raspberry, and strawberry flavors |
| Flintstones® Plus Iron [OTC] | 2500 | 1.05 | 1.2 | 1.05 | 4.5 | 60 | 400 | 15 | Fe 15 mg, folic acid 0.3 mg, niacin 13.5 mg; grape, orange, peach-apricot, raspberry, and strawberry flavors |
| My First Flintstones® [OTC] | 2500 | 1.05 | 1.2 | 1.05 | 4.5 | 60 | 400 | 15 | Folic acid 0.3 mg, niacin 13.5 mg; cherry, grape, and orange flavors |
| One-A-Day® Kids Bugs Bunny and Friends Complete [OTC] | 3000 | 1.5 | 1.7 | 2 | 6 | 60 | 400 | 30 | Biotin 40 mcg, Ca 100 mg, Cu 2 mg, Fe 18 mg, folic acid 0.4 mg, iodine 150 mcg, Mg 20 mg, niacin 15 mg, pantothenic acid 10 mg, phosphorus 100 mg, Zn 12 mg; **contains phenylalanine**: sugar free, fruity flavors |
| One-A-Day® Kids Bugs Bunny and Friends Plus Extra C [OTC] | 2500 | 1.05 | 1.2 | 1.05 | 4.5 | 250 | 400 | 15 | Folic acid 0.3 mg, niacin 13.5 mg, **contains phenylalanine**: sugar free, fruity flavors |
| One-A-Day® Kids Extreme Sports [OTC] | 3000 | 1.5 | 1.7 | 2 | 6 | 60 | 400 | 30 | Biotin 40 mcg, Ca 100 mg, Cu 2 mg, Fe 18 mg, folic acid 0.4 mg, iodine 150 mcg, Mg 20 mg, niacin 15 mg, pantothenic acid 10 mg, phosphorus 100 mg, Zn 12 mg; **contains phenylalanine** |
| One-A-Day® Kids Scooby-Doo! Complete [OTC] | 3000 | 1.5 | 1.7 | 2 | 6 | 60 | 400 | 30 | Biotin 40 mcg, Ca 100 mg, Cu 2 mg, Fe 18 mg, folic acid 0.4 mg, iodine 150 mcg, Mg 20 mg, niacin 15 mg, pantothenic acid 10 mg, phosphorus 100 mg, Zn 12 mg; **contains phenylalanine**: fruity flavors |

*(continued)*

| Product | A (int. units) | B$_1$ (mg) | B$_2$ (mg) | B$_6$ (mg) | B$_{12}$ (mcg) | C (mg) | D (int. units) | E (int. units) | Additional Information |
|---|---|---|---|---|---|---|---|---|---|
| One-A-Day® Kids Scooby-Doo! Fizzy Vites [OTC] | 1500 | 0.75 | 0.85 | 1 | 3 | 170 | 200 | 15 | Biotin 20 mcg, Ca 50 mg, Cu 1 mg, Fe 9 mg, folic acid 0.2 mg, iodine 75 mcg, Mg 10 mg, niacin 7.5 mg, pantothenic acid 5 mg, phosphorus 50 mg, sodium 20 mg, Zn 6 mg; **contains phenylalanine**: crazy grape, orange pucker, and wild cherry flavors |
| One-A-Day® Kids Scooby-Doo! Plus Calcium [OTC] | 2500 | 1.05 | 1.2 | 1.05 | 4.5 | 60 | 400 | 15 | Ca 200 mg, folic acid 0.3 mg, niacin 13.5 mg; **contains phenylalanine**: fruity flavors |
| Poly-Vi-Flor® 0.25 mg | 2500 | 1.05 | 1.2 | 1.05 | 4.5 | 60 | 400 | 15 | Fluoride 0.25 mg, folic acid 0.3 mg, niacin 13.5 mg; fruity flavor |
| Poly-Vi-Flor® 0.5 mg | 2500 | 1.05 | 1.2 | 1.05 | 4.5 | 60 | 400 | 15 | Fluoride 0.5 mg, folic acid 0.3 mg, niacin 13.5 mg; fruity flavor |
| Poly-Vi-Flor® 1 mg | 2500 | 1.05 | 1.2 | 1.05 | 4.5 | 60 | 400 | 15 | Fluoride 1 mg, folic acid 0.3 mg, niacin 13.5 mg; fruity flavor |
| Poly-Vi-Flor® 0.25 mg With Iron | 2500 | 1.05 | 1.2 | 1.05 | 4.5 | 60 | 400 | 15 | Fluoride 0.25 mg, Cu 1 mg, folic acid 0.3 mg, iron 12 mg, niacin 13.5 mg, Zn 10 mg; fruity flavor |
| Poly-Vi-Flor® 0.5 mg With Iron | 2500 | 1.05 | 1.2 | 1.05 | 4.5 | 60 | 400 | 15 | Fluoride 0.5 mg, Cu 1 mg, folic acid 0.3 mg, iron 12 mg, niacin 13.5 mg, Zn 10 mg; fruity flavor |

Key: Ca = calcium, Cr = chromium, Cu = copper, Fe = iron, Mg = magnesium, Mn = manganese, Mo = molybdenum, Se = selenium, Zn = zinc.

## Prenatal Formulations

| Product | A (int. units) | B₁ (mg) | B₂ (mg) | B₆ (mg) | B₁₂ (mcg) | C (mg) | D (int. units) | E (int. units) | Additional Information |
|---|---|---|---|---|---|---|---|---|---|
| **Caplet** | | | | | | | | | |
| PreCare® Prenatal | | 3 | 3.4 | 50 | 12 | 50 | 6 mcg | 3.5 mg | Ca 250 mg, Cu 2 mg, Fe 40 mg, folic acid 1 mg, Mg 50 mg, Zn 15 mg; dye free |
| StrongStart™ | 1000 | 3 | 3 | 20 | 12 | 100 | 400 | 30 | Ca 200 mg, Fe 29 mg, folic acid 1 mg, niacinamide 15 mg, pantothenic acid 7 mg, Zn 20 mg; docusate sodium 25 mg |
| **Capsule** | | | | | | | | | |
| Anemagen™ OB | | 1.6 | 1.8 | 20 | 12 | 60 | 400 | 30 | Ca 200 mg, Fe 28 mg, folic acid 1 mg; docusate calcium 25 mg |
| Chromagen OB® | | 1.6 | 1.8 | 20 | 12 | 60 | 400 | 30 | Ca 200 mg, Cu 2 mg, Fe 28 mg, folic acid 1 mg, Mn 2 mg, niacinamide 5 mg, Zn 25 mg; docusate calcium 25 mg |
| Prenatal H | | 10 | 6 | 5 | 15 | 200 | | | Cu 0.8 mg, Fe 106 mg, folic acid 1 mg, Mg 6.9 mg, Mn 1.3 mg, niacinamide 30 mg, pantothenic acid 10 mg, Zn 18.2 mg |
| Prenatal U | | 10 | 6 | 5 | 15 | 200 | | | Cu 0.8 mg, Fe 106.5 mg, folic acid 1 mg, Mn 1.3 mg, niacinamide 30 mg, pantothenic acid 10 mg |
| **Powder** | | | | | | | | | |
| Obegyn® (per 4 level tsp/8.25 g) | 2500 (as palmatate) 2500 (as beta-carotene) | 1.7 | 2 | 10 | 12 | 120 | 400 | 60 | Biotin 300 mcg, Ca 455 mg, Cu 2 mg, Fe 18 mg, folic acid 1 mg, iodine 150 mcg, Mg 150 mg, niacin 20 mg, pantothenic acid 10 mg, Zn 25 mg; **phenylalanine 84 mg/8.25 g**; orange flavor (495 g/60 doses) |
| **Tablet** | | | | | | | | | |
| A-Free Prenatal | | 2 | 2 | 1 | 2 | 33.3 | 133.3 | 10 | Calcium 333.3 mg, biotin 10 mcg, Cu 0.1 mg, Fe 9 mg, folic acid 266.6 mcg, Mg 33.3 mg, Mn 0.1 mg, niacinamide 10 mg, pantothenic acid 5 mg, Zn 7.5 mg |
| Advanced NatalCare® | 2700 | 3 | 3.4 | 20 | 12 | 120 | 400 | 30 | Ca 200 mg, Cu 2 mg, Fe 90 mg, folic acid 1 mg, Mg 30 mg, niacinamide 20 mg, Zn 25 mg; docusate sodium 50 mg |

*(continued)*

| Product | A (int. units) | B₁ (mg) | B₂ (mg) | B₆ (mg) | B₁₂ (mcg) | C (mg) | D (int. units) | E (int. units) | Additional Information |
|---|---|---|---|---|---|---|---|---|---|
| Aminate Fe-90 | 4000 | 3 | 3.4 | 20 | 12 | 120 | 400 | 30 | Ca 250 mg, Cu 2 mg, Fe 90 mg, folic acid 1 mg, iodine 150 mcg, niacinamide 20 mg, Zn 25 mg; docusate sodium 50 mg |
| Cal-Nate™ | 2700 | 3 | 3.4 | 20 | | 120 | 400 | 30 | Ca 125 mg, Cu 2 mg, Fe 27 mg, folic acid 1 mg, odine 150 mcg, niacinamide 20 mg, Zn 25 mg; docusate calcium 50 mg |
| Citracal® Prenatal Rx | 2700 | 3 | 3.4 | 20 | | 120 | 400 | 30 | Ca 125 mg, Cu 2 mg, Fe 27 mg, folic acid 1 mg, iodine 150 mcg, niacinamide 20 mg, Zn 25 mg; docusate sodium 50 mg |
| Duet® | 3000 | 1.8 | 4 | 25 | 12 | 120 | 400 | 30 | Ca 200 mg, Cu 2 mg, Fe 29 mg, folic acid 1 mg, Mg 25 mg, niacinamide 20 mg, Zn 25 mg |
| KPN Prenatal | 2666.6 | 2 | 2 | 1 | 2 | 33.3 | 133.3 | 10 | Ca 333.3 mg, biotin 10 mcg, Cu 0.1 mg, Fe 9 mg, folic acid 266.6 mcg, Mg 33.3 mg, Mn 0.1 mg, niacinamide 10 mg, pantothenic acid 5 mg, Zn 7.5 mg |
| NatalCare® CFe 60 [DSC] | 1000 | 2 | 3 | 10 | 12 | 120 | 400 | 11 | Fe 60 mg, folic acid 1 mg, niacinamide 20 mg |
| NatalCare® GlossTabs™ | 2700 | 3 | 3.4 | 20 | 12 | 120 | 400 | 10 | Biotin 30 mcg, Ca 200 mg, Cu 2 mg, Fe 90 mg, folic acid 1 mg, Mg 30 mg, niacinamide 20 mg, pantothenic acid 6 mg, Zn 15 mg; docusate sodium 50 mg |
| NatalCare® PIC | 4000 | 2.43 | 3 | 1.64 | 3 | 50 | 400 | | Ca 125 mg, folic acid 1 mg, niacinamide 10 mg, polysaccharide-iron complex 60 mg, Zn 18 mg |
| NatalCare® PIC Forte | 5000 | 3 | 3.4 | 4 | 12 | 80 | 400 | 30 | Ca 250 mg, Cu 2 mg, folic acid 1 mg, iodine 200 mcg, Mg 10 mg, niacinamide 20 mg, polysaccharide-iron complex 60 mg, Zn 25 mg |
| NatalCare® Plus | 4000 | 1.84 | 3 | 10 | 12 | 120 | 400 | 22 | Ca 200 mg, Cu 2 mg, Fe 27 mg, folic acid 1 mg, niacinamide 20 mg, Zn 25 mg |
| NatalCare® Rx | 2000 | 0.75 | 0.8 | 2 | 1.25 | 40 | 200 | 7.5 | Biotin 15 mcg, Ca 100 mg, Cu 1.5 mg, folate 0.5 mg, Fe 27 mg, Mg 50 mg, niacin 8.5 mg, pantothenic acid 3.75 mg, Zn 12.5 mg |
| NatalCare® Three | 3000 | 1.8 | 4 | 25 | 12 | 120 | 400 | 22 | Ca 200 mg, Cu 2 mg, Fe 28 mg, folic acid 1 mg, Mg 25 mg, niacinamide 20 mg, Zn 25 mg |
| NataFort® | 1000 | 2 | 3 | 10 | 12 | 120 | 400 | 11 | Fe 60 mg, folic acid 1 mg, niacinamide 20 mg |

*(continued)*

| Product | A (int. units) | B$_1$ (mg) | B$_2$ (mg) | B$_6$ (mg) | B$_{12}$ (mcg) | C (mg) | D (int. units) | E (int. units) | Additional Information |
|---|---|---|---|---|---|---|---|---|---|
| NataTab™ CFe | 4000 | 3 | 3 | 3 | 8 | 120 | 400 | 30 | Ca 200 mg, Fe 50 mg, folic acid 1 mg, iodine#150 mcg, niacin 20 mg, Zn 15 mg |
| NataTab™ FA | 4000 | 3 | 3 | 6 | 8 | 120 | 400 | 30 | Ca 200 mg, Fe 29 mg, folic acid 1 mg, iodine 150 mcg, niacin 20 mg, Zn 15 mg |
| NataTab™ Rx | 4000 | 3 | 3 | 3 | 8 | 120 | 400 | 30 | Biotin 30 mcg, Ca 200 mg, Cu 3 mg, Fe 29 mg, folic acid 1 mg, iodine 150 mcg, Mg 100 mg, niacin 20 mg, pantothenic acid 7 mg, Zn 15 mg |
| Nestabs® CBF | 4000 | 3 | 3 | 3 | 8 | 120 | 400 | 30 | Ca 200 mg, Fe 50 mg, folic acid 1 mg, iodine 150 mcg, niacin 20 mg, Zn 15 mg |
| Nestabs® FA | 4000 | 3 | 3 | 3 | 8 | 120 | 400 | 30 | Ca 200 mg, Fe 29 mg, folic acid 1 mg, iodine 150 mcg, niacin 20 mg, Zn 15 mg |
| Nestabs® RX | 4000 | 3 | 3 | 3 | 8 | 120 | 400 | 30 | Biotin 30 mcg, Ca 200 mg, Cu 3 mg, Fe 29 mg, folic acid 1 mg, iodine 150 mcg, Mg 100 mg, niacin 20 mg, pantothenic acid 7 mg, Zn 15 mg |
| Niferex®-PN | 4000 | 2.43 | 3 | 1.64 | 3 | 50 | 400 |  | Ca 125 mg, folic acid 1 mg, niacinamide 10 mg, polysaccharide-iron complex 60 mg, Zn 18 mg |
| Niferex®-PN Forte | 5000 | 3 | 3.4 | 4 | 12 | 80 | 400 | 30 | Ca 250 mg, Cu 2 mg, folic acid 1 mg, iodine 200 mcg, Mg 10 mg, niacinamide 20 mg, polysaccharide-iron complex 60 mg, Zn 25 mg |
| OB-20 | 2000 | 43 | 0.5 | 2.5 | 2 | 30 | 100 | 15 | Biotin 37.5 mcg, Ca 125 mg, Cr 6.25 mcg, Fe 12.5 mg, folic acid 2.5 mg, Mg 37.5 mg, Mn 1.25 mg, niacinamide 5 mg, pantothenic acid 2.5 mg, Se 6.25 mcg, Zn 6.2 mg |
| PreCare® Conceive™ |  | 3 | 3.4 | 50 | 12 | 60 |  | 30 | Ca 200 mg, Cu 2 mg, Fe 30 mg, folic acid 1 mg, Mg 100 mg, niacinamide 20 mg, Zn 15 mg |
| Prenatal 1-A-Day | 4000 | 2 | 3 | 3 | 10 | 100 | 400 | 15 | Biotin 100 mcg, Ca 200 mg, Cu 2 mg, Fe 27 mg, folic acid 800 mcg, Mg 60 mg, Mn 2 mg, niacinamide 20 mg, pantothenic acid 10 mg, Zn 15 mg |
| Prenatal AD | 2700 | 3 | 3.4 | 12 | 120 | 120 | 400 | 30 | Ca 200 mg, Cu 2 mg, Fe 90 mg, folic acid 1 mg, Mg 30 mg, niacinamide 20 mg, Zn 25 mg; docusate sodium 50 mg |

*(continued)*

| Product | A (int. units) | B$_1$ (mg) | B$_2$ (mg) | B$_6$ (mg) | B$_{12}$ (mcg) | C (mg) | D (int. units) | E (int. units) | Additional Information |
|---|---|---|---|---|---|---|---|---|---|
| Prenatal MR 90 Fe™ | 4000 | 3 | 3.4 | 20 | 12 | 120 | 400 | 30 | Ca 250 mg, Cu 2 mg, Fe 90 mg, folic acid 1 mg, iodine 150 mcg, niacinamide 20 mg, Zn 25 mg; docusate sodium 50 mg |
| Prenatal MRT with Selenium | 5000 | 3 | 3.4 | 10 | 12 | 120 | 400 | 30 | Biotin 30 mcg, Ca 200 mg, Cr 25 mcg, Cu 2 mg, Fe 27 mg, folic acid 1 mg, iodine 150 mcg, Mg 25 mg, Mn 5 mg, Mo 25 mcg, niacinamide 20 mg, pantothenic acid 10 mg, Se 20 mcg, Zn 25 mg |
| Prenatal Plus | 4000 | 1.8 | 3 | 10 | 12 | 120 | 400 | 22 | Ca 200 mg, Cu 2 mg, Fe 27 mg, folic acid 1 mg, niacinamide 20 mg, Zn 25 mg |
| Prenatal Rx 1 | 4000 | 1.5 | 1.6 | 4 | 2.5 | 80 | 400 | 15 | Biotin 30 mcg, Ca 200 mg, Cu 3 mg, Fe 60 mg, folic acid 1 mg, Mg 100 mg, niacinamide 17 mg, pantothenic acid 7 mg, Zn 25 mg |
| Prenatal Z | 3000 | 1.5 | 1.6 | 2.2 | 2.2 | 70 | 400 | 10 | Ca 200 mg, Fe 65 mg, folic acid 1 mg, iodine 175 mcg, Mg 100 mg, niacin 17 mg, Zn 15 mg |
| Prenate Elite™ | | 3 | 3.4 | 20 | 12 | 120 | 400 | 10 | Biotin 300 mcg, Ca 200 mg, Cu 2 mg, Fe 90 mg, folate 1 mg, Mg 30 mg, niacinamide 20 mg, pantothenic acid 6 mg, Zn 15 mg; docusate sodium 50 mg |
| Prenate GT™ | 2700 | 3 | 3.4 | 20 | 12 | 120 | 400 | 10 | Biotin 30 mcg, Ca 200 mg, Cu 2 mg, Fe 90 mg, folic acid 1 mg, Mg 30 mg, niacinamide 20 mg, pantothenic acid 6 mg, Zn 15 mg; docusate sodium 50 mg |
| Stuartnatal® Plus 3™ | 3000 | 1.8 | 4 | 25 | 12 | 120 | 400 | 22 | Ca 200 mg, Cu 2 mg, Fe 28 mg, folic acid 1 mg, Mg 25 mg, niacinamide 20 mg, Zn 25 mg |
| Stuart Prenatal® | 4000 | 1.8 | 1.7 | 2.6 | 8 | 120 | 400 | 30 | Ca 200 mg, Fe 28 mg, folic acid 0.8 mg, niacin 20 mg, Zn 25 mg |
| Trinate | 3000 | 1.8 | 4 | 25 | 12 | 120 | 400 | 22 | Ca 200 mg, Cu 2 mg, Fe 28 mg, folic acid 1 mg, Mg 25 mg, niacin 20 mg, Zn 25 mg |

*(continued)*

| Product | A (int. units) | B₁ (mg) | B₂ (mg) | B₆ (mg) | B₁₂ (mcg) | C (mg) | D (int. units) | E (int. units) | Additional Information |
|---|---|---|---|---|---|---|---|---|---|
| Ultra NatalCare® | 2700 | 3 | 3.4 | 20 | 12 | 120 | 400 | 30 | Ca 200 mg, Cu 2 mg, Fe 90 mg, folic acid 1 mg, iodine 150 mcg, niacinamide 20 mg, Zn 25 mg; docusate sodium 50 mg |
| **Tablet, Chewable** | | | | | | | | | |
| Duet® | 3000 | 1.8 | 4 | 25 | 12 | 120 | 400 | 30 | Ca 100 mg, Cu 2 mg, Fe 29 mg, folic acid 1 mg, Mg 25 mg, niacinamide 20 mg, Zn 25 mg; **phenylalanine 15 mg/tablet** |
| NataChew™ | 1000 | 2 | 3 | 10 | 12 | 120 | 400 | 11 | Fe 29 mg, folic acid 1 mg, niacinamide 20 mg; peanut extract, wild berry flavor |
| NutriNate® | 1000 | 2 | 3 | 10 | 12 | 120 | 400 | 11 | Fe 29 mg, folic acid 1 mg, niacinamide 20 mg; wild berry flavor |
| PreCare® | | | | 2 | | 50 | 6 mcg | 3.5 mg | Ca 250 mg, Cu 2 mg, Fe 40 mg, folic acid 1 mg, Mg 50 mg, Zn 15 mg |
| StrongStart™ | 1000 | 1 | 3 | 20 | 15 | 100 | 400 | 30 | Ca 200 mg, Fe 29 mg, folic acid 1 mg, niacinamide 15 mg, pantothenic acid 7 mg, Zn 20 mg; **phenylalanine 6 mg/tablet** |
| **Combination Package** | | | | | | | | | |
| CareNate™ 600 (tablet) | 3500 | 2 | 3 | 3 | 12 | 60 | 400 | 30 | Cu 2 mg, Fe 60 mg, folic acid 1 mg, Mg 25 mg, Zn 20 mg; dioctylsulfosuccinate sodium 50 mg Packaged with chewable tablets containing Ca 600 mg; wild berry flavor |
| Duet™ DHA (tablet) | 3000 | 1.8 | 4 | 25 | 12 | 120 | 400 | 30 | Ca 200 mg, Cu 2 mg, Fe 29 mg, folic acid 1 mg, Mg 25 mg, niacinamide 20 mg, Zn 25 mg Packaged with capsules containing Omega-3 fatty acids ≥ DHA 200 mg |

Key: Ca = calcium, Cr = chromium, Cu = copper, Fe = iron, Mg = magnesium, Mn = manganese, Mo = molybdenum, Se = selenium, Zn = zinc.

## Vitamin B Complex Combinations

| Product | B₁ (mg) | B₂ (mg) | B₆ (mg) | B₁₂ (mcg) | C (mg) | E (int. units) | Additional Information |
|---|---|---|---|---|---|---|---|
| **Caplet** | | | | | | | |
| Allbee® with C [OTC] | 15 | 10.2 | 5 | | 300 | | Niacinamide 50 mg, pantothenic acid 10 mg |
| Allbee® C-800 [OTC] | 15 | 17 | 25 | 12 | 800 | 45 | Niacinamide 100 mg, pantothenic acid 25 mg |
| Allbee® C-800 + Iron [OTC] | 15 | 17 | 25 | 12 | 800 | 45 | Fe 27 mg, folic acid 0.4 mcg, niacinamide 100 mg, pantothenic acid 25 mg |
| **Capsule** | | | | | | | |
| Trinsicon® | | | | 15 | | | C 75 mg, Fe 110 mg, folic acid 0.5 mg, liver-stomach concentrate (containing intrinsic factor and other vitamin B complex factors) 240 mg |
| **Liquid** | | | | | | | |
| Apatate® [OTC] (per 5 mL) | 15 | | 0.5 | 25 | | | Cherry flavor (120 mL) |
| Gevrabon® [OTC] (per 30 mL) | 5 | 2.5 | 1 | 1 | | | Choline 10 mg, Fe 15 mg, iodine 100 mcg, Mg 2 mg, Mn 2 mg, niacinamide 60 mg, pantothenic acid 10 mg, Zn 2 mg; alcohol, benzoic acid; sherry wine flavor (480 mL) |
| **Softgel** | | | | | | | |
| Nephrocaps® | 1.5 | 1.7 | 10 | 6 | 100 | | Biotin 150 mcg, folic acid 1 mcg, niacinamide 20 mg, pantothenic acid 5 mg |

*(continued)*

| Product | B₁ (mg) | B₂ (mg) | B₆ (mg) | B₁₂ (mcg) | C (mg) | E (int. units) | Additional Information |
|---|---|---|---|---|---|---|---|
| **Tablet** | | | | | | | |
| Diatx™ | 1.5 | 1.5 | 50 | | 60 | | Biotin 300 mcg, cobalamin 1 mg, folacin 5 mg, niacinamide 20 mg, pantothenic acid 10 mg [dye free, lactose free, sugar free] |
| DiatxFe™ | 1.5 | 1.5 | 50 | | 60 | | Biotin 300 mcg, cobalamin 1 mg, ferrous fumarate 304 mg, folacin 5 mg, niacinamide 20 mg, pantothenic acid 10 mg [dye free, lactose free, sugar free] |
| NephPlex® Rx | 1.5 | 1.7 | 10 | 6 | 60 | | Biotin 300 mcg, folic acid 1 mg, niacinamide 20 mg, pantothenic acid 10 mg, zinc 12.5 mg |
| Nephro-Vite® | 1.5 | 1.7 | 10 | 6 | 60 | | Biotin 300 mcg, folic acid 0.8 mcg, niacinamide 20 mg, pantothenic acid 10 mg |
| Nephro-Vite® Rx | 1.5 | 1.7 | 10 | 6 | 60 | | Biotin 300 mcg, folic acid 1 mcg, niacinamide 20 mg, pantothenic acid 10 mg |
| Nephron FA® | 1.5 | 1.7 | 10 | 6 | 40 | | Biotin 300 mcg, docusate sodium 75 mg, ferrous fumarate 200 mg, folic acid 1 mg, pantothenic acid 10 mg |
| Olay® Vitamins Essential Folic Acid w/B₁₂ Complex [OTC] | | 25 | 25 | 200 | | 200 | Folic acid 600 mcg, Se 50 mcg |
| Olay® Vitamins Super B-Stress Defense [OTC] | 10 | 10 | 5 | 12 | 500 | 30 | Biotin 100 mcg, folic acid 400 mcg, niacin 100 mg, pantothenic acid 20 mg |
| Stresstabs® B-Complex [OTC] | 10 | 10 | 5 | 12 | 500 | 30 | Biotin 45 mcg, folic acid 0.4 mcg, niacinamide 100 mg, pantothenic acid 20 mg |
| Stresstabs® B-Complex + Iron [OTC] | 10 | 10 | 5 | 12 | 500 | 30 | Biotin 45 mcg, Fe 18 mg, folic acid 0.4 mcg, niacinamide 100 mg, pantothenic acid 20 mg |
| Stresstabs® B-Complex + Zinc [OTC] | 10 | 10 | 5 | 12 | 500 | 30 | Biotin 45 mcg, Cu 3 mg, folic acid 0.4 mcg, niacinamide 100 mg, pantothenic acid 20 mg, Zn 23.9 mg |
| Surbex-T® [OTC] | 15 | 10 | 5 | 10 | 500 | | Ca 20 mg, niacinamide 100 mg |
| Z-Bec® [OTC] | 15 | 10.2 | 10 | 6 | 600 | 45 | Niacinamide 100 mg, pantothenic acid 25 mg, Zn 22.5 mg |
| **Tablet, Chewable** | | | | | | | |
| Apatate® [OTC] | 15 | | 0.5 | 25 | | | Cherry flavor |

Key: Ca = calcium, Cr = chromium, Cu = copper, Fe = iron, Mg = magnesium, Mn = manganese, Mo = molybdenum, Se = selenium, Zn = zinc

# INDICATION / THERAPEUTIC CATEGORY INDEX

## ACROMEGALY

## ACUTE CORONARY SYNDROME

## ADAMS-STOKES SYNDROME

## ADDISON DISEASE

## ADENOSINE DEAMINASE DEFICIENCY

## ADRENOCORTICAL FUNCTION ABNORMALITIES

## AGE-RELATED MACULAR DEGENERATION (AMD)

## ALCOHOL DEPENDENCE

## ANESTHESIA (GENERAL)

## ANESTHESIA (LOCAL)

## Local Anesthetic, Amide Derivative

## Local Anesthetic, Injectable

# ANESTHESIA (OPHTHALMIC)

## Local Anesthetic

# ANGINA PECTORIS

## Antilipemic Agent, HMG-CoA Reductase Inhibitor

## Antiplatelet Agent

## Beta-Adrenergic Blocker

## ANGIOEDEMA (HEREDITARY)

## ANGIOGRAPHY (OPHTHALMIC)

## ANTHRAX

### Cardiac Glycoside

### Cholinergic Agent

### Hydantoin

### Theophylline Derivative

## ARSENIC POISONING

### Chelating Agent

## ARTHRITIS

### Analgesic, Nonnarcotic

## Analgesic, Topical

## Antiinflammatory Agent

## Antineoplastic Agent

## Antirheumatic, Disease Modifying

## Chelating Agent

## Gastric Acid Secretion Inhibitor

## Gold Compound

## Immunosuppressant Agent

## Monoclonal Antibody

## Nonsteroidal Antiinflammatory Drug (NSAID)

## Gastric Acid Secretion Inhibitor

## Nonsteroidal Antiinflammatory Drug (NSAID)

# CACHEXIA

## Antineoplastic Agent

## Vitamin

## Vitamin, Fat Soluble

# CEREBRAL PALSY

## Skeletal Muscle Relaxant

# CEREBROVASCULAR ACCIDENT (CVA)

## Antiplatelet Agent

## Fibrinolytic Agent

## Nonsteroidal Antiinflammatory Drug (NSAID)

# CHICKENPOX

## Antiviral Agent

## Vaccine, Live Virus

## COLITIS (ULCERATIVE)

### 5-Aminosalicylic Acid Derivative

### Antiinflammatory Agent

## COLLAGEN DISORDERS

### Adrenal Corticosteroid

## COLONIC EVACUATION

### Laxative

## CONDYLOMA ACUMINATUM

### Antiviral Agent

### Biological Response Modulator

### Immune Response Modifier

### Keratolytic Agent

## CONGENITAL SUCRASE-ISOMALTASE DEFICIENCY

### Enzyme

## CONGESTION (NASAL)

### Adrenergic Agonist Agent

## Antihistamine

# CONJUNCTIVITIS (ALLERGIC)

**Laxative, Stimulant**

**Stool Softener**

## CONTRACEPTION

### Contraceptive

### Contraceptive, Implant (Progestin)

### Contraceptive, Oral

## Contraceptive, Progestin Only

## Estrogen and Progestin Combination

## Progestin

## Spermicide

# COPROPORPHYRIA

## Antiarrhythmic Agent, Class II

## Beta-Adrenergic Blocker

# CORNEAL EDEMA

## Lubricant, Ocular

# COUGH

## Antihistamine

## Antihistamine/Antitussive

## Antihistamine/Decongestant/Antitussive

## Antihistamine/Decongestant Combination

## Antitussive

## Antitussive/Decongestant

## Antitussive/Decongestant/Expectorant

## DEBRIDEMENT OF CALLOUS TISSUE

### Keratolytic Agent

## DEBRIDEMENT OF ESCHAR

### Protectant, Topical

## DECUBITUS ULCERS

### Enzyme

### Enzyme, Topical Debridement

### Protectant, Topical

### Topical Skin Product

## DEEP VEIN THROMBOSIS (DVT)

### Anticoagulant (Other)

### Factor Xa Inhibitor

### Low Molecular Weight Heparin

## DEMENTIA

### Acetylcholinesterase Inhibitor

### Antidepressant, Tricyclic (Tertiary Amine)

### Benzodiazepine

### Cholinergic Agent

### Ergot Alkaloid and Derivative

### Phenothiazine Derivative

### Topical Skin Product

## DENTAL CARIES (PREVENTION)

### Mineral, Oral

## DEPRESSION

### Antidepressant

### Antidepressant, Alpha-2 Antagonist

### Antidepressant, Aminoketone

### Antidepressant, Miscellaneous

### Antidepressant, Monoamine Oxidase Inhibitor

### Antidepressant, Phenethylamine

### Antidepressant/Phenothiazine

### Antidepressant, Selective Serotonin Reuptake Inhibitor

### Antidepressant, Serotonin/Norepinephrine Reuptake Inhibitor

### Antidepressant, Tetracyclic

### Antidepressant, Triazolopyridine

### Antidepressant, Tricyclic (Secondary Amine)

### Antidepressant, Tricyclic (Tertiary Amine)

### Antipsychotic Agent, Thienobenzodiaepine

### Benzodiazepine

## DEPRESSION (RESPIRATORY)

### Respiratory Stimulant

## DERMATITIS

### Antidepressant, Tricyclic (Tertiary Amine)

### Antipsoriatic Agent

### Antiseborrheic Agent, Topical

### Dietary Supplement

### Topical Skin Product

## DERMATOLOGIC DISORDERS

### Adrenal Corticosteroid

## DERMATOMYCOSIS

### Antifungal Agent

## DERMATOSIS

### Adrenal Corticosteroid

### Anesthetic/Corticosteroid

### Antibiotic, Topical

## Corticosteroid, Topical

## DIABETES INSIPIDUS

### Hormone, Posterior Pituitary

### Vasopressin Analog, Synthetic

## DIABETES MELLITUS, INSULIN-DEPENDENT (IDDM)

### Antidiabetic Agent

### Antidiabetic Agent, Parenteral

## DIABETES MELLITUS, NONINSULIN-DEPENDENT (NIDDM)

### Antidiabetic Agent

### Antidiabetic Agent, Incretin Mimetic

### Antidiabetic Agent, Oral

## DRY MOUTH

### Gastrointestinal Agent, Miscellaneous

## DRY SKIN

### Topical Skin Product

### Vitamin, Fat Soluble

### Vitamin, Topical

## DUCTUS ARTERIOSUS (CLOSURE)

### Nonsteroidal Antiinflammatory Drug (NSAID)

## DUCTUS ARTERIOSUS (TEMPORARY MAINTENANCE OF PATENCY)

### Prostaglandin

## DUODENAL ULCER

### Antacid

### Antibiotic, Macrolide Combination

### Antibiotic, Penicillin

### Antiflatulent

### Electrolyte Supplement, Oral

### Gastric Acid Secretion Inhibitor

### Nonsteroidal Antiinflammatory Drug (NSAID), COX-2 Selective

## DYSTONIA

### Neuromuscular Blocker Agent, Toxin

## DYSURIA

### Analgesic, Urinary

### Antispasmodic Agent, Urinary

## EAR WAX

### Otic Agent, Analgesic

### Otic Agent, Ceruminolytic

## EATON-LAMBERT SYNDROME

### Cholinergic Agent

## ECLAMPSIA

### Anticonvulsant

### Barbiturate

### Benzodiazepine

## ECZEMA

### Adrenal Corticosteroid

### Antifungal/Corticosteroid

### Corticosteroid, Intranasal

### Corticosteroid, Topical

## EDEMA

### Antihypertensive Agent, Combination

### Diuretic, Combination

### Diuretic, Loop

## Contraceptive, Progestin Only

## Hormone, Posterior Pituitary

## Progestin

# END-STAGE RENAL DISEASE (ESRD)

## Phosphate Binder

# ENURESIS

## Antidepressant, Tricyclic (Tertiary Amine)

## Antispasmodic Agent, Urinary

## Vasopressin Analog, Synthetic

# EPICONDYLITIS

## Analgesic, Nonnarcotic

## Gastric Acid Secretion Inhibitor

## Nonsteroidal Antiinflammatory Drug (NSAID)

## EPIDERMAL GROWTH FACTOR RECEPTOR (EGFR)

### Antineoplastic Agent, Monoclonal Antibody

### Epidermal Growth Factor Receptor (EGFR) Inhibitor

## EPILEPSY

### Anticonvulsant

### Anticonvulsant, Miscellaneous

### Anticonvulsant, Sulfonamide

### Barbiturate

## Antibiotic, Ophthalmic

# EYE IRRITATION

## Adrenergic Agonist Agent

## Ophthalmic Agent, Miscellaneous

## EYELID INFECTION

### Antibiotic, Ophthalmic

### Pharmaceutical Aid

## FABRY DISEASE

### Enzyme

## FACTOR VIII DEFICIENCY

### Blood Product Derivative

### Hemophilic Agent

## FACTOR IX DEFICIENCY

### Antihemophilic Agent

## FAMILIAL ADENOMATOUS POLYPOSIS

### Nonsteroidal Antiinflammatory Drug (NSAID), COX-2 Selective

## FATTY ACID DEFICIENCY

### Intravenous Nutritional Therapy

### Nutritional Supplement

## FEBRILE NEUTROPENIA

### Colony-Stimulating Factor

## Quinolone

## FEVER

### Antipyretic

## FIBROCYSTIC BREAST DISEASE

### Androgen

## FIBROCYSTIC DISEASE

### Vitamin, Fat Soluble

### Vitamin, Topical

## FIBROMYOSITIS

### Antidepressant, Tricyclic (Tertiary Amine)

## FOLLICLE STIMULATION

### Ovulation Stimulator

## FUNGUS (DIAGNOSTIC)

### Diagnostic Agent

## GAG REFLEX SUPPRESSION

### Analgesic, Topical

### Local Anesthetic

## GALACTORRHEA

### Anti-Parkinson Agent

### Ergot Alkaloid and Derivative

## GALL BLADDER DISEASE (DIAGNOSTIC)

### Diagnostic Agent

## GAS PAINS

### Antiflatulent

## GASTRIC ULCER

### Antacid

### Antiflatulent

### Histamine H₂ Antagonist

### Prostaglandin

## GASTRITIS

### Antacid

### Histamine H₂ Antagonist

## GASTROESOPHAGEAL REFLUX DISEASE (GERD)

### Cholinergic Agent

### Gastric Acid Secretion Inhibitor

### Gastrointestinal Agent, Prokinetic

### Histamine H₂ Antagonist

## GOUT

### Antigout Agent

### Nonsteroidal Antiinflammatory Drug (NSAID)

### Uricosuric Agent

### Xanthine Oxidase Inhibitor

## GRAFT VS HOST DISEASE

### Immunosuppressant Agent

## GRAM-NEGATIVE INFECTION

### Acne Products

### Aminoglycoside (Antibiotic)

## HEADACHE (VASCULAR)

### Analgesic, Nonnarcotic

### Antiarrhythmic Agent, Class II

## HYPERLIPIDEMIA

### Antihyperlipidemic Agent, Miscellaneous

### Antilipemic Agent, HMG-CoA Reductase Inhibitor

### Bile Acid Sequestrant

### HMG-CoA Reductase Inhibitor

### Vitamin, Water Soluble

## HYPERMAGNESEMIA

### Diuretic, Loop

### Electrolyte Supplement, Oral

## HYPERMENORRHEA (TREATMENT)

### Contraceptive, Oral

### Contraceptive, Progestin Only

## HYPERPARATHYROIDISM

### Calcimimetic

### Vitamin D Analog

## HYPERPHOSPHATEMIA

### Electrolyte Supplement, Oral

### Phosphate Binder

## HYPERPIGMENTATION

### Topical Skin Product

## HYPERPLASIA, VULVAR SQUAMOUS

### Estrogen Derivative

## HYPERPROLACTINEMIA

### Anti-Parkinson Agent

### Ergot Alkaloid and Derivative

### Ergot-like Derivative

## HYPERTENSION

### Adrenergic Agonist Agent

## Beta-Adrenergic Blocker

## Calcium Channel Blocker

## Diagnostic Agent

## Diuretic, Combination

## INFLAMMATORY BOWEL DISEASE

### 5-Aminosalicylic Acid Derivative

## INFLUENZA

### Antiviral Agent

### Antiviral Agent, Inhalation Therapy

### Antiviral Agent, Oral

### Vaccine, Inactivated Virus

## INFLUENZA A

### Antiviral Agent

## INSOMNIA

### Anticonvulsant

### Antihistamine

### Barbiturate

### Benzodiazepine

### Hypnotic

## Vitamin, Fat Soluble

## Vitamin, Topical

## Vitamin, Water Soluble

# MALODORS

## Gastrointestinal Agent, Miscellaneous

# MANIA

## Anticonvulsant

## Antimanic Agent

## Phenothiazine Derivative

# MAPLE SYRUP URINE DISEASE

## Vitamin, Water Soluble

# MARFAN SYNDROME

## Rauwolfia Alkaloid

# MAROTEAUX-LAMY SYNDROME

## Enzyme

## Antihypertensive Agent, Combination

## Antineoplastic Agent

## Diuretic, Loop

## Diuretic, Miscellaneous

## Diuretic, Thiazide

## Immunosuppressant Agent

# NEPHROTOXICITY (CISPLATIN-INDUCED)

## Antidote

# NERVE BLOCK

## Analgesic, Topical

## Local Anesthetic

## NEUROGENIC BLADDER

### Antispasmodic Agent, Urinary

## NEUROLOGIC DISEASE

### Adrenal Corticosteroid

## NEUTROPENIA

### Colony-Stimulating Factor

## NIPPLE CARE

### Topical Skin Product

## NOCTURIA

### Antispasmodic Agent, Urinary

## OBESITY

### Amphetamine

### Anorexiant

### Lipase Inhibitor

## OBSESSIVE-COMPULSIVE DISORDER (OCD)

### Antidepressant, Selective Serotonin Reuptake Inhibitor

### Antidepressant, Tricyclic (Tertiary Amine)

## OPHTHALMIC SURGICAL AID

### Ophthalmic Agent, Miscellaneous

## OPIATE WITHDRAWAL (NEONATAL)

### Analgesic, Narcotic

## OPIOID DEPENDENCE

### Analgesic, Narcotic

## OPIOID POISONING

### Antidote

## ORGANOPHOSPHATE PESTICIDE POISONING

### Anticholinergic Agent

### Antidote

## ORGAN REJECTION

### Immunosuppressant Agent

## ORGAN TRANSPLANT

### Immunosuppressant Agent

## OSTEOARTHRITIS

### Analgesic, Nonnarcotic

## Analgesic, Topical

## Gastric Acid Secretion Inhibitor

## Nonsteroidal Antiinflammatory Drug (NSAID)

## Nonsteroidal Antiinflammatory Drug (NSAID), COX-2 Selective

## Prostaglandin

## OSTEODYSTROPHY

### Vitamin D Analog

# OVARIAN FAILURE

## Estrogen and Androgen Combination

## Estrogen and Progestin Combination

## Estrogen Derivative

# OVERACTIVE BLADDER

## Anticholinergic Agent

# OVULATION INDUCTION

## Gonadotropin

## Ovulation Stimulator

# PAGET DISEASE OF BONE

## Bisphosphonate Derivative

## Polypeptide Hormone

# PAIN

## Analgesic Combination (Narcotic)

## Analgesic, Miscellaneous

## Analgesic, Narcotic

## Analgesic, Nonnarcotic

## Calcium Channel Blocker, N-Type

## PAIN (ANOGENITAL)

### Anesthetic/Corticosteroid

### Local Anesthetic

## PAIN (BONE)

### Radiopharmaceutical

## PAIN (DIABETIC NEUROPATHY NEURALGIA)

### Analgesic, Topical

## PAIN (LUMBAR PUNCTURE)

### Analgesic, Topical

## PAIN (MUSCLE)

### Analgesic, Topical

## PAIN (SKIN GRAFT HARVESTING)

### Analgesic, Topical

## PAIN (VENIPUNCTURE)

### Analgesic, Topical

## PANCREATIC EXOCRINE INSUFFICIENCY

### Enzyme

## PANCREATIC EXOCRINE INSUFFICIENCY (DIAGNOSTIC)

### Diagnostic Agent

## PANCREATITIS

### Anticholinergic Agent

## PANIC ATTACKS

### Benzodiazepine

## PANIC DISORDER (PD)

### Antidepressant, Selective Serotonin Reuptake Inhibitor

## PARACOCCIDIOIDOMYCOSIS

### Antifungal Agent

## PARALYTIC ILEUS (PROPHYLAXIS)

### Gastrointestinal Agent, Stimulant

## PARKINSONISM

### Anti-Parkinson Agent

### Anti-Parkinson Agent, COMT Inhibitor

### Antiviral Agent

### Dopaminergic Agent (Anti-Parkinson)

## PLAGUE

### Antibiotic, Aminoglycoside

### Antitubercular Agent

### Vaccine, Inactivated Bacteria

## PLANTARIS

### Keratolytic Agent

## PLANTAR WARTS

### Topical Skin Product

## PLATELET AGGREGATION (PROPHYLAXIS)

### Antiplatelet Agent

### Vasodilator

## PNEUMOCYSTIS CARINII

### Antibiotic, Miscellaneous

### Antiprotozoal

### Sulfonamide

### Sulfone

## PNEUMONIA

### Aminoglycoside (Antibiotic)

### Antibiotic, Carbapenem

### Antibiotic, Ketolide

### Antibiotic, Miscellaneous

## PNEUMONIA, COMMUNITY-ACQUIRED

### Antibiotic, Quinolone

## POISON IVY

### Protectant, Topical

## POISON OAK

### Protectant, Topical

## POISON SUMAC

### Protectant, Topical

## POLIOMYELITIS

### Vaccine, Live Virus and Inactivated Virus

## POLYCYTHEMIA VERA

### Antineoplastic Agent

## POLYMYOSITIS

### Antineoplastic Agent

### Immunosuppressant Agent

## POLYPS, NASAL

### Adrenal Corticosteroid

## PSEUDOGOUT

## PSEUDOHYPOPARATHYROIDISM

## PSORIASIS

## Immunosuppressant Agent

## Keratolytic Agent

## RESPIRATORY DISTRESS SYNDROME (RDS)

### Lung Surfactant

## RESPIRATORY SYNCYTIAL VIRUS (RSV)

### Antiviral Agent

### Monoclonal Antibody

## RESPIRATORY TRACT INFECTION

### Aminoglycoside (Antibiotic)

### Antibiotic, Carbacephem

### Antibiotic, Macrolide

### Antibiotic, Miscellaneous

### Antibiotic, Penicillin

### Antibiotic, Quinolone

### Cephalosporin (First Generation)

### Cephalosporin (Second Generation)

### Cephalosporin (Third Generation)

## ROUNDWORMS

### Anthelmintic

## RUBELLA

### Vaccine, Live Virus

## SALIVATION (EXCESSIVE)

### Anticholinergic Agent

## SARCOIDOSIS

### Corticosteroid, Topical

## Antiseborrheic Agent, Topical

## Keratolytic Agent

## SKIN PROTECTANT

**Pharmaceutical Aid**

**Protectant, Topical**

## SKIN ULCER

**Enzyme**

## SLEEPING SICKNESS

**Antiprotozoal**

**Topical Skin Product**

## SMALLPOX

**Vaccine**

## SMOKING CESSATION

**Antidepressant, Monoamine Oxidase Inhibitor**

**Smoking Deterrent**

## SOFT TISSUE INFECTION

**Aminoglycoside (Antibiotic)**

**Antibiotic, Carbacephem**

**Antibiotic, Carbapenem**

**Antibiotic, Miscellaneous**

**Antifungal Agent, Topical**

**Antifungal/Corticosteroid**

**Antiseborrheic Agent, Topical**

**Disinfectant**

# TISSUE GRAFT

## Immunosuppressant Agent

# TOOTHACHE

## Local Anesthetic

# TOPICAL ANESTHESIA

## Local Anesthetic

## TOURETTE DISEASE

### Antipsychotic Agent, Butyrophenone

### Neuroleptic Agent

### Phenothiazine Derivative

## TOXICITY, NONSPECIFIC (TREATMENT)

### Antacid

### Antidote

### Diuretic, Osmotic

### Electrolyte Supplement, Oral

### Laxative

## Laxative

## Prostaglandin

# ZOLLINGER-ELLISON SYNDROME (DIAGNOSTIC)

## Diagnostic Agent

# QUICK LOOK DRUG BOOK

## Image Guide to Tablets and Capsules

The Quick Look Drug Book 2006 image insert displays actual color photographs of the most commonly prescribed tablets and capsules.

Drugs are listed alphabetically by generic name, and, where applicable, the trade name is listed. Dosages appear under each individual image.

Use the white scale at the bottom of each image to determine the actual size. The distance between each division on the scale is equivalent to 1/8 inch or 3.175 mm.

## Acetaminophen and Codeine

### (generic)

300/15 mg     300/30 mg

300/60 mg

## Acetaminophen and Tramadol

### Ultracet™

37.5  mg

## Acyclovir

### (generic)

200 mg     400 mg

800  mg

## Alendronate

### Fosamax®

5 mg     10 mg

35 mg     40 mg

70 mg

## Allopurinol

### (generic)

100 mg     300 mg

## Alprazolam

### (generic)

0.5 mg     1 mg

2 mg

## Amitriptyline

### (generic)

10 mg

25 mg

50 mg

75 mg

100 mg

150 mg

## Amlodipine

### Norvasc®

2.5 mg

5 mg

10 mg

## Amlodipine and Benazepril

### Lotrel®

2.5/10 mg

5/10 mg

5/20 mg

10/20 mg

## Amoxicillin

### (generic)

250 mg

500 mg

### Trimox®

250 mg

500 mg

## Amoxicillin and Clavulanate Potassium

### (generic)

200/28.5 mg

400/57 mg

500/125 mg

875/125 mg

## Atenolol

### (generic)

25 mg

50 mg

## Atomoxetine

### Strattera™

10 mg

18 mg

25 mg

40 mg

60 mg

## Atorvastatin

### Lipitor®

10 mg

20 mg

40 mg

80 mg

## Azithromycin

### Zithromax®

250 mg

500 mg

## Benazepril

### (generic)

5 mg

10 mg

20 mg      40 mg

## Bisoprolol and Hydrochlorothiazide

**(generic)**

2.5/6.25 mg      5/6.25 mg

10/6.25 mg

## Bupropion

**(generic)**

75 mg      100 mg

### Wellbutrin SR®

100 mg      200 mg

### Wellbutrin XL®

150 mg      300 mg

## Buspirone

**(generic)**

5 mg      10 mg

## Butalbital Compound

**(generic)**

40/50/325 mg

## Captopril

**(generic)**

12.5 mg      25 mg

| 50 mg | 100 mg |

## Carisoprodol

### (generic)

350 mg

## Carvedilol

### Coreg®

| 3.125 mg | 6.25 mg |
| 12.5 mg | 25 mg |

## Celecoxib

### Celebrex™

| 100 mg | 200 mg |

400 mg

## Cephalexin

### (generic)

| 250 mg | 500 mg |

## Cetirizine

### Zyrtec®

| 5 mg | 10 mg |

### Zyrtec-D 12 Hour™

5 mg

## Ciprofloxacin

**(generic)**

250 mg     500 mg

750 mg

## Citalopram

**Celexa™**

10 mg     20 mg

40 mg

## Clindamycin

**(generic)**

150 mg     300 mg

## Clonazepam

**(generic)**

0.5 mg     1 mg

2 mg

## Clonidine

**(generic)**

0.1 mg     0.2 mg

0.3 mg

## Clopidogrel

**Plavix®**

75 mg

## Cyclobenzaprine

### (generic)

10 mg

## Desloratadine

### Clarinex®

5 mg

## Dextroamphetamine and Amphetamine

### Adderall XR™

| 5 mg | 15 mg |

## Diazepam

### (generic)

| 2 mg | 5 mg |

10 mg

## Diclofenac

### (generic)

| 25 mg | 50 mg |

## Digoxin

### (generic)

| 125 mcg | 250 mcg |

### Lanoxin®

| 0.125 mg | 0.25 mg |

## Diltiazem

### (generic)

120 mg

180 mg          300 mg

### Cartia XT™

120 mg          180 mg

240 mg          300 mg

## Donepezil

### Aricept®

5 mg

## Doxazosin

### (generic)

1 mg          2 mg

4 mg          8 mg

## Doxycycline

### (generic)

50 mg          100 mg

## Enalapril

### (generic)

2.5 mg          5 mg

10 mg

## Escitalopram

### Lexapro™

10 mg      20 mg

## Estradiol

### (generic)

0.5 mg      1 mg

2 mg

## Estradiol and Norgestimate

### Tri-Sprintec™ 28

multiple dosages

## Estrogens (Conjugated/Equine)

### Premarin®

0.3 mg      0.45 mg

0.625 mg      0.9 mg

1.25 mg      2.5 mg

## Ethinyl Estradiol and Drospirenone

### Yasmin®

0.03/3 mg

## Ethinyl Estradiol and Levonorgestrel

### Aviane™ 28

0.02/0.1 mg

## Ethinyl Estradiol and Norgestimate

### Ortho Tri-Cyclen® LO

multiple dosages     multiple dosages

## Ezetimibe

### Zetia™

10 mg

## Famotidine

### (generic)

20 mg          40 mg

## Fenofibrate

### Tricor®

54 mg          67 mg

145 mg         160 mg

200 mg

## Fexofenadine

### Allegra®

30 mg          60 mg

180 mg

## Fexofenadine and Pseudoephedrine

### Allegra-D®

60/120 mg

## Fluconazole

### (generic)

100 mg | 200 mg

### Diflucan®

50 mg | 100 mg

150 mg | 200 mg

## Fluoxetine

### (generic)

10 mg | 20 mg

## Folic Acid

### (generic)

400 mcg | 1 mg

## Fosinopril

### Monopril®

10 mg | 20 mg

## Furosemide

### (generic)

20 mg | 40 mg

80 mg

## Gabapentin

### Neurontin®

100 mg | 300 mg

400 mg | 600 mg

800 mg

## Gemfibrozil

**(generic)**

600 mg

## Glimepiride

**Amaryl®**

1 mg

2 mg

4 mg

## Glipizide

**(generic)**

2.5 mg

5 mg

5 mg

10 mg

10 mg

## Glyburide

**(generic)**

1.5 mg

2.5 mg

3 mg

5 mg

6 mg

## Hydrochlorothiazide

**(generic)**

25 mg

50 mg

# Hydrochlorothiazide and Triamterene

## (generic)

25/37.5 mg

25/50 mg

50/75 mg

# Hydrocodone and Acetaminophen

## (generic)

7.5/750 mg

# Hydroxyzine

## (generic)

10 mg

25 mg

50 mg

# Ibuprofen

## (generic)

200 mg

400 mg

600 mg

800 mg

# Irbesartan

## Avalide®

150/12.5 mg

## Avapro®

75 mg

150 mg

300 mg

## Isosorbide Mononitrate

### (generic)

| 30 mg | 60 mg |
|-------|-------|

120 mg

## Lamotrigine

### Lamictal®

| 25 mg | 100 mg |
|-------|--------|
| 150 mg | 200 mg |

## Lansoprazole

### Prevacid®

| 15 mg | 30 mg |
|-------|-------|

## Levofloxacin

### Levaquin®

| 250 mg | 500 mg |
|--------|--------|

750 mg

## Levothyroxine

### (generic)

| 25 mcg | 25 mcg |
|--------|--------|
| 50 mcg | 100 mcg |
| 125 mcg | 300 mcg |

### Levothroid®

| 25 mcg | 50 mcg |
|--------|--------|

| | |
|---|---|
| 75 mcg | 88 mcg |
| 100 mcg | 112 mcg |
| 125 mcg | 137 mcg |
| 150 mcg | 150 mcg |
| 200 mcg | 300 mcg |

## Levoxyl®

| | |
|---|---|
| 25 mcg | 50 mcg |
| 75 mcg | 88 mcg |

| | |
|---|---|
| 100 mcg | 112 mcg |
| 125 mcg | 137 mcg |
| 150 mcg | 175 mcg |
| 200 mcg | 300 mcg |

## Synthroid®

| | |
|---|---|
| 25 mcg | 50 mcg |
| 75 mcg | 88 mcg |
| 100 mcg | 112 mcg |

| | |
|---|---|
| 125 mcg | 137 mcg |
| 150 mcg | 175 mcg |
| 200 mcg | 200 mcg |

## Lisinopril

### (generic)

| | |
|---|---|
| 2.5 mg | 5 mg |
| 10 mg | 20 mg |
| | 40 mg |

## Lisinopril and Hydrochlorothiazide

### (generic)

| | |
|---|---|
| 10/12.5 mg | 20/12.5 mg |
| | 20/25 mg |

## Lorazepam

### (generic)

| | |
|---|---|
| 0.5 mg | 1 mg |
| | 2 mg |

## Losartan

### Cozaar®

| | |
|---|---|
| 25 mg | 50 mg |

100 mg

## Losartan and Hydrochlorothiazide

### Hyzaar®

50/12.5 mg      100/25 mg

## Lovastatin

### (generic)

10 mg      20 mg

40 mg

## Loxapine

### (generic)

5 mg

## Meclizine

### (generic)

12.5 mg      25 mg

## Meclofenamate

### (generic)

50 mg

## Medroxyprogesterone

### (generic)

2.5 mg      5 mg

10 mg

## Meloxicam

### Mobic®

7.5 mg      15 mg

## Metaxalone

### Skelaxin®

400 mg      800 mg

## Metformin

### (generic)

500 mg      850 mg

1000 mg

## Methotrexate

### (generic)

2.5 mg      5 mg

10 mg

## Methylphenidate

### Concerta®

18 mg      27 mg

36 mg      54 mg

## Methylprednisolone

### (generic)

4 mg

## Metoclopramide

### (generic)

5 mg          10 mg

## Metoprolol

### (generic)

50 mg          100 mg

### Toprol XL®

25 mg          50 mg

100 mg          200 mg

## Metronidazole

### (generic)

250 mg          500 mg

## Minocycline

### (generic)

50 mg          100 mg

## Mirtazapine

### (generic)

15 mg          30 mg

45 mg

## Montelukast

### Singulair®

4 mg      5 mg

10 mg

## Naproxen

### (generic)

250 mg      375 mg

500 mg

## Niacin

### Niaspan®

500 mg      750 mg

1000 mg

## Nifedipine

### (generic)

60 mg      90 mg

## Nitrofurantoin

### (generic)

50 mg      100 mg

## Nortriptyline

### (generic)

10 mg      25 mg

50 mg      75 mg

## Olanzapine

### Zyprexa®

| | |
|---|---|
| 2.5 mg | 5 mg |
| 7.5 mg | 10 mg |

| | |
|---|---|
| 15 mg | 20 mg |

## Olmesartan

### Benicar™

| | |
|---|---|
| 5 mg | 20 mg |
| | 40 mg |

## Omeprazole

### (generic)

| | |
|---|---|
| 10 mg | 20 mg |

## Oxycodone

### Oxycontin®

| | |
|---|---|
| 10 mg | 20 mg |
| 40 mg | 80 mg |

## Oxycodone and Acetaminophen

### (generic)

| | |
|---|---|
| 5/325 mg | 5/500 mg |

### Endocet®

7.5/500 mg          10/650 mg

## Pantoprazole

### Protonix®

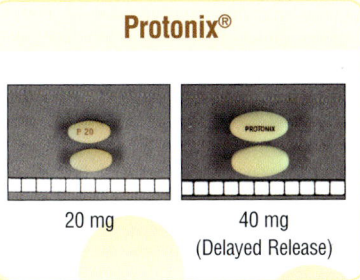

20 mg          40 mg
(Delayed Release)

## Paroxetine

### (generic)

10 mg          20 mg

30 mg          40 mg

### Paxil® CR

12.5 mg          25 mg

37.5 mg

## Penicillin V Potassium

### (generic)

250 mg          500 mg

## Phenytoin

### Dilantin® Kapseals®

30 mg          100 mg

## Pioglitazone

### Actos™

15 mg          30 mg

45 mg

# Potassium Chloride

## (generic)

8 mEq      10 mEq

750 mg

## Klor-Con® 8

8 mEq

## Klor-Con® 10

10 mEq

# Pravastatin

## Pravachol®

10 mg      20 mg

40 mg      80 mg

# Prednisone

## (generic)

1 mg      2.5 mg

5 mg      10 mg

20 mg      50 mg

# Promethazine

## (generic)

25 mg      50 mg

## Propoxyphene and Acetaminophen

### (generic)

65/650 mg 100/650 mg

## Propranolol

### (generic)

10 mg 20 mg

40 mg 60 mg

80 mg 120 mg

160 mg

## Quetiapine

### Seroquel®

25 mg 100 mg

200 mg 300 mg

## Quinapril

### Accupril®

5 mg 10 mg

20 mg 40 mg

## Quinine

### (generic)

200 mg          325 mg

325 mg

## Rabeprazole

### Aciphex®

20 mg

## Raloxifene

### Evista®

60 mg

## Ramipril

### Altace™

1.25 mg          2.5 mg

5 mg          10 mg

## Ranitidine

### (generic)

75 mg          150 mg

300 mg

## Risedronate

### Actonel®

5 mg          30 mg

35 mg

## Risperidone

### Risperdal®

0.25 mg          0.5 mg

1 mg          3 mg

4 mg

## Rosiglitazone

### Avandia®

2 mg          4 mg

8 mg

## Rosuvastatin

### Crestor®

5 mg          10 mg

20 mg          40 mg

## Sertraline

### Zoloft®

25 mg          50 mg

100 mg

## Sildenafil

### Viagra™

25 mg          50 mg

100 mg

## Simvastatin

**Zocor®**

5 mg

10 mg

20 mg

40 mg

80 mg

## Spironolactone

**(generic)**

25 mg

50 mg

100 mg

## Sulfamethoxazole and Trimethoprim

**(generic)**

400/80 mg

800/160 mg

## Sumatriptan

**Imitrex®**

25 mg

50 mg

100 mg

## Tamsulosin

**Flomax®**

0.4 mg

## Temazepam

### (generic)

| 15 mg | 30 mg |

## Terazosin

### (generic)

| 1 mg | 2 mg |
| 5 mg | 10 mg |

## Tizanidine

### (generic)

| 2 mg | 4 mg |

## Tolterodine

### Detrol® LA

| 2 mg | 4 mg |

## Topiramate

### Topamax®

| 15 mg | 25 mg |
| 100 mg | 200 mg |

## Tramadol

### (generic)

| 50 mg |

# Trazodone

## (generic)

50 mg      100 mg

150 mg

# Valacyclovir

## Valtrex®

500 mg      1000 mg

# Valdecoxib

## Bextra™

10 mg      20 mg

# Valproic Acid and Derivatives

## Depakote®

125 mg      250 mg

500 mg

# Valsartan

## Diovan™

80 mg      160 mg

# Valsartan and Hydrochlorothiazide

## Diovan HCT®

80/12.5 mg      160/12.5 mg

160/25 mg

## Venlafaxine

### Effexor XR®

37.5 mg     75 mg

150 mg

## Verapamil

### (generic)

180 mg     240 mg

360 mg

## Warfarin

### (generic)

1 mg     2.5 mg

3 mg     4 mg

5 mg     6 mg

7.5 mg

## Zolpidem

### Ambien®

5 mg     10 mg